KB152081

MEDICAL ETYMOLOGY

ETYMOLOGY

Based on
ENGLISH ETYMOLOGY

SECOND EDITION

의학어원론

머리말

수의 세계는 어떻게 생겼을까? 어느 현자가 그린 대로 모양, 색깔, 감촉, 움직임을 갖는 풍경의 세계일까?

어떻게 생겼든, 현자가 아닌 우리는 수의 세계를 숫자와 기호로 이루어진 메타언어로 표현한다. 그러니 수의 세계를 여행하려는 자, 이 메타언어를 깨달아야 한다.

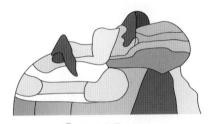

ⓒ Daniel Tammet

수의 세계. 사반트(*savant*)인 다니엘 타멧이 원주율 π를 소수점 이하 19자리까지 그의 '수 언어'로 '썼다'. (F. savant, E. *sapient* < L. sapiens < L. sapĕre *to taste, to perceive*)

소리의 세계는 어떻게 생겼을까? 듣지도 못하는 절대 고독의 작곡가에게처럼, 어루만지고 쓰러뜨리며 따뜻하게 해주기도 하고 얼어붙게 하기도 하는 바람의 세계일까?

어떻게 생겼든, 절대 고독을 모르는 우리는 소리의 세계를 음표와 기호로 이루어진 메타언어로 표현한다. 그러니 소리의 세계를 여행하려는 자, 이 메타언어를 깨달아야 한다.

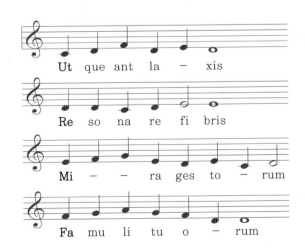

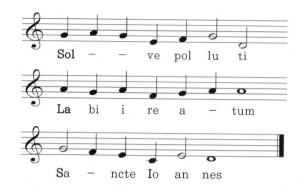

소리의 세계. 위 가사 마디의 첫음절이 우리의 메타언어인 계명 Ut (> Do), Re, Mi, Fa, Sol, La, Si가 되었다. '성 요한이시여, 종들이 당신께서 행하신 신비를 편한 목소리로 노래할 수 있도록 더렵혀진 입술로 범한 죄를 씻어 주십시오.'

생명의 세계는 어떻게 생겼을까? 달걀처럼 생겼을까, 올챙이처럼 생겼을까, 아니면, 거시기처럼 생겼을까, 머시기처럼 생겼을까?

어떻게 생겼든, 아는 것보다 모르는 것이 더 많은 우리는 생명의 세계를 인간의 언어로 이루어진 메타언어로 표현한다. 메타언어 대신 학술용어라는 낱말을 사용할 따름이다. 그러니 생명의 세계를 여행하려는 자, 먼저 인간의 언어를 깨달아야 한다.

Caenorhabditis elegans (예쁜꼬마선충). 새로운(L. caeno- < G. kainos *new*) 막대벌레(L. rhabditis < G. rhabdos *rod*)로서 우아한(L. elegans < L. eligĕre *to elect*) 몸짓으로 움직인다. 모델 생명체의 하나이다.

언어는 생각의 도구이다. 언어를 깨닫는 자, 생각이 자유스럽다. 생각이 자유스러운 자, 새로운 생각을 만든다. - 언어가 너희를 자유롭게 하리라.

Language Will Free You
LINGUA LIBERABIT VOS
Ἡ ΓΛΩΣΣΑ ΛΥΣΕΙ ΥΜΑΣ

이 책의 이름은 잘못되었다. 〈의학 어원론〉이 아니라 〈생명과학 어원론〉이다.

Biological Etymology
ETYMOLOGIA BIOLOGICA
Ἡ ΒΙΟΛΟΓΙΚΗ ΕΤΥΜΟΛΟΓΙΑ

〈생명과학 어원론〉으로 바꾸어도 잘못되기는 마찬가지이다. 〈영어 어원론〉이다.

English Etymology
ETYMOLOGIA ANGLICA
Ἡ ΑΓΓΛΙΚΗ ΕΤΥΜΟΛΟΓΙΑ

첫째판이 나온 해부터 전남대학교 의과대학 교과과정에 의학어원론이 포함되었고 정교재로 사용하고 있다. 지금까지 열네 해를 학생들과 함께 공부하면서 내용을 숙성시켰다. 숙성된 내용을 더해 개정판으로 내놓는다.

전남대학교 의과대학이 부분적으로 의학전문대학원 제도를 병행하고 있을 때였다. 대학의 부탁으로 대학원 신입생을 위해 해마다 입학 전 특별수업을 하였다. 신입생들은 전국 각지의 타 대학을 이미 졸업하였거나 졸업 예정이었다. 수업 후 학생들이 말하였다. 세상에, 이런 과목도 있었답니까?!

대학을 떠나서도 생명과학과 언어학을 공부하고 있다. 그게 가능한 것은 어원론이 뒤받쳐 주기 때문이라고 확신한다. 생소한 낱말도 어원으로 접근하면 알고 있던 말무리에 쉬이 합쳐진다. *Jesus the Christ*께서 친히 사용하셨다는 낱말 중 하나(마테오 5:18)를 빌려오자면, 처음 보는 낱말이 금방 좆(*jot*)만 해지는 것이다.

서문이라고 하는 *preface*의 어원은 라틴어 praefatio(< prae- *before, beyond* + fari *to speak*) - '먼저 말하기'이다. '운명'이라는 영어 낱말 *fate*(< L. fatum *what is spoken* < L. fari *to speak*)와 뿌리를 같이 한다.

돌이켜보면, 나는 이 책을 쓰게끔 운명 지워져 있었다.

언어 때문에 상처받는 사람이 없기를 바라며 (이 책의 존재 목적이다),
센트럴파크의 메타세쿼이아 숲 속 현미경 판독실에서,
마이클과 함께 정상우 쓰다.

차례

약어와 기호

abl.	*ablative* (탈격)		F.	*French* (프랑스어)
acc.	*accusative* (대격)		G.	*Greek* (그리스어)
dat.	*dative* (여격)		IE.	*Indo-European root*
f.	*feminine* (여성)			(인도유럽어 말뿌리)
gen.	*genitive* (속격)		It.	*Italian* (이탈리아어)
m.	*masculine* (남성)		L.	*Latin* (라틴어)
n.	*neuter* (중성)		Sp.	*Spanish* (스페인어)
nom.	*nominative* (주격)		>, <	파생어나 합성어가 만들어진 방향
pl.	*plural* (복수)		+	파생어나 합성어 성분의 결합
sing.	*singular* (단수)		∞	동족어
voc.	*vocative* (호격)		†	사망, 사어
D.	*Deutsch* (독일어)		*	추정 낱말
E.	*English* (영어)		~	생략, 반복

m. (*masculine*, 남성), f. (*feminine*, 여성), n. (*neuter*, 중성), sing. (*singular*, 단수), pl. (*plural*, 복수) 등의 문법 용어는, 뜻을 얼른 드러내기 위해, 일부러 약자를 사용하지 않은 곳이 있다. *noun* (명사), *pronoun* (대명사), *adjective* (형용사), *verb* (동사), *adverb* (부사), *preposition* (전치사), *present* (현재), *past* (과거), *future* (미래), *personal* (인칭) 등의 문법 용어는, 역시 뜻을 얼른 드러내기 위해, 처음부터 약자를 사용하지 않았다. *Sanskrit* (산스크리트어), *Hindi* (힌디어), *Sinhalese* (스리랑카어), *Iranian* (이란어), *Persian* (페르시아어), *Avestan* (아베스타어), *Tocharian* (토카라어), *Illyrian* (일리리아어), *Oscan* (오스칸어), *Celtic* (켈트어), *Gaulish* (골어), *Gaelic* (게일어), *Irish* (아일랜드어), *Germanic* (게르만어), *Old Norse* (고대 스칸디나비아어), *Swedish* (스웨덴어), *Dutch* (네덜란드어), *Portuguese* (포르투갈어), *Slavic* (슬라브어), *Russian* (러시아어), *Etruscan* (에트루리아어), *Iberian* (이베리아어), *Semitic* (셈어), *Sumerian* (수메르어), *Akkadian* (아카드어), *Hebrew* (헤브라이어), *Aramaic* (아람어), *Arabic* (아라비아어), *Hamitic* (함어), *Egyptian* (이집트어), *Coptic* (콥트어), *Hungarian* (헝가리어), *Dravidian* (드라비다어), *Malayan* (말레이어), *Chinese* (중국어), *Japanese* (일본어), *Korean* (한국어), 원주민 언어 등 간혹 나오는 언어 이름은 약자를 사용하지 않았다.

이 책을 어떻게 할까요?

차례를 보고서,

1. 제1부 어원론 편을 읽습니다.
2. 제2부 라틴어 편의 역사, 알파벳과 발음을 읽습니다.
3. 제2부 라틴어 편의 각 품사별 설명 부분을 읽습니다.
4. 제3부 그리스어 편의 역사, 알파벳과 발음, 자역을 읽습니다.
5. 제3부 그리스어 편의 각 품사별 설명 부분을 읽습니다.
6. 제5부 학명을 읽습니다. 학명은 문법을 연습하기 위한 좋은 도구입니다.
   문법 순서대로 나오기 때문입니다.

영어 색인을 보고서,

7. 수시로 알고 싶은 어원의 단어를 영어 색인에서 찾습니다.
   알고 싶은 단어의 어원이 무엇인지, 동족어 무리에는 어떤 단어들이 있는지 봅니다.
   무리 중에 이미 알고 있는 단어가 있으면 연결시켜 놓습니다.
   익숙해지면 라틴어와 그리스어에 대해 조금 더 관심을 갖습니다.

표제어 순서는,

표제어를 품사별로, 같은 품사 내에서는 변화 종류별로, 같은 변화 내에서는 알파벳 순서로 실었습니다. 뜻이나 꼴의 비교가 가능한 경우에는 한데 모았습니다. 그러나, 한 표제어 안에 나오는 동족어 단어들의 품사나 변화의 종류가 무시로 달라지기 때문에 표제어의 순서는 큰 의미 없습니다. 단, 제4부 용어 비교에서는 뜻에 따라 표제어를 실었고, 제5부 학명에서는 문법에 따라 학명을 실었습니다.

제 1 부

어원론

Etymology

Etymologia

제 1 장 학문과 언어

학문과 어원론

옷, 밥과 국, 집 등 생존에 필요한 첫 낱말이 무슨 뜻에서 어떻게 시작했는지는 전혀 모르거나 기껏해야 짐작할 수 있을 따름이다. 그러나 옷, 밥과 국, 집이 의식주라는 문화의 단계가 되고 복식학, 식품학, 건축학이라는 학문의 단계가 되면 낱말이 무슨 뜻에서 어떻게 만들어졌는지, 어떻게 변해 왔는지 알 수 있다.

문화와 학문의 단계에서 만들어지는 낱말은 새로운 내용을 표현하기 위해서이다. 새로운 내용을 표현하기 위해 만들어진 낱말은 내용에 가장 잘 어울려야 살아남으며 그렇지 않은 낱말은 변하거나 사라지고 만다. 적자생존과 진화의 법칙이 낱말에도 적용되는 것이니, 낱말의 다윈주의이다.

문화와 학문의 단계에서 만들어진 낱말로서 현재 살아남은 낱말은, 지금까지는, 내용에 가장 잘 어울리는 낱말이기 때문에 살아남아 있다. 따라서 내용을 알면 낱말은 덩달아 알아지도록 되어 있다. 학문을 이해하면 학술용어는 뒤따라 이해되고 외우려 하지 않아도 외워지게끔 되어 있는 것이다.

우리나라 생명과학도들이 맞닥뜨리는 가장 큰 난관은 용어 문제이다. 내용을 다 이해해 놓고도 새판잡이로 용어를, 암호라도 되는 양, 외워재껴야 한다. 단연코 용어는 암호가 아니며 외워재껴야 하는 대상이 아닌데도 그러하다. 용어의 뿌리인 어원(*etymon*)과 어원으로부터 그렇게 만들어질 수밖에 없었던 길, 즉 어원론(*etymology*)을 모르기 때문이다.

어원과 어원론을 모르면 하나하나의 용어를 따로따로 머리 속에 쑤셔 넣어야 한다. 그러나 어원과 어원론을 알면 용어들이, 반짝이는 물고기 떼처럼, 무리지어 머리 속으로 헤엄쳐 들어온다. 나아가, 아직 사전에 오르지 않은 새로운 용어라 할지라도 만든 사람이 어떤 생각에서 그리 만들었는지, 잘 만들었는지 잘못 만들었는지 알 수 있다.

생명과학도가 어원과 어원론을 공부하는 것은 용어의 장벽을 무너뜨리고자 함이다. 그러나 거기에는 훨씬 깊은 뜻이 들어 있다. 생각의 지평을 넓게 된다는 점이다. 언어는 표현의 수단일 뿐 아니라 생각의 도구이다. 용어의 장벽을 무너뜨리면 생각은 그 이상으로 자유스러워진다. 자유를 위하여!

학술어로서 영어

현재 유일한 국제공용어는 영어이며, 가시적 시간 안에 다른 언어가 영어를 제치고 새로운 국제공용어로 될 가능성은 없다. 지구촌 시대에서 영어는, 모국어와 함께, 생존을 위한 언어가 되어 있는 것이다. 학문의 세계에서도 국제공용어는 영어이다.

영어가 국제공용어가 된 데에는 세계사적 이유도 있지만, 속을 들여다보면, 영어만큼 세계어에 적합한 언어도 없다는 것을 알 수 있다.

영어의 모태가 되는 앵글로·색슨족의 문화는 세계의 중심 문화였던 그리스·라틴 문화에 비해 변방의 문화였다. 따라서 영어에는 본디부터 영어였던 '쓸 만한' 낱말이 그리 많지 않았다. 또한 영어는, 처음에는 그렇지 안했지만, 어순(*word order*)과 관사·대명사·조동사·전치사·접속사 등 기능어(*function word*)에 따라 문법이 결정되는 분석어(*analytic language*)로 틀을 바꿨다. 분석어 자체는, 접근하기 쉽고 저항감 없이 바깥 낱말을 받아들일 수 있으나, 낱말의 변신이 제한적이며, 제한적인 만큼 파생이나 합성어를 만드는 데에 한계가 있다.

영어의 이 두 가지 결함을, 즉 깊지 않는 문화적 배경과 약한 조어력을 필연으로 뒤따르는 것은 어휘의 빈한함이었다. 그러나 영어는, 조어력이 강한 굴절어(*inflectional language*)이면서 오랫동안 세계의 중심 문화어였던 라틴어와 그리스어 낱말을 폭넓게 받아들임으로써 빈한한 어휘의 문제를 해결하였을 뿐 아니라 분석어이면서도 조어력까지 강한 언어로 발전하였다.

심장 또는 마음을 가리키는 영어 *heart*, 라틴어 cor, 그리스어 kardia에서부터 기원한 영어 낱말들을 예로 들어보자. 본디 영어 *heart*에서부터 만들어진 낱말에는 *hearty, heartful, heartless, hearten* 정도와 *heartbeat*나 *heartburn, heart-stopper, heart-to-heart, heart attack, heart failure* 등의 표현이 있다. 이에 비해 라틴어로부터는 cor에서 만들어진 *courage, cordate, cordial,* *concord, discord, misericord, accord, record* 등이 들어와 있고, 그리스어로부터는 kardia에서 만들어진 *cardiac, cardioid, electrocardiogram, pericardium, endocardium, myocardium, epicardium, bradycardia, tachycardia, dextrocardia* 등이 들어와 있다. 나아가 이들 낱말은 다시 더 많은 파생어와 합성어를 만들어 내고 표현한다. 라틴어와 그리스어에서부터 기원한 낱말이 얼마나 많이 영어 속에 들어와 있으며 라틴어와 그리스어의 조어력이 얼마나 대단한지를 얼른 알 수 있다. (그리스어 kardia는 καρδια를 로마자로 자역(字譯)한 것이다. 특별한 경우가 아니면, 다른 어원론에서처럼, 그리스어 낱말을 자역해 실었다.)

심장 또는 마음에 관한 영어 낱말을 보면 본디 영어 낱말은 일상용(日常用) 구어(口語)이고, 라틴어 기원의 영어 낱말은 격식용(格式用) 문어(文語)이며, 그리스어 기원의 영어 낱말은 기술용(技術用) 전문어(專門語)임을 알 수 있다. 라틴어 기원의 영어 낱말이 격식용이 된 것은 1066년 노르만의 영국 정복 이후 약 삼백 년 동안 라틴어의 후예인 프랑스어가 영국 지배층의 언어이었으며, 서구 식자층에서는 천년 넘도록 라틴어가 쓰였기 때문이다. 그리스어 기원의 영어 낱말이 기술용이 된 것은, 라틴어의 어휘가 풍부하고 조어력이 강하다 하지만 그리스어에는 미치지 못하며, 로마 의학이 그리스 의학의 재포장품이었듯, 라틴 문화는 그리스 문화의 중계자적 계승자이었기 때문이다.

이와 같은 영어 낱말의 기원에 따른 용도상 차이는 물론 절대적인 것은 아니다. 그러나, 본디 영어 낱말로 돌아가자는 언어 순수주의(*linguistic purism*)가 오랫동안 꿈틀대왔음에도 불구하고, 오늘날에도 적용할 수밖에 없는 차이이다.

학문의 세계에서는 하나의 대상에 대해 일상용 낱말과, 격식용 낱말과, 기술용 낱말을 모두 사용한다. 기술용 낱말 말고도 격식용 낱말과 일상용 낱말을 함께 사용하는 것은 라틴어가 오랫동안 널리 쓰였으며 영어가 보편화되었기 때문이다. 요즈음 학문 세계에서는 대중성까지 강조되고 있다. 또한, 같은 뜻이라고 하더라도 이런 때는 영어 기원의 낱말을 사용하고 저런 때는 라틴어 기원의 낱말을 사용하며 그런 때는 그리스어 기원의 낱말을 사용하는 등, 어원에 따라 사용처가 다르다. 따라서, 학문하는 사람은 하나의 대상에 대해 영어와 라틴어와 그리스어 기원의 낱말을 모두 알아야 한다는 말이 된다. 쉬운 문제는 아니지만 그렇다고 어려운 문제도 아니다. 세 언어가 뿌리를 같이 하며 나름대로 흐름을 따라 발전해 왔기 때문이다. 열쇠는 어원론 안에 있다.

영어 낱말의 어원

인도유럽조어

영어 *heart*, 라틴어 cor, 그리스어 kardia를 곰곰 들여다보면 어딘지 닮은 데가 있다. 영어가 속하는 게르만어파나 라틴어가 속하는 이탈리아어파, 그리스어가 속하는 헬라어파의 언어 모두가, 인도의 산스크리트어와 함께, 하나의 인도유럽조어(祖語, *Proto-Indo-European* 또는 *Indo-European*)에서 비롯되었기 때문이다. 영어 *heart*, 라틴어 cor, 그리스어 kardia의 인도유럽어 말뿌리(*Indo-European root*)는 *kerd-이며, *heart*, cor, kardia는 동족어(同族語, *cognate*)이고, 그로부터 기원한 영어 낱말들은 동족어 무리인 것이다. (*kerd-의 위첨자 별표(*)는 어원론 학자들이 기록상 확인하지 못했으나 존재하였으리라고 추론하는 낱말임을 나타낸다. 인도유럽조어는 기록된 것이 없어 모두 위첨자 별표를 붙이게 되므로 인도유럽조어임이 분명할 때에는, 이 책에서처럼, 붙이지 않기도 한다.)

IE. kerd- (원형) *heart*

　> IE. kerd-en- (접미사 첨가형)

　　> E. **heart**

　　　> E. *hearty, heartful, heartless, hearten*

　> IE. krd- (모음 탈락형)

　　> L. cor, cordis, n. 심장, 마음, 의지, 용기, 지혜　　**E** *(suggested)* **core**

　　　> L. cordatus, cordata, cordatum 심장 모양의, 현명한　　**E** *cordate*

　　　> L. cordialis, cordiale 마음에서 우러나는　　**E** *cordial*

　　　> L. *coraticum, *coratici, n. 용기, 열정, 욕망, 분노　**E** *courage, encourage*

　　　> L. praecordium, praecordii, n. (< prae *before, beyond*)

　　　　전흉부(前胸部), 명치부위　　**E** *precordium*

　　　　> L. praecordialis, praecordiale 전흉부의, 명치부위의　**E** *precordial*

　　　> L. concors, (gen.) concordis (< con- < cum *with, together*)

　　　　한마음의, 합치하는, 일치하는, 화목하는　　**E** *concord*

> L. discors, (gen.) discordis (< dis- *apart from, down, not*)
어긋나는, 상반되는, 불목하는   **E** *discord*

> L. misericors, (gen.) misericordis (< miser *wretched*)
자비로운   **E** *misericord*

> L. accordo, **accordavi**, accordatum, accordare (< ac- < ad *to,
toward, at, according to*) 일치시키다, 상응시키다   **E** *accord*

> L. recordor, recordatus sum, recordari (< re- *back, again*)
기억하고 있다   **E** *record*

> IE. krd-ya- (접미사 첨가형)

   > G. kardia, kardias, f. *heart, mind, soul*

     E *cardi(o)-, electrocardiogram (ECG),* (D. Elektrokardiogramm >)
EKG, cardiomegaly

     > G. kardiakos, kardiakē, kardiakon (< + -akos *adjective
suffix*) *of heart*

       > L. cardiacus, cardiaca, cardiacum 심장의, 심장병의;
(*on the heart side of the body* >) 위(胃)의, 위병
(胃病)의, 들문(~門)의   **E** *cardiac*

     > G. kardioeidēs, kardioeidēs, kardioeides (< + eidos
shape) *heart-shaped*   **E** *cardioid*

     > G. perikardios, perikardia, perikardion (< peri *around,
near, beyond, on account of*) *pericardial*

       > L. pericardium, pericardii, n. 심장막,
심낭(心囊)   **E** *pericardium, pericardial*

     > L. endocardium, endocardii, n. (< G. end(o)- < endon
within) 심장속막, 심내막   **E** *endocardium, endocardial*

     > L. myocardium, myocardii, n. (< G. my(o)- < mys, myos,
m. *mouse, muscle*) 심근층   **E** *myocardium, myocardial*

     > L. epicardium, epicardii, n. (< G. epi *upon*) 심장바깥막,
심외막   **E** *epicardium, epicardial*

     > L. bradycardia, bradycardiae, f. (< G. bradys *slow*) 느린
맥, 서맥(徐脈)   **E** *bradycardia, bradycardiac*

     > L. tachycardia, tachycardiae, f. (< G. tachys *swift*) 빠른
맥, 빈맥(頻脈)   **E** *tachycardia, tachycardiac*

     > L. dextrocardia, dextrocardiae, f. (< L. dexter, dextra,
dextrum *right*) 우심증   **E** *dextrocardia*

> IE. kred-dhə- (< + IE. dhə- *to do, to place*) (합성형) *to place trust*

   > L. credo, **credidi**, creditum, credĕre 믿다, 맡기다

     E (*first personal singular, present indicative, active 'I believe'* >) *credo,*
(credo >) *creed, grant* (< *'consent to support'*)

     > L. creditum, crediti, n. 신뢰, 신용, 영예, 남에게 맡겨놓은 (빌려
준) 것   **E** *credit, accredit*

> L. credentia, credentiae, f. 신뢰, 신임   **E** *credence*
> > L. credentialis, credentiale 신뢰의, 신임의   **E** *credential*
> L. credibilis, credibile 믿을 만한, 신용할 만한   **E** *credible*
> > L. credibilitas, credibilitatis, f. 신뢰성, 신용   **E** *credibility*
> > L. incredibilis, incredibile (< in- *not*) 믿을 수 없는,
> > 믿어지지 않는   **E** *incredible*
> > > L. incredibilitas, incredibilitatis, f. 믿을 수 없음   **E** *incredibility*
> L. credulus, credula, credulum 쉽게 믿는   **E** *credulous*
> > L. credulitas, credulitatis, f. 쉽게 믿음, 경신(輕信),
> > 맹신(盲信)   **E** *credulity*
> > L. incredulus, incredula, incredulum (< in- *not*) 의심
> > 많은, 회의적인   **E** *incredulous*
> > > L. incredulitas, incredulitatis, f. 의심 많음, 회의   **E** *incredulity*

인도유럽조어의 재구성

기록이 없는 인도유럽조어를 추론할 수 있는 것은 인도유럽어족(*Indo-European family*)에 속하는 언어를 비교해 봄으로써 가능하다. 비교법(*comparative method*)이라고 한다. 먼저 시작해 볼 수 있는 낱말은 '부모형제'와 같은 친족관계의 명사, '나·너'와 같이 가까운 대상을 가리키는 대명사, 1부터 10까지의 수사 등 변화가 작은 핵심 어휘(*core vocabulary*)들이다.

Sanskrit (Indo-Iranian)	Greek (Hellenic)	Latin (Italic)	†Gothic (East Germanic)	Swedish (North Germanic)	Deutsch (High West Germanic)	English (Low West Germanic)
pita	patēr	pater	fadar	fader	Vater	father

'아버지'를 예로 들면 게르만어파에 속하는 언어의 기록을 조사해 '아버지'의 게르만어 말뿌리(*Proto-Germanic root*) fadar를 찾으며, 같은 방법으로 '아버지'에 관한 이탈리아어파 말뿌리(*Proto-Italic root*), 헬라어파 말뿌리(*Proto-Hellenic root*), 발트·슬라브어파 말뿌리(*Balto-Slavic root*), 켈트어파 말뿌리(*Proto-Celtic root*), 인도이란어파 말뿌리(*Proto-Indo-Iranian root*) 등을 찾고 마지막으로 인도유럽어 말뿌리 pəter-를 찾는다.

일단 핵심 어휘의 낱말에 대한 말뿌리가 조사되면 자음과 모음의 변화에 대한 규칙을 알 수 있다. 다시 '아버지'를 예로 들면 인도유럽어 말뿌리 pəter-가 게르만어로 전해지면서 'p'는 'f'로 변하였음을 알 수 있는 것이다. (독일어 Vater의 'V'는 'f'로 발음한다.) 그리고 이러한 규칙을 '발'의 인도유럽어 말뿌리 ped-와 그리스어 pod-, 라틴어 ped-, 영어 foot에서도 확인해 볼 수 있다.

위와 같은 비교법으로 인도유럽조어 학자들은 많은 인도유럽어 말뿌리를 재구성해 놓았을 뿐 아니라, 인도유럽조어의 문법까지도 재구성해 놓았다. 재구성된 문법은 인도유럽조어가 고도의 굴절어였음을 보여준다.

그림의 법칙

인도유럽조어의 파열음(폐쇄음)이 게르만어계에서 보이는 규칙적 변화를 그림의 법칙(Grimm's law)이라고 한다. 동화집으로 잘 알려진 언어학자 그림 형제 중 형인 야코프 그림(Jacob Grimm, 1785-1863)의 이름에서 비롯했다. 대자음추이(Great Consonant Shift)라고도 한다. 법칙은 무성 파열음의 마찰음화(摩擦音化), 유성 파열음의 무성음화(無聲音化), 기음 파열음의 비기음화(非氣音化) 세 가지의 연쇄추이로 이루어져 있다. 연쇄추이의 순서에 대해서는 아직 정설이 없다.

마찰음화(spirantization): IE. /p/, /t/, /k/		>	Germanic /f/, /θ/, /h/	
IE. pəter-	>	G. patēr	L. pater	E. *father*
IE. trei-	>	G. treis	L. tres	E. *three*
IE. kerd-	>	G. kardia	L. cor	E. *heart*

무성음화(devoicing):	IE. /b/, /d/, /g/	>	Germanic /p/, /t/, /k/	
IE. bak-	>	G. baktron	L. baculum	E. *peg*
IE. dekṃ	>	G. deka	L. decem	E. *ten*
IE. gnō-	>	G. gignōskein	L. gnoscĕre	E. *know*

비기음화(deaspiration):	IE. /bh/, /dh/, /gh/	>	Germanic /b/, /d/, /g/	
IE. bhrāter–	>	G. phratēr	L. frater	E. *brother*
IE. dhe–	>	G. thema	L. factum	E. *deed*
IE. gher–	>	G. choros	L. hortus	E. *garden*

인도유럽조어의 파열음 앞에 다른 자음이 위치할 경우에는 변화가 일어나지 않았다.

IE. ster–	>	G. astēr	L. stella	E. *star*

마찰음화와 무성음화는 게르만어계에서 일어난 변화이며 그리스어와 라틴어에서는 변화가 없었다. 그러나 비기음화는 그리스어와 라틴어에서도 일어나 인도유럽조어의 /bh/, /dh/, /gh/가 그리스어에서는 /ph/, /th/, /ch/로, 라틴어에서는 /f/, /f/, /h/로 바뀌었다.

그림의 법칙이 단어의 첫 자음에만 적용되는 것은 아니다. 그러나 첫 자음 이외의 자음은 그림의 법칙이 적용된 후 추가로 다른 변화를 겪은 경우가 상당히 있어 겉보기에 법칙으로부터 벗어난 것처럼 보일 수 있다.

그림의 법칙을 알면 영어에서 영어 고유어와 라틴어·그리스어로부터의 차용어가 동족어 관계에 있음을 쉽게 알게 되어 어휘의 이해 폭이 확장된다. *heart, cordial, cardiac*이 기본 뜻 심장이라는 동족어이며, *peg, bacillus, bacterium*이 기본 뜻 막대기라는 동족어이고, *deed, fact, theme*이 기본 뜻 세워 놓은 것이라는 동족어임을 바로 알 수 있는 것이다.

인도유럽조어와 라틴어와 그리스어와 영어

영어 낱말은 인도유럽어의 말뿌리를 중심으로 한 동족어 무리 안에서 이해하는 것이 좋다. 그렇다고 해서 인도유럽어 말뿌리나 중간 단계를 모두 알고 있어야 한다는 말은 아니다. 하나의 인도유럽어 말뿌리에서 비롯한 동족어에는 무엇이 있고 그 동족어로부터 어떤 영어 낱말이 만들어졌는가를 이해하는 정도라면 충분하다. '심장' 또는 '마음'을 예로 들면 다음 중 밑줄 친 부분이 눈여겨볼 부분 인 것이다. (이 책에서는 인도유럽어 말뿌리와 라틴어, 그리스어 낱말들은 왼쪽 에 푸른색으로 적었고 거기서 만들어진 영어 낱말은 오른쪽 글상자 안에 붉은색 으로 적었다.)

IE. kerd- *heart*   **E** *heart, hearty, heartful, heartless, hearten*

> L. cor, cordis, n. 심장, 마음, 의지, 용기, 지혜   **E** *(suggested)* **core**

> L. cordatus, cordata, cordatum 심장 모양의, 현명한   **E** *cordate*

> L. cordialis, cordiale 마음에서 우러나는   **E** *cordial*

··· ··· ···

> L. recordor, recordatus sum, recordari (< re- *back, again*) 기억하고 있다   **E** *record*

> G. kardia, kardias, f. *heart, mind, soul*   **E** *cardi(o)-*

> G. kardiakos, kardiakē, kardiakon (< + -akos *adjective suffix*) *of heart*

> L. cardiacus, cardiaca, cardiacum 심장의, 심장병의; (*on the heart side of the body* >) 위(胃)의, 위병(胃病)의, 들문(~門)의   **E** *cardiac*

> G. kardioeidēs, kardioeidēs, kardioeides (< + eidos *shape*) *heart-shaped*   **E** *cardioid*

> G. perikardios, perikardia, perikardion (< peri *around, near, beyond, on account of*) *pericardial*

> L. pericardium, pericardii, n. 심장막, 심낭(心囊)   **E** *pericardium, pericardial*

> L. endocardium, endocardii, n. (< G. end(o)- < endon *within*) 심장속막, 심내막   **E** *endocardium, endocardial*

··· ··· ···

> L. dextrocardia, dextrocardiae, f. (< L. dexter, dextra, dextrum *right*) 우심증   **E** *dextrocardia*

> IE. kred-dhə- (< + IE. dhə- *to do, to place*) *to place trust*

> L. credo, credidi, creditum, credĕre 믿다, 맡기다

E *(first personal singular, present indicative, active 'I believe'* >) **credo**, (credo >) **creed**, **grant** (< *'consent to support'*)

> L. creditum, crediti, n. 신뢰, 신용, 영예, 남에게 맡겨놓은 (빌려 준) 것   **E** *credit, accredit*

··· ··· ···

어원론에서 핵심 부분은 영어 낱말들이다. 따라서 알고자 하는 영어 낱말을 확 인한 후 그 낱말의 어원과 동족어 무리의 영어 낱말들을 훑어보면 족하다. 어원

론은 영어 어원을 이해하기 위함이지 라틴어나 그리스어를 이해하고자 함이 아니기 때문이다. 그러나, 그렇게 해서 어원에 재미를 붙이게 되면 어원론과 친해지고 싶고, 친해지고 싶은 만큼 라틴어와 그리스어를 한 번 더 들여다보게 되며, 그러는 사이 자신도 모르게 라틴어와 그리스어에 입문해 있음을 발견하게 될 것이다. (사실은, 영어든 독일어든 프랑스어든 스페인어든 포르투갈어든, 인도유럽어족의 언어를 '잘' 하기 위해서는 어원론과 어원론을 위한 라틴어 및 그리스어 입문이 절대 필요하다.)

••• 영어 동족어 무리의 표제어

영어 동족어 무리 중 낯선 낱말은 낯익은 낱말을 통해 쉽게 가까워질 수 있다. 따라서 사용하지 않는 인도유럽어 말뿌리는 표제어로서 마땅치 않다. 영어 고유어의 경우, 학술용어의 수가 많지 않고 어휘형성의 원리가 라틴어나 그리스어와는 다르다. 역시 표제어로는 마땅치 않다.

라틴어와 그리스어의 경우, 그리스어 기원보다는 라틴어 기원의 낱말이 낯익은 경우가 더 많다. 또한 그리스어에서 기원한 영어 낱말은, 그리스어의 철자나 문법을 따르는 것이 아니라, 라틴어화라는 통과의례를 거친 후에야 영어에 들어올 수 있다. (요즘은 지켜지지 않는 경우도 어느 정도 있지만.) 지금도, 식물이든 동물이든 미생물이든, 학명은 라틴어 낱말이나 라틴어화한 그리스어 낱말을 라틴어 문법에 따라 적게 되어 있다. 따라서 이 책에서는, 원래 라틴어 낱말이면 물론이거니와, 그리스어 낱말이라고 하더라도 라틴어화한 적이 있으면 라틴어화한 꼴을 표제어로 삼아 〈어원론을 위한 라틴어〉 편에 실었다. '심장' 또는 '마음'과 '동맥'의 어원 및 영어 동족어 무리를 〈어원론을 위한 라틴어〉 편에 다음과 같이 실어 놓았다는 말이다. 왼쪽의 괄호 안 숫자는 다음에 기술할 '통합 기초 문법'과 '어휘형성'에서 참조하기 위해 붙여 놓은 임시 줄번호이다.

(1) cor, cordis, n. 심장, 마음, 의지, 용기, 지혜　　　　　　　E *cord(i)-, (suggested) core*

(2) 　　　> cordatus, cordata, cordatum 심장 모양의, 현명한　　E *cordate*

(3) 　　　> cordialis, cordiale 마음에서 우러나는　　　　　　E *cordial*

(4) 　　　> *coraticum, *coratici, n. 용기, 열정, 욕망, 분노　　E *courage, encourage*

(5) 　　　> praecordium, praecordii, n. (< prae *before, beyond*) 전흉부
　　　　　　(前胸部), 명치부위　　　　　　　　　　　　　　E *precordium*

(6) 　　　　　> praecordialis, praecordiale 전흉부의, 명치부위의　E *precordial*

(7) 　　　> concors, (gen.) concordis (< con- < cum *with, together*) 한

마음의, 합치하는, 일치하는, 화목하는　　　　　　　　**E** *concord*

(8)　　　> discors, (gen.) discordis (< dis- *apart from, down, not*) 어긋나는,
　　　　　상반되는, 불목하는　　　　　　　　　　　　　**E** *discord*

(9)　　　> misericors, (gen.) misericordis (< miser *wretched*) 자비로운　**E** *misericord*

(10)　　> accordo, **accordavi**, accordatum, accordare (< ac- < ad *to, toward,*
　　　　　at, according to) 일치시키다, 조화시키다, 상응시키다　　**E** *accord*

(11)　　> recordor, recordatus sum, recordari (< re- *back, again*) 기억하고
　　　　　있다　　　　　　　　　　　　　　　　　　**E** *record*

(12)　< IE. kerd- *heart*

> **E** *heart, hearty, heartful, heartless, hearten; heartbeat, heartburn,*
> *heart-stopper, heart-to-heart, heart attack, heart failure*

(13)　　> G. kardia, kardias, f. *heart, mind, soul*

> **E** *cardi(o)-, electrocardiogram (ECG),* (D. Elektrokardiogramm >) *EKG,*
> *cardiomegaly*

(14)　　　> G. kardiakos, kardiakē, kardiakon (< + -akos *adjective*
　　　　　　suffix) *of heart*

(15)　　　　> L. cardiacus, cardiaca, cardiacum 심장의, 심장병의;
　　　　　　　(*on the heart side of the body* >) 위(胃)의, 위
　　　　　　　병(胃病)의, 들문(~門)의　　　　　　　　**E** *cardiac*

(16)　　　> G. kardioeidēs, kardioeidēs, kardioeides (< + eidos *shape*)
　　　　　　heart-shaped　　　　　　　　　　　　　**E** *cardioid*

(17)　　　> G. perikardios, perikardia, perikardion (< peri *around, near,*
　　　　　　beyond, on account of) *pericardial*

(18)　　　　> L. pericardium, pericardii, n. 심장막,
　　　　　　　심낭(心囊)　　　　　　　　　　**E** *pericardium, pericardial*

(19)　　　> L. endocardium, endocardii, n. (< G. end(o)- < endon *within*)
　　　　　　심장속막, 심내막　　　　　　　　　**E** *endocardium, endocardial*

(20)　　　> L. myocardium, myocardii, n. (< G. my(o)- < mys, myos, m.
　　　　　　mouse, muscle) 심근층　　　　　**E** *myocardium, myocardial*

(21)　　　> L. epicardium, epicardii, n. (< G. epi *upon*) 심장바깥막,
　　　　　　심외막　　　　　　　　　　　　**E** *epicardium, epicardial*

(22)　　　> L. bradycardia, bradycardiae, f. (< G. bradys *slow*) 느린
　　　　　　맥, 서맥(徐脈)　　　　　　　　　**E** *bradycardia, bradycardiac*

(23)　　　> L. tachycardia, tachycardiae, f. (< G. tachys *swift*) 빠른
　　　　　　맥, 빈맥(頻脈)　　　　　　　　　**E** *tachycardia, tachycardiac*

(24)　　　> L. dextrocardia, dextrocardiae, f. (< L. dexter, dextra,
　　　　　　dextrum *right*) 우심증　　　　　　　　**E** *dextrocardia*

(25)　　> IE. kred-dhə- (< + IE. dhə- *to do, to place*) *to place trust*

(26)　　　> L. credo, **credidi**, creditum, credĕre 믿다, 맡기다

> **E** (*first personal singular, present indicative, active 'I believe'*
> >) *credo,* (credo >) *creed, grant* (< '*consent to support*')

(27)　　　　　　　　　　　> L. creditum, crediti, n. 신뢰, 신용, 영예, 남에게 맡겨
　　　　　　　　　　　　　놓은 (빌려준) 것　　　　　　　　　**E** *credit, accredit*

(28)　　　　　　　　　　　> L. credentia, credentiae, f. 신뢰, 신임　　　**E** *credence*

(29)　　　　　　　　　　　　> L. credentialis, credentiale 신뢰의, 신임의　**E** *credential*

(30)　　　　　　　　　　　> L. credibilis, credibile 믿을 만한, 신용할 만한　**E** *credible*

(31)　　　　　　　　　　　　> L. credibilitas, credibilitatis, f. 신뢰성, 신용　**E** *credibility*

(32)　　　　　　　　　　　　> L. incredibilis, incredibile (< in- *not*) 믿을 수
　　　　　　　　　　　　　없는, 믿어지지 않는　　　　　　　　**E** *incredible*

(33)　　　　　　　　　　　　　> L. incredibilitas, incredibilitatis, f.
　　　　　　　　　　　　　　믿을 수 없음　　　　　　　　　**E** *incredibility*

(34)　　　　　　　　　　　> L. credulus, credula, credulum 쉽게 믿는　**E** *credulous*

(35)　　　　　　　　　　　　> L. credulitas, credulitatis, f. 쉽게 믿음, 경신
　　　　　　　　　　　　　(輕信), 맹신(盲信)　　　　　　　　**E** *credulity*

(36)　　　　　　　　　　　　> L. incredulus, incredula, incredulum (< in-
　　　　　　　　　　　　　not) 의심 많은, 회의적인　　　　　**E** *incredulous*

(37)　　　　　　　　　　　　　> L. incredulitas, incredulitatis, f. 의심
　　　　　　　　　　　　　　많음, 회의　　　　　　　　　　**E** *incredulity*

(38) **arteria, arteriae, f.** 동맥(動脈)　　　**E** *artery, arterial, arteri(o)-, arteriovenous*

(39)　　　　　　　　　　　> arteriola, arteriolae, f. (< + -ola *diminutive suffix*)
　　　　　　　　　　　세동맥(細動脈)　　　**E** *arteriole, arteriolar, arteriol(o)-*

(40)　　　　　　　　　　　> *metarteriola, *metarteriolae, f. (< *arterial*
　　　　　　　　　　　　capillary < G. met- < meta *between,*
　　　　　　　　　　　　along with, across, after) 메타세동맥　**E** *metarteriole*

(41)　　　　　　　< G. artēria, artērias, f. *windpipe, artery, vein*

(42)　　　　　　　　　　> L. arteritis, arteritidis, f. (< G. artēria *artery* + -itis
　　　　　　　　　　　noun suffix denoting inflammation) 동맥염　**E** *arteritis*

(43)　　　　　　　　　　> L. endarteritis, endarteritidis, f. (< G. end(o)-
　　　　　　　　　　　< endon *within*) 동맥속막염,
　　　　　　　　　　　동맥내막염　　　　　　　　　　　**E** *endarteritis*

(44)　　　　　　< G. airein (aeirein) *to raise; (passive) to rise*

(45)　　　　　　　　> G. aortē, aortēs, f. *aorta*

(46)　　　　　　　　　> L. aorta, aortae, f. 대동맥　　　　**E** *aorta, aortic*

(47)　　　　　　　> G. eōra, eōras, f. *suspension, string*

(48)　　　　　　　　　> G. meteōros, meteōros, meteōron (< met- (< meta)
　　　　　　　　　　between, along with, across, after + eōra) *lifted*
　　　　　　　　　　up, in air　　　　　　　　　　　**E** *meteorology*

(49)　　　　　　　　　> G. meteōron, meteōrou, n. *meteor*

(50)　　　　　　　　　　> L. meteorum, meteori, n.
　　　　　　　　　　운석(隕石)　　　　　　　　**E** *meteor, meteorite*

(51)　　　< IE. wer- *to raise, to lift, to hold suspended*

그리스어 낱말로서 라틴어화해 본 적이 없거나 라틴어화해 본 적이 있다 하더라도 그리스어 문법을 설명하기 위해서는 그리스어 낱말을 표제어로 삼아 〈어원론을 위한 그리스어〉 편에 실었다.

(52) hōra, hōras, f. *limited time, period, time, year, season, hour;* ((pl.) Horai)
    (*Greek mythology*) *goddesses of orderly life*

(53) > L. hora, horae, f. 시간; ((pl.) Horae) (로마 신화) 계절과 질서의
    여신들   **E** *hour, Horae*

(54)   > L. horarius, horaria, horarium 시간의, 시간을 나타내는 **E** *horary*

(55) > hōroskopos, hōroskopou, m. (< hōra *time, hour* + skopos *watcher*)
    observer of the hour of nativity, caster of nativities, nativity

(56)   > L. horoscopus, horoscopi, m. 점성가, 출생 시간을 가리키는
    별의 위치, 12궁도   **E** *horoscope*

(57) < IE. yer- *year, season*   **E** *year*

모든 영어 낱말이 인도유럽조어에서부터 기원한 것은 아니며, 모든 영어 낱말의 어원이 밝혀져 있는 것도 아니다. 어원이 밝혀져 있는 낱말은 밝혀져 있는 데까지, 그렇지 않은 낱말은 아무런 표기 없이 〈어원론을 위한 라틴어〉 편 또는 〈어원론을 위한 그리스어〉 편에 실어 놓았다.

〈어원론을 위한 라틴어〉 편의 예:

(58) caeremonia, caeremoniae, f. (caerimonia, caerimoniae, f.)
    종교적 예식, 경외심, 신성함   **E** *ceremony*
(59) < (*probably*) *Of Etruscan origin*

〈어원론을 위한 그리스어〉 편의 예:

(60) mimos, mimou, m. *imitator, actor*   **E** *mime*
(61) > pantomimos, pantomimou, m. (< *all-imitator* < panto- < pas,
    pasa, pan *all*) *a theatrical performer who played by gestures
    and actions without words*
(62)   > L. pantomimus, pantomimi, m. 무언극 배우 **E** *pantomime*
(63) > mimikos, mimikē, mimikon *of mime*
(64)   > L. mimicus, mimica, mimicum 흉내 내는, 모조의 **E** *mimic, mimicry*
(65) > mimeisthai (*middle*) *to imitate*
(66)   > mimēsis, mimēseōs, f. *imitation, copy*
(67)   > L. mimesis, mimesis, f. 모방, 모사(模寫), 모의(模擬);

(생물) 의태(擬態) **E** *mimesis*

(68)   > mimētikos, mimētikē, mimētikon

imitative   **E** *mimetic, sympathomimetic, parasympathomimetic*

(69)   > L. mimus, mimi, m. 풍자극 배우, 풍자극

(70)   > L. mimosus, mimosa, mimosum 흉내 내는

(71)   > L. mimosa, mimosae, f. (< *mimicking the sensitivity of an animal* < herba mimosa *mimicking herb*)

미모사, 함수초(含羞草)   **E** *mimosa*

(72)   [용례] Mimosa pudica 미모사, 함수초   **E** Mimosa pudica

(문법) mimosa 미모사: 단수 주격

pudica 부끄러워하는: 형용사, 여성형

단수 주격 < pudicus, pudica, pudicum

부끄러워하는, 정숙한, 순결한 < pudeo,

pudui, puditum, pudēre 부끄러워하다,

부끄럽게 하다

(73) G. astēr, asteros, m. *star*

(74)   > L. aster, asteris, m. 별; (생물학) 성상체;

(Aster) (식물) Aster속(屬)   **E** *aster, asteroid*

(75)   > G. asteriskos, asteriskou, m. (< + -iskos *diminutive suffix*)

little star

(76)   > L. asteriscus, asterisci, m. 작은 별, 별표   **E** *asterisk*

(77)   < IE. ster- *star*

제3장 어원론을 위한 통합 기초 문법

하나의 인도유럽어 말뿌리에서부터 갈래가 다른 영어, 라틴어, 그리스어 낱말들이 만들어지는 경우가 많다. 또한 각 낱말들은, 명사, 형용사, 동사 등 품사가 다르며, 같은 품사라 하더라도 변화의 종류가 다른 경우가 많다. 게다가 수시로 그리스어 낱말을 라틴어 낱말로 바꾸어준다. 이렇다 보니 어원론을 시작하기 위해서는 라틴어와 그리스어 문법을, 문턱 만큼, 미리 알고 있어야 한다.

이 책은 어원론에 꼭 필요한 최소한의 라틴어와 그리스어 문법을 〈차례〉에 나오는 각 항목의 첫 부분에서 설명하고 있다. 먼저 이를 알아두는 것도 방법이다. 그러나 실제 그리 해보면 앞부분을 이해하기 위해서는 뒷부분을 이해하고 있어야 하고 뒷부분을 이해하기 위해서는 앞부분을 이해하고 있어야 한다는 '자기 꼬리물기'가 된다.

라틴어 문법과 그리스어 문법은, 세부적으로는 많이 다르지만, 뼈대에 있어서는 같다. 따라서 통합 기초 문법이 가능하다. 다음은 자기 꼬리를 물지 않고 시작하기 위해 필요한 라틴어와 그리스어의 통합 기초 문법이다. 문법 용어는, 라틴어와 그리스어 문법에 고유한 경우를 제외하고는, 영문법 용어를 사용하였다.

품사

어원론에서 중요한 라틴어와 그리스어 품사는 명사, 형용사, 동사, 전치사이다. 명사, 형용사, 동사는 꼴을 바꿈으로써 문장 안에서 역할을 달리하는 변화 품사이며, 전치사는 불변화 품사이다.

어간과 어미

라틴어와 그리스어 품사 중 변화 품사는 낱말의 앞부분을 그대로 둔 채 뒷부분을 바꾼다. 바뀌지 않는 앞부분을 낱말의 줄기, 어간(語幹, *stem*)이라고 하고 바뀌는 뒷부분을 낱말의 꼬리, 어미(語尾, *ending*)라고 한다. 다음 예에서 하이픈의 앞 밑줄친 부분이 어간이고 뒤가 어미이다. (라틴어 명사 주격 cor는 어미 없이 어간만 있는 꼴이다.) 명사와 형용사의 어간은, 정식으로는, 하나이며, 동사의 어간은, 정식으로도, 더 많다.

(1) L. cor, cord-is, n. 심장, 마음, 의지, 용기, 지혜   **E** *(suggested)* **core**

(2)　　> L. cordat-us, cordat-a, cordat-um 심장 모양의, 현명한   **E** **cordate**

(10)　　> L. accord-o, accordav-i, accordat-um, accord-are (< ac- < ad *to, toward, at, according to*) 일치시키다, 조화시키다, 상응시키다   **E** **accord**

(13) G. kardi-a, kardi-as, f. *heart, mind, soul*   **E** **cardi(o)-**

(14)　　> G. kardiak-os, kardiak-ē, kardiak-on *of heart*   **E** **cardiac**

명사와 형용사의 변화

라틴어와 그리스어에서 명사 또는 형용사의 어미 바꿈을 변화 또는 곡용(曲用)이라고 한다. 영어로는 *declension*(< L. declinatio < declinare *to decline*)이라고 하며 으뜸꼴인 주격으로부터 '굽어져 나온 꼴'이란 뜻이다. 이 책에서는 영문법 우리말 용어를 따라 변화라고 하였다.

라틴어와 그리스어의 명사는 성(性)이 있으며, 수(數)와 격(格)에 따라 어미가 바뀐다. 형용사도 수식하는 명사의 성, 수, 격에 따라 어미가 바뀐다. 명사 및 형용사에서 성, 수, 격의 종류와 약자는 다음과 같다.

성(性, *gender*):　　남성(男性, *masculine*)　　m.

　　　　　　　　　여성(女性, *feminine*)　　f.

　　　　　　　　　중성(中性, *neuter*)　　n.

수(數, *number*):	단수(單數, *singular*)	sing.
	복수(複數, *plural*)	pl.
격(格, *case*):	주격(主格, *nominative*)	nom.
	속격(屬格, *genitive*)	gen.
	여격(與格, *dative*)	dat.
	대격(對格, *accusative*)	acc.
	탈격(奪格, *ablative*)	abl.
	호격(呼格, *vocative*)	voc.

그리스어에는 탈격이 없고, 그 대신, 속격과 여격이 탈격의 역할을 분담한다. 어원론에서는 그리스어 낱말이라고 하더라도 라틴어화한 다음 라틴어 문법을 적용하므로 우선은 이 부분을 잊어도 좋다.

어원론은 성을 필요로 한다. 수와 격에 있어서는 단수 주격과 단수 속격을 필요로 하며, 부분적으로 단수 탈격, 복수 주격, 복수 속격을 필요로 한다. 어원론에서 별 볼일 없는 격은 회색으로 적었다.

라틴어·그리스어 명사의 성은 자연의 성을 따르는 낱말이 많지만 엉뚱한 성을 갖는 낱말도 있다. 인도유럽조어를 사용하던 사람들의 정령(精靈) 신앙 때문이다. 그래도, 경험하다 보면, 성을 결정짓는 나름대로 흐름이 있음을 알게 된다.

동사의 변화

동사는 태(능동태·(중간태)·수동태), 법(직설법·가정법·명령법·부정법), 시제(현재 등), 수(단수·복수), 인칭(일인칭·이인칭·삼인칭) 등에 따라 어미가 바뀌는데, 동사의 어미 바꿈을 활용(活用)이라고 한다. 영어 낱말 *conjugation*(< L. conjugatio < conjugare *to join together*)이란 어미 바꿈에 의해 태, 법, 시제, 수, 인칭이 하나로 묶임을 뜻한다. 이 책에서는, 명사와 형용사 변화 (*declension*)에서와 마찬가지로, 활용(*conjugation*)도 영문법 용어를 따라 변화라고 하였다.

*declension*과 *conjugation*을 합하여 굴절(屈折, *inflection*)이라고 한다. 영어 낱말 *inflection*(< L. inflexio < inflectĕre *to bend into*)은 주격 또는 능동태 직설법 현재의 꼴에서부터 '굽은' 꼴이란 뜻이다. 라틴어와 그리스어 같은 언어를 굴절어(*inflectional language*)라고 부르는 이유이다.

명사

라틴어와 그리스어 명사는 단수 주격, 단수 속격, 성을 보아 무슨 변화를 하는지 알 수 있고, 단수 속격을 보아 어간이 무엇인지 알 수 있다. 따라서 명사라면 라틴어나 그리스어 사전 모두 이 셋을 순서대로 제시하며, 어원론에서도 이 셋이 필요하다.

(1) L. cor, cord-is, n. 심장, 마음, 의지, 용기, 지혜   **E** *cord(i)-*

: 단수 주격은 cor, 단수 속격은 cordis 인 중성 명사이며, 어간은 단수 속격 cord-is 에서 어미 -is 를 떼어내고 남은 cord- 이다. 제3변화 제2식 b 명사이다.

(13) G. kardi-a, kardi-as, f. *heart, mind, soul*   **E** *cardi(o)-*

: 단수 주격은 kardia, 단수 속격은 kardias 인 여성 명사이며, 어간은 단수 속격 kardi-as 에서 어미 -as 를 떼어내고 남은 kardi- 이다. 제1변화 제1식 명사이다.

라틴어 명사

라틴어의 명사변화에는 다음과 같은 종류가 있다. '제 x 변화 제 y 식' 보다도 굵게 표시한 대표 명사를 알아 두는 것이 좋다.

••• 제1변화

단수의 주격 어미가 -a, 속격 어미가 -ae인 여성 또는 남성 명사. 성은 거의 여성이다. 단수 주격의 어간과 단수 속격의 어간이 같다.

cellul-a, cellul-ae, f. 세포

••• 제2변화

단수 속격의 어미가 -i인 남성, 여성, 중성 명사. 단수 주격의 어간과 단수 속격의 어간이 같다.

제1식   단수 주격 어미가 -us, 속격 어미가 -i인 남성 또는 여성 명사. 성은 거의 남성이다.

nucle-us, nucle-i, m. 핵

제2식   단수 주격이 어미 없이 -er로 끝나며 속격 어미가 -i인 남성 명사.

faber, fabr-i, m. 목수

제3식   단수 주격 어미가 -um, 속격 어미가 -i인 중성 명사.

ov-um, ov-i, n. 알

••• 제3변화

단수 속격의 어미가 -is인 남성, 여성, 중성 명사. 원칙적으로 단수 주격의 어간과 단수 속격의 어간이 다르다. 속격어간이 정식 어간이다.

제1식 a   단수 속격의 음절수가 많아지며 어간 끝에 자음이 하나만 있는 남성, 여성 명사.

homo, homin-is, m. 사람

제1식 b   단수 속격의 음절수가 많아지며 어간 끝에 자음이 하나만 있는 중성 명사.

caput, capit-is, n. 머리

제2식 a   단수 속격의 음절수가 많아지며 어간 끝에 자음이 둘 이상 있는
         남성, 여성 명사.

         dens, dent-is, m. 이, 치아

제2식 b   단수 속격의 음절수가 많아지며 어간 끝에 자음이 둘 이상 있는
         중성 명사.

         cor, cord-is, n. 심장, 마음

제2식 c   단수 주격과 단수 속격의 음절수가 같은 남성, 여성 명사.

         aur-is, aur-is, f. 귀

제3식   단수 주격이 -al, -ar, -e로 끝나는 중성 명사.

         mar-e, mar-is, n. 바다

●●● 제4변화

단수 속격의 어미가 -us인 남성, 여성, 중성 명사. 단수 주격의 어간과 단수
속격의 어간이 같다.

제1식   단수 주격 어미가 -us, 속격 어미도 -us인 남성과 여성 명사.
         성은 거의 남성이다.

         man-us, man-us, f. 손

제2식   단수 주격 어미가 -u, 속격 어미가 -us인 중성 명사.

         corn-u, corn-us, n. 뿔

●●● 제5변화

단수의 주격 어미가 -es이고 속격 어미가 -ei인 남성 또는 여성 명사. 성은
거의 여성이다. 단수 주격의 어간과 단수 속격의 어간이 같다.

di-es, di-ei, m. 날; f. 날짜

그리스어 명사

그리스어의 명사변화에는 다음과 같은 종류가 있다. 라틴어 명사변화에 빗대어, 라틴어 명사변화에서처럼 '제 x 변화 제 y 식'보다도 굵게 표시한 대표 명사를 알아 두는 것이 좋다.

●●● 제 1 변화

> 단수의 주격 어미가 -a 또는 -ē 로 끝나는 여성 명사와 단수의 주격 어미가 -ēs 또는 -as 로 끝나는 남성 명사. 단수 주격의 어간과 단수 속격의 어간이 같다. 라틴어 명사의 제1변화(cellul-a, cellul-ae, f. 세포)에 해당한다.

제 1 식   단수 주격 어미가 -a, 어간의 끝이 -e, -i, -r 인 여성 명사. 단수 속격 어미는 -as 이다.

hōr-a, hōr-as, f. *time, hour*

제 2 식   단수 주격 어미가 -a, 어간의 끝이 -e, -i, -r 가 아닌 여성 명사. 단수 속격 어미는 -ēs 이다.

dox-a, dox-ēs, f. *opinion, glory*

제 3 식   단수 주격이 -ē 인 여성 명사. 단수 속격 어미는 -ēs 이다.

graph-ē, graph-ēs, f. *drawing, writing*

제 4 식   단수 주격 어미가 -ēs 로 끝나는 남성 명사. 단수 속격 어미는 -ou 이다.

poiēt-ēs, poiēt-ou, m. *maker, creator, poet*

제 5 식   단수 주격 어미가 -as 로 끝나는 남성 명사. 단수 속격 어미는 -ou 이다.

neani-as, neani-ou, m. *young man, youth*

● ● ● 제 2 변화

단수의 주격 어미가 –os 로 끝나는 남성 또는 여성 명사와 –on 으로 끝나는 중성 명사. 단수 속격 어미는 –ou 이다. 단수 주격의 어간과 단수 속격의 어간이 같다.

제 1 식 단수의 주격 어미가 –os 로 끝나는 남성 또는 여성 명사. 주로 남성 명사이다. 라틴어 명사의 제2변화 제1식(nucle-us, nucle-i, m. 핵)에 해당한다.

log-os, log-ou, m. *word, speech*

제 2 식 단수 주격 어미가 –on 으로 끝나는 중성 명사. 라틴어 명사의 제2변화 제3식(ov-um, ov-i, n. 알)에 해당한다.

dōr-on, dōr-ou, n. *gift*

● ● ● 제 3 변화

단수 주격 어미는 변화 방식에 따라 다르며 단수 속격 어미가 –os (–eōs, –ous)인 남성, 여성, 중성 명사. 원칙적으로 단수 주격의 어간과 단수 속격의 어간이 다르다.

제 1 식 a 단수 속격의 어간이 치음 자음(d, t, th), 연구개음 자음(g, k, ch), 순음 자음(b, p, ph)으로 끝나는 남성 또는 여성 명사. 라틴어 명사의 제3변화 제1식 a(homo, hominis, m. 사람)에 해당한다.

gerōn, geront-os, m. *oldness, old man*

제 1 식 b 단수 속격의 어간이 자음으로 끝나는 중성 명사. 라틴어 명사의 제3변화 제1식 b(caput, capitis, n. 머리)에 해당한다.

onoma, onomat-os, n. *name*

제 2 식 단수 속격의 어간이 유음 자음(l, r)이나 비음 자음(m, n)으로 끝나는 남성 또는 여성 명사.

anēr, andr-os, m. *man, male*

제 3 식   단수 속격의 본디 어간이 치음 자음(s)으로 끝나는 명사 또는 이와 같은 명사. 주로 중성 명사이다.

gen-os, gen-ous, n. (genes- *original stem*) *race, family, kind*

제 4 식   단수 속격의 본디 어간이 모음(i, y, eu)으로 끝나는 남성 또는 여성 명사. 라틴어 명사의 제 3 변화 제 2 식 c(auris, auris, f. 귀)에 해당한다.

poli-s, pol-eōs, f. (poli- *original stem*) *city*

형용사

라틴어와 그리스어 형용사는, 명사와 달리, 남성형·여성형·중성형 셋의 단수 주격을 보아 무슨 변화를 하는지, 어간이 무엇인지 알 수 있다. 따라서 라틴어나 그리스어 사전은 형용사의 남성형·여성형·중성형의 단수 주격을 순서대로 제시한다. 남·여성형의 단수 주격이 같은 꼴이고 중성형의 단수 주격만 다른 꼴인 경우에는 남·여성형의 단수 주격과 중성형의 단수 주격을 제시한다. 단수 주격에서 어미를 떼어내고 남은 부분이 어간이다.

라틴어 형용사 중 제 3 변화 제 3 식 형용사는 남·여·중성형의 단수 주격이 같으며, 단수 주격의 어간과 단수 속격의 어간이 다르다. 이 경우 라틴어사전은 단수 주격과 함께 단수 속격을 제시해 어간을 밝히며 속격 앞에다 (gen.)이라고 써 놓는다. 그리스어 형용사 중 제 3 변화와 제 1·3 변화의 일부 형용사는 단수 주격만으로는 어간을 찾을 수 없는 경우가 있다. 이 경우에는 사전의 도움이 필요하다.

(2) L. cordatus, cordata, cordatum 심장 모양의, 현명한   E *cordate*

: 남성형은 cordatus, 여성형은 cordata, 중성형은 cordatum이며, 어간은 주격 어미 -us, -a, -um을 떼어내고 남은 cordat-이다. 제 1·2 변화 형용사이다.

(3) L. cordialis, cordiale 마음에서 우러나는   E *cordial*

: 남·여성형은 cordialis, 중성형은 cordiale 이며, 어간은 주격 어미 –is, –e를 떼어내고 남은 cordial– 이다. 제3변화 제2식 형용사이다.

(7) L. concors, (gen.) concordis 한마음의, 합치하는, 일치하는, 화목하는 　　　E concord

: 남·여·중성형 모두 주격은 concors 이며 속격은 concordis 이다. 어간은 속격 어미 –is를 떼어내고 남은 concord– 이다. 제3변화 제3식 형용사이다.

(14) G. kardiakos, kardiakē, kardiakon (< + –akos *adjective suffix*)
　　　 of heart 　　　E cardiac

: 남성형은 kardiakos, 여성형은 kardiakē, 중성형은 kardiakon 이며, 어간은 주격 어미 –os, –ē, –on 을 떼어내고 남은 kardiak– 이다. 제1·2 변화 형용사이다.

라틴어 형용사

　　라틴어 형용사변화에는 다음과 같은 종류가 있다. '제 x 변화 제 y 식'보다도 굵게 표시한 대표 형용사를 알아 두는 것이 좋다.

●●● 제1·2변화

> 남성형 변화는 명사의 제2변화 제1식 또는 제2식을 따르며, 여성형 변화는 명사의 제1변화를 따르고, 중성형 변화는 명사의 제2변화 제3식을 따른다. 단수 주격의 어미를 떼어내고 남은 부분이 어간이다.

제1식　　　남성형의 변화가 명사 제2변화 제1식을 따른다.

　　　　　　bon–us, bon–a, bon–um 좋은

제2식　　　남성형의 변화가 명사 제2변화 제2식을 따른다.

　　　　　　niger, nigr–a, nigr–um 검은

제3변화 명사에서처럼 남·여·중성형의 단수 속격 어미가 –is로 끝난다. 단수 주격의 꼴에 따라 세 가지로 나눈다.

제1식   단수 주격이 남성형은 –er, 여성형은 –is, 중성형은 –e로 끝난다. 단수 주격의 어미를 떼어내고 남은 부분이 어간이다.

             acer, acr–is, acr–e 신, 날카로운, 혹독한

제2식   단수 주격이 남·여성형은 –is, 중성형은 –e로 끝난다. 남성형과 여성형의 어미변화가 같으므로 사전은 남·여성형과 중성형 두 가지만의 단수 주격을 제시한다. 단수 주격의 어미를 떼어내고 남은 부분이 어간이다.

             omn–is, omn–e 모든

제3식   남·여·중성형에서 단수 주격은 주격끼리, 단수 속격은 속격끼리 같으며 단수 속격의 음절수가 많아진다. 단수 주격의 끝음절이 –ns, –s, –x, –l, –r로 끝나는 형용사이다. 사전은 단수 주격과 단수 속격을 제시한다. 단수 속격의 어미를 떼어내고 남은 부분이 어간이다.

             potens, (gen.) potent–is 힘 있는, 능력 있는

그리스어 형용사

그리스어사전은 형용사의 남·여·중성형 단수 주격 세 가지를 순서대로 제시한다. 남·여성형이 같은 꼴이고 중성형이 다른 꼴인 경우 남·여성형과 중성형 두 가지만을 제시한다. 그러나 그런 경우에도 이 책에서는, 보기 편하도록, 남·여·중성형 세 가지를 모두 제시하였다.

그리스어의 형용사변화에는 다음과 같은 종류가 있다. 라틴어 형용사변화에 빗대어, 라틴어 형용사변화에서처럼 '제 x 변화 제 y 식'보다도 굵게 표시한 대표 형용사를 알아 두는 것이 좋다.

●●● 제1 · 2 변화

남성형과 중성형은 제2변화 남성 명사와 중성 명사의 변화를 따르고, 여성형은 제1변화 여성 명사의 변화를 따른다. 여성형 형용사의 어간이 -e, -i, -r로 끝나면 단수 주격 어미는 -a가 되고 그렇지 않으면 -ē가 된다. 단수 주격의 어미를 떼어내고 남은 부분이 어간이다. 라틴어 형용사의 제1 · 2변화 제1식(bon-us, bon-a, bon-um 좋은)에 해당한다.

kathar-os, kathar-a, kathar-on *clean, pure*

dynamik-os, dynamik-ē, dynamik-on *powerful*

●●● 제2 변화

남성형, 여성형, 중성형이 각각 제2변화 남성, 여성, 중성 명사의 변화를 따른다. 제2변화 남성 명사와 여성 명사의 변화가 똑같기 때문에 형용사도 남성형과 여성형의 변화가 똑같다. 앞에 다른 낱말이 붙은 파생 형용사나 합성 형용사가 주로 제2변화를 한다. 단수 주격의 어미를 떼어내고 남은 부분이 어간이다.

atom-os, atom-os, atom-on *uncut, indivisible*

●●● 제3 변화

남성형, 여성형, 중성형 모두 제3변화 명사변화를 따르는 형용사이다. 여성 명사처럼 변하는 형용사와 남성 명사처럼 변하는 형용사 두 가지가 있다. 단수 속격의 어미를 떼어내고 남은 부분이 어간이다.

hygi-ēs, hygi-ēs, hygi-es *healthy*

piōn, piōn, pion *fat, plump, fertile, rich*

●●● 제1 · 3 변화

남성형과 중성형은 제3변화 남성과 중성의 명사변화를 따르고, 여성형은 제1변화 여성 명사의 변화를 따른다. 단수 속격의 어미를 떼어내고 남은 부분이 어간이다.

pas, pasa, pan *all*

명사와 형용사의 일치

　라틴어든 그리스어든 형용사의 성·수·격은 수식하는 명사나 대명사의 성·수·격과 일치하여야 한다. 학술용어도 라틴어 형용사나 라틴어화한 그리스어 형용사가 라틴어 문법을 따라야 한다고 규정해 놓고 있다. 학술용어에서 명사는 대부분 단수 주격으로 사용되므로 형용사도 단수 주격이 대부분이다.

　라틴어 형용사는 수식하는 명사의 앞뒤 어디에다 놓아도 좋으나 뒤에 놓는 후치수식이 일반적이다. '동물의 감수성을 흉내 내는, 부끄러워하는 풀꽃'의 학명을 예로 들면 다음과 같다.

(72)　[용례] Mimosa pudica 미모사, 함수초(含羞草)
　　　　(문법) mimosa 미모사: 명사, 단수 주격 < mimosa, mimosae, f.
　　　　pudica 부끄러워하는: 형용사, 여성형 단수 주격
　　　　　　< pudicus, pudica, pudicum 부끄러워하는, 정숙한, 순결한
　　　　　< pudeo, pudui, puditum, pudēre 부끄러워하다, 부끄럽게 하다

동사

　라틴어 동사는 현재부정법과 직설법 현재 단수 일인칭을 보아 무슨 변화를 하는지 알 수 있고, 그리스어 동사는 현재부정법을 보아 무슨 변화를 하는지 알 수 있다.

(10) L. accordo, accordavi, accordatum, accordare (< ac- (< ad) *to, toward, at, according to*) 일치시키다, 조화시키다, 상응시키다　　`E accord`

　　: 능동태 현재부정법이 어미 -are, 직설법 현재 단수 일인칭이 어미 -o 로 끝나는 정형 제1변화 동사이다.

(11) L. recordor, recordatus sum, recordari (< re- *back, again*) 기억하고 있다　　`E record`

　　: 현재부정법이 어미 -ari, 직설법 현재 단수 일인칭이 어미 -or 로 끝나는 탈형 제1변화 동사이다.

(26) L. credo, credidi, creditum, credĕre 믿다,
맡기다

: 능동태 현재부정법이 어미 –ĕre, 직설법 현재 단수 일인칭이 어미 –o 로 끝나는 정형 제3변화 A식 동사이다.

(44) G. airein (aeirein) *to raise;* (*passive*) *to rise*

: 능동태 현재부정법이 어미 –ein 으로 끝나는 정형동사이다.

(65) G. mimeisthai (*middle*) *to imitate*

: 중간태 현재부정법이 어미 –eisthai 로 끝나는 정형동사이다.

라틴어 정형(定形)동사란 능동태와 수동태의 구분이 분명한 동사이며 대부분의 동사가 정형동사이다. 탈형(脫形, *deponent*)동사란 꼴이 수동태이지만 뜻은 능동태인 동사이다. 이태(異態)동사라고도 한다. 영어 *deponent*(< L. deponĕre *to put apart*)도 꼴을 '제쳐놓은' 동사라는 뜻이다.

그리스어 정형동사에는, 능동태와 수동태 외에, 주어의 행위가 다시 주어에 미치는 태가 있다. 능동태와 수동태의 가운데 태라는 뜻에서 중간태(*middle*)라고 한다. 탈형동사는 꼴이 중간태 또는 수동태이나 뜻이 능동태인 동사이다. 라틴어에서와 마찬가지로 대부분의 동사가 정형동사이다.

그리스어 정형동사에서 태를 밝히는 경우는 중간태나 수동태가 되면서 뜻이 중간태나 수동태가 아닌 다른 뜻으로 바뀌는 경우이다. 앞의 예에서 '일으키다'의 동사 airein 의 수동태가 '일어나다'라는 자동사의 뜻을 갖는 것이 예이다. 따라서, 이런 경우까지 고려하면, 어원론의 관점에서는 그리스어 동사의 종류를 정형 능동태, 정형 중간태, 정형 수동태, 그리고 탈형 능동태의 네 가지로 정리하는 것이 편리하다.

라틴어 동사

라틴어사전은 동사변화에 필요한 기본꼴을 제시한다. 정형동사의 경우에는 네 가지 기본꼴, 즉 능동태 직설법 현재 단수 일인칭, 능동태 직설법 완료 단수 일

인칭, 능동태 목적분사, 그리고 능동태 현재부정법을 차례대로 제시한다. (이 가운데, 어원론에 필요한 꼴은 능동태 직설법 현재 단수 일인칭, 능동태 목적분사, 능동태 현재부정법의 세 가지이다. 능동태 직설법 완료 단수 일인칭의 색깔을 달리 한 이유이다.) 탈형동사의 경우에는 세 가지 기본꼴, 즉 직설법 현재 단수 일인칭, 직설법 완료 단수 일인칭 남성형, 현재부정법을 차례대로 제시한다. (어원론에서 필요한 꼴도 이 세 가지이다.)

동사변화에는 다음과 같은 종류가 있다. '정형 또는 탈형 제 x 변화 제 y 식'보다도 굵게 표시한 대표 동사를 기억해 두는 것이 좋다.

정형동사의 변화

●●● 제 1 변화

능동태 현재부정법이 -are로 끝나는 동사.

am-o, **amav**-i, **amat**-um, **am**-are 사랑하다

●●● 제 2 변화

능동태 현재부정법이 -ēre로 끝나는 동사.

hab-eo, **habu**-i, **habit**-um, **hab**-ēre 가지다

●●● 제 3 변화 A식

능동태 현재부정법이 -ĕre로 끝나며 능동태 직설법 현재 단수 일인칭이
-o로 끝나는 동사.

leg-o, **leg**-i, **lect**-um, **leg**-ĕre 모으다, 뽑다, 읽다

●●● 제 3 변화 B식

능동태 현재부정법이 -ĕre로 끝나며 능동태 직설법 현재 단수 일인칭이
-io로 끝나는 동사.

cap-io, **cep**-i, **capt**-um, **cap**-ĕre 잡다, 붙잡다, 획득하다

••• 제 4 변화

능동태 현재부정법이 -ire로 끝나는 동사.

aud-io, audiv-i (audi-i), audit-um, aud-ire 듣다

탈형동사의 변화

••• 제 1 변화

현재부정법이 -ari로 끝나는 동사.

imit-or, imitat-us sum, imit-ari 모방하다, 본받다

••• 제 2 변화

현재부정법이 -eri로 끝나는 동사.

tu-eor, tuit-us (tut-us) sum, tu-eri 지켜보다, 주시하다, 보살피다

••• 제 3 변화 A식

현재부정법이 -i로 끝나며 직설법 현재 단수 일인칭이 -or로 끝나는 동사.

loqu-or, locut-us sum, loqu-i 말하다

••• 제 3 변화 B식

현재부정법이 -i로 끝나며 직설법 현재 단수 일인칭이 -ior로 끝나는 동사.

pat-ior, pass-us sum, pat-i 당하다, 견디다, 참다, 고통받다, 내버려 두다

••• 제 4 변화

현재부정법이 -iri로 끝나는 동사.

ori-or, ort-us sum, or-iri 돋다, 나다, 출현하다

라틴어 동사의 기본꼴은 동사를 활용하는데 필요하다. 어원론을 이해하기 위해 필요한 꼴은 동사의 현재부정법 (*present infinitive*), 현재분사 (*present participle*), 수동형 미래분사(*gerundive*), 과거분사(*past participle*)의 네 가지다. 분사는 기본꼴로부터 쉽게 만들어진다. 그 방법은 라틴어 동사편에 기술되어 있다.

그리스어 동사

그리스어사전은 정형 능동태, 정형 중간태, 정형 수동태, 또는 탈형 능동태의 직설법 현재 단수 일인칭을 표제어로 제시함으로써 동사의 어간과 뜻을 밝힌다. 정형 능동태의 직설법 현재 단수 일인칭의 어미는 -ō 아니면 -mi이다. (이에 따라 정형 능동태를 가지는 동사를 ō 동사와 mi 동사의 두 가지로 구분한다. 일반적으로 동사는 ō 동사이며 어미변화가 규칙적이다.) 정형 중간태, 정형 수동태, 탈형 능동태의 직설법 현재 단수 일인칭의 어미는 -omai이다.

이 책에서는, 그리스어사전과는 달리, 현재부정법을 제시함으로써 어간과 뜻을 밝혀 놓았다. 대부분의 어원론에서 제시하는 형식이기 때문이다. 현재부정법의 어미는 (1) 정형 능동태 ō 동사의 경우에는 -ein이고, (2) 정형 능동태 mi 동사의 경우에는 -nai이며, (3) 정형 중간태, 정형 수동태, 탈형 능동태 동사의 경우에는 -esthai이다.

정형 능동태 ō 동사의 어간이 -e-, -a-, -o-로 끝나는 동사는, 단축의 원리에 따라, 현재부정법 어미가 -ein (< -e-ein), -an (< -a-ein), -oun (< -o-ein)으로 단축된다. 이런 단축동사의 정형 중간태와 정형 수동태의 현재부정법 어미는 각각 -eisthai, -asthai, -ousthai가 되며 이런 꼴의 탈형동사 현재부정법 어미도, 탈형동사의 정의상, 마찬가지이다.

이상을 간추리면, 그리스어사전이 제시하는 직설법 현재 단수 일인칭의 어미와 어원론이 제시하는 현재부정법의 어미에는 (1) -ō/-ein (-ein, -an, -oun), (2) -mi/-nai, (3) -omai/-esthai (-eisthai, -asthai, -ousthai)의 세 가지가 있는 것이다.

그리스어사전과 어원론에서 표시하는 동사 어미의 종류

형	태	ō, mi 동사	직설법 현재 단수 일인칭 (그리스어사전)	현재부정법 (어원론)	
정형	능동태	ō 동사	–ō	–ein	
				–ein	< –e-ein
				–an	< –a-ein
				–oun	< –o-ein
		mi 동사	–mi	–nai	
	중간태, 수동태	ō, mi 동사	–omai	–esthai	
				–eisthai	< –e-esthai
				–asthai	< –a-esthai
				–ousthai	< –o-esthai
탈형	능동태	(해당 안 됨)	–omai	–esthai	
				–eisthai	< –e-esthai
				–asthai	< –a-esthai
				–ousthai	< –o-esthai

그리스어 낱말의 라틴어화

학술용어에서는, 다음 용례처럼, 라틴어나 라틴어화한 그리스어를 라틴어 문법
에 맞춰 써 왔다. 전에 비하면 조금 더 영어답게 바뀐 용어도 있지만 지금도 마
찬가지이며, 앞으로도 학명에는 라틴어와 라틴어화한 그리스어를 쓰지 않을 수
없다.

[용례] L. status epilepticus 뇌전증 지속상태
  (문법) L. status 상태: 단수 주격
    < L. status, status, m. 상태, 현상, 체질, 신분, 지위
    < L. sto, steti, statum, stare 서다, 서 있다, 오래가다
  L. epilepticus 뇌전증의: 형용사, 남성형 단수 주격
    < L. epilepticus, epileptica, epilepticum 뇌전증의

< G. epilēptikos, epilēptikos, epilēptikon *of epilepsy*
< G. epilambanein (< ep(i)– *upon* + lambanein *to seize*) *to seize upon*

라틴어와 그리스어는 각각 이탈리아어파와 헬라어파에 속해 파가 다르지만 인도유럽어족 안에서는 가장 가까운 사이이다. 문법의 뼈대가 같고, 상당 부분 어휘를 공유한다. 역사적으로도 두 언어는 매우 밀접하다. 따라서 로마 시대부터 이미 라틴어는 선발 언어인 그리스어의 어휘를 라틴어화하여 써 왔으며 그때 라틴어화하는 규칙이 지금껏 내려오고 있다. 학술용어에서 라틴어화해서 쓰는 그리스어 낱말은 명사와 형용사가 주를 이룬다.

철자의 라틴어화

그리스어 낱말을 라틴어화할 때에는 그리스어 철자를 해당하는 라틴어 철자로 바꿔준다. 달라지는 철자는 다음 두 가지이다.

••• 자음 k의 라틴어화

라틴어는 날카로운 발음을 싫어하므로 그리스어 자음 'k'를 'c'로 바꾼다. 다음 예에서, 그리스어의 형용사 어간 kardiak–는 cardiac–로 라틴어화한다. (어미 –os, –ē, –on의 라틴어화는 '문법의 라틴어화'를 따른다.) 그러나 날카로운 발음이 필요할 때에는 바꾸지 않는다. 그리스어 형용사 leukos와 명사 plax가 만든 라틴어 합성어는, 'k'를 날카롭게 발음해야 하므로, leucoplacia('류꼬플라치아')가 아닌 leukoplakia('류코플라키아')이다.

(14) G. **kardiak–os, kardiak–ē, kardiak–on** *of heart*

(15) > L. **cardiac–us, cardiac–a, cardiac–um** 심장의, 심장병의;
   (*on the heart side of the body* >) 들문의, 위(胃)의, 위병의 **E** *cardiac*

L. **leukoplakia, leukoplakiae,** f. (< G. leukos *bright, white* + plax,
   plakos, f. *plaque, slab*) 백색판증 **E** *leukoplakia*
   < IE. leuk– *light, brightness* + IE. plak– *to be flat*

영어는 그리스어 낱말을 라틴어화한 다음 들여왔다. 그 전통에 따라, 라틴어화한 적이 없는 그리스어 낱말을 차용할 때에도 영어는 그리스어의 'k'를 'c'로 바꾼다. *tocopherol*이나 *oxytocin*이 그 예이다. 근래에는 그리스어 'k'를 'c'로 바꾸지 않고 'k' 그대로 표기하는 경향이 있다. *enkephalin*이 그 예이다. 그러다보니, 'c'와 'k'를 혼용하기도 한다. *procaryote/prokaryote*와 *eucaryote/eukaryote*가 그 예이다.

G. tokos, tokou, m. *birth, offspring* 　　　　E *tocology, tocopherol, tocolytic*

　　　> G. eutokia, eutokias, f. (< eu- *well) normal childbirth*

　　　　　> L. eutocia, eutociae, f. 순산(順産), 정상분만 　　E *eutocia*

　　　> G. dystokia, dystokias, f. (< dys- *bad) difficult childbirth,*
　　　　　painful childbirth

　　　　　> L. dystocia, dystociae, f. 난산(難産) 　　E *dystocia*

　　　> G. oxytokia, oxytokias, f. (< oxys *quick) quick delivery* 　E *oxytocin*

　> IE. tek- *to beget, to give birth to*

G. enkephalos, enkephalou, m. (< *which is within the head* < en- *in*
　　　+ kephalē *head) brain* 　　E *encephal(o)-, encephalitis, enkephalin*

　　　< G. kephalē, kephalēs, f. *head* 　　E *cephalic, -cephalic; cephalad*

　< IE. ghebh-el- *head*

G. karyon, karyou, n. *nut*

　　　E *cary(o)- (kary(o)-),* (pro- *'before, in front'* >) *procaryote (prokaryote),*
　　　(eu- *'well'* >) *eucaryote (eukaryote)*

　< IE. kar-, ker- *hard, things with hard shells*

　　　> G. karkinos, karkinou, m. *crab*

　　　> L. cancer, cancri, m. (cancer, canceris, m.) 게

••• 이중모음 'ai', 'oi'의 라틴어화

그리스어 이중모음 'ai', 'oi'는 'ae', 'oe'로 라틴어화한다. 고전 라틴어의 이중모음 'ae', 'oe'의 발음은 그리스어 이중모음 'ai', 'oi'와 같았기 때문이다.

G. haima, haimatos, n. *blood*

　　　> L. haemat(o)- (피에 관한 파생어나 합성어를 만드는 연결형)
　　　　피의, 혈액의 　　E *haemat(o)- (hemat(o)-)*

　　　> L. -aemia, -aemiae, f. (피에 관한 파생어나 합성어를 만드는
　　　　연결형) 혈액의 ~상태 　　E *-aemia (-emia)*

　　　> G. haimorrhagia, haimorrhagias, f. (< + -rrhagia < -rrhag-

stem of rhēgnynai *to break, to burst* + -ia) *hemorrhage*
> L. haemorrhagia, haemorrhagiae, f.

출혈(出血)　　　**E** *haemorrhage (hemorrhage), hemorrhagic*

< IE. sai- *thick fluid*

G. oisophagos, oisophagou, m. (< oisein (*future infinitive of* pherein
to carry) + phagein *to eat*) *gullet*
> L. oesophagus, oesophagi, m.

식도(食道)　**E** *oesophagus (esophagus), esophageal, esophagogastric*

< IE. bhag- *to share out, apportion, also to get a share*

영국식 영어에서는 라틴어화한 'ae', 'oe'를 그대로 사용한다. 미국식 영어에서는 'ae'와 'oe'를, 현대영어의 발음을 따라, 모두 'e'로 줄인다. *haematology* (*hematology*), *haemorrhage* (*hemorrhage*), *oesophagus* (*esophagus*) 등에서 잘 드러난다. 이 책에서는 어원에 충실한 영국식 영어 낱말을 먼저 적고 발음 따라 바뀐 미국식 영어 낱말을 괄호 안에 적었다. 그러나 그로부터 만들어진 파생어나 합성어는 미국식 영어를 따라 적었다.

'ae'와 'oe'를 모두 'e'로 줄이다 보면 오해가 생긴다. kainos (*new*), koinos (*common*), kenos (*empty*) 모두 ceno- 또는 keno-로 옮겨질 수 있는 것이다. 근래에는, 오해 사지 않으려고, 그리스어의 이중모음을 그대로 표기하는 경향이 조금 있다. *koilocyte, koilonychia*가 그 예이다.

G. kainos, kainē, kainon *new,*

strange　　**E** *Caenozoic (Cenozoic, Cainozoic), -cene, kainite*

< IE. ken- *fresh, new, young*

G. koinos, koinē, koinon *common, public*　**E** *coenobite (cenobite), epicene, Koine*

< IE. kom *beside, near, by, with*

G. kenos, kenē, kenon *empty*　　　　　　　　　　　**E** *cenotaph*

< IE. ken- *empty*

G. koilos, koilē, koilon *hollow*　　　　**E** *coel(o)- (cel(o)-), koilocyte*

> G. koilia, koilias, f. *hollow of the belly, belly, womb,*

body cavity　　**E** *-coele (-cele, -coel), blastocoele*

> G. koiliakos, koiliakē, koiliakon *of body cavity, belonging*

to the belly, suffering in the bowels

> L. coeliacus, coeliaca, coeliacum

복강(腹腔)의　　　　　　　　　　　　　　　E *coeliac (celiac)*

> G. koilōma, koilōmatos, n. *cavity*

> L. coeloma, coelomatis, n.

체강(體腔)　　　　　　　　E *coelom (celom), coelomic (celomic)*

> L. coelacanthus, coelacanthi, m. (< *hollow spine*

< + G. akantha *thorn, thistle*) 실러캔스　　　E *coelacanth*

> L. koilonychia, koilonychiae, f. (< *hollow nail*

< + G. onyx *nail*) 숟가락손발톱 (*spoon nail*)　　E *koilonychia*

< IE. keuə- *to swell; vault, hole*

●●● 학명의 전통성

학명은 어원을 충실히 따르는 것을 원칙으로 한다. 다음 예에서 혈우병은 흔히 미국식 영어를 써서 *hemophilia*라고 하나 인플루엔자균의 학명으로는 어원에 충실한 Haemophilus influenzae가 강력하게 추천된다.

G. haima, haimatos, n. *blood*

> L. haemophilia, haemophiliae, f. (< + G. philia *affection*)

혈우병(血友病)　　E *haemophilia (hemophilia), hemophiliac, hemophilic*

> L. Haemophilus, Haemophili, m. (< *requiring growth factors*

present in blood < + G. philos *affecting*) (세균)

헤모필루스속(屬)　　　　　　　　E *haemophilus (hemophilus)*

[용례] Haemophilus influenzae (Hemophilus influenzae)

인플루엔자균　　　　　　　E Haemophilus influenzae

(문법) Haemophilus (Hemophilus) 헤모필루스속(屬): 단수 주격

influenzae 인플루엔자의: 단수 속격

< influenza, influenzae, f.

< IE. sai- *thick fluid*

문법의 라틴어화

그리스어 명사나 형용사를 라틴어로 바꿀 때에는 상응하는 변화의 명사나 형용사로 바꾸는 것이 원칙이다. 〈어원론을 위한 라틴어〉 편의 맞대보기는 이에 대한 규칙과 예외를 담고 있다.

••• 그리스어 명사의 라틴어화

제1변화 명사의 예

(52) G. hōr–a, hōr–as, f. *limited time, period, time, year, season, hour;* ((pl.) Horai) (*Greek mythology*) *goddesses of orderly life*

(53)   > L. hor–a, hor–ae, f. 시간; ((pl.) Horae) (로마 신화) 계절과 질서의 여신들

제2변화 명사의 예

(49) G. meteōr–on, meteōr–ou, n. *meteor*

(50)   > L. meteor–um, meteor–i, n. 운석(隕石)

제3변화 명사의 예

(66) G. mimēs–is, mimēs–eōs, f. *imitation, copy*

(67)   > L. mimes–is, mimes–is, f. 모방, 모사(模寫), 모의(模擬); (생물) 의태(擬態)

••• 그리스어 형용사의 라틴어화

제1·2변화 형용사의 예

(14) G. kardiak–os, kardiak–ē, kardiak–on *of heart*

(15)   > L. cardiac–us, cardiac–a, cardiac–um 심장의, 심장병의; (*on the heart side of the body* >) 들문(~門)의, 위(胃)의, 위병의

(63) G. mimik–os, mimik–ē, mimik–on *of mime*

(64)   > L. mimic–us, mimic–a, mimic–um 흉내 내는, 모조의

제 4 장　어휘형성

어휘(語彙, *lexicon*)란 한 언어 또는 한 분야의 낱말 전체를 가리킨다. 생명과학 분야의 영어 어휘는 라틴어와 그리스어 기원의 낱말이 압도하고 나머지를 영어 고유 낱말이 채운다. 독일어와 프랑스어로부터 들어온 낱말도 대부분 그 바탕은 라틴어와 그리스어이다.

라틴어 · 그리스어의 어휘형성

의존형태소와 자립형태소

영어 *cordial*의 어원인 라틴어 cordialis는 명사 cor의 속격어간 cord-에다 발음의 편의상 -i-를 끼워 넣은 후 -alis를 붙여 만든 형용사이다. 영어 *concord*의 어원인 라틴어 concors는 명사 cor의 주격어간 cor의 앞에 con-을 붙여 만든 형용사이다. 영어 *discord*의 어원인 라틴어 discors는 명사 cor의 주격어간 cor의 앞에 dis-를 붙여 만든 형용사이다.

라틴어 cordialis를 구성하는 cord-와 -alis, concors를 구성하는 con-과 -cor, discors를 구성하는 dis-와 -cor는 더 이상 나누어지지 않는 최소 의미단위이다. 형태소(形態素, *morpheme*)라고 한다.

(1)　L. **cor, cord–is, n.** 심장, 마음, 의지, 용기, 지혜　　　　　　　　E *(suggested)* **core**

(3)　　　　> cord-i-alis, cord-i-ale 마음에서 우러나는　　　　　　　E *cordial*

(7)　　　　> con-cors, (gen.) con-cordis (< con- (<cum) *with, together*) 한

　　　　　　 마음의, 합치하는, 일치하는, 화목하는　　　　　　　　E **concord**

(8)　　　　> dis-cors, (gen.) dis-cordis (< dis- *apart from, down, not*) 어긋나는,

　　　　　　 상반되는, 불목하는　　　　　　　　　　　　　　　E *discord*

(12)　　< IE. kerd- *heart*　　　　　E *heart, hearty, heartful, heartless, hearten*

형태소에는 두 가지가 있다. 명사 어간의 뒤에 붙어 관계 또는 속성의 형용사를 만드는 -alis나 명사, 형용사, 동사 앞에 붙어 뜻을 부정하는 dis-처럼 혼자서는 어휘를 만들지 못하는 형태소를 의존형태소(*bound morpheme*)라고 한다. 이에 비해 명사 cor나 con-의 원형인 전치사 cum처럼 혼자서도 어휘를 만드는 형태소를 자립형태소(*free morpheme*)라고 한다. 의존형태소는 자립형태소에 붙어야만 어휘를 만들 수 있다.

파생어

파생어(派生語, *derivative*)는 있는 낱말에 의존형태소를 붙여 만든 새로운 어휘이다. 라틴어 cred-i-bilis 및 in-cred-i-bilis와 arteri-ola는 동사 cred-ĕre와 명사 arteri-a의 파생어들이고, 그리스어 mim-ē-sis와 aster-iskos는 동사 mim-eisthai와 명사 astēr의 파생어들이다.

(1) L. cor, cord-is, n. 심장, 마음, 의지, 용기, 지혜　　　E *(suggested) core*

(12)　　< IE. kerd- *heart*　　　E *heart, hearty, heartful, heartless, hearten*

(25)　　　　> IE. kred-dhə- (< + IE. dhə- *to do, to place*) *to place trust*

(26)　　　　　> L. cred-o, credid-i, credit-um, cred-ĕre 믿다, 맡기다　　E *grant*

(30)　　　　　　> L. cred-i-bilis, cred-i-bile 믿을 만한, 신용할
만한　　　E *credible, credibility*

(32)　　　　　　> L. incred-i-bilis, incred-i-bile (< in- *not* 믿을
수 없는, 믿어지지 않는　　　E *incredible*

(38) L. arteri-a, arteri-ae, f. 동맥(動脈)　　　E *artery, arterial, arteri(o)-*

(39)　　> L. arteri-ola, arteri-olae, f. (< + -ola *diminutive suffix*)
세동맥(細動脈)　　　E *arteriole, arteriolar, arteriol(o)-*

(65) G. mim-eisthai (*middle*) *to imitate*

(66)　　> G. mim-ē-sis, mim-ē-seōs, f. (< -sis *noun suffix*) *imitation, copy*　　E *mimesis*

(73) G. astēr, aster-os, m. *star*

(74)　　　> L. aster, aster-is, m. 별; (생물학) 성상체;
(Aster) (식물) Aster속(屬)　　　E *aster, asteroid*

(75)　　　> G. aster-iskos, aster-iskou, m. (< + -iskos *diminutive suffix*)
little star

(76)　　　　　　　　　> L. aster-iscus, aster-isci, m. 작은 별, 별표　　　　E *asterisk*

(77)　　　< IE. ster- *star*

••• 접미사와 접두사

의존형태소 중 어간 또는 어근 뒤에 붙어 원래 낱말의 뜻이나 역할을 바꾸어 주는 형태소가 접미사(接尾辭, *suffix*)이다. 접미사 중 파생어를 만드는 접미사를 파생접미사(*derivational suffix*), 굴절 어미의 역할을 하는 접미사를 굴절접미사(*inflectional suffix*)라고 한다.

위의 예에서 라틴어 cred-i-bilis의 -bilis는 동사의 어간이나 어근에 붙어 형용사를 만드는 접미사이며, 그리스어 mim-ē-sis의 -sis는 동사 어근에 붙어 명사를 만드는 접미사이다. 라틴어 명사 arteri-ola는 명사 arteri-a의 어간에 라틴어 지소 접미사 -ola를 붙여 만든 지소사(指小辭, *diminutive*)이고, 그리스어 명사 aster-iskos는 명사 astēr의 어간에 그리스어 지소 접미사 -iskos를 붙여 만든 지소사이다.

접두사(接頭辭, *prefix*)는 다른 낱말의 앞에 붙어 낱말의 뜻을 바꿔주는 의존형태소이다. in-credibilis의 in-은 뒤에 오는 낱말을 부정한다.

이 책의 라틴어편과 그리스어편에서는 '지소사', '명사를 만드는 방법', '형용사를 만드는 방법'에서 어원론에 필요한 접미사들을 정리해 놓았다. 〈용어 비교〉편에서는 비교가 필요한 접두사와 접미사들을 대비해 놓았다.

합성어

합성어(合成語, *compound*)는 둘 이상의 자립형태소를 붙여 만든 새로운 어휘이다.

심장벽의 세 층을 영어로 *endo-cardi-um, myo-cardi-um, epi-cardi-um*이라고 한다. 그리스어에서 비롯한 라틴 합성어를 차용한 용어이다. 각각 전치사·명사·접미사, 명사·명사·접미사, 전치사·명사·접미사로 이루어져 있어 자립형태소가 둘 이상이다. 이 경우 접미사는 어휘 형성의 측면에서 보면 파생접미사가 되고 굴절의 측면에서 보면 굴절접미사가 된다.

(1) cor, cord–is, n. 심장, 마음, 의지, 용기, 지혜　　　E *cord(i)–, (suggested) core*

(9)　　　　　> miser–i–cors, (gen.) miser–i–cordis (< miser *wretched*)

　　　　자비로운　　　　　　　　　　　　　　　　　　　E *misericord*

(12)　　< IE. kerd– *heart*

　　　　　　　　E *heart, hearty, heartful, heartless, hearten; heartbeat, heartburn, heart-stopper, heart-to-heart, heart attack, heart failure*

(13)　　　　　> G. kardi–a, kardi–as, f. *heart, mind, soul*

　　　　　　　　E *cardi(o)–, electrocardiogram (ECG),* (D. Elektrokardiogramm >) *EKG, cardiomegaly*

(19)　　　　　> L. endo-cardium, endo-cardii, n. (< G. end(o)– < endon

　　　　within) 심장속막, 심내막　　　　E *endocardium, endocardial*

(20)　　　　　> L. myo-cardium, myo-cardii, n. (< G. my(o)– < mys, myos, m.

　　　　mouse, muscle) 심근층　　　　　E *myocardium, myocardial*

(21)　　　　　> L. epi-cardium, epi-cardii, n. (< G. ep(i)– < epi *upon*)

　　　　심장바깥막, 심외막　　　　　　　　E *epicardium, epicardial*

연결형

　　파생어와 합성어의 정의는 영어에서도 마찬가지이다. 영어 *hearty, heartful, heartless, hearten*은 파생어가 되고 *heartbeat, heart-stopper, heart attack*은 합성어가 된다.

　　파생어나 합성어에서 영어 형태소는 떨어지자마자 원래의 모습으로 되돌아간다. 그러나 라틴어나 그리스어의 자립형태소 성분은 떨어지고 나서도 원래 모습으로 되돌아가지 않는다. 영어의 파생어나 합성어가 물리적 변화의 결과라면 라틴어와 그리스어의 파생어나 합성어는 화학적 변화의 결과인 셈이다. 분석어와 굴절어의 차이이다.

　　라틴어와 그리스어에서 파생어나 합성어를 만드는 형태소 성분을 연결형(連結形, *combining form*)이라고 한다.

　　라틴어 miser-i-cors 나 my-o-cardium 을 보면 두 성분 사이에 연결모음(*combining vowel*)이 삽입되어 있다. 발음의 편의성 때문이다. 연결형은 음편의 –i– 나 –o– 까지를 포함한다. miseri– 나 myo– 까지를 합성어 성분으로 보는 것이다.

　　심근층은 myo-cardium 이고 근육통은 my-algia 이다. 그리스어로 근육을 뜻하는 myo-의 -o-가 자음으로 시작하는 형태소 앞에는 붙고 모음으로 시작하는 형태소 앞에는 붙지 않는다. 따라서 연결형을 표기할 때에는 연결모음을 괄호 안에 넣어 표기한다. my(o)-라고 표기하는 것이다.

그리스어 전치사인 endon이나 epi의 연결형 end(o)- 또는 ep(i)-도 모음으로 시작하는 형태소 앞에서 끝 모음이 탈락함을 보여준다.

우측핵규칙

파생어나 합성어의 성분 중에서 가장 오른쪽 성분이 핵심어라는 것이 우측핵규칙(*righthand head rule*)이다.

파생어 cred-i-bilis는 오른쪽 성분 -bilis에 의해 품사가 동사에서 형용사로 결정되며 '할 수 있는'이라는 뜻을 갖는다. 합성어 endo-cardium과 myo-cardium, epi-cardium은 오른쪽 성분인 -cardium의 층을 구분하기 위해 endo-, myo-, epi-가 수식해준다.

우측핵규칙의 개념은 파생어나 합성어의 뜻을 이해하기 위해서도 필요하지만, 모음탈락과 같은 꼴을 이해하기 위해서도 필요하다.

라틴어·그리스어 어휘형성과 어간

명사와 형용사의 어간

●●● 속격어간 (어간)

라틴어 명사 'cor, cordis, n.'로부터 만들어진 형용사 cord-atus는 명사의 단수 속격 어간 cord-에다 형용사를 만드는 접미사 -atus를 붙여 만든 파생어이고, 동사 ac-cord-are는 같은 속격 어간에다 정형 제1변화 동사를 만드는 접미사 -are를 붙여 *cord-are를 만든 다음 그 앞에 '~에게'의 뜻을 갖는 전치사의 연결형 ac-를 붙여 만든 합성어이다. 그리스어 명사 'kardia, kardias, f.'로부터 만들어진 형용사 kardi-akos는 명사의 단수 속격 어간 kardi-에다 형용사를 만드는 접미사 -akos를 붙여 만든 파생어이다. 'kardia, kardias, f.'의 경우, 단수 주격 어간과 단수 속격 어간이 같기 때문에 얼른 드러나지 않을 따름이다. 라틴어 형용사 'potens, (gen.) potent-is'나 'impotens, (gen.) impotent-is'로부터 만들어진 명사 potentia나 impotentia도 마찬가지이다. 형용사의 단수 속격 어간에다 명사를 만드는 접미사 -ia를 붙여 만들었다.

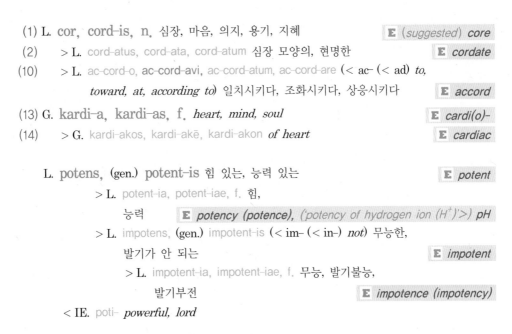

(1) L. cor, cord-is, n. 심장, 마음, 의지, 용기, 지혜　　　E (suggested) core
(2)　 > L. cord-atus, cord-ata, cord-atum 심장 모양의, 현명한　　E cordate
(10)　 > L. ac-cord-o, ac-cord-avi, ac-cord-atum, ac-cord-are (< ac- (< ad) to, toward, at, according to) 일치시키다, 조화시키다, 상응시키다　　E accord
(13) G. kardi-a, kardi-as, f. heart, mind, soul　　　E cardi(o)-
(14)　 > G. kardi-akos, kardi-akē, kardi-akon of heart　　E cardiac

　 L. potens, (gen.) potent-is 힘 있는, 능력 있는　　　E potent
　　 > L. potent-ia, potent-iae, f. 힘, 능력　　E potency (potence), ('potency of hydrogen ion (H⁺)'>) pH
　　 > L. impotens, (gen.) impotent-is (< im- (< in-) not) 무능한, 발기가 안 되는　　　E impotent
　　　 > L. impotent-ia, impotent-iae, f. 무능, 발기불능, 발기부전　　　E impotence (impotency)
　 < IE. poti- powerful, lord

　이처럼, 라틴어이든 그리스어이든, 명사 또는 형용사에 붙여 파생어나 합성어를 만들 때에는 단수 속격의 어간에다 붙여 만드는 것이 원칙이다. 라틴어와 그리스어 있어서 명사와 형용사의 단수 속격 어간은, 변화의 축이 될 뿐 아니라, 파생어와 합성어를 만드는 데 있어서도 축이 되는 것이다. 따라서 명사와 형용사의 어간이라 함은 바로 단수 속격 어간, 줄여서, 속격어간을 가리킨다. 그리스어 문법에서 속격을 '낳다'는 뜻의 genikē ptōsis라고 한 이유가 여기에 있다. (그리스어 문법의 genikē ptōsis를 라틴어 문법이 genitivus casus라고 옮겼다. 영문법의 genitive case는 라틴어 문법 용어를 그대로 갖다 놓은 용어이다. 우리말이 소유격(所有格)이라고 하지 않고 속격(屬格)이라고 옮긴 데에도 낱말의 속(屬)을 대표한다는 뜻이 녹아 있다.)

　라틴어와 그리스어에 있어서 명사나 형용사 모두 제3변화에서만 단수 주격의 어간과 속격어간이 다르며, 제3변화 일부와 그 외의 변화 양식에서는 단수 주격의 어간과 속격어간이 같다.

●●● 주격어간

그리스어 '빛'은 단수 주격이 어미 없이 어간만 있는 phōs, 단수 속격이 phōtos 이다. 따라서 속격어간은 phōt-가 되며, 광자(光子)는 photon(< phot- + -on *a termination of Greek neuter nouns and adjectives*)이 되고, 광합성은, 발음의 편의상 -o-를 끼워 넣어, photosynthesis(< phot-o- + synthesis)가 된다. 그러나 '빛을 나르는' 샛별 Phosphorus나 화학 원소 인(燐) phosphorus는 주격어간 phos-에다 '나르는'이라는 뜻의 형용사 -phoros(남성형)를 붙인 후 라틴어 남성 명사로 바꿔준 낱말이다.

L. **phasis**, phasis, f. 상(相), 위상(位相), (변화·발달의) 단계   **E** *phase*
     < G. phasis, phaseōs, f. *appearance*
  < IE. bha- *to shine*
     > G. phōs, phōt-os, n. *light*   **E** *phot(o)-, photon*
       > L. photosynthesis, photosynthesis, f. (< + G. syn- *with, together* + tithenai *to put*) 광합성   **E** *photosynthesis*
       > L. Phosphorus, Phosphori, m. (< *light-bearer* < + G. -phoros, -phoros, -phoron *carrying, bearing*) 샛별; (phosphorus) 인(燐)   **E** *Phosphor, phosphorus (P)*

phosphorus처럼 주격어간을 이용해 파생어나 합성어를 만드는 예는, 원칙이 아니므로, 적다. 그러나 원칙이 아니면서도 쓰이고 있을 정도로 완강하다. 몇몇 '유명한' 낱말들이 그러하다.

▌동사의 어간

라틴어와 그리스어 동사도, 명사나 형용사처럼, 어간을 그대로 둔 채 어미를 바꿈으로써 문장 안에서의 역할을 달리한다. 다음 예에서 하이픈의 앞부분이 동사 어간이고 뒷부분이 어미이다.

(26) L. cred-o, credid-i, credit-um, cred-ĕre 믿다, 맡기다

(65) G. mim-eisthai (*middle*) *to imitate*

　'동사'의 영어 낱말 *verb*가 '말', '낱말'이란 뜻의 라틴어 verbum에서 기원했듯이, '말' 하면 '동사'이며 동사로부터는 많은 파생어와 합성어가 만들어진다. 이때에도 물론, 어간이 축의 역할을 한다.

●●● 라틴어 동사의 어간

　명사와 형용사의 어간은 정식으로는 속격어간 하나이나, 동사의 어간은 정식으로도 더 많다. 어원론에서 필요로 하는 동사 어간은, 정형 동사의 경우, 능동태 현재부정법 또는 능동태 직설법 현재 단수 일인칭에서 어미를 떼어낸 현재어간과 능동태 목적분사에서 어미를 떼어낸 능동태 목적분사 어간이다. 능동태 목적분사는 문법상의 이름이며 실제적으로는 과거분사의 어간을 보여주는 기능을 한다. 그래서 능동태 목적분사 어간을 과거분사 어간이라고도 한다. 능동태 직설법 완료 단수 일인칭에서 어미를 떼어낸 완료어간은, 어원론에서는, 무시해도 좋을 정도이다.

(26) L. cred-ĕre　　(능동태 현재부정법)　　　　　　　　현재어간

　　　 cred-o　　　(능동태 직설법 현재 단수 일인칭)　현재어간

　　　 credid-i　　 (능동태 직설법 완료 단수 일인칭)　완료어간

　　　 credit-um　(능동태 목적분사)　　　　　　　　능동태 목적분사 어간

　　　　　　　　　　　　　　　　　　　　　　　　　(과거분사 어간)

　정형 동사 cred-ĕre의 어원론에서 필요한 두 어간과 거기에서 비롯한 낱말들은 다음과 같다.

(26) L. cred-o, credid-i, credit-um, cred-ĕre 믿다, 맡기다

　　　　> L. cred- (현재어간)

(28)　　　　> L. credentia, credentiae, f. 신뢰, 신임　　　　**E** *credence, credential*

(30)　　　　> L. credibilis, credibile 믿을 만한, 신용할 만한　**E** *credible, credibility*

　　　　> L. credit- (능동태 목적분사 어간 (과거분사 어간))

(27)　　　　> L. creditum, crediti, n. 신뢰, 신용, 영예, 남에게 맡겨놓은

　　　　　　(빌려준) 것　　　　　　　　　　　　　　　　**E** *credit, accredit*

탈형동사의 경우에는 현재부정법 또는 직설법 현재 단수 일인칭에서 어미를 떼어낸 현재어간과 직설법 완료 단수 일인칭에서 어미를 떼어낸 완료어간의 두 가지가 있다. 둘 다 어원론에서 필요로 하는 어간이다. 탈형동사에서는 완료어간이 과거분사의 어간까지 보여준다. 탈형동사 pat-i의 두 어간과 거기에서 비롯한 낱말들은 다음과 같다.

L. pat-i   (현재부정법)   현재어간

pat-ior   (직설법 현재 단수 일인칭)   현재어간

pass-us sum   (직설법 완료 단수 일인칭)   완료어간

(과거분사 어간)

L. **patior, passus sum, pati** 당하다, 견디다, 참다, 고통받다, 내버려 두다
> L. pat- (현재어간)
　> L. patiens, (gen.) patientis (*present participle*) 참는, 괴로움 당
　　하는, 병 앓는, 꿋꿋한　　　　　　　　　　　　　　**E** *patient*
　　> L. patientia, patientiae, f. 인내　　　　　　　**E** *patience*
　　> L. impatiens, (gen.) impatientis (< im- (< in-) *not* +
　　　patiens *patient*) 참지 못하는　　　　　　　　**E** *impatient*
　　　> L. impatiens, impatientis, f. (< *the ripe seed-pods*
　　　　readily burst open when touched) 봉숭아속(屬)
　　　　의 식물　　　　　　　　　　　　　　　　　　**E** *impatiens*
　　　　> L. impatientia, impatientiae, f. 참지 못함, 성
　　　　　급함, 조바심, 안달　　　　　　　　　　　　**E** *impatience*
> L. pass- 완료어간 (과거분사 어간)
　> L. passio, passionis, f. 수난, 격정　　　　　**E** *passion, passionate*
　> L. passivus, passiva, passivum 당하는, 수동적인, 피동의, 소극
　　적인; (문법) 수동태의　　　　　　　　　　　　　**E** *passive*

•◦◦ 그리스어 동사의 어간

그리스어 동사 중 규칙적 변화를 하는 동사의 경우에는 현재어간이 중요하다. 현재어간은 현재부정법 또는 직설법 현재 단수 일인칭에서 어미를 떼어내고 남은 부분이다. 그리스어 동사 mim-eisthai의 현재어간과 거기에서 비롯한 낱말들은 다음과 같다.

(65) G. **mim-eisthai** (현재부정법) (*middle*) *to imitate*

> G. mim- (현재어간)

(66)　　　　> G. mimēsis, mimēseōs, f. (< -sis *noun suffix*) *imitation, copy*

(67)　　　　　　> L. mimesis, mimesis, f. 모방, 모사(模寫), 모의(模擬); (생물)
　　　　　　　의태(擬態)　　　　　　　　　　　　　　　　　　　**E** *mimesis*

(68)　　　　> G. mimētikos, mimētikē, mimētikon (< -tikos *adjective suffix*)
　　　　　imitative　　　　**E** *mimetic, sympathomimetic, parasympathomimetic*

　　그리스어 동사 중 불규칙변화를 하는 동사는 부정과거(不定過去, *aorist*)의 어
간을 보아야 본디 어간을 알 수 있다. 본디 어간이 현재 시제에서는 바뀌었으나
부정과거 시제에서는 바뀌지 않고 쓰여 왔기 때문이다. 그리스어사전은 불규칙
변화를 하는 동사의 부정과거형을 제시해주나 영어사전은, 필요할 때에만, 부정
과거어간을 제시해준다. 다음은 '배우다'라는 동사 manthan-ein의 파생어와 합
성어가 현재어간 manthan-이 아니라 부정과거어간 math-을 축으로 만들어졌음
을 보여준다.

G. **manthan-ein** (math- *aorist stem*) *to learn*
　　　> G. mathē, mathē, f. *learning*
　　　　　> G. polymathēs, polymathēs, polymathes (< polys *much*)
　　　　　　having learnt much　　　　　　　**E** *polymath*
　　　> G. mathēma, mathēmatos, n. (< -ma *resultative noun suffix*)
　　　　　what is learned, the act of learning, learning, knowledge
　　　　　> G. mathēmatikos, mathēmatikē, mathēmatikon (< -ikos
　　　　　　adjective suffix) *inclined to learn, mathematical*　**E** *mathematics*
　< IE. mendh- *to learn*

어간의 확장

　　라틴어 동사 cred-ĕre의 현재어간은 cred-이고, cred-에서 비롯한 명사
credentia의 속격어간은 credenti-이며, credenti-에서 비롯한 형용사
credentialis의 속격어간은 credential-이다. cred-ĕre의 현재어간 cred-에서 비
롯한 형용사 credibilis의 속격어간은 credibil-이며, credibil-에서 비롯한 명사
credibilitas의 속격어간은 credibilitat-이다. 그리스어 명사 kardi-a의 속격어
간은 kardi-이고, kardi-에서 비롯한 형용사 kardiakos의 속격어간은 kardiak-

이며, kardi-에서 비롯한 형용사 perikardios의 속격어간은 perikardi-이다. 이처럼, 라틴어나 그리스어 낱말은 파생어나 합성어를 만들면서 어간이 확장되게끔 되어 있으며 확장된 어간을 축으로 해서 또다시 새로운 파생어나 합성어가 만들어지게 되어 있다. 어간 확장은 굴절어가 가지는 조어력의 바탕이 된다.

(26) L. cred-o, credid-i, credit-um, cred-ĕre 믿다, 맡기다
      > L. cred- (현재어간)
(28)   > L. credenti-a, credenti-ae, f. 신뢰, 신임   **E** *credence*
(29)   > L. credential-is, credential-e 신뢰의, 신임의   **E** *credential*
(30)   > L. credibil-is, credibil-e 믿을 만한, 신용할 만한   **E** *credible*
(31)   > L. credibilitas, credibilitat-is, f. 신뢰성, 신용   **E** *credibility*

(13) G. kardi-a, kardi-as, f. *heart, mind, soul*   **E** *cardi(o)-*
(14)   > G. kardiak-os, kardiak-ē, kardiak-on *of heart*   **E** *cardiac*
(17)   > G. perikardi-os, perikardi-a, perikardi-on (< peri- < peri *around, near, beyond, on account of*) *pericardial*   **E** *pericardium, pericardial*

어근

    몇몇 동족어 무리의 낱말은 어간의 윗단계 말뿌리까지 확인해 올라갈 수 있다. 추정상의 인도유럽어 말뿌리보다는 한참 아래이나 어떤 어간보다도 위에 있는 말뿌리이다. 어근(語根, *root*)이라고 한다. 어근은 동사와 밀접하게 관계되어 있지만 동사 외에도 명사, 형용사, 부사 등을 만들어낸다. (언어 형태론에서는 아무런 형태소가 덧붙지 않은 기본 형태소를 어근이라고 한다. 어원론에서 말하는 어근과는 다르다.)

    어근의 꼴은 동사의 꼴과 한참 다를 수 있다. 그런 경우 사전은 별도로 어근을 보여준다. 라틴어 동사 sequi(뒤따르다)의 어근 sec-, 그리스어 동사 tithenai(두다)의 어근 the-를 예를 들면 다음과 같다.

    L. sequor, secutus sum, sequi (sec- *root of* sequi *to follow*) 뒤따르다,
       잇따르다, 추구(追求)하다, 누구에게 (유산·상속으로) 돌아가다, 누구의
       차지가 되다   **E** *sequent, sue, suit, suite*
         > L. sequentia, sequentiae, f. 후속, 연속, 결과, 순서,
           연쇄   **E** *sequence, sequential*

> L. sequela, sequelae, f. 후속, 결과, 귀결, (군대를) 따라 다니는

　　사람, 후유증　　　　　　　　　　**E** *sequela*, (pl.) *sequelae, sequel*

> L. secundus, secunda, secundum (< sec- *root* + -undus, -unda,

　　-undum *adjective suffix*) 뒤따르는, 순조로운, 둘째의

> **E** *secund, second* (< *'following'*), (secunda minuta *'second minute'*
> >) *second*

> L. secondarius, secondaria, secondarium 2차적인,

　　부차적인, 속발한, 제2기의　　　　　　　　**E** *secondary*

< IE. sek^w- *to follow*

G. tithenai (the- *root of* tithenai) *to put, to place*

> G. thesis, theseōs, f. (< + -sis *noun suffix*) *placing*

> L. thesis, thesis, f. 논제　　　　　　**E** *thesis*, (pl.) *theses*

> G. thema, thematos, n. (< + -ma *resultative noun suffix*)

what is placed down

> L. thema, thematis, n. 주제, 제목　　　　　　**E** *theme*

< IE. dhe- *to put, to set*

라틴어·그리스어 어휘형성과 발음의 편의성

　　라틴어와 그리스어에서는 파생어나 합성어를 만들 때, 음편(音便, *euphony*)을 위해, 모음을 삽입하거나 탈락 또는 전환시키며, 자음을 삽입하거나 탈락 또는 동화시킨다.

　　어원론을 이해하기 위한 좋은 방법 중 하나는 파생어나 합성어를 분해해 보는 것이다. 분해는 모음탈락, 자음탈락, 모음전환, 자음동화 등 눈에 잘 띄지 않는 변화를 지적할 줄 알아야 가능해진다. 모음삽입과 자음삽입은 눈에 잘 띄는 편이다.

모음삽입

　　파생어나 합성어를 만들 때 앞부분 끝 발음과 뒷부분 첫 발음이 부딪히면 그 사이에 연결 모음을 끼워 넣는다. 대개는 자음끼리 부딪힐 때이다. 라틴어에서는,

miser-i-cors와 cred-i-bilis에서처럼, -i-를 끼워 넣는 것이 일반적이며, 그리스어에서는, my-o-cardium과 phot-o-synthesis에서처럼, -o-를 끼워 넣는 것이 일반적이다. 품사 변화에 있어서 라틴어 어미에는 -i-가 많이 들어가며 그리스어 어미에는 -o-가 많이 들어가기 때문에 생긴 버릇이다. 다음 예 중 연결형 my(o)-와 phot(o)-는 모음 앞에서는 my-와 phot- 꼴로, 자음 앞에서는 myo-와 photo- 꼴로 연결됨을 뜻한다.

(9) L. miser-i-cors, (gen.) miser-i-cordis (< miser *wretched* + cor, cordis, n. *heart*) 자비로운　　　　　　　　　　　　　　　　E *misericord*

(30) L. cred-i-bilis, cred-i-bile 믿을 만한, 신용할 만한　　　　E *credible*

(20) L. my-o-cardium, my-o-cardii, n. (< G. my(o)- < mys, myos, m. *mouse, muscle*) 심근층　　　　　　　　　　　E *myocardium, myocardial*

L. phot-o-synthesis, phot-o-synthesis, f. (< G. phot(o)- (< phōs, phōtos, n.) + syn- *with, together* + tithenai *to put*) 광합성　E *photosynthesis*

모음탈락

파생어나 합성어를 만들 때 앞부분의 끝과 뒷부분의 처음이 모음이면 모음 하나를 탈락시킨다. 모음충돌에 의한 발음의 단절(모음단절, *hiatus*)을 피하기 위해서이다. 의미가 좀 더 약한 쪽의 모음을 탈락시키는데 앞부분의 끝 모음이다. 즉, 우측핵규칙이 적용되는 것이다.

영어 *endarteritis*는 그리스어 기원의 연결형 end(o)-가 end-의 꼴로 붙은 합성어이고 *meteorology*는 그리스어 기원의 연결형 met(a)-가 met-의 꼴로 붙은 합성어이다.

(43) L. endarteritis, endarteritidis, f. (< G. end(o)- < endon *within* + artēria *artery* + -itis *noun suffix denoting inflammation*) 동맥속막염, 동맥내막염　　　　　　　　　　　　　　E *endarteritis*

(48) G. meteōros, meteōros, meteōron (< G. met(a)- < meta *between, along with, across, after* + eōra *suspension*) *lifted up, in air*　E *meteorology*

모음탈락은 라틴어에서는 잘 지켜지지 않는 경향이 있고, 그리스어에서도 예외가 있다. 그리스어 전치사의 연결형 amphi-, peri-, pro-와 형용사의 연결형

hemi-, poly-가 대표적 예외이다.

G. amphi (*preposition, adverb*) *on both sides, around*
> G. amphi- *on both sides, around*   **E** *amphi-, amphibian, amphiaster*
< IE. ant-bhi- *from both sides*

G. peri (*preposition, adverb*) *around, near, beyond, on account of*
> G. peri- *around, near, beyond,*
on account of   **E** *peri-, periodic, periodontal, periosteal*
< IE. per *basic meanings of 'forward', 'through'*

G. pro (*preposition, adverb*) *before, in front, for, instead of*
> G. pro- *before, in front*   **E** *pro-, proenzyme*
< IE. per *basic meanings of 'forward', 'through'*

G. hēmisys, hēmiseia, hēmisy *half*
> G. hemi- *half*   **E** *hemi-, hemialgia*
< IE. semi- *half, as first member of a compound*

G. polys, pollē, poly *many, much, frequent*
> G. poly- *many, much, frequent*   **E** *poly-, polyuria*
< IE. pelə- *to fill*

자음삽입

파생어나 합성어를 만들 때 모음단절을 피하는 다른 방법은 자음삽입이다. 영어에서 첫 발음이 모음인 명사 앞의 부정관사를 '*a*'가 아닌 '*an*'으로 하는 것과 진배없다.

라틴어에서 회복 또는 반복을 뜻하는 접두사로 re-와 red-가 있다. 자음으로 시작하는 동사 앞에서는 re-가 쓰이고 모음으로 시작하는 동사 앞에서는 red-가 쓰인다. red-는 후기 라틴어에서 re-로 합쳐졌다.

L. curro, cucurri, cursum, currĕre 달리다
> L. recurro, recurri, recursum, recurrĕre (< re- *back, again* +
currĕre *to run*) 원래의 자리로
돌아가다   **E** *recur, recurrent, recurrence, recursive*
< IE. kers- *to run*

L. emo, emi, emptum, emĕre 획득하다, 사다

> L. redimo, **redemi**, redemptum (redemtum), redimĕre (< red-
back, again + emĕre *to take, to obtain, to buy*) 되사다, 몸
값을 치르고 구해내다, 대가를 지불하고 사다,
속죄하다　　　　　　　　　　　　　**E** *redeem, redemption (ransom)*

< IE. em- *to take, to distribute*

그리스어에서 부정(否定)을 뜻하는 접두사 a-와 an-도 마찬가지이다. 자음으로
시작하는 낱말 앞에서는 a-가 쓰이고 모음으로 시작하는 낱말 앞에서는 an-이
쓰인다.

G. mnasthai *to remember*

> G. amnēstein (amnēsteein) (< a- *not* + mnasthai *to remember*)
to fall into oblivion

> G. amnēstia, amnēstias, f. *oblivion*

> L. amnestia, amnestiae, f. 사면　　　　　　　**E** *amnesty*

> G. amnēsia, amnēsias, f. *forgetfulness*

> L. amnesia, amnesiae, f. 기억상실, 건망증　　　**E** *amnesia*

< IE. men- *to think*

G. archein *to lead, to rule*

> G. archos, archou, m. *leader, chief*

> G. anarchia, anarchias, f. (< an- *not*) *state without a chief
or head*

> L. anarchia, anarchiae, f. 무정부상태　　　**E** *anarchy*

그리스어에서 rh-로 시작하는 낱말(강한 숨표가 붙는 ρ 로 시작하는 낱말) 앞에
모음으로 끝나는 낱말이 붙으면 rh-는 -rrh-가 된다. 역시 발음의 편의성 때문
이다. 단, 앞의 낱말이 이중모음(ai, au, ei, eu, oi, ou)으로 끝나면 예외로 한다.

G. arrhythmia, arrhythmias, f. (< a- *not*) *arrhythmia*

> L. arrhythmia, arrhythmiae, f. 부정맥(不整脈)　**E** *arrhythmia*

< G. rhythmos, rhythmou, m. *rhythm, measure*

> L. rhythmus, rhythmi, m. 주기적 운동, 박자, 운율,
리듬　　　　　　　　　　**E** *rhythm, rhythmic, rhythmical*

> G. eurhythmia, eurhythmias, f. (< eu- *well*)
eurhythmia

> L. eurhythmia, eurhythmiae, f. 조화(調和)리듬,
조화성　　　　　　　　　**E** *eurhythmia*

> L. dysrhythmia, dysrhythmias, f. (< G. dys- *bad*)

리듬장애, 율동장애 　　　　　E *dysrhythmia*

< G. rhein (rheein) *to flow*

> G. rhoia, rhoias, f. *flow, flux*

> G. diarrhoia, diarrhoias, f. (< di(a)- *through,*
thoroughly, apart)

> L. diarrhoea, diarrhoeae, f.

설사(泄瀉) 　　　　　E *diarrhoea (diarrhea), diarrheal*

< IE. sreu- *to flow*

자음탈락

　　파생어나 합성어를 만들 때 자음충돌을 피하기 위해 자음을 탈락시키기도 한다. 라틴어 기원의 ex-가 자음 s로 시작하는 낱말과 합성어를 만들 때나 그리스어 기원의 syn-이 's + 자음'으로 시작하는 낱말과 합성어를 만들 때가 그 예이다.

　　L. exspiro, exspiravi, exspiratum, exspirare (< ex- *out of, away*
from + spirare *to breathe*)

> L. expiro, expiravi, expiratum, expirare 숨을 내쉬다, 만기가
되다, 숨이 끊어지다 　　　E *expire, expiration, expiratory, expiry*

< L. spiro, spiravi, spiratum, spirare 입김을 내불다, 호흡하다, 발산
하다, 생각하다, 갈망하다

< IE. (s)peis- *to blow*

　　L. exsudo, exsudavi, exsudatum, exsudare (< ex- *out of, away from*
+ sudare *to sweat*)

> L. exudo, exudavi, exudatum, exudare 땀으로 나오다, 스며
나오다, 삼출(滲出)하다 　　　　　E *exude, exudate*

< L. sudo, sudavi, sudatum, sudare 땀 흘리다, 적시다, 방울방울
떨어뜨리다

< IE. sweid- *sweat, to sweat*

　　G. systolē, systolēs, f. *shortening, contraction*

> L. systole, systoles, f. 음절단축(장음절을 짧게 함),
수축(收縮), 수축기(收縮期) 　　　E *systole, systolic*

< G. systellein (< sy- (< syn) *with, together* + stellein) *to*
draw, to shorten, to contract 　　　E *systaltic*

< G. stellein *to put in order, to prepare, to send, to make compact*
(with o-grade and zero-grade forms stol- *and* stal-*)*

< IE. stel- *to put, to stand; with derivatives referring to a standing*
object or place

그리스어에서 강한 숨표가 붙은 모음을 발음할 때에는 [ㅎ] 음이 들어가므로 자역할 때에도 'h'를 덧붙이나 그 앞에 다른 낱말이 붙는 경우에는 더 이상 [ㅎ] 음이 들어가지 않게 되어 'h'를 덧붙이지 않는다. 정확하게는 발음탈락이지만 마치 자음탈락처럼 보인다. 지금은 일부러 'h'를 덧붙여 어원을 분명히 해두려는 경향이 있다.

G. anaimia, anaimias, f. (< an- *not* + haima + -ia *noun suffix*) *anemia*

> L. anaemia, anaemiae, f. (anemia, anemiae, f.)

빈혈(貧血)　　　　　　　**E** *anaemia (anemia), anaemic (anemic)*

< G. haima, haimatos, n. *blood*

< IE. sai- *thick fluid*

G. anōmalia, anōmalias, f. (< + -ia *noun suffix*) *unevenness, unequality*

> L. anomalia, anomaliae, f. 이례(異例), 변칙,
이상(異常), 기형(畸形)　　　**E** *anomaly*

< G. anōmalos, anōmalos, anōmalon (< an- *not*)
uneven, unequal

< G. homalos, homalē, homalon *even*

< G. homos, homē, homon *of the same, common*

< IE. sem- *one; also adverbially 'as one', together with*

G. hidrōs, hidrōtos, m. *sweat, perspiration*

> G. hidrōsis, hidrōseōs, f. (< + -sis *noun suffix*) *sweating*

> L. hidrosis, hidrosis, f. 발한(發汗)　　**E** *hidrosis*

> L. osmidrosis, osmidrosis, f. (< + G. osmē *smell*)
땀악취증　　　　**E** *osmidrosis (bromidrosis)*

> L. anidrosis, anidrosis, f. (< G. an- *not*)
땀없음증　　　　**E** *anidrosis (anhidrosis)*

> L. bromidrosis, bromidrosis, f. (< G. brōmos *bad
smell*) 땀악취증　**E** *bromidrosis (bromhidrosis) (osmidrosis)*

> L. hyperidrosis, hyperidrosis, f. (< G. hyper- *over*)
땀과다증　　　　**E** *hyperidrosis (hyperhidrosis)*

< IE. sweid- *sweat, to sweat*

모음전환

파생어나 합성어를 만들면서 뒤에 오는 낱말의 모음이 변하는 경우 본디 낱말의 꼴을 짐작하기 어렵게 만든다. 그러나 여기에도 나름대로 규칙이 있다.

라틴어에서 파생어나 합성어를 만들 때, 뒤에 오는 낱말의 단모음 'a'나 단모음 'e' 다음에 자음이 하나만 있으면 'a'나 'e'는 'i'로 바뀐다. 다음 예에서, caput의 'a'는 단모음이고 그 다음의 'p'는 자음 하나이므로 occiput가 되고, tenēre의 맨앞 'e'는 단모음이고 그 다음의 'n'은 자음 하나이므로 continēre가 된다. 영어 *enemy, insipid, navigate, deficient* 등도 모음전환된 라틴어 낱말에서 비롯하였다. *enemy*가 좀 다르게 보이는 것은 라틴어 inimicus가 프랑스어를 거쳐 영어에 들어왔기 때문이다. 그렇지 않은 형용사 *inimical*과 대비된다.

    L. caput, capitis, n. 머리   **E** *capital*
        > L. occiput, occipitis, n. (< oc- (< ob) *before, toward(s), over,*
            against, away + caput *head*) 뒤통수, 후두(後頭)   **E** *occiput*
    < IE. kaput- *head*

    L. teneo, tenui, tentum, tenēre 잡다, 지키다, 소유하다,
        깨닫다   **E** *tenet, tenant, ...*
        > L. contineo, continui, contentum, continēre (< con- (< cum)
        with, together; intensive + tenēre *to hold*) 포함하다, 붙잡아
        두다, 억제하다   **E** *contain, containment, countenance*
            > L. continens, (gen.) continentis (*present participle*) 붙어
                있는; 자제력 있는, 절제하는
                E (terra continens >) *continent, continental, subcontinent;*
                continent (< 'holding together, restraining oneself)
    < IE. ten- *to stretch*

    L. amicus, amica, amicum 친구의, 우호적인
        > L. amicus, amici, m. 친구   **E** Sp. *amigo*
        > L. inimicus, inimica, inimicum (< in- *not* + amicus *friendly*)
        비우호적인, 원수의   **E** *enemy, inimical*
    < IE. am- (*Latin and Celtic root*) '*various nursery words*'

    L. sapio, sapivi (sapii, sapui), –, sapĕre 맛있다, 맛을 알다, 알다,
        지혜롭다

> L. sapidus, sapida, sapidum 맛있는   **E** *sapid*

> L. insipidus, insipida, insipidum (< in- *not* + sapidus *sapid*
맛없는   **E** *insipid*

< IE. sep-, sap- *to taste, to perceive*

L. navigo, navigavi, navigatum, navigare (< navis *ship* + agĕre *to
drive, to do*) 항해하다   **E** *navigate*

< IE. ag- *to drive, to draw, to move*

L. deficio, defeci, defectum, deficĕre (< de- *apart from, down, not* +
facĕre *to make*) 떨어져 나가다, 모자라다, 결핍되다

E *(third personal singular, present indicative, active 'it is lacking'>)*
deficit, deficient, defect, defective

< IE. dhe- *to put, to set*

라틴어에서 파생어나 합성어를 만들 때, 뒤에 오는 낱말의 단모음 'a' 다음에
자음이 둘 있으면 단모음 'a'는 'e'로 바뀐다. 다음 예에서, annus의 'a'는 단모음
이고 그 다음의 'nn'은 자음이 둘이므로 biennium, millennium이 되는 것이다.

L. annus, anni, m. 해, 년(年)   **E** *annual*

> L. biennium, biennii, n. (< bis *twice* + annus *year*) 2년, 2년의
기간

> L. biennalis, biennale 2년간의, 2년마다의   **E** *biennial*, lt. *biennale*

> L. millennium, millennii, n. (< mille *thousand* + annus *year*)
천년   **E** *millennium*

< IE. at-, atno- *to go* > *the period gone through, the revolving year*

라틴어에서 파생어나 합성어를 만들 때, 뒤에 오는 낱말의 'ae'는 'i'로 바뀌
고, 'au'는 'u'로 바뀐다.

L. caedo, cecidi, caesum, caedĕre 베다, 후려치다, 도살하다

> L. incido, incidi, incisum, incidĕre (< in- *in, on, into, toward* +
caedĕre *to cut, to kill*) 베다, 칼로 새기다, 베어내다   **E** *incise, incisive*

> L. incisio, incisionis, f. 베어냄, 절개(切開)   **E** *incision*

> L. incisura, incisurae, f. 베어낸 자리, 패임, 절흔(切痕)   **E** *incisure*

> L. incisor, incisoris, m. 베어내는 사람, 앞니, 절치(切齒)   **E** *incisor*

< IE. kaəid- *to strike*

L. claudo, clausi, clausum, claudĕre 닫다, 막다   **E** *close, closet, clause*

> L. concludo, **conclusi**, conclusum, concludĕre (< con- (< cum)

with, together + claudĕre *to shut*) 종결하다,

결론짓다   **E** *conclude, conclusive*

> L. conclusio, conclusionis, f. 종결, 결론   **E** *conclusion*

< IE. klau- (*possibly*) *hook, peg*

그리스어에서는 동사에서 명사나 형용사를 만들 때 동사 어간의 'e'가 'o'로 바뀐다. 그리스어의 명사나 형용사는 단독으로 쓰이기보다도 파생어나 합성어를 만들 때 많이 쓰이므로 마치 동사에서부터 파생어나 합성어가 만들어지면서 모음전환이 일어난 것처럼 보인다.

G. legein *to pick, to gather, to speak*

> G. lexis, lexeōs, f. *speech, word*

> G. lexikos, lexikē, lexikon *of speech, of word*

> L. lexicon, lexici, n. (< G. lexikon biblion *word*

book) 사전, 어휘   **E** *lexicon*

> G. logos, logou, m. *word, speech, discourse, reason, account,*

ratio, proportion   **E** *logic, logical, ...*

< IE. leg- *to collect; with derivatives meaning 'to speak'*

G. trepein *to turn, to turn away*

> G. tropē, tropēs, f. *turning, turn, solstice, flight, defeat, victory,*

change   **E** *tropism, ..., entropy*

> G. tropaion, tropaiou, n. *sign of victory, trophy*

> L. tropaeum, tropaei, n. (trophaeum, trophaei, n.)

전승기념물 (기둥 위에 전리품을 걸었음), 전리품,

승리   **E** *trophy*

< IE. trep- *to turn*

자음동화

라틴어나 그리스어에서 자음으로 끝나는 낱말이 자음으로 시작하는 낱말과 파생어나 합성어를 만들 때 앞 낱말의 끝 자음은 다음에 오는 자음에 동화한다. 자음 동화를 가리키는 영어 *assimilation*의 *as-*도 라틴어의 전치사 연결형 ad-의 -d-가 다음 자음 s-에 동화한 결과이다.

L. similis, simile 비슷한

> **E** (*neuter* sing. >) **simile**, (Fac simile! *'Make a similar thing!'* >) **facsimile**, (facsimile >) **fax**

> L. similo, similavi, similatum, similare 비슷해지다, 닮다

> L. assimilo, assimilavi, assimilatum, assimilare (< as-
(< ad) *to, toward, at, according to* + similare *to seem,
to be like*) 비슷하게 만들다, 같게 하다　**E** *assimilate, dissimilate*

> L. assimilatio, assimilationis, f. 비슷하게 만듦, 같게
함, 동화(同化), 동화작용　**E** *assimilation, dissimilation*

< IE. sem- *one; also adverbially 'as one', together with*

이 책에서는 라틴어편과 그리스어편의 전치사 항에서 동화형과 모음 탈락형
및 자음 탈락형을 다음처럼 예와 함께 정리해 놓았다.

L. ad (대격지배) (장소, 시간) ~에, ~으로, ~까지, ~에게로, ~ 부근에, (관계)
관해서, (수반) ~따라, (목적) 위하여

> L. ad-, ac- (*before* c, k, q), af- (*before* f), ag- (*before* g), al-
(*before* l), an- (*before* n), ap- (*before* p), ar- (*before* r), as-
(*before* s), at- (*before* t), a- (*before* sc, scr, sp, st) *to, toward,
at, according to*

E *ad- (ac-, af-, ag-, al-, an-, ap-, ar-, as-, at-, a-), add, accent,
acquire, affair, aggressive, ally, announce, appear, arrive,
associate, attract, ascend, ascribe, aspect, astringent*

> L. -ad *toward*　　**E** *-ad, ...*

< IE. ad- *to, near, at*

G. ana (대격지배) ~ 위로, ~ 가운데

> G. an(a)- *up, upward; again, throughout; back, backward; against;
according to, similar to*　**E** *an(a)-, anabolism, cathode, cation*

< IE. an- *on*

G. kata (속격지배) ~ 아래로, ~에 대항하여; (대격지배) ~에 의해서, ~을 따라서

> G. kat(a)-, kath- (*before aspirate*) *down, mis-, according to,
along, thoroughly*　**E** *cat(a)- (cath)-, catabolism, cathode, cation*

< IE. kat- *down*

G. syn (여격지배) ~와 함께

> G. syn-, syl- (*before* l), sym- (*before* m, b, p, ph), sy- (*before*
s + consonant, z) *with, together*

E *syn- (syl-, sym-, sy-), syndrome, syllable, symmetry, symbiosis,
symptom, symphysis, systolic, syzygy*

< IE. ksun *preposition and preverb meaning 'with'*

그리스어에서 동사 어근에 붙어 명사를 만드는 접미사 -ma, -mos, -sis 앞의 파열음은 접미사의 첫 자음에 동화한다. graph-ma가 gramma가 되고, leg-sis 가 lexis가 되는 것은 이 때문이다.

G. gramma, grammatos, n. (< graph- + -ma *resultative noun suffix*)
  thing written, letter of alphabet   **E** *-gram, ...*
  > L. gramma, grammatis, n. (< *what is drawn or written*)
   그램(무게 단위), 작은 무게   **E** *gramme (gram, g)*
 < G. graphein *to scratch, to draw, to write*
< IE. gerbh- *to scratch*

G. lexis, lexeōs, f. (< leg- + -sis *noun suffix*) *speech, word*
  > G. lexikos, lexikē, lexikon *of speech, of word*
   > L. lexicon, lexici, n. (< G. lexikon biblion *word
    book*) 사전, 어휘   **E** *lexicon*
 < G. legein *to pick, to gather, to speak*
< IE. leg- *to collect; with derivatives meaning 'to speak'*

언어의 순혈주의

파생어나 합성어를 보면 영어는 영어끼리, 라틴어는 라틴어끼리, 그리스어는 그리스어끼리 붙여 만듦을 알 수 있다. 언어의 순혈주의(純血主義, *in-breeding*) 이다. 형용사를 예로 들면 본디 영어 낱말 *heart-y, heart-ful, heart-less*의 *-y, -ful, -less*은 모두 영어 접미사이며, 라틴어에서 비롯한 영어 낱말 *cord-ate, cord-i-al*의 *-ate*와 *-al*은 모두 라틴어 유래 접미사이고, 그리스어에 비롯한 영어 낱말 *cardi-ac*의 *-ac*는 그리스어 유래 접미사이다.

(1) cor, cordis, n. 심장, 마음, 의지, 용기, 지혜 **E** *(suggested) core*
(2) > cordatus, cordata, cordatum 심장 모양의, 현명한 **E** *cordate*
(3) > cordialis, cordiale 마음에서 우러나는 **E** *cordial*
(12) < IE. kerd- *heart* **E** *heart, hearty, heartful, heartless, hearten*
(13) > G. kardia, kardias, f. *heart, mind, soul*

(14)   > G. kardiakos, kardiakē, kardiakon (< + -akos *adjective suffix*) *of heart*

(15)   > L. cardiacus, cardiaca, cardiacum 심장의, 심장병의;
(*on the heart side of the body* >) 위(胃)의, 위병(胃病)의, 들문(~門)의   **E** *cardiac*

(17)   > G. perikardios, perikardia, perikardion (< peri– < peri *around, near, beyond, on account of*) *pericardial*

(18)   > L. pericardium, pericardii, n. 심장막, 심낭(心囊)   **E** *pericardium, pericardial*

(20)   > L. myocardium, myocardii, n. (< G. my(o)– < mys, myos, m. *mouse, muscle*) 심근층   **E** *myocardium, myocardial*

영어 *pericardium*이 비롯한 라틴어 pericardium은 그리스어의 형용사 중성형 perikardion을 라틴어화한 낱말이다. 당연히 언어의 순혈주의를 따르고 있다. 뿐만 아니다. 영어 *myocardium*이 비롯한 라틴어 myocardium은, 그런 그리스어 낱말이 있었던 것도 아니고 꼴도 라틴어꼴인 -um으로 되어 있지만, 그리스어 기원의 my(o)–에 그리스어 기원의 -cardium을 붙여 순혈주의를 지켰다. 한 술 더 떠서, 영어 *a-cardia*(무심장증), *electro-cardi-o-gram*(심전도), *cardi-o-megaly*(심장비대) 등은, 그런 그리스어 낱말도 없었고 그런 라틴어 낱말도 없었으나 모두 그리스어 기원의 성분을 갖다 붙임으로써 역시 순혈주의를 지켰다.

예외가 없는 것은 아니지만 언어의 순혈주의는 상당히 엄격하게 지켜지고 있으며, 지키는 것이 바람직하다. 학명도 언어의 순혈주의를 따르도록 강력히 권장하고 있다.

언어의 순혈주의를 따르기 위해서는 낱말의 국적을 알아야 하나 어원론을 공부하다보면 절로 알아지게 되어 있다. 심근병증을 가리키는 *cardiomyopathy*에서 *cardio-*가 그리스어 기원이므로 *myo-* 및 *-pathy*도, 예외가 아닌 이상, 그리스어 기원이라고 미루어 알 수 있고, 나아가, 공감을 가리키는 *sympathy*의 *sym-*도 그리스어 기원이라고 미루어 알 수 있는 것이다.

혼종어

dextrocardia는 라틴어 형용사 dextr–와 그리스어 명사 kardia의 혼종어로서 언어의 순혈주의에 위배된다. 이와 같은, 국적이 다른 낱말끼리의 파생어나 합성어를 혼종어(混種語, *hybrid word*)라고 한다. 바람직하지는 않지만 관례에 따라 또는 대안이 없어 부분적으로 사용하고 있다.

혼종어에 있어서도 학술용어에서는 라틴어와 그리스어 사이의 혼종어가 많은데 그런 경우 그리스어적 성향이 좀 더 우세하다. dextr-o-cardia에서도 그리스어적 연결 모음 -o-를 끼워 넣었다.

(24) L. dextrocardia, dextrocardiae, f. (< L. dexter, dextra, dextrum *right*
+ G. kardia *heart*) 우심증   <u>E</u> *dextrocardia*

국제학술어휘

오른쪽을 그리스어로는 dexios 또는 dexiteros라고 하므로 우심증의 올바른 합성어는 dexiocardia 또는 dexiterocardia이며 의학사전에는 dexiocardia가 올라 있다. 그러나 dexiocardia는 사용하지 않을 뿐 아니라 있는지조차도 잘 알려져 있지 않다. 그리스어 dexios의 동족어인 라틴어 dexter를 사실상의 국제 표준처럼 사용하기 때문이다.

학술용어에서는 언어의 순혈주의를 사수해야 한다고 주장할 수 없다. 편광을 오른쪽으로 선회시키는 우선성 *dextrorotatory*의 dextr(o)-를, 경우에 따라서 dexi(o)-로 해야 한다고 주장하게 되기 때문이다. 좌선성 *levorotatory*의 lev(o)-(라틴어)와 lai(o)-(그리스어)의 관계도 마찬가지이다. 학술용어는 하나의 사실에 대해서 하나의 낱말이 있어야 하는 것을 원칙으로 하고 있고, 그 원칙은 맞다.

L. dexter, dextra, dextrum (dexter, dextera, dexterum) 오른쪽의,
길조의, 오른손잡이의, 솜씨 좋은

> <u>E</u> *dexter, dextrous (dexterous), dextr(o)-, dextrorotatory* (D-), *(dextro-rotatory glucose >) dextrose, dextrin (< 'the property of turning the plane of polarization 138.68° to the right'), dextran*

> dextra, dextrae, f. (dextera, dexterae, f.) 오른손,
오른편   <u>E</u> *dextrad (< + -ad 'toward')*
> dextralis, dextrale 오른손의, 오른편의, 오른편에 있는   <u>E</u> *dextral*
> dextrorsum (< dextrovorsum < dexter + vortĕre (vertĕre) *to turn*)
(부사) 오른쪽으로   <u>E</u> *dextrorse*

> dexteritas, dexteritatis, f. 능숙, 다행   **E** *dexterity*

> ambidexter, ambidextra, ambidextrum (< amb(i)- *on both sides,*

    around) 양손잡이의, 솜씨가 비상한, 언행이 다른,

    표리부동한   **E** *ambidexter, ambidexterity*

< IE. deks- *right*

> G. dexios, dexia, dexion (dexiteros, dexitera, dexiteron)

    right   **E** *dexiocardia, dexiotropic*

L. laevus, laeva, laevum 왼쪽의, 서투른, 흉조의

    E *laev(o)- (lev(o)-), levorotatory* (L-), *levulose* (< *'formerly, levorotatory*

    glucose; now, the naturally occurring (levorotatory) form of fructose')

< IE. laiwo- *left*

> G. laios, laia, laion *left*   **E** *lai(o)-, laiose*

학술용어에서 dextr(o)-와 lev(o)-는 오른쪽과 왼쪽을 가리키는 공인어이다. 학술상의 국제어인 셈이다. 이런 어휘를 국제학술어휘(*International Scientific Vocabulary*, ISV)라고 한다.

국제학술어휘는 언어의 순혈주의를 초월한다. 그러나 어원론의 관점에서 보면 그것은 예외 규정이며, 다행히도 그 범위는 제한적이다.

영어의 어휘형성

영어 어휘형성의 기본은 파생어와 합성어이다. 파생어와 합성어의 정의는 라틴어·그리스어에서의 정의와 같다. 혼종어의 정의도 같다.

학술 라틴어나 학술 그리스어와 달리 영어는 일상의 삶에 바탕을 둔 생동하는 언어이다. 그러다보니 라틴어나 그리스어에서 흔치 않은 조어법이 영어에서는 활발하다. 단축어, 혼성어, 역성어, 인명 및 지명 유래어, 두문자어 및 두문자약어 등이다.

파생어

파생어(派生語, *derivative*)는 있는 낱말에 의존형태소를 붙여 만든 새로운 낱말이다. *heart*의 파생어 *hearty, heartful, heartless, hearten*은 영어 고유어

heart에다 역시 영어에 고유한 의존형태소 -y, -ful, -less, -en을 붙여 만들었다.

파생어를 만들 때 영어가 영어에 고유한 성분만 이용하란 법은 없다. 이미 영어에 들어와 있는 낱말과 의존형태소를 이용할 수 있다. 영어 globule은 구(球)를 뜻하는 라틴어 globus에 의존형태소인 지소접미사 -ulus가 붙은 globulus에서 비롯했다. 소구(小球)라는 뜻을 갖는다. 그 globule에다 라틴어·그리스어에서 형용사를 만드는 접미사 중 하나(L. -inus, -ina, -inum; G. -inos, -inē, -inon)인 의존형태소 -in을 붙이면 영어 파생어 globulin (글로불린)이 된다. -in은 globulin과 같은 단백질 외에도 지질, 약제와 같은 화학물질의 명칭을 만든다. prostaglandin, penicillin 등이다.

-in과 기원이 같지만 염기성 또는 그에 준하는 물질과 조염원소의 이름에다는 -ine을 붙여 파생어를 만든다. adenine, amine, asparagine, caffeine, iodine 등이다.

합성어

합성어(合成語, compound)는 둘 이상의 자립형태소를 붙여 만든다. 영어 고유어 heartbeat, heartburn, heart-stopper, heart-to-heart, heart attack, heart failure는 자립형태소들을 가져다 놓기만 하면 되는 게르만어계 언어의 합성어 형성을 잘 보여준다.

합성어의 자립형태소가 heartbeat와 heartburn의 경우 붙어 있고, heart-stopper의 경우 하이픈으로 연결되어 있으며, heart attack과 heart failure의 경우 떨어져 있는데 두 성분의 결합강도를 반영한다. heart-to-heart에서처럼 구(句) 합성어는 하이픈으로 연결한다.

husband, woman, lady, window 등은 하나의 자립형태소로 보이지만 기실 합성어이다. 이런 깜찍한 합성어를 융합형 합성어(amalgamated compound)라고 한다.

파생어에서와 마찬가지로 합성어를 만들 때에도 이미 영어에 들어와 있는 자립형태소를 이용할 수 있다. 직무(L. munus)에서 면제된(L. in- not), 즉 면역의 뜻을 갖는 연결형 immuno-에다 globulin을 가져다 붙이면 immunoglobulin (면역글로불린)이란 합성어가 된다. hematoglobulin (혈색소)은 혈액(G. haima, haimatos, n.)이라는 뜻의 그리스어 연결형 *hemato-*에 *globulin*을 붙여 만든 합성어이다.

혼종어

혼종어(混種語, *hybrid*)는 국적이 다른 낱말끼리의 파생어나 합성어이다. 라틴어와 그리스어 사이의 혼종어가 많다. 합성어 *hematoglobulin*은 그리스어와 라틴어의 혼종어이기도 하다.

혼종어를 이루는 성분은 국제학술어휘인 경우가 많다. *hemato-*와 *globulin* 모두 국제학술어휘에 속한다.

단축어

단축어(短縮語, *clipping, shortening*)는 짧게 줄인 낱말이다. *phone*(전화)은 *telephone*의 앞을 줄였고, *lab*(실험실)은 *laboratory*의 뒤를 줄였으며, *flu*(독감)는 *influenza*의 앞뒤를 줄였고, *fancy*(환상)는 *fantasy*의 앞뒤를 남기면서 가운데를 줄였다.

hemoglobin(혈색소)은 합성어 *hemato-globulin*의 두 성분 각각에서 가운데 한 음절씩을 줄였다. 지금은, *hematoglobulin*이 일부 사전에 올라 있기는 해도, 전적으로 *hemoglobin*이란 단축어를 사용한다. *myoglobin*(근색소)은 *myohemoglobin*의 가운데를 줄인 단축어이다. *hemoglobin*과 마찬가지로 *myoglobin* 분자 안에도 *heme*이 들어 있다는 것을 어원은 보여준다. *heme*은, *hemoglobin*에서처럼, *myoglobin*의 기능상 핵심 성분이다.

혼성어

혼성어(混成語, *blend, portmanteau word*)는 두 낱말을 단축시킨 후 합성해 만든 새 낱말이다. *brunch*(브런치)는 영어 고유어 *breakfast*와 *lunch*가 만든 혼성어이고 *spam*(스팸)은 라틴어에서 온 영어 *spice*와 영어 고유어 *ham*이 만든 혼종어이자 혼성어이다.

학술용어 중에도 혼성어가 상당수 만들어져 있으며 앞으로도 계속 만들어질 것이다. *urinalysis*(소변검사)는 라틴어에서 온 영어 *urine*과 그리스어에서 온 영어 *analysis*가 만들었고, 현대인이 치루고 있는 두 역병 *diabesity*(당뇨병과 비만증)는 그리스어에서 온 영어 *diabetes*와 라틴어에서 온 영어 *obesity*가 만들었다.

역성어

역성어(逆成語, *back-formation*)란 파생어 또는 합성어 꼴의 낱말로부터 구성 성분을 떼어내 만든 새 낱말을 말한다. 라틴어나 그리스어로부터 들어온 낱말에서부터 만들어진 경우가 많다.

완두를 뜻하는 라틴어 pisum이 *pease*의 꼴로 영어에 들어왔다가 복수로 오인받아 새로 만들어진 *pea*가 역성어이다. 그리스어 tēle(멀리)와 라틴어 visio(보기)의 혼종어인 명사 *television*에서부터 새로 만들어진 동사 *televise*도 역성어이다. 합성어 *hematoglobulin*의 단축어인 *hemoglobin*으로부터 새로이 만들어진 *heme*과 *globin* 역시 역성어이다.

인명유래어

인명유래어(人名由來語, *eponym*)란 사람 이름에서 따온 낱말이다. 본디는 낱말이 비롯한 사람을 가리키지만, 실제는 사람에서 비롯한 낱말을 가리키는 경우가 더 많다.

인명유래어는 *parkinsonism*(파킨슨증)의 *James Parkinson*(영국)처럼 처음 기술하였거나 크게 공헌한 사람의 이름을 따온다. 그러나 꼭 그런 것만도 아니다. 새치기한 이름도 나돌고 따와서는 안 될 이름도 나돈다.

인명유래어중 환자 이름을 따온 용어는 환자명유래어(*autoeponym*)이다. *Lou Gehrig's disease, Christmas factor, JC virus, BK virus* 등이 있지만 손가락으로 헤아리는 정도이다.

인명유래어이지만 귀띔해주지 않으면 눈치 채지 못할 정도로 익숙해진 낱말도 있다. 철자도 소문자화 해버렸다. 아일랜드 소작인들의 배척운동 때문에 만들어진 *boycott*, 미국 치안판사의 체벌 때문에 만들어진 *lynch* 등이 그렇다. 향미료를 넣은 포도주 *hippocras*는 히포크라테스로부터 유래한다.

지명유래어

지명유래어(地名由來語, *toponym*)는 지중해 섬나라 *Malta*의 지명에서 유래한 *Maltese dog*(몰타 개), *Maltese cat*(몰타 고양이), *Maltese cross*(몰타 십자)처럼 땅이름에서 유래한다. 영국 제4대 샌드위치 백작의 카드놀이 때문에 만들어진 *sandwich*도, 인명유래어가 아니라, 지명유래어이다. 제4대 샌드위치 백작의 샌드위치는 영지 이름이고 백작 이름은 따로 있다. *John Montagu*이다.

지명유래어를 곧잘 만나는 곳은 바이러스, 세균, 곰팡이, 기생충 등의 감염성 질환명이다. *norovirus*(노로바이러스)는 미국 오하이오 주의 작은 도시 *Norwalk*를 연고지로 하고, *coxsackievirus*(콕사키바이러스)는 미국 뉴욕 주의 작은 도시 *Coxsackie*를 연고지로 한다.

동식물과 미생물의 학명은 인명·지명을 자주 인용한다. 물론 인용은 인명과 지명 모두를 라틴어화한 후 라틴어 문법에 따른다는 국제 규약을 준수한다.

우리나라 토박이인 개나리의 학명 Forsythia koreana는 스코틀랜드 원예가 *William Forsyth*의 이름과 우리나라 지명을 인용하였다. 브루셀라증을 일으키는 대표 세균의 학명 Brucella melitensis는 스코틀랜드 출신의 영국 군의관 *David Bruce*의 이름과 지중해 *Malta*섬의 라틴어명 Melita를 인용하였다.

라틴어 꼴을 한 학명은 그 꼴 그대로 영어 안에 들어온다. 인명이나 지명을 인용한 학명은 라틴어로 단장한 인명·지명유래어인 셈이다.

두문자어와 두문자약어

둘 이상의 낱말이 만든 표현에서 두문자를 모아 다루기 좋은 낱말을 만들 수 있다. 병명 *acquired immune deficiency syndrome*(후천 면역결핍 증후군)의

*AIDS*나 균명 *human immunodeficiency virus*(사람 면역결핍 바이러스)의 *HIV* 등이다.

*AIDS*처럼 두문자를 따온 낱말이 영어의 음소배열(*English phonotactics*)에 합당하면 두문자어(*acronym*)라고 하고, 일반 낱말인양 발음한다. HIV처럼 그렇지 않으면 두문자약어(*initialism*)라고 하고, 알파벳 하나하나씩 발음한다.

두문자어는 일반 낱말의 꼴을 하고 있기 때문에 *Aids*같이 첫 문자만 대문자를 쓰고 나머자는 소문자를 쓰기도 한다. 익숙해져서 아예 소문자로만 쓰는 두문자어도 있다. *laser*(*light amplification by stimulated emission of radiation*)가 그러하다.

분자생물학의 발달로 새로운 유전자와 단백질이 규명되면서 너무하다 싶을 정도로 많은 두문자어와 두문자약어가 만들어지고 있다. 잘못하면 알파벳의 미로 속에 갇히고 말 정도이다. 갇히지 않기 위한 유일한 방법은, 물론, 어원의 이해이다.

영어·라틴어·그리스어 기원 학술용어의 의미 차이

학문의 세계에서는 하나의 대상에 대해 영어와 라틴어와 그리스어 기원의 용어를 모두 사용한다. 그러나 각각 사용처가 다르다.

(1) cor, cordis, n. 심장, 마음, 의지, 용기, 지혜

(2)　　　　 > cordatus, cordata, cordatum 심장 모양의, 현명한　　　　　E *cordate*

(12)　　 < IE. kerd- *heart*　　　　　　　　　　　　　　　　　　　　E *heart*

(13)　　　　 > G. kardia, kardias, f. *heart, mind, soul*

E *cardi(o)-, electrocardiogram (ECG)*, (D. Elektrokardiogramm >) *EKG, cardiomegaly*

(16)　　　　 > G. kardioeidēs, kardioeidēs, kardioeides (< + eidos *shape*)
　　　　　　 heart-shaped　　　　　　　　　　　　　　　　　　　 E *cardioid*

(22)　　　　 > L. bradycardia, bradycardiae, f. (< G. bradys *slow*) 느린
　　　　　　 맥, 서맥(徐脈)　　　　　　　　　　　　　E *bradycardia, bradycardiac*

(23)　　　　 > L. tachycardia, tachycardiae, f. (< G. tachys *swift*) 빠른
　　　　　　 맥, 빈맥(頻脈)　　　　　　　　　　　　E *tachycardia, tachycardiac*

너무 단순화시킴으로써 오류를 범하는 무리를 무릅쓰고라도 도구적 유용성을 위해 요약해 보면, 본디 영어 용어는 대상 하나만을 직접적으로 표현하고자 할 때 사용한다. 라틴어 기원의 영어 용어는 대상을 다른 대상과 대비시켜 표현하고자 할 때 사용한다. 그리스어 기원의 영어 용어는 대상을 전문적 측면에서 표현하고자 할 때 사용한다. *heart-shaped*라 하면 그냥 심장 모양이다. 그러나 *cordate*라고 하면 머리 모양(*capitate*), 꼬리 모양(*caudate*), 이빨 모양(*dentate*), 톱니 모양(*serrate*) 등에 비교하였을 때의 심장 모양이고, *cardioid*는 극좌표에서 방정식 $\rho(\theta) = 2r(1 - \cos\theta)$로 주어지는 심장 모양의 도형이다.

　　영어나 라틴어 기원의 영어 용어는 구체적 대상을 다룬다. 이에 비해 그리스어 기원의 영어 용어는 개념적 대상을 다룬다. 큰 척추동물의 심장에 있는 '심장의 뼈'(E.) *bone of the heart* 또는 (L.) os cordis는 육체의 눈으로 보는 구체적 대상이다. 그러나 그리스어 기원의 '느린맥' *bradycardia*나 '빠른맥' *tachycardia*는 생각의 눈으로 보는 개념적 대상이다.

　　앞에서 예를 든 라틴어와 그리스어 기원의 영어 용어를 모두 본디 영어 낱말로 바꿔놓을 수 있다. *capitate*는 *head-shaped*, *caudate*는 *tail-shaped*, *dentate*는 *tooth-shaped*, *serrate*는 *saw-tooth-shaped*, *cordate*와 *cardioid*는 *heart-shaped*, *bradycardia*는 *slow heartbeat*, *tachycardia*는 *fast heartbeat*가 된다. 그러나 그렇게 하지 않는다. 첫째는 주변 용어들과의 연계성 때문이다. *cardi(o)*-를 모두 '*heart-*'로 대치시키려고 할 때 *electrocardiogram*, *cardiomegaly* 등 동족어 무리의 다른 용어는 처리하기 곤란하다. 둘째는 본디 영어 낱말로 대치하였을 경우, 그 다음 확장성이 매우 제한되기 때문이다. *tachycardia*로부터는 매우 그리스어적으로 자연스럽게 *tachycardiac*이란 형용사가 파생한다. 그러나 *fast heartbeat*로는 어려운 이야기이다. 언젠가 빠른맥을 늦추는 약을 개발한 사람이 '항빈맥제'라는 뜻의 용어를 만들고 싶을 때에는 어떠할 것인가? *antitachycardiac drug*는 듣는 순간 자연스럽다. 그러나 *fast heartbeat*로는 … 막막하다. 용어를 만들 때에는 확장성도 고려하는 것이다.

　　라틴어와 그리스어 기원의 영어 용어를 모두 본디 영어 낱말로 바꿔놓을 수 없는 세 번째 이유는 언어의 순혈주의 때문이다. 학술용어에서는 국제학술어휘와 혼종어를 사용할 수밖에 없고 사용해야 한다. 그렇지만 그것은 제한적이고 제한적이어야 한다. 혼란을 막고 뜻을 분명히 해두기 위해서이다.

언어의 순혈주의는 합성어를 만들 때뿐 아니라 의존형태소인 접두사나 접미사 등 접사를 붙여 파생어를 만들 때에도 적용된다. 학술용어에는 라틴어나 그리스어 기원의 접사를 붙여 만든 용어들이 많이 있는데, 그런 용어도 라틴어 기원의 접사는 라틴어 낱말에다 붙이고 그리스어 기원의 접사는 그리스어 낱말에다 붙이는 것이다. 예를 들면, 상태를 가리키는 *-osis*, 염증을 가리키는 *-itis*, 종양을 가리키는 *-oma* 등은 그리스어 기원의 접미사이므로 그 앞에 붙는 낱말도 그리스어 기원의 낱말이어야 한다. 동맥(*artery* < G. artēria)의 염증은 *arteritis*가 되는 것이 당연하며, 정맥(*vein* < L. vena)의 염증은 *phlebitis*(< G. phleps, phlebos, f. *vein*)가 되는 것이 당연하다.

이상을 간추려 보자면, 용어를 하나씩 보면 예외가 있지만 본디 영어 용어는 구체적 대상 하나만을 직접적으로 가리킬 때 사용한다. 연계성, 확장성, 언어의 순혈주의 때문에 라틴어와 그리스어 기원의 영어 용어를 사용할 수밖에 없는데, 라틴어 기원의 영어 용어는 본디 영어 용어가 가리킨 구체적 대상을 다른 구체적 대상과 대비시켜 가리킬 때 사용하며, 그리스어 기원의 영어 용어는 그 대상의 전문적, 개념적 특성을 가리킬 때 사용한다. 하나의 대상에 대해 본디부터 영어인 용어와 라틴어, 그리스어 기원의 영어 용어가 모두 사용되며 각각의 용어는 사용처가 다른 것이다. 그리고, 이 의미상 차이를 느끼게 해주는 것도 어원론이다.

이런 의미상 차이는 어원은 달라도 뜻이 같은 용어들 사이에서도 실존한다. 정상 모습과 동떨어져 있는 모습을 인도유럽어는 '나쁜' 모습이라고 하는데, 영어판으로는 *bad shape*이 되고, 라틴어판으로는 *malformation*이 되며, 그리스어판으로는 *dysplasia*가 된다. 그러나, '나쁜' 모습이라는 뜻이 같아도 사용처가 다르다. *bad shape*은 눈에 거슬리는 정서적 기형이고, *malformation*(기형)은 육체의 눈으로 보는 구체적 기형이며, *dysplasia*(형성이상, 이형성)는 생각의 눈으로 보는 개념적 기형이다.

제 5 장 영어사전의 어원 표기

　어원 중심으로 영어 낱말을 다룬 사전도 있다. 일반 영어사전들도 표제어의 발음 바로 다음이나 뜻풀이 끝에다 별도의 난을 두어 어원을 밝히는 것이 일반적이다. (우리나라에서 발간된 영한사전은, 큰 사전을 빼놓고는, 어원을 밝히지 않는 것이 일반적이다.)

　영어 어원사전이든 일반 영어사전이든 '좋은' 어원 표기란, 표제어의 말뿌리와 그 말뿌리에서 비롯한 동족어를 보여주고, 그 동족어에서부터 비롯한 영어 낱말 무리에는 무엇이 있으며 그 중 표제어는 꼴과 뜻이 어떻게 진화해서 지금처럼 되었는가를 보여주는 것이다. 그러나 '그렇게까지 좋은' 사전은 하나도 없다. 어원론의 사실상 표준인 〈Oxford English Dictionary〉도 그렇게까지 좋지 않기는 매한가지이다. 궁색하지만 좋게 해석해, 지면의 여유가 없기 때문이리라. 지면의 제약을 받지 않는 전자사전의 경우도, 아직까지는, 마찬가지이다. 종이 사전을 옮겨놓았기 때문이다.

　영어사전의 어원 표기 방식에는 아직도 통일된 기준이 없다. 〈Oxford English Dictionary〉의 표기 방식은 다른 사전들과는 또 다르다. 격을 한 단계 높였다고나 할까?

　어원 표기 방식에 통일된 형식이 없어 좀 혼란스럽게 생각되겠지만, 이 책의 내용을 알고 나면 어떤 형식의 어원 표기라도 좇아갈 수 있다. 물론 〈Oxford English Dictionary〉도 포함된다.

　다음은 영어사전들이 어원을 표기하는 일반 형식이다.

표제어

　사전은 같은 철자의 낱말이라고 하더라도 어원이 다르면 표제어를 달리 한다. 구분은 어깨번호로 한다.

E. temple^1 [L. *templum* consecrated place] 신전

E. temple^2 [L. *tempora* temples] 관자놀이

E. temple^3 [L. *templum* a contrivance for keeping cloth stretched to
its proper width in the loom, originally the same word
as TEMPLE^2] (베틀에서 베를 팽팽하게 당겨 주는) 쳇발

어원란의 글꼴

어원란의 라틴어, 그리스어, 그 외 외국어는 모두 영어 본문과는 다른 글꼴이다. 영어가 아니라는 것을 얼른 눈에 띄도록 하기 위한 배려이다. 영어 문장 중에 나오는 학명을 다른 글꼴로 하는 것과 같다.

영어사전의 본문은 반듯한 글꼴이다. 로마체라고도 한다. 반듯한 글꼴과 쉽게 구분되는 글꼴은 기운 글꼴이다. 따라서 영어사전의 어원란에 나오는 라틴어, 그리스어 등은 기운 글꼴로 쓰여 있다. 기운 글꼴을, 정확한 표현은 아닌지만, 이탤릭체라고도 한다. 진짜 이탤릭체는, 그냥 기운 글꼴이 아니라, 멋부린 기운 글꼴이다. 다음은 영어사전의 예이다.

E. type [L. *typus* < G. *typos* blow, mold, die < G. *typtein* to strike]
형(型), 활자(活字), 표준

영어 본문이 기운 글꼴이면 본문 중 외국어는 바른 글꼴이 된다. 이 책에서는 약자를 제외한 영어 낱말을 기운 글꼴로, 라틴어, 그리스어, 그 외 외국어를 바른 글꼴로 썼다. 단, 이 부분, '영어사전의 어원 표기'는 예외이다. 영어사전에 나와 있는 꼴 그대로를 보여주기 위함이다. 다음은 이 책의 예이다.

G. etymos, etymos, etymon *real, actual, true*
> G. etymon, etymou, n. *the 'true' literal sense of a word
according to its origin, its 'true' or original form*
> L. etymon, etymi, n. 낱말의 원형, 어원(語源), 말밑   **E** *etymon*
> G. etymologia, etymologias, f. (< + -logia *study*)
etymology
> L. etymologia, etymologiae, f. 어원론, 어원학   **E** *etymology*
< IE. es- *to be*

명사 표기

라틴어나 그리스어 명사에서 비롯한 영어 낱말의 어원을 이해하기 위해서는 기본 꼴인 단수 주격이 필요하고 어간을 찾기 위한 단수 속격이 필요하다.

영어사전은, 라틴어이든 그리스어이든, 기본 꼴인 단수 주격을 제시한다. 어간은 주격어간과 속격어간이 다른 경우에만, 그것도 밝혀야 할 필요가 있을 때에만 제시한다. 어간을 제시하는 대신 단수 속격이나 단수 대격을 제시하는 경우도 있다. 이런 경우에는 속격 또는 대격의 어미를 떼어내 어간을 찾아낸다.

> E. noun [L. *nomen* name] 명사
>
> : 단수 주격(L. *nomen*)만 제시

> E. onomatopoeia [G. *onoma, onomat-* name + G. *-poiia* making
>   < G. *poiein* to make] 의성어 만들기, 의성어
>
> : 단수 주격(G. *onoma*, G. *-poiia*)과 속격어간
>   (G. *onomat-*)을 제시

영어사전을 포함한 일반 사전은 라틴어나 그리스어 명사의 성을 제시하지 않는다. 그러나 관용구를 이해하기 위해서는 성이 필요하며 특히 학술용어를 다루기 위해서는 더욱 그러하다.

> [용례] xeroderma pigmentosum 색소성 건피증(乾皮症)
>   (문법) xeroderma 건피증
>   pigmentosum 색깔이 많은 (< 색소가 많은)

사전이 라틴어나 그리스어 명사의 성을 제시하지 않는다고 하더라도 라틴어의 기초 문법 정도만 알고 있으면 관용구나 학술용어에서 쉽고 정확하게 명사의 성을 알 수 있다. 색소성 건피증 xeroderma pigmentosum에서 pigmentosum은, 뜻으로 보아, xeroderma를 수식하는 형용사이고 형용사인 이상 중성형 단수임이 분명하다. pigmentosum이 형용사 중성형 단수인 이상 xeroderma는 중성 명사 단수일 수밖에 없다.

> [용례] xeroderma pigmentosum 색소성 건피증(乾皮症)

(문법) xeroderma 건피증: 중성 명사, 단수 주격

     < xeroderma, xerodermatis, n.

pigmentosum 색깔이 많은 (< 색소가 많은): 형용사, 중성형 단수 주격

     < pigmentosus, pigmentosa, pigmentosum

(관용구나 학술용어는 어원론을 즐길 수 있는 좋은 노리개이다. 예를 들자면, pigmentosum이 형용사 중성형 단수이기에 -osum이 라틴어 형용사 접미사임을 알 수 있고, -osum이 라틴어 기원이므로 pigment-도 라틴어 기원임을 알 수 있다. 중성 명사 단수 -derma는 -a로 끝나면서도 여성 명사가 아니니까 -ma라는 접미사가 붙은 그리스어 기원의 명사임을 알 수 있고, 따라서 당연하게, 속격어간은 -dermat-가 되고 복수 주격은 -dermata가 됨을 알 수 있다. xeroderma pigmentosum의 복수 주격은, 쓰이지 않지만 즐기기 위해 만들어 보자면, xerodermata pigmentosa가 된다.)

형용사 표기

라틴어나 그리스어 형용사에서 비롯한 영어 낱말의 어원을 이해하기 위해서는 남성형, 여성형, 중성형의 단수 주격이 필요하다. 형용사의 경우에는 남성형, 여성형, 중성형의 단수 주격을 보고서 속격어간을 찾을 수 있다.

영어사전은, 라틴어이든 그리스어이든, 남성형 단수 주격 하나만을 제시한다. 명사에서처럼, 어간은 주격어간과 속격어간이 다른 경우에만, 그것도 어간을 밝혀야 할 필요가 있을 때에만, 별도로 제시한다. 어간을 제시하는 대신 남성형의 단수 속격이나 단수 대격을 제시하는 경우도 있다.

     E. adjective [L. *adjectivus* < L. *adjicĕre* to throw to] 형용사

       : 남성형 단수 주격(L. *adjectivus*)만 제시

     E. nominal [L. *nominalis* < L. *nomen, nomin-* name] 이름의, 명칭상의;
             (문법) 명사의

       : 남성형 단수 주격(L. nominalis)만 제시 (남·여성형이 동일함)

     E. potent [L. *potens, potent-* being powerful, being able] 힘 있는, 능력 있는

: 남성형 단수 주격(L. potens)과 속격어간(L. potent-)을 제시
(남·여·중성 형이 동일함)

E. xer(o)- [G. *xēros* dry] '건조한'이라는 뜻의 연결형
: 남성형 단수 주격(G. xēros)만 제시

동사 표기

라틴어 동사에서 비롯한 영어 낱말의 어원을 이해하기 위해서는 동사의 현재부정법 (*present infinitive*), 현재분사 (*present participle*), 수동형 미래분사 (*gerundive*), 과거분사(*past participle*)의 네 가지 꼴이 필요하다.

영어 낱말이 라틴어 동사의 현재부정법이나 현재분사에서 비롯한 경우에는 현재부정법 하나를 보여주고, 수동형 미래분사나 과거분사 어간에서 비롯한 경우에는 현재부정법과 함께 분사의 어간을 보여주는 사전이 많다. 사전에 따라서는 현재부정법 대신 직설법 현재 단수 일인칭을 보여주기도 한다. (라틴어나 그리스어 사전에서는 직설법 현재 단수 일인칭이 동사의 표제어이다.) 분사는 남성형 하나를 보여주는 것이 일반적이나 경우에 따라 여성형이나 중성형 하나를 보여주기도 한다.

E. infinitive [L. *infinitivus* indefinite < L. *in-* not + L. *finitivus* definite <
L. *finitus* past participle of *finire* to finish] 부정사의, 부정사
: 현재부정법(L. *finire*)과 과거분사 남성형(L. *finitus*)을 제시

그리스어 규칙 동사의 경우에 영어사전은 현재부정법 하나를 보여준다. 불규칙 동사의 경우에는 현재부정법 옆에 어간이나 어근을 곁들인다.

E. genesis [L. *genesis* < G. *genesis* birth, origin, creation < G. *gignesthai*
(*gen-* root of *gignesthai*) to be born, to become] 탄생, 생성, 발생,
형성; (Genesis) 창세기
: 현재부정법(G. *gignesthai*)과 어근(G. *gen-*)을 제시

그 외 품사의 표기

영어사전에서 어원이 되는 부사, 전치사, 접속사 등 불변화 품사의 표기는 단순하다. 낱말과 뜻만을 제시하기 때문이다. 전치사가 합성어를 이룰 경우에는 연결형을 제시한다. 대명사는 변화 품사이기는 하나 영어사전은 해당하는 낱말 하나와 뜻을 보여준다.

E. adverb [L. *adverbium* < L. *ad-* to, toward, at, according to +
　　　　　L. *verbum* word, verb] 부사

　: 전치사(L. *ad*)의 연결형(L. *ad-*)을 제시

E. preposition [L. *praepositio* < L. *prae-* before + L. *ponĕre* to put,
　　　　　　to place] 전치사

　: 전치사(L. *prae*)의 연결형(L. *prae-*)을 제시

E. pronoun [L. *pronomen* < L. *pro-* before, forward; for; instead of +
　　　　　L. *nomen* name] 대명사

　: 전치사(L. *pro*)의 연결형(L. *pro-*)을 제시

E. nostrum [L. *nostrum* (something) our own making < L. neuter of
　　　　　noster our < L. *nos* we] 비약(秘藥), 만병통치약

　: 소유대명사(L. *noster*)와 인칭대명사(L. *nos*)를 제시

어원론을
위한
라틴어

Etymological Latin

Lingua Latina
Etymologica

제1장 역사

　라틴어(Lingua Latina)는 이탈리아 반도의 중서부에 위치한 라티움(Latium) 지방의 라틴족 언어이었다. 라틴족은 산발적인 도시국가들로 시작하였으나 그 중 가장 강했던 로마를 중심으로 공화정을 결성, 북쪽의 에트루리아(Etruria)와 남쪽의 그리스 식민도시를 축출하고 제국의 틀을 갖추었다. 그러면서 에트루리아에 들어온 그리스어 알파벳을 빌려 라틴어 알파벳, 곧 로마 문자를 가지게 되었는데 이 때부터 공화정 말기 이전까지의 라틴어를 고 라틴어(*Old Latin*)라고 한다.

　로마공화정 말기부터 제정로마 전반기까지, 이른바 라틴문학의 전성기를 고전 라틴어 시기라고 하며, 이 시기의 문어(文語)가 고전 라틴어(*Classical Latin*)이다. 고전이라는 이름은 이 때에 활동한 루크레티우스(Lucretius), 베르길리우스(Vergilius), 호라티우스(Horatius), 오비디우스(Ovidius) 등의 운문과 키케로(Cicero), 카이사르(Gaius Julius Caesar) 등의 산문이 훗날까지 라틴어 문장의 전형으로 여겨졌기 때문에 붙여진 이름이다. 고전 라틴어 시기의 구어(口語)는 민중 라틴어(*Vulgar Latin*)로서 문어와는 차이가 있었다.

　제정로마 후반기인 후기 라틴어 시기에 제국이 동서로 나뉘고 서로마제국이 멸망하면서 라틴어는 일반인과 학계 및 교회에 의해 계승되었다. 일반인에 의해 계승된 라틴어는 민중 라틴어로서 그 후 로망스 제어(諸語)로 분화해 현재의 이탈리아어, 스페인어, 포르투갈어, 프랑스어, 루마니아어를 이루었다.

　학계와 교회에 의해 계승된 라틴어는 고전 및 민중 라틴어로서 학계는 고전 라틴어를, 교회는 민중 라틴어를 근간으로 전개하여 각각 학술 라틴어(*Academic Latin*)와 교회 라틴어(*Ecclesiastical Latin*)를 이루었다. 중세 때에는 교회 라틴어의 전개 폭이 컸고, 문예부흥 때에는 학술 라틴어의 전개 폭이 컸다. 그런 중에도 교회 라틴어와 학술 라틴어 모두 고전 라틴어에 맞추어 왔으므로 둘 사이에는 다른 점보다도 같은 점이 훨씬 더 많다.

이 책은, 당연히, 현대 학술 라틴어(*Modern Academic Latin*)를 따랐다. 지금의 학술용어가 그러하기 때문이다. 다음 표는 라틴어의 시대구분을 보여준다.

~ 75 yr BCE Old L.	~ 3c CE Classical L.	3c ~ 6c Late L.	6c ~ 14c Medieval L.	14c ~ 16c Renaissance L.	16c ~ Present Modern L.*,**
Written	Written (Classical)	Academic Latin			
		Ecclesiastical Latin			
Spoken	Spoken (Vulgar)	Romance Languages (Italian, Spanish, Portuguese, French, Romanian)			

* *Modern Latin*을 *New Latin* 또는 *Neo-Latin*이라고도 한다.

** 학술 라틴어가 공용어에서 물러난 19세기 말부터를 현재 라틴어(*Contemporary Latin*)라고 세분하기도 한다.

학술 라틴어는 19세기 전반까지 서구의 공식 학술어이었다. 천문학의 코페르니쿠스(Copernicus)와 케플러(Kepler), 철학의 베이컨(Bacon), 물리학의 뉴턴(Newton), 수학의 가우스(Gauss), 분류학의 린네(Linne), 의학의 베살리우스(Vesalius)와 하비(Harvey) 등이 학술 라틴어로 저서를 남겼다. 문학작품으로는 에라스무스(Erasmus)의 〈바보 예찬〉과 모어(More)의 〈유토피아〉 등이 있다. 현재에도 많은 학술용어를 라틴어로 만들거나, 라틴어가 아닌 경우, 라틴어화하여 만든다.

라틴어를 모르는 사람들은 라틴어를 사어(死語)라고 한다. 아는 사람들에게는, 라틴어가 살아 있는 언어이다. 살아 있는 언어이기 때문에 미니스커트(*miniskirt*)를 가리키는 tunicula minima, 핫팬츠(*hot pants*)를 가리키는 brevissimae bracae femineae 같은 일상용어들이 돌아다니고 있지 않겠는가?

학술 라틴어와 교회 라틴어는 고전 라틴어의 영향을 많이 받아왔다. 따라서 고전 라틴어, 학술 라틴어, 교회 라틴어는 서로 소통 가능하다. 이 책에서는 고전 라틴어 저술가들의 문장 또한 만날 수 있다.

알파벳과 발음

현대 학술 라틴어의 알파벳은 영어와 똑같은 대소문자로 표기하며, w 글자가 없으므로, 모두 25글자이다. 25글자는 6글자의 모음과 19글자의 자음으로 이루어져 있다. 모음 y과 자음 k 및 z 는 그리스어 낱말을 차용하기 위해 그리스어 알파벳에서 가져온 글자이다. 25글자의 이름과 대소문자는 다음과 같다.

글자이름	대문자	소문자
a	A	a
be	B	b
ce	C	c
de	D	d
e	E	e
ef	F	f
ge	G	g
ha	H	h
i	I	i
iod	J	j
kappa	K	k
el	L	l
em	M	m
en	N	n
o	O	o
pe	P	p
cu	Q	q
er	R	r
es	S	s
te	T	t
u	U	u
vu	V	v
ix	X	x
ipsilon	Y	y
zeta	Z	z

고전 라틴어와 현대 라틴어는 알파벳과 발음에서 조금 다르다. 고전 라틴어에는, w 외에도, j와 u의 두 글자가 없었다. j의 발음은 짧은 [ㅣ]이었기 때문에 i가 j를 대신하였고, v의 발음은 [ㅜ]이었기 때문에 u의 자리에 v가 쓰였다.

라틴어 알파벳은 소리 나는 대로 읽는 표음문자이다.

현대 라틴어 모음의 소리값은 단순하다. 고전 라틴어는 모라박자언어(*mora-timed language*)로써 모음의 장단 구분이 중요하였으나 현대 라틴어는 음절박자언어(*syllable-timed language*)로써 장단 대신 음절 구분과 그에 따른 강세가 중요하다.

a [ㅏ]로 소리 낸다.
   (보기) familia (파밀리아, 가족), mater (마떼르, 어머니), pater (빠떼르, 아버지)

e [ㅔ]로 소리 낸다.
   (보기) ego (에고, 나), equus (에쿠우스, 말)

i [ㅣ]로 소리 낸다.
   (보기) filius (필리우스, 아들), filia (필리아, 딸)

o [ㅗ]로 소리 낸다.
   (보기) domus (도무스, 집)

u [ㅜ]로 소리 낸다.
   (보기) puer (뿌에르, 소년), puella (뿌엘라, 소녀)

y [ㅣ]로 소리 낸다.
   (보기) lympha (림파, 림프)
   (고전 라틴어에서의 소리값은 [ㅟ]이다)

이중모음에는 au, ei, ui, ae, oe, eu가 있다. au, ei, ui는 각각의 소리값을 가지나 앞모음에 뒷모음을 약하게 붙여 소리 낸다. 그러나 ae와 oe는 하나의 소리값을 가지며, eu는 각각의 소리값을 가지거나 하나의 소리값을 가진다.

ae [ㅐ, ㅔ]로 소리 낸다. 각각의 소리값을 갖는 경우에는 분음부호를 붙여 aë로 표기하고
[ㅏㅔ]로 소리 낸다.
(보기) aequus (애쿠우스, 같은), aër (아에르, 공기)
(고전 라틴어에서의 소리값은 [아이]이다)

oe [ㅚ, ㅔ]로 소리 낸다. 각각의 소리값을 갖는 경우에는 분음부호를 붙여 oë로 표기하고
[ㅗㅔ]로 소리 낸다.
(보기) poena (뾔나, 벌), poëta (뽀에따, 시인)
(고전 라틴어에서의 소리값은 [오이]이다)

eu [ㅔㅜ]를 단음절처럼 소리 낸다. 라틴어화한 그리스어 낱말의 eu는 [ㅠ]로 소리 낸다.
(보기) seu (세우, 또는), euthanasia (유타나시아, 안락사)

현대 라틴어 자음의 소리값은 기본적으로 영어에서와 같다. 고전 라틴어의 발
음과 다른 점은 구개음화(*palatalization*)나 유성음화(*voicing*) 등, 현대 라틴어
로 오면서 일어난 음운변화 때문이다. 다음은 영어 또는 고전 라틴어 자음과는
다른 소리값을 가진 자음들이다.

s [ㅅ]로 소리 낸다. s가 두 모음 사이에 있거나 낱말의 끝에 있으면서 그 앞이 유성
자음일 때에는 유성음화가 일어나 약한 [ㅈ] 소리가 섞인다.
(보기) stella (스뗄라, 별), testis (떼스띠스, 증언, 불알)
miser (미세르, 불쌍한), mors (모르스, 죽음)
(고전 라틴어에서의 소리값은 맑은 [ㅅ] 하나이다)

sc [ㅅㄲ]로 소리 낸다. 전설모음 e, i, y, ae, oe 앞에서는 구개음화가 일어나 영어의
경구개음 [ʃ]처럼 소리 낸다.
(보기) scala (스깔라, 사다리), sciens (시엔스, 아는)
(고전 라틴어에서의 소리값은 맑은 [ㅅㄲ] 하나이다)

t [ㄸ]로 소리 낸다. ti가 강세를 받지 않으면서 다음에 모음이 오면 i가 반모음화되면
서 구개음화가 일어나므로 경구개음 [찌]로 소리 낸다. ti가 강세를 받거나 ti 앞에 s,
x, t가 있으면 본래대로 소리 낸다.
(보기) stella (스뗄라, 별), testis (떼스띠스, 증언, 불알)
natio (나찌오, 나라), scientia (시엔찌아, 과학), quaestio (퀘스띠오, 질문)
(고전 라틴어에서의 소리값은 [ㄸ] 하나이다)

c   후설모음 a, o, u나 자음 앞에서는 [ㄲ]로, 전설모음 e, i, y, ae, oe 앞에서는 구개
    음화가 일어나 경구개음 [ㅊ]로 소리 낸다.
    (보기) caput (까뿌뜨, 머리), crista (끄리스따, 능선), circum (치르꿈, 빙둘러, 가까이),
          caecus (채꾸스, 눈먼, 막힌)
    (고전 라틴어에서의 소리값은 [ㄲ] 하나이다)

g   후설모음 a, o, u나 자음 앞에서는 [ㄱ]로, 전설모음 e, i, y, ae, oe 앞에서는 구개
    음화가 일어나 경구개음 [ㅈ]로 소리 낸다.
    (보기) gallus (갈루스, 수탉), glomus (글로무스, 실타레), gingiva (진지바, 잇몸)
    (고전 라틴어에서의 소리값은 [ㄱ] 하나이다)

j   영어의 반모음 [j]처럼 소리 낸다.
    (보기) jejunus (예유누스, 공복의), jugum (유굼, 멍에), jus (유스, 법)
    (고전 라틴어에서는 i로 표기한다)

v   영어의 [v]처럼 소리 낸다.
    (보기) virus (비루스, 바이러스)
    (고전 라틴어에서의 소리값은 [ㅜ]이다)

ch [ㅋ]로 소리 낸다. 그리스어 알파벳 χ (chi)를 라틴어화할 때 쓴다.
    (보기) chaos (카오스, 혼돈), chiasma (키아스마, 교차), chorda (코르다, 줄)

ph 영어의 [f]처럼 소리 낸다. 그리스어 알파벳 φ (phi)를 라틴어화할 때 쓴다.
    (보기) pharmacia (파르마치아, 약국), physis (피시스, 자연, 피조물)
    (고전 라틴어에서의 소리값은 [ㅍ + ㅎ]이다)

rh 영어의 [r]처럼 소리 낸다. 낱말의 처음에 나와 [h]음과 함께 발음되는 그리스어 알파벳
    ρ (rho)를 라틴어화할 때 쓴다.
    (보기) rheuma (류마, 흐름)
    (고전 라틴어에서의 소리값은 [ㄹ + ㅎ]이다)

th [ㅌ]로 소리 낸다. 그리스어 알파벳 θ (theta)를 라틴어화할 때 쓴다.
    (보기) thema (테마, 주제), thrombus (트롬부스, 혈전)

라틴어의 분철과 강세

●●● 분철

음절은 모음을 핵(*nucleus*)으로 한다. 핵 앞에는 개시 자음(*onset*)이, 뒤에는 종

결 자음(*coda*)이 올 수 있다.

낱말의 음절을 구분하는 것을 분철(*syllabification*)이라고 한다. 분철의 기준은 철자가 아니라 발음이다. 분철은 인위적인 것이 아니라 음운론적 현상인 것이다.

- 파생어나 합성어는 연결형 사이에서 분철한다.
- 모음과 모음, 모음과 이중모음 사이는 분철한다.
- 모음 사이에 자음이 하나이면 다음 음절로 분철한다.
- 단모음은 보통 다음 자음을 끌어올린다.
- 모음 사이에 자음이 둘 이상이면 끝 자음만 다음 음절로 분철한다.
- 파열음(폐쇄음) 다음에 유음이 오면 하나의 자음으로 취급, 분철하지 않는다.
- qu, ch, ph, rh, th는 발음상 하나의 자음이다. x는 발음상 두 자음이다.

분철의 보기가 아래에 있다. 강세규칙은 분철을 전제로 하므로 분철이 중요하다.

(보기)			
conjunctiva (결막)	>	ˌcon·junc·ˈti·va	
duodenum (십이지장)	>	ˌdu·o·ˈde·num	
appendix (부속물, 충수)	>	ap·ˈpen·dix	
appendicitis (충수염)	>	ap·ˌpen·di·ˈci·tis	
nucleus (핵)	>	ˈnu·cle·us	
nucleolus (핵소체)	>	nu·ˈcle·o·lus	
vertebra (척추뼈)	>	ˈver·te·bra	

(주) 국제음성기호(IPA) 표기법에 따라 제1강세(ˈ)와 제2강세(ˌ)를 표시한다. 강세는 음절의 모음에만 주어지는 것이 아니라 음절 전체에 주어진다.

음절을 헤아릴 때에는 오른쪽 끝음절부터 헤아린다. 맨 오른쪽 끝음절이 *ult* (*ultimate*), *ult*의 앞 음절이 *penult*, *penult*의 앞 음절이 *antepenult*, *antepenult*의 앞 음절이 *preantepenult*이다. 왼쪽 첫째 음절은 *initial*이라고 한다.

••• 강세

한 음절 낱말은 낱말 자체에 강세가 주어지고 두 음절 낱말은 첫음절(*initial*)에 강세가 주어진다. 세 음절 이상의 낱말은 *penult*가 장모음이거나, 장모음에 해당하는 이중모음이거나, 자음으로 끝나면 *penult*에 강세가 주어진다. 그렇지 않으면 *antepenult*에 강세가 주어진다.

강세음절 앞에 둘 이상의 음절이 있으면 똑같은 방법으로 두 번째 강세음절을 찾고 제1강세, 제2강세로 구분한다. 제2강세의 정도는 제1강세보다 낮다.

앞의 보기를 보면, ap·ˈpen·dix에서는 *penult*가 자음으로 끝나므로 *penult*에 강세가 주어진다. appendix의 어간 appendic-에 염증을 뜻하는 접미사 ‑itis가 붙은 ap·pen·di·ˈci·tis에서는 *penult*인 ‑itis의 ‑i‑가 장모음이므로 역시 *penult*에 강세가 주어진다. 이때 강세음절 앞의 음절수가 둘 이상 되니까 같은 방법으로 제2강세를 찾으면 ap·ˌpen·di·ˈci·tis가 된다. nucleus의 ‑eus는 형용사 접미사로서 ‑e‑가 단모음이기 때문에 *antepenult*에 강세가 주어져 ˈnu·cle·us가 된다. nucleus의 어간 nucle‑에 지소 접미사 ‑olus를 붙인 nucleolus는 ‑o‑가 단모음이기 때문에 nu·ˈcle·o·lus가 된다.

••• 라틴어화한 그리스어의 분철과 강세

그리스어 낱말의 분철과 강세주기는 라틴어와 다르다. 그러나 라틴어화한 그리스어 낱말에다는 라틴어식 방식을 적용한다. ch, ph, rh, th 등, 이중자(二重字, *digraph*) 자음을 주의하면 충분하다.

(보기)	G. korōnē	>	corona (왕관)	>	co·ˈro·na
	G. museion	>	museum (박물관)	>	mu·ˈse·um
	G. kranion	>	cranium (머리뼈)	>	ˈcra·ni·um
	G. nekrōsis	>	necrosis (괴사)	>	ne·ˈcro·sis
	G. karkinōma	>	carcinoma (암종)	>	ˌcar·ci·ˈno·ma
	G. synthesis	>	synthesis (합성)	>	ˈsyn·the·sis
	G. philadelphia	>	philadelphia (형제애)	>	ˌphil·a·ˈdel·phi·a

(주) 그리스어 낱말은 로마자로 자역해 실었다.

라틴어는 사전이 아니면 모음의 장단을 표시하지 않는다. 그러나 그리스어가 라틴어화한 경우에는 *penult*의 음절핵이 장모음인지 아닌지 원래 그리스어를 보아 알 수 있다. corona의 *penult*는 그리스어 korōnē의 *penult*가 장모음이므로 당연히 장모음이 되고, museum의 *penult*는 그리스어 museion의 *penult*가 이중모음이므로 당연히 장모음이 된다. 그리스어의 상태 접미사 -ōsis, 종양 접미사 -ōma는 라틴어화한 -osis와 -oma의 *penult* 역시 장모음일 수밖에 없음을 보여준다. 이들 낱말의 *penult*에 강세가 위치하는 이유를 어원이 말해주고 있는 것이다.

라틴어 낱말의 영어 발음

라틴어 낱말이 일단 영어에 들어오면 차용어가 되고 영어식으로 발음한다. 그 발음은 고전 라틴어보다는 현대 라틴어의 발음에 더 가깝다. 이 책이 현대 라틴어를 따르는 이유 중 하나이다. 영어나 현대 라틴어 모두 구개음화와 유성음화가 일어나는 언어이다. (이 항목에서 라틴어라 함은 라틴어화한 그리스어를 포함한다.)

> (보기) Caesar (사람 이름)
>> 고전 라틴어 [카이사르], 현대 라틴어 [채사르], 영어 [시저]
>
> vagina (질, 집)
>> 고전 라틴어 [우아기나], 현대 라틴어 [바지나], 영어 [버자이너]
>
> virus (바이러스)
>> 고전 라틴어 [우이루스], 현대 라틴어 [비루스], 영어 [바이러스]
>
> cirrhosis (경화증)
>> 고전 라틴어 [키로시스], 현대 라틴어 [치로시스], 영어 [시로시스]

명사 어미의 영어 발음

영어가 라틴어로부터 직접 차용한 학술용어는 명사가 대부분이다. 명사를 수식하는 낱말을 함께 차용하기도 한다.

영어 학술용어에 자주 쓰이는 라틴어 명사 단·복수 주격과 속격, 단수 탈격 어미의 영어 발음을 알파벳순으로 적으면 다음과 같다. 명사 수식어의 어미변화는 명사의 어미변화를 답습하므로 따로 언급할 필요가 없다.

(보기)	어미	발음	어미	발음
	−a	[−ə]·	−is	[−is]
	−ae	[−i:]	−ium	⁴[−iəm]
	−arum	[−ˈarəm]	−o	[−ou]
	−e	[−i]	−orum	[−ˈorəm]
	−ei	[−iai]	−u	[−ju:]
	−erum	[−ˈerəm]	−ua	[−juə]
	−es	[−i:z]	−um	[−əm]
	−i	[−ai], [−i(:)]	−us	[−əs]
	−ia	[−iə]	−uum	[−juəm]

(주) −arum과 −erum, −orum의 *penult*는 강세음절이다.
     −i의 발음은 [−ai]이다. 단수 속격 −i의 발음은 가끔 [−i(:)]라고도 한다.

영어 *ride, code, huge, breathe*의 어말 −*e*는 발음하지 않는다. *silent* ⟨*e*⟩라고 한다. 후기중세영어와 초기현대영어 때 일어난 발음소실 때문이다.

묵음이라고 하지만 *silent* ⟨*e*⟩는 중요한 기능을 한다. *ride*와 *code*가 이중모음을 가지고, *huge*가 이중모음과 경구개음을 가지며, *breathe*가 장모음과 유성 자음을 가지면서 품사가 동사로 바뀌는 것은 모두 *silent* ⟨*e*⟩ 때문이다.

라틴어 명사 어미 −*e*는 굴절접미사로서 문법적 기능을 하며 *silent* ⟨*e*⟩와는 출생부터 다르다. 영어에 차용된 후에도 발음된다. 영어에 들어온 *Aphrodite*의 어말 −*e*는 [ㅓ]로 발음하는 것이다. 동사의 굴절접미사 −*e*도 마찬가지이다. 영어에 차용되고 나면 명사 어미의 발음에 준하여 [ㅓ]로 발음한다. 명령법 현재 단수 이인칭 *recipe*(받으십시오)의 발음은 [ˈresəpi]가 되는 것이다.

영어 강세

영어는 강세박자언어(*stress-timed language*)이다. 강세음절은 보다 높게, 보다 크게, 보다 길게, 보다 분명하게 발음한다. 비강세음절은 모음을 약하게(*bowel reduction*), 자음을 부드럽게(*consonant lenition*), 결과적으로 조금 더 빠르게 발음한다. 자연스런 힘주기와 자연스런 힘빼기의 조화이다.

영어 낱말을 기원에 따라 영어 고유어, 프랑스어 차용어, 라틴어 차용어로 크게 나누어볼 수 있다. 프랑스어 차용어는 프랑스어화한 라틴어인 경우가 대부분이다. 라틴어 차용어는 다른 언어를 경유하지 않고 직접 영어 안으로 들어온 라틴어이며, 현대 학술용어의 다수가 이에 해당한다.

프랑스어나 현대 라틴어는 음절박자언어이지만 영어 안에 차용된 낱말은 강세박자의 영향권 안에 놓이게 된다. 그만큼 강세가 더 중요해지는 것이다.

영어의 강세주기에는 영어식, 프랑스어식, 라틴어식의 세 방식이 있다.

영어 고유어는 첫 번째 자립형태소의 첫음절이 강세를 받는다. 이는 게르만계 언어의 특징 중 하나이다. ˈfa·ther, ˈfa·ther·ly, ˈfa·ther·li·ness, for·ˈget, for·ˈget-ta·ble, ˌun·for·ˈget·ta·ble 등이다. 영어의 고유 접두사는 몇 개 안 되므로 고유어 대부분이 첫 음절 강세를 갖는다고 볼 수 있다.

프랑스어는 끝음절 강세어이다. 영어의 프랑스어 차용어도 끝음절 강세를 보인다. ca·ˈnal, re·ˈport, ma·ˈchine, po·ˈlice 등이다. 강세어말(*tonic ending*)을 갖는 em·ploy·ˈee, ro·ˈsette, an·ˈtique 등도 마찬가지이다. 이 부분에서 예를 든 낱말들은 모두 라틴어나 라틴어화한 그리스어 기원이다.

영어의 라틴어 차용어는 차용된 후에도 앞에 기술한 라틴어 강세 위치를 그대로 유지한다.

위의 강세주기는 사람 이름의 강세주기에도 마찬가지로 적용된다.

ˈPar·kin·son, ˈAlz·hei·mer 등 게르만계 이름은 영어식 강세주기를 따라가고, Des·ˈcartes, Pas·ˈcal, Pas·ˈteur 등 프랑스계 이름은 프랑스어식 강세주기를 따라가며, ˌLe·o·ˈnar·do da ˈVin·ci, Gal·ˈva·ni 등 라틴계 이름은 라틴어식 강세주기를 따라간다.

현대영어에서는 영어식 첫음절 강세주기가 좀 더 세지고, 프랑스어식 끝음절 강세주기가 좀 약해져 있다. 강세를 왼쪽으로 잡아끄는 힘이 더 세진 것이다(*stress advancement*). 그래도 라틴어 기원의 학술용어는 흔들림 없이 라틴어식 강세주기를 지키고 있다.

ap·ˈpen·dix / ap·ˌpen·di·ˈci·tis 나 ˈnu·cle·us / nu·ˈcle·o·lus 같은 낱말 쌍을 영어의 시선에서 보면 강세 위치가 변덕부리는 것처럼 보인다. 그렇지만 라틴어의 시선으로 보면 강세 위치는 제자리이다.

영어 ˈpho·to·graph 와 pho·ˈto·gra·phy 의 강세는 라틴어식 강세주기를 따랐다. ˌpho·to·ˈgra·phic 의 강세는 강세어말(*tonic ending*)인 –*ic* 때문이며 프랑스어식 강세주기의 영향이다. 영어의 세 가지 강세 주는 방법은 현재에도 재현되는 통시성(*diachrony*)을 갖는 것이다.

영어 강세는 일차적으로 낱말의 본적, 즉 어원에 의해 결정된다. 어원을 알면 영어 낱말의 강세음절이 더 쉽게 파악된다.

대모음추이

고대영어에 라틴 알파벳을 전한 사람들은 선교사였으며 발음은 구개음화되어 있었다. 고대영어의 [아ː], [베ː], [체ː]는 중세영어 때 프랑스어의 영향을 받아 마찰음화를 일으켜 [아ː], [베ː], [세ː]가 되었고, [아ː], [베ː], [세ː]는 중세영어 말과 현대영어 초에 걸쳐 일어난 대모음추이(*Great Bowel Shift*)의 영향을 받아 현대영어의 [에이], [비ː], [시ː]가 되었다. 영어 알파벳의 나머지 문자 이름도, 이름에 강세장모음이 들어 있으면, 같은 길을 밟았다.

시기	A	B	C	음운변화
고전 라틴어	[a:]	[be:]	[ke:]	
고대영어	[a:]	[be:]	[tse:]	구개음화
중세영어	[a:]	[be:]	[se:]	마찰음화
현대영어	[ei]	[bi:]	[si:]	대모음추이

대모음추이란 강세장모음의 상승과 이중모음화로 구성되어 있다. 발음할 때 혀의 위치가 상대적으로 낮은 [e:]에서 그보다 높은 [i:]로 바뀌는 것이 모음상승의 예이고, [a:]가 (모음상승 후) [ei]로 바뀌는 것이 이중모음화의 예이다.

대모음추이는 역사적 사건으로 끝나고 만 것이 아니라 지금도 적용되는 규칙이다. 다음 보기는 대모음추이가 영어에 들어온 라틴어 차용어의 강세장모음에도 적용됨을 보여준다.

(보기)	conjunctiva (결막)	>	ˌcon·junc·ˈti·va	이중모음화	[ai]
	duodenum (십이지장)	>	ˌdu·o·ˈde·num	모음상승	[i:]
	appendicitis (충수염)	>	ap·ˌpen·di·ˈci·tis	이중모음화	[ai]
	nucleus (핵)	>	ˈnu·cle·us	이중모음화	[ju:]
	corona (왕관)	>	co·ˈro·na	이중모음화	[ou]
	museum (박물관)	>	mu·ˈse·um	모음상승	[i:]
	necrosis (괴사)	>	ne·ˈcro·sis	이중모음화	[ou]
	carcinoma (암종)	>	ˌcar·ci·ˈno·ma	이중모음화	[ou]

(주) 밑줄 친 음절의 모음이 강세장모음으로서 대모음추이의 적용을 받는다.

영어 학술용어에 자주 등장하는 염증의 접미사 *-itis*, 상태의 접미사 *-osis*, 종양의 접미사 *-oma*는 모두 그리스어에서 비롯했고, *penult*가 장모음이므로 제1강세를 받으며, 발음은 대모음추이에 의해 이중모음화 된다.

삼음절 단음화

강세 장모음 또는 이중모음을 갖는 영어 낱말이 파생어나 합성어를 만들면서 강세음절 뒤로 두 음절 늘어나 세 음절이 되면 강세음절은 단음화한다. 삼음절 단음화(*trisyllabic shortening, trisyllabic laxing*)라고 한다.

(보기)	ˈho·ly (거룩한)	[hou·]	>	ˈhol·i·day	[hol·]
	ˈwild (야생의)	[waild]	>	ˈwil·der·ness	[wil·]
	ˈtype (전형)	[taip]	>	ˈtyp·i·cal	[tip·]
	ˈna·ture (자연)	[nei·]	>	ˈnat·u·ral	[næt·]
	vas·cu·ˈli·tis (혈관염, 단수)	[·lai·]	>	vas·cu·ˈlit·i·des (복수)	[·lit·]
	len·ˈti·go (흑색점, 단수)	[·tai·]	>	len·ˈtig·i·nes (복수)	[·tidz·]

(주) 밑줄 친 음절이 단음화한다. 단음화된 모음은 다음 자음을 끌어올려 분철된다.
(예) ˈho·ly > ˈhol·i·day

음소배열

영어 *know*의 첫 자음 *k*, *lamb*의 끝 자음 *b*, *often*의 *f* 다음 자음 *t*는 발음하지 않는다. 초기현대영어에서 일어난 자음군단순화(*consonant cluster simplification*)라는 음운변화 때문이다.

뜻의 차이를 일으키는 최소의 음성단위가 음소(*phoneme*)이다. 어두음의 경우, *knight*의 음소 /k/ 는 발음하지 않지만 *spring*의 음소 /spr/ 는 아무 걸림 없이 발음한다. 연속된 어두 음소가 발음되기 위한 제약과 허용이 있는 것이다. 허용되는 음소배열은 한 언어의 음운체계 안에서 결정된다. 이에 대한 이론이 음소배열론 (*phonotactics*)이다.

그리스어의 음운체계에는 영어에서 허용하지 않는 음소배열이 있다. 그런 음소 배열을 갖는 낱말이 영어에 들어오면 일부 자음이 묵음 처리된다.

영어 낱말의 어두에서 자음 두 개가 연속될 때에는 첫 음이 파열음(폐쇄음)이거나 /s/를 제외한 마찰음이면 두 번째 음은 유음 또는 활음 중 하나이어야 두 자음모두 발음된다. *play, twin, cue, fly, thwart, hue* 에서와 달리, /pt-/, /ps-/, /pn-/, /ks-/, /gn-/, /ft-, fθ -/ 등은 허용되지 않는 것이다.

영어 낱말의 어두에서 자음 두 개가 연속될 때 첫 음이 비음이면 두 번째 음은활음이어야 두 자음 모두 발음된다. *music*은 허용되나 /mn-/ 은 허용되지 않는다.

다음 보기는 라틴어화한 그리스어의 영어 차용어로서 허용되지 않는 어두 자음군의 첫 자음이 묵음 처리됨을 보여준다.

(보기)				
	pterosaurus (익룡)	[te-]	xenon (제논)	[zi:-]
	ptosis (처짐)	[tou-]	xylophone (목금)	[zai-]
	psychosis (정신병)	[sai-]	gnosis (앎)	[nou-]
	pseudonym (가명)	[sʲu:-]	phthisis (황폐증)	[θai-]
	pneumonia (폐렴)	[nʲu:-]	mnemonics (기억술)	[ni-]

위의 음소배열에 관한 제한은 어두에서의 제한이다. 파생어나 합성어를 만들면서 어두 자음이 어중으로 들어가게 되면 발음은 허용된다. *helicopter, proptosis, diagnosis* 등에서는 낱말 가운데의 /-pt-/, /-gn-/ 가 발음되는 것이다. *hel·i·cop·ter, prop·to·sis, di·ag·no·sis* 등, 연속 자음이 앞뒤 음절로나뉘면서 발음상 더 이상 연속되지 않기 때문이다.

낱말의 강세와 발음에도 규칙이 있다. 규칙을 알면 언어가 쉬워진다. 언어는과학이다.

제3장 품사

라틴어에도 영어에서처럼 8품사가 있다. 명사, 대명사, 형용사, 동사, 부사, 전치사, 접속사, 감탄사이다. 8품사 중 어미변화를 하는 품사는 명사, 대명사, 형용사, 동사이다.

명사

명사변화

라틴어 명사는 어간을 그대로 둔 채 어미를 바꿈으로써 수와 격을 드러낸다. 명사변화라고 한다. 정식 어간은, 단수 속격에서 어미를 떼어내고 남은 속격어간이며, 명사변화뿐 아니라 파생어나 합성어를 만들 때에도 축의 역할을 한다. 따라서, 라틴어 명사를 알아둘 때에는, 뜻과 어간을 알기 위해 단수 주격과 단수 속격을 함께 알아두어야 한다.

형용사나 형용사에 준하는 분사로 명사를 수식할 때에는 명사의 성·수·격에 형용사나 분사의 성·수·격을 일치시켜야 한다. 따라서 명사 단수의 주격 및 속격과 함께 성까지 알아둘 필요가 있다. 라틴어사전도 단수 주격, 단수 속격, 성의 세 가지를 차례대로 제시한다.

● ● ● 제1변화

단수의 주격 어미가 -a, 속격 어미가 -ae; 복수의 주격 어미가 -ae, 속격 어미가 -arum 인 남성 또는 여성 명사. 단수 주격의 어간과 단수 속격의 어간이 같다. 성은 거의 여성이다.

cellula, cellulae, f. 세포

	단 수	복 수	
주격	cellul-a	cellul-ae	~이, ~가, ~은, ~는, ~께서
속격	cellul-ae	cellul-arum	~의
여격	cellul-ae	cellul-is	~게, ~에게, ~께, ~한테
대격	cellul-am	cellul-as	~을, ~를
탈격	cellul-a	cellul-is	~에서, ~로부터, ~으로부터
호격	cellul-a	cellul-ae	~여, ~이여

cellula, cellulae, f. (< + -ula *diminutive suffix*) 작은 방, 노예 골방, 비둘기 집, 벌집; 세포(細胞)

> **E** *cell*, *(cellule + -ose 'glucose' > 'carbohydrate which is the main structural constituent of plant cell walls' >)* **cellulose, Cellophane**® *(< 'transparent material made from regenerated cellulose')*

> cellularis, cellulare 작은 방으로 된, 구획 방식의;

　세포의　　　　　　　　　**E** *cellular, subcellular, unicellular, multicellular*

　　> intracellularis, intracellulare (< intra- *inside*) 세포 안의　　**E** *intracellular*

　　> *extracellularis, *extracellulare (< extra- *outside*) 세포 바깥의　　**E** *extracellular*

　　> *intercellularis, *intercellulare (< inter- *between, among*) 세포

　　　사이의　　　　　　　　　**E** *intercellular*

　　> *cellularitas, *cellularitatis, f. 세포밀도, 세포충실성　　**E** *cellularity*

> cellulosus, cellulosa, cellulosum 작은 칸이 많은

> cellulitis, cellulitidis, f. (< *inflammation of areolar tissue (loose connective tissue)* < + -itis *noun suffix denoting inflammation*) 연조직염(軟組織炎),

　봉와염(蜂窩炎), 봉소염(蜂巢炎), 벌집염　　**E** *cellulitis, (cellulitis >) cellulite*

< cella, cellae, f. 광　　　　　　　　　　**E** *cellar*

< IE. kel- *to cover, to conceal, to save*

> **E** *hall* (< *'covered place'*), *hallmark* (< *'London assay office at Goldsmith's Hall'*), *hull* (< *'husk, pod' < 'that which covers'*), *hell* (< *'concealed place'*), *helmet, holster, hole, hollow*

> L. celo, celavi, celatum, celare 숨기다

　> L. color, coloris, m. 색, 외모, 음색(音色), 가식(假飾)　　**E** *color (colour); colorimeter*

　　> L. coloro, coloravi, coloratum, colorare 채색하다　　**E** *colorant, coloration*

　　　> L. coloratura, coloraturae, f. 화려한 기교적 선율　　**E** *coloratura*

　　　> L. discoloro, discoloravi, discoloratum, discolorare (< dis- *apart from, down, not* + colorare *to color*) 변색시키다, 변색

　　　하다　　　　　　**E** *discolor (discolour), discoloration*

　> L. clam (부사) 숨어서, 몰래

　　> L. clandestinus, clandestina, clandestinum (< *apparently on the pattern of* intestinus) 비밀리의, 내밀한　　**E** *clandestine*

　> L. concelo, concelavi, concelatum, concelare (< con- (< cum) *with, together;*

intensive + celare *to hide*) 숨기다   **E** *conceal*

> L. occulo, **occului**, occultum, occulĕre (< oc- (< ob) *before, toward(s), over against, away* + celare *to hide*) 숨기다   **E** *occult*

[용례] spina bifida occulta 잠재이분척추, 숨은 척추갈림증   **E** *spina bifida occulta*
    (문법) spina 척추: 단수 주격 < spina, spinae, f. 가시, 등마루
        bifida 두 갈래의: 형용사, 여성형 단수 주격
           < bifidus, bifida, bifidum
        occulta 숨겨진: 과거분사, 여성형 단수 주격
           < occultus, occulta, occultum

> L. cilium, cilii, n. (< *that which covers*) 눈꺼풀, 속눈썹; 섬모(纖毛)   **E** *cilium, (pl.) cilia*
  > L. ciliaris, ciliare 눈꺼풀의, 속눈썹의;
    섬모의   **E** *ciliary (< 'of eyelids, eyelashes, or cilia')*

[용례] corpus ciliare (< *a ring-like body the plicated part of which resembles white eyelashes (cilia) surrounding the lens when viewed from behind*) 섬모체(纖毛體),
모양체(毛樣體)   **E** *ciliary body, ciliary (< 'of ciliary body')*
    (문법) corpus 몸, 체(體): 단수 주격 < corpus, corporis, n.
      ciliare: 형용사, 중성형 단수 주격

> L. *ciliatus, *ciliata, *ciliatum 섬모가 있는   **E** *ciliate, ciliated*
> L. supercilium, supercilii, n. (< super- *above* + cilium *eyelash*) 윗눈썹; (건축)
상인방(上引枋); 꼭대기, 자부심, 엄격함   **E** *superciliary*
  > L. superciliosus, superciliosa, superciliosum 엄격한, 도도한   **E** *supercilious*
> L. kinocilium, kinocilii, n. (< G. kin(o)- (< kinein *to move*) + L. cilium *eyelash*) 운동섬모   **E** *kinocilium, (pl.) kinocilia*
> L. stereocilium, stereocilii, n. (< *nonmotile, cilium-like long microvillus* < G. stereos *solid* + L. cilium *eyelash*) 부동섬모   **E** *(pl.) stereocilia*
> G. kalyptein *to cover, to conceal*
  > G. Kalypsō, Kaplypsōnos, f. (< *she who conceals*) (*Greek mythology*) *a nymph who kept Odysseus on her island, Ogygis, for seven years*
    > L. Calypso, Calypsonis, f. (Calypso, Calypsus, f.) (그리스 신화) 칼립소   **E** *Calypso*
  > G. kalyptos, kalyptē, kalypton *covered, covering*
    > L. eucalyptus, eucalypti, m. (< *being well-covered; the flower before it opens being protected by a sort of cap* < G. eu- *well* + kalyptos) 유칼립투스   **E** *eucalyptus*
  > G. apokalyptein (< ap(o)- *away from, from* + kalyptein) *to uncover, to disclose, to reveal*
    > G. apokalypsis, apokalypseōs, f. *revelation*
      > L. apocalypsis, apocalypsis, f. 계시, 묵시, 예언   **E** *apocalypse*
> G. koleos, koleou, m. (koleon, koleou, n.) *sheath (of a sword)*

E (koleos + ptilon *'feather'* >) *coleoptile*, (koleos + rhiza *'root'* >) *coleorhiza*, (koleos + pteron *'wing'* >) *coleoptera*

> L. coleus, colei, m. (< *the connate staminal filaments*) (식물) 콜레우스　　**E** *coleus*

> (*probably*) L. caulis, caulis, f. (caules, calulis, f.) (관목이나 초본식물의 속이 빈) 줄기,

대; 줄기처럼 생긴 것; 양배추 뿌리　　**E** *caulis*, (pl.) *caules, caul(i)-, cauliflower, kale (kail)*

> L. -caulis, -caule ~줄기의, ~줄기처럼 생긴

∞ (*probably*) G. kaulos, kaulou, m. *stalk, stem; shaft (of a spear), hilt (of a sword)*　　**E** *caul(o)-*

> IE. klep- *to steal*

> G. kleptein *to steal*　　**E** *cleptomania (kleptomania)*

aqua, aquae, f. 물　　**E** *aqua-, aquaculture, aquaporin, aquarelle*

　　　[용례] aqua regia 왕수(王水)

　　　　　(문법) aqua 물: 단수 주격

　　　　　　　regia 왕의: 형용사, 여성형 단수 주격

　　　　　　　　　< regius, regia, regium < rex, regis, m. 왕

　　　[용례] aquae ductus (aquaeductus) 물길, 수로, 수도관　　**E** *aqueduct*

　　　　　(문법) aquae 물의: 단수 속격

　　　　　　　ductus 도관: 단수 주격 < ductus, ductus, m.

　　> *aqueus, *aquea, *aqueum 물의, 물을 함유한, 수용성의　　**E** *aqueous*

　　> aquarius, aquaria, aquarium 물의, 물에 관한

　　　　> aquarius, aquarii, m. 물 긷는 사람; (Aquarius) (천문) 물병자리　　**E** *Aquarius*

　　　　> aquarium, aquarii, n. 어항, 수족관　　**E** *aquarium*

　　> aquaticus, aquatica, aquaticum 물속이나 물 주위에 사는, 물기 있는　　**E** *aquatic*

　　> *exaquaria, *exaquariae, f. (< ex- *out of, away from*)

　　　　배수로　　**E** *sewer, (sewer >) sewerage, (sewer >) sewage*

< IE. akʷa- *water*　　**E** *island (< 'water land')*

alea, aleae, f. 주사위

　　> aleator, aleatoris, m. 도박꾼

　　　　> aleatorius, aleatoria, aleatorium 운수 보기의, 도박의　　**E** *aleatory*

algebra, algebrae, f. 대수학(代數學)　　**E** *algebra, algebraic*

< (*Arabic*) al-jabr *reunion of broken parks, restoration of parts to make a whole (from the*
compendium on calculation by restoring and balancing*)*

barba, barbae, f. 수염, 턱수염; (동물·식물) 수염 같은 구조물　　**E** *barber, barb*

　　> barbatus, barbata, barbatum (동물·식물) 수염이 있는, 수염 모양의 술이 있는　　**E** *barbate*

　　> barbella, barbellae, f. (< + -ella *diminutive suffix*) (동물·식물) 짧고 빳빳한 털　　**E** *barbellate*

< IE. bhardh-a- *beard*　　**E** *beard*

barca, barcae, f. 작은 배　　**E** *barque (bark), barge, embark, disembark*

< (*disputed*) Of Celtic or Coptic origin

beriberia, beriberiae, f. 각기(脚氣)

  < (*Sinhalese*) beri *weakness*　　　　　　　　**E** *beriberi* (< *'the reduplication of* beri, *being intensive'*)

bestia, bestiae, f. 짐승　　　　　　　　　　　　　　　　　　　　　　　　　　　　**E** *beast*

    > bestialis, bestiale 짐승의, 야수의　　　　　　　　　　　　　　　　　　**E** *bestial*

      > bestialitas, bestialitatis, f. 수성(獸性), 수욕(獸慾), 수간(獸姦)　　　**E** *bestiality*

    > bestiarium, bestiarii, n. (인간 풍자의) 동물 우화집　　　　　　　　　**E** *bestiary*

bracae, bracarum, f. (pl.) 가랑이 넓은 바지　　　　　　　　　　　　　　　**E** *bracket*

  < (*Germanic*) brak- *trousers*　　　　　　　　　　　　　　　　**E** *breeches, breech*

bractea, bracteae, f. 금속박편, 금박, 은박, 목재박편; 포엽(苞葉)　　**E** *bract, bracteal, bracteate*

    > bracteola, bracteolae, f. (< + -ola *diminutive suffix*) 금박; 포(苞)　　**E** *bracteole, bracteolate*

bulla, bullae, f. 거품, 낭포(囊胞), 큰 공기집, 기포(氣疱), 물집, 수포(水疱); (대문에 박아 놓는)
동그란 장식용 징, 장식용 장치; 귀족 아이의 목에 걸어주던 호부(護符) 달린 패물; (밀랍
또는 납으로 봉인한) 교황의 대교서, 대칙서

    E *bulla,* (pl.) *bullae; bullet* (< *'small ball'*)*, bowling* (< *'the wooden ball rolled at the target
ball'*)*,* Sp. *bola; bulletin, bill, billet* (< *'a short written order for soldier's food and lodging'*)

    > bullosus, bullosa, bullosum 거품이 많은, 물집이 만들어지는, 수포성의　　**E** *bullous*

    > bullio, bullivi, bullitum, bullire (< *to bubble*) 부글부글

        끓다　　　　　　**E** *boil, bullion* (< *'melted metal'*)*, budge* (< *'to stir', 'to boil'*)

      > ebullio, ebullivi, ebullitum, ebullire (< e- *out of, away from* + bullire *to boil*)

        끓어오르다, 비등(沸騰)하다　　　　　　　　　　**E** *ebullient, ebullition*

 < IE. beu-, bheu- *probably imitative root, appearing in words loosely associated with the
notion 'to swell'*

    E *pocket* (< *'bag'*)*, pouch, pouchitis, pucker, pock* (< *'pustule'*)*,* (pocks >) *pox, smallpox*
(< *'compared to pox proper or great pox (syphilis)'*)*, chickenpox* (< *'mildness compared
to smallpox'*)*, poxvirus* (< *'originally, the causative agent of cowpox or smallpox; in later
use, any member causing the pox diseases in general'*)*, puff, puffy, puffer, boil* (<
'pustule')*, boast, bud, bug*

    > (*possibly*) L. bucca, buccae, f. 볼, 뺨, 구강　　　　　　　　　　　**E** *buccal*

      > L. buccula, bucculae, f. (< + -ula *diminutive suffix*) 작은 볼; (양쪽 볼을 가려
        주는) 투구의 턱받이　　　　　　　　　　　　　　　　　**E** *buckle*

    > G. boubōn, boubōnos, m. *abdomen, groin, a swelling in the groin, swollen gland*

      > L. bubo, bubonis, m. 가래톳　　　　　　　　　　　　　　**E** *bubo, bubonic*

        > L. bubonulus, bubonuli, m. (< + -ulus *diminutive suffix*)

        가래톳　　　　　　　　　　　　　　**E** *bubonulus,* (pl.) *bubonuli*

    > (*probably*) G. bōlos, bōlou, f. *clod of earth*

      > L. bolus, boli, m. 덩어리, 음식덩이, 약덩이　　　　　　　　　**E** *bolus*

cabanna, cabannae, f. (capanna, capannae, f.) 오두막집, 움막　　　　　**E** *cabin, cabinet*

caeremonia, caeremoniae, f. (caerimonia, caerimoniae, f.) 종교적 예식, 경외심,
　　신성함　　　　　**E** *ceremony*
　< (*probably*) *Of Etruscan origin*

calumnia, calumniae, f. 속임수, 무고, 허위 진술　　　　　**E** *calumny, challenge*
　　　　　> calumnior, calumniatus sum, calumniari 무고하다, 비방하다　　**E** *calumniate*
　　　< calvor, –, calvi 속이다
　< IE. kel- *to deceive, to trick*

calvaria, calvariae, f. 해골(骸骨), 두개골(頭蓋骨), 머리덮개뼈　　**E** *calvaria,* (calvaria >) *calvarial*
　　　< calvus, calva, calvum 대머리의, 매끈매끈한
　< IE. klə-wo- *bald*

camphora, camphorae, f. 장뇌(樟腦), 캠퍼　　　　　**E** *camphor*
　　　< (*Arabic*) kafur
　　　< (*Sanskrit*) karpura
　< (*probably*) *Of Austroasiatic origin*

casa, casae, f. 오막살이, 초가집, 막사　　**E** (It. casa > It. casino (*diminutive*) >) *casino*

catena, catenae, f. 사슬, 결박, 속박　　　　　**E** *chain, catenin*
　　　> cateno, catenavi, catenatum, catenare 사슬로 매다, 결박하다, 속박하다, 사슬로 잇다,
　　　　연결시키다　　　　　**E** *catenate*
　　　　　> concateno, concatenavi, concatenatum, concatenare (< con- (< cum) *with,*
　　　　　　together + catenare *to chain*) 함께 묶다, 잇다, 연결시키다　　**E** *concatenate*

ciphra, ciphrae, f. 영(零); 아라비아 숫자, 기호　　　　**E** *cipher (cypher), decipher*
　　　< (*Arabic*) cifr *the arithmetical symbol 'zero' or 'nought', written in Indian and Arabic*
　　　　numeration　　　　　**E** *zero*
　< (*Sanskrit*) sunya *empty*

cloaca, cloacae, f. 하수도, 총배출강(總排出腔), 부골누관(腐骨瘻管)　**E** *cloaca,* (pl.) *cloacae, cloacal*
　< IE. kleuə- *to wash, to clean*
　　　> G. klyzein *to wash*
　　　　> G. klysis, klyseōs, f. *washing*
　　　　　> L. clysis, clysis, f. 씻기, 관장(灌腸), 주액(注液)　　**E** *clysis*

> G. klystēr, klystēros, m. *washer, clyster, syringe*

    > L. clyster, clysteris, m. 관장제, 관장   **E** *clyster*

> G. kataklyzein (< kat(a)- *down, mis-, according to, along, thoroughly*) *to wash
down, to deluge*

    > G. kataklysmos, kataklysmou, m. *deluge*

      > L. cataclysmos, cataclysmi, m. 대홍수, 격변   **E** *cataclysm*

clocca, cloccae, f. 종, 종시계, 시계

> **E** *clock, o'clock (< 'of or according to the clock: used to express time, after a numeral
indicating the hour'), clockwise, counterclockwise; cloak (< 'bell-shaped'), cloche (<
'bell-shaped')*

< *Of imitative origin*

corrigia, corrigiae, f. (< cor- (< cum) *with, together* + *rig-) 가죽끈, 구두끈,
말채찍

> **E** (ex- *'intensive'* + corrigia *'thong, whip'* >) *scourge*

< IE. reig- *to bind*   **E** *rig*

coxa, coxae, f. 고관절(股關節), 엉덩관절, 고관절부(股關節部), 관골부(臗骨部), 엉덩이,
볼기

> **E** *coxa, cuisse, cushion*

< IE. koksa- *body part, hip, thigh*

culcita, culcitae, f. 매트리스, 요, 보료   **E** *quilt*

culpa, culpae, f. 탓, 잘못   **E** *culpable, culprit*

cura, curae, f. 조심, 신중, 노력, 정성, 걱정, 보살핌, 치료

> **E** *(noun) cure, curette, curettage,* (manus *'hand'* + cura *'care'* >) *manicure,* (sine cura
'without care' >) *sinecure*

> curiosus, curiosa, curiosum 세심한 주의를 기울이는, 호기심 많은   **E** *curious*

    > curiositas, curiositatis, f. 호기심   **E** *curiosity, (curiosity >) curio*

> curo, curavi, curatum, curare 돌보다, 마음 쓰다, 조치하다, 치료하다

> **E** *(verb) cure, curative, curable,* (pes, ped- *'foot'* + curare *'to take care'* >) *pedicure*

> curator, curatoris, m. 돌보는 사람, 후견인, 담당자, 관리인, 감독   **E** *curator*

> accuro, accuravi, accuratum, accurare (< ac- (< ad) *to, toward, at, according
to* + curare *to take care*) 정성들여 하다, 정확하게 하다   **E** *accurate, accuracy*

> excuro, excuravi, excuratum, excurare (< ex- *out of, away from* + curare
to take care) 정성들여 보살피다, 공들이다, 깨끗이 하다   **E** *scour*

> procuro, procuravi, procuratum, procurare (< pro- *before, forward, for,
instead of* + curare *to take care*) 돌보다, 관리하다, 대리하다   **E** *procure*

> procuratio, procurationis, f. 관리, 처리, 대리   **E** *procuracy, (procuracy >) proxy*

> procurator, procuratoris, m. 대리인; (로마 역사)

행정 장관　　　　　　　　　　　　　　　**E** *procurator, (procurator >) proctor*

> securus, secura, securum (< se- *apart, without* + cura *care*) 안심하는,

안전한　　　　　　　　　　**E** *secure, sure, assure, reassure, ensure, insure, insurance*

> securitas, securitatis, f. 안심, 안전　　　　　　　**E** *security, surety*

> insecurus, insecura, insecurum (< in- *not* + securus *free from care*) 불안한,

자신이 없는, 불안전한　　　　　　　　　　　　　　　**E** *insecure*

fala, falae, f. (창・화살 등을 던지거나 쏘는) 목제 망대, (pl.) 원형 경기장의 경주로 표시 기둥

위에 세운 작은 원추탑　　　　**E** *(probably) catafalque, (catafalque >) scaffold*

fimbria, fimbriae, f. (띠・옷단 등의) 술, 들쭉날쭉한 가장자리, 채(綵)　**E** *fimbria, (pl.) fimbriae, fimbrin*

> fimbriatus, fimbriata, fimbriatum 술 달린, 가장자리가 들쭉날쭉한　　　**E** *fimbriate*

> (*metathetic alteration*) *frimbia, *frimbiae, f. 술, 가두리장식, 들쭉날쭉함, 가장자리　**E** *fringe*

fistula, fistulae, f. 대롱, 관(管), (Pan 신의) 악기(syrinx); 누(瘻), 누관(瘻管),

샛길　　　　　　　　　　　　　　　**E** *fistula, fistular, fistulous, fester*

forma, formae, f. (< *possibly via Etruscan*) 모양, 형태, 모형, 도형, 형, 형식,

방식　　　　　　　　　　　　　　　**E** *form, platform (< 'flat form')*

[용례] F. forme fruste (< *worn-down form*) 불완전형(不完全形)　　**E** *forme fruste*

(문법) forme 형(形): 여성 명사, 단수 주격

< F. forme, f. < L. forma, formae, f.

fruste 마멸된, 닳은: 형용사, 여성형 단수 주격

< F. fruste *used, defaced* < It. frusto *use*

> formula, formulae, f. (< + -ula *diminutive suffix*) 형식, 공식, 처방,

조성　　　　　**E** *formula, (pl.) formulae (formulas), formulary, (formula >) formulate*

> -formis, -forme 모양의, 형(形)의

> **E** *-form, uniform, biform, claviform, cribriform, cruciform, cuneiform, ensiform, falciform, filiform, fungiform, funiform, fusiform, lentiform, moniliform, morbilliform, oviform, pampiniform, panduriform, piliform, piriform (pyriform), pisiform, plexiform, reniform, retiform, storiform, vermiform, verruciform; coliform, dendriform, herpetiform, hydatidiform, spongiform*

> multiformis, multiforme (< multus *many*) 여러 모양의, 다형(多形)의　**E** *multiform*

> deformis, deforme (< de- *apart from, down, not*) 볼품없는, 변형된,

기형의

> deformitas, deformitatis, f. 볼품없음, 변형, 기형　　　**E** *deformity*

> formalis, formale 형식을 갖춘, 형식적인　　　　**E** *formal, (formal >) informal*

> formosus, formosa, formosum 잘생긴, 아름다운　　　　　**E** *Formosa*

> formo, **formavi**, formatum, formare 모양을 만들다, 형성하다

E *form, formative, (form >)* **malformed** *(< 'badly formed; affected by physical abnormality, especially by congenital anomaly')*

[용례] liber formatus 만들어 놓은 책　　　　　　　　　　　**E** *format*

　　(문법) liber 책: 남성 명사, 단수 주격 < liber, libri, m.

　　　　formatus 만들어 놓은: 과거분사, 남성형 단수 주격

　　　　　< formatus, formata, formatum

> formatio, formationis, f. 형성, 형체

E *formation, (formation >)* **malformation** *(< 'bad formation; physical abnormality, especially congenital anomaly')*

> conformo, **conformavi**, conformatum, conformare (< con- (< cum) *with, together* + formare *to form*) 꼴을 만들다, (각 부분을 균형 잡아) 배치시키다, (규칙에) 들어맞게 하다, 순응시키다, (기준을) 충족시키다, (형상·성질을) 일치시키다　　　　　　　　　　**E** *conform*

　　> conformatio, conformationis, f. 구조, (각 부분의 균형 잡힌) 배치, 적합, 순응, 일치　　　　　　　　　**E** *conformation*

> deformo, **deformavi**, deformatum, deformare (< de- *apart from, down, not* + formare *to form*) 볼품없이 만들다, 기형으로 만들다, 변형시키다　　**E** *deform*

　　> deformatio, deformationis, f. 볼품없이 만듦, 기형, 변형　　**E** *deformation*

> informo, **informavi**, informatum, informare (< in- *in, on, into, toward* + formare *to form*) 모양을 만들다, 묘사하다, 알려주다, 정보를 주다　　**E** *inform*

　　> informatio, informationis, f. 형성, 소묘(素描), 보고, 정보　　　　　　　　　　**E** *information, informatics*

> reformo, **reformavi**, reformatum, reformare (< re- *back, again* + formare *to form*) 본래의 모양을 되찾다, 다른 모양으로 바꾸다, 개조하다, 개혁하다　　　　　　　　　　　**E** *reform*

　　> reformatio, reformationis, f. 개조, 개혁　　**E** *reformation*

> transformo, **transformavi**, transformatum, transformare (< trans- *over, across, through, beyond* + formare *to form*) 변형시키다, 전환시키다　　　　　　　　**E** *transform, transformant*

　　> transformatio, transformationis, f. 변형, 전환, 형질전환　　**E** *transformation*

< G. morphē, morphēs, f. *form, shape, appearance, beauty*

E **morpheme** *(< 'on the pattern of phoneme')*, **monomorphic (monomorphous)** *(< 'of a single form')*, **dimorphic** *(< 'of two forms')*, **polymorphic (polymorphous)** *(< 'two or more forms in one species, as the castes of social insects')*, **pleomorphic** *(< 'two or more forms in one life cycle')*, **dysmorphic** *(< 'malformed')*, **enantiomorphic** *(< 'of an opposite form')*, **amorphous** *(< 'shapeless')*, **allomorphism, polymorphism, morphology, morphogeny** *(morphogenesis)*, *(morphogeny >)* **morphogenic; polymorphonuclear** *(< 'having a nucleus with lobules of various shapes, specifically designating a neutrophil')*

> G. amorphia, amorphias, f. (< a- *not* + morphē + -ia) *unsightedness, ugliness*

　　> (*perhaps aphetic*) L. morphea, morpheae, f. 국소 피부경화증　　**E** *morphea*

> G. dysmorphos, dysmorphos, dysmorphon (< dys- *bad*) *deformed*

> G. dysmorphōsis, dysmorphōseōs, f. (< + -ōsis *condition*) *malformation*

> L. dysmorphosis, dysmorphosis, f. 기형　　　　　E *dysmorphosis*

> G. metamorphoun (metamorphoein) (< met(a)- *between, along with, across, after*) *to transform*

> G. metamorphōsis, metamorphōseōs, f. (< + -ōsis *condition*) *transformation*

> L. metamorphosis, metamorphosis, f. 탈바꿈, 변형, 변태(變態)　　　　　E *metamorphosis*

> L. Morpheus, Morphei, m. (< *Ovid's name for the god of dreams, with reference to his ability to take on the form of any person*) (로마 신화) 꿈의 신 (잠의 신 Somnus의 아들)

E *morphine* (< '*the drug's sleep-inducing properties*'), (*endogenous morphine* > '*any of endogenous neuropeptides with morphine-like activity*' >) *endorphin(s)*

> L. morphogenesis, morphogenesis, f. (< + G. genesis *birth*) (발생) 형태발생, 형태형성　　　　E *morphogenesis* (*morphogeny*), (*morphogenesis* >) *dysmorphogenesis*

furca, furcae, f. 두 가닥 갈퀴(쇠스랑·작살), 지겟작대기, 까치발; Y자 모양으로 가랑이진 기둥 머리에 목을 달아 거는) 형틀; 분지(分枝), 음차(音叉)　　　　E *fork,* F. *fourchette*

> bifurcatus, bifurcata, bifurcatum (< bi- *two* + furca *fork*) 두 갈래로 된　　　E *bifurcate*

gemma, gemmae, f. 식물의 새싹, 움, 보석　　　　　E *gemma, gem, gemstone*

> gemmula, gemmulae, f. (< + -ula *diminutive suffix*) 작은 싹, 작은 보석　　E *gemmule*

> gemmo, **gemmavi**, gemmatum, gemmare 싹이 트다, 발아(發芽)하다, 보석으로 장식되다　　　　E *gemmate*

< IE. gembh- *nail, tooth*　　　　　E *comb, cam*

> G. gomphos, gomphou, m. *nail, peg, bolt, tooth*

> L. gomphosis, gomphosis, f. (< + G. -ōsis *condition*) 못박이관절　　E *gomphosis*

gloria, gloriae, f. 영광, 명예　　　　　E *glory*

> gloriosus, gloriosa, gloriosum 영광스러운, 명예로운　　　　E *glorious*

> ingloriosus, ingloriosa, ingloriosum (< in- *not*) 명예스럽지 못한, 이름 없는　E *inglorious*

> glorifico, glorificavi, glorificatum, glorificare (< gloria *glory* + -ficare (< facĕre) *to make*) 영광을 돌리다, 명예롭게 하다　　　　E *glorify*

gunna, gunnae, f. 모피, 모피로 만든 겉옷　　　　　E *gown*

gutta, guttae, f. (액체의) 방울, 물방울, 반점(斑點), 얼룩점

E *gutta, gutter, gout* (< '*from the notion of the 'dropping' of a morbid material from the blood in and around the joints*'), *gouty*

> guttatus, guttata, guttatum 물방울 모양의 얼룩이 있는, 반점이 있는　　E *guttate, guttated*

lacrima, lacrimae, f. 눈물
> lacrimalis, lacrimale 눈물의　　　　　　　　　　　　　　　E *lacrimal (lachrymal)*
> lacrimo, lacrimavi, lacrimatum, lacrimare 눈물 흘리다, 울다　　E *lacrimation, lacrimator*
< (*Archaic Latin*) dacruma 눈물
< IE. dakru- *tear*　　　　　　　　　　　　　　　　　　　　　　E *tear*
> G. dakryon, dakryou, n. *tear*　　　　　　　　　E *dacry(o)-, dacryon, dacryocyst*

lacuna, lacunae, f. 웅덩이, 구덩이　　　　　　　E *lacuna,* (pl.) *lacunae, lacunar, lagoon*
< lacus, lacus, m. (lacus, laci, m.) 못, 호수;
통　　　　　　　　　　E *lake, lacustrine* (< *'on the pattern of palustrine'*)
< IE. laku- *body of water, lake, sea*　　　　　　　　　　　E (*Gaelic*) *loch*
> G. lakkos, lakkou, m. *pond, cistern, hole, pit*

lamina, laminae, f. 켜, 판(板), 층(層), 박(箔), 엽(葉), (척추뼈의) 고리판
E *lamina,* (pl.) *laminae,* (*lamina* >) *laminar, bilaminar, trilaminar, laminin, lamin; laminectomy*

[용례] lamina cribrosa 체판(~板), 사판(篩板), 사상판(篩狀板)　　　　E *lamina cribrosa*
(문법) lamina 판: 단수 주격
cribrosa 체[篩] 모양의, 체처럼 작은 구멍이 많은: 형용사, 여성형 단수 주격
< cribrosus, cribrosa, cribrosum < cribrum, cribri, n. 체[篩]

> lamella, lamellae, f. (< + -ella *diminutive suffix*) 얇은 막, 박판(薄板), 층판(層板),
판(板)　　　　E *lamella,* (pl.) *lamellae,* (*lamella* >) *lamellar, omelet;* (pl.) *lamellipodia*
> lamellatus, lamellata, lamellatum 얇은 판으로 된, 얇은 판 모양의, 납작한　E *lamellate*
> laminaria, laminariae, f. (< *a thin, flat, brown seaweed*) 다시마　　E *laminaria*
> lamino, laminavi, laminatum, laminare 얇은 판으로 만들다, 얇은 판을 포개어 합판을
만들다, 얇은 판이 되다, 얇게 갈라지다　　　　　　　　　E *laminate, lamination*

lancea, lanceae, f. (자루 중간에 가죽고리가 달린) 창　　　E *lance, lanciform, lancet*
> lanceola, lanceolae, f. (< + -ola *diminutive suffix*) 작은 창　　　E *lanceolar*
> lanceolatus, lanceolata, lanceolatum (*past participle of* (*obsolete*) lanceolare)
작은 창으로 무장한, 창 모양으로 된　　　　　　　　　E *lanceolate*
> lanceo, lanceavi, lanceatum, lanceare 창을 던지다　　　　　E *launch*
< *Of Celtic origin*

larva, larvae, f. 유령, 탈, 가면; 애벌레, 유충(幼蟲), 유생(幼生)　E *larva,* (pl.) *larvae, larval, larvicide*
< (*probably*) *Of Etruscan origin*
> L. lar, laris, m. 가정, 도시의 수호신; 고향, 본거지　　　　E *lar,* (pl.) *lares*

libra, librae, f. 저울, 천평, 로마시대의 무게 단위(1파운드에 해당), 수준,

수평　　　　　　　　　　　　　　　　　　　　**E** *Libra,* (libra pondo *'by pound weight'* >) *lb. (£),* It. *lira*

> libella, libellae, f. (< + -ella *diminutive suffix*) 작은 무게, 수평기　　　**E** *level*

> aequilibrium, aequilibrii, n. (< aequus *equal* + libra *balance*)

　　평형(平衡)　　　　　　　　　　　**E** *equilibrium,* (equilibrium >) *disequilibrium*

> aequilibro, aequilibravi, aequilibratum, aequilibrare (< aequus *equal* + libra

　　balance) 평형시키다, 평형하다　　　**E** *equilibrate,* (equilibrate >) *disequilibrate*

> delibero, deliberavi, deliberatum, deliberare (< de- *apart from, down, not; intensive*

　　+ libra *balance*) (주의 깊게 무게를 달다 >) 깊이 생각하다, 결정하다　**E** *deliberate*

< (*Mediterranean word*) lithra *scale*

> G. litra, litras, f. 그리스의 무게 단위(1파운드에 해당)　　　**E** *litre (liter)*

litera, literae, f. (littera, litterae, f.) 글자; (pl.) 편지, 문서, 문학,

　　학문　　　　　　　　　**E** *letter,* (Dutch) *letter,* (litera >) *transliterate*

> literalis, literale 글자의, 글자대로의　　　　　　**E** *literal, literally*

> literatim (부사) 글자 그대로, 한 자 한 자씩, 축자적(逐字的)으로　**E** *literatim*

> literarius, literaria, literarium 문학의, 문어의　　　　**E** *literary*

> literatura, literaturae, f. 문학, 문헌　　　　　　**E** *literature*

> literatus, literata, literatum 글을 읽고 쓸 수 있는,

　　학식 있는　　　　　　　　　　**E** *literate,* (literate >) *literacy*

> illiteratus, illiterata, illiteratum (< il- (< in-) *not*) 문맹의,

　　무학의　　　　　　　　　　**E** *illiterate,* (illiterate >) *illiteracy*

> literatus, literati, m. 학자, 문학자, 지식인　**E** *literatus,* (pl.) *literati*

> alliteratio, alliterationis, f. (< *on the pattern of* obliteratio < al- (< ad)

　　to, toward, at, according to + litera *letter*) 두운(頭韻),

　　두운법　　　　　　　　　**E** *alliteration,* (alliteration >) *alliterate*

> oblitero, obliteravi, obliteratum, obliterare (< ob- *before, toward(s), over,*

　　over, against, away + litera *letter*) 지우다, 제거하다, 말소하다　**E** *obliterate*

　　[용례] thromboangiitis obliterans 폐쇄혈전혈관염　**E** *thromboangiitis obliterans*

　　(문법) thromboangiitis 혈전혈관염: 단수 주격

　　　　< thromboangiitis, thromboangiitidis, f.

　　　　obliterans (혈관 내강을) 지우는: 현재분사, 남·여·

　　　　중성형 단수 주격 < obliterans, (gen.) obliterantis

> obliteratio, obliterationis, f. 제거, 말소　　　**E** *obliteration*

< (*possibly*) G. diphthera, diphtheras, f. *prepared hide, leather (used to write on)*

> L. diphtheria, diphtheriae, f. (< *formation of false membrane* < G.

　　diphthera + -ia *noun suffix*) 디프테리아　　**E** *diphtheria, diphtheric*

< G. dephein *to tan hides*

< IE. deph- *to stamp*

lympha, lymphae, f. 맑은 물, 샘물; 림프 (림프액)

E *lymph, lymph(o)-, lymphoid* (< 'resembling or pertaining to lymph or lymphatic tissue'), *lymphocyte* (< 'a cell found in the lymph'), *lymphoblast, endolymph* (< 'the fluid contained within the membranous labyrinth of the inner ear'), *perilymph* (< 'the fluid contained within the bony labyrinth of the inner ear, surrounding the membranous labyrinth'), *cortilymph* (< 'the fluid filling the intercellular spaces of the organ of Corti')

> lymphaticus, lymphatica, lymphaticum 림프의   **E** *lymphatic*

> lymphoma, lymphomatis, n. (< + G. -ōma *noun suffix denoting tumor*)

    림프종   **E** *lymphoma*

> lymphoedema, lymphoedematis, n. (< + G. oedēma *swelling*)

    림프부종   **E** *lymphoedema (lymphedema)*

< (*altered spelling due to pseudo-etymological association with* G. nymphē, nymphēs, f. *bride, maiden, nymph*) *limpa, *limpae, f. 맑은 물

> limpidus, limpida, limpidum 맑은, 투명한   **E** *limpid*

macula, maculae, f. 반(斑), 점(點), 반점, 오점, 그물코

E *macula (macule),* (pl.) *maculae (macules), macular, mail* (< 'mail armor, denoting the individual metal elements'), (tri- three + macula net > 'a kind of fishing-net' >) *trammel*

> maculo, maculavi, maculatum, maculare 반점을 만들다, 얼룩지게 하다,

    더럽히다   **E** *maculate, immaculate*

< IE. sme- *to smear, to smear on, to stroke on*   **E** *smite*

> (*possibly*) G. smēchein *to wipe, to cleanse*

> G. smēgma, smēgmatos, n. *detergent, soap*

> L. smegma, smegmatis, n. 세척제; 귀두지(龜頭脂), 구지(垢脂),

    치구(恥垢)   **E** *smegma, smegmatic*

mala, malae, f. 위턱, 빰

> malaris, malare 위턱의, 빰의   **E** *malar*

> maxilla, maxillae, f. (< + -illa *diminutive suffix*) 위턱뼈,

    상악골(上顎骨)   **E** *maxilla,* (pl.) *maxillae*

> maxillaris, maxillare 위턱뼈의, 상악골의   **E** *maxillary*

< maxla, maxlae, f. 위턱, 빰

mappa, mappae, f. 식탁보, 상보, (던져서 경기 시작을 알리던) 신호깃발

E (mappa mundi 'sheet of the world' >) *map, napkin* (< 'a tablecloth'), (a napron 'a tablecloth' > (wrong division) >) *apron*

< *Of Semitic origin*

massa, massae, f. 덩어리, 질량   **E** *mass, massive, amass,* F. *en masse* (< 'in a mass')

< G. maza, mazēs, f. *(kneaded) lump, barley cake*

< IE. mag-, mak- *to knead, to fashion, to fit*

> **E** *make, mason, (mason >) masonry, freemason, match (< 'mate, spouse' < 'one who is fitted with (another)'), crossmatch, mismatch, mingle, intermingle, among (< 'mixture, crowd'), mongrel*

> L. macero, **maceravi**, maceratum, macerare 반죽하다, 물에 담가 부드럽게 하다, 약
하게 하다, 시달리게 하다   **E** *macerate*

> G. massein *to knead*   **E** *massage*

> G. magma, magmatos, n. *unguent*

> L. magma, magmatis, n. 향유의 찌꺼기; 정니(晶泥), 유제(乳劑), 마그마   **E** *magma*

mola, molae, f. 맷돌, 방아, (제사용 동물 위에 뿌리던 거칠고 소금 친) 밀가루(mola salsa *salted meal*), 기태(奇胎)   **E** *mill,* F. *moulin, mole*

> molaris, molare 맷돌의, 갈아 바수는, 기태의   **E** *molar*

> molaris, molaris, m. (< molaris dens *grinding tooth*) 어금니,
구치(臼齒), 대구치(大臼齒)   **E** *molar, premolar, retromolar*

> immolo, **immolavi**, immolatum, immolare (< im- (< in) *in, on, into, toward*) (잡으
려는) 희생동물에 소금 섞은 밀가루를 뿌리다, 제물로 바치다, 희생시키다   **E** *immolate*

< IE. melə-, mel- *to crush, to grind; with derivatives referring to various ground or crumbling substances (such as flour) and to instruments for grinding or crushing (such as millstones)*   **E** *meal, oatmeal,* (probably) *mellow*

> L. milium, milii, n. 조[粟]; (*small keratin-filled subepidermal cyst*) 비립종(粃粒腫),
좁쌀종   **E** *millet; milium,* (pl.) *milia*

> L. miliaceus, miliacea, miliaceum 조의, 좁쌀의

> L. miliarius, miliaria, miliarium 조의, 좁쌀의; 퍼진, 속립성(粟粒性)의   **E** *miliary*

> L. miliaria, miliariae, f. (*originally, any disease characterized by the presence of a miliary skin rash*) 땀띠, 한진(汗疹)

> L. malleus, mallei, m. 망치, 망치뼈, 추골(鎚骨); (망치 >) 마비저(馬鼻疽, *glanders*)

> **E** *malleus, mallet, pall-mall (< 'a game in which players use a mallet to drive a boxwood ball* (It. *palla) through an iron ring suspended at the end of a long alley'), mall (< 'a tree-bordered walk in St. James's Park, London, formerly the site of a pall-mall alley')*

> L. malleolus, malleoli, m. (< + -olus *diminutive suffix*) 작은 망치,
복사, 복사뼈, 과(踝)   **E** *malleolus,* (pl.) *malleoli, (malleolus >) malleolar*

> L. malleo, **malleavi**, malleatum, malleare 망치질하다   **E** *malleable*

> G. mylē, mylēs, f. (mylos, mylou, m.) *mill, millstone, molar*   **E** *myl(o)-*

> G. mylos, mylē, mylon *milled*

> G. amylon, amylou, n. (< *thing not ground at a mill* < a- *not* + mylon
milled) starch, fine meal

> L. amylum, amyli, n. 앙금, 녹말, 전분(澱紛)

> **E** *amylum, amyloid (< 'stained with iodine, like starch'), amylase, amyl,* (amylon + -ose (< *glucose*) > *'a water-soluble non-congealing glycan of starch' >) amylose,* (amylon + pēktos *'congealed' > 'a water-insoluble congealing glycan of starch' >) amylopectin*

> L. amylaceus, amylacea, amylaceum 녹말의, 전분의   **E** *amylaceous*

[용례] corpora amylacea (pl.) 전분질체

(澱紛質體)   **E** *(pl.) corpora amylacea*

(문법) corpora 몸, 체(體): 복수 주격

< corpus, corporis, n.

amylacea: 형용사, 중성형 복수 주격

Moneta, Monetae, f. (로마 신화) 경고의 여신(주노 여신의 별칭, 골족의 로마 침입을 여신 신전의
거위를 통해 경고하였음)

> moneta, monetae, f. 조폐소(재화의 수호신이기도 한 주노 여신의 로마 신전에서 화폐가
주조되었음), 화폐   **E** *mint, mintage, money, moneyed (monied)*

> monetarius, monetaria, monetarium 화폐의, 금융의   **E** *monetary*

< (*probably*) *Of Etruscan origin*

mora, morae, f. 지연, 유예, 휴지, 장애; (단음절에 해당하는)
운율 단위   **E** *mora, demur, remora (< 'regarded as ship delayers')*

> moratorius, moratoria, moratorium 지연하는, 유예하는   **E** *moratory, moratorium*

< IE. merə- *to delay, to hinder*

mumia, mumiae, f. 미라, 미라로 만든 가루약   **E** *mummy, mummify*

< (*Arabic*) mumiya(h) *embalmed body, mummy*

< (*Persian*) mum *wax*

myrrha, myrrhae, f. 미르라, 몰약(沒藥, 동부 아프리카 및 아라비아 지방의 감람과(橄欖科)
Commiphora속(屬) 식물에서 채취하는 방향성 수지(樹脂)·향료·약용); (Myrrha)
(그리스 신화) Cinyras (또는 Theias) 왕의 딸 (아버지와 불륜관계에서 임신,
아라비아로 피신하여 Adonis를 낳고 몰약나무로 변신함)   **E** *myrrh*

> (*Portuguese*) mirra *myrrh*

> (*Japanese*) ミイラ 木乃伊

> (*Korean*) 미라 (미이라)

< G. myrrha, myrrhas, f. *myrrh;* (Myrrha) (*Greek mythology*) *a daughter of the
king Cinyras of Cyprus (or the king Theias of Assyria) and the mother of
Adonis by her father*

< (*Arabic*) murr *bitter, myrrh*

< *Of Semitic origin*

> G. myrtos, myrtou, f. *myrtle*

> L. myrtus, myrti, f. (myrtus, myrtus, f.) 도금양(桃金孃)나무   **E** *myrtle*

> G. myrsinē, myrsinēs, f. (myrrhinē, myrrhinēs, f.) *ancient Greek names for the myrtle*

naphtha, naphthae, f. 나프타 기름, 석뇌유(石腦油), (특히 바빌론 부근에서 산출되던) 인화성이

강한 역청(瀝靑)

> **E** *naphtha, naphthalene, (naphthenate + palmitate >) napalm, (naphthalic >) phthalic, phthalein, phenolphthalein, (phthalimidoglutarimide >) thalidomide*

< G. naphtha, naphthas, f. *naphtha*

< *Of Oriental origin*

nebula, nebulae, f. 안개, 김, 구름, 성운; 각막박영(角膜薄影),

각막백탁(角膜白濁)　　　　　　　　　　　　　　**E** *nebula, nebular, nebulize, nebulin*

> nebulosus, nebulosa, nebulosum 안개 낀, 희미한, 모호한　　**E** *nebulous*

< IE. nebh- *cloud*　　　　　　　　　　　　　　　　　　**E** *Niflheim, Nibelung*

> L. nimbus, nimbi, m. 먹구름, 소나기, 후광　　　　　　　　**E** *nimbus*

> G. nephelē, nephelēs, f. *cloud, darkness, bird-net*　　　**E** *nephelometer*

> G. nephos, nephous, n. *cloud, darkness, bird-net*　　　**E** *nephology*

nonna, nonnae, f. 유모, 기르는 사람; 수녀　　　　　　**E** *nun, (nun >) nunnery*

< IE. nana *child's word for a nurse or female adult other than its mother, whence little old man, dwarf*

> *(possibly)* G. nanos, nanou, m. *dwarf*

> L. nanus, nani, m. 난쟁이　　　　　　　　　　　**E** *nan(o)-, nanism, nano*

> L. nanus, nana, nanum 난쟁이의, 작은

nucha, nuchae, f. 목덜미, 항(項)　　　　　　　　　　　**E** *nucha*

[용례] ligamentum nuchae 목덜미인대, 항인대　　　　　　**E** *ligamentum nuchae*

(문법) ligamentum 인대: 단수 주격 < ligamentum, ligamenti, n.

nuchae 목덜미의: 단수 속격

> nuchalis, nuchale 목덜미의　　　　　　　　　　　　**E** *nuchal*

< *(Arabic)* nuka *spinal marrow (confused with* nuqra *nape of the neck)*

pandura, pandurae, f. 기타 모양의 3선 악기, 삼현금(三絃琴)　**E** *pandurate, panduriform*

< G. pandoura, pandouras, f. *three-stringed lute*

< *(probably)* *(Persian)* tanbur

perna, pernae, f. 넓적다리, 절인 돼지고기, 훈육(燻肉), 햄; *(from the shape of the peduncle >)*

조개　　　　　　　　　　**E** *(perna > *pernula > perula, perla >) pearl*

> pernio, pernionis, m. (< perna *leg* + -io *noun suffix*) 발(발뒤꿈치)의 동상(凍傷),

동상　　　　　　　　　　　　　　　　　　　　　　**E** *pernio*

< IE. persna- *heel*

pluma, plumae, f. 깃털; 깃털 모양의 것, 솟아오르는 연기(구름·물·맨틀 융기)

    < IE. pleus- *to pluck; a feather, fleece*

E *plume, plumage*
E *fleece*

provincia, provinciae, f. 통치권, 관할권, 직분; (이탈리아 본토 이외 로마의 총독이 통치한)
    주(州), 주민, 영역

    > provicialis, proviciale 주(州)의, 지방의

E *province*
E *provincial*

petechia, petechiae, f. 점출혈(點出血)

E *petechia, petechial*

purpura, purpurae, f. 자(홍)색의 권패류 (특히 소라): 자줏빛, 황제, 고관; (의학) 자색반
    (紫色斑)

E **purpura, purpuric,** (purpura > (dissimilated) >) **purple**

    < G. porphyra, porphyras, f. *shellfish yielding purple dye, purple, purple cloth*

        E *(haematoporphyrin >)* **porphyrin(s)** *(< 'deep-red or purple fluorescent crystalline pigments'),* **protoporphyrin, uroporphyrin, coproporphyrin,** *(porphyrin >)* **porph(o)-**

        > G. porphyreos, porphyrea, porphyreon (porphyrous, porphyrē, porphyroun)
            purple

        > L. porphyria, porphyriae, f. (< *porphyrin* + -ia) 포르피린증

E *porphyria*

pustula, pustulae, f. 거품, 물집; 농포(膿疱), 고름물집

    > pustulo, pustulavi, pustulatum, pustulare 농포를 생기게 하다, 농포가 생기다

E *pustule, pustular*
E *pustulation*

  < IE. pu-, phu- *to blow, to swell; echoic of blowing out cheeks, puffing*

    > L. praeputium, praeputii, n. (< prae- *before, beyond* + put- (< IE. pu-) *penis*)
        포피(包皮), 음경꺼풀

E *preputium (prepuce)*

    > G. physa, physēs, f. *bellows, bladder, bubble*

        > G. physan (physaein) *to blow*

            > G. emphysan (emphysaein) (< em- (< en) *in*) *to blow in*

                > G. emphysēma, emphysēmatos, n. *inflation*

                    > L. emphysema, emphysematis, n. 공기증, 폐공기증, 기종
                        (氣腫), 폐기종

E *emphysema, emphysematous*

        > G. physallis, physalleōs, f. *bladder, bubble*

            > L. physalis, physalis, f. 거품; 꽈리

E *physalis, physaliphorous (physalipherous)*

        > L. physostigma, physostigmatis, n. (< *the style of the flower becomes inflated*
            above the stigma < + G. stigma *tattoo-mark, brand*) (나이지리아 지방)
            칼라바르 콩(*Calabar bean*)

            E **physostigmine,** *(physostigmine >)* **neostigmine,** *(physostigma >)* **stigmasterol**
            (< 'a sterol present in Calabar beans')

    > (*suggested*) G. pygē, pygēs, f. *rump, buttock*

E *pyg(o)-, -pygia (-pyga)*

        > L. pygidium, pygidii, n. (< G. pygē + -idion *diminutive suffix*) 항문상판(肛門
            上板), 미부(尾部)

E *pygidium*

> L. dipygus, dipygi, m. (< G. di- *two* + pygē) 두골반체(體)　　　　**E** *dipygus*

rima, rimae, f. 틈, 틈새, 균열, 열(裂)　　　　**E** *rima, rimose*

  [용례] rima glottidis 성대틈새, 성문열(聲門裂)　　　　**E** *rima glottidis*

  (문법) rima 틈새, 열(裂): 단수 주격

     glottidis 성문(聲門)의, 성대문(聲帶門)의: 단수 속격 < glottis, glottidis, f.

< IE. rei- *to scratch, to tear, to cut; hypothetical base of various extended*

  forms　　　**E** *rive, rift, rifle, reap, ripe* (< '*ready for reaping*'), *ripen, rife, row, rope*

  > L. ripa, ripae, f. (< *that which is cut out by a river*)

    강변　　　**E** *river*, (ad '*to*' + ripa '*shore*' >) *arrive*

Roma, Romae, f. 로마　　　　**E** *Roma (Rome)*

  > Romanus, Romana, Romanum 로마의, 로마인의, 로마식의　　　**E** *Roman, Romanize*

    > Romanicus, Romanica, Romanicum 로마의; (언어) 로망스어의; (미술·건축)

     로마네스크 양식의

      E *Romance* (< '*of a Romance language*'); *romance* (< '*stories written or recited in a Romance language*'), *romantic, romanticism*

sagina, saginae, f. 살찌우는 먹이, 석죽과의 풀

  > sagino, **saginavi**, saginatum, saginare 살찌우다

    > saginatus, saginata, saginatum (*past participle*) 살찐　　　**E** *saginate*

sagitta, sagittae, f. 화살　　　　**E** *sagittate*

  > sagittarius, sagittaria, sagittarium 화살의

    > sagittarius, sagittarii, m. 궁수; (Sagittarius) (천문) 사수좌(射手座), 인마궁

     (人馬宮)　　　**E** *Sagittarius*

    > sagittalis, sagittale (두개골) 시상봉합(矢狀縫合)의　　　**E** *sagittal*

saphena, saphenae, f. 복재(伏在)정맥, 두렁정맥　　　　**E** *saphenous*

  < (*Arabic*) safin *hidden* (*vein*)

scarlata, scarlatae, f. 선홍색 옷, 선홍색　　　　**E** *scarlet*

  > scarlatina, scarlatinae, f. 성홍열(猩紅熱)　　　**E** *scarlatina*

  < (*Arabic*) siqillat *fine cloth*

scintilla, scintillae, f. 불꽃, 섬광(閃光)

  E *scintilla, scintillation*, (*scintillation* >) *scinti-, scintiscan, scintigram, stencil, tinsel*

< IE. skai- *to gleam softly*　　　　　　　　　　　　　　　　E *shine, sheer*

　　> G. skēnē, skēnēs, f. *stage, scene building, theater, tent, covered place*

　　　　> L. scaena, scaenae, f. (scena, scenae, f.) 무대, 극장, 천막, 장면, 현장　　E *scene*

　　　　　　> L. scaenarius, scaenaria, scaenarium (scenarius, scenaria, scenarium)

　　　　　　　　무대의, 연극의　　　　　　　E It. *scenario*, (It. scenario >) *scenery*

　　　　> G. skēnikos, skēnikē, skēnikon *belonging to the stage, theatrical*

　　　　　　> L. scaenicus, scaenica, scaenicum (scenicus, scenica, scenicum)

　　　　　　　　무대의, 연극의, 연극 같은　　　　　　　E *scenic*

　　　　> G. proskēnion, proskēniou, n. (< pro- *before, in front*) *the stage area in front*
　　　　　　of the scene building

　　　　　　> L. proscenium, proscenii, n. 앞무대

　　　　　　　　　　　　　　　　　　　　　　　　E *proscenium*

　　> G. skia, skias, f. *shadow, outline, ghost*　　　　E *skiascope*

　　　　> G. skiouros, skiourou, m. (< *shadow tailed* < skia *shadow* + oura *tail*) *squirrel*

　　　　　　> L. sciurus, sciuri, m. 다람쥐　　E *sciurus*, (sciurus >) *squirrel*

spina, spinae, f. 가시; 등마루, 척추(脊椎), 척주(脊柱)
　　　　　　　　　　　　　　　　　　　　　　E *spine, spiny*

　　> spinosus, spinosa, spinosum 가시 많은, 가시의, 뾰족한, 까다로운　　E *spinous*

　　> spinalis, spinale 등마루의, 척추의; 척수(脊髓)의　　E *spinal, bulbospinal*

　　> infraspinatus, infraspinata, infraspinatum (< infra- *below, beneath*) 가시 아래의

　　> supraspinatus, supraspinata, supraspinatum (< supra- *above*) 가시 위의

< IE. spei- *sharp point*　　　　　E *spitz, spire* (< *'slender stalk'*), *spoke*

　　> L. spica, spicae, f. (spicum, spici, n.) 뾰족한 끝, 이삭　　E *spica, spike*, (probably) *spigot*

　　　　> L. spicula, spiculae, f. (< + -ula *diminutive suffix*) 침상체(針狀體), 침골
　　　　　　(針骨), 가시　　　　　　　E *spicula* (*spicule*), (pl.) *spiculae, spicular*

　　　　> L. spiculum, spiculi, n. (< + -ulum *diminutive suffix*) (벌 · 전갈의) 독침,
　　　　　　창, 화살끝, 창, 바늘, 가시　　　E *spiculum*, (pl.) *spicula, spicular*

　　　　　　> L. spiculo, spiculavi, spiculatum, spiculare 뾰족하게 하다　　E *spiculate*

spuma, spumae, f. 거품, 포말(泡沫)
　　　　　　　　　　　　　　　　　　　　　　　　E *spume*
< IE. (s)poi-mo- *foam*　　　　　　　　　　　　　　　　E *foam*

　　> L. pumex, pumicis, m. (< *spongelike appearance*) 속돌, 경석(輕石), 부석(浮石)　　E *pumice*

squama, squamae, f. 조잡 > 얇은 껍질, 비듬, (어류 · 파충류의)
　　　　　　비늘　　　　　　　　　　　E *squama* (*squame*), (pl.) *squamae*

　　> squamosus, squamosa, squamosum 비늘 많은, 비늘 있는　　E *squamous, squamosal*

　　> squamatus, squamata, squamatum 비늘 덮인　　　　　　E *squamate*

　　> desquamo, desquamavi, desquamatum, desquamare (< de- *apart from, down,*
　　　　not + squama *scale*) 비늘을 벗기다, 껍질을 벗기다　　E *desquamate, desquamative*

　　< squaleo, −, −, squalēre 거칠다, 불결하다

　　　　> squalor, squaloris, m, 조잡, 불결
　　　　　　　　　　　　　　　　　　　　　　　　E *squalor*

> squalidus, squalida, squalidum 거친, 불결한 **E** *squalid*

stella, stellae, f. 별 **E** *stellar*
    > stellatus, stellata, stellatum 별 모양의, 별표의, 별이 총총한 **E** *stellate*
    > constellatio, constellationis, f. (< con- (< cum) *with, together* + stella *star*) 별자리,
        성좌(星座) **E** *constellation*
  < IE. ster- *star* **E** *star, starry;* (Hebrew) *Esther*
    > G. astēr, asteros, m. *star*
        > L. aster, asteris, m. 별; (생물학) 성상체; (Aster) (식물)
            Aster속(屬) **E** *aster, asteroid, amphiaster (diaster)*
        > G. astron, astrou, n. *constellation, star*
            E *astrology, astronomy, astronaut, astrocyte (< 'a star-shaped glial cell'), astrovirus (< 'a star-like appearance with five or six points')*
          > L. astrum, astri, n. 성좌, 별 **E** *disaster (< 'ill-starred event'), disastrous*
            > L. astralis, astrale 별의 **E** *astral*
        > G. asteriskos, asteriskou, m. (< + -iskos *diminutive suffix*) *little star*
          > L. asteriscus, asterisci, m. 작은 별, 별표 **E** *asterisk*
        > G. asterios, asteria, asterion *starry*
          > L. asterion, asterii, n. 별모양점, 성상점(星狀點) **E** *asterion*

storia, storiae, f. (storea, storeae, f.) 골풀로 만든 자리, 거적 **E** *storiform*

synovia, synoviae, f. (*probably arbitrarily formed by Paracelsus, applied to the nutritive fluid peculiar to the several parts of the body, and also to the gout, but limited by later physicians to the fluid of the joints*) 활액(滑液) **E** *synovia, synovial*

talea, taleae, f. 싹, 꺾꽂이 가지, 나뭇가지, 막대기, 부신(符信) **E** *tally*
    > talio, -, -, taliare 가지를 쳐내다, 자르다
    E *tailor, detail (< 'piece by piece'), retail (< 'a piece cut off'), entail (< 'to allot a piece')*
  < IE. tal- *to grow, to sprout*

tenebrae, tenebrarum, f. (pl.) 어두움
    > tenebrosus, tenebrosa, tenebrosum 어두운 **E** *tenebrous*
  < IE. teme- *dark*
    > L. temere (부사) 아무렇게나, 생각 없이
        > L. temeritas, temeritatis, f. 무모, 저돌 **E** *temerity*
        > L. temerarius, temeraria, temerarium 무모한, 저돌적인 **E** *temerarious*

terra, terrae, f. (< *dry land*) 땅, 지구; (Terra) (로마 신화) 땅의 여신

E *terrace, inter, disinter, terrier* (< 'earth dog'), (terra merita 'deserved earth' >) *turmeric*, (terra cocta 'cooked earth' >) It. **terra cotta**

> terreus, terrea, terreum 땅의, 흙으로 된

> terrenus, terrena, terrenum 땅의, 현세의　　　**E** *terrene*, (terrenum >) *terrain*

> mediterraneus, mediterranea, mediterraneum (< medius *middle* + terra *land*) 내륙의,

　　육지로 둘러싸인; (Mediterraneus) 지중해(地中海)의　　**E** *Mediterranean*

> terrestris, terrestre 땅의, 지구의, 지상의, 현세의　　**E** *terrestrial, extraterrestrial*

> terrarium, terrarii, n. 길로 쓰는 둑, 성토(盛土); 육생생물 생태관　**E** *terrarium*

> territorium, territorii, n. 영토, 지역, 관할구역　　**E** *territory*

　　> territorialis, territoriale 영토의, 지역의, 토지의　**E** *territorial*

< IE. ters- *to dry*　　　　　　　　　　　　　　　**E** *thirst*

> L. torreo, **torrui**, tostum, torrēre 말리다, 굽다, 태우다

E *torrent, torrid, toast* (< 'a slice or piece of bread browned at the fire: often put in wine, water, or other beverage')

> G. tarsos, tarsou, m. *frame of wickerwork (originally for drying cheese), mat of reeds; hence a flat surface, blade or flat of the oar, sole of the foot (the flat of the foot between the toes and the heel), ankle*

　　> L. tarsus, tarsi, m. 발목, 족근(足根), 발목뼈, 족근골(足根骨); 눈꺼풀판, 검판(瞼板)　**E** *tarsus*

　　　　> L. tarsalis, tarsale 발목의, 발목뼈의; 눈꺼풀판의　**E** *tarsal*

　　　　> L. metatarsus, metatarsi, m. (< G. met(a)- *between, along with, across, after* + tarsos *sole of the foot*) 발허리, 중족(中足), 발허리뼈, 중족골 (中足骨)

　　　　　　　　　　　　　　　　　E *metatarsus, metatarsal*

tibia, tibiae, f. (*earlier*) 피리; 정강뼈, 경골(脛骨)　　**E** *tibia*

　　> tibialis, tibiale 정강뼈의, 경골의, 정강이의　　**E** *tibial*

∽ (*suggested*) G. siphōn, siphōnos, m. *pipe, tube, siphon*　**E** *siphon*

turba, turbae, f. 소란, 군중

　　> turbo, turbinis, m. 소용돌이, 팽이, 소라　　**E** *turbine, turbo*

　　　　> turbinatus, turbinata, turbinatum (뱅뱅 돌린) 원뿔꼴의　**E** *turbinate*

　　> turbidus, turbida, turbidum 어지러운, 탁한　　**E** *turbid, trouble*

　　　　> turbiditas, turbiditatis, f. 혼란, 혼탁　　**E** *turbidity*

　　> turbulentus, turbulenta, turbulentum 소용돌이치는　**E** *turbulent*

　　　　> turbulentia, turbulentiae, f. 혼란, 동요, 교란, 난기류　**E** *turbulence*

　　> turbo, turbavi, turbatum, turbare 휘젓다, 어지럽히다

　　　　> disturbo, disturbavi, disturbatum, disturbare (< dis- *apart from, down, not* + turbare *to whorl*) 어지럽히다, 방해하다, 교란시키다, 장애를 일으키다

　　　　　　　　　　　　　　　E *disturb, disturbance*

　　　　> perturbo, perturbavi, perturbatum, perturbare (< per- *through, thoroughly* + turbare *to whorl*) 어지럽히다　**E** *perturb, perturbable, imperturbable, perturbation*

< IE. (s)twer- *to turn, to whorl*

E *stir, storm*

ulna, ulnae, f. 팔꿈, 팔꿈치, 아래팔; 한 발(길이); 자뼈, 척골(尺骨)　　　　**E** *ulna*

> ulnaris, ulnare 자뼈의, 척골의　　　　**E** *ulnar*

< IE. el- *to bend, elbow,*

forearm　　　**E** *ell (< 'unit of length' < 'length of forearm'), elbow (< 'forearm bend')*

> G. ōlenē, ōlenēs, f. *elbow, forearm*

> G. ōlekranon, olēkranou, n. (< ōlenē + kranion *skull, upper part*
of the head) *point of the elbow*

> L. olecranon, olecrani, n. 팔꿈치머리, 주두(肘頭)　　　**E** *olecranon*

< IE. elei- *to bend*

> L. obliquus, obliqua, obliquum (< ob- *before, toward(s), over, against, away*)
비스듬한　　　**E** *oblique*

> L. obliquitas, obliquitatis, f. 기울기, 경사, 경사도, 모호, 사악(邪惡)　　**E** *obliquity*

> (*suggested*) L. licium, licii, n. 꼰 양털실, (천·그물 등의) 씨줄, 실, 줄

> L. trilix, (gen.) trilicis (< tri- *three* + licium *a thread of the warp*) 세 줄
실로 짠, 천 세 겹의, 천이 질긴　　　**E** *trellis*

unda, undae, f. 물결, 파도

> undula, undulae, f. (< + -ula *diminutive suffix*) 작은 물결, 작은 파도

> *undulo, *undulavi, *undulatum, *undulare 물결치다, 파상(波狀)으로
일렁거리다　　　**E** *undulate, undulant*

> undo, undavi, undatum, undare 물결치다, 파상(波狀)으로 일렁거리다, 넘치다

> abundo, abundavi, abundatum, abundare (< ab- *off, away from* + undare
to surge) 넘치다, 풍부하다　　　**E** *abundant, abound*

> inundo, inundavi, inundatum, inundare (< in- *in, on, into, toward* +
undare *to surge*) 잠기게 하다, 넘치다　　　**E** *inundate*

> redundo, redundavi, redundatum, redundare (< red- *back, again* +
undare *to surge*) 넘치다, 넘치도록 많다,
지나치게 많다　　　**E** *redundant, redundance (redundancy)*

> superundo, superundavi, superundatum, superundare (< super- *above* +
undare *to surge*) 넘치다, 에워싸다　　　**E** *surround, surroundings*

< IE. wed- *water, wet*　　　**E** *water, watery, wet, wash, winter, otter (< 'water creature')*

> G. hydōr, hydatos, n. *water*

E *hydr(o)- (< 'water or hydrogen'); hydraulic, hydrodynamic, hydrostatic, hydrant,
hydrophilic, hydrophilia, hydrophobic, hydrophobia, hydrate, (hydrate >)
hydration, dehydrate, dehydration; hydrous, anhydrous, hydride(s),
anhydride(s), hydronium (< 'on the pattern of ammonium'); hydrogen (H),
hydrochloric acid (HCl, chlorhydric acid), (chlorhydric acid >) achlorhydria*

> G. hydra, hydras, f. *water-serpent, hydra;* (Hydra) (*Greek mythology*)
*the fabulous many-headed snake of the marshes of Lerna, whose
heads grew again as fast as they were cut off, said to have been
at length killed by Hercules*　　　**E** *hydra; Hydra*

> G. hydatis, hydatidos, f. *a drop of water, watery*

vesicle   **E** *hydatid* (< 'a cyst containing a clear watery fluid'); *hydatidiform*

> L. hydroa, hydratis, n. 물집증, 수포증 ·   **E** *hydroa*

> L. hydrargyrum, hydrargyri, n. (< + G. argyros, argyrou, m. *silver*)

    수은(水銀)   **E** *hydrargyrum (Hg), hydrargyria (hydrargyrism)*

> (*probably*) (*Via Etruscan*) L. uter, uteris, m. (물 · 포도주를 담는) 가죽부대

   > L. utriculus, utriculi, m. (< + -culus *diminutive suffix*) 작은

     가죽부대, 타원낭, 소실(小室)   **E** *utricle,* (utriculus >) *utricular*

> (*Old Irish*) uisce 물   **E** *usquebaugh (whisky, whiskey)* (< 'water of life')

> (*Russian*) voda 물

   > (*Russian*) vodka (< voda *water* + -ka *diminutive suffix*) 보드카   **E** *vodka*

< IE. awed- *to moisten, to flow*

> IE. euə-dh-r *udder*   **E** *udder*

 > L. uber, uberis, n. 젖, 동물의 젖통, 풍요

  > L. uber, (gen.) uberis 살찐, 풍요한

   > L. ubertas, ubertatis, f. 풍요, 다산   **E** *uberty*

   > L. ubero, uberavi, uberatum, uberare 풍요롭게 하다, 풍요하다

    > L. exubero, exuberavi, exuberatum, exuberare (< ex- *out*

     of, away from + uberare *to bear abundantly*) 우거지게

     하다, 우거지다   **E** *exuberant*

> IE. we-r- (ur-) *water, liquid, milk*

 > L. urina, urinae, f. 오줌, 요(尿), 소변(小便)

  E *urine,* (urine analysis >) *urinalysis, uriniferous, uric,* (purum + uricum 'pure and urine' >) *purine, uric acid, urate*

  > L. urinarius, urinaria, urinarium 오줌의   **E** *urinary*

  > L. urinalis, urinale 오줌의   **E** *urinal*

  > L. urino, urinavi, urinatum, urinare 오줌 누다   **E** *urinate*

   > L. urinatio, urinationis, f. 배뇨   **E** *urination*

> IE. wers- (ur-) *to rain, to drip*

 > G. ouron, ourou, n. *urine*

  E *ur(o)-, urology, -uria, -uric, urea* (< 'nitrogenous breakdown product of protein in urine'), *uracil (U), uridine (U), uronic acid* (< 'occurring naturally in the urine')

  > G. ourēthra, ourēthras, f. (< + -thra *noun suffix*)

   > L. urethra, urethrae, f. 요도(尿道)   **E** *urethra, urethral*

  > G. ourein *to urinate*

   > G. ourētēr, ourētēros, m. *ureter*

    > L. ureter, ureteris, m. 요관(尿管)   **E** *ureter, ureteric (ureteral)*

   > G. ourēsis, ourēseōs, f. *urination*

    > L. diuresis, diuresis, f. (< G. di(a)- *through, thoroughly, apart*) 이뇨(利尿)   **E** *diuresis, diuretic, antidiuretic, natriuresis*

    > L. enuresis, enuresis, f. (< *involuntary discharge of urine, often occurring during sleep at night* < G. en- *in*)

유뇨증(遺尿症), 야뇨증(夜尿症)　　　　　　　　　　　　　**E** *enuresis*

> L. anuria, anuriae, f. (< G. an- *not* + -uria) 무뇨(無尿),
　무뇨증(無尿症)　　　　　　　　　　　　　　　　**E** *anuria*

> L. oliguria, oliguriae, f. (< G. oligos *few, little* + -uria) 핍뇨(乏尿),
　핍뇨증(乏尿症)　　　　　　　　　　　　　　　**E** *oliguria*

> L. polyuria, polyuriae, f. (< G. polys *much* + -uria) 다뇨(多尿),
　다뇨증(多尿症)　　　　　　　　　　　　　　　**E** *polyuria*

> L. glycosuria, glycosuriae, f. (< F. glycose *old variant of* F. glucose
　(< G. glykys *sweet*) *glucose* + -uria)
　당뇨(糖尿)　　　　**E** *glycosuria (glucosuria), glycosuric (glucosuric)*

> L. proteinuria, proteinuriae, f. (< *protein* + -uria) 단백뇨(蛋白尿)　**E** *proteinuria*

> L. haematuria, haematuriae, f. (< G. haima, haimatos, n. *blood* + -uria)
　혈뇨(血尿)　　　　　　　　　　　　　　**E** *haematuria (hematuria)*

> L. pyuria, pyuriae, f. (< G. pyon, pyou, n. *pus* + -uria) 농뇨(膿尿),
　고름뇨　　　　　　　　　　　　　　　　　　**E** *pyuria*

> L. dysuria, dysuriae, f. (< G. dys- *bad* + -uria) 배뇨통　**E** *dysuria*

> L. nocturia, nocturiae, f. (< L. nox, noctis, f. *night* + -uria)
　nycturia, nycturiae, f. (< G. nyx, nyktos, f. *night* + -uria)
　야간뇨, 야뇨증　　　　　　　　　　　　**E** *nocturia (nycturia)*

> L. ischuria, ischuriae, f. (< G. ischein *to hold* + -uria) 요정체　**E** *ischuria*

> L. uremia, uremiae, f. (< G. ouron + haima, haimatos, n. *blood* + -ia)
　요독증(尿毒症)　　　　　　　　　　**E** *uraemia (uremia), uremic*

urna, urnae, f. 항아리, 단지, 납골호(納骨壺)　　　　　　　**E** *urn*
　< *(probably) Of* non-IE. *origin*

vespa, vespae, f. 말벌; 장의사 일꾼　　　　　　**E** *vespa, vespiary*
　< IE. wopsa- *wasp*　　　　　　　　　　　　　　　**E** *wasp*

victima, victimae, f. (산 제물로 바쳐지는 동물) 제물, 희생물　**E** *victim*
　< IE. weik- *consecrated, holy*

Vesta, Vestae, f. (< *a household goddess*) (로마신화) 화로불의 여신　**E** *Vesta*
　< *(probably)* IE. wes- *to live, to dwell, to pass the night, with derivatives meaning 'to be'*　**E** *was, were*
　　> *(possibly)* G. asty, asteōs (asteos), n. *city, capital; town (as opposed to country)*
　　　> L. astus, astus, m. (< *practiced in town*) 영리함, 교묘함, 책략
　　　　> L. astutus, astuta, astutum 영리한, 능란한, 교활한　**E** *astute*

villa, villae, f. 농장, 별장, 공공건물　　　　　　　　　**E** *villa*
　> villanus, villana, villanum 농장의, 별장의　　　　**E** *villain*

> villaticus, villatica, villaticum 농장의, 별장의 | **E** village

< IE. weik- *clan (social unit above the household)*

> L. vicus, vici, m. 부락, 전답, 도시의 한 구역

> L. vicinus, vicina, vicinum 이웃의, 인근의, 부근의, 근처의 | **E** vicinage

> L. vicinalis, vicinale 이웃의, 인접한 | **E** vicinal

> L. vicinitas, vicinitatis, f. 부근, 근처 | **E** vicinity

> G. oikos, oikou, m. (oikia, oikias, f., oikion, oikiou, n.) *house, household, family, home*

E *oecology (ecology)* (< 'study of the environment as a house'), (an- 'not' + oikos 'home' + -sis 'feminine noun suffix' > 'homelessness' > 'apoptosis due to absence of cell and matrix interactions' >) *anoikis, monoecious (monecious), dioecious (diecious), dioicous), autoecism (autecism), heteroecism (heterecism)*

> G. oikēsis, oikēseōs, f. *dwelling, administration* | **E** *ecesis*

> G. oikein (oikeein) *to dwell; (middle) to inhabit*

> G. oikoumenē, oikoumenēs, f. (*present participle of middle voice*) *inhabited world, civilized world* | **E** *ecumenical*

> G. oikonomos, oikonomou, m. (< oikos *house* + nomos *management* (< nemein *to manage*)) *householder, steward*

> G. oikonomia, oikonomias, f. *household management, thrift*

> L. oeconomia, oeconomiae, f. 가정(家政), 재산관리, 경영, 경제 | **E** *economy*

> G. oikonomikos, oikonomikē, oikonomikon *of a household, economical*

> L. oeconomicus, oeconomica, oeconomicum 가정(家政)에 관한, 경제상의, 경제적인

E *economic* (< 'of or pertaining to economy'), *economical* (< 'thrifty')

> G. paroikia, paroikias, f. (< G. par(a)- *beside, along side of, beyond* + oikos *house*) *sojourn, community of sojourners; parish*

> L. parochia, parochiae, f. 교구 내의 소교구, 성당 구역 | **E** *parish, parochial*

> L. gynoecium, gynoecii, n. (< G. gynē, gynaikos, f. *woman* + oikion *house*) (식물) 꽃의 자성(雌性)기관, 암술 | **E** *gynoecium (gynecium)*

> L. androecium, androecii, n. (< G. anēr, andros, m. *man, male* + oikion *house*) (식물) 꽃의 웅성(雄性)기관, 수술 | **E** *androecium (andrecium)*

> (*Sanskrit*) visah *dwelling, house*

> (*Sanskrit*) vaisya *peasant, laborer* | **E** *Vaisya*

맞대보기 1 어미 -a, -ē 로 끝나는 그리스어 제1변화 여성 명사는 -a로 끝나는 라틴어 여성 명사가 되어 위의 변화(제1변화)를 따른다.

---

academia, academiae, f. 아카데미아 (아테네 근처 아카데무스의 정원에 있던 플라톤의

학원)   **E** *academy, academic*

< G. akadēmia, akadēmias, f. (*more properly* akadēmeia, *adjective of*
   Akadēmos) *the grove of Academus, a garden near Athenae, where Plato*
   taught

 < G. Akadēmos, Akadēmou, m. *a hero of ancient Greek legend*

arteria, arteriae, f. 동맥(動脈)   **E** *artery; arteriovenous*

  > arterialis, arteriale 동맥의   **E** *arterial*

  > arteriola, arteriolae, f. (< + -ola *diminutive suffix*)

    세동맥(細動脈)   **E** *arteriole, arteriolar*

    > *metarteriola, *metarteriolae, f. (< *arterial capillary* < G. met(a)-
      between, along with, across, after) 메타세동맥   **E** *metarteriole*

 < G. artēria, artērias, f. *windpipe* > *artery, vein*

  > L. arteritis, arteritidis, f. (< G. artēria + -itis *noun suffix denoting*
    inflammation) 동맥염   **E** *arteritis*

   > L. endarteritis, endarteritidis, f. (< G. end(o)- < endon *within*)

    동맥속막염, 동맥내막염   **E** *endarteritis*

< G. airein (aeirein) *to raise; (passive) to rise*

 > G. aortē, aortēs, f. *aorta*

  > L. aorta, aortae, f. 대동맥   **E** *aorta, aortic*

 > G. eōra, eōras, f. *suspension, string*

  > G. meteōros, meteōros, metēoron (< met(a)- *between, along with, across*
    after + eōra) *lifted up, in air*   **E** *meteorology*

   > L. meteorum, meteori, n. 운석(隕石)   **E** *meteor, meteorite*

< IE. wer- *to raise, to lift, to hold suspended*

lyra, lyrae, f. 리라, 7현금, 노래, 서정시   **E** *lyre*

 < G. lyra, lyras, f. *lyre*

  > G. lyrikos, lyrikē, lyrikon *of lyre*

   > L. lyricus, lyrica, lyricum 리라의, 서정시의, 서정의   **E** *lyric, (lyric >) lyrical*

nausea, nauseae, f. 뱃멀미, 구역질, 욕지기   **E** *nausea, nauseate, (suggested) noise*

 < G. nausia, nausias, f. (nautia, nautias, f.) *seasickness*

 < G. naus, neōs, f. *ship*

  > G. nautēs, nautou, m. *sailor*

   > L. nauta, nautae, m. 뱃사공   **E** *astronaut (cosmonaut)*

  > G. nautikos, nautikē, nautikon *of or belonging to ships, seafaring*

   > L. nauticus, nautica, nauticum 선원의, 항해의, 해사(海事)의   **E** *nautical*

  > G. nautilos, nautilou, m. *sailor, seaman; paper nautilus*

   > L. nautilus, nautili, m. 낙지의 일종(*paper nautilus*), 앵무조개   **E** *nautilus*

> G. Argonautēs, Argonautou, m. (*Greek mythology*) *one of the legendary heroes who accompanied Jason in the Argo in his quest of the Golden Fleece*
> L. Argonauta, Argonautae, m. (그리스 신화) Argo호의 선원

`E argonaut`

< IE. nau- *boat*
> L. navis, navis, f. 배, 주(舟), 선박

`E nave, navy, naval`

> L. navicula, naviculae, f. (< navis, navis, f. *ship* + -cula *diminutive suffix*) 작은 배
> L. navicularis, naviculare 작은 배의, 배의, 주상(舟狀)의

`E navicular`

> L. navigo, navigavi, navigatum, navigare (< navis, navis, f. *ship* + agěre *to drive, to do*) 항해하다

`E navigate`

> L. navigatio, navigationis, f. 항해

`E navigation`

bursa, bursae, f. 주머니, 윤활낭, 점액낭

`E bursa, purse, reimburse, sporran`

> bursaria, bursariae, f. 금고, 회계

`E bursary`

< G. byrsa, byrsēs, f. *hide, wine-skin*

coryza, coryzae, f. 코감기

`E coryza`

< G. koryza, koryzēs, f. *running at the nose, catarrh*

machina, machinae, f. 기계, 장치, 음모

`E machine, machinery`

> machinor, machinatus sum, machinari 제작하다, 고안하다, 음모하다

`E machinate`

< G. (*Doric*) machana, machanēs, f. (< *that which enables*) *device*
(*Attic*) mēchanē, mēchanēs, f. *device*
> G. mēchanikos, mēchanikē, mēchanikon *ingenious, inventive, clever*

`E mechanic, mechanics, mechanical`

> L. mechanismus, mechanismi, m. 기전(機轉), 기작(機作), 기서(機序), 기제(機制)

`E mechanism`

< IE. magh- *to be able, to have power*

`E may, dismay, might, main (< 'power')`

> (*Old Persian*) magus (< *mighty one*) *member of a priestly caste*
> G. magos, magou, m. *magus*
> L. magus, magi, m. 페르시아의 현자, 마술사

`E magic, magician`

chorda, chordae, f. (corda, cordae, f.) 현(弦), 줄, 끈, 삭(索)

`E chord (cord), notochord, cordon`

> Chordata, Chordatorum, n. (pl.) 척삭동물문(脊索動物門); 척삭동물(脊索動物)

`E Chordata, chordate`

< G. chordē, chordēs, f. *gut, gut string, string, chord*
> G. akrochordōn, akrochordōnos, m. (< akros *extreme, topmost, terminal* + chordē *chord*) *a wart with a thin neck*

`E acrochordon`

< IE. gherə- *gut, entrail*

`E yarn`

> L. hernia, herniae, f. 헤르니아, 탈장, 탈출,

이탈   **E** *hernia, (hernia >) herniated, (hernia >) herniation, herniorrhaphy*

> L. haruspex, haruspicis, m. (< *inspector of entrails* < haru- (*of Etruscan origin*)

+ -spex, -spicis, m. *observer*) (희생동물의 내장을 보고 점치는) 장복(臟卜)

점쟁이   **E** *haruspex*

> G. chorion, choriou, n. *intestinal membrane, fetal membrane, afterbirth*

> L. chorion, chorii, n. 융모막(絨毛膜)   **E** *chorion, chorionic*

[용례] chorion frondosum 거친융모막, 번생융모막, 융모융모막   **E** *chorion frondosum*

chorion laeve 평활융모막, 무융모융모막   **E** *chorion laeve*

(문법) chorion 융모막: 단수 주격

frondosum 잎새 많은, 번생(繁生)하는: 형용사, 중성형 단수 주격

< frondosus, frondosa, frondosum

laeve 매끈한, 평활(平滑)한, 갈고 닦은, 유창한: 형용사, 중성형

단수 주격 < laevis, laeve

> L. choroideus, choroidea, choroideum (chorioideus, chorioidea, chorioideum)

(< + G. eidos *shape*) 융모막 모양의, 혈관이 얼기설기한, 맥락(脈絡)의

(Vide CHOROIDEA; *See* E. *choroid*)

hypha, hyphae, f. 균사(菌絲)   **E** *hypha, (pl.) hyphae, hyphal*

< G. hyphē, hyphēs, f. *web*

< IE. webh- *to weave, also to move quickly*

E *weave, woof, weft, web, webster, wafer, waffle; wave (< 'to move back and forth as in weaving'), microwave, waver (< 'to flicker'), wobble (< 'to move from side to side, to move away')*

schola, scholae, f. 수업, 학교, 학파   **E** *school*

> scholaris, scholare 학교의   **E** *scholar*

< G. scholē, scholēs, f. *holding back, stop, rest, leisure, employment of leisure in disputation, school*

< G. schein *to get*

> G. scholazein *to be at leisure, to devote one's leisure (to learning)*

> G. scholastikos, scholastikē, scholastikon *studious, learned*   **E** *scholastic*

< IE. segh- *to hold*

> L. severus, severa, severum 엄격한, 심한   **E** *severe*

> L. severitas, severitatis, f. 엄격, 심각, 중증도(重症度)   **E** *severity*

> L. perseverus, persevera, perseverum (< per- *through, thoroughly* + severus *severe*) 대단히 엄격한, 심한

> L. persevero, **perseveravi**, perseveratum, perseverare 고수하다, 고집하다, 견디어 내다   **E** *persevere, perseverate*

> L. perseverantia, perseverantiae, f. 참을성, 불굴의 노력   **E** *perseverance*

> L. perseveratio, perseverationis, f. 고집(증), 이상언행
반복증
E *perseveration*

> G. echein (*root* sch–) *to hold, to possess, to be in a certain condition*

> G. hexis, hexeōs, f. *condition, state, behavior, habit*

> G. hektikos, hektikē, hektikon *habitual, consumptive*

> L. hecticus, hectica, hecticum 소모성의, 결핵성의
E *hectic*

> G. kachexia, kachexias, f. (< kakos, kakē, kakon *bad, evil*) *cachexia*

> L. cachexia, cachexiae, f. 불건전한 정신상태, 도덕의 타락, 카켁시아
악액질(惡液質), 종말증
E *cachexia, cachectic*

> G. schēma, schēmatos, n. *holding, form, figure*

> L. schema, schematis, n. 태도, 형, 안(案), 계획, 도해(圖解), 도표,
개요(槪要)
E *schema, (pl.) schemata, scheme, schematic*

> G. epechein (< ep(i)– *upon* + echein *to hold*) *to arrest, to stop, to take a position*

> G. epochē, epochēs, f. *stoppage, station, position (of a planet), fixed point of time*

> L. epocha, epochae, f. (특정의) 시기, (특별한) 때, 신기원, 획기적
사건
E *epoch*

> G. synechein (< syn– *with, together* + echein *to hold*) *to hold together*

> G. synecheia, synecheias, f. *continuity, perseverance*

> L. synechia, synechiae, f. 유착(癒着)
E *synechia, (pl.) synechiae*

> G. ourachos, ourachou, m. (< G. ouron *urine* + echein *to hold*) *a canal in the fetus that connects the urinary bladder with the allantois and, after birth, becomes a fibrous cord*

> L. urachus, urachi, m. 요막관(尿膜管)
E *urachus, urachal*

> G. eunouchos, eunouchou, m. (< eunē, eunēs, f. *bed, marriage bed, bedroom* + och– (< echein) *to hold*) *bedroom guard, chamberlain, eunuch*

> L. eunuchus, eunuchi, m. 내시(內侍), 환관(宦官),
고자(鼓子)
E *eunuch, eunuchism, eunuchoid*

> G. ischein *to hold*

> G. ischaimos, ischaimos, ischaimon (< G. ischein *to hold* + haima *blood*) *holding blood*

> L. ischaemia, ischaemiae, f. 허혈(虛血),
국소빈혈
E *ischaemia (ischemia), ischemic*

> G. sthenos, sthenous, n. *strength*
E *thrombosthenin, calisthenics*

> G. asthenēs, asthenēs, asthenes (< a– *not*) *weak, sick*
E *asthenic*

> G. astheneia, astheneias, f. *weakness, sickness*

> L. asthenia, astheniae, f. 무력(증)(無力(症))

E *asthenia, -asthenia, somasthenia, psychasthenia, neurasthenia, thrombasthenia*

> L. myasthenia, myastheniae, f. (< G. my(o)– *muscle*) 근육

무력증(筋肉無力症)

E *myasthenia*

[용례] myasthenia gravis 중증(重症)
근육무력증

E *myasthenia gravis*

(문법) myasthenia 근육무력증: 단수 주격
gravis 무거운, 심한: 형용사, 남·여성형
단수 주격 < gravis, grave

> L. sthenia, stheniae, f. (< *on the pattern of* asthenia) 강장(强壯), 항진(亢進) E *sthenia*

zona, zonae, f. 허리띠, (여자) 정조, (남자) 전대(錢帶), 대(帶), (기후에 따라 나눈 지구의)
지대(地帶), 지역

E *zone, zonation*

[용례] zona glomerulosa 토리층, 사구대(絲毬帶), 구상대(毬狀帶) E *zona glomerulosa*
zona fasciculata 다발층, 속상대(束狀帶) E *zona fasciculata*
zona reticularis 그물층, 망상대(網狀帶) E *zona reticularis*
(문법) zona 대(帶): 단수 주격
glomerulosa 토리 모양의: 형용사, 여성형 단수 주격
< glomerulosus, glomerulosa, glomerulosum
fasciculata 다발 모양의: 형용사, 여성형 단수 주격
< fasciculatus, fasciculata, fasciculatum
reticularis 그물 모양의: 형용사, 남·여성형 단수 주격
< reticularis, reticulare

> zonula, zonulae, f. (< + -ula *diminutive suffix*) 작은 지대, 작은 띠,
소대(小帶) E *zonula (zonule), zonular*
> zonalis, zonale (zonarius, zonaria, zonarium) 띠의, 전대의 E *zonal (zonary)*
< G. zōnē, zōnēs, f. *belt, girdle; waist, loins*
< G. zōnnynai *to gird*
< IE. yos- *to gird*
> G. zōstēr, zōstēros, m. *girdle, belt, especially as worn by men*
> L. zoster, zosteris, m. 허리띠; 대상포진(帶狀疱疹), 띠헤르페스 E *zoster*

맞대보기 2 어미 -ēs, -istēs으로 끝나는 그리스어 제1변화 명사는 -a로 끝나는 라틴어 명사가
되어 위의 변화(제1변화)를 따른다.

---

charta, chartae, f. 종잇조각, 표지, 문서,
판(板) E *chart, charter, card, discard, carton, cartoon, cartridge, cartel*

[용례] Magna Charta (영국사) 대헌장
(문법) magna 큰: 형용사, 여성형 단수 주격 < magnus, magna, magnum
charta 문서: 단수 주격

< G. chartēs, chartou, m. *leaf of paper, layer of papyrus*
< (*probably*) *Of Egyptian origin*

sophista, sophistae, m. 학자, 철학교사, 궤변가

      < G. sophistēs, sophistou, m. *crafty man, prudent man, teacher of wisdom, sophist*
       > G. sophistikos, sophistikē, sophistikon *sophistic*
        > L. sophisticus, sophistica, sophisticum 궤변의
         > L. sophistico, **sophisticavi**, sophisticatum, sophisticare 궤변을 부리다, 복잡하게 하다, 정교하게 하다

       < G. sophizesthai (*middle*) *to become wise, to become learned, to devise*
        > G. sophisma, sophismatos, n. *clever device*

      < G. sophizein *to make wise, to teach*
     < G. sophos, sophē, sophon *clever, skillful, learned, wise*
      > G. sophia, sophias, f. *cleverness, skill, knowledge, wisdom*

       > G. philosophia, philosophias, f. (< philein (phileein) *to love* + sophia *wisdom*) *philosophy*
        > L. philosophia, philosophiae, f. 철학

       > G. philosophos, philosophou, m. (< philein (phileein) *to love* + sophia *wisdom*) *philosopher*
        > L. philosophus, philosophi, m. 철학자

맞대보기 3 어미 -ē 또는 -ēs로 끝나는 그리스어 제1변화 명사 중 관례상 그대로 쓰는 라틴어 낱말은 일부 격만 그리스어 명사 변화를 따르며 그 외는 위의 변화(제1변화)를 따른다.

---

aloë, aloës, f. 알로에[蘆薈]

    < G. aloē, aloēs, f. *aloe*
   < (*Arabic*) alloch *aloe*

diabetes, diabetae, m. 수도관, 파이프; 당뇨병

    [용례] diabetes mellitus 당뇨병(糖尿病)

      diabetes insipidus 요붕증(尿崩症)

     (문법) diabetes: 단수 주격
       mellitus (꿀처럼) 달콤한: 형용사, 남성형 단수 주격
        < mellitus, mellita, mellitum
       insipidus 맛없는: 형용사, 남성형 단수 주격

< insipidus, insipida, insipidum

< G. diabētēs, diabētou, m. (< di(a)- *through, thoroughly, apart* + bainein)

passer through, siphon

< G. bainein *to go*

< IE. g^wa-, g^wem- *to go, to come* (Vide VENIRE: *See* E. *venue*)

●●● 제2변화

단수 속격의 어미가 –i인 남성, 여성, 중성 명사. 단수 주격의 어간과 단수 속격의 어간이 같다.

●●● 제2변화 제1식

단수 주격 어미가 -us, 속격 어미가 –i; 복수 주격 어미가 –i, 속격 어미가 –orum인 남성 또는 여성 명사. 성은 거의 남성이다.

nucleus, nuclei, m. 핵

	단 수	복 수	
주격	nucle-us	nucle-i	~이, ~가, ~은, ~는, ~께서
속격	nucle-i	nucle-orum	~의
여격	nucle-o	nucle-is	~게, ~에게, ~께, ~한테
대격	nucle-um	nucle-os	~을, ~를
탈격	nucle-o	nucle-is	~에서, ~로부터, ~으로부터
호격	nucle-e	nucle-i	~여, ~이여

nucleus, nuclei, m. 핵(核), 중심

E *nucleus*, (pl.) *nuclei, nuclear, nucleate, anucleate, multinucleate, enucleate, nucleopore, nucleic acid, nuclease, nucleoside(s)* (< 'a glycoside'), *nucleotide(s)* (< 'perhaps on the pattern of peptide'); *nucleoplasm, nucleosome*

> nucleolus, nucleoli, m. (< + -olus *diminutive suffix*)

핵소체(核小體)　**E** *nucleolus*, (pl.) *nucleoli, nucleolar; nucleolonema*

< (*syncopated variant*) nuculeus, nuculea, nuculeum (< + -eus *adjective suffix*) 작은 견과의

< nucula, nuculae, f. (< + -ula *diminutive suffix*) 작은 견과

< nux, nucis, f. 견과(堅果)

< IE. kneu- *nut*

           E *nougat, nucellus*

           E *nut, nutmeg (< 'musky nut'), doughnut (donut)*

acervus, acervi, m. 더미, 덩어리, 뭉치

> acervo, **acervavi**, acervatum, acervare 쌓다, 축적하다, 개괄적으로 모아놓다

    > coacervo, **coacervavi**, coacervatum, coacervare (< co- (< cum) *with, together*

      + acervare *to heap*) 쌓아올리다, 누적하다

           E *coacervate*

angulus, anguli, m. 모퉁이, 구석, 각(角)

           E *angle*

> angularis, angulare 각의, 각이 있는, 모난

           E *angular*

> -angulus, -angula, -angulum 각이 있는

    > triangulum, trianguli, n. (< tri- *three*) 삼각형

           E *triangle, triangular*

    > quadrangulum, quadranguli, n. (< quadri- *four*) 사각형 **E** *quadrangle, quadrangular*

    > rectangulus, rectangula, rectangulum (< rectus *right*) 직각의; (rectangulum

      quadrangulum *rectangular quadrangle* >) 구형(矩形)의, 장방형(長方形)의,

      직사각형의   **E** *rectangular*, (rectangulum quadrangulum >) *rectangle*

< IE. ank-, ang- *to bend*

E *angle (< 'fish-hook'), England (< 'land of the Angles' < 'the shape of their original homeland, the Angel district of Schleswig'), ankle*

> L. Angli, Anglorum, m. (pl.) (< *the Angel district of Schleswig*) 앵글족(族)

           E *Anglo-*

    > L. Anglia, Angliae, f. 영국

      > L. Anglicus, Anglica, Anglicum 앵글족의, 영국의, 영어의

           E *Anglicize*

        > L. Anglicanus, Anglicana, Anglicanum 영국의, 영국 국교의

           E *Anglican*

> L. uncus, unci, m. 갈고리, 구(鉤)

           E *uncus, unciform*

    > L. uncinus, uncini, m. 작은 갈고리, 낚싯바늘

      > L. uncinatus, uncinata, uncinatum 갈고리의, 구(鉤)의, 구상(鉤狀)의 **E** *uncinate*

> G. onkos, onkou, m. *barb, grabble-hook*

    > L. Onchocerca, Onchocercae, f. (< + G. kerkos, kerkou, f. *tail*)

    (사상충 絲狀蟲) 옹코서카속(屬)

           E *Onchocerca, onchocerciasis*

> G. ankylos, ankylē, ankylon *crooked, curved*

           E *ancyl(o)- (ankyl(o)-)*

    > G. ankyloun (ankyloein) *to crook, to stiffen*

      > G. ankylōsis, ankylōsēos, f. (< + -ōsis *condition*) *ankylosis*

        > L. ankylosis, ankylosis, f. 관절굳음(증),

        강직(强直)   **E** *ankylosis, (ankylosis >) ankylose*

    > L. Ancylostoma, Ancylostomatis, n. (< + G. stoma, stomatos, n. *mouth*)

    (선충 線蟲) 구충속(鉤蟲屬)

           E *Ancylostoma, ancylostomiasis*

> G. ankōn, ankonōs, m. *curve, bend, elbow*

    > L. ancon, anconis, m. 곱자, 곱척; 팔꿈치

           E *ancon*

      > L. anconeus, anconea, anconeum 팔꿈치의

           E *anconeus, anconeal*

> G. ankyra, ankyras, f. *anchor, support*

           E *ankyrin*

    > L. ancora, ancorae, f. 닻, 피난처, 의지할 곳

           E *anchor, anchorage*

annus, anni, m. 해, 년(年)

> annuus, annua, annuum 일년의, 매년의, 연례의

> annuitas, annuitatis, f. 연금   **E** *annuity*

> semiannuus, semiannua, semiannuum (< semi- *half* + annuus *yearly*)

반년의   **E** *semiannual*

> annualis, annuale 해마다의, 한 해의   **E** *annual, biannual* (< 'semiannual or, rarely, biennial')

> annalis, annale 해[年]의, 연한에 관한   **E** *annals*

> anniversarius, anniversaria, anniversarium (< annus *year* + versus *turning*) 해마다

돌아오는   **E** *anniversary*

> biennium, biennii, n. (< bis *twice* + annus *year*) 2년, 2년의 기간

> biennalis, biennale 2년간의, 2년마다의   **E** *biennial,* lt. *biennale*

> millennium, millennii, n. (< mille *thousand* + annus *year*) 천년   **E** *millennium*

> perennis, perenne (< per- *through, thoroughly* + annus *year*) 1년간 내내 계속되는,

끊임없는, 영구한   **E** *perennial*

< IE. at-, atno- *to go* > *the period gone through, the revolving year*

avus, avi, m. 할아버지

> avunculus, avunculi, m. (*diminutive*) 외삼촌   **E** *avuncular, uncle*

> atavus, atavi, m. (*uncertain*; < IE. ati- *beyond*; < IE. atto- (*nursery word*) *father*)

고조부의 아버지

> atavismus, atavismi, m. 격세유전(隔世遺傳)   **E** *atavism, atavistic*

< IE. awo- *an adult male relative other than one's father*

beccus, becci, m. 부리, 닭 주둥이   **E** *beak*

> Sp. pico *sharp point, peak, beak, little bit*   **E** *pico-, picornavirus*

< *Of Celtic origin*

carpus, carpi, m. 손목, 수근(手根), 손목뼈, 수근골(手根骨)   **E** *carpus*

> carpalis, carpale 손목의, 손목뼈의   **E** *carpal*

< G. karpos, karpou, m. *wrist*

> G. metakarpion, metakarpiou, n. (< met(a)- *between, along with, across,*

after + karpos *wrist* + -ion *diminutive suffix*)

> L. metacarpium, metacarpii, n.

> (*altered*) L. metacarpus, metacarpi, m. 손허리, 중수(中手), 손허리

뼈, 중수골(中手骨)   **E** *metacarpus, metacarpal*

< IE. kwerp- *to turn*

Cartesius, Cartesii, m. (< L. Renatus Cartesius) 데카르트

> Cartesianus, Cartesiana, Cartesianum 데카르트의   **E** *Cartesian*

< F. René Descartes (1596-1650) (< *a family name originated in the Reformation period denoting support for the compromise of religious charters for each municipality* < *of the charters* < L. charta < G. chartēs) 데카르트

catinus, catini, m. 접시, 사발, 도가니
> catillus, catilli, m. 작은 접시, 쟁반 **E** *kettle*
< (*probably*) *Of Mediterranean origin*
∞ (*perhaps*) G. kotylē, kotylēs, m. *small cup (nearly half a pint), socket of the hip joint* **E** *cotyloid*
> G. kotylēdōn, kotylēdōnos, m. *a cup-shaped cavity, the sucker of an octopus, socket of the hip joint;* (*botany*) Cotyledon *navelwort*
> L. cotyledon, cotyledonis, m. (식물) Cotyledon umbilicus, 태반엽(胎盤葉), 떡잎, 자엽(子葉) **E** *cotyledon, monocotyledon (monocot), dicotyledon (dicot)*

cirrus, cirri, m. 곱슬머리 타래; (식물) 덩굴손, 새털구름, 권운(卷雲); (*slender and filamentous, usually flexible, appendages* >) 모상돌기(毛狀突起), (편충의) 음경(陰莖) **E** *cirrus,* (pl.) *cirri, cirr(i)- (cirro-), cirrose (cirrous), cirrate*

Confucius, Confucii, m. 공구(孔丘), 공자(孔子), 공부자(孔夫子) **E** *Confucius, Confucian, Confucianism*
< (*Chinese*) K'ung Futsze(孔夫子)

culmus, culmi, m. (초본의) 줄기, 대, 짚 **E** *culm, culmiferous*
< IE. kolə-mo- *grass, reed* **E** *haulm*
> G. kalamos, kalamou, m. *reed, cane, writing-reed*
> L. calamus, calami, m. (초본의) 줄기, 갈대, 갈대 펜
E *calamus, calamite,* ((*suggested*) calamellus (*diminutive*) >) *caramel, caramelize*

cuniculus, cuniculi, m. 토끼, 토끼굴, 땅굴, 수로, 비밀 계략; 충도(蟲道) **E** *cuniculus, coney (cony)*
< (*probably*) *Of Iberian origin*

dominus, domini, m. 주인 **E** *domino,* It. *don (Don),* Sp. *don (Don)*
[용례] Quo vadis, Domine? 주여, 어디로 가시나이까?
(문법) quo 어디로: 의문 부사
vadis 너는 간다, 당신은 가십니다: 능동태 직설법 현재 단수 이인칭
< vado, vasi, vasum, vadĕre 가다
Domine: 주인이시여, 주여: 단수 호격
[용례] Anno Domini (A.D.) 주님의 해에, 서기(西紀)로 **E** *Anno Domini (A.D.)*
(문법) Anno 해에: 시간의 탈격 (단수 탈격) < annus, anni, m.
Domini 주님의: 단수 속격

> domina, dominae, f. 안주인

> **E** *dame;* It. *donna,* (prima domina *'first lady'* >) It. *prima donna,* (mea domina *'my lady'* >) It. *madonna;* (mea domina *'my lady'* >) F. *madame,* (pl.) *mesdames*

> dominicella, dominicellae, f. (< + -ella *diminutive suffix*) 처녀

> **E** (mea dominicella *'my young lady'* >) F. *mademoiselle,* (pl.) *mesdemoiselles;* *damsel*

> dominium, dominii, n. 소유권, 소유지, 소유, 지배, 영역   **E** *domain*

> dominio, dominionis, f. 주권, 지배권, 통치권   **E** *dominion, dungeon*

> *domininarium, *domininarii, n. †지배, †지배권, †지배영역; 위험, 위험 요인   **E** *danger* (< *'power to harm'*)

> condominium, condominii, n. 공동 주관   **E** *condominium (condo)*

> dominor, dominatus sum, dominari 주인노릇하다, 다스리다   **E** *dominate*

> dominans, (gen.) dominantis (*present participle*) 지배적인, 우세한, 우성(優性)의   **E** *dominant,* (dominant >) *codominant,* (dominant >) *dominance*

> praedominor, praedominatus sum, praedominari (< prae- *before, beyond* + dominari *to rule*) 지배하다, 우월하다   **E** *predominate, predominant*

< domus, domus, f. (domus, domi, f.) 집, 고향, 본국, 가족

> domesticus, domestica, domesticum 집안의, 국내의   **E** *domestic*

> domestico, **domesticavi**, domesticatum, domesticare 길들이다   **E** *domesticate*

> domicilium, domicilii, n. (< domus *house* + colĕre *to cultivate, to dwell*) 거처, 주소   **E** *domicile*

< IE. dem- *house, household*   **E** *timber*

> G. dōma, dōmatos, n. *house, household, palace, temple*   **E** *dome*

fiscus, fisci, m. 바구니, 금고, 국고

> fiscalis, fiscale 국고의, 국가 재정의   **E** *fiscal*

> confisco, **confiscavi**, confiscatum, confiscare (< con- (< cum) *with, together* + fiscus *basket, chest, treasury*) 국고에 귀속시키다, 몰수하다   **E** *confiscate*

< IE. bheidh- *to weave, to tie*

fumus, fumi, m. 연기, 김, 증기

> **E** (*noun*) *fume,* (fumus terrae (Fumaria officinalis) *'smoke of the earth; so called from its smell'* >) *fumitory*

> fumaria, fumariae, f. 현호색과(玄胡索科)의 식물(괴불주머니 비슷한, 향기 나는 꽃이 핌); (Fumaria) 푸마리아속(屬)   **E** *fumaric acid* (< *'found in* Fumaria officinalis*'*), *fumarate*

> fumo, **fumavi**, fumatum, fumare 연기가 나다, 연기를 내다, 김이 나다, 김을 내다   **E** (*verb*) *fume,* (per- *'through, thoroughly'* + fumare *'to smoke'* >) *perfume*

> fumatorium, fumatorii, n. 훈증실(燻蒸室)   **E** *fumatory*

> fumigo, **fumigavi**, fumigatum, fumigare (< fumus *smoke* + agĕre *to drive, to do*) 연기를 내다, 연기를 쐬다   **E** *fumigate, fumigant*

< IE. dheu-, dheue- *the base of a wide variety of derivatives meaning 'to rise in a cloud', as dust, vapor, or smoke, and related to semantic notions of breath, various color adjectives, and forms denoting defective perception or wits*

E *dust, down* (< *'bird's down'* < *'fine like dust'*), *dusk, dun, dizzy, dizziness, doze, dull, deaf, dumb, dumbbell* (< *'an apparatus, like that for swinging a church-bell, but without the bell itself, and thus making no noise, in the 'ringing' of which bodily exercise was taken'*), (*dumb* >) *dummy, dwell* (< *'to remain in a place'* < *'to lead astray'*), *indwell* (< *'originally translating* L. *inhabitare to inhabit'*); *dove* (< *'dark-colored bird'*); *deer* (< *'breathing creature'*), *reindeer* (< *'horned animal'*), (*wild deer* > *'land inhabited only by wild animals'* >) *wilderness*

> L. fuscus, fusca, fuscum 어둠침침한, 가무잡잡하게 그을린, 갈색의　　**E** *fuscous, lipofuscin*

　　> L. fusco, fuscavi, fuscatum, fuscare 어둡게 하다

　　　　> L. offusco, offuscavi, offuscatum, offuscare (obfusco, obfuscavi, ob-
　　　　　　fuscatum, obfuscare (< of- (< ob) *before, toward(s), over, against, away*) 어둡게 하다, 혼란시키다　　**E** *obfuscate*

> (*possibly*) L. foeteo, –, –, foetēre (feteo, –, –, fetēre) 악취를 풍기다, 썩다

　　> L. foetor, foetoris, m. (fetor, fetoris, m.) 악취, 입냄새　　**E** *fetor*

　　> L. foetidus, foetida, foetidum (fetidus, fetida, fetidum) 악취를 풍기는　　**E** *fetid*

> (*possibly*) L. furo, furui, –, furère 미쳐 날뛰다, 격정에 사로잡히다, 격분하다

　　> L. furia, furiae, f. 광란, 격분, 흑사병; (Furiae) (로마 신화) 복수의 세 여신　**E** *fury, Furies*

　　　　> L. furiosus, furiosa, furiosum 미쳐 날뛰는　　**E** *furious*

　　　　> L. infurio, infuriavi, infuriatum, infuriare (< in- *in, into, onto, toward* +
　　　　　　furia *fury*) 격분시키다　　**E** *infuriate*

　　> L. furor, furoris, m. 광포, 벅찬 감격, 미친 듯한 열정　　**E** *furor*

> (*possibly*) L. februm, febri, n. 청정(淸淨), 재계(齋戒); (pl.) (고대 로마에서 2월에 거행한)
　　속죄의 제사

　　> L. Februarius, Februaria, Februarium 속죄 제사의,
　　　　2월의　　**E** (Februarius mensis *'month of expiation'* >) *February*

> G. typhein *to smoke*

　　> G. typhos, typhou, m. *smoke, steam, stupor*

　　　　> L. typhus, typhi, m. 티푸스(열병으로 머리가 멍해지는 것), 발진티푸스,
　　　　　　질부사(窒扶斯)

　　　　E *typhus, typhous, typhoid, typhoidal, paratyphoid* (< *'infection due to any of the Salmonella serotypes except* S. typhi'), *stove, stew*

> G. theion, theiou, n. *brimstone, sulfur*　**E** *thi(o)-, thiamine, thiol-, thion-, methionine (Met, M)*

> G. thyein *to burn (incense), to offer burnt-sacrifice*

　　> G. thyia, thyias, f. *a kind of resinous tree or a juniper*

　　　　> L. thuja, thujae, f. (< thuia) 향나무, 생명의 나무 (arbor vitae); (Thuja)
　　　　　　측백(側柏)나무속(屬)　　**E** *thuja*

　　> G. thymos, thymou, m. *spirit, mind, courage*　　**E** *-thymia, dysthymia*

　　> G. thymon, thymou, n. (thymos, thymou, m.) (< *plant having a strong smell*)
　　　　thyme

> L. thymum, thymi, n. (thymus, thymi, m.) 백리향(百里香)　　　E *thyme*

> G. thyein *to rage, to seethe*

> G. ekthyein *to break out as heat or humors*

> G. ekthyma, ekthymatos, n. (< ek- *out of, away from*) *ecthyma*

> L. ecthyma, ecthymatis, n. 고름궤양증, 농창(膿瘡)　　E *ecthyma*

> G. typhlos, typhlē, typhlon *blind*　　　E *typhl(o)-, typhlology*

> G. typhlon, typhlou, n. *cecum*

> L. typhlon, typhli, n. 맹장(盲腸)　　　E *typhlitis*

fundus, fundi, m. 바닥, 토지, 토대, 기저(基底)　　　E *fundus, fundic, fund*

> fundo, fundavi, fundatum, fundare 토대를 세우다　　　E *found*

> fundatio, fundationis, f. 토대, 기초　　　E *foundation*

> fundamentum, fundamenti, n. 토대, 기초　　　E *fundament, fundamental*

> profundus, profunda, profundum (< pro- *before, forward, for, instead of*)
깊은　　　E *profound, profundity*

> latifundium, latifundii, n. (< latus *broad* + fundus *estate*) 대지주(大地主)의
토지　　　E *latifundium, (pl.) latifundia*

< IE. bhudh-, budh- *bottom, base*　　　E *bottom*

> G. abyssos, abyssou, m. (< a- *without* + byssos, byssou, m. *bottom*) *bottomless
chasm*　　　E *abyss*

gibbus, gibbi, m. (gibba, gibbae, f.) 혹, 곱사등, 육봉(肉峰)　　　E *gibbous, gibbosity*

gladius, gladii, m. 검(劍)

> gladiolus, gladioli, m. (< + -olus *diminutive suffix*) 작은 검, 글라디올러스, 흉골체
(胸骨體)　　　E *gladiolus*

> gladiator, gladiatoris, m. 검투사　　　E *gladiator*

< IE. kel- *to strike, to cut; with derivatives referring to something broken or cut off, piece of
wood, twig*

E ((*Gaelic*) claidheamh mor *'sword great'* >) **claymore, hilt, Hilda** (< *'battle'*), **Matilda** (<
'mighty in battle')

> L. calamitas, calamitatis, f. 재난　　　E *calamity, calamitous*

> G. kolaphos, kolaphou, m. *blow with the fist*

> L. colaphus, colaphi, m. 주먹으로 한 대 침, 손바닥으로 때림, 뺨 때림

E F. *coup*, F. *contrecoup* (< *'counterblow'*), **cope** (< *'to deal effectively with
something difficult'*), **coupon** (< *'a detachable portion of a stock certificate' <
'piece cut off'*), **recoup**

> G. kolobos, kolobē, kolobon *curtailed*　　　E *colobus monkey* (< *'shortened thumbs'*)

> G. kolobōma, kolobōmatos, n. (< + -ōma *resultative noun suffix*) *the part
removed in mutilation*

> L. coloboma, colobomatis, n. 결손

E *coloboma*

> G. klan (klaein) *to break*

> G. klasis, klaseōs, f. *breaking*

E *-klasis*

> G. klasma, klasmatos, n. *breaking*

E *iconoclasm*

> G. klastēs, klastou, m. *breaker*

E *-clast, iconoclast (< 'image breaker'), osteoclast (< 'bone breaker'), chondroclast (< 'cartilage breaker')*

> G. klastos, klastē, klaston *broken*

E *clastic, -clastic, pyroclastic (< 'broken in fragments by fire'), leukocytoclastic (< 'of leukocytic (neutrophilic) fragments')*

> G. klados, kladou, m. *branch, shoot, olive-branch (wound round with wool and presented with suppliants*

E *clade, clad(o)-, cladogram (< 'a dendrogram illustrating the supposed evolutionary relationship between clades')*

> G. klōn, klōnos, m. *twig, shoot, sprout*

E *clone, clonal, clonality, monoclonality, polyclonality*

> L. Clonorchis, Clonorchis, f. (< + G. orchis *testis*) (흡충) 간흡충속(屬); 간디스토마

E *Clonorchis, clonorchiasis*

> G. klēros, klērou, m. *lot, drawing lots (many officials at Athens obtained their offices by lot), share, the clergy (as opposed to the laity)*

E *clerk, clerical, clergy*

> IE. kleg- *to cry, to sound*

E *laugh, laughter*

hortus, horti, m. 정원

E *horticulture*

> hortensis, hortense 정원의, 정원 재배의

< IE. gher- *to grasp, to enclose; with derivatives meaning 'enclosure'*

E *gird, girdle, girth, garden, kindergarten, Asgard (< 'god's yard'), yard (< 'enclosure'), orchard (< 'god's yard')*

> G. choros, chorou, m. *dancing-place, dancing in a ring, choral dance, chorus*

> L. chorus, chori, m. 무도, 윤무, 가무, 합창

E *chorus, choir, choral*

> G. choreia, choreias, f. *dance*

E *choreographer, choreomania*

> L. chorea, choreae, f. 춤, 무도병

E *chorea, choreic, choreatic; choreiform*

> G. choraulēs, choraulou, m. (< choros *dance* + aulos *flute*) *flute player who accompanied the dance*

> L. choraules, choraulae, m. 합창 반주의 플루트 주자

E *carol*

> L. cohors, cohortis, f. (< co- (< cum) *with, together*) 울안, 떼; (로마) 보병대 (Legio의 10분의 1)

E *cohort, court, courteous, courtesy, (courtesy >) curtsy (curtsey), (*cohortitiana >) courtesan, courtship*

humerus, humeri, m. 어깨, 위팔, 상완(上腕); 위팔뼈, 상완골(上腕骨)

E *humerus*

> *humeralis, *humerale 어깨의, 위팔의; 위팔뼈의, 상완골의

E *humeral*

< IE. om(e)so- *shoulder*

> G. ōmos, ōmou, m. *shoulder, upper arm*　　　　　　　　　**E** *om(o)-*

> G. akrōmion, akrōmiou, n. (< akros *extreme* + ōmos + -ion *diminutive suffix*)

point of the shoulder　　　　　　　　**E** *acromion, acromial*

jocus, joci, m. 농담, 장난, 놀이

> **E** *joke, joker, jewel, jewellery (jewelry)*, (jocus partitus *'divided play or game, even game'* > *'uncertain chance, uncertainty'* >) *jeopardy, jeopardize*

> joculus, joculi, m. (< + -ulus *diminutive suffix*) 우스갯소리, 장난감

> jocularis, joculare 우스꽝스러운, 익살맞은　　　　　　　　**E** *jocular*

> joculor, joculatus, sum, joculari 장난하다, 익살부리다　　　　**E** *juggle*

< IE. yek- *to speak*

lectus, lecti, m. (lectus, lectus, m.) 침상, (고대 로마의)

식탁　　　　　　　　　**E** *litter, littermate, coverlet, wagon-lit*

< IE. legh- *to lie, to lay*

> **E** *lie, underlie, lay, allay* (< *'to lay aside, to lay down'*), *inlay, onlay, layer, lair*, D. *Lager* (< *'a store for keeping'*), *ledge, ledger, low* (< *'lying flat'*), (comparative) *lower*, (IE. ambhi *'around'* > *bi- *'at, by'* >) *below, law* (< *'that which is set down'*), *bylaw* (< *'local ordinance'*), (IE. peku- *'wealth, movable property, livestock'* + IE. legh- > *'business partner'* >) *fellow*, (D. Anlage *'laying on, for the first'* >) *anlage*

> G. lochos, lochou, m. *place for lying in wait, ambush, childbirth*

> G. locheios, locheia, locheion *of child*

birth　　　　　**E** *(neuter pl.) lochia* (< *'vaginal discharge after childbirth'*)

locus, loci, m. 장소, 지방, 자리, 유전자 자리, 유전자좌(遺傳子座)

> **E** *locus*, (pl.) *loci, locoregional, locomotion, locomotor, lieu*, (locum tenens *'holding the place (of another)'* >) *lieutenant*, (medius locus *'middle place'* >) *milieu*

> localis, locale 장소의, 지역적인, 국소(局所)의

> **E** *local*, (local >) *localize*, (F. local >) *locale* (< *'respelled to indicate stress on the final syllable'*)

> localitas, localitatis, f. 장소, 지역, 현장, 자리잡기　　　　**E** *locality*

> loculus, loculi, m. (< + -ulus *diminutive suffix*) 작은 장소, 칸막이한 동물의

우리 하나, 소방(小房), 소강(小腔), 소실(小室)　**E** *loculus (locule)*, (pl.) *loculi*

> locularis, loculare 칸막이한, 방이

있는　　　　　　**E** *locular, unilocular, bilocular, multilocular*

> loculatus, loculata, loculatum 칸막이한, 방이 있는　　　　**E** *loculate*

> loco, locavi, locatum, locare 놓다　　　　**E** *locate*, (locate >) *relocate*

> locatio, locationis, f. 배치, 위치,

임대　　　**E** *location*, (location >) *translocation*, (translocation >) *translocate*

> alloco, **allocavi**, allocatum, allocare (< al- (< ad) *to, toward, at, according to*) 할당하다, 배분하다, 배당하다, 배치하다　　**E** *allocate*

　　> allocatio, allocationis, f. 할당, 배분, 배당, 배치　　**E** *allocation*

> colloco, **collocavi**, collocatum, collocare (< col- (< cum) *with, together* + locare *to place*) 나란히 놓다, 배치하다; (문법) 연어(連語)를 이루다　　**E** *collocate, couch*

　　> collocatio, collocationis, f. 배치; (문법) 연어　　**E** *collocation*

> disloco, **dislocavi**, dislocatum, dislocare (< dis- *apart from, down, not* + locare *to place*) 자리를 바꾸다, 전위(轉位)하다, 탈구(脫臼)하다　　**E** *dislocate*

　　> dislocatio, dislocationis, f. 어긋남, 이탈, 전위, 탈구　　**E** *dislocation (luxation)*

< (*probably*) IE. stlokos *place*

< IE. stel- *to put, to stand; with derivatives referring to a standing object or place*　　**E** *still, stall, stallion, forestall, pedestal* (< '*foot stall*'), *stale, stalemate, stalk, stilt, stout*

> L. stallum, stalli, n. 마구간의 한 칸, 합창대 석

> **E** *install* (< '*to instate in an office, rank, etc. with the customary ceremonies or formalities*' < '*to invest with an office or dignity by seating in a stall or official seat, as the choir-stall of a canon in a cathedral, or that of a Knight of the Garter or Bath in the chapel of his order, the throne of a bishop, etc.*')

> L. stolidus, stolida, stolidum (< *firm-standing*) 우둔한, 뜻 없는　　**E** *stolid*

> L. stultus, stulta, stultum (< *unmovable, uneducated*) 어리석은　　**E** *stultify*

> G. stēlē, stēlēs, f. *pillar, post, headstone*　　**E** *stele,* (pl.) *stelai*

　　> L. stela, stelae, f. 기둥, 석탑, 묘비　　**E** *stela,* (pl.) *stelae*

> G. stellein *to put in order, to prepare, to send, to make compact* (*with o-grade and zero-grade forms* stol- *and* stal-)

　　> G. apostellein (< ap(o)- *away from, from*) *to send away*

　　　　> G. apostolos, apostolou, m. *messenger, apostle*

　　　　　　> L. apostolus, apostoli, m. 사도　　**E** *apostle, apostolic*

　　> G. epistellein (< ep(i)- *upon*) *to send to, to send a message*

　　　　> G. epistolē, epistolēs, f. *message, order, letter*

　　　　　　> L. epistola, epistolae, f. (epistula, epistulae, f.) 편지, 문서　　**E** *epistle, epistolary*

　　> G. diastellein (< di(a)- *through, thoroughly, apart*) *to put away, to separate, to dilate*

　　　　> G. diastolē, diastolēs, f. *putting away, separation, dilatation*

　　　　　　> L. diastole, diastoles, f. 음절연장(단음절을 길게 함); 확장(擴張), 확장기(擴張期), 이완(弛緩), 이완기(弛緩期)　　**E** *diastole, diastolic*

　　> G. systellein (< sy- (< syn) *with, together*) *to draw, to shorten, to contract*　　**E** *systaltic*

　　　　> G. systolē, systolēs, f. *putting together, shortening, contraction*

　　　　　　> L. systole, systoles, f. 음절단축(장음절을 짧게 함); 수축(收縮), 수축기(收縮期)　　**E** *systole, systolic*

> L. asystole, asystoles, f. (< G. a- *not*)

무수축(無收縮)　　　　　　　　　　　　　　**E** *asystole (asystolia), asystolic*

> G. peristellein (< peri- *around, near, beyond, on account of*) *to wrap up;*

(*passive, in medical context*) *to be contracted round*　　　　**E** *peristaltic*

> L. peristalsis, peristalsis, f. 꿈틀운동,

연동(蠕動)　　　　　　　　　　**E** *peristalsis, antiperistalsis, aperistalsis*

lumbus, lumbi, n. 허리, 요부(腰部), (가축) 등심;

성욕의 자리　　　　　**E** *lumbus (loin), loin,* (super + lumbus *'above the loin'* >) *sirloin*

> lumbaris, lumbare 허리의, 요부의　　　　　　　　　　　　**E** *lumbar*

> lumbago, lumbaginis, f. 요통, 허리통증　　　　　　**E** *lumbago, lumbaginous*

< IE. lendh- *loin*

mucus, muci, m. 점액, 콧물　　　　**E** *mucus, muc(o)-, mucin(s), mucinous; mucinogen*

> mucilago, mucilaginis, f. (식물성) 점액　　　　　　**E** *mucilage, mucilaginous*

> mucosus, mucosa, mucosum 점액이 많은, 점액을 분비하는, 점액의, 점액성의　　　**E** *mucous*

[용례] tunica mucosa (< *mucous membrane*) 점막(粘膜)

(문법) tunica 막: 단수 주격 < tunica, tunicae, f. 층, 막

mucosa: 형용사, 여성형 단수 주격

> mucosa, mucosae, f. 점막(粘膜)　　　　　　　　　**E** *mucosa, mucosal*

[용례] lamina propria mucosae (점막) 고유판　　　　**E** *lamina propria*

lamina muscularis mucosae 점막 근(육)판　　　**E** *muscularis mucosae*

(문법) lamina 판: 단수 주격 < lamina, laminae, f. 판, 층

propria 고유한: 형용사, 여성형 단수 주격

< proprius, propria, proprium 자기 자신에게 속한, 고유한

muscularis 근의, 근육의: 형용사, 남·여성형 단수 주격

< muscularis, musculare

mucosae 점막의: 단수 속격

> mucidus, mucida, mucidum 곰팡 난, 쉰,

코 흘리는　　　　**E** *moist,* (*moist* >) *moisture,* (*moisture* >) *moisturize, musty*

> mucor, mucoris, m. 곰팡이; (Mucor) (곰팡이) 털곰팡이속(屬)　　　**E** *mucor*

< IE. meug- *slimy, slippery; with derivatives referring to various wet or slimy substances*

and conditions. **E** *smuggle (< 'to slip contraband through'), mold (mould), moldy (mouldy), meek*

> G. myxa, myxas, f. *mucus, lamp wick*

E *myx(o)-, myxoid, myxovirus (< 'the viruses with a particular affinity for certain mucins'), orthomyxovirus, paramyxovirus, match (< 'wick of a candle' ' 'lamp wick')*

> L. myxoma, myxomatis, n. (< *myxoid tumor of primitive connective tissue*

cells < + G. -ōma *noun suffix denoting tumor*) 점액종　　　**E** *myxoma*

> L. myxoedema, myxoedematis, n. (< *myxoid edema due to glycosaminoglycan*

deposition < + G. oidēma *swelling*) 점액부종   **E** *myxoedema (myxedema)*

> G. mykēs, mykētos, m. *mushroom*   **E** *myc(o)-, mycet(o)-, mycology*

>> L. -myces, -mycetis, m. 버섯,

곰팡이   **E** *-myces,* (pl.) *-mycetes, -mycete, -mycetin, -mycin*

>> L. saccharomyces, saccharomycetis, m. (< G. sakcharon *sugar*)

사카로미세스, 효모균   **E** *saccharomyces,* (pl.) *saccharomycetes*

>> L. schizosaccharomyces, schizosaccharomycetis, m. (< G.

schizein *to split*) 분열사카로미세스,

분열효모균   **E** *schizosaccharomyces,* (pl.) *schizosaccharomycetes*

>> L. streptomyces, streptomycetis, m. (< G. streptos *twisted*)

스트렙토미세스   **E** *streptomyces, streptomycin*

>> L. mycelium, mycelii, n. (< *on the pattern of* epithelium)

균사체(菌絲體)   **E** *mycelium,* (pl.) *mycelia, mycelial*

>> L. mycosis, mycosis, f. (< + G. -ōsis *condition*) 진균증(眞菌症),

곰팡이병   **E** *mycosis, mycotic, -mycosis, -mycotic*

>> L. mycobacterium, mycobacterii, n. (< *moldlike growth on the surface of*

liquid media + bacterium) 마이코박테륨   **E** *mycobacterium, mycobacterial*

∞ IE. meus- *damp; with derivatives referring to swampy ground and vegetation and to*

figurative qualities

of wetness   **E** *mire, moss,* (IE. wel- 'to see' + IE. meus- > 'moss used in dyeing' >) *litmus*

> L. mustus, musta, mustum 풋, 햇, 새, 신선한

>> L. mustum, musti, n. (발효 전의) 포도즙, 햇포도주

E *mustard* (< 'originally prepared by making the ground seeds of certain cruciferous plants into a paste with must')

> G. mysos, mysous, m. *uncleanness*   **E** *mysophobia*

musculus, musculi, m. (< + -culus *diminutive suffix*) 작은 쥐, 근육, 근, 섭조개, (성곽 포위

작전에 쓰는) 이동식 엄폐물   **E** *muscle, mussel,* (musculus >) *musculature*

[용례] musculus soleus 가자미근   **E** *soleus (muscle)*

musculus serratus anterior 앞톱니근   **E** *serratus anterior (muscle)*

musculus uvulae 목젖근   **E** *musculus uvulae*

musculus orbicularis oculi 눈둘레근   **E** *orbicularis oculi (muscle)*

musculus orbicularis oris 입둘레근   **E** *orbicularis oris (muscle)*

musculi lumbricales 벌레근   **E** *lumbrical muscles*

musculus masseter 깨물근   **E** *masseter (muscle)*

musculus extensor digitorum longus (< *long extensor of toes*)

긴발가락폄근   **E** *extensor digitorum longus (muscle)*

musculus levator palpebrae superioris (< *levator of upper eyelid*)

위눈꺼풀올림근, 상안검거근   **E** *levator palpebrae superioris (muscle)*

(문법) musculus 근육, 근: 단수 주격

soleus 가자미 모양의: 형용사, 남성형 단수 주격

< soleus, solea, soleum

serratus 톱니 자국의: 과거분사, 남성형 단수 주격

  < serratus, serrata, serratum

  < serro, serravi, serratum, serrare 톱으로 켜다, 자르다

anterior 앞의: 형용사, 남·여성형 단수 주격

  < anterior, anterior, anterius ((gen.) anterioris)

uvulae 목젖의: 명사, 단수 속격 < uvula, uvulae, f.

orbicularis 둘레의: 형용사, 남·여성형 단수 주격

  < orbicularis, orbiculare

oculi 눈의: 명사, 단수 속격 < oculus, oculi, m.

oris 입의: 명사, 단수 속격 < os, oris, n.

musculi 근육들: 복수 주격

lumbricales 지렁이 모양의: 형용사, 남·여성형 복수 주격

  < lumbricalis, lumbricale

masseter 깨물근: 명사, 단수 주격 (musculus와 동격)

  < masseter, masseteri, m.

extensor 폄근: 명사, 단수 주격 (musculus와 동격)

  < extensor, extensoris, m.

digitorum 발가락들의: 명사, 복수 속격 < digitus, digiti, m.

longus 긴: 형용사, 남성형 단수 주격 < longus, longa, longum

levator 올림근: 명사, 단수 주격 (musculus와 동격)

  < levator, levatoris, m.

palpebrae 눈꺼풀의: 명사, 단수 속격 < palpebra, palpebrae, f.

superioris 위의: 형용사, 남·여·중성형 단수 속격

  < superior, superior, superius ((gen.) superioris)

> muscularis, musculare 근육의   **E** *muscular, intramuscular, neuromuscular*

< mus, muris, m., f. ((gen. pl.) murium) 쥐, 생쥐

> murinus, murina, murinum 쥐의, 생쥐의   **E** *murine*

< IE. mus- *mouse; also a muscle, from the resemblance of a flexing muscle to the movements of a mouse*   **E** *mouse*

> G. mys, myos, m. *mouse, muscle*   **E** *my(o)-, myoblast, myocyte, myofiber, myofibril, myosin, myoid*

> G. myosōtis, myosōtidos, f. (< ous, ōtos, n. *ear*) *a plant with leaves like a mouse's ears*

> L. myosotis, myosotidis, f. 물망초; (Myosotis) 물망초속(屬)   **E** *myosotis*

> L. endomysium, endomysii, n. (< G. end(o)- < endon *within*) 근육내막, 근육속막   **E** *endomysium, endomysial*

> L. perimysium, perimysii, n. (< G. peri- *around, near, beyond, on account of*) 근육다발막   **E** *perimysium, perimysial*

> L. epimysium, epimysii, n. (< G. ep(i)- *upon*) 근육외막, 근육바깥막   **E** *epimysium, epimysial*

> G. myōn, myōnos, m. *muscle, cluster of muscles*

> (*probably*) G. myelos, myelou, m. *bone marrow; spinal marrow* (< *the spinal cord seen within the spinal column's vertebral canal resembles the bone marrow within the medullary cavities of long bones*)

> **E** **myel(o)-;** (*myel(o)- 'bone marrow'* >) **myeloblast, myelocyte, myeloid, osteomyelitis;** (*myel(o)- 'spinal marrow'* >) **myelin** (< *'peripheral nerve marrow apparently identical to what could be found in the spinal cord'*), **myelinate, demyelinate, unmyelinated, myelinize, encephalomyelitis, poliomyelitis, -myelia**

> (*Sanskrit*) muska *scrotum*

> **E** **musk** (< *'from the similarity in shape of the sac on the abdomen of a male musk deer in which musk is produced'*), **musky, nutmeg** (< *'musky nut'*)

nervus, nervi, m. 힘줄, 활시위, 현(弦), 기력; 신경

E **nerve,** (*nerve* >) **innervate, denervate, reinnervate**

> nervosus, nervosa, nervosum 힘줄이 많은, 억센; 신경의, 신경성의, 신경과민의

E **nervous**

< IE. (s)neu- *sinew*

> G. neuron, neurou, n. *nerve, sinew, muscle*

E **neur(o)-, neural** (< *'of nerves, or of the nervous system'*), **endoneural** (< *'within a nerve'*), **perineural** (< *'around a nerve'*), **neurite** (< *'neuronal process'*), **neurotize** (< *'to reinnervate'* < *'with unexplained insertion of -t-'*); (*neural stem cell* >) **nestin, neuraminic acid** (< *'an amino sugar: a cleavage product of a brain lipoid'*), (*neuraminic acid* > (*probably*) *'on the pattern of hyaluronidase'* >) **neuraminidase**

> L. neuron, neuri, n. 신경세포, 신경원(神經元)

E **neuron, neuronal,** (*internuncial neuron* >) **interneuron**

> L. neurula, neurulae, f. (< G. neuron *nerve* + L. -ula *diminutive suffix*) 신경배(神經胚)

E **neurula,** (*neurula* >) **neurulation**

> L. neurosis, neurosis, f. (< G. neuron *nerve* + -ōsis *condition*) 신경증(神經症)

E **neurosis, neurotic,** D. Neurose

> L. aponeurosis, aponeurosis, f. (< *broadened sinew* < G. ap(o)- *away from, from* + neuron *sinew* + -ōsis *condition*) 널힘줄, 건막(腱膜)

E **aponeurosis, aponeurotic**

> L. endoneurium, endoneurii, n. (< G. end(o)- *within*) 신경내막, 신경속막

E **endoneurium, endoneurial**

> L. perineurium, perineurii, n. (< G. peri- *around, near, beyond, on account of*) 신경다발막

E **perineurium, perineurial**

> L. epineurium, epineurii, n. (< G. ep(i)- *upon*) 신경외막, 신경바깥막

E **epineurium, epineurial**

< IE. (s)ne- *to spin, to sew*

E **needle**

> G. nēma, nēmatos, n. *thread*

E **nemat(o)-, nem(o)- (nema-), nemaline** (< *'thread-like'*), **-nema (-neme), axoneme** (< *'axial thread'*), **plectonemic** (< *'of twisted thread'*), **synaptonemal** (< *'of conjoined threads'*); **nucleolonema**

> L. Nemathelminthes, Nemathelminthium, m. (pl.) (< + G. helmins, helminthos, m. *parasitic worm*) (기생충) 선형동물문(線形動物門)　　　**E** *nemathelminth*

> L. Nematoda, Nematodorum, n. (pl.) (< + G. -ōdēs *like, resembling*) (선형 동물) 선충강(線蟲綱)　　　**E** *nematode*

> L. treponema, treponematis, n. (< G. trepein *to turn*) (세균) 트레포네마균　　　**E** *treponema, treponemal*

numerus, numeri, m. 수, 다수, 서민, 종류, (전체에 대한)

　　부분　　　**E** *number,* (numero (abl.) *'in number'* >) *No.*

> numeralis, numerale 수의, 수를 표시하는　　　**E** *numeral*

> numerarius, numeraria, numerarium 수의, 수에 관한

　　> supernumerarius, supernumeraria, supernumerarium (< super- *above*) 과잉의, 과다한　　　**E** *supernumerary*

> numericus, numerica, numericum 수의, 수로 표시된　　　**E** *numeric (numerical)*

> numerosus, numerosa, numerosum 수많은　　　**E** *numerous*

> numero, **numeravi,** numeratum, numerare 세다, 계산하다　　　**E** *numerate, numerator, numeracy* (< *'on the model of literacy'*)

　　> numerabilis, numerabile 셀 수 있는　　　**E** *numerable*

　　　> innumerabilis, innumerabile (< in- *not*) 셀 수 없는, 무수한　　　**E** *innumerable*

　　> enumero, **enumeravi,** enumeratum, enumerare (< e- *out of, away from* + numerare *to count*) 셈하다, 열거하다　　　**E** *enumerate*

< IE. nem- *to assign, to allot;*

　　to take　　　**E** *numb* (< *'to take', 'to seize'*), *benumb, nimble* (< *'quick to seize'*)

> G. nemein *to assign, to allot, to manage, to regulate, to graze, to drive to pasture*

　　> G. nemesis, nemeseōs, f. *vengeance*　　　**E** *Nemesis*

　　> G. nomos, nomou, m. *usage, custom, management, regulation, law*

　　　E *nomo-, nomogenesis* (< *'evolution determined by law'*), *nomogram (nomograph)* (< *'a graphic table for computation' < 'laws'*), *-nomy, antinomic, metronome* (< *'measure of regulation'*)

　　> G. anomos, anomos, anomon (< a- *not*) *lawless*

　　　> G. anomia, anomias, f. *lawlessness*

　　　　> L. anomia, anomiae, f. 무규범 상태, 아노미 현상　　　**E** *anomy (anomie)*

　　> G. autonomos, autonomos, autonomon (< autos *self*) *having or making one's own laws, independent*　　　**E** *autonomous; heteronomous* (< *'on the pattern of autonomous'*)

　　　> G. autonomia, autonomias, f. *the having or making of one's own laws, independence*

　　　　> L. autonomia, autonomiae, f. 자율(自律), 자치(自治)

　　　　　E *autonomy, autonomic, dysautonomia; heteronomy* (< *'on the pattern of autonomy'*)

　　> G. astronomos, astronomos, astronomon (< astron *star*) *star-arranging*

> G. astronomia, astronomias, f. *astronomy*

> L. astronomia, astronomiae, f. 천문학   **E** *astronomy*

> G. oikonomos, oikonomou, m. (< oikos *house*) *householder, steward*

> G. oikonomia, oikonomias, f. *household management, economy*

> L. oeconomia, oeconomiae, f. 가정경제 관리, 재산 관리,

경영, 경제   **E** *economy*

> G. taxonomia, taxonomias, f. (< taxis *arrangement* + -nomia *manage-*

ment) *taxonomy*

> L. taxonomia, taxonomiae, f. 분류법, 분류학   **E** *taxonomy*

> G. nomizein *to adopt as a usage*

> G. nomisma, nomismatos, n. *usage, custom, current coin,*

money   **E** *numismatic*

> G. nomimos, nomimos, nomimon *legal*

> L. nummus, nummi, m. 주화(鑄貨)   **E** *nummulite*

> L. nummulus, nummuli, m. (< + -ulus *diminutive suffix*)

보조 주화   **E** *nummular*

> G. nomas, nomados, m., f. *roaming about for pasture, nomad*   **E** *nomad*

oculus, oculi, m. 눈알, 안구(眼球); (식물) 눈[芽]   **E** *oculus, (pl.) oculi, oculomotor*

> ocularis, oculare 눈알의

> **E** *ocular, intraocular, extraocular, (cornu *anteoculare >) antler, monocular, (bini 'two together' >) binocular, pinochle (< 'binocular')*

> inoculo, inoculavi, inoculatum, inoculare (< in- *in, on, into, toward* + oculus *eye,*

bud) 눈접을 붙이다, 심중에 박아주다, 접종(接種)하다   **E** *inoculate*

> inoculum, inoculi, n. 접종물(接種物), 접종원(接種原)   **E** *inoculum*

< IE. ok^w- *to see*   **E** *eye, eyeball, eyelid, eyelash, eyebrow, daisy (< 'day's eye'), window (< 'wind eye')*

> G. ōps, ōpos, f. *eye, face*   **E** *-ops; -opia, -opic*

> G. Kyklōps, Kyklōpos, m. (< *round-eyed* < kyklos *circle* + ōps) (*Greek mythology*)

Cyclops

> L. Cyclops, Cyclopis, m. (그리스 신화) 외눈박이 거인족의 하나; (cyclops)

단안체, 물벼룩 (< *having one eye (apparently single, but really double)*

situated in the middle of the front of the head)   **E** *Cyclops, cyclops*

> L. cyclopia, cyclopiae, f. 외눈증, 단안증   **E** *cyclopia*

> G. hydrōps, hydrōpos, m. (< *water face* < hydōr *water* + ōps) *edema*

> L. hydrops, hydropis, m. 부종(浮腫), 수종(水腫)   **E** *hydrops*

> L. hydropisis, hydropisis, f. (hydropisia, hydropisiae, f.) 부종,

수종   **E** *hydropsy, (hydropsy >) dropsy*

> (*suggested*) G. anthrōpos, anthrōpou, m. (< *human-faced* < anēr, andros, m.

man, male + ōps) *human being (as opposed to gods and beasts)*   **E** *anthrop(o)-*

> G. prosōpon, prosōpou, n. (< pros- *towards, near, beside(s)* + ōps) *face,*

appearance, mask (worn by actors), person   **E** *prosop(o)-*

> L. diprosopus, diprosopi, m. (< G. di- *two* + prosōpon *face*)

두얼굴체(體)　　　　　　　　　　　　　　**E** *diprosopus*

> L. photopia, photopiae, f. (< G. phōs, phōtos, n. *light* + ōps + -ia *noun*

suffix) 명소시(明所視), 광순응　　　　　　　**E** *photopia*

> L. scotopia, scotopiae, f. (< G. skotos *darkness* + ōps + -ia *noun suffix*)

암소시(暗所視), 암순응　　　　　　　　　　**E** *scotopia*

> L. emmetropia, emmetropiae, f. (< G. emmetros *in measure* (< em- (< en)

in + metron *measure*) + ōps + -ia *noun suffix*) 정시(正視)　　**E** *emmetropia*

> L. hypermetropia, hypermetropiae, f. (< G. hypermetros *beyond measure*

(< hyper- *over* + metron *measure*) + ōps + -ia *noun suffix*)

원시(遠視)　　　　　　　　**E** *hypermetropia (hyperopia)*

> L. myopia, myopiae, f. (< G. myein *to close the eyes* + ōps + -ia *noun*

suffix) 근시(近視)　　　　　　　　　　　　**E** *myopia*

> L. presbyopia, presbyopiae, f. (< G. presbys *old man, elder* + ōps + -ia

noun suffix) 노시안(老視眼), 노안(老眼)　　　**E** *presbyopia*

> L. isopia, isopiae, f. (< G. isos *equal* + ōps + -ia *noun suffix*)

양안등시각(兩眼等視覺)　　　　　　　　　　**E** *isopia*

> L. anisopia, anisopiae, f. (< G. anisos *unequal* (< an- *not* + isos *equal*)

+ ōps + -ia *noun suffix*) 부등시(不等視)　　　**E** *anisopia*

> L. isometropia, isometropiae, f. (< G. isos *equal* + metron *measure* + ōps

+ -ia *noun suffix*) 양안굴절동등　　　　　　　**E** *isometropia*

> L. anisometropia, anisometropiae, f. (< G. anisos *unequal* (< an- *not* + isos

equal) + metron *measure* + ōps + -ia *noun suffix*) 굴절부등　　**E** *anisometropia*

> L. amblyopia, amblyopiae, f. (< G. amblys *blunt, dull, dim* + ōps + -ia *noun*

suffix) 약시(弱視)　　　　　　　　　　　　**E** *amblyopia*

> L. diplopia, diplopiae, f. (< G. diploos *double* + ōps + -ia *noun suffix*)

복시(複視), 겹보임　　　　　　　　　　　　**E** *diplopia*

> L. nyctalopia, nyctalopiae, f. (< G. nyx *night* + alaos *blind* + ōps + -ia

noun suffix) 밤소경증, 야맹증　　　　　　　**E** *nyctalopia*

> L. hemeralopia, hemeralopiae, f. (< G. hēmera *day* + alaos *blind* + ōps

+ -ia *noun suffix*) 주간맹, 낮소경　　　　　**E** *hemeralopia*

> L. protanopia, protanopiae, f. (< *blindness to red, considered the first of the*

primary colors < G. prōtos *first* + an- *not* + ōps + -ia *noun suffix*) 적색맹,

제일색맹　　　　　　　　　　　　　　　　**E** *protanopia*

> L. deuteranopia, deuteranopiae, f. (< *blindness to green, considered the second*

of the primary colors < G. deuteros *second* + an- *not* + ōps + -ia *noun suffix*)

녹색맹, 제이색맹　　　　　　　　　　　　　**E** *deuteranopia*

> L. tritanopia, tritanopiae, f. (< *blindness to blue, considered the third of the*

primary colors < G. tritos *first* + an- *not* + ōps + -ia *noun suffix*) 청색맹,

제삼색맹　　　　　　　　　　　　　　　　**E** *tritanopia*

> G. opsis, opseōs, f. *seeing, view, appearance*

> G. synopsis, synopseōs, f. (< syn- *with, together*) *general view*

> L. synopsis, synopsis, f. 개관(槪觀), 개요(槪要), 줄거리   **E** *synopsis, synoptic*

> L. stereopsis, stereopsis, f. (< G. stere(o)- *solid, three-dimensional*)

입체시(立體視)   **E** *stereopsis*

> G. -opsia, -opsias, f. *seeing*

> G. autopsia, autopsias, f. (< autos *self*) *seeing with one's own eyes, eye-witnessing*

> L. autopsia, autopsiae, f. 부검(剖檢), 시체해부   **E** *autopsy (necropsy)*

> L. hemianopsia, hemianopsiae, f. (< G. hemi- *half* + an- *not*)

반맹(半盲)   **E** *hemianopsia*

> L. *parachromatopsia, *parachromatopsiae, f. (< G. par(a)- *beside, along side of, beyond* + chrōma, chrōmatos, n. *color*)

색맹(色盲)   **E** *parachromatopsia*

> G. optos, optē, opton *seen, visible*

> G. optikos, optikē, optikon *of or pertaining to sight*

> L. opticus, optica, opticum 시각(視覺)의, 시력의,

광학의   **E** *optic, optics, panoptic,* (optic >) *optical*

> G. dioptra, dioptras, f. (< di(a)- *through, thoroughly, apart* + optos *visible* + -tra *instrumental suffix*) *an optical instrument for measuring light refraction to determine heights, levelling, etc.*

> L. dioptra, dioptrae, f. 디옵터   **E** *dioptre (diopter), dioptric*

> G. ophthalmos, ophthalmou, m. (*taboo deformation*)

eye   **E** *ophthalmic, ophthalmology, ophthalm(o)-, -ophthalmos (-ophthalmus)*

> G. ophthalmia, ophthalmias, f. *inflammation of the eye, eye disease*

> L. ophthalmia, ophthalmiae, f. 안염(眼炎),

안구증(眼球症)   **E** *ophthalmia, -ophthalmia*

> L. xerophthalmia, xerophthalmiae, f. (< G. xēros *dry*) 안구건조증,

안건조증   **E** *xerophthalmia*

> L. enophthalmos, enophthalmi, m. (enophthalmus, enophthalmi, m.)

(< G. en- *in*) 안구함몰   **E** *enophthalmos (enophthalmus)*

> L. exophthalmos, exophthalmi, m. (exophthalmus, exophthalmi, m.)

(< G. ex- *out of, away from*) 안구돌출   **E** *exophthalmos (exophthalmus)*

> L. buphthalmos, buphthalmi, m. (buphthalmus, buphthalmi, m.) (< *ox eye, enlargement of the eyeball owing to increased intra-ocular pressure* < G. bous, boos, m., f. *ox, cow*) 우안(牛眼), 소눈증   **E** *buphthalmos (buphthalmus)*

> L. lagophthalmos, lagophthalmi, m. (lagophthalmus, lagophthalmi, m.)

(< *being unable to close the eyes, as the hare was supposed to* < G.
lagōs, lagō, m. *hare*) 토안(兎眼), 토끼눈증   **E** *lagophthalmos (lagophthalmus)*

> G. opē, opēs, f. *hole, opening*

> G. metōpon, metōpou, n. (< met(a)- *between, along with, across, after*)
forehead, front   **E** *metopic*

pampinus, pampini, m. 포도나무순, 덩굴손   **E** *pampiniform*

   < *Of* non-IE. *origin*

populus, populi, m. 국민, 백성   **E** *people, populism, populace*

> popularis, populare 국민의, 동포의, 대중의, 대중의 환심을 사는   **E** *popular*

> popularitas, popularitatis, f. 인구, 동포, 대중성, 인기   **E** *popularity*

> populo, **populavi**, populatum, populare 거주하게 하다, 거주하다   **E** *populate*

> populatio, populationis, f. 주민수, 인구; (생물) 개체군(群), (통계) 모집단   **E** *population*

> publicus, publica, publicum 공공의, 널리 알려진,
국가에 관한   **E** *public, (public house >) pub, publicity, republic*

> publico, **publicavi**, publicatum, publicare 공유재산으로 만들다, 공포하다,
공개하다, 매음하다, 출판하다   **E** *publish, publication*

pulvinus, pulvini, m. 방석, 베개; (식물) 엽침(葉枕),
(곤충) 부착반(附着盤)   **E** *pulvinus, (pl.) pulvini, pillow*

> pulvillus, pulvilli, m. (< + -ulus *diminutive suffix*) 작은 방석, 작은 베개;
(곤충) 부착반(附着盤)   **E** *pulvillus, (pl.) pulvilli*

> pulvinaris, pulvinare 방석의, 베개의

> pulvinare, pulvinaris, n. 방석, 베개; 시상(視床)베개, 시상침(視床枕)   **E** *pulvinar*

> pulvinatus, pulvinata, pulvinatum 방석 모양을 한, 베개 모양을 한; (식물) 엽침이 있는,
(곤충) 부착반이 있는   **E** *pulvinate*

rivus, rivi, m. 개울, 물길   **E** *rivulet*

> rivalis, rivale 개울의, 개울을 같이 사용하는, 경쟁상대의   **E** *rival, rivalry*

> derivo, **derivavi**, derivatum, derivare (< de- *apart from, down, not* + rivus *stream*)
끌어오다, 유도하다, 파생시키다   **E** *derive*

> derivativus, derivativa, derivativum 끌어온, 유도된, 파생된   **E** *derivative*

< IE. reiə- *to flow, to run*

> **E** *run, runny, rennet* (< 'it causes milk to run (together), to coagulate'), (rennet > 'milk-
curdling enzyme of rennet' >) *rennin, random* (< 'at great speed'), *randomize*

> (*Gaulish*) Renos *river*   **E** *Rhine, D. Rhein*

Sclavus, Sclavi, m. 슬라브족 사람 (유럽의 중부와 동부에 사는 아리안계 사람)

E *Slav, slave* (< 'Many Slavs were taken captive and sold into slavery'), **slavery,** (Sclavus 'your obedient slave' >) *ciao*

< G. Sklabos, Sklabou, m. *Slav*

< (*Slavic*) Sloveninu *Slav*

sirupus, sirupi, m. 시럽, 사리별(舍利別)

E *syrup (sirup), syrupy*

< (*Arabic*) sharab *wine or other beverage, syrup*

E *sherbet*

somnus, somni, m. 잠; (Somnus) (로마 신화) 잠의 신(밤의 여신 Nox의 아들, 죽음의 신 Mors의 형제, 그리스 신화의 Hypnos에 해당)

E *Somnus, somniloquism (somniloquy), somnambulism*

> somnium, somnii, n. 꿈

> somnolentus, somnolenta, somnolentum 몹시 졸리는

E *somnolent*

> somnolentia, somnolentiae, f. 몹시 졸림

E *somnolence*

> insomnia, insomniae, f. (< in- *not*) 잠자지 않음, 불면증

E *insomnia*

> somnifer, somnifera, somniferum (< somnus *sleep* + -fer (< ferre *to carry, to bear*) *carrying, bearing*) 잠 오게 하는

E *somniferous*

< IE. swep- *to sleep*

> L. sopor, soporis, m. 깊은 잠

E *soporous*

> L. *soporificus, *soporifica,*soporificum (< sopor *sleep* + -ficus (< facĕre) *making*) 졸리게 하는, 최면(催眠)의

E *soporific*

> G. hypnos, hypnou, m. *sleep, sleepiness;* (Hypnos) (*Greek mythology*) *the god of sleep (son of Nyx 'night', brother of Thanatos 'death')*

E *Hypnos, hypn(o)-, hypnagogue, hypnagogic, hypnozoite*

> G. hypnoun (hypnoein) *to put to sleep*

E *hypnotic, hypnotism*

> G. *hypnōsis, *hypnōseōs, f. (< + -ōsis *condition*) *putting to sleep*

> L. hypnosis, hypnosis, f. 최면

E *hypnosis*

sonus, soni, m. 소리

E *sound,* (sonus 'sound' >) *sonic, supersonic, transonic* (< 'on the pattern of supersonic'), (sonic >) *sonicate, sonnet, sone* (< 'a unit of subjective loudness'), (sound navigation and ranging >) *sonar, infrasound, ultrasound, ultrasonic, ultrasonography*

> sono, sonui, sonitum, sonare 소리 나다, 소리를 내다

E *sonant,* It. *sonata*

> sonor, sonoris, m. 소리, 음향, 반향

> sonorus, sonora, sonorum 소리 나는, 울려 퍼지는, 공명하는

E *sonorous,* (sonorous >) *sonorant*

> sonoritas, sonoritatis, f. 울려 퍼짐, 공명

E *sonority*

> assono, assonui, −, assonare (< as- (< ad) *to, toward, at, according to* + sonare *to sound*) 소리로 응답하다, 메아리치다, 공명하다

E *assonant, assonance*

> consono, consonui, −, consonare (< con- (< cum) *with, together* + sonare *to sound*) 함께 소리 나다, 화음을 이루다

E *consonant, consonantal, consonance*

> dissono, dissonui, dissonitum, dissonare (< dis- *apart from, down, not* +

sonare *to sound*) 다른 소리가 나다, 조화되지 않다 **E** *dissonant, dissonance*

> resono, resonavi (resonui), –, resonare (< re- *back, again* + sonare *to sound*) 울리다, 공명하다, 공진하다 **E** *resound, resonate, resonant, resonance*

> unisonus, unisona, unisonum (< unus *one* + sonus *sound*) 한 소리만 나는, 같은 음의 **E** *unison*

< IE. swen-, swenə- *to sound* **E** *swan* (< *'singer'*)

sparus, spari, m. (sparum, spari, n.) (갈고리를 단) 작은 창(槍)

< IE. sper- *spear, pole, rod*

> **E** *spear, spearmint* (< (*probably*) *'from the appearance of the flowers on the stem'*), *spareribs* (< *'ribs on a spear'*), *spar* (< *'raft, beam'*)

talus, tali, m. 발목, 목말뼈, 거골(距骨); 놀이골패, 주사위 **E** *talus, talon, talipes, talin*

> talaris, talare 발목의, 목말뼈의 **E** *talar*

terminus, termini, m. 경계, 한계, 종말, 만기, 기간, 용어 **E** *terminus,* (pl.) *termini, term, preterm*

> terminalis, terminale 경계선에 있는, 마지막의 **E** *terminal*

> terminologia, terminologiae, f. (< + G. -logia *study*) 용어론, (총칭) 용어 **E** *terminology*

> termino, terminavi, terminatum, terminare 경계를 정하다, 끝내다 **E** *terminate*

> interminabilis, interminabile (< in- *not*) 끝없는, 무한한 **E** *interminable*

> determino, determinavi, determinatum, determinare (< de- *apart from, down, not; intensive* + terminare *to set bounds to*) 경계를 정하다, 결정하다 **E** *determine, determinant, determination*

> extermino, exterminavi, exterminatum, exterminare (< ex- *out of, away from* + terminare *to set bounds to*) 경계 밖으로 쫓아내다, 제거하다, 말살하다 **E** *exterminate*

< IE. ter- *root of derivatives meaning peg, post, boundary marker, goal*

titulus, tituli, m. 표제, 제목, 항, 직위 **E** *title, entitle, tittle* (< *'mark over a vowel'*)

> titularis, titulare 칭호가 있는, 이름뿐인 **E** *titular*

> F. titre *title, standard* **E** *titre (titer), titrate,* (*titrate* >) *titration*

< IE. tel- *ground, floor, board*

> L. tellus, telluris, f. 땅, 지구, 지면; (Tellus) (로마 신화) 양육의 여신

> **E** *tellurian, telluric, tellurium (Te)* (< *'in contrast to uranium* (< G. ouranos *'heaven'*), *discovered nine years earlier'*)

> (*suggested*) L. tabula, tabulae, f. 판, 글판, 화폭, 게시판, 표 **E** *table, tablet, tabloid, tablature*

> L. tabularis, tabulare 판의, 표의 **E** *tabular*

> L. tabulo, –, –, tabulare 평판 모양으로 하다, 표로 만들다 **E** *tabulate*

tophus, tophi, m. (tofus, tofi, m.) 응회석(凝灰石); 통풍결절(痛風結節) **E** *tophus,* (pl.) *tophi*

> tophaceus, tophacea, tophaceum 응회석의; 통풍결절의　　　　　**E** *tophaceous*

umbilicus, umbilici, m. 배꼽, 가운데　　　　　**E** *umbilicus, (umbilicus >) umbilicate, nombril*

　　　> L. umbilicalis, umbilicale 배꼽의　　　　　**E** *umbilical*

　< IE. nobh–, ombh– *navel; later also central knob, boss of a shield, hub of*

　　a wheel　　　　　**E** *navel, nave, (nauger 'nave (of a wheel) drill' > (wrong division) >) auger*

　　　> L. umbo, umbonis, m. 방패의 두드러진 부분, 팔꿈치, 곶　　　　　**E** *umbo*

　　　> G. omphalos, omphalou, m. *navel, knob or boss of a shield, center*

　　　　　E *omphalos, omphal(o)–, omphalocele (< 'umbilical hernia'), omphaloscepsis (omphaloskepsis)*

uterus, uteri, m. (배[腹] >) 자궁　　　　　**E** *uterus*

　　　[용례] corpus uteri 자궁체　　　　　**E** *corpus uteri*

　　　　　　cervix uteri 자궁목　　　　　**E** *cervix uteri*

　　　　　(문법) corpus 몸, 체(體): 단수 주격 < corpus, corporis, n.

　　　　　　　cervix 목, 경(頸): 단수 주격 < cervix, cervicis, f.

　　　　　　　uteri 자궁의: 단수 속격

　　　[용례] in utero 자궁 안에서, 자궁내　　　　　**E** *in utero*

　　　　　(문법) in (소재) ~ 안에: 전치사, 탈격지배

　　　　　　　(방향) ~ 안으로: 전치사, 대격지배

　　　　　　　utero 단수 탈격

　　　> uterinus, uterina, uterinum 자궁의　　　　　**E** *uterine, intrauterine, extrauterine*

　< IE. udero– *abdomen, womb, stomach; with distantly similar forms (perhaps taboo*

　　deformations) in various languages

　　　> (*perhaps taboo deformation*) L. venter, ventris, m. 배[腹], 복부(腹部),

　　　　위　　　　　**E** *ventrad, ventriloquism, eventration*

　　　　　> L. ventralis, ventrale 배의, 배쪽의, 복부의　　　　　**E** *ventral*

　　　　　> L. ventriculus, ventriculi, m. (< + –culus *diminutive suffix*) 작은 배[腹], 실(室),

　　　　　　심실(心室), 뇌실(腦室), 위　　　　　**E** *ventricle, intraventricular, interventricular*

　　　　　　> L. *ventricularis, *ventriculare 작은 배의, 실(室)의, 심실의, 뇌실의,

　　　　　　　위의　　　　　**E** *ventricular*

　　　> (*perhaps taboo deformation*) L. vesica, vesicae, f. 가죽주머니, 방광(膀胱), 낭(囊),

　　　　수포(水胞), 물집　　　　　**E** *vesica, vesic(o)–*

　　　　　> L. vesicalis, vesicale 낭의, 방광의　　　　　**E** *vesical*

　　　　　> L. vesicula, vesiculae, f. (< + –ula *diminutive suffix*) 작은 가죽주머니, 작은

　　　　　　방광, 소낭(小囊), 소포(小胞), 수포(水胞), 잔물집　　　　　**E** *vesicle, vesiculate*

　　　　　　> L. vesicularis, vesiculare 소낭의, 소포의, 수포의,

　　　　　　　잔물집의　　　　　**E** *vesicular, multivesicular*

　　　　　> L. vesico, vesicavi, –, vesicare 물집이 생기다　　　　　**E** *vesicate, vesicant, vesication*

　　　> G. hystera, hysteras, f. *womb*　　　　　**E** *hyster(o)–*

　　　　　> G. hysterikos, hysterikē, hysterikon *belonging to the womb, suffering in*

the womb, hysterical (< Women being much more liable than men to
this disorder, it was originally thought to be due to a disturbance of
the uterus and its functions)

> L. hystericus, hysterica, hystericum 히스테리아성의, 병적으로
홍분한 **E** *hysteric, hysterical*
> L. hysteria, hysteriae, f. 히스테리아, 병적 홍분 **E** *hysteria*

Volcanus, Volcani, m. (*later* **Vulcanus, Vulcani, m.**) (로마 신화) 불과 대장장이의 신,
Jupiter 신과 Juno 여신의 아들, Venus 여신의 남편 (Aetna 산에 살면서 Jupiter 신의
번개를 만들었음) **E** *Vulcan, volcano, volcanic, vulcanize*

pinus, pini, f. (**pinus, pinus, f.**) 소나무 **E** *pine (< 'yielding a resin'), pineapple*

> pinea, pineae, f. 솔방울
> pinealis, pineale 솔방울
모양의 **E** (glandula pinealis *'pineal gland'* >) *pineal; pinealocyte*
< IE. peiə- *to be fat, to swell* **E** *fat, fatty, fatten;* (Celtic) *Eire (Ireland)*
> L. pituita, pituitae, f. 수액(樹液), 점액(粘液), 콧물, 피고름 **E** *pip*
> L. pituitarius, pituitaria, pituitarium (< *believed to secrete nasal mucus*) (점액을
분비하는 >) 뇌하수체의
E *pituitary; pituicyte (< 'a glial cell of the posterior pituitary'), hyperpituitarism, hypopituitarism*
> L. pinguis, pingue 기름기 도는, 살찐 **E** *pinguid*
> L. pinguiculus, pinguicula, pinguiculum 조금 살찐, 토실토실한
> L. pinguecula, pingueculae, f. 결막황반(結膜黃斑), 검열반(瞼裂斑) **E** *pinguecula*
> G. piōn, piōn, pion *fat, plump; fertile; rich*
E (pro- *'before, in front'* + piōn >) *propionic acid (< 'being the first in the order of the carboxylic acid series to form fatty compounds (formic (methanoic) and acetic (ethanoic) acids, which precede it in the series, lack this property'), propane, propyl, propylene, ((incorrectly named) iso- + pr(opyl)ene >) isoprene, isoprenoid*
> G. Pieria, Pierias, f. *a region of Macedonia, the reputed home of Muses* **E** *Pierian*

vannus, vanni, f. 키, 풍구, 바람개비 **E** *fan*
< IE. wet- *to blow, to inspire, to arouse spiritually*
E *Odin (Woden),* (G. hēmera Hermou *'day of* Hermēs', L. dies Mercurii *'day of* Mercurius' > *'Odin's day, Woden's day'* >) *Wednesday*
> G. atmos, atmou, m. (atmis, atmidos, f.) *breath, vapor, steam, smoke*
> L. atmosphaera, atmosphaerae, f. (< G. atmos *vapor* + sphaira *ball, globe*)
대기(大氣), 기압, 분위기 **E** *atmosphere, atmospheric*
> (*Sanskrit*) atman *breath, soul,*
essence **E** *atman,* (maha *'great'* + atman *'soul'* > mahatman *'great soul'* >) *mahatma*

vulgus, vulgi, n. (**m.**) (복수 없음) 평민, 서민, 민중

> vulgaris, vulgare 서민적, 일반적, 보통의, 통속적, 저속한   **E** *vulgar*

> vulgo, **vulgavi**, vulgatum, vulgare 퍼뜨리다, 책을 출간하다   **E** *Vulgate*

  > divulgo, **divulgavi**, divulgatum, divulgare (< di- (< dis-) *apart from, down, not* + vulgare *to make public, to publish*) 세상에 퍼뜨리다, 공포하다   **E** *divulge*

    > (*suggested*) promulgo, **promulgavi**, promulgatum, promulgare (< pro- *before, forward, for, instead of* + vulgare *to make public, to publish*) 퍼뜨리다, 공포(公布)하다   **E** *promulgate*

algorismus, algorismi, m. 아라비아식 기수법(記數法), 아라비아숫자 산법(算法), 산술(算術)   **E** *algorism, (algorism >)* **algorithm** *(< 'affected by G. arithmos number')*

  < (*Arabic*) al-Khwarizmi *the native of Khwarazm (modern Khiva in Uzbekistan), surname of the Arab mathematician (Abu Ja'far Muhammad ibn Musa al-Khwarizmi), who flourished early in the 9th century, and through the translation of whose work on algebra, the Arabic numerals became generally known in Europe*

맞대보기 1   어미 –os로 끝나는 그리스어 제2변화 명사는 –us로 끝나는 라틴어 명사가 되어 위의 변화(제2변화 제1식)를 따른다. 따라서 명사 접미사 -mos(결과), –smos (결과), –ismos(결과, 상태, 주의)로 끝나는 그리스어 기원의 학술용어는 –mus, –smus, –ismus로 끝나는 제2변화 제1식의 라틴어 명사가 된다.

Cadmus, Cadmi, m. (그리스 신화) 카드무스

  E *Cadmus, Cadmean,* (G. Kadmeia gē *'Cadmean earth, so called because found near Thebes, home of Cadmus' >*) *cadmium (Cd),* (G. Kadmeia gē *'Cadmean earth' >*) *calamine*

  < G. Kadmos, Kadmou, m. (*Greek mythology*) *Cadmus, the legendary founder of Thebes in Boeotia, and introducer of the alphabet into Greece*

Cerberus, Cerberi, m. (그리스 신화) 서버러스(케르베로스)   **E** *Cerberus*

  < G. Kerberos, Kerberou, m. (*Greek mythology*) *the watch-dog which guarded the entrance of the infernal regions, represented as having three heads*

Rhesus, Rhesi, m. Thracia의 왕   **E** *(rhesus monkey ('arbitrary use') >)* **rhesus (Rh)**

  < G. Rhēsos, Rhēsou, m. *a mythical king of Thrace*

angelus, angeli, m. 사자(使者), 천사(天使)   **E** *angel*

  < G. angelos, angelou, m., f. *messenger (used by the Septuagint to translate (Hebrew) malak, in full (Hebrew) malak-yehowah messenger of Jehovah), envoy, angel*

    > G. archangelos, archangelou, m. (< archos *chief*) *archangel*

> L. archangelus, archangeli, n. 대천사(大天使)　　　　　　**E** *archangel*

> G. euangelion, euangeliou, n. (< eu- *well*) *good news, gospel*

> L. evangelium, evangelii, n. 복음　　　　　　**E** *evangel*

< *Of Oriental origin*

beryllus, berylli, m. 녹주석(綠柱石)　　　　　　**E** *beryl, (perhaps) brilliant*

> L. beryllium, beryllii, n. 베릴륨　　　　　　**E** *beryllium (Be), berylliosis*

< G. bēryllos, bēryllou, f. *beryl*

< *Of Dravidian origin*

bombus, bombi, m. 붕붕대는 소리, 웅성거리는

소리　　　　　　**E** *(probably) bomb, bombard, (perhaps) bound, rebound*

< G. bombos, bombou, m. *deep and hollow sound*

< *Of echoic origin*　　　　　　**E** *boom*

bulbus, bulbi, m. 구근식물, 양파, 망울, 팽대; 연수(延髓, 숨뇌, medulla oblongata); (bulbus

oculi >) 안구(眼球)　　　　　　**E** *bulb, (bulb >) bulbar; bulbospinal; retrobulbar*

> bulbosus, bulbosa, bulbosum 구근이 있는　　　　　　**E** *bulbous*

> syringobulbia, syringobulbiae, f. (< G. syrinx *water cavity* + L. bulbus

medulla oblongata) 숨뇌구멍증, 연수공동증(延髓空洞症)　　　　　　**E** *syringobulbia*

< G. bolbos, bolbou, m. *bulbous root, onion*

byssus, byssi, f. 아마(亞麻), 아마포, 면(綿), 붕대포　　　　　　**E** *byssus, byssocausis*

< G. byssos, byssou, f. *fine linen, cotton, byssus*

> G. byssinos, byssinē, byssinon *made of byssus*

> L. byssinosis, byssinosis, f. (< + G. -ōsis *condition*) 면폐증(綿肺症)　　**E** *byssinosis*

< *(Semitic)* b-w-tz *to be white*

coccus, cocci, m. 낱알, 씨, 장과(漿果); 알균,

구균(球菌)　　　　　　**E** *coccus, (pl.) cocci, coccal, -coccus, (pl.) -cocci, -coccal*

< G. kokkos, kokkou, m. *kernel, grain, berry; scarlet berry* (< *the insect bodies were*

mistaken for grains or berries)

> L. coccum, cocci, n. 낱알, 씨, 장과(漿果); 연지벌레, 연지벌레 암컷으로 만든

붉은 염료, 심홍색　　　　　　**E** *cocoon*

> L. coccineus, coccinea, coccineum 심홍색의　　　　　　**E** *cochineal*

> G. *kokkidion, *kokkidiou, n. (< + -idion, -idiou, n. *diminutive suffix*) *small*

coccus

> L. †Coccidium, †Coccidii, n. †콕시디움 포자충의 한 속(屬) (현재는 다른

속으로 재분류됨)　　　　　　**E** *coccidiosis*

> L. Coccidioides, Coccidioidis, f. (< + G. eidos *shape*) (병원성
불완전 진균) 콕시디오이데스속(屬)   **E** Coccidioides, *coccidioidomycosis*

condylus, condyli, m. (불거진) 손가락 마디, (갈대·대나무) 마디; 과상(顆狀)돌기,
관절융기   **E** *condyle,* (condylus >) *condylar, condyloid*
> epicondylus, epicondyli, m. (< G. ep(i)- *upon*) 위관절융기   **E** *epicondyle*
< G. kondylos, kondylou, m. *knuckle (originally, hard lump, knob)*
> G. kondylōma, kondylōmatos, n. (< *a knuckle-like growth* < + -ōma *noun*
suffix denoting tumor) *condyloma*
> L. condyloma, condylomatis, n.
콘딜로마   **E** *condyloma,* (pl.) *condylomata (condylomas)*

[용례] condyloma acuminatum, (pl.) condylomata acuminata 첨형(尖形)
콘딜로마   **E** *condyloma acuminatum,* (pl.) *condylomata acuminata*
condyloma latum, (pl.) condylomata lata 편평(扁平)
콘딜로마   **E** *condyloma latum,* (pl.) *condylomata lata*
(문법) condyloma 콘딜로마: 단수 주격
acuminatum 뾰쪽한, 첨형(尖形)의: 형용사, 중성형 단수 주격
< acuminatus, acuminata, acuminatum
latum 넓은: 형용사, 중성형 단수 주격
< latus, lata, latum
condylomata 콘딜로마: 복수 주격
acuminata 뾰쪽한, 첨형(尖形)의: 형용사, 중성형 복수 주격
lata 넓은: 형용사, 중성형 복수 주격

embolus, emboli, m. 색전(塞栓)   **E** *embolus,* (pl.) *emboli, embolic*
< G. embolos, embolou, m. (embolon, embolou, n.) *anything put in,*
stopper, wedge, tongue of land between two rivers, wedge-shaped
order of battle, beak or ram of a ship
> G. embolizein *to embolize*   **E** *embolize*
> G. embolismos, embolismou, m. *embolism*
> L. embolismus, embolismi, m.
색전증(塞栓症)   **E** *embolism, thromboembolism*
< G. emballein (< em- (< en) *in* + ballein) *to throw in, to insert*
> G. emblēma, emblēmatos, n. *inlaid work, raised ornament on a vessel*   **E** *emblem*
< G. ballein (bol-, bal- *stem*) *to throw, to cast*
> G. bolē, bolēs, f. *throw, shot*
> G. amphibolos, amphibolos, amphibolon (< amphi- *on both sides, around*
+ ballein) *thrown or hitting on both sides, ambiguous*
E *amphibolic, amphibole* (< *'in allusion to the protean variety in composition and*
appearance')

> G. proballein (< pro *forward* + ballein) *to throw forward*

    > G. problēma, problēmatos, n. (< *thing thrown forward*) *question*

        proposed for solution, set task

        > L. problema, problematis, n. 문제, 과제   **E** *problem, problematic*

> G. symballein (< sym- (< syn) *with, together* + ballein) *to throw together,*

    to compare

    > G. symbolon, symbolou, n. *symbol, token, treaty*

        > L. symbolum, symboli, n. 장표, 상징, 부호,

        기호   **E** *symbol, symbolic, symbolism, symbolize, symbology*

> G. diaballein (< *to throw across* < di(a)- *through, thoroughly, apart* + ballein)

    to slander

    > G. diabolē, diabolēs, f. *slander, false accusation*

    > G. diabolos, diabolou, m. *slanderer, fiend,*

        devil   **E** *devil, diabolic, diabolism, diabolize*

> G. hyperballein (< hyper- *over* + ballein) *to throw over*

    > G. hyperbolē, hyperbolēs, f. *passing over, excess*

        > L. hyperbola, hyperbolae, f. 과장; (수학)

        쌍곡선   **E** *hyperbole, hyperbola, hyperbolic*

> G. paraballein (< par(a)- *beside, along side of, beyond* + ballein) *to throw*

    beside, to compare

    > G. parabolē, parabolēs, f. *throwing (placing) side by side, comparison,*

        parable

        > L. parabola, parabolae, f. 비교, 비유, 우화, 설교, 대치(對置); (수학)

        포물선

        E *parable, parabola, parabolic, parole* (< *'formal promise'* < *'speech'*)

        > L. parabolo, parabolavi, parabolatum, parabolare

        담화하다   **E** *parlor (parlour), parlance, parliament*

> G. metaballein (< met(a)- *between, along with, across, after* + ballein) *to*

    change, to exchange

    > G. metabolē, metabolēs, f. *change,*

        exchange   **E** *metabolize, metabolism, metabolic, metabolite*

> G. anaballein (< an(a)- *up, upward; again, throughout; back, backward;*

    against; according to, similar to + ballein) *to throw up*

    > G. anabolē, anabolēs, f. *mound, cloak, delay*   **E** *anabolism, anabolic, anabolite*

> G. kataballein (< kat(a)- *down, mis-, according to, along, thoroughly* + *ballein*)

    to throw down, to destroy, to pay down

    > G. katabolē, katabolēs, f. *attack,*

        payment   **E** *catabolize, catabolism, catabolic, catabolite*

> G. ballizein *to jump about,*

    to dance **E** *ball* (< *'dance'*)*, ballet* (< *'dance to music'*)*, ballad* (< *'song to dance to'*)

    > G. ballismos, ballismou, m. *act of jumping about, dance*

> L. ballismus, ballismi, m.

도리깨질증   **E** *ballismus (ballism), hemiballismus (hemiballism)*

> L. ballista, ballistae, f. 암석 투척기, 노포(弩砲), 쇠뇌   **E** *ballistic, ballistics*

< IE. gʷelə- *to throw, to reach, with further meaning to pierce*   **E** *kill, quell (< 'to kill')*

> (*suggested*) G. boulē, boulēs, f. (< *throwing forward of the mind*) *will,*
advice, project

> L. aboulia, abouliae, f. (abulia, abuliae, f.) 의지상실증   **E** *aboulia (abulia)*

> G. belonē, belonēs, f. *point of an arrow, needle*   **E** *belonephobia*

∽ IE. gʷel- *to fly, wing* (Vide VOLARE; *See* E. *volant*)

ginglymus, ginglymi, m. 경첩관절   **E** *ginglymus, (pl.) ginglymi*

< G. ginglymos, ginglymou, m. *hinge*

gyrus, gyri, m. 회전(回轉), 선회(旋回), 회(回), 뇌회(腦回), 이랑

E *gyrus, (pl.) gyri, agyria (lissencephaly), gyroscope (< 'an instrument designed to illustrate the dynamics of rotating bodies, including the earth')*

> gyro, **gyravi**, gyratum, gyrare 회전하다, 선회하다   **E** *gyrate*

< G. gyros, gyrou, m. *ring, circle*

< G. gyros, gyra, gyron *curved, round*

isthmus, isthmi, m. 지협(地峽), 협부(峽部), 잘룩   **E** *isthmus, isthmic*

< G. isthmos, isthmou, m. *narrow passage, a neck of land between two seas, specially the Isthmus of Corinth connecting the Peloponnesus with northern Greece*

lemniscus, lemnisci, m. 리본, 장식띠; (해부) 섬유띠, 섬유대   **E** *lemniscus, (pl.) lemnisci, lemniscate*

< G. lēmniskos, lēmniskou, m. *ribbon*

pessus, pessi, m. (pessum, pessi, n.) (부드러운 양털로 만든) 자궁전(子宮栓)

> pessarium, pessarii, n. 자궁전(子宮栓), 질좌제(膣座劑), 페서리   **E** *pessary*

< G. pessos, pessou, m. *an oval stone used in playing a game like draughts, a medicated plug (from its shape)*

rhonchus, rhonchi, m. 코 고는 소리, 쿨럭거리는 소리; 뻑뻑거림,

건성수포음(乾性水泡音)   **E** *rhonchus, (pl.) rhonchi, rhonchal (rhonchial)*

< G. rhonchos, rhonchou, m. *snoring*

< G. rhenchein *to snore, to snort*

< IE. srenk- *to snore*

> G. rhynchos, rhynchou, m. *snout, bill, beak*

> L. rhynchus, rhynchi, m. 주둥이　　　　　　　　　　　**E** *rhynch(o)-, -rhynchus*

thesaurus, thesauri, m. 보고, (사전 등) 지식의 보고, 보물　　**E** *thesaurus, treasure, treasury*

　　< G. thēsauros, thēsaurou, m. *treasury, treasure*

thrombus, thrombi, m. 혈전(血栓)　　　　　　　　　　　**E** *thrombus,* (pl.) *thrombi*

　　< G. thrombos, thrombou, m. *lump, piece, curd of milk, blood clot*

< IE. dherebh- *to coagulate* (Vide *TROPHICUS; See E. *trophic*)

thymus, thymi, m. 가슴샘, 흉선(胸腺)

　　E *thymus, thymic,* (thymic T-lymphocytes >) *thymocyte, thymine (T)* (< 'obtained by the action of dilute sulphuric acid on thymic nucleic acid'), *thymidine (T), athymic*

　　< G. thymos, thymou, m. *warty excrescence*

topus, topi, m. 장소, 토지

　　E *topology, topography, topoisomer, isotope* (< 'an element occupying the same place in the periodic table'), *epitope* (< 'an area on the surface of an antigen recognized by the immune system; an antigenic determinant'), *paratope* (< 'an epitope-binding site of an antibody'), *biotope (biotop)* (< 'the smallest subdivision of a habitat, characterized by a high degree of uniformity in its environmental conditions and in its plant and animal life')

　　< G. topos, topou, m. *place*　　　　　　　　　　　**E** *toponym* (< 'place name')

　　　> G. topion, topiou, n. (< + -ion *diminutive suffix*) *field,* (pl.) *ornamental gardening*

　　　　> L. topia, topiorum, n. (pl.) 원예, 풍경화

　　　　　> L. topiarius, topiaria, topiarium 원예에 관한, 풍경화에 관한　**E** *topiary*

　　　> G. topikos, topikē, topikon *of or pertaining to a place; local, or concerning commonplaces*

　　　　E (ta topika 'matters concerning commonplaces' >) *topic, topical, somatotopic* (< 'related to particular areas of the body')

　　　> G. atopos, atopos, atopon (< G. a- *not*) *out of place, unusual*

　　　　> G. atopia, atopias, f.

　　　　unusualness　　　　　　　**E** *atopy* (< 'atopic hyper-sensitiveness'), *atopic*

　　　> G. ektopos, ektopos, ektopon (< G. ek- *out of, away from*) *out of place*

　　　　> L. ectopia, ectopiae, f. 이소증(異所症), 딴곳증,

　　　　　전위(轉位), 편위(偏位)　　　　　　　　**E** *ectopia (ectopy), ectopic*

　　　> L. heterotopia, heterotopiae, f. (< G. heteros *different*) 이소증(異所症), 딴곳증,

　　　　전위(轉位), 편위(偏位)　　　　　　　　**E** *heterotopia, heterotopic*

　　　> L. Utopia, Utopiae, f. (< *no place, land of nowhere* < G. ou *not* + topos + -ia)

　　　　유토피아, 이상향

E *Utopia (< 'no place'), utopian, Eutopia (< 'good place'), Cacotopia (< 'bad place'), dystopia (< 'bad place')*

    < IE. top- *to arrive, goal*

tyrannus, tyranni, m. 폭군, 전제군주; (그리스 역사) 참주(僭主)   **E** *tyrant; tyrannous, tyrannicide*

    < G. tyrannos, tyannou, m. *tyrant, absolute monarch*

        > G. tyrannikos, tyrannikē, tyrannikon *tyranny*

            > L. tyrannicus, tyrannica, tyrannicum 폭군의, 전제군주의;

              참주의   **E** *tyrannic (tyrannical)*

        > G. tyrannia, tyrannias, f. *tyranny*

            > L. tyrannia, tyranniae, f. 폭정   **E** *tyranny*

        > L. Tyrannosaurus, Tyrannosauri, m. (< G. tyrannos + sauros *lizard*)

            티라노사우루스속(屬)   **E** *tyrannosaurus (tyrannosaur)*

rhythmus, rhythmi, m. 주기적 운동, 박자, 운율, 리듬   **E** *rhythm*

    < G. rhythmos, rhythmou, m. *rhythm, measure*

        > G. rhythmikos, rhythmikē, rhythmikon *rhythmic*

            > L. rhythmicus, rhythmica, rhythmicum 주기적인   **E** *rhythmic, rhythmical*

        > G. arrhythmia, arrhythmias, f. (< a- *not* + rhythmos) *arrhythmia*

            > L. arrhythmia, arrhythmiae, f. 부정맥(不整脈)   **E** *arrhythmia, hypsarrhythmia*

        > G. eurhythmia, eurhythmias, f. (< eu- *well* + rhythmos) *eurhythmia*

            > L. eurhythmia, eurhythmiae, f. 조화(調和)리듬, 조화성   **E** *eurhythmia*

        > L. dysrhythmia, dysrhythmiae, f. (< G. dys- *bad* + rhythmos) 리듬장애,

            율동장애   **E** *dysrhythmia*

    < G. rhein (rheein) *to flow*

        > G. rheos, rheou, m. *current*   **E** *rheo-, rheostat*

        > G. rheuma, rheumatos, n. *flow, discharge, humor of the body*

          E *rheum, rheumatic (< 'suffering from abnormal fluid discharge'), rheumatoid, rheumatism*

        > G. rhoia, rhoias, f. *flow, flux*

            > G. diarrhoia, diarrhoias, f. (< di(a)- *through, thoroughly, apart*)

              > L. diarrhoea, diarrhoeae, f. 설사(泄瀉)   **E** *diarrhoea (diarrhea), diarrheal*

        > G. gonorrhoia, gonorrhoias, f. (< *supposed to be a discharge of semen*

            < gonē, gonēs, f. ((*ancient Greek*) gonos) *begetting, birth, origin;*

            offspring, seed) *gonorrhea*

            > L. gonorrhoea, gonorrhoeae, f. 임질(淋疾)

          E *gonorrhoea (gonorrhea), gonorrheal, (gonorrhoea >) gonococcus*

        [용례] Neisseria gonorrh(o)eae 임균(淋菌)   **E** Neisseria gonorrh(o)eae

        (문법) Neisseria (세균) 나이세리아속(屬): 단수 주격

            < Neisseria, Neisseriae, f.

< Albert Ludwig Sigesmund Neisser (1855-1916),

German physician

gonorrh(o)eae 임질의: 단수 속격

> L. pyorrhoea, pyorrhoeae, f. (< G. pyon *pus*) 농루(膿漏), 고름흐름,
줄고름   **E** *pyorrhoea (pyorrhea)*

> L. leukorrhoea, leukorrhoeae, f. (leucorrhoea, leucorrhoeae, f.)
(< G. leukos *bright, white*) (백색) 질분비(膣分泌),
백대하(白帶下)   **E** *leukorrhoea (leukorrhea, leucorrhea)*

> L. galactorrhoea, galactorrhoeae, f. (< G. gala, galaktos, n. *milk*)
젖흐름증, 젖분비과다   **E** *galactorrhoea (galactorrhea)*

> L. otorrhoea, otorrhoeae, f. (< G. ous, ōtos, n. *ear*)
귓물, 이루(耳漏)   **E** *otorrhoea (otorrhea), otorrheal*

> L. rhinorrhoea, rhinorrhoeae, f. (< G. rhis, rhinos, f. *nose*)
콧물, 비루(鼻漏)   **E** *rhinorrhoea (rhinorrhea), rhinorrheal*

> L. sialorrhoea, sialorrhoeae, f. (< G. sialon *saliva*)
침과다증   **E** *sialorrhoea (sialorrhea)*

> L. seborrhoea, seborrhoeae, f. (< L. sebum *suet, grease*)
지루(脂漏), 기름흐름   **E** *seborrhoea (seborrhea), seborrheic*

> L. steatorrhoea, steatorrhoeae, f. (< G. stear, steatos, m. *solid fat,
suet, tallow*) 지방변증(脂肪便症)   **E** *steatorrhoea (steatorrhea), steatorrheal*

> G. rhoos, rhoou, m. (rhous, rhoou, m.) *stream*

> G. haimorrhois, haimorrhoidos, f. (< haima, haimatos, n. *blood*) *blood
discharging*

> L. haemorrhoida, haemorrhoidae, f.
치핵(痔核)   **E** *haemorrhoid (hemorrhoid), hemorrhoidal*

> G. katarrhein (katarrheein) (< kat(a)- *down, mis-, according to, along,
thoroughly*) *to flow down, to fall down*

> G. katarrhous, katarrhoou, m. *running down, rheum*

> L. catarrhus, catarrhi, m. 카타르(점막의 염증), 감기 **E** *catarrh, catarrhal*

< IE. sreu- *to flow*   **E** *stream*

borborygmus, borborygmi, m. 창자가스소리, 복명(腹鳴)   **E** *borborygmus*

< G. borborygmos, borborygmou, m. *a rumbling in the bowels*

< G. borboryzein *to rumble*

< *Of imitative origin*

nystagmus, nystagmi, m. 안진(眼震), 안구진탕(眼球震盪), 눈떨림   **E** *nystagmus*

< G. nystagmos, nystagmou, m. *drowsiness, nodding*

< G. nystazein *to be sleepy, to nod*

< IE. sneud(h)- *to be sleepy*

∞ IE. sner– *expressive root of various verbs for making noises*   **E** *sneer, snarl, snorkel* (< *'to snore'*)

∞ (*Germanic root*) snu– *imitative beginning of words connected with the nose*

> **E** *snout, snuff, snuffle, sniff,* (*sniff* > (*frequentative*) >) *sniffle, snivel, snub* (< *'to turn one's nose at'*), *snap, snip, snatch*

spasmus, spasmi, m. 경련수축(痙攣收縮), 경축(痙縮), 연축(攣縮)   **E** *spasm*

> < G. spasmos, spasmou, m. (spasma, spasmatos, n.) *spasm*
>> < G. span (spaein) *to draw, to tug, to tear, to rend, to drain*
>>> < IE. (s)pen– *to draw, to stretch, to spin* (Vide PENDĒRE: *See* E. *poise*)

embolismus, embolismi, m. 색전증(塞栓症)   **E** *embolism, thromboembolism*

> < G. embolismos, embolismou, m. *embolism*
>> < G. embolizein *embolize*   **E** *embolize*
>>> < G. embolos, embolou, m. *anything put in*
>>>> < G. emballein (< em– (< en) *in* + ballein) *to throw in, to insert*
>>>>> < G. ballein *to throw, to cast*
>>>>>> < IE. gʷelə– *to throw, to reach, with further meaning to pierce* (Vide EMBOLUS: *See* E. *embolus*)

syllabus, syllabi, m. 장부, 목록, 요목   **E** *syllabus*

> < L. (*misprinted*) sittyba, sittybae, f. 장부, 목록, 요목
>> < G. sittyba, sittybas, f. *parchment label, table of contents*
>>> < *Of unknown origin*

맞대보기 2   어미 –os로 끝나는 그리스어 제2변화 명사이나 관례상 그대로 쓰는 라틴어 낱말은 단수 주격만 –os가 되며 위의 변화(제1변화)를 따른다.

---

cosmos, cosmi, m. (정연한) 질서, 조화; (질서 정연한 일체로서의) 세계, 우주; 코스모스

> **E** *cosm(o)–, cosmopolis, cosmopolite, cosmopolitan, cosmonaut; cosmos* (< *'its elegant foliage'*)

> < G. kosmos, kosmou, m. *order, harmony; world, universe* (< *so called by Pythagoras or his disciples, who regarded the physical world as a perfectly ordered and harmonious system*); *ornament, adornment*
>> > G. kosmikos, kosmikē, kosmikon *of the world, of the universe*
>>> > L. cosmicus, cosmica, cosmicum 우주의, 세계의   **E** *cosmic*
>> > G. kosmein (kosmeein) *to arrange, to adorn*
>>> > G. kosmētikos, kosmētikē, kosmētikon *skilled in arranging*   **E** *cosmetic, cosmetician*

제2변화 제2식

단수 주격이 어미 없이 -er로 끝나며 속격 어미가 -i; 복수의 주격 어미가 -i, 속격 어미가 -orum인 남성 명사.

faber, fabri, m. 목수

	단 수	복 수	
주격	faber	fabr-i	~이, ~가, ~은, ~는, ~께서
속격	fabr-i	fabr-orum	~의
여격	fabr-o	fabr-is	~게, ~에게, ~께, ~한테
대격	fabr-um	fabr-os	~을, ~를
탈격	fabr-o	fabr-is	~에서, ~로부터, ~으로부터
호격	faber	fabr-i	~여, ~이여

faber, fabri, m. 목수   **E** Homo faber (< 'Man the Maker'), *forge, forgery*
   > fabrica, fabricae, f. 제작소, 구조물, 정교한 기술, 계교   **E** *fabric*
     > fabrico, **fabricavi**, fabricatum, fabricare 제작하다, 계교를 꾸미다   **E** *fabricate*
      > fabricatio, fabricationis, f. 제작, 계교; 날조, 위조, 허구증   **E** *fabrication*
  < IE. dhabh- *to fit together*   **E** *daft*

liber, libri, m. 나무의 속껍질, 책
    > librarius, libraria, librarium 책의   **E** *library, librarian*
    > libellus, libelli, m. (< + -ellus *diminutive suffix*) 소책자, 문서   **E** *libel, (libel >) libelous*
  < IE. leup-, lep- *to peel off, to break off, to scale*

   E *leaf, leaflet; lift, loft, aloft; lodge* (< 'sheltered place' < 'leafy arbor'), *dislodge, logistics* (< 'to lodge'), *lobby* (< 'roof made from bark, shelter')

   > L. (*suggested*) lapis, lapidis, m. 돌, 경계석, 이정표석(로마를 기점으로 1000 passus
     (약 1.5 Km)마다 세웠음), 기념비석, 묘석, 보석
    > L. lapidarius, lapidaria, lapidarium 돌의, 보석의, 석공의, 보석 세공의   **E** *lapidary*
    > L. dilapido, **dilapidavi**, dilapidatum, dilapidare (< di- (< dis-) *apart from,*
      down, not + lapis *stone*) 여기저기 마구 던지다, 낭비하다, 망가뜨리다   **E** *dilapidate*
   > G. lepein *to peel off*
    > G. lepis, lepidos, f. *scale, rind, shell*   **E** *lepidic*
     > G. lepros, lepra, lepron *scaly, rough*
      > G. lepra, lepras, f. *leprosy*

> L. lepra, leprae, f. 나병(癩病), 한센병 (< Gerhard Henrik
Armauer Hansen (1841-1912), *Norwegian physician*)　**E** *leper*
> L. leprosus, leprosa, leprosum 나병의,
한센병의　**E** *leprosy, leprotic*
> L. leprosarium, leprosarii, n. 나병원, 한센병
병원　**E** *leprosarium*
> L. leproma, lepromatis, n. (< + G. -ōma *noun suffix*
denoting tumor) 나종(癩腫), 나결절(癩結節), 한센병종,
한센병결절
E ***leproma, lepromatous, lepromin*** *(< 'a purified homogenate*
of lepromatous tissue')
> L. Lepidoptera, Lepidopterorum, n. (pl.) (< + G. pteron *wing*)
(나비·나방 등) 인시류목(鱗翅類目)의 곤충　**E** *lepidopteran*
> L. Hymenolepis, Hymenolepidis, f. (< *membranous rind* < G. hymēn,
hymenos, m. *thin skin, membrane*) (촌충) 히메노레피스속(屬)　**E** Hymenolepis
> G. lemma, lemmatos, n. *rind, husk*
> L. plasmalemma, plasmalemmatis, n. (< G. plasma, plasmatos, n.
something molded) 세포막　**E** *plasmalemma, plasmalemmal*
> L. sarcolemma, sarcolemmatis, n. (< G. sarx, sarkos, f. *flesh*)
횡문근형질막, 근초(筋鞘), 근섬유막　**E** *sarcolemma, sarcolemmal*
> L. oolemma, oolemmatis, n. (< G. ōon, ōou, n. *egg*)
난자형질막, 난막(卵膜)　**E** *oolemma, oolemmal*
> G. leptos, leptē, lepton *cleaned of the husks, thin, slender,*
delicate　**E** *lept(o)-, leptomeninx, leptotene, leptospira, leptin*
> G. laparos, lapara, laparon *thin, weak, soft*
> G. lapara, laparas, f. *flank, loins*　**E** *laparotomy, laparoscope*
> G. lapassein *to empty, to evacuate*
> G. lapaxis, lapaxeōs, f. *evacuation*　**E** *litholapaxy*

puer, pueri, m. 소년, 어린이
> puerilis, puerile 소년의, 어린이의　**E** *puerile*
> puerilitas, puerilitatis, f. 소년기, 어린이다움, 유치함　**E** *puerility*
> puerpera, puerperae, f. (< + -pera < -para < parĕre *to bring forth, to bear*)
산후부(産後婦), 산후녀, 산욕부(産褥婦)　**E** *puerpera, puerperal*
> puerperium, puerperii, n. (< + -perium < -parus < parĕre *to bring forth, to*
bear) 산욕기(産褥期), 산후기(産後期)　**E** *puerperium*
> puera, puerae, f. 소녀
> puella, puellae, f. (< + -ella *diminutive suffix*) 소녀
< IE. pau-, pou- *little, few*　**E** *few, foal, filly*
> L. putus, puti, m. 사내아이　**E** (It.) *putto*, (pl.) *putti*

> L. pullus, pulli, m. 동물의 새끼   **E** *pullet, poultry, pony*

> L. parvus, parva, parvum 작은; 적은   **E** *parvovirus (< 'small virus'); parvicellular (< 'of few cells')*

>> L. parum (부사) 조금, 모자라게

>>> **E** *(parum 'little' + affinis 'closely related, akin' > 'neutral quality and low chemical reactivity' >) paraffin*

> L. paucus, pauca, paucum 적은, 소수의, 드문   **E** *paucicellular, pauciarticular*

>> L. paucitas, paucitatis, f. 소수   **E** *paucity*

> L. paulus, paula, paulum 얼마 안 되는, 적은, 근소한   **E** *Paul*

> L. pauper, (gen.) pauperis (< IE. pau- + IE. perə- *to produce, to procure*)

가난한   **E** *pauper, poor, impoverish*

>> L. paupertas, paupertatis, f. 가난   **E** *poverty*

> L. (*probably*) pubes, (gen.) puberis (puber, (gen.) puberis) 사춘기의, 성년이 된,

병역 적령의; (잎·줄기·열매가) 솜털이 있는, 싱싱한   **E** *puberal*

>> L. pubes, pubis, f. 수염, 털, 성년, 청춘, 음모, 음부, 두덩   **E** *pubic (< 'of pubic region')*

>>> L. pubis, pubis, f. (< os pubis *pubic bone*)

치골(恥骨)   **E** *pubic (< 'of pubic bone')*

>> L. pubertas, pubertatis, f. 사춘기, (성년의 표시인) 수염, 음모(陰毛),

젊은이   **E** *puberty, pubertal, prepubertal, postpubertal*

>> L. pubesco, pubui, -, pubescĕre (< + -escĕre *suffix of inceptive (inchoative)*

verb) 사춘기에 접어들다, 성년이 되다, 무르익다, 온통 뒤덮이다   **E** *pubescent*

> G. pais, paidos, m., f. *child*

>> **E** *paed(o)- (ped(o)-), paediatric (pediatric), pediatrics, pediatrician, pedagogue, paedophilia (pedophilia)*

>> G. paideia, paideias, f. *child-rearing, teaching, education, knowledge*

>>> **E** *(enkyklios paideia 'all-round education' > 'encyclical arts and sciences considered by the Greeks as essential to a liberal education' >) encyclopaedia (encyclopedia), (orthos 'upright, straight, correct' + paideia 'the treatment and prevention of physical deformities, especially in children' >) orthopaedics (orthopedics)*

cancer, cancri, m. (cancer, canceris, m.) 게; (*meaning from a translation of* G. karkinos

(*crab, carcinoma*) (*Aulus Cornelius Celsus*) >) 암(癌); (Cancer) (성좌) 게자리

E *cancer, chancre (< 'a destructive sore'), chancroid (< 'chancre-like, soft chancre'), canker, cancer phobia (cancerphobia, cancerophobia) (< 'irrational fear of cancer')*

> cancrosus, cancrosa, cancrosum (cancerosus, cancerosa, cancerosum)

암(癌)의   **E** *cancerous, precancerous*

> cancrum, cancri, n. 괴저(壞疽)   **E** *cancrum*

< IE. kar-, ker- *hard, things with hard shells*   **E** *hard, hardness, hardy, -ard (< 'bold, hardy'), drunkard*

> L. carina, carinae, f. 빠개놓은 호도껍질, 빠개놓은 호도껍질 모양으로 오목하게 생긴

것, 배의 밑바닥, 배의 용골(龍骨)   **E** *carina, careen*

>> L. carino, carinavi, carinatum, carinare 용골(龍骨)을 대다   **E** *carinate*

> G. karyon, karyou, n. *nut*

> L. karyopyknosis, karyopyknosis, f. (< + G. pyknos *dense* + -ōsis *condition*)

  핵농축, 핵위축

> L. karyorrhexis, karyorrhexis, f. (< + G. rhēxis *breaking*) 핵붕괴,

  핵파괴

> L. karyolysis, karyolysis, f. (< + G. lysis *loosening*) 핵용해

> G. karkinos, karkinou, m. *crab*

  > G. karkinōma, karkinōmatos, n. (< *(suggested)* *the swollen veins surrounding*
    the part affected bear a resemblance to the limbs of a crab (Galen of
    Pergamon) < karkinos + -ōma *noun suffix denoting tumor*) carcinoma
    > L. carcinoma, carcinomatis, n. 암종(癌腫); 암(癌)

      > L. carcinomatosis, carcinomatosis, f. 암종증(癌腫症)

> G. kratos, kratous, n. *strength, might, power, rule*

  > G. dēmokratia, dēmokratias, f. (< dēmos *the people* + kratos)
    popular government

  > G. autokratēs, autokratēs, autokrates (< autos *self* + kratos) *ruling by oneself,*
    absolute

  > G. Hippokratēs, Hippokratous, m. (< *one superior in horses* < hippos *horse*
    + kratos) *Hippocrates*

    > L. Hippocrates, Hippocratis, m. 히포크라테스

      > L. Hippocraticus, Hippocratica, Hippocraticum
        히포크라테스의

        [용례] Corpus Hippocraticum 히포크라테스 전집 **E** *Hippocratic Corpus*
        vinum Hippocraticum (< *wine strained through a filter*
          called Hippocrates' sleeve) 히포크라테스 포도주 **E** *hippocras*
        (문법) corpus 전집: 단수 주격 < corpus, corporis, n.
            몸, 체(體), 몸통, 전집(全集)
            vinum 포도주: 단수 주격 < vinum, vini, n.
            Hippocraticum: 형용사, 중성형 단수 주격

  > G. Sōkratēs, Sōkratous, m. (< *having safe might* < sōs *safe* + kratos)
    Socrates
    > L. Socrates, Socratis, m. 소크라테스

> G. akrateia, akrateias, f. (akrasia, akrasias, f.) (< a- *not* + kratos) *incontinence,*
  intemperance

cancer, cancri, m. 격자, 창살

> cancellus, cancelli, m. (< + -ellus *diminutive suffix*) 격자, 창살, 난간   **E** *cancellous*

   > cancello, **cancellavi**, cancellatum, cancellare 격자 모양으로 만들다, 발을
치다, 울타리를 두르다; (글씨를) 북북 그어 지우다, 취소하다   **E** *cancel*

    > cancellatio, cancellationis, f. 취소, 말소   **E** *cancellation (cancelation)*

   > cancellarius, cancellarii, m. (< *originally a court official stationed at
the grating separating public from judges*) (황제나 장관의) 문지기
겸 비서장, (중세에 궁중의 공문서를 다룬) 상서(尙書)   **E** *chancellor*

< carcer, carceris, m. 감옥

   > incarcero, **incarceravi**, incarceratum, incarcerare (< in- *in, on, into, toward*
+ carcer *prison* + -are) 감금(監禁)하다   **E** *incarcerate*

    > incarceratio, incarcerationis, f. 감금, 감돈(嵌頓)   **E** *incarceration*

< (*probably*) *Borrowed from an unidentified source*

●●● 제 2 변화 제 3 식

단수 주격 어미가 –um, 속격 어미가 –i; 복수의 주격 어미가 –a, 속격 어미가 –orum 인
중성 명사. 단수 및 복수에서 주격, 대격, 호격이 똑같다.

ovum, ovi, n. 알

	단 수	복 수	
주격	ov-um	ov-a	~이, ~가, ~은, ~는, ~께서
속격	ov-i	ov-orum	~의
여격	ov-o	ov-is	~게, ~에게, ~께, ~한테
대격	ov-um	ov-a	~을, ~를
탈격	ov-o	ov-is	~에서, ~로부터, ~으로부터
호격	ov-um	ov-a	~여, ~이여

ovum, ovi, n. 알, 난(卵), 난자(卵子),
난세포(卵細胞)   **E** *ovum,* (pl.) *ova, ov(i)-, oviparous, oviposit, oviform; ovoid*

> ovalis, ovale 난형의, 난원형의   **E** *oval*

> ovatus, ovata, ovatum (밑부분이 더 큰) 달걀꼴의   **E** *ovate*

   > obovatus, obovata, obovatum (< ob- *before, toward(s), over, against,
away*) (끝부분이 더 큰) 거꿀달걀꼴의   **E** *obovate*

> ovulum, ovuli, n. (< + -ulum *diminutive suffix*) 작은 알, 난포내

난자   **E** *ovule;* (ovulum >) *ovulate,* (ovulate >) *ovulation, ovulatory, anovulatory*

> ovarium, ovarii, n. 난소(卵巢), 자방(子房)   **E** *ovary, ovarian*

> mesovarium, mesovarii, n. (< G. mesos *middle* + L. ovarium *ovary*)

난소간막, 난소사이막   **E** *mesovarium*

> oviductus, oviductus, m. (< ovum *egg* + ductus *duct*) 난관(卵管),

수란관(輸卵管)   **E** *oviduct*

< IE. owyo-, oyyo- *egg*   **E** *egg,* (cock's egg >) *cockney*

> G. ōion, ōiou, n. (ōon, ōou, n.) *egg*

E *oo-, oogenesis, oogonium, oocyte, ootid* (< 'on the pattern of spermatid'), *oospore*

> L. oolemma, oolemmatis, n. (< G. lemma *rind*) 난자형질막, 난막   **E** *oolemma*

> L. oophoron, oophori, n. (< + G. -phoros, -phoros, -phoron *carrying, bearing*) 난소   **E** *oophoritis, oophorectomy*

> (*Persian*) khaviyar (khaya *egg* + -dar *bearing*) 캐비아   **E** *caviar, caviare*

< IE. awi- *bird* (Vide AVIS: *See* E. *avian*)

verbum, verbi, n. 말, 낱말; (문법) 동사   **E** *verbiage, verb, preverb*

> verbalis, verbale 말의, 말뿐인; (문법) 동사의, 동사에서 파생한   **E** *verbal*

> verbatim (부사) 말 그대로, 한마디 한마디씩, 축어적(逐語的)으로   **E** *verbatim*

> adverbium, adverbii, n. (< ad- *to, toward, at, according to* + verbum *verb*)

부사   **E** *adverb, adverbial*

> proverbium, proverbii, n. (< pro- *before, forward, for, instead of* + verbum *word*)

속담, 격언   **E** *proverb, proverbial*

< IE. werə-, wer- *to speak*   **E** *word*

> G. eirein *to say, to speak, to order*

> G. eirōn, eirōnos, m. *dissembler in speech*

> G. eirōneia, eirōneias, f. *dissimilation, disguise*

> L. ironia, ironiae, f. 반어(反語), 풍자(諷刺)   **E** *irony, ironic*

> G. rhētōr, rhētoros, m. *orator, public speaker*

> G. rhētorikos, rhētorikē, rhētorikon *oratorical, rhetorical*   **E** (rhētorikē technē >) *rhetoric, rhetorical*

amuletum, amuleti, n. 부적(符籍), 호부(護符)   **E** *amulet*

azzurum, azzuri, n. (azolum, azoli, n.) 청금석(青金石),

천람석(天藍石)   **E** *azure, azurophilic* (< 'staining readily with blue aniline dyes')

< (*Arabic*) al-lazaward *lapis lazuli, blue color*

< (*Persian*) lazward *lapis lazuli, blue color*

> L. lazulum, lazuli, n. (lazurus, lazuri, m.) 청금석(青金石)

bellum, belli, n. 전쟁

> Bellona, Bellonae, f. (로마 신화) 전쟁의 여신, 군신 Mars의 자매　　**E** *Bellona*

> bellicus, bellica, bellicum 전쟁의

　　> bellicosus, bellicosa, bellicosum 전쟁이 많은, 호전적인　　**E** *bellicose, bellicosity*

> belligero, belligeravi, belliǵeratum, belligerare (< bellum *war* + gerěre *to*

　bear) 전쟁하다　　**E** *(belligerant >) belligerent*

> rebellis, rebelle (< re- *back, again* + bellum *war*) 투항했다가 다시 도전하는,

　반란하는, 반항하는　　**E** *rebel, revel (< 'to rise up in rebellion')*

　　> rebellio, rebellionis, f. 도전, 반란, 반항　　**E** *rebellion, rebellious*

< duellum, duelli, n. (*archaic*) 전쟁, 결투　　**E** *duel*

< IE. dau-, deu- *to injure, to destroy, to burn*

caenum, caeni, n. 진흙탕, 오물

> (*suggested*) obscaenus, obscaena, obscaenum (obscenus, obscena, obscenum)

(< obs- (< ob) *before, toward(s), over, against, away* + caenum *filth*) 불길한,

더러운, 외설한　　**E** *obscene*

> obscaenitas, obscaenitatis, f. (obscenitas, obscenitatis, f.) 불길, 외설　　**E** *obscenity*

< IE. kwei- *muck, filth*

callum, calli, n. (피부) 굳은살, 경결(硬結); (골절) 애벌뼈, 가골(假骨); 둔감　　**E** *callus*

> callosus, callosa, callosum 굳은살의, 못이 박힌, 굳은살 빛깔의, 애벌뼈의, 둔감한　　**E** *callous*

[용례] corpus callosum 뇌들보, 뇌량(腦梁)　　**E** *corpus callosum, callosal*

(문법) corpus 몸, 체(體): 단수 주격 < corpus, corporis, n.

callosum 굳은살 같은: 형용사, 중성형 단수 주격

> callositas, callositatis, f. 굳은살, 못, 둔감　　**E** *callosity*

< IE. kal- *hard*　　**E** *Excalibur*

chininum, chinini, n. 키니네, 금계랍(金鷄蠟)

< Sp. quina

E *(quina >)* **quinic acid,** *(quina >)* **quinine,** *(quinic acid + -one (< ketone) >)* **quinone(s),** *(hydrogenated quinone >)* **hydroquinone,** *(ubiquitous quinone >)* **ubiquinone,** *(chloroplast quinone >)* **plastoquinone,** *(quinine >)* **quinoline,** *(chlorinated quinoline >)* **chloroquine,** *(prime chloroquine >)* **primaquine**

> (*Dutch*) kinine *quinine*, 키니네, 금계랍(金鷄蠟)

< (*Quechua*) kina *bark, the bark of various species of cinchona and remigia, used largely in medicine as a febrifuge, tonic, and antiperiodic, chiefly in the form of the salt, sulphate of quinine, which is popularly termed quinine*

cocainum, cocaini, n. 코카인

　　　　　< Sp. coca　　　　　　　　　　　　　　　　　　　　　　　　E *cocaine*

　　< (*Peruvian*) cuca *the name in Bolivia of* Erythroxylum coca; *hence, applied to its dried*
　　　　leaves, which have been employed from time immemorial, with powdered lime, as a
　　　　masticatory, appeaser of hunger, and stimulant of the nervous system

colostrum, colostri, n. 첫젖, 초유(初乳)　　　　　　　　　　　　　　E *colostrum*

colum, coli, n. (< *wickerwork*) 여과기, 체
　　　　> colo, colavi, colatum, colare 거르다, 여과하다　　　　　E *portcullis* (< '*sliding door*')
　　　　　　> colatorium, colatorii, n. 여과기　　　　　　　　　　E *colander*
　　　　　　> percolo, percolavi, percolatum, percolare (< per- *through, thoroughly*) 거르다,
　　　　　　　여과하다, 스며들게 하다　　　　　　　　　　　　　　E *percolate*
　　< IE. kagh- *to catch, to seize; wickerwork, fence*　　　　　　E *hedge, quay*
　　　　> L. cohum, cohi, n. 쟁기 자루와 멍에를 매어주는 가죽 끈
　　　　　　> L. inchoo, inchoavi, inchoatum, inchoare (< incohare < in- *in, on, into, toward*
　　　　　　　+ cohum *strap fastening a plow beam to the yoke*) 시작하다　E *inchoate*
　　　　　　　　> L. inchoativus, inchoativa, inchoativum (문법) 동작의 개시를 뜻하는,
　　　　　　　　　기동동사(起動動詞)의　　　　　　　　　　　　　E *inchoative*

damnum, damni, n. (배상해야 할) 손해, 손실, 손상　　　　　　　E *damage*
　　　　> damno, damnavi, damnatum, damnare 유죄판결을 내리다, 처벌하다,
　　　　　비난하다　　　　　　　　　　　　　　　　　　　E *damn,* (*damn* >) *darn*
　　　　　　>condemno, condemnavi, condemnatum, condemnare (< con- (< cum)
　　　　　　　with, together; intensive + damnare *to damage*) 유죄판결을 내리다, 처벌
　　　　　　　하다, 비난하다　　　　　　　　　　　　　　　　　E *condemn*
　　　　> indemnis, indemne (< in- *not* + damnum *damage, loss*) 손상받지 않은, 손해 보지
　　　　　않은, 면책받는　　　　　　　　　　　　　　　　　　E *indemnify*
　　　　　　> indemnitas, indemnitatis, f. 배상, 보상, 면책　　　　E *indemnity*
　　< IE. dap- *to apportion* (*in exchange*)

mendum, mendi, n. (menda, mendae, f.) 신체적 결함, 흠, 오류
　　　　> mendicus, mendica, mendicum 빈궁한, 거지의, 구걸하는　E *mendicant*
　　　　> emendo, emendavi, emendatum, emendare (< e- *out of, away from* + mendum
　　　　　fault, blemish) (잘못을) 고치다　　　　　　　　E *emend, amend,* (*amend* >) *mend*
　　< IE. mend- *physical defect, fault*
　　　　> L. mendax, (gen.) mendacis 속이는　　　　　　　　　E *mendacious*
　　　　　　> L. mendacitas, mendacitatis, f. 거짓, 허위　　　　E *mendacity*

dorsum, dorsi, n. 등, 뒤, 등 쪽, 배부(背部)　　　E *dorsum, dorsad* (<+ -*ad* '*toward*'), *dorsiflexion*

> dorsalis, dorsale 등의, 등 쪽의, 배부의　　　　　　　　　　　　**E** *dorsal*

> indorso, **indorsavi**, indorsatum, indorsare (< in- *in, on, into, toward*) 배서(背書)

하다, 시인하다　　　　　　　　　　　　　　　　　　　　　**E** *endorse*

fanum, fani, n. 성역, 신전

> fanaticus, fanatica, fanaticum 신전의, 신들린, 광신적인, 열광적인　　**E** *fanatic (fan)*

> profanus, profana, profanum (< *outside the temple* < pro- *before, forward, for,*

instead of + fanum *temple*) 신성하지 못한, 속된, 문외한의, 신성모독의　**E** *profane*

> profanitas, profanitatis, f. 신성모독, 모독　　　　　　**E** *profanity*

< IE. dhes- *root of words in religious concepts*

> L. (*archaic*) fesia > feria, feriae, f. 제일, 축제일, 휴일　　**E** *feria, fair (< 'holiday')*

> L. festus, festa, festum 축제의　　　　　**E** *feast, festoon (< 'decoration for a feast')*

> L. festivus, festiva, festivum 축제의　　　　**E** *festive, festival, festivity*

> G. theos, theou, m., f. *god, goddess*　**E** *theology, monotheism, polytheism, henotheism, atheism*

> G. theios, theia, theion *of a god, sacred to a god*

> G. pantheios, pantheios, pantheion (< pan- *all*) *of all gods, sacred to*

all gods　　　　　　　　　　　　　　　　　　**E** *pantheon*

> G. entheos, entheos, entheon (< en- *in*) *possessed by a god, inspired*

> G. enthousia, enthousias, f. *possession by a god, inspiration*　**E** *enthusiasm*

> L. Theobroma, Theobromatis, n. (< G. theos *god* + brōma *food*) 카카오나무

속(屬)　　　　　　　　　　　　　　　**E** (Theobroma cacao >) *theobromine*

fascinum, fascini, n. (fascinus, fascini, m.) (음경 모양의) 부적, 주문, 마력, 매혹

> fascino, **fascinavi**, fascinatum, fascinare 호리다, 매혹하다, 황홀케 하다　**E** *fascinate*

gypsum, gypsi, n. 석고(*calcium sulfate dihydrate, CaSO₄ · 2H₂O*), 깁스, 석고상　**E** *gypsum*

< G. gypsos, gypsou, f. *chalk, gypsum*

< *Of Semitic origin*

hilum, hili, n. (< *little thing, trifle; thought to have originally meant 'that which adheres*

to a bean) (흔히 부정사(否定詞)와 함께) 보잘 것 없는 것, 사소한 것; 씨앗의 배꼽 (태좌

(胎座)에 붙은 부분); (혈관·신경이 드나드는 내장의) 문(門)　　**E** *hilum,* (pl.) *hila, hilar*

> hilus, hili, m. (혈관·신경이 드나드는 내장의) 문(門)　　　　**E** *hilus,* (pl.) *hili*

> nihilum, nihili, n. (< ne- *not* + hilum *little thing, trifle*) 무(無)

> nihil, n. (불변화) 아무것도 ~ 아니, 무(無) (Vide NON: *See* E. *non-*)

letum, leti, n. (lethum, lethi, n.) (죽임에 의한) 죽음, 파멸

> letalis, letale (lethalis, lethale) 치명적인　　　　　　　　　**E** *lethal, sublethal*

< IE. olə- *to destroy*

lucrum, lucri, n. 이득, 벌이

> lucror, lucratus sum, lucrari 득이 되다

< IE. lau- *gain, profit*

E *lucre*
E *lucrative*
E *guerdon*

mantellum, mantelli, n. (mantelum, manteli, n.) 식탁수건, 손수건, 외투, 싸개, 구실, 핑계

E *mantle, dismantle, mantel,* F. *manteau,* (portare *'to carry' > 'traveling bag' >*) *portmanteau*

< (*perhaps*) *Of Celtic origin*

naucum, nauci, n. (naucus, nauci, m.) 호도의 보늬, (과실의) 껍질, 하찮은 것

E (flocci- *'flock'* + nauci- *'trifle'* + nihili- *'nothing'* + pili- *'hair'* + -fication > *'words signifying at a small price or at nothing' >*) *floccinaucinihilipilification*

otium, otii, n. 한가, 휴식

> negotium, negotii, n. (< neg- *not* + otium, otii, n. *ease*) 분주함, 일, 사업

> negotior, negotiatus sum, negotiari 사업하다, 거래하다
E *negotiate, negotiable*

Palatium, Palatii, n. 옛 로마의 일곱 언덕의 하나 (신전과 궁전이 있었음); (palatium) 궁전,

관저, 저택
E *palace* (< *'imperial residence or temple on the Palatine hill'*), *palatial*

> Palatinus, Palatina, Palatinum 팔라틴 언덕의; (palatinus) 황제의
E *palatine*

palatum, palati, n. 입천장, 구개(口蓋), 미각, 천공(天空)

E *palate, palatal, palatable, palatalize* (< *'to modify a speech sound into a palatal sound'*)

> palatinus, palatina, palatinum 입천장의, 구개의
E *palatine*

< (*perhaps*) *Of Etruscan origin*

praedium, praedii, n. 토지, 부동산
E *praedial*

< praes, praedis, m. 보증인, 보증인의 재산

< IE. wadh- *pledge, to pledge*

E *wed, wedlock, wage, wager, gage, engage, mortgage* (< *'dead pledge; the debt becomes dead when the pledge was redeemed'*)

pretium, pretii, n. 값, 보수, 가치
E *price, prize,* F. *prix*

> pretiosus, pretiosa, pretiosum 값비싼, 귀중한
E *precious*

> pretio, −, −, pretiare 값을 매기다, 평가하다
E *praise*

> appretio, **appretiavi**, appretiatum, appretiare (< ap- (< ad) *to, toward, at, according to*) 값을 매기다, 평가하다,

가치를 인정하다
E *appraise, appraisal, reappraisal, appreciate*

> depretio, **depretiavi**, depretiatum, depretiare 가치를 떨어뜨리다 (< de-
apart from, down, not)   **E** *depreciate*

< IE. per- *to traffic in, to sell; a verbal root belonging to the group of* IE. per *forward,*
through

> L. interpres, interpretis, m., f. (< inter- *between, among*) 중재자, 해석자, 통역자

> L. interpretor, interpretatus sum, interpretari 중재하다, 해석하다, 설명하다,
통역하다   **E** *interpret, interpreter, interpretation*

> G. pernanai *to sell*

> G. pornē, pornēs, f. *prostitute*   **E** *pornography (porno)*

pulpitum, pulpiti, n. (pulpitus, pulpiti, m.) 발판, 연단, 설교단, 무대   **E** *pulpit*

serum, seri, n. 유장(乳漿), 혈청(血清)

E *serum,* (pl.) *sera, serosanguineous, serology, seropositive, seronegative, seroconversion;*
serotype (serovar), **serovar** (< *'on the pattern of cultivar'*)

> serosus, serosa, serosum 장액성(漿液性)의, 혈청의   **E** *serous*

> serositas, serositatis, f. 장액성   **E** *serosity*

< IE. ser- *to stream*

> G. oros, orou, m. *whey*   **E** *orotic acid* (< *'discovered in milk'*)

> (*suggested*) G. rhis, rhinos, f. *nose,* (pl.) *nostrils*

E *rhin(o)-, rhinoceros, rhinology, rhinovirus, rhinal, entorhinal* (< *'interior to the rhinal*
sulcus')

Sodoma, Sodomorum, n. (pl.) 소돔(사해 남단에 있던 팔레스타인의 옛 도시)   **E** *Sodom*

> sodomia, sodomiae, f. 계간(鷄姦), 수간(獸姦)   **E** *sodomy*

< G. Sodoma, Sodomōn, n. (pl.) *Sodom*

< (*Hebrew*) sədom *Sodom*

solum, soli, n. 바닥, 터전, 땅; 발바닥

> solea, soleae, f. 실내용 샌들; 가자미   **E** *sole, (sole >) insole*

> soleus, solea, soleum 가자미 모양의   **E** *soleus (muscle)*

< IE. sel- *human settlement*

> (*Germanic*) sal- *room*   **E** *salon, saloon*

spolium, spolii, n. 짐승의 가죽, 약탈품, 전리품

> spolio, **spoliavi**, spoliatum, spoliare (가죽을) 벗기다, 약탈하다, 전리품으로 차지하다

E *spoil* (< *'to mar or to impair the quality of'* < *'to damage or to injure to make unfit or*
useless'), ***spoilage***

> despolio, **despoliavi**, despoliatum, despoliare (< de- *apart from, down, not;*
intensive + spoliare *to strip of clothing, to rob, to spoil*) 약탈하다,

빼앗다   **E** *despoil*

  < IE. spel- *to split, to break off*   **E** *spill* (< *'shedding blood'* < *'to destroy, to kill'*)

     > IE. (s)plei- *to split, to splice*

        E *split, splint, splinter, flint* (< *'stone splinter'*), *flinders, splice* (< *'to join by untwisting and interweaving the strands of the ends so as to form one continuous length'*), (*splice* + *-o-* + *-some 'body'* >) *spliceosome*

        > (*suggested*) G. sphallein *to make fall, to injure*

          > G. asphalton, asphaltou, n. (< *binding material assuring the solidity of walls* < a- *not* + *sphaltos *able to make fall*) *asphalt*

            > L. asphaltum, asphalti, n. 아스팔트   **E** *asphalt*

sputum, sputi, n. 가래, 객담   **E** *sputum*

     < spuo, spui, sputum, spuĕre 침 뱉다, 뱉어내다

  < IE. sp(y)eu- *to spit, to spew*   **E** *spit, spittle, spew, spout*

     > G. ptyein *to spit*

       > G. ptysis, ptyseōs, f. *spitting*   **E** *-ptysis* (< *'expectoration'*)

         > L. haemoptysis, haemoptysis, f. (< G. haima, haimatos, n. *blood*)

          객혈(喀血)   **E** *haemoptysis (hemoptysis)*

       > G. ptyalon, ptyalou, n. *spittle,*

        saliva   **E** *ptyal(o)-, ptyalism (sialism), ptyalin* (< *'salivary amylase'*)

     > G. sialon, sialou, n. *spittle, saliva*

        E *sial(o)-, sialism (ptyalism), sialic acid(s)* (< *'isolated from the salivary glands of cattle; an N-acyl derivative of neuraminic acid'*), *sialogram* (< *'radiograph of salivary ducts'*)

talcum, talci, n. 활석(滑石, *hydrated magnesium silicate*, $Mg_3Si_4O_{10}(OH)_2$)

    탈크   **E** *talcum (talc), talcosis*

     < (*Arabic*) talq *various transparent, translucent, or shining minerals, as talc proper, mica, selenite, etc*

   < *Of Persian origin*

templum, templi, n. 경계를 둘러친 공간, 제한된 구역, 점쟁이가 지팡이로 공중에 그은 공간,

    눈에 들어오는 구역, 경내(境內), 성역, 성전, 신전   **E** *temple, Templar*

     > contemplor, contemplatus sum, contemplari (< con- (< cum) *with, together; intensive* + templum *place for observation*) 자세히 보다, 숙고하다, 명상하다   **E** *contemplate, contemplative*

  < IE. tem-, temə- *to cut*

     > L. tondeo, totondi, tonsum, tondēre 베어내다, 깎다, 이발하다

       > L. tonsura, tonsurae, f. 삭발, 벌목   **E** *tonsure*

       > L. tonsor, tonsoris, m. 이발사, 정원사, 비평가   **E** *tonsorial*

     > G. temnein *to cut*

E *-tomy* (< 'cutting, dividing'), **rhizotomy** (< 'cutting a root'), **dichotomy** (< 'dividing in two'), **lithotomy** (< 'incision of a duct or organ, especially of the urinary bladder, for removal of stone'), *-tome* (< 'cutting instrument, segment'), **microtome** (< 'cutting instrument to make thin sections'), **Mammotome**® (< 'cutting instrument of breast tissue'), **sclerotome** (< 'hard tissue segment'), **myotome** (< 'muscle segment'), **dermatome** (< 'skin segment')

> G. tomos, tomē, tomon *cut, divide*

　　> G. atomos, atomos, atomon (< a- *not*) *uncut, indivisible*

　　　　> G. atomos, atomou, f. *a hypothetical body, so infinitely small as to be incapable of further division; and thus held to be one of the ultimate particles of matter, by the concourse of which, according to Leucippus and Democritus, the universe was formed*

　　　　　　> L. atomus, atomi, f. 원자(原子)　　　**E** *atom, (atom >) atomic*

　　> G. entomos, entomos, entomon (< en- *in*) *cut up, cut into pieces*　　**E** (G. zōion entomon *'segmented animal'* >) *entomology*

> G. tomos, tomou, m. *piece cut off, slice, section*　　**E** *tomography* (< *'recording of cut section'*)

> G. tomē, tomēs, f. *cutting, dividing*

　　> G. anatomē, anatomēs, f. (< *cutting up* < G. an(a)- *up, upward; again, throughout; back, backward; against; according to, similar to) cutting up, dissection*

　　　　> L. anatomia, anatomiae, f. 해부, 분해, 해부학　　　**E** *anatomy*

　　　　> G. anatomikos, anatomikē, anatomikon *anatomic*

　　　　　　> L. anatomicus, anatomica, anatomicum
　　　　　　해부(학)의　　　**E** *anatomic (anatomical)*

　　> G. ektomē, ektomēs, f. (< G. ek- *out of, away from) cutting out, excision*　　　**E** *-ectomy*

> G. tmēsis, tmēseōs, f. *cutting*　　**E** *-tmesis, neurotmesis*

> G. diatemnein (< di(a)- *through, thoroughly, apart) to cut through*

　　> G. diatomos, diatomos, diatomon *cut through, cut in half*

　　　　> L. diatoma, diatomae, f. 규조(珪藻)　　**E** *diatom, diatomaceous*

> G. epitemnein (< ep(i)- *upon) to make an incision into, to abridge*

　　> G. epitomē, epitomēs, f. *abridgement, summary*

　　　　> L. epitome, epitomes, f. (epitoma, epitomae, f.) 개요, 요약　　　**E** *epitome, (epitome >) epitomize*

velum, veli, n. 돛, 범(帆), 장막, 가리개, 덮개, 천장　　**E** *velum, velar, ((neuter pl.) vela >) veil, voile*

> vexillum, vexilli, n. (< + -illum *diminutive suffix*) (고대 로마의) 군기, 군기 밑의 부대　　　**E** *vexillum*

> velo, velavi, velatum, velare 가리다, 덮다, 둘러싸다

> velamen, velaminis, n. 가리개, 덮개, 막(膜)　　　　　**E** *velamen*

> velamentum, velamenti, n. 가리개, 덮개, 막(膜)　　　　**E** *velamentous*

> revelo, **revelavi**, revelatum, revelare (< re- *back, again* + velare *to veil*)

　　(감추어진 것을) 드러내다, 묵시하다　　　　　　　　**E** *reveal, revelation*

< IE. weg- *to weave a web*

∽ IE. wokso- *wax (< (perhaps) that which grows)*　　**E** *wax (< 'beeswax, earwax')*

venum, veni, n. (venus, venus, m.) 판매, 매매

> venalis, venale 파는, 돈과 바꾸는　　　　　　　　　　**E** *venal*

> vendo, **vendidi**, venditum, venděre (< venum *sale* + dare *to give*) 팔다　　**E** *vend*

< IE. wes- *to buy, to sell*

> (*perhaps*) L. vilis, vile 싼, 값어치 없는, 천한　　　　**E** *vile*

> L. vilifico, −, −, vilificare (< vilis *vile* + -ficare (< facěre) *to make*) 얕보다,

　　헐뜯다　　　　　　　　　　　　　　　　　　　　　**E** *vilify*

> L. vilipendo, −, −, vilipenděre (< vilis *vile* + penděre *to weigh, to consider*)

　　얕보다, 헐뜯다　　　　　　　　　　　　　　　　　　**E** *vilipend*

> G. ōneisthai *to buy*

> (*Persian*) bazar *sale-traffic*　　　　　　　　　　　**E** *bazaar*

vinum, vini, n. 포도주, 술

> **E** *wine, (wine + -ery (< -arius '-ary') >) winery, (vinum acre 'acrid wine' >) vinegar, (vinum + -yl > 'a radical derived from ethylene which is related to ethanol in wine' >) vinyl*

> vinea, vineae, f. 포도나무, 포도원　　　　　　　　　　**E** *vine*

> vindemia, vindemiae, f. (< vinum *wine* + deměre *to remove*) 포도 추수, 추수, 수확 **E** *vintage*

< (*Italic noun, (probably) of Mediterranean origin*) wino- *wine*

> G. oinos, oinou, m. *wine*　　　　　　　　　　　　　**E** *oenophilist*

vitium, vitii, n. 흠, 결점, 악습　　　　　　　　　　　**E** *vice*

> vitiosus, vitiosa, vitiosum 흠 있는, 나쁜　　　　　　　**E** *vicious*

> vitiligo, vitiliginis, f. (< *blemish*) 백반증(白斑症)　　**E** *vitiligo*

> vitio, vitiavi, vitiatum, vitiare 손상시키다, 더럽히다, 무효화하다　　**E** *vitiate*

> vitupero, vituperavi, vituperatum, vituperare (< vitium *fault* + parare *to make*

　　ready) 질책하다　　　　　　　　　　　　　　　　　**E** *vituperate*

< IE. wei- *vice, fault, guilt*

맞대보기 1 어미 -on 으로 끝나는 그리스어 제2변화 중성 명사는 -um 으로 끝나는 라틴어
중성 명사가 되어 위의 변화(제2변화 제3식)를 따른다.

---

antrum, antri, n. 굴, 공동(空洞)　　　　　　　　　　**E** *antrum, antral*

< G. antron, antrou, n. *cave, cavern*

asylum, asyli, n. (불가침의) 피신처   **E** *asylum*

     < G. asylon, asylou, n. (< a- *not* + sylon *seizure, right to seizure*) *refuge, sanctuary*

centrum, centri, n. (< *that point of the compass around which the other describes the circle*)

         중심, 중추, 센터

> **E** *centrum, centre (center), centr(i)-, centrifugal, centripetal, hypocenter* (< '*the deep center*')

     > centralis, centrale 중심의, 중추의   **E** *central*

     > centriolum, centrioli, n. (< *body within the centrosome* < -olum *diminutive suffix*) 중심소체(中心小體)   **E** *centriole*

     > *concentro, *concentravi, *concentratum, *concentrare (< con- (< cum) *with, together*) 중심에 모으다, 집중하다, 농축하다   **E** *concentrate*

         > concentratio, concentrationis, f. 집중, 농축; (화학) 농도   **E** *concentration*

   < G. kentron, kentrou, n. *prick, sting, goad,*

       spur, pain   **E** *centr(o)-, centrosome* (< '*central body*'), *centromere* (< '*central part*')

       > G. kentrikos, kentrikē, kentrikon *pertaining to the center*

> **E** *centric; -centric;* ('*having (such) a centre*'>) *concentric, eccentric;* ('*having a specified centre*'>) *egocentric, ethnocentric, linguocentric;* ('*having the centromere attached at a specified point*'>) *metacentric, submetacentric, telocentric, acrocentric*

       > G. epikentros, epikentros, epikentron (< ep(i)- *upon*) *situating upon a center*

         > L. epicentrum, epicentri, n. (< *the point over the center*) 진앙(震央) **E** *epicenter*

  < IE. kent- *to prick, to jab*

    > G. kentein (kenteein) *to prick*

      > G. kentēsis, kentēseōs, f. *pricking*

        > L. centesis, centesis, f. 천자(穿刺), 찌름, 뚫음

> **E** *centesis, -centesis, thoracocentesis (thoracentesis), peritoneocentesis, amniocentesis*

        > G. parakentēsis, parakentēseōs, f. (< par(a)- *beside, along side of, beyond*) *piercing at the side, couching a cataract, tapping for dropsy*

          > L. paracentesis, paracentesis, f. 천자   **E** *paracentesis*

    > G. kestos, kestē, keston *embroidered* (< *stitched*)

      > G. kestos, kestou, m. *belt, girdle (particularly that worn by a bride in ancient times)*   **E** *cestus*

        > L. Cestoda, Cestodorum, n. (pl.) (< + G. -ōdēs *like, resembling*) 조충강(條蟲綱)   **E** *cestode*

ischium, ischii, n. 좌골(坐骨), 궁둥뼈   **E** *ischium, ischial*

    < G. ischion, ischiou, n. *hip, hip joint, socket of the hip bones*

      > G. ischias, ischiados, f. *pain in the hip*

        > G. ischiadikos, ischiadikē, ischiadikon *of pain in the hip, of the ischium*

          > L. ischiadicus, ischiadica, ischiadicum 좌골신경통의, 좌골의,

궁둥이의   **E** *ischiadic*

> (*corrupted*) L. sciaticus, sciatica, sciaticum 좌골신경통의,

좌골의   **E** *sciatic,* (sciatica passio *'sciatic passion'* >) *sciatica*

metallum, metalli, n. 광산, 광물, 금속, 채석장   **E** *metal, metallic, metallurgy,* (metal >) *mettle*

< G. metallon, metallou, n. *mine, quarry, pit*

organum, organi, n. 도구, 기관(器官), 장기(臟器), 기(器), 오르간

> organulum, organuli, n. (< + -ulum *diminutive suffix*) 작은 오르간

> organella, organellae, f. (< + -ella *diminutive suffix*) 소기관(小器官),

세포내기관   **E** *organelle, organellar*

> organismus, organismi, m. 유기체(有機體), 생명체, 생체, 생물,

미생물   **E** *organism, microorganism*

> organizo, **organizavi,** organizatum, organizare 체계를 형성하다   **E** *organize, organizer*

> organizatio, organizationis, f. 조직, 체제, 기구, 단체, 조직화,

기질화(基質化)   **E** *organization*

< G. organon, organou, n. *tool, instrument, implement*   **E** *organ*

> G. organikos, organikē, organikon *of or relating to an organ, instrumental*

> L. organicus, organica, organicum 기관의, 장기의, 기질적(基質的)인,

유기적(有機的)인, 조직적인   **E** *organic, inorganic*

< IE. werg- *to do*

E *work, wrought, wright, irk* (< *'to work'*), *irksome, bulwark* (< *'plank work'*), *boulevard* (< *'plank work'*)

> G. orgia, orgiōn, n. (pl.) *secret rites, worship* (< *service*)   **E** *orgy*

> G. orgiazein *to celebrate orgies*

> G. orgiastēs, orgiastou, m. *one who celebrates orgies*

> G. orgiastikos, orgiastikē, orgiastikon *of orgies*   **E** *orgiastic*

> G. ergon, ergou, n. *deed, work*

E *erg, -ergic, adrenergic, cholinergic, endergonic, exergonic, ergonomics,* (allos *'other'* + -ergeia *'reactivity'* > *'altered reactivity'* >) *allergy, allergic,* (meta *'across'* + ergon > *'change of function'* >) *metergasis*

> G. ergastikos, ergastikē, ergastikon *laborious,*

industrious   **E** *ergastoplasm* (< *'basophilic fibrillar formations in gland cells'*)

> G. geōrgos, geōrgou, m. (< gē *earth*) *farmer*   **E** *georgic*

> G. -ourgos, -ourgou, m. *worker*   **E** *-urge, dramaturge*

-ourgia, -ourgias, f. *working*   **E** *-urgy, metallurgy, thaumaturgy*

> G. cheirourgia, cheirourgias, f. (< cheir, cheiros, f. *hand*) *manual*

labor, craft   **E** *surgery, surgical, surgeon*

> G. leitourgia, leitourgias, f. (< leito- (< leōs) *people*) *public service,*

expenditure for the state, public service to the gods   **E** *liturgy*

> G. energeia, energeias, f. (< en- *in*) *activity*

> L. energia, energiae, f. 원기(元氣), 힘,
에너지　　**E** *energy* (< *'workable contents, kinetic or potential'*)

> G. synergein (< syn- *with, together*) *to work together*

> G. synergia, synergias, f. *working together*

> L. synergia, synergiae, f. 협동작용, 상승작용, 상승효과　　**E** *synergy*

> L. dyssynergia, dyssynergiae, f. (< G. dys- *bad*)
근육협동장애　　**E** *dyssynergy*

> G. anergos, anergos, anergon (< an- *not*) *inactive*

> G. anergia, anergias, f. *idleness*　　**E** *anergy*

> G. argos, argos, argon (< a- *not*) *idle*　　**E** *argon (Ar)* (< *'its chemical inertness'*)

> G. lēthargia, lēthargias, f. (< lēthē, lēthēs, f. *forgetting* + *argos*)
forgetfulness

> L. lethargia, lethargiae, f. 졸음증, 기면(嗜眠)　　**E** *lethargy, lethargic*

saccharum, sacchari, n. (Persia · Arabia · India 등지에서 사탕갈대에 칼자국을 내어 흘러
나오는 즙을 모은) 약용 당밀; 사탕, 설탕, 당분

E *sacchar(o)-, saccharide(s), monosaccharide(s), disaccharide(s), oligosaccharide(s), polysaccharide(s)* (glycan(s)), *mucopolysaccharide(s)* (now called glycosamino-glycan(s)), (mucopolysaccharide >) *mucopolysaccharidosis; saccharine, saccharin*

< G. sakcharon, sakcharou, n. *sugar*

< (*Persian*) sakar *sugar*

> (*Arabic*) sukkar *sugar*

> F. sucre *sugar*　　**E** *sucrose, sugar*

< (*Sanskrit*) sarkara *sugar, akin to* sarkarah *pebble*

sesamum, sesami, n. 참깨　　**E** *sesame, sesamoid*

< G. sēsamon, sēsamou, n. *sesame*

< *Of Oriental origin*

perineum, perinei, n. 회음(會陰), 샅　　**E** *perineum, perineal*

< G. perinaion, perinaiou, n. (< peri- *around, near, beyond, on account of* + inan
(inaein) *to evacuate, to defecate*) *region of evacuation*

tartarum, tartari, n. 주석(酒石), 치석(齒石)　　**E** *tartar, tartaric acid, tartrate*

< G. tartaron, tartarou, n. *tartar encrusting the sides of casks*

theatrum, theatri, n. 극장, 무대, 연극, 관객, 그리스 의회의 의원이 모이던 계단식 강단, 활동
범주　　**E** *theatre (theater)*

< G. theatron, theatrou, n. *theatre, stage, play, spectators*

> G. amphitheatron, amphitheatrou, n. (< amphi- *on both sides, around*)
amphitheatre

> L. amphitheatrum, amphitheatri, n. 원형극장,

원형경기장   **E** *amphitheatre (amphitheater)*

< G. theasthai *to look on, to view, to contemplate*

> G. theōros, theōrou, m. *spectator, looker-on, ambassador sent to a festival or oracle*

> G. theōria, theōrias, f. *a looking at, viewing, contemplation, speculation, theory, also a sight, a spectacle*

> L. theoria, theoriae, f. 이론, 학설, 철학적 사변, 학리(學理)   **E** *theory*

> G. theōrein (theōreein) *to be a spectator, to look at, to inspect*

> G. theōrēma, theōrēmatos, n. *spectacle, speculation, theory, (in Euclid) a proposition to be proved*

> L. theorema, theorematis, n. 정리(定理), 공식(公式)   **E** *theorem*

> G. theōrētikos, theōrētikē, theōrētikon *contemplative*

> L. theoreticus, theoretica, theoreticum 이론의, 이론적,

학리의, 사변적   **E** *theoretic (theoretical)*

< IE. dhau- *to see*

> G. thauma, thaumatos, n. *miracle, wonder*   **E** *thaumatology, thaumaturgy*

맞대보기 2   어미 on으로 끝나는 그리스어 제2변화 중성 명사이나 관례상 그대로 쓰는 라틴어 낱말은 단수 주격만 -on으로 되며 위의 변화(제2변화 제3식)를 따른다.

---

colon, coli, n. 결장(結腸), 잘록창자; 대장(大腸), 큰창자   **E** *colon, colonic, megacolon*

[용례] Escherichia coli 대장균

> **E** **Escherichia coli,** (E. coli >) *coliform,* (E. coli + -cin (< caedĕre *'to cut, to kill'*) > *'an antibiotic produced by some coliform bacteria'* >) *colicin*

(문법) Escherichia (세균) 대장균속(屬): 단수 주격

< Escherichia, Escherichiae, f.

< Theodor Escherich (1857-1911), *German pediatrician and bacteriologist*

coli 대장의: 단수 속격

> colistinus, colistina, colistinum

대장의   **E** *colistin* (< *'antibiotic produced by* Bacillus polymyxa *var.* colistinus*'*)

> mesocolon, mesocoli, n. (< *mesentery of the colon* < G. mesos *middle*) 결장

간막(結腸間膜), 잘록창자간막   **E** *mesocolon*

< G. kolon, kolou, n. (kōlon, kōlou, n.) *food, meat, large intestine*

> G. kolikos, kolikē, kolikon *of large intestine*

> L. colicus, colica, colicum 배앓이의, 복통의   **E** *colicky*

> L. colica, colicae, f. 배앓이, 복통, 급통증(急痛症), 산통(疝痛)   **E** *colic*

skeleton, skeleti, n. (< G. skeleton sōma *dried body, mummy*) 뼈대, 골격, 해골

> **E** *skeleton, skeletal, cytoskeleton, cytoskeletal, endoskeleton, exoskeleton*

  < G. skeletos, skeletē, skeleton *dried up*

   < G. skellesthai (*passive*) *to be dried up*

  < G. skellein *to dry*

< IE. skelǝ- *to parch, to wither*

 > G. sklēros, sklēra, sklēron *dry, hard*   **E** *scler(o)-, sclerous*

  > G. sklēroun (sklēroein) *to harden*

   > G. sklērōsis, sklērōseōs, f. (< -ōsis *condition*) *hardness*

    > L. sclerosis, sclerosis, f. 경화증(硬化症), 경화(硬化)

> **E** *sclerosis, sclerotic, (sclerosis >) sclerosed, (sclerosed >) sclerose,
-sclerosis*

     > L. arteriosclerosis, arteriosclerosis, f. (< G. artēria *artery*)

      동맥경화증   **E** *arteriosclerosis*

     > L. atherosclerosis, atherosclerosis, f. (< G. athērē *groats,
gruel*) 죽상(粥狀)경화증, 죽(粥)경화증   **E** *atherosclerosis*

     > L. arteriolosclerosis, arteriolosclerosis, f. (< arteriola
arteriole) 세동맥(細動脈)경화증   **E** *arteriolosclerosis*

   > L. sclera, sclerae, f. 공막(鞏膜)   **E** *sclera, scleral*

    > L. episclera, episclerae, f. (< G. ep(i)- *upon*) 겉공막,
상공막   **E** *episclera, episcleral*

   > L. sclerema, sclerematis, n. (< *on the pattern of* oedema) 경화   **E** *sclerema*

   > L. scleroedema, scleroedematis, n. (< + G. oidēma *swelling*)
경화부종   **E** *scleroedema (scleredema)*

   > L. scleroderma, sclerodermatis, n. (< + G. derma *skin*) 피부경화증   **E** *scleroderma*

●●● 제 3 변화

단수 속격의 어미가 -is인 남성, 여성, 중성 명사. 원칙적으로 단수 주격의 어간과 단수
속격의 어간이 다르다.

●●● 제 3 변화 제 1 식 a

단수 속격의 음절수가 많아지며 어간 끝에 자음이 하나만 있는 남성, 여성 명사. 단수의
속격 어미는 -is; 복수의 주격 어미는 -es, 속격 어미는 -um이 된다.

homo, hominis, m. 사람

	단 수	복 수	
주격	homo	homin-es	~이, ~가, ~은, ~는, ~께서
속격	homin-is	homin-um	~의
여격	homin-i	homin-ibus	~게, ~에게, ~께, ~한테
대격	homin-em	homin-es	~을, ~를
탈격	homin-e	homin-ibus	~에서, ~로부터, ~으로부터
호격	homo	homin-es	~여, ~이여

homo, hominis, m. 사람　　　　　　　　　　　　　　　　　　E *homo*

[용례] Homo homini lupus (est). 인간은 인간에게 늑대(이다)

(문법) homo 인간은: 단수 주격

homini 인간에게: 단수 여격

lupus 늑대: 단수 주격 < lupus, lupi, m.

est 이다: esse 동사, 직설법 현재 단수 삼인칭

> homunculus, homunculi, m. (< homun- (< homin-) + -culus *diminutive suffix*)

난쟁이, 축소인간, 변변치 못한 사람, 정자미인(精子微人)　　E *homunculus*, (pl.) *homunculi*

> hominaticum, hominatici, n. 군신관계의 서약, (신하로서의) 경의, 존경　　E *homage*

> homicida, homicidae, m. (< + caedĕre *to cut, to kill*) 살인자　　E *homicide*

> homicidium, homicidii, n. (< + caedĕre *to cut, to kill*) 살인　　E *homicide*

> Hominidae, Hominidarum, f. (pl.) 사람과(科)의 인류 (현생인류와 화석인류를 포함)　　E *hominid*

< IE. dhghem- *earth, earthling*　　　　　　E *bridegroom* (< '*earthling (man) of the bride*')

> L. humanus, humana, humanum 사람의, 사람다운　　E *human, humane*

> L. humus, humi, f. 땅, 흙　　　E *humus, inhume, exhume, transhumance*

> L. humilis, humile 낮은, 비천한, 겸손한　　　E *humble*

> L. humilitas, humilitatis, f. 비천, 겸손, 겸허　　　E *humility*

> L. humilio, humiliavi, humiliatum, humiliare 낮추다, 비하시키다, 모욕하다　E *humiliate*

> G. chthōn, chthonos, f. *soil, ground, earth, country*

> G. autochthōn, autochthonos, f. (< autos *self*) *a being sprung from that land itself*　　E *autochthonous*

> G. chamai (*adverb*) *on the ground, on the soil, dwarf*

> G. chamaileōn, chamaileontos, m. (< + leōn *lion*) *chameleon*

> L. chamaeleon, chamaeleontis, m. (chamaeleon, chamaeleonis, m.)

카멜레온　　　E *chamaeleon (chameleon)* (< '*lion on the ground*')

cardo, cardinis, m. 문지도리, 경첩, 축(軸)

> cardinalis, cardinale 문지도리의, 주요한, 기본적인　　　E *cardinal* (< '*pivotal*')

> cardinalis, cardinalis, m. (< episcopus cardinalis *chief bishop*) 추기경(樞機卿)

    E *cardinal* (< 'pivot of church life', 'of the color of a cardinal's cassock; deep scarlet')

< IE. (s)ker- *to leap, to jump out*   **E** *scherzo*

> G. kordylē, kordylēs, f. *bump, swelling, club*

    > L. Cordyceps, Cordycipitis, f. (< *club-headed* < + -ceps < caput *head*) (자낭
진균 子囊眞菌) 동충하초속(冬蟲夏草屬)   **E** *Cordyceps*

ordo, ordinis, m. (< *originally a row of threads in a loom*) 열(列), 계급, 순서, 질서, 규정;

(가톨릭) 수도회; (분류) 목(目)   **E** *order, suborder*

> ordinalis, ordinale 순서를 표시하는   **E** *ordinal*

> ordinarius, ordinaria, ordinarium 순서대로의, 정규의, 통상적인, 평범한   **E** *ordinary, extraordinary*

> ordino, ordinavi, ordinatum, ordinare 배열하다, 정돈하다, 관리하다, 규정하다, 임명
하다   **E** *ordain, disorder*

    > ordinatus, ordinata, ordinatum (*past participle*) 배열된,
질서 잡힌   **E** (linea ordinata applicata *'line applied parallel'* >) *ordinate*

        > inordinatus, inordinata, inordinatum (< in- *not*) 무질서한, 멋대로의   **E** *inordinate*

    > ordinantia, ordinantiae, f. (국왕·정부 등 권력 기관이 발하는)
포고(布告)   **E** *ordinance*, (ordinance >) *ordnance* (< 'military provision')

    > subordino, subordinavi, subordinatum, subordinare (< sub- *under, up from
under* + ordinare *to arrange*) 종속시키다   **E** *subordinate*

    > *coordino, *coordinavi, *coordinatum, *coordinare (< co- (< cum) *with,
together* + ordinare *to arrange*) 함께 배열하다, 균형 잡히게 하다, 대등하게
하다, 조정하다   **E** *coordinate, coordinator*

        > coordinatio, coordinationis, f. 협조, 협동, 조화,
조정   **E** *coordination, incoordination*

< (*Italic root of uncertain origin*) ord- *to arrange, arrangement*

> L. ordior, orsus sum, ordiri 베틀에 날을 날다, 베를 짜기 시작하다, 짜다, 시작하다

    > L. primordium, primordii, n. (< primus *first* + ordiri *to begin* + -ium *noun
suffix*) 시작, 최초, 원본, 원기(原基)   **E** *primordium*, (pl.) *primordia*

        > L. primordialis, primordiale 최초의, 원시의   **E** *primordial*

> L. orno, ornavi, ornatum, ornare 장비하다, 꾸미다   **E** *ornate*

    > L. ornamentum, ornamenti, n. 장비, 장식, 장식품 **E** *ornament, ornamental, ornamentation*

    > L. adorno, adornavi, adornatum, adornare (< ad- *to, toward, at, according
to* + ornare *to deck*) 장비를 갖추다, 꾸미다   **E** *adorn, adornment*

    > L. suborno, subornavi, subornatum, subornare (< sub- *under, up from under*
+ ornare *to deck*) 비밀리에 준비시키다, 사주하다, 위증시키다   **E** *suborn, subornation*

carbo, carbonis, m. 숯, 석탄

> carbunculus, carbunculi, m. (< carbun- (< carbon-) + -culus *diminutive suffix*)

작은 석탄, 홍옥(紅玉), 탄저(炭疽), 큰 종기(腫氣)　　　**E** *carbuncle, carbuncular*

< IE. ker- *heat, fire*　　　**E** *hearth*

> L. cremo, **cremavi,** crematum, cremare 불사르다, 화장하다　　**E** *cremate*

> (*possibly*) G. keramos, keramou, m. *potter's clay, pottery*

> G. keramikos, keramikē, keramikon *of clay, of pottery*　　**E** *ceramic*

caupo, cauponis, m. 소매상인, 주막 주인　　　**E** *cheap, chapman,* (chapman >) *chap*

histrio, histrionis, m. 배우

> histrionicus, histrionica, histrionicum 배우의, 연기의, 극적인　　**E** *histrionic*

< *Of Etruscan origin*

latro, latronis, m. 용병, 호위병, (서양장기의) 말; 강도

> latrunculus, latrunculi, m. (< latro *bandit* + -culus *diminutive suffix*) (서양장기의)

말, 졸; 바늘도둑, 소매치기

> latrocinium, latrocinii, n. 신변경호직; 절도 행위　　**E** *larceny*

> Latrodectus, Latrodecti, m. (< latro *bandit* + G. daknein *to bite*) (독거미)

라트로덱투스속(屬)　　**E** *Latrodectus, latrodectism, latrotoxin*

< IE. le- *to get*

> G. latreia, latreias, f. *hired labor, service (for pay), duties,*

worship　　**E** *-latry, iconolatry, idolatry, ophiolatry, plutolatry, pyrolatry*

> G. -latrēs, -latrou, m. *worshipper*　　**E** *-later*

pulmo, pulmonis, m. 허파, 폐(肺)　　**E** *pulmonic* (< 'pulmonary, of pulmonary artery'), *pulmonology*

> pulmonarius, pulmonaria, pulmonarium 폐질환의, 폐의　　**E** *pulmonary*

> pulmonalis, pulmonale 폐의

[용례] cor pulmonale 폐성심(肺性心)　　**E** *cor pulmonale*

(문법) cor 심장: 단수 주격 < cor, cordis, n. 심장, 마음

pulmonale 폐의: 형용사, 중성형 단수 주격

< IE. pleu- *to flow*

> G. pleumōn, pleumonos, m. *lung*

  > G. pneumōn, pneumonos, m. (< *influenced by* pneuma, pneumatos, n.
    breath) *lung*   **E** *pneumon(o)- (pneum(o)-), pneumonocyte (pneumocyte)*

    > G. pneumonia, pneumonias, f. (< *inflammation of the parenchyma of*
      the lung, especially of infectious (chiefly bacterial) origin < -ia *noun*
      suffix) pneumonia

      > L. pneumonia, pneumoniae, f. 폐렴   **E** *pneumonia*

        [용례] Streptococcus pneumoniae 폐렴 사슬알균,
          폐렴 연쇄구균   **E** Streptococcus pneumoniae
          Mycoplasma pneumoniae
          폐렴 마이코플라즈마   **E** Mycoplasma pneumoniae
          (문법) streptococcus 사슬알균, 연쇄구균: 단수 주격
            < streptococcus, streptococci, m.
          mycoplasma 마이코플라즈마: 단수 주격
            < mycoplasma, mycoplasmatis, n.
          pneumoniae 폐렴의: 단수 속격

    > L. pneumonitis, pneumonitidis, f. (< *inflammation of the parenchyma*
      of the lung, especially of non-infectious (allergic, physical, chemical,
      etc.) origin < -itis *noun suffix denoting inflammation*) 폐렴 **E** *pneumonitis*

    > G. pneumonikos, pneumonikē, pneumonikon *of the lungs, affected with*
      lung disease

      > L. pneumonicus, pneumonica, pneumonicum 폐의, 폐렴의 **E** *pneumonic*

    > L. pneumonoconiosis, pneumonoconiosis, f. (pneumoconiosis, pneumo-
      coniosis, f.) (< + G. konis *dust* + -ōsis *condition*)
      진폐증(塵肺症)   **E** *pneumonoconiosis (pneumoconiosis)*

    > L. pneumococcus, pneumococci, m. (< + G. kokkos *grain, berry*) 폐렴
      알균, 패렴구균(肺炎球菌)

      E *pneumococcus* (< '*an individual organism of the species* Sreptococcus
      pneumoniae'), (pl.) *pneumococci*

> L. pluit, pluvit (pluit), −, pluĕre (비인칭동사) 비 오다

  > L. pluvia, pluviae, f. 비   **E** *pluvial*

    > L. pluviosus, pluviosa, pluviosum 비가 많이 (자주) 오는 **E** *pluvious (pluviose)*

> (*probably*) L. palus, paludis, f. 습지

  E *paludal, paludism* (< '*malaria, as formerly thought to be caused by noxious marsh gas*')

  > L. paluster, palustris, palustre (palustris, (gen.) palustre) 습지의 **E** *palustrine*

> G. ploutos, ploutou, m. (< *overflowing*) *wealth, riches* **E** *plutocracy, plutolatry, Plutarch*

  > G. Ploutōn, Ploutōnos, m. (*Greek mythology*) *the giver of wealth, the god*
    of the lower world (also called Hades)

    > L. Pluto, Plutonis, m. (로마 신화) 지하의 신;
      명왕성(冥王星)   **E** *Pluto, plutonium (Pu)* (< '*on the pattern of uranium*')

> G. pyelos, pyelou, f. *trough, basin*   **E** *pyel(o)-*

titio, titionis, m. 불씨

> *intitio, *intitiavi, *intitiatum, *intitiare (< in- *in, on, into, toward* + titio *firebrand*)
불붙이다, 꾀다   **E** *entice*

humor, humoris, m. 물기, 습기, 물, 액체, 체액(體液)

> **E** *humor (humour) (< 'mental disposition' < 'bodily fluid' < 'moisture'), humorous, humoresque*

> humoralis, humorale 체액의, 체액성의   **E** *humoral*

< humeo, −, −, humēre 젖다

> humecto, **humectavi**, humectatum, humectare 젖게 하다   **E** *humectant*

> humidus, humida, humidum 젖은, 습한   **E** *humid, (humid >) humidify*

> humiditas, humiditatis, f. 습기, 습도   **E** *humidity*

< IE. weg^w- *wet*

> G. hygros, hygra, hygron *wet*   **E** *hygr(o)-, hygrometer, hygroscopic*

> L. hygroma, hygromatis, n. (< + G. -ōma *noun suffix denoting tumor*)
물주머니   **E** *hygroma*

odor, odoris, m. 냄새   **E** *odor (odour), malodor*

> odorus, odora, odorum 향내 나는, 코를 찌르는, 예리한 후각의   **E** *odorous, malodorous*

> odoro, **odoravi**, odoratum, odorare 냄새피우다, 방향(芳香)을
풍기다   **E** *odorant, malodorant, deodorant*

> odorifer, odorifera, odoriferum (< odor *smell* + -fer (< ferre *to carry, to bear*)
carrying, bearing) 방향(芳香)을 풍기는, 향료(香料)를 만들어내는   **E** *odoriferous*

< IE. od- *to smell*

> L. oleo, olui, −, olēre (*with -l- for -d- representing a Sabine borrowing*) 냄새 나다,
냄새를 풍기다

> L. redoleo, **redolui**, −, redolēre (< red- *back, again* + olēre *to smell*)
냄새를 풍기다   **E** *redolent*

> L. olfacio, **olfeci**, olfactum, olfacĕre (< olēre *to smell* + facĕre *to make*)
냄새를 맡다   **E** *olfaction*

> L. olfactorius, olfactoria, olfactorium 후각의, 냄새 맡는   **E** *olfactory*

> G. ozein *to smell*   **E** *ozone (< 'a bluish toxic gas with a sharp odor, O_3')*

> L. ozostomia, ozostomiae, f. (< + G. stoma *mouth* + -ia) 입냄새증, 구취증
(口臭症)   **E** *ozostomia*

> G. osmē, osmēs, f. *smell*

> **E** *osmic, osmics, geosmin (< 'earth smell'); osmium (Os) (< 'pungent smell of osmium tetroxide, OsO_4'), (osmium > osmium tetroxide >) osmic acid, osmiophilic*

> L. osmidrosis, osmidrosis, f. (< + G. hidrōsis *sweating*)
땀악취증   **E** *osmidrosis (bromidrosis)*

> L. anosmia, anosmiae, f. (< G. an- *not*) 후각상실증   **E** *anosmia*

> L. *parosmia, *parosmiae, f. (< G. par(a)- *beside, along side of, beyond*)

이상후각   **E** *parosmia*

> G. -ōdēs, -ōdēs, -ōdes *smelling*   **E** *cacodyl* (< 'disgusting garlic odor')

rumor, rumoris, m. 철썩거리는 소리, 떠들썩함, 소문, 세평(世評)   **E** *rumor (rumour)*

< IE. reu- (*probably echoic*) *to bellow*

> L. rugio, rugivi (rugii), rugitum, rugire 으르렁대다, 울부짖다, 포효하다, (뱃속에서)

쪼르륵 소리 나다   **E** *riot, rut,* (probably) *bruit*

> L. rugitus, rugitus, m. 포효; 창자가스소리, 복명(腹鳴)   **E** *rugitus*

> L. rugo, −, ructum, rugĕre 트림하다

> L. ructus, ructus, m. 트림   **E** *ructus*

> L. raucus, rauca, raucum 목쉰, 귀에 거슬리는   **E** *raucous*

torpor, torporis, m. 둔감(鈍感), 지둔(遲鈍)   **E** *torpor*

< torpeo, −, −, torpēre 빳빳해지다, 무디어지다   **E** *torpid, torpidity, torpedo*

< IE. ster- *stiff*

E *stark, starch* (< 'stiff'), *stern* (< 'firm'), *start* (< 'to move stiffly, to move briskly'), *startle* (< 'to cause to react with fear' < 'to move quickly (typically said of cattle'), *starve* (< 'to die' < 'to become stiff'), (starve >) *starvation, stare* (< 'having fixed eyes, rigid'), *stork* (< 'probably from the stiff movements of the bird'), *strut* (< 'to stand out stiffly'), *stretch, straight*

> L. stirps, stirpis, f. 나무등걸, 풀뿌리

> L. ex(s)tirpo, ex(s)tirpavi, ex(s)tirpatum, ex(s)tirpare 뿌리째 뽑아버리다, 제거

하다   **E** *extirpate, extirpation*

> G. stereos, sterea, stereon *stiff, stark, solid, constant*

E *stere(o)-* (< 'of firm and solid forms having three dimensions'), *stereotype* (< 'a duplicate solid plate of an original typographical element, used for printing instead of the original'), *stereoscope, stereophone, stereo; cholesterol* (< 'first found in gallstones'), (cholesterol >) *sterol(s), -sterol,* (sterol >) *steroid(s),* (testis + sterol + -one (< ketone) >) *testosterone,* (aldehyde + steroid + -one (< ketone) >) *aldosterone, -sterone; steric* (< 'pertaining or relating to the arrangement in space of the atoms in a molecule'), (allos 'other' >) *allosteric*

> G. stērixis, stērixeōs, f. *fixed position*   **E** *asterixis*

> L. strenuus, strenua, strenuum 튼튼한; 활기찬   **E** *strenuous*

∞ G. strēnēs, strēnēs, strēnes *hard, strong, rough*

> IE. (s)ter-n- *name of thorny plants*   **E** *thorn*

calor, caloris, m. 열, 더위   **E** *calor,* F. *calorie, calorimetry*

< caleo, calui, −, calēre 뜨겁다, 따뜻하다, 흥분하다   **E** (Sp. calentura 'fever' >) *calenture*

> calidus, calida, calidum (caldus, calda, caldum) 뜨거운, 따뜻한, 열렬한

> calidarius, calidaria, calidarium (caldarius, caldaria, caldarium) 데우는,

온탕의   **E** Sp. *caldera, caldron (cauldron)*

> excaldo, excaldavi, excaldatum, excaldare (< ex- *out of, away from* +

calidus *hot*)   `E scald`

> calefacio, **calefeci**, calefactum, calefacĕre (calfacio, **calfeci**, calfactum, calfacĕre)

(< calēre *to be hot* + facĕre *to make*) 뜨겁게 하다, 따뜻하게 하다, 흥분

시키다   `E chauffeur (< 'one who fuels the fire of a steam engine')`

< IE. kelə- *warm*   `E lee (< 'covering, protection'), lukewarm`

rubor, ruboris, m. 적색, 홍안, 부끄러움, 발적(發赤)   `E rubor`

     < ruber, rubra, rubrum 붉은

< IE. reudh- *red, ruddy* (Vide RUBER: *See* E. *rubric*)

tumor, tumoris, m. 부음, 붓는 병, 종기, 종양, 분노, 오만   `E tumor (tumour), tumorlet (< 'minute tumor')`

> tumorosus, tumorosa, tumorosum 종양의   `E tumorous`

< tumeo, −, −, tumēre 부풀다, 붓다, 화나다, 오만하다

> tumulus, tumuli, m. 흙더미, 언덕; 무덤   `E tumulus, (pl.) tumuli`

> tumultus, tumultus, m. (tumultus, tumulti, m.) 소란   `E tumult`

     > tumultuosus, tumultuosa, tumultuosum 소란스러운   `E tumultuous`

> tumesco, **tumuli**, −, tumescĕre (< tumēre *to swell* + -escĕre *suffix of*

inceptive (inchoative) verb) 부풀어 오르다, 부어오르다,

화가 치밀다   `E tumescent, intumescent`

> tumefacio, **tumefeci**, tumefactum, tumefacĕre (< tumēre *to swell* + facĕre

to make) 부풀게 하다, 붓게 하다   `E tumefy, tumefacient, tumefactive, tumefaction`

> tuber, tuberis, n. 혹, 종기; 매듭, 나무의 옹이, 괴경(塊莖)   `E tuber, truffle`

> tuberalis, tuberale 융기한

> tuberosus, tuberosa, tuberosum 혹이 많은, 괴경형(塊莖形)의,

결절(結節)의   `E tuberous`

     > tuberositas, tuberositatis, f. 융기, 결절; 조면(粗面)   `E tuberosity`

> tuberculum, tuberculi, n. (< + -culum *diminutive suffix*) 구근(球根),

융기(隆起), 결절(結節); 종기(腫氣),

결핵(結核)   `E tuberculum, tubercle, tuberculous, tuberculin`

     > tuberculosis, tuberculosis, f. (< + G. -ōsis *condition*) 결핵   `E tuberculosis`

> protubero, **protuberavi**, protuberatum, protuberare (< pro- *before,*

forward, for, instead of) 불룩이 내밀다, 돌출(突出)하다, 돌기(突起)

하다   `E protuberant, protuberance`

> contumelia, contumeliae, f. (< con- (< cum) *with, together; intensive*) (언동의)

오만함, 무례, 모욕   `E contumely`

< IE. teuə-, teu- *to swell, to be strong*   `E thousand (< 'swollen hundred'), thumb, thimble, thigh, thole`

> L. turgeo, **tursi**, −, turgēre 부풀다, 과장되다   `E turgid`

> L. turgor, turgoris, m. 팽창, 팽압   `E turgor`

> L. turgesco, −, −, turgescĕre (< turgēre *to swell* + -escĕre *suffix of inceptive*

(inchoative) verb) 부어오르다, 격렬하게

되다   E *turgescent, turgescence, deturgescence*

> L. tomentum, tomenti, n. (솜·털·짚 등의) 쿠션 속   E *tomentum,* (pl.) *tomenta*

    > L. tomentosus, tomentosa, tomentosum 부드러운 털이

빽빽이 난   E *tomentose (tomentous)*

> L. obturo, **obturavi**, obturatum, obturare (< *stopped up* < *swollen, coagulated* < ob-
before, toward(s), over, against, away + *-turare) 막다, 마개를 박다, 밀폐하다;

시장기를 풀다   E *obturate*

    > L. obturator, obturatoris, m. 막는 것, 닫개, 폐쇄물, 전색자(栓塞子), 전자(栓子)   E *obturator*

> G. tylos, tylou, m. (tylē, tylēs, f.) *lump, knob, callus, nail, peg,*

penis   E *tylectomy, tylosis, gonotyl*

> G. tyros, tyrou, m. (< *swelling, coagulating*)

cheese   E *tyrosine (Tyr, Y)* (< *'first discovered in casein'*)

    > G. boutyron, boutyrou, n. (< bous, boos, m., f. *ox, cow* + tyros *cheese / but*
perhaps of Scythian or other barbarous origin) *butter*

      > L. butyrum, butyri, n. 버터, 우락(牛酪)

E *butter, butyric, gamma-aminobutyric acid (GABA), butyl,* (butyl + -anus
'adjective suffix' >) *butane, butterfly*

> G. tymbos, tymbou, m. *mound; tomb, grave*   E *tomb*

> G. sōros, sōrou, m. *heap, file*

    > L. sorus, sori, m. (식물) (양치식물의) 자낭군(子囊群);

(동물) 꽁치(의 일종)   E *sorus,* (pl.) *sori*

> G. sōma, sōmatos, n. *body*

    > L. soma, somatis, n. 몸, 신체, 체(體), 몸통, 구간(軀幹), 체간(體幹), 세포체(細胞體)

E *soma,* (pl.) *somata, somite* (< *'body segment'*), *somat(o)-, somatization,
somatotropin* (growth hormone), *somatomedin(s)* (< *'intermediary in
somatotropin action'*), *somatostatin* (< *'an inhibitor of the release of
somatotropin and other hormones'*), *-some, lysosome* (< *'richness in hydrolytic
enzymes'*), *endosome* (< *'endocytosed bodies'*), *phagosome,* (peroxide >)
peroxisome, microsome (< *'small bodies (fragments) of endoplasmic
reticulum'*), *ribosome, polyribosome (polysome), chromosome* (< *'chromatic
bodies'*), *autosome* (< *'the non-aberrant chromosomes previously called
ordinary chromosomes, unlike allosomes (sex chromosomes)'*), *episome* (<
'particle additional to a chromosome' < *'(now obsolete) a small particle which
together with a larger 'protosome' constitutes a gene, and which by its
absence causes gene mutation'*), *acrosome, melanosome, -somy* (< *'numerical
state of a chromosome'*), *monosomy, trisomy; nucleosome*

    > G. sōmatikos, sōmatikē, sōmatikon *of body*   E *somatic*

> G. sōs, sōs, sōon (< *swollen, strong*) *safe, healthy*

    > G. sōzein *to save*

E (kreas 'flesh' + sōzein 'to save' >) *creosote,* (creosote >) *creosol (cresol)*

    > G. sōtēr, sōtēros, m. *preserver, savior*

      > G. sōtēria, sōtērias, f. *preservation, salvation*   E *soteriology*

> G. Sōkratēs, Sōkratous, m. (< *having safe might* < sōs + kratos *might*)

Socrates

> L. Socrates, Socratis, m. 소크라테스   **E** *Socrates*

dolor, doloris, m. 아픔, 고통   **E** *dolor (dolour),* F. *douloureux*

    < doleo, dolui, dolitum, dolēre 아프다, 괴로워하다   **E** *doleful*

      > dolens, (gen.) dolentis (*present participle*) 아픈, 괴로운   **E** *dolent*

        > indolens, (gen.) indolentis (< in- *not*) 무통성의; 나태한   **E** *indolent*

          > indolentia, indolentiae, f. 무통; 나태   **E** *indolence*

      > condoleo, **condolui,** condolitum, condolēre (< con- (< cum) *with, together* + dolēre *to grieve*) 겹쳐서 아프다, 고통을 함께 나누다   **E** *condole*

        > condolens, (gen.) condolentis (*present participle*) 겹쳐서 아픈, 고통을 함께 나누는   **E** *condolent*

          > *condolentia, *condolentiae, f. 애도, 조위   **E** *condolence*

   < IE. del(ə)- *to split, to carve, to cut*

      > G. dēleisthai (*middle*) *to hurt, to damage, to destroy*

        > G. dēlētēr, dēlētēros, m. *destroyer*

          > G. dēlētērios, dēlētēria, dēlētērion *noxious*

            > L. deleterius, deleteria, deleterium 해로운   **E** *deleterious*

algor, algoris, m. 냉기, 한기   **E** *algor*

    [용례] algor mortis 사후체온하강   **E** *algor mortis*

      (문법) algor 체온하강: 단수 주격

        mortis 주검의: 단수 속격 < mors, mortis, f. 죽음, 주검

    < algeo, alsi, −, algēre 춥다

      > algidus, algida, algidum 추운, 찬   **E** *algid*

   < IE. algh- *frost, cold*

Caesar, Caesaris, m. Julia 씨족의 가문명;

    Gaius Julius Caesar (100–44 B.C.E.)   **E** *Caesar,* D. *Kaiser,* (*Russian*) *Tsar (Tzar, Czar)*

      > Caesareus, Caesarea, Caesareum Gaius Julius Caesar의, 제왕의   **E** *caesarean (cesarean)* (< '*figuratively*')

   < (*probably*) *Of Etruscan origin*

imber, imbris, m. 소나기, 폭우, 빗발침   **E** (ignis '*fire*' + imber '*shower of rain*' + -ite >) *ignimbrite*

    > imbrex, imbricis, f. 수키와, 손바닥을 오목하게 하여 치는 박수

      > imbrico, **imbricavi,** imbricatum, imbricare 기와로 덮다, 기왓장처럼 겹쳐 놓다   **E** *imbricate*

   < IE. ombh-ro- *rain*

      > (*possibly*) L. imbuo, **imbui,** imbutum, imbuēre 적시다, 더럽히다, 물들이다, 가르치다   **E** *imbue*

passer, passeris, m. 참새

    > passerinus, passerina, passerinum 참새의, 참새 종류의   **E** *passerine*

vomer, vomeris, m. 쟁기, 보습, 보습뼈, 서골(鋤骨)   **E** *vomer*

    < IE. wogʷh-ni- *plowshare, wedge*   **E** *wedge*

pecten, pectinis, m. 빗, 가리비, 즐(櫛), 음모(陰毛), 음부(陰部), 두덩   **E** *pecten*

    > pectineus, pectinea, pectineum 빗 모양의, 빗살 모양의, 두덩근의, 치골근

      (恥骨筋)의   **E** *pectineal, pectineus (muscle)* (< *'its arising at the pecten pubis'*)

    > pectinatus, pectinata, pectinatum 빗 모양을 한, 빗살 모양을 한   **E** *pectinate*

    < pecto, **pexi,** pexum (pexitum), pectĕre 빗다, 빗질하다

  < IE. pek- *to pluck the hair, to fleece, to comb*   **E** *fight*

    > G. pektein *to clip, to shear*

    > G. kteis, ktenos, m. (< kten- < *pkten-) *comb*   **E** *cten(o)-, ctenoid, ctenophore*

      > G. ktenidion, ktenidiou, n. (< + -idion *diminutive suffix*) *comb-like*

        structure   **E** *ctenidium*

pes, pedis, m. 발, 족[足]

    E *pedestal* (< *'foot stall'*), *pioneer* (< *'foot soldier who prepares the way for an army'*), ((Anglo-Norman) pe de grue *'foot of crane'* > *'the clawlike, three-branched mark used in genealogy to show succession'* >) *pedigree, ped(i)-*, (ped- *'foot'* + curare *'to take care'* >) *pedicure, -pede*, (ab ante *'away before'* + pes *'foot'* >) *vamp, (vamp >) revamp*

    > pedalis, pedale 발의   **E** *pedal*

    > pedester, pedestris, pedestre 걸어가는, 보행(步行)의, 산문적(散文的)인   **E** *pedestrian*

    > pediculus, pediculi, m. (< + -culus *diminutive suffix*) 작은 발, 꼭지, 족(足), 각(脚),

      경(莖), 병(柄)   **E** *pedicle*

      > pedunculus, pedunculi, m. (< *alteration of* pediculus) 작은 발, 꼭지, 족(足),

        각(脚), 경(莖), 병(柄)   **E** *peduncle, pedunculate*

      > pedicellus, pedicelli, m. (< + -ellus *diminutive suffix*) 작은 발, 족돌기(足突起) **E** *pedicel*

      > petiolus, petioli, m. (< + -olus *diminutive suffix*) 작은 발, 꼭지, 잎자루   **E** *petiole*

    > pedica, pedicae, f. 올가미, 덫

      > impedico, impedicavi, impedicatum, impedicare (< im- (< in) *in, on, into,*

        toward + pedica *fetter*) 올가미로 걸다, 덫으로 잡다   **E** *impeach*

    > impedio, impedivi (impedii), impeditum, impedire (< im- (< in) *in, on, into, toward* +

      pes *foot*) 족쇄를 채우다, 방해하다   **E** *impede, (impede >) impedance*

    > expedio, expedivi (expedii), expeditum, expedire (< ex- *out of, away from* + pes

      foot) 놓아주다, (장애물·난관 등을 제거하고) 개척하다, 진척시키다,

      재빨리 해치우다   **E** *expedite, expeditious, expedient*

      > expeditio, expeditionis, f. 출정, 원정, 탐험   **E** *expedition*

    > talipes, talipedis, m. (< *walking on the ankles, walking lamely* < talus *ankle* +

pes *foot*) 휜발, 조막발, 기형족(畸形足), 만곡족(彎曲足)　　　　　**E** *talipes*

> quadrupes, (gen.) quadrupedis (< quadru- (< quattuor) *four* + pes *foot*) 네발 달린,
네발로 다니는　　　　　**E** *quadruped*

> multipes, (gen.) multipedis (< multus *many* + pes *foot*) 발 많이 가진,
다족(多足)의　　　　　**E** *multiped*

> centipeda, centipedae, f. (< centum *hundred* + pes *foot*) 지네　　　　**E** *centipede*

> millipeda, millipedae, f. (< mille *thousand* + pes *foot*) 노래기　**E** *millipede (milliped, millepede)*

< IE. ped- *foot*　　　　　**E** *foot, fetter*

> G. pous, podos, m. *foot, (unit of distance) foot*

E *pod(o)-, podalic* (< 'on the pattern of cephalic'), *podiatry, podocyte, -pod, antipodal* (< 'in direct opposite' < 'having the feet opposite')

> G. podion, podiou, n. (< + -ion, -iou, n. *diminutive suffix*) *little foot*

> L. podium, podii, n. 발판, 대(臺), 단(壇); 작은 발을 닮은 구조　**E** *podium, pew*

> L. pseudopodium, pseudopodii, n. (< G. pseudēs *false*) 헛다리,
위족(僞足)　　　　**E** *pseudopodium (pseudopod)*, (pl.) *pseudopodia*

> L. lamellipodium, lamellipodii, n. (< lamella *small plate*)
라멜리포듐　　　　**E** (pl.) *lamellipodia*

> L. filopodium, filopodii, n. (< filum *thread*) 사족(絲足), 사상
가족(絲狀假足)　　　**E** (pl.) *filopodia*

> G. kalopodion, kalopodiou, n. (< kalon, kalou, n. *wood*) *little wooden
foot, shoemaker's last*

> (Arabic) qalib *shoemaker's last, mold*

E (probably) *caliber (calibre)*, (caliber >) *calibrate*, (caliber >) *calipers (callipers)*

> G. podagra, podagras, f. (< + agra *seizure*) *foot disease, gout, trap for the feet*

> L. podagra, podagrae, f. 무지통풍(拇趾痛風)　　　**E** *podagra*

> G. Oidipous, Oidipodos, m. (< *swollen-footed* < oidein *to swell*) *Oedipus*

> L. Oedipus, Oedipodis, m. (Oedipus, Oedipi, m.) 오이디푸스　**E** *Oedipus*

> G. tripous, tripodos, m. (< tri- (< treis) *three*) *three-footed structure*

> L. tripus, tripodis, m. 삼각 그릇, 삼각대, 세발 의자;
세발 쌍둥이　　**E** *tripod; tripus* (< 'conjoined twins having three feet')

> G. tetrapous, tetrapodos, m. (< tetr(a)- (< tessares) *four*) *four-footed
structure, four-footed animal*

> L. tetrapus, tetrapodis, m. 테트라포드, 네발 동물　　**E** *tetrapod*

> G. octōpous, octōpodos, m. (< octō *eight*) *eight-footed animal*　**E** *octopod*

> L. octopus, octopi, m. 낙지, 문어, 팔각류 동물　　　**E** *octopus*

> G. polypous, polypodos, m. (< polys *many*) *many-footed animal*　**E** *polypod*

> L. polypus, polypi, m. (동물) 폴립 (강장동물 중 착생 생활을 하는 개체);
(의학) 용종(茸腫)　　　　**E** *polyp, polypoid*

> L. polyposis, polyposis, f. (< + G. -ōsis *condition*)
용종증　　　　　**E** *polyposis*

[용례] polyposis coli 대장용종증　　　　　　　　　　**E** *polyposis coli*

    (문법) polyposis 용종증: 단수 주격

      coli 대장의: 단수 속격 < colon, coli, n. 대장

> G. antipodes, antipodōn, m. (pl.) (< ant(i)- *before, against, instead of*) *the inhabitants of opposite sides of the earth*

  > L. antipodes, antipodum, m. (pl.) 대척지(對蹠地)의 사람들, 대척지, 대극(對極)

    E *antipodes,* (antipodes >) *antipode,* (antipodes >) *antipodean,* (antipodes >) *antipodal*

> L. Decapoda, Decapodorum, n. (pl.) (< G. deka *ten*) (동물) (게 · 새우 등) 십각류목(目)　　　　　　　　**E** *decapod*

> L. Cephalopoda, Cephalopodorum, n. (pl.) (< G. kephalē *head*) (동물) (오징어 · 문어 등) 두족류강(綱)　　**E** *cephalopod,* (cephalopod + toxin >) *cephalotoxin*

> L. Xenopus, Xenopi, m. (< *clawed toad* < *strange toad which has claws on its digits* < G. xenos *strange*) (두꺼비) 세노푸스속(屬)　　**E** *Xenopus*

> L. Rhizopus, Rhizopi, m. (< *in allusion to the form of its rhizoids* < G. rhiza *root*) (곰팡이) 리조푸스속(屬)　　　　**E** *Rhizopus*

> G. peza, pezēs, f. *foot, end, top*

  > G. trapeza, trapezēs, f. (< tra- < tetr(a)- *four*) *table, dining table, money-changer's table*

    > G. trapezion, trapeziou, n. (< + -ion *diminutive suffix*) *little table*

      > L. trapezium, trapezii, n. 사다리꼴　　**E** *trapeze*

        > L. trapezius, trapezia, trapezium 사다리꼴의, 마름모양의, 능형(菱形)의

        [용례] os trapezium (< *an irregular four-sided figure*) 큰마름뼈, 대능형골(大菱形骨)　　　　　**E** *trapezium*

          (문법) os 뼈: 단수 주격 < os, ossis, n.

            trapezium: 형용사, 중성형 단수 주격

        [용례] musculus trapezius (< *each of a pair of large flat triangular muscles, together forming the figure of a trapezium*) 등세모근, 승모(僧帽)근　　**E** *trapezius (muscle)*

          (문법) musculus 근육, 근: 단수 주격 < musculus, musculi, m.

            trapezius: 형용사, 남성형 단수 주격

      > G. trapezoeidēs, trapezoeidēs, trapezoeides (< + eidos *shape*) *table-shaped*

        > L. trapezoideus, trapezoidea, trapezoideum 사다리꼴 모양의

          [용례] os trapezoideum (< *small trapezium*) 작은마름뼈, 소능형골(小菱形骨)　　　　　**E** *trapezoid*

            (문법) os 뼈: 단수 주격 < os, ossis, n.

> G. pedilon, pedilou, n. *sandal, shoe, boot, slipper*

>> L. cypripedium, cypripedii, n. (< *Venus' shoe, lady's slipper: in reference to the inflated pouch formed by the labellum* < G. Kypris *Aphrodite* + pedilon *slipper*) 개불알꽃 **E** *cypripedium*

> G. pedon, pedou, n. *ground, soil* **E** *ped(o)-*

> G. pēdon, pēdou, n. *blade of an oar* **E** *pilot*

>> G. pēdalion, pēdaliou, n. *rudder*

> G. pēdan (pēdaein) *to leap, to throb*

>>> G. diapēdan (diapēdaein) (< di(a)- *through, thoroughly, apart* + pēdan) *to ooze through*

>>>> G. diapēdēsis, diapēdēseōs, f. *oozing*

>>>>> L. diapedesis, diapedesis, f. 누출, 누출성 출혈 **E** *diapedesis*

> (*Persian*) pai *foot, leg*   **E** (pl.) *pajamas* (< '*leg clothing*'), *teapoy* (< '*three-legged*', '*tripod*')

> (*verbal root*) IE. ped- *to walk, to stumble, to fall* **E** *fetch*

>> L. pejor, pejor, pejus ((gen.) pejoris) (비교급) 더 나쁜

>>> L. pejoro, pejoravi, pejoratum, pejorare 악화시키다, 악화하다 **E** *pejorate, pejorative*

>>>> L. pejoratio, pejorationis, f. 악화, (가치의) 하락; (언어) (뜻의) 타락 **E** *pejoration*

>>>> L. *impejoro, *impejoravi, *impejoratum, *impejorare (< im- (< in) *in, on, into, toward* + pejorare *to make worse*) 해치다, 손상시키다 **E** *impair, impairment*

>> L. pessimus, pessima, pessimum (최상급) 가장 나쁜 **E** *pessimism*

>> L. pecco, peccavi, peccatum, peccare (비틀거리다, 잘못하다 >) 죄를 짓다

E (*first personal singular, perfect indicative, active 'I have sinned'* >) *peccavi, peccant*

>>> L. peccabilis, peccabile 죄를 짓기 쉬운 **E** *peccable*

>>>> L. impeccabilis, impeccabile (< im- (< in-) *not*) 죄를 짓지 않는, 흠 없는 **E** *impeccable*

hospes, hospitis, m., f. (< IE. ghos-pot- *guest master, one who symbolizes the relationship of reciprocal obligation* < + IE. poti- *powerful, lord*) 손님 맞는 집주인, 손님, 낯선 사람 **E** *host* (< '*in charge of the stranger*')

> hospitium, hospitii, n. (서로 접대하도록 되어 있는 개인이나 국가 사이의) 우호관계, 주객지의(主客之誼), 정중한 접대, 환대 **E** *hospice*

> hospitalis, hospitale 손님의, 손님을 접대하는

>> hospitale, hospitalis, n. 병원, 구호소, (pl.) 응접실 **E** *hospital, hospitalize, hostel, hotel, (motor + hotel >) motel*

> hospitalitas, hospitalitatis, f. 접대, 환대 **E** *hospitality*

> hospitó, hospitavi, hospitatum, hospitare 환대하다 **E** *hospitable*

< IE. ghos-ti- *guest, host, stranger; properly 'someone with whom one has reciprocal duties of hospitality'* **E** *guest*

> L. hostis, hostis, m., f. 이방인, 적   **E** *host* (< 'multitude of armed men')

    > L. hostilis, hostile 비우호적인, 적(敵)의   **E** *hostile*

       > L. hostilitas, hostilitatis, f. 적의(敵意), 적대행위   **E** *hostility*

> G. xenos, xenē, xenon *strange, foreign*

    E *xenon (Xe)* (< 'the hitherto unknown inert gas'), *xenobiotic* (< 'designating a substance foreign to the body'), *xenophilia, xenophobia*

limes, limitis, m. (논·밭의) 두렁길, 샛길, 지경(地境), 한계(限界)   **E** *(noun) limit, lintel*

    > limito, limitavi, limitatum, limitare 경계를 긋다, 제한하다,

    한정하다   **E** *(verb) limit, limited, (in- > il- 'not' >) illimited*

      > limitatio, limitationis, f. 제한, 한정   **E** *limitation*

      > delimito, delimitavi, delimitatum, delimitare (< de- *apart from, down, not; intensive*) 경계를 짓다, 구획하다   **E** *delimit*

< IE. (e)lei-, (e)li- *to bend*   **E** *limb* (< 'a part of a body')

    > L. limen, liminis, n. 문턱, (상하) 인방(引枋), 출입문, 역(閾)   **E** *limen, liminal, subliminal*

      > L. elimino, eliminavi, eliminatum, eliminare (< e- *out of, away from* + limen *threshold, lintel*) 문 밖으로 내쫓다, 제거하다   **E** *eliminate*

      > L. praeliminaris, praeliminare (< *before the threshold* < prae- *before, beyond* + limen *threshold, lintel*) 예비의   **E** *preliminary*

      > L. sublimis, sublime (< *up to the lintel* < sub- *under, up from under* + limen *threshold, lintel*) 공간에 매달린, 높은, 고상한   **E** *sublime*

        > L. sublimitas, sublimitatis, f. 높은 곳, 고상, 숭고, 초월   **E** *sublimity*

        > L. sublimo, sublimavi, sublimatum, sublimare 높이다, 고상하게 하다, 승화시키다, 승화하다   **E** *sublimate*

          > L. sublimatio, sublimationis, f. 높임, 승화   **E** *sublimation*

satelles, satellitis, m., f. 근위병, 수행원, 공범자; 위성   **E** *satellite*

< *Of Etruscan origin*

nepos, nepotis, m. 손자, 조카   **E** *nephew, nepotism*

< IE. nepot- *grandson, nephew*

    > (*feminine*) IE. nepti- *granddaughter, niece*

      > L. neptis, neptis, f. 손녀, 조카딸   **E** *niece*

cinis, cineris, m., f. 재[灰], 잿더미, 폐허, 무덤, 시체 태운 재, 유골, 죽음

    > cinereus, cinerea, cinereum 재[灰]의, 잿빛의   **E** *cinereous*

    [용례] tuber cinereum 회색융기   **E** *tuber cinereum*

      (문법) tuber 혹: 단수 주격 < tuber, tuberis, n.

        cinereum: 형용사, 중성형 단수 주격

    > cinerarius, cineraria, cinerarium 재의, 유골의   **E** *cinerary*

    > incinero, -, -, incinerare (< in- *in, on, into, toward* + cinis *ashes*) 재를 바르다,

재를 뿌리다; 태워서 재로 만들다, 화장하다, 재가 되다   **E** *incinerate*

    < IE. keni- *dust, ashes*

       > G. konis, koneōs, f. (konia, konias, f.) *dust*

          > G. konidion, konidiou, n. (< + -idion, -idiou, n. *diminutive suffix*)

             > L. conidium, conidii, n. 분생(分生) 홀씨

                 E *conidium (conidiospore)*, (pl.) *conidia, conidiophore* (< 'the branch of a mycelium of a fungus that bears conidia')

          > L. otoconium, otoconii, n. (< G. ous, ōtos, n. *ear*) 평형모래, 평형사(平衡砂), 이석(耳石)

            statoconium, statoconii, n. (< G. statos *standing*) 평형모래, 평형사, 이석

                 E *otoconium (statoconium) (otolith, statolith)*, (pl.) *otoconia (statoconia) (otoliths, statoliths)*

          > L. pneumonoconiosis, pneumonoconiosis, f. (pneumoconiosis, pneumoconiosis, f.)

            (< G. pneumōn, pneumonos, m. *lung* + konis + -ōsis *condition*) 진폐증 (塵肺症)   **E** *pneumonoconiosis (pneumoconiosis)*

funus, funeris, m. 장례, 장례식

       > funereus, funerea, funereum 장례식의, 장례식 같은   **E** *funereal*

       > funeralis, funerale 장례의, 장례식의   **E** *funeral*

   < IE. dheuə- *to close, to finish, to come full circle*   **E** *down* (< '(from) hill'), *dune* (< 'sandy hill'), *town* (< 'fortified place')

   ∽ IE. dheu-, dheuə- *to die*   **E** *die, dead, death, dwindle*

honos, honoris, m. (honor, honoris, m.) 명예, 존경   **E** *honor (honour)*

       > honorarius, honoraria, honorarium 명예상의, 무보수의   **E** (honorarium donum 'honorary gift' >) *honorarium, honorary*

       > honoro, **honoravi**, honoratum, honorare 존경하다, 경의를 표하다

          > honorabilis, honorabile 명예로운, 존경할 만한   **E** *honorable*

       > honorificus, honorifica, honorificum (< + -ficus (< facĕre) *making*) 명예롭게 하는, 경의를 표하는   **E** *honorific*

       > honestus, honesta, honestum 존경받을 만한, 품위 있는, 정직한   **E** *honest*

          > honestas, honestatis, f. 명예, 품위, 정직   **E** *honesty*

mos, moris, m. 풍습, (pl.) 도덕   **E** (pl.) *mores*

       > moralis, morale 도덕적   **E** *moral*

   < IE. me- *expressing certain qualities of mind; to strive strongly, to be energetic*   **E** *mood*

ros, roris, m. 이슬   **E** (ros marinus 'marine dew' >) *rosemary*

   < IE. ros- *dew*

       > G. drosos, drosou, f. *dew*

> G. droseros, drosera, droseron *dewy*

> L. drosera, droserae, f. (< *the glistening hairs on the leaves*) 끈끈이
주걱 종류의 식충식물   **E** *drosera (sundew)*

> L. Drosophila, Drosophilae, f. (< + G. philos *loving*) 초파리속(屬);
초파리   **E** *Drosophila (fruit fly)*

sal, salis, m., n. 소금   **E** *sal, salad (< 'salted'),* It. *salami, saltpeter*

> salinus, salina, salinum 소금의   **E** *saline, ('saline' >) salinity*

> salarius, salaria, salarium 소금의, 소금에 관한

> salarium, salarii, n. (로마 군인들에게 소금값으로 주던) 급여금, 봉급   **E** *salary*

> salio, **salii,** salitum (salsum), salire 소금 치다, 짜게 하다, 소금에 절이다

E *sauce (< 'salted'), (sauce > 'vessel for holding sauce' >) saucer, (saucer >) saucerization,*
sausage (< 'salted'), Sp. *salsa*

< IE. sal- *salt*   **E** *salt, salty, saltwort,* D. *Salzburg, silt (< 'salt marsh')*

> G. hals, halos, m. *salt*

E *hal(o)-, halogen(s), halide(s), (halogen + ethane >) halothane, (hals 'salt' > 'living in a*
saline habitat' >) halobiont, halophilic

> G. hals, halos, f. *salt water, sea*

sol, solis, m. 해, 태양, 햇빛; (Sol) (로마 신화) 태양신

E *sol, Sol, turnsole, (parare 'to make ready' + sol 'sun' > 'making ready against the sun'*
>) parasol

> solaris, solare 해의, 해에 관한, 태양의   **E** *solar*

> solarium, solarii, n. 일광욕실, 해시계   **E** *solarium*

> solanum, solani, n. (< *nightshade; originally, sun plant*) 가지과의 식물   **E** *solanine*

> solstitium, solstitii, n. (< sol *sun* + sistĕre *to make to stand*) (하지·동지의) 지점
(至點), 전환점   **E** *solstice*

> insolo, **insolavi,** insolatum, insolare (< in- *in, on, into, toward*) 햇볕에 쬐다, 일광
소독하다   **E** *insolate*

> insolatio, insolationis, f. 햇볕에 말림, 일광욕, 일광소독, 일사병   **E** *insolation*

< IE. saə wel- *sun*

E *sun, (G.* hēmera Hēliou *'day of* Helios', L. dies Solis *'day of the sun' >) Sunday,*
south (< 'sunside'), southern

> G. hēlios, hēliou, m. *sun, sunlight;* (Hēlios) (*Greek mythology*) *the sun god*

E *Helios, helium (He) (< 'its existence deduced from the solar spectrum'), heli(o)-,*
heliotaxis, heliotropism

> G. hēliotropion, hēliotropiou, n. *heliotrope*

> L. heliotropium, heliotropii, n. 향일성 식물, 헬리오트로프   **E** *heliotrope*

> L. helianthus, helianthi, m. 해바라기 (H. annuus), 뚱딴지 (돼지감자, H. tuberosus) **E** *helianthus*

rex, regis, m. 왕   **E** *Rex, regicide, viceroy*

> regina, reginae, f. 여왕 　　　　　　　　　　　　　　　　　　　　**E** *Regina*

< IE. reg- *to move in a straight line* (Vide REGĔRE: *See* E. *regent*)

codex, codicis, m. 책, 기록부, 장부(帳簿), 대장(臺帳), 법전, (성서·고전의) 사본(寫本)

　　　　E *code, (code + -on 'a termination of Greek neuter nouns and adjectives' >) codon, anticodon, encode, decode, codify*

　　　< caudex, caudicis, m. 통나무, 등걸, 널빤지, 책, 대장(臺帳), 멍청이

　　< *caudĕre *to strike, to beat*

　　　> cudo, **cudi**, cusum, cudĕre 두들기다, 금속을 두들겨서 (화폐를) 만들다

　　　　> incudo, **incudi**, incusum, incudĕre (< in- *in, on, into, toward* + cudĕre
　　　　　to forge) (화폐에) 각인을 찍다　　　　　　　　　　　　　**E** *incuse*

　　　　　> incus, incudis, f. 모루, 철침(鐵砧), 꾸준한 노력; (해부) 모루뼈,
　　　　　　　침골(砧骨)　　　　　　　　　　　　　　　　　　　　　　**E** *incus*

< IE. kau- *to hew, to strike*　　　　　　　**E** *hew, hay (< 'cut grass'), hacksaw, hoe*

　　> (*suggested*) L. causa, causae, f. 까닭, 원인　　　**E** *(noun) cause, (by cause >) because*

　　　> L. causalis, causale 원인의, 인과(因果)관계의　　　　　　　　**E** *causal*

　　　> L. causo, **causavi**, causatum, causare 원인이 되다, (원인이 되어)
　　　　일으키다　　　　　　　　　　　　　　　　　　　　**E** *(verb) cause, causative*

　　　　> L. causatio, causationis, f. 핑계, 인과관계, 인과작용　　**E** *causation*

　　　　> L. accuso, **accusavi**, accusatum, accusare (< ac- (< ad) *to, toward, at,*
　　　　according to + causare *to cause*) 탓으로 돌리다, 비난하다, 고소하다　**E** *accuse*

　　　　　> L. accusativus, accusativa, accusativum 고발에 관한; 원인이 되는,
　　　　　　(결과를) 만들어 내는; (문법) 대격(對格)의　　　**E** *accusative (acc.)*

　　　　> L. excuso, **excusavi**, excusatum, excusare (< ex- *out of, away from*
　　　　+ causare *to cause*) 변명하다, 용서하다, 면제해 주다　　　**E** *excuse*

pollex, pollicis, m. 엄지손가락　　　　　　　　　　　　　　　　　　**E** *pollex*

hallux, hallucis, m. 엄지발가락　　　　　　　　　　　　　　　　　**E** *hallux*

alcohol, alcoholis, m. 알코올, 주정(酒精)

　　　E *alcohol (< 'fluids of the idea of sublimation: an essence, quintessence, or 'spirit', obtained by distillation or rectification' < 'any fine impalpable powder produced by trituration, or especially by sublimation' < 'the fine-metallic powder used in the East to stain the eyelids'), (alcohol dehydrogenatus 'alcohol dehydrogenated' >) aldehyde(s), (aldehyde, 'with a euphonic insertion of -an- > 'synthesized from acetaldehyde and ammonia with hydrogen cyanide' >) alanine (Ala, A), phenylalanine (Phe, F), (dioxyphenylalanine 'former name of 3,4-dihydroxyphenylalanine' >) dopa, (dopa + amine >) dopamine, (alcohol >) -ol, (ethane + -ol >) ethanol, ((G.) -ene + -ol >) enol, (aldehyde + -ol >) aldol, aldolase*

　　> alcoholicus, alcoholica, alcoholicum 알코올성의, 주정의　　**E** *alcoholic*

> alcoholismus, alcoholismi, m. 알코올 중독, 음주벽　　　　　　　　　　E *alcoholism*
< (*Arabic*) al-kuhl *collyrium, the fine metallic powder used in the East to stain the eyelids*

imago, imaginis, f. 모상, 초상, 상(像), 모습; (곤충) 성충(成蟲)　E *imago, (pl.) imagines (imagoes), image*
　　> imaginor, imaginatus sum, imaginari 상상하다　　　　　E *imagine, imagination*
　　　　> imaginativus, imaginativa, imaginativum 상상력이 풍부한　　　E *imaginative*
　　> imaginarius, imaginaria, imaginarium 가상적인, 비실제적인　　　E *imaginary*
　　> imaginabilis, imaginabile 상상할 수 있는　　　　　　　E *imaginable*
< IE. aim- *to copy*
　　> L. aemulus, aemula, aemulum 같아지려고 하는, 지지 않으려고 하는, 겨루는　E *emulous*
　　　　> L. aemulor, emulatus sum, aemulari 겨루다　　　　　E *emulate*
　　> L. imitor, imitatus sum, imitari 모방하다, 본받다　　　E *imitate, imitable, inimitable*

margo, marginis, f. 가장자리, 테두리, 여지　　　　　　　　　E *margin*
　　> marginalis, marginale 가장자리의, 테두리의　　　　　　E *marginal*
　　> margino, marginavi, marginatum, marginare 테를 두르다, 에워싸다, 깃을 달다　E *marginate*
< IE. merg- *boundary, border*
　　E *mark, birthmark, hallmark (< 'London assay office at Goldsmith's Hall'), landmark, marker, marked, markedly, demarcation, (demarcation >) demarcate, remark, remarkable, remarkably*
　　> L. marcha, marchae, f. 변경(邊境), 변방(邊方)　E *marquis (< 'prefect of frontier town'), marquise*

soror, sororis, f. 자매, 누이　　　　　　　　E *sororal, sorority (< 'on the pattern of fraternity')*
< IE. swesor- (< *woman of one's own kin group in an exogamous society* < (*perhaps*) IE.
　s(w)e- *pronoun of the third person and reflexive, one's own* + IE. esor *woman*)
　sister　　　　　　　　　　　　　　　　　E *sister*
　　> L. sobrinus, sobrini, m. 사촌형제
　　　　> L. consobrinus, consobrini, m. (< con- (< cum) *with, together*) 이종사촌형제　E *cousin*

uxor, uxoris, f. (< *she who gets accustomed to the new household after patrilocal marriage*)
　　아내　　　　　　　　　　　　　　　E *uxorial, uxorious, uxoricide*
< IE. euk- *to become accustomed*

hereditas, hereditatis, f. 상속, 유전　　　　　　　　　E *heredity*
　　　> hereditarius, hereditaria, hereditarium 상속의, 유전의, 유전성의　　E *hereditary*
　　　> heredito, hereditavi, hereditatum, hereditare 상속하다, 상속받다　E *heritage, heritable*
　　　　> inheredito, inhereditavi, inhereditatum, inhereditare (< in- *in, on, into,*
　　　　　　toward + hereditare *to make heir, to receive as heir*)
　　　　　　상속받다　　　　　　　　　　E *inherit, inheritance, inheritable*
　　< heres, heredis, m., f. 상속인　　　　　　　　　E *heir*
< IE. ghe- *to release, to let go, to leave behind; (in the middle voice) to be released, to go,*

to be empty   **E** *go, ago, gait, forgo* (< *'to go without'*)

> G. chōros, chōrou, m. *open area, locality, place*   **E** *chorography, kinetochore*

> G. chōris (*adverb, preposition*) *apart, separate*   **E** *choripetalous*

> G. chōrizein *to part, to separate*

> G. chōristos, chōristē, chōriston *parted, separated*

> L. choristoma, choristomatis, n. (< + G. -ōma *noun suffix*

denoting tumor) 분리종, 이소종(異所腫)   **E** *choristoma*

> (*Sanskrit*) hina- *inferior, verbal adjective of* jahati *he leaves, he lets go*   **E** *Hinayana*

quies, quietis, f. 쉼, 고요함, 영면

> requies, requietis, f. (< re- *back, again* + quies *rest*) 휴식, 안식

> **E** (*Requiem aeternam dona eis, Domine... 'Eternal rest give to them, O Lord...'* (*the Introit in the Mass of the Dead*) >) *requiem*

> quiesco, **quievi**, quietum, quiescĕre (< + -escĕre *suffix of inceptive (inchoative) verb*) 쉬다, 고요해지다

> **E** (quiescens (*present participle*) >) *quiescent*, (quietus (*past participle*) >) *quiet*, (quietus >) *quit*, (quietus >) *coy*, (quit >) *quite*, (quit >) *requite*, (requite >) *requital*, (quiet >) *disquiet*

> quietudo, quietudinis, f. 고요함, 평정   **E** *quietude*

> acquiesco, **acquievi**, acquietum, acquiescĕre (< ac- (< ad) *to, toward, at, according to* + quiescĕre *to become quiet*) 쉬다, 마음 놓고 믿다, 묵인하다   **E** *acquiesce, acquiescent*

> acquiescentia, acquiescentiae, f. 평정, 납득, 묵인   **E** *acquiescence*

> requiesco, **requievi**, requietum, requiescĕre (< re- *back, again* + quiescĕre *to become quiet*) 쉬다, 고요해지다, 영면하다

> **E** (*third personal singular, present subjunctive, active 'he/she may rest'* >) *requiescat*

> quieto, -, -, quietare 쉬게 하다, 고요하게 하다   **E** *acquit*

< IE. kʷeiə- *to rest, to be quiet*   **E** *while, whilom*

> L. tranquillus, tranquilla, tranquillum (< tran- (< trans) *over, across, through, beyond*) 고요한, 평온한   **E** *tranquil, tranquillize (tranquilize)*

> L. tranquillitas, tranquillitatis, f. 고요, 평온   **E** *tranquillity (tranquility)*

cassis, cassidis, f. 투구

< (*perhaps*) IE. kadh- *to shelter, to cover*   **E** *hat, hood, heed*

cuspis, cuspidis, f. (화살·창 등의) 날카로운 끝, (벌의) 침, 첨(尖), 첨두(尖頭)

> **E** *cuspis (cusp)*, (pl.) *cuspides*, *cuspid* (< *'pointed'*), *bicuspid* (< *'two-pointed'*), *tricuspid* (< *'three-pointed'*)

> cuspidatus, cuspidata, cuspidatum 끝이 뾰족한, 돌기가 있는   **E** *cuspidate*

fraus, fraudis, f. 속임수, 사기   **E** *fraud*

     > fraudulentus, fraudulenta, fraudulentum 속이는, 사기적인   **E** *fraudulent*

     > frustra (부사) 속여, 속아, 헛되이

         > frustror, frustratus sum, frustrari 속이다, 헛되게 하다, 좌절시키다   **E** *frustrate*

             > frustratio, frustrationis, f. 속임, 허탕, 좌절   **E** *frustration*

   < IE. dhwer- *to trick, to injure*   **E** *(probably) dwarf, dwarfism*

laus, laudis, f. 칭찬, 예찬, 찬미   **E** *(noun) laud*

     > laudo, laudavi, laudatum, laudare 칭찬하다, 예찬하다, 찬미하다   **E** *(verb) laud, laudable*

         > allaudo, –, –, allaudare (< al- (< ad) *to, toward, at, according to* + laudare *to*

             praise) 칭찬하다   **E** *allow (< 'reinforced by* allocare *to place'), allowable, allowance*

   < IE. leu- *echoic root*   **E** D. *Lied, Volkslied*

vis, viris, f. 힘   **E** *vim*

     > violentus, violenta, violentum 난폭한   **E** *violent*

       > violentia, violentiae, f. 난폭, 폭력   **E** *violence*

     > violo, violavi, violatum, violare 난폭하게 다루다, 어기다   **E** *violate, violable, inviolable*

   < IE. weiə- *to go after something, to pursue with vigor, to desire, with noun forms meaning*

     force, power   **E** *gain, rowen*

     > IE. wi-ro- *man*   **E** *werewolf, world (< 'life or age of man')*

         > L. invito, invitavi, invitatum, invitare (< in- *in, on, into, toward*) 권유하다,

            초대하다   **E** *invite, vie*

            > L. invitatio, invitationis, f. 권유, 초대   **E** *invitation*

         > L. vir, viri, m. 어른, 남자 어른, 장부   **E** *vir*

            > L. virilis, virile 어른의, 성인 남자의, 남성의; 용감한   **E** *virile, virilize, virilism*

               > L. virilitas, virilitatis 남성다움, (남성의) 생식력   **E** *virility*

            > L. virtus, virtutis, f. 남자의 품격, 능력, 덕성   **E** *virtue*

               > L. virtuosus, virtuosa, virtuosum 힘 있는,

                   덕스러운   **E** It. *virtuoso (< 'skilled'), virtuosity, virtuous*

               > L. virtualis, virtuale 힘 있는; 실질적, 사실상; 잠재적   **E** *virtual*

            > L. eviro, eviravi, eviratum, evirare (< e- *out of, away from*) 거세하다   **E** *eviration*

forfex, forficis, f. 가위, 집게발, (가위 모양의) 전투 대열   **E** *forficate*

   < (*possibly*) IE. bherdh- *to cut*   **E** *board, border, borderline*

cicatrix, cicatricis, f. 흉터, 반흔(瘢痕), 상흔(傷痕)   **E** *cicatrix, ('cicatrical' >) cicatricial, cicatrize*

radix, radicis, f. 뿌리, 무, 근본   **E** *radix, (pl.) radices, radish, horseradish*

     > radicalis, radicale 뿌리의, 근본의   **E** *radical*

     > radicula, radiculae, f. (< + -cula *diminutive suffix*) 작은 뿌리, 잔뿌리, 무   **E** *radicle, radicular*

     > radico, radicavi, –, radicare (radicor, radicatus sum, radicari) 뿌리박다,

뿌리내리다 　　　　　　　　　　　　　　　　　　　　　E *irradicable* *(ineradicable)*

　　> eradico, eradicavi, eradicatum, eradicare (< e- *out of, away from*) 근절

　　　　시키다 　　　　　　　　　　　　　E *eradicate, eradicable, ineradicable (irradicable)*

< IE. wrad- *root, branch* 　　　　　　　　　　　　　　　E *root, rootlet, wort*

　> L. ramus, rami, m. 가지[枝] 　　　　　　　　　　　　E *ramus,* (pl.) *rami*

　　> L. ramosus, ramosa, ramosum 가지가 많은, 여러 갈래로 갈라진 　　　E *ramose*

　　> L. ramifico, ramificavi, ramificatum, ramificare (< + -ficare (< facĕre)

　　　to make) 가지를 내다, 가지 치다 　　　　　　　　　　　　E *ramify*

　　> L. ramulus, ramuli, m. (< + -ulus *diminutive suffix*) 잔가지,

　　　여린 가지 　　　　　　　　　　　　　　　　E *ramulus,* (pl.) *ramuli*

　　　　> L. ramulosus, ramulosa, ramulosum 잔가지가 많은, 여린 가지가 많은　E *ramulose*

　> G. rhiza, rhizēs, f. *root; stem, origin* 　　　　E *rhiz(o)-, rhizophagous, rhizotomy*

　　> G. rhizousthai *to take root*

　　　> G. rhizōma, rhizōmatos, n. (< -ma *resultative noun suffix*) *a prostrate*

　　　　or subterranean root-like stem emitting roots and usually producing

　　　　leaves at its apex; a rootstock

　　　　> L. rhizoma, rhizomatis, n. (식물) 근경(根莖),

　　　　　지하경(地下莖) 　　　　　　　　　　　　　E *rhizoma (rhizome)*

　　> G. glykyrrhiza, glykyrrhizēs, f. (< glykys *sweet*) *the rhizome of the plant*

　　　Glycyrrhiza glabra

　　　> L. glycyrrhiza, glycyrrhizae, f. 감초(甘草) 　　　　E *licorice (liquorice)*

　　> L. rhizobium, rhizobii, n. (< + G. bios *life*) 뿌리혹세균, 근류균(根瘤菌)　E *rhizobium*

　　> L. Rhizopus, Rhizopi, m. (< *in allusion to the form of its rhizoids* < + G. pous

　　　foot) (곰팡이) 리조푸스속(屬) 　　　　　　　　　　　E Rhizopus

> (*possibly*) L. radius, radii, m. 막대기, 자막대기, 수레바퀴의 살, 반지름; (*the bone*

　acting like the radius of a circle when the forearm is rotated while the elbow

　is fixed) 노뼈, 요골(橈骨); 빛살, 광선

　　E *radius,* (pl.) *radii, radian, radio-* (< 'of radial bone'); *ray,* (radioactive >) *radium*
　　(Ra), (radium >) *radon (Rn)*

　> L. radialis, radiale 반지름의; 요골의, 노뼈의; 광선의, 방사형(放射形)의 　E *radial*

　> L. radio, radiavi, radiatum, radiare (수레바퀴에) 살을 대다; 빛살을 뻗치다,

　　(빛·열이) 방사(放射)하다 　　　　　　　　　　E *radiate, radiant, radiator*

　　> L. radiatus, radiata, radiatum (*past participle*) (바퀴에) 살을 댄; 빛을

　　　발산한, 방사한

　　　[용례] corona radiata (뇌, 난소의) 부챗살관, 방사관 　　　E *corona radiata*

　　　　(문법) corona 관(冠): 단수 주격 < corona, coronae, f.

　　　　　radiata: 과거분사, 여성형 단수 주격

　　> L. radiatio, radiationis, f. 방사(放射), 방사선

　　　E *radiation, radi(o)-* (< 'of radiation'), (radiotelephony >) *radio,* (radio
　　　detection and ranging >) *radar, radiology, radiograph, radiodensity,*
　　　radiolucent, radiopaque, radioactive, radioisotope, radiosensitive,
　　　radioresistant

> L. irradio, irradiavi, irradiatum, irradiare (< ir- (< in) *in, on, into, toward*) 빛나다, 빛을 방사하다, 조사(照射)하다　**E** *irradiate*
> L. *irradiatio, *irradiationis, f. 조사(照射)　**E** *irradiation*

pix, picis, f. 목(木) 타르, 불에 그을린 수지(樹脂), 피치

> **E** *pitch, (pitch 'black' + blende 'to blind, to deceive' > 'a black ore resembling a lead mineral' >) pitchblende, (pix + oleum 'oil' + -ine 'chemical suffix' > 'isolated from coal tar oil' >) picoline, (picoline >) picolinic acid, dipicolinic acid*

< IE. pik- *pitch*
> G. (*Ionic*) pissa, pissēs, f.; (*Attic*) pitta, pittēs, f.) *pitch*

vernix, vernicis, f. (veronix, veronicis, f.) 베레니케산(産) 수지(樹脂), 수지막(樹脂膜), 바니시, (ワニス) 와니스, (ワニス > ニス) 니스　**E** *varnish*

[용례] vernix caseosa 태아기름막, 태지(胎脂)　**E** *vernix caseosa*
　(문법) vernix: 단수 주격
　　caseosa 치즈 같은: 형용사, 여성형 단수 주격
　　　< caseosus, caseosa, caseosum 치즈가 많은, 치즈의, 치즈 같은
< G. Berenikē, Berenikēs, f. *Benghazi in Libya* (현재 지명)

(vix), vicis, f. (주격 없음) 차례, 대신(代身)　**E** (vice (abl.) *'in place of'* >) *vice-*

[용례] vice versa 바뀐 차례로, 역으로　**E** *vice versa*
　[문법] vice 차례로: 단수 탈격
　　versa 바뀐: 과거분사, 여성형 단수 탈격
　　　< versus, versa, versum
　　　< verto, versi, versum, vertere 돌리다, 돌다, 바꾸다
> vicarius, vicaria, vicarium 대신하는, 대리하는, 보좌의　**E** *vicarious, vicar*
> vicissim (부사) 다음 차례로, 번갈아, 바꾸어
　> vicissitudo, vicissitudinis, f. 교대, 교체, (한 상태에서 다른 상태로) 변화, 변천　**E** *vicissitude*
< IE. weik-, weig- *to bend, to wind*

> **E** *wych-, wicker, wicket (< 'door that turns'), weak (< 'pliant'), weakness, week (< 'a turning, series')*
> L. vicia, viciae, f. (< *twining plant*) 살갈퀴속(屬)의 콩과 식물　**E** *vetch*

vox, vocis, f. 목소리, 언어　**E** *voice, (voice >) voiced, (voice >) voiceless*

[용례] vox populi 백성의 소리, 인심
　(문법) vox 소리: 단수 주격
　　populi 백성의: 단수 속격 < populus, populi, m.
> vocalis, vocale 목소리의, 발성의　**E** *vocal, vowel, semivowel*

> voco, **vocavi**, vocatum, vocare 부르다   **E** *vouch (< 'to call to court to prove title to property')*

> vocatio, vocationis, f. 부름, 소환, 소명, 천직   **E** *vocation*

> vocativus, vocativa, vocativum 부르는데 쓰이는, 호칭의; (문법)

호격(呼格)의   **E** *vocative (voc.)*

> vocabulum, vocabuli, n. 명칭, 용어

> vocabularium, vocabularii, n. 자전(字典)   **E** *vocabulary*

> advoco, **advocavi**, advocatum, advocare (< ad- *to, toward, at, according to*

+ vocare *to call*) 의견·도움·사건처리를 위해 부르다   **E** *avow, disavow*

> advocatus, advocati, m. 법률고문, 변호인, 옹호자, 지지자   **E** *advocate*

> convoco, **convocavi**, convocatum, convocare (< con- (< cum) *with, together*

+ vocare *to call*) 함께 부르다, 불러 모으다, 소집하다   **E** *convoke*

> evoco, **evocavi**, evocatum, evocare (< e- *out of, away from* + vocare *to call*)

불러내다, 유발(誘發)하다   **E** *evoke, evocative*

> invoco, **invocavi**, invocatum, invocare (< in- *in, on, into, toward* + vocare

to call) (구원·보호를 청하여 또는 증인으로 신을) 부르다, (법의 힘 등에)

호소하다   **E** *invoke, invocation*

> provoco, **provocavi**, provocatum, provocare (< pro- *before, forward, for,*

instead of) 불러일으키다, 유발(誘發)하다, 도발(挑發)하다, 야기(惹起)

하다   **E** *provoke, provocative*

> provocatio, provocationis, f. 유발, 도발, 야기   **E** *provocation*

> revoco, **revocavi**, revocatum, revocare (< re- *back, again* + vocare *to call*)

다시 불러들이다, 소환하다, 취소하다   **E** *revoke, revocable, irrevocable*

> aequivocus, aequivoca, aequivocum (< aequus *equal* + vox *voice*) 같은 뜻으로 들

리는, 애매한   **E** *equivocal, unequivocal, equivocate*

< IE. wek^w- *to speak*

> G. ops, opos, f. *voice*   **E** *Calliope (< 'beautiful-voiced')*

> G. epos, epeos, n. *word, legend, song*   **E** *epos*

> G. epikos, epikē, epikon *epic*

> L. epicus, epica, epicum 서사적, 서사시의   **E** *epic*

lux, lucis, f. 빛   **E** *lux*

> luceo, **luxi**, –, lucēre 빛나다, 드러나다, 명백하다   **E** *lucent, radiolucent*

> lucidus, lucida, lucidum 빛나는, 밝은, 투명한, 또렷한   **E** *lucid*

> pellucidus, pellucida, pellucidum (< pel- (< per) *through, thorough*)

+ lucidus *bright*) 투명한, 밝은, 명료한   **E** *pellucid*

[용례] zona pellucida 투명띠, 투명대(透明帶), 투명층   **E** *zona pellucida*

(문법) zona 허리띠, 대(帶), 지역: 단수 주격

< zona, zonae, f.

pellucida 투명한: 형용사, 여성형 단수 주격

[용례] septum pellucidum 투명중격, 투명사이벽   **E** *septum pellucidum*

(문법) septum (공간을 나누는) 중격(中隔), 사이벽: 단수 주격

< septum, septi, n. (saeptum, saepti, n.) 울타리

pellucidum 투명한: 형용사, 중성형 단수 주격

> elucido, elucidavi, elucidatum, elucidare (< e- *out of, away from* +
lucidus bright) 빛나게 하다, 빛을 비추다, 밝히다, 설명하다   **E** *elucidate*

> transluceo, -, -, translucēre (< trans- *over, across, through, beyond* +
lucēre to shine) 꿰뚫어 비치다, 투명하다   **E** *translucent*

> lucifer, lucifera, luciferum (< lux, lucis, f. *light* + -fer (< ferre *to carry, to bear*)
carrying, bearing) 빛을 가져다주는, 빛을 지니는   **E** *luciferin, luciferase*

> Lucifer, Luciferi, m. (< (*probably*) G. Phōsphoros) 샛별; 마왕 루시퍼   **E** *Lucifer*

< IE. leuk- *light, brightness*

> **E** *light, alight, lightning, enlighten,* (*light amplification by stimulated emission of radiation* >) *laser, lea* (< '*where light shines*')

> L. lumen, luminis, n. 빛, 촛불; (창, 틈, 구멍 >) 내강(內腔)

> **E** *lumen, luminophore* (<'*light radical*'), *luminol, superluminal; lumen,* (pl.) *lumina, luminal, intraluminal, adluminal, abluminal*

> L. lumino, luminavi, luminatum, luminare 비추다, 조명하다, 밝게 하다

> L. illumino, illuminavi, illuminatum, illuminare (< in- *in, on, into, toward* + luminare *to cast light*) 비추다, 조명하다, 밝게 하다

> **E** *illuminant, illuminati, illuminate,* (*illuminate* >) *transilluminate, illumination*

> L. *luminesco, *luminui, -, *luminescĕre (< + -escĕre *suffix of inceptive (inchoative) verb*) 냉광(冷光)을 내다   **E** *luminescence, luminescent, luminesce*

> L. lustrum, lustri, n. 정화(淨化), (고대 로마의 5년마다 호구조사를 끝낸 다음 행한)
재계(齋戒), (고대 로마의) 인구조사, 5년간, 회계연도   **E** *lustrum*

> L. lustro, lustravi, lustratum, lustrare 정화하다, 두루 살피다   **E** *lustrate, lustre (luster)*

> L. illustro, illustravi, illustratum, illustrare (< il- (< in) *in, on, into, toward* + lustrare *to purify, to make bright*) 밝히다, 명백하게 하다,
비추다   **E** *illustrate*

> L. luna, lunae, f. (하늘의) 달   **E** F. *demilune*

> L. lunaris, lunare 달의, 음력의   **E** *lunar*

> L. semilunaris, semilunare (< semi- *half*) 반달의   **E** *semilunar*

> L. sublunaris, sublunare (< sub- *under, up from under*) 달 아래의,
지상의   **E** *sublunary*

> L. lunula, lunulae, f. (< + -ula *diminutive suffix*) 반달, 손톱 및 발톱 반월,
조반월(爪半月)   **E** *lunula,* (pl.) *lunulae*

> L. lunatus, lunata, lunatum 반달 모양의, 초승달 모양의, 월상(月狀)의   **E** *lunate*

> L. lunaticus, lunatica, lunaticum 달의 영향을 받는, 미친   **E** *lunatic* (<'*moonstruck*')

> G. leukos, leukē, leukon *bright, white*

> **E** *leuc(o)- (leuk(o)-), leucocyte (leukocyte), leukotriene(s)* (<'*originally isolated from leucocytes, which contain three conjugated double bonds*'), *interleukin(s)* (<'*ability to act as communication signals between different populations of leukocytes*'), *leucine (Leu, L)* (< '*a white matter*'), *isoleucine (Ile, I)*

> L. leukaemia, leukaemiae, f. (< G. leukos *white* + haima *blood* + -ia)

백혈병(白血病)　　　　　　　　　　　　　　　　　　E *leukaemia (leukemia), leukemic, leukemoid*

> L. leukosis, leukosis, f. (< G. leukos *white* + -ōsis *condition*) 백혈증(白血症)　　E *leukosis*

fauces, faucium (< faucum), f. (pl.) ((sing.) faux, faucis, f.) 목구멍, 구협(口峽)　　E *fauces, faucial*

> suffoco, suffocavi, suffocatum, suffocare (< suf- (< sub) *under, up from under* +

facuces *throat*) 목을 조르다, 질식(窒息)시키다　　　　　　　　E *suffocate, suffocant*

맞대보기 1　그리스어 제3변화 제1식과 제2식의 남성 또는 여성 명사는 위의 변화(제3변화 제1식 a)를 따르는 라틴어 명사가 되며 성은 그리스어의 성을 따르는 것을 원칙으로 한다.

Ammon, Ammonis, m. 암몬　　　　　　　　　　　　　　　E *Ammon, ammonite*

[용례] cornu Ammonis (CA) (< *Ammon's horn*) 암몬의 뿔　　E *cornu Ammonis (CA)*
(문법) cornu 뿔: 단수 주격 < cornu, cornus, n.
Ammonis 암몬의: 단수 속격

> L. ammoniacus, ammoniaca, ammoniacum 암몬의

[용례] sal ammoniacum (< *sal ammoniac, NH₄Cl*) 암몬의 소금

E *ammonia, ammoniacal, (ammonia >) ammonium, (ammonia >) amide(s), (ammonia >) amine(s), (amine >) amino, (amide >) imide(s), (amine >) imine(s), (imine >) imino, (vita 'life' + amine >⁺ vitamine 'a mistaken belief about the chemical nature of the compounds'>) vitamin(s), (cobalt + vitamin >) cobalamin, cyanocobalamin (< 'a cobalamin derivative with a cyanide ion')*

(문법) sal 소금: 단수 주격 < sal, salis, n.
ammoniacum 암몬의: 형용사, 중성형 단수 주격

< G. Ammōn, Ammōnos, m. *Ammon*

< (*Egyptian*) a-m-n *the hidden (one)*

Pharao, Pharaonis, m. 파라오　　　　E *Pharaoh (< final -h after the Hebrew form), Pharaonic*

< G. Pharaō, Pharaōnos, m. *Pharaoh*

< (*Hebrew*) parōh *Pharaoh*

< (*Egyptian*) pr-o *the great house*

aër, aëris, m. 공기, 안개　　　　　E *air, airway, aer(o)- (aeri-), aerial, aerosol*

> L. aëror, aëratus sum, aërari 공기를 쐬다, 통기시키다　　E *aerate, aeration*

> It. aria *air*　　　　　　　　　　　　　　　　　　　　　E *aria*

> It. mala aria (< L. mala *bad*) *bad air*

> It. mal' aria (< *contracted form*) *bad air*

> L. malaria, malariae, f. 말라리아, 학질(瘧疾),

학(瘧)   **E** *malaria, malarial*

< G. aēr, aeros, m., f. *air, mist*

E *aer(o)-, aerobe, aerobic, aerobics, anaerobe, anaerobic, aerophagia (aerophagy)*

< G. aēnai *to blow, to breathe*

> G. aura, auras, f. *air, breath, breeze, draught*

> L. aura, aurae, f. 미풍, 기(氣),

조짐   **E** *aura, aural,* (*exaurare *'to rise into the air'* >) *soar*

< IE. we- *to blow*   **E** *wind, window* (< *'wind eye'*)*, wing, weather*

> L. ventus, venti, m. 바람, 역경, 허풍; 통풍구, 출구   **E** *vent*

> L. ventulus, ventuli, m. (< + -ulus *diminutive suffix*) 산들바람

> L. ventilo, **ventilavi**, ventilatum, ventilare 바람을 일으키다,

선동하다   **E** *ventilate, ventilator, ventilatory*

> L. ventilatio, ventilationis, f.

환기   **E** *ventilation; hyperventilation, hypoventilation*

> (*Sanskrit*) nirvana (< nirva *to blow out* < nis- *out* + va *to blow*) *blowing out,*
extinction, disappearance   **E** *nirvana*

cremaster, cremasteris, m. 고환올림근, 고환거근(擧筋)   **E** *cremaster, cremasteric*

< G. kremastēr, kremastēros, m. *hanger, suspender*

< G. kremannynai *to hang, to hang up*

sphincter, sphincteris, m. 조임근, 괄약근(括約筋)   **E** *sphincter, sphincteral*

[용례] musculus sphincter ani 항문조임근   **E** *sphincter ani (muscle)*

musculus sphincter pupillae 동공조임근,

축동근(縮瞳筋)   **E** *sphincter pupillae (muscle)*

(문법) musculus 근육, 근: 단수 주격 < musculus, musculi, m.

sphincter: 단수 주격 (musculus와 동격)

ani 항문의: 단수 속격 < anus, ani, m.

pupillae 동공의: 단수 속격 < pupilla, pupillae, f.

< G. sphinktēr, sphinktēros, m. *sphincter*

< G. sphingein *to grow close, to draw tight*

> G. Sphinx, Sphingos, f. (< *strangler*) (*Greek mythology*) *Sphinx*

> L. Sphinx, Sphingis, f. (그리스 신화) 스핑크스

E *Sphinx, sphingosine* (< *'enigmatic as Sphinx,' with irregular -s-'*)*,*
(*sphingosine* >) **sphingolipid(s)**, (*sphingosine* > *'sphingolipid found*
in myelin sheath' >) **sphingomyelin(s)**

< IE. spheig- *to flourish, to grow thick, to expand, to succeed*

< IE. spe- *to flourish, to grow thick, to expand, to succeed*　　　**E** *spare, speed*

　　> L. spes, spei, f. ((pl. nom.) spes, speres) 희망

　　　　> L. spero, **speravi**, speratum, sperare 희망하다　　**E** *('Dr. Hoping-one' >) Esperanto*

　　　　　　> L. despero, **desperavi**, desperatum, desperare (< de- *apart from, down,*

　　　　　　　　not + sperare *to hope*) 실망하다　　　　　**E** *despair, desperate*

　　　　> L. prosper (prosperus), prospera, prosperum (< pro- *before, forward, for,*

　　　　　　instead of + sper- *stem of* spes) 소원대로 되는, 번영하는　　**E** *prosperous*

　　　　　　> L. prosperitas, prosperitatis, f. 소원대로 됨, 행운, 번영　　**E** *prosperity*

　　　　　　> L. prospero, **prosperavi**, prosperatum, prosperare 소원대로 되게 하다,

　　　　　　　　행운을 안겨주다, 번영하게 하다　　　　　　　　**E** *prosper*

　　> (*suggested*) L. spatium, spatii, n. 공간, 간격, 동안　　　**E** *space, interspace*

　　　　> L. spatialis, spatiale 공간의　　　　　　　　　　**E** *spatial*

　　　　> L. spatiosus, spatiosa, spatiosum 광활한, 웅대한, 오랜　　**E** *spacious*

　　> (*suggested*) L. spissus, spissa, spissum 빽빽한, 조밀한, 농축된, 힘겨운

　　　　> L. spisso, **spissavi**, spissatum, spissare 빽빽하게 하다, 조밀하게 하다, 조이다,

　　　　농축하다

　　　　　　> L. inspisso, **inspissavi**, inspissatum, inspissare (< in- *in, on, into,*

　　　　　　　　toward + spissare *to thicken*) 빽빽하게 하다, 조밀하게 하다, 조이다,

　　　　　　　　농축하다　　　　　　　　　　　　　　　**E** *inspissate*

anthrax, anthracis, f. 탄저병(炭疽病)　　　　　　　　　　**E** *anthrax*

　　[용례] Bacillus anthracis 탄저균(炭疽菌)　　　　　　**E** Bacillus anthracis

　　　(문법) Bacillus 바실루스속(屬): 단수 주격

　　　　　　< bacillus, bacilli, m. 작은 막대기, 막대균, 간균(桿菌), 바실루스;

　　　　　　　(Bacillus) (세균) 바실루스속(屬)

　　　　　　< baculus, baculi, m. (baculum, baculi, n.) 지팡이, 막대기

　　　　anthracis 탄저병의: 단수 속격

　　< G. anthrax, anthrakos, m. *coal, (burning coal* >)

　　　carbuncle　　**E** *anthracene* (< *'from coal-tar'*), (phen(o)- + anthracene >) *phenanthrene*

　　　> L. anthracosis, anthracosis, f. (< *deposition of carbon particles in the lungs*

　　　　< + G. -ōsis *condition*) 탄분증(炭粉症), 석탄가루증　　**E** *anthracosis*

calyx, calycis, m. 잔, 배(杯); 꽃받침, 악(萼); 신배(腎杯)

　　E *calyx*, (pl.) *calyces*, *calyceal*, *calycectasis* (*calicectasis*, *caliectasis*), *glycocalyx* (<
　　'sugar coat')

　　　> L. calyculus, calyculi, m. (< + -ulus *diminutive suffix*)

　　　　작은 잔　　　　　　　**E** *calyculus* (*caliculus*), (pl.) *calyculi* (*caliculi*)

　　< G. kalyx, kalykos, f. *cup, husk, shell, bud,* (pl.) *earings*

< IE. kal- *cup*

　　> L. calix, calicis, m. 잔, 컵; 성배(聖杯); 신배(腎杯)

E *calix,* (pl.) *calices, chalice, calicivirus* (< *'virus which has a capsid with cup-shaped depressions'), calicectasis (caliectasis) (calycectasis)*

> L. caliculus, caliculi, m. (< + –ulus *diminutive suffix*) 작은 잔, 작은 컵, 작은

컵 모양의 구조　　　　　　　**E** *caliculus (calyculus),* (pl.) *caliculi (calyculi)*

> G. kylix, kylikos, f. *drinking cup*　　　　　　　**E** *kylix*

lichen, lichenis, m. 지의(地衣), 태선(苔癬)　　　　　**E** *lichen, lichenoid, lichenify*

　　[용례] lichen planus 편평태선(扁平苔癬)　　　　**E** *lichen planus*

　　(문법) lichen 태선: 단수 주격

　　　　planus 편평한: 형용사, 남성형 단수 주격

　　　　　< planus, plana, planum 편평한, 평평한, 납작한, 평이한, 명확한

　　　　< G. leichēn, leichēnos, m. *tree moss*

　　< G. leichein *to lick*

< IE. leigh– *to lick*　　　　　　**E** *lick, lecher* (< *'to live in debauchery'*)

　　> L. lingo, linxi, linctum, lingĕre 핥다

　　　　> L. cunnilingus, cunnilingi, m. (< cunnus *vulva*) 외음핥기　**E** *cunnilingus*

　　　　> L. anilingus, anilingi, m. (< anus *anus*) 항문핥기　　**E** *anilingus*

ascaris, ascaridis, f. 회충(蛔蟲)　　　　　**E** *ascaris, ascariasis, ascarid*

　　< G. askaris, askaridos, f. *intestinal worm*

ephelis, ephelidis, f. 주근깨　　　　　　**E** *ephelis,* (pl.) *ephelides*

　　< G. ephēlis, ephēlidos, f. *freckle*

iris, iridis, f. (iris, iris, f.) 무지개; (Iris) (그리스 신화) 무지개의 여신, 붓꽃과의 식물

　　　　(붓꽃·꽃창포·제비붓꽃 등); (*different colors* >) 홍채(虹彩)

　　　　E *Iris, iridescent, iridium (Ir)* (< *'compounds of various colors'); iris, iridial, iridocorneal*

　　< G. iris, iridos, f. *rainbow; (Iris) (Greek mythology) Goddess of the rainbow and messenger of the gods*

　< IE. wei–, weiə– *to turn, to twist; with derivatives referring suppleness or binding*　　　　　　**E** *wire, garland*

　　> L. vieo, –, vietum, viēre 구부리다, 잡아매다, 엮다

　　　　> L. vimentum, vimenti, n. 가는 나뭇가지, 울짱,

　　　　　사립짝　　**E** *vimentin* (< *'arrays of flexible rods, ordered or nonordered'*)

　　　　> L. vitis, vitis, f. 포도넝쿨, 포도나무　**E** *viticulture, vise (vice)* (< *'that which winds'*)

　　> L. vincio, vinxi, vinctum, vincire 매다, 엮다, 묶다

　　　　> L. vinculum, vinculi, n. 끈, 유대, 속박　　**E** *vinculum,* (pl.) *vincula, vinculin*

　　　　> (*suggested*) L. vinca, vincae, f. 빈카

E (Vinca rosea (*now,* Catharanthus roseus) > *vincaleukoblastine* >) **vinblastine**, (*vinblastine* + (*perhaps*) crista '*crest*' >) **vincristine**

> G. is, inos, f. *sinew, nerve, muscle; strength, force*

E *inosine* (< '*found in meat and meat extracts*'), *inositol* (< '*isolated from heart muscle extracts*'), **inotropic** (< '*affecting the force of muscle contractions*'), (a- '*not*' + makros '*long, large*' + in- (< is, inos, f.) '*sinew*' >) **amacrine**

> G. inion, iniou, n. (< + -ion *diminutive suffix*) *nape of the neck, occipital bone*

> L. inion, inii, n. 뒤통수점, 외후두융기정점

E *inion*

pyramis, pyramidis, f. 피라미드, 모뿔, 각추(角錐), 추체(錐體)

E *pyramid*

> pyramidalis, pyramidale 피라미드 모양의, 모뿔의, 각추의, 추체의

E *pyramidal*

< G. pyramis, pyramidos, f. *pyramid*

< (*Egyptian*) pimar *pyramid*

psoas, psoatis, m. 허리근, 요근(腰筋)

E *psoas*

> iliopsoas, iliopsoatis, m. (< ilium *ilium*) 엉덩허리근, 장요근(腸腰筋)

E *iliopsoas*

< (*erroneously*) G. psoas (acc. pl.) *a muscle of the loin*

< G. psoa, psoas, f. *a muscle of the loin*

맞대보기 2　염증의 명사 접미사 –itis로 끝나는 그리스어 기원의 학술용어는 위의 변화(제3변화 제1식 a)를 따르는 라틴어 여성 명사가 된다. (단수 속격은 –itidis가 되고, 복수 주격은 –itides가 된다)

---

meningitis, meningitidis, f. (< G. mēninx, mēningos, f. *membrane* + -itis *noun suffix denoting inflammation* < -itēs *adjective suffix*)

수막염(髓膜炎)

E *meningitis,* (pl.) *meningitides, meningitic*

[용례] Neisseria meningitidis 수막염균

E Neisseria meningitidis

(문법) Neisseria (세균) 나이세리아속(屬): 단수 주격

< Neisseria, Neisseriae, f.

< Albert Ludwig Sigesmund Neisser (1855-1916), *German physician*

meningitidis 수막염의: 단수 속격

< IE. mems- *flesh, meat* (Vide MEMBRANA; *See* E. *membrane*)

otitis, otitidis, f. (< G. ous, ōtos, n. *ear* + -itis) 이염(耳炎)

E *otitis*

[용례] otitis media 중이염(中耳炎)

E *otitis media*

(문법) otitis 이염(耳炎): 단수 주격

media 가운데의: 형용사, 여성형 단수 주격 < medius, media, medium

< IE. ous- *ear* (Vide AURIS: *See* E. *aural*)

polyarteritis, polyarteritidis, f. (< G. polys *many* + artēria *artery* + -itis) 다발성동맥염
(多發性動脈炎)   **E** *polyarteritis*

   [용례] polyarteritis nodosa 결절성 다발성동맥염   **E** *polyarteritis nodosa*
       (문법) polyarteritis 다발성동맥염: 단수 주격
           nodosa 매듭이 많은: 형용사, 여성형 단수 주격
               < nodosus, nodosa, nodosum < nodus, nodi m. 매듭

●●● 제3변화 제1식 b

> 단수 속격의 음절수가 많아지며 어간 끝에 자음이 하나만 있는 중성 명사. 단수의 속격
> 어미는 -is; 복수의 주격 어미는 -a, 속격 어미는 -um 이 된다. 단수 및 복수에서 주격,
> 대격, 호격이 똑같다.

caput, capitis, n. 머리

	단 수	복 수	
주격	caput	capit-a	~이, ~가, ~은, ~는, ~께서
속격	capit-is	capit-um	~의
여격	capit-i	capit-ibus	~게, ~에게, ~께, ~한테
대격	caput	capit-a	~을, ~를
탈격	capit-e	capit-ibus	~에서, ~로부터, ~으로부터
호격	caput	capit-a	~여, ~이여

caput, capitis, n. 머리

> **E** *cape, chief, chef, kerchief* (< *'a cloth used to cover the head, formerly a woman's head-dress'*), *(kerchief* >) *handkerchief,* (F. a chief *'to a head'* > *'to finish'* >) *achieve, mischief, mischievous, cadet* (< *'little chief'*), *(cadet* >) *caddie (caddy),* (suggested) *cabbage,* (suggested) *capsize* (< *'to sink by the head'*)

   [용례] caput medusae 메두사 머리   **E** *caput medusae*
       (문법) caput: 단수 주격
           medusae 메두사의: 단수 속격 < Medusa, Medusae, f.

   > capitaneus, capitanea, capitaneum 으뜸가는, 주요한, 현저한   **E** *captain, chieftain*
   > capitalis, capitale 머리의, 생명에 관계되는, 으뜸가는   **E** *capital*
       > capital, capitalis, n. (capitale, capitalis, n.) (사형에 처할 만한) 중죄, (제관의)

고깔; (*principal money laid out* >) 자본

> **E** *cattle* (< '*live stock*'), *chattel* (< '*article other than live stock*'), *capital* (< '*fund of money*'), *capitalism*

> capitatus, capitata, capitatum 머리가 있는, 머리 모양을 한 **E** *capitate*

> capitatio, capitationis, f. 인원별 계산, 인두세 **E** *capitation*

> capitulum, capituli, n. 작은 머리, 기둥머리, 장(章), 작은 머리
모양의 뼈 **E** *capitulum, capitular, chapter*

> capitulo, **capitulavi**, capitulatum, capitulare 장(章)으로 분류하다, 조건을 정리
하다 **E** *capitulate*

> recapitulo, **recapitulavi**, recapitulatum, recapitulare (< re- *back, again*
+ capitulare *to draw up in heads or chapters, to arrange conditions*)
요점을 다시 설명하다, 어린 동물이 선조의 발달단계를 되풀이하다,
재연하다 **E** *recapitulate*

> capitellum, capitelli, n. 기둥머리 **E** *capitellum, capital*

> (*suggested*) capillus, capilli, m.
머리털 **E** (dis- '*apart from, down, not*' + capillus '*hair*' > '*disordered hair*' >) *disheveled*

> capillaris, capillare 머리털의, 머리털 같은; 모세관의,
모세혈관의 **E** *capillary, (capillary* >) *capillarity*

> choriocapillaris, choriocapillare (< chorion *fetal membrane;*
highly vascularized tissue) 맥락막 모세혈관의

> occiput, occipitis, n. (< oc- (< ob) *before, toward(s), over, against, away* + caput
head) 뒤통수, 후두(後頭) **E** *occiput*

> occipitalis, occipitale 뒤통수의, 후두의 **E** *occipital*

> sinciput, sincipitis, n. (< *senciput < semi- *half* + caput *head*) 이마 **E** *sinciput, sincipital*

> biceps, (gen.) bicipitis (< bi- (< bis) *two* + caput *head*) 머리 둘 가진 **E** *biceps, bicipital*

[용례] musculus biceps brachii 위팔두갈래근, 상완이두근 **E** *biceps brachii (muscle)*
musculus biceps femoris 넓적다리두갈래근, 대퇴이두근 **E** *biceps femoris (muscle)*
(문법) musculus 근육, 근: 단수 주격 < musculus, musculi, m.
biceps 머리 둘 가진: 형용사, 남·여·중성형 단수 주격
brachii 위팔의, 상완의: 단수 속격 < brachiium, brachii, n.
femoris 넓적다리의, 대퇴부의: 단수 속격 < femur, femoris, n.

> triceps, (gen.) tricipitis (< tri- (< tres) *three* + caput *head*) 머리 셋 가진 **E** *triceps, tricipital*

[용례] musculus triceps brachii 위팔세갈래근, 상완세갈래근 **E** *triceps brachii (muscle)*
musculus triceps surae 장딴지세갈래근 **E** *triceps surae (muscle)*
(문법) musculus 근육, 근: 단수 주격 < musculus, musculi, m.
triceps 머리 셋 가진: 형용사, 남·여·중성형 단수 주격
brachii 위팔의, 상완의: 단수 속격 < brachium, brachii, n.
surae 장딴지의: 단수 속격 < sura, surae, f.

> quadriceps, (gen.) quadricipitis (< quadri- (< quattuor) *four* + caput *head*) 머리
넷 가진 **E** *quadriceps, quadricipital*

[용례] musculus quadriceps femoris 넓적다리네갈래근,

　　　대퇴사두근 **E** *quadriceps femoris (muscle)*

　　(문법) musculus 근육, 근: 단수 주격 < musculus, musculi, m.

　　　quadriceps 머리 넷 가진: 형용사, 남·여·중성형 단수 주격

　　　femoris 넓적다리의, 대퇴부의: 단수 속격 < femur, femoris, n.

> praeceps, (gen.) praecipitis (< prae- *before, beyond* + caput *head*) 곤두박이는,

가파른 **E** *precipitous*

　　> praecipitium, praecipitii, n. 낭떠러지, 벼랑; 위기, 추락, 몰락 **E** *precipice*

　　> praecipito, **praecipitavi**, praecipitatum, praecipitare 곤두박이게 하다, (급속히)

　　　거꾸로 떨어지다, 아래로 떨어지다, 침전(沈澱)하다

E *precipitate, precipitant, precipitation, coprecipitate, immunoprecipitation, cryoprecipitation, precipitin*

> decapito, **decapitavi**, decapitatum, decapitare (< de- *apart from, down, not* +

caput *head* + -are) 목을 베다, 참수하다, 해임하다 **E** *decapitate*

> (*perhaps*) cappa, cappae, f. 두건, 모자, 망토, 두건 달린 외투

E *cap, (three hands, holding the bets, in a cap >) handicap, cape, chaperon (chaperone) (< 'a person, especially a married or elderly woman, who, for the sake of propriety, accompanies a young unmarried lady in public, as guide and protector' < 'hood'), escape (< 'to leave one's cloak behind'); (Capuchin > 'the color of the coffee resembles that of a Capuchin's habit' >) cappuccino*

　　> cappella, cappellae, f. (< + -ella *diminutive suffix*) 작은 망토, 소성당

E *chapel (< 'the cappella or cloak of St. Martin, preserved by the Frankish kings as a sacred relic, the name was applied to the sanctuary in which this was preserved, and thence to any private sanctuary or holy place'), chaplain*

< IE. kaput- *head* **E** *head, forehead, behead*

inguen, inguinis, n. 샅, 사타구니, 샅고랑, 샅굴, 서혜부(鼠蹊部); 아랫배, 음부(陰部); 가래톳;

가지가 줄기에 붙은 부분

　　> inguinalis, inguinale 샅의, 사타구니의, 샅고랑의, 샅굴의, 서혜부의 **E** *inguinal*

< IE. eng^w- *groin, internal organ*

　> G. adēn, adenos, n. *acorn, gland*

E *aden(o)-, adenine (A) (< 'isolated from the pancreatic gland of the ox'), adenosine (A)*

　　> G. adenoeidēs, adenoeidēs, adenoeides (< + eidos *shape*) *gland-like*

E *adenoid, adenovirus (< 'isolated from the human adenoids (pharyngeal tonsils)'*

　　> L. adenitis, adenitidis, f. (< + -itis *noun suffix denoting inflammation*) 샘염,

　　　선염(腺炎) **E** *adenitis, sialadenitis, lymphadenitis*

　　> L. adenoma, adenomatis, n. (< + G. -ōma *noun suffix denoting tumor*) 샘종,

　　　선종(腺腫) **E** *adenoma, adenomatous*

　　> L. adenocarcinoma, adenocarcinomatis, n. (< + G. karkinos *crab* + -ōma

　　　noun suffix denoting tumor) 샘암종, 선암종(腺癌腫) **E** *adenocarcinoma*

nomen, nominis, n. 이름, 명목; (문법) 명사

E *noun, anomia* (< *'a form of aphasia characterized by inability to recall the names of objects, on the pattern of aphasia, but etymologically incorrect'*)

> nominalis, nominale 이름의, 이름에 관한, 명목상의; (문법) 명사의　　　　E *nominal*

> nomino, **nominavi**, nominatum, nominare 이름 부르다, 명명하다, 지명하다,

　　임명하다　　　　　　　　　　　　E *(verb)* **nominate, nominee, misnomer, renown**

　　　> nominatus, nominata, nominatum (*past participle*) 명명된, 유명한　E *(adjective)* **nominate**

　　　　　> innominatus, innominata, innominatum (< in- *not*) 이름 없는,

　　　　　　　무명의　　　　　　　　　　　　　　　E *innominate*

　　　　　> nominativus, nominativa, nominativum 지명된, 기명의;

　　　　　　　(문법) 주격(主格)의　　　　　　　　E *nominative (nom.)*

　　　　　> denomino, **denominavi**, denominatum, denominare (< de- *apart from, down,*

　　　　　　　not; intensive) 이름을 따서 붙이다, 이름을 밝히다,

　　　　　　　지명하다　　　　　　　　　　　　E *denominate, denominator*

　　　　　　　> denominativus, denominativa, denominativum 이름을 나타내는; (문법)

　　　　　　　　　명사(형용사) 유래의　　　　　　　E *denominative*

> nomenclatura, nomenclaturae, f. (< nomen *name* + calatus (< calare *to call*) *called*)

　　명명법, 학명, 학술어　　　　　　　　　　　E *nomenclature*

> pronomen, pronominis, n. (< pro- *before, forward, for, instead of* + nomen *name*

　　< G. antōnymia *pronoun*) (문법) 대명사　　　E *pronoun*

> ignominia, ignominiae, f. (< *loss of a name* < in- *not* + nomen *name*) 불명예,

　　치욕　　　　　　　　　　　　　　　　　E *ignominy*

　　　> ignominiosus, ignominiosa, ignominiosum 불명예스러운, 치욕적인　E *ignominious*

> binominis, binomine (binomius, binomia, binomium) (< bi- *two* + nomen *name*) 두

　　이름의, 두 이름 가진

　　E *binominal; binomial, multinomial* (< *'on the pattern of binomial'*), *polynomial* (< *'on the pattern of multinomial'*); *binomen*

> trinominis, trinomine (trinomius, trinomia, trinomium) (< tri- *three* + nomen *name*)

　　세 이름의, 세 이름 가진　　　　　　　　　E *trinominal; trinomen*

< IE. no-men- *name*　　E *name,* (suggested by supernomen *'above the name'* >) *surname, unnamed*

> G. onoma, onomatos, n. ((*Aeolic*) onyma, onymatos, n.) *name*

E *onomatomania, synonym, antonym, homonym, acronym, eponym* (< *'(the one) upon a name'*), *toponym* (< *'place name'*), *pseudonym, cryptonym, patronymic, metronymic (matronymic), matronymic* (< *'on the pattern of patronymic'*)

> G. onomatopoiia, onomatopoiias, f. (< + G. -poiia *making* < poiein *to make*)

　　word-making

　　　> L. onomatopoeia, onomatopoeiae, f. 의성어 만들기, 의성어　E *onomatopoeia*

> G. anōnymos, anōnymos, anōnymon (< an- *not*) *nameless, of unknown name*

　　　> L. anonymus, anonyma, anonymum 무명의, 익명의, 서명하지 않은　E *anonymous*

　　　　　> L. *anonymitas, *anonymitatis, f. 무명, 익명, 불명　E *anonymity*

> G. homōnymos, homōnymos, homōnymon (< homos *of the same*) *of the*

same name

> L. homonymus, homonyma, homonymum 같은 이름의, 동명이인(同名
異人)의, 동음이의(同音異意)의; (안과) 같은 (이름) 쪽의,
동측의　　　　　　　　　　　　　　　**E** *homonym, homonymous*

> G. heterōnymos, heterōnymos, heterōnymon (< heteros *different*)

of different names

> L. *heteronymus, *heteronyma, *heteronymum 다른 이름의, 동철이음이의
(同綴異音異意)의; (안과) 다른 (이름) 쪽의, 반대측의　**E** *heteronym, heteronymous*

> G. ‾ōnymia, ‾ōnymias, f. *naming*

> G. metōnymia, metōnymias, f. (< met(a)‾ *between, along with, across,*
after) *change of name*

> L. metonymia, metonymiae, f. 환치(換置),
환유(換喩)　　　　　　　**E** *metonymy, (metonymy >) metonym*

---

omen, ominis, n. 축원, 징조　　　　　　　　　　　　　　　**E** *omen*

> ominosus, ominosa, ominosum 미리 알리는, 흉조의　　　　**E** *ominous*

> ominor, ominatus sum, ominari 축원하다, 점치다, (전조로) 예견하다

> abominor, abominatus sum, abominari 흉조를 물리치다, 몹시 싫어하다,
혐오하다　　　　　　　　　　　　　　　　　　**E** *abominate*

> abominabilis, abominabile 혐오스러운　　　　　**E** *abominable*

< IE. o‾ *to believe, to hold as true*

---

pollen, pollinis, n. 고운 가루, 밀가루, 꽃가루　**E** *pollen, pollinate, pollinosis*

< IE. pel‾ *dust, flour*

> L. pulvis, pulveris, m., f. 가루,
먼지　　　　**E** *powder,* (F. poudre *'powder'* > *'application of powder'* >) *poudrage*

> L. pulverizo, –, pulverizatum, pulverizare 가루로 만들다, 빻다　**E** *pulverize*

> (*probably*) L. pulpa, pulpae, f. 과육(果肉), 속살, 수(髓)　　　**E** *pulp*

> L. pulposus, pulposa, pulposum 과육이 많은, 속살의, 수(髓)의

[용례] nucleus pulposus 속질핵, 수핵(髓核)　　　**E** *nucleus pulposus*

(문법) nucleus 핵: 단수 주격 < nucleus, nuclei, m.
pulposus: 형용사, 남성형 단수 주격

> G. palē, palēs, f. *fine meal, fine dust*

> G. palynein *to sprinkle*　　　　　　　　　**E** *palynology*

> (*probably*) G. poltos *porridge*

> (*probably*) L. puls, pultis, f. 죽　　　　**E** *poultice, pultaceous*

---

stapes, stapedis, n. (stapes, stapitis, n.) 등자뼈, 등골(鐙骨)　　**E** *stapes*

> stapedius, stapedia, stapedium 등자뼈의　　　**E** *stapedius, stapedial*

< stapia, stapiae, f. 등자(鐙子)

< *Of Germanic origin*

crus, cruris, n. 아랫다리, 다리, 각(脚), 다리 같은 구조, 살   **E** *crus,* (pl.) *crura*
> cruralis, crurale 다리의, 각부(脚部)의   **E** *crural*

jus, juris, n. 법
> juro, juravi, juratum, jurare 선서하다   **E** *jury, juror*
>> abjuro, abjuravi, abjuratum, abjurare (< ab- *off, away from* + jurare *to swear*)
>> (서약하면서) 부인하다   **E** *abjure*
>> adjuro, adjuravi, adjuratum, adjurare (< ad- *to, toward, at, according to* +
>> jurare *to swear*) 덧붙여 서약하다, (서약하면서) 간청하다, 명하다   **E** *adjure*
>> conjuro, conjuravi, conjuratum, conjurare (< con- (< cum) *with, together* +
>> jurare *to swear*) 함께 선서하다, 모의하다   **E** *conjure*
>> perjuro, perjuravi, perjuratum, perjurare (< *(breaking) through justice* < per-
>> *through, thoroughly* + jurare *to swear*) 위증하다   **E** *perjure, perjury, perjurer*
> judex, judicis, m. (< jus, juris, n. *law* + dicĕre *to say*) 재판관, 심판자   **E** (noun) *judge*
>> judico, judicavi, judicatum, judicare 재판하다,
>> 판단하다   **E** (verb) *judge, judgement (judgment)*
>> judicium, judicii, n. 재판, 심리, 판단   **E** *judicious*
>>> judiciarius, judiciaria, judiciarium 재판의, 사법의   **E** *judiciary*
>>> judicialis, judiciale 재판의, 사법의   **E** *judicial*
>>> praejudicium, praejudicii, n. (< prae- *before, beyond* + judicium *judge-*
>>> *ment*) 선입견, 예단(豫斷), 편견   **E** *prejudice*
> jurisdictio, jurisdictionis, f. (< jus, juris, n. *law* + dictio (<dicĕre *to say*) *saying*)
> 재판권, 사법권   **E** *jurisdiction*
> jurisprudentia, jurisprudentiae, f. (< jus, juris, n. *law* + prudentia *foreseeing, knowledge*)
> 법학, 법리학, 법철학   **E** *jurisprudence*
> injurius, injuria, injurium (< in- *not*) 불법적인, 불의한, 부당한
>> injuria, injuriae, f. 불법, 불의, 모욕, 침해, 손상   **E** *injury*
>>> injuriosus, injuriosa, injuriosum 불법의, 모욕의, 손상 끼치는   **E** *injurious*
>>> injurior, injuriatus sum, injuriari 모욕하다, 폭행하다   **E** *injure*
< IE. yewes- *law*
> L. justus, justa, justum 법을 잘 지키는, 정의로운   **E** *just,* (just >) *unjust*
>> L. justitia, justitiae, f. 정의   **E** *justice*
>> L. justifico, justificavi, justificatum, justificare (< justus *just* + -ficare (< facĕre)
>> *to make*) 정당화하다   **E** *justify*
>>> L. justificatio, justificationis, f. 정당화   **E** *justification*
>> L. injustus, injusta, injustum (< in- *not*) 불법적인, 불의한, 부당한   **E** †*injust*
>>> L. injustitia, injustitiae, f. 불법, 불의, 부당   **E** *injustice*

jus, juris, n. 국, 국물, 수프, 액(液), 즙(汁)　　　　　　　　　　　　　　**E** *juice, juicy*

< IE. yeuə- *to blend, to mix food*

  > G. zymē, zymēs, f. *leaven, corruption*　　　　**E** *zym(o)-, zymase, zymology, zymogen*

    > G. enzymos, enzymos, enzymon (< en- *in*) *leavened*

> **E** *enzyme, -enzyme (-zyme), enzymatic (enzymic), proenzyme (< 'before' enzyme), apoenzyme (< 'enzyme without prosthetic group' < 'away' enzyme), coenzyme (< 'organic nonprotein prosthetic group for apoenzyme' < 'with' enzyme), holoenzyme (< 'whole' enzyme), isoenzyme (isozyme) (< 'equal' enzyme), lysozyme (muramidase) (< 'an enzyme present in the tissues and secretions of the body, which is capable of rapidly dissolving certain bacteria' < 'lytic' enzyme), (ribonucleic enzyme >) ribozyme*

pus, puris, n. 고름, 농(膿); 독살스러운 인간　　　　　　　　　　　　　**E** *pus*

  > purulentus, purulenta, purulentum 고름이 가득한, 곪은　　　　　**E** *purulent*

  > puteo, putui, –, putēre 썩다, 악취가 나다

    > puter, putris, putre (putris, putre) 썩은

      > putreo, putrui, –, putrēre 썩어 있다, 노쇠하다

        > putridus, putrida, putridum 썩은　　　**E** *putrid, potpourri (< 'rotten pot')*

        > putresco, putrui, –, putrescĕre (< + -escĕre *suffix of inceptive (inchoative) verb*) 썩기 시작하다, 푸석해지다　　**E** *putrescent*

      > putrefacio, putrefeci, putrefactum, putrefacĕre (< puter *putrid* + facĕre *to make*) 썩게 하다, 썩히다, 부패시키다　　**E** *putrefy, putrefactive*

        > putrefactio, putrefactionis, f. 부패　　　　　　　**E** *putrefaction*

  > suppuro, suppuravi, suppuratum, suppurare (< sub- *under, up from under* + pus *pus*) 곪다, 곪게 하다　　　　　　　　　**E** *suppurate, suppurative*

    > suppuratio, suppurationis, f. 곪음, 화농(化膿)　　　**E** *suppuration*

< IE. pu- *to rot, to decay*　　　　**E** *foul, foil, defile, filth, fuzzy (< 'sponge')*

  > G. pyon, pyou, n. *pus*　　　　　　　　　　　　　　　**E** *py(o)-*

    > G. empyein (< em- (< en) *in* + pyon) *to suppurate*

      > G. empyema, empyematos, n. (< + -ma *resultative noun suffix*) *suppuration, gathering*

        > L. empyema, empyematis, n. 축농(蓄膿), 고름집; 농흉(膿胸), 가슴고름집

> **E** *empyema (< 'a collection of pus within a naturally existing anatomical cavity'), empyemic*

    > G. hypopyon, hypopyou, n. (< hyp(o)- *under* + pyon) *matter under the cornea*

      > L. hypopyon, hypopyi, n. 앞방고름, 앞방축농　　　**E** *hypopyon*

  > L. pyogenes, (gen.) pyogenis (< + G. -genēs, -genēs, -genes *producing*) 고름을 만드는, 화농성의

  > L. pyogenicus, pyogenica, pyogenicum (< + G. -genēs, -genēs, -genes *producing*) 고름을 만드는, 화농성의　　　　　　　　　　　　　**E** *pyogenic*

rus, ruris, n. (< *open land*) 시골

> ruralis, rurale 시골의   **E** *rural*

> rusticus, rustica, rusticum 시골풍의, 소박한, 거친   **E** *rustic*

< IE. reuə- *to open, space*   **E** *room, rummage* (< *'ship's hold'*)

onus, oneris, n. 짐, 부담, 책임, 수고   **E** *onus*

> onerosus, onerosa, onerosum 짐스러운, 부담이 따르는, 수고로운   **E** *onerous*

> onero, **oneravi**, oneratum, onerare 짐 지우다, 책임을 맡기다, 힘들게 하다

> exonero, **exoneravi**, exneratum, exnerare (< ex- *out of, away from* + onerare
to burden) 짐을 부리다, 면제하다   **E** *exonerate*

< IE. en-es- *burden*

opus, operis, n. 일, 작품   **E** *opus,* (pl.) *opera,* It. *operetta*

> opusculum, opusculi, n. (문학·음악 등의) 소품   **E** *opuscule*

> operor, operatus sum, operari 일하다, 작용하다

> **E** *operate, operative, preoperative, intraoperative, postoperative,* (oper- + -on *'a*
termination of Greek neuter nouns and adjectives' > *'a working unit'* > *'a group of*
genes whose expression is coordinated by an operator' >) **operon,** (manu operari *'to*
work by hand' >) **maneuver (manoeuvre),** (manu operari *'to cultivate'* >) **manure,**
(in operibus *'in works'* >) **inure (enure)**

> operans, (gen.) operantis (*present participle*) 일하는, 작용하는   **E** *operant*

> operatio, operationis, f. 작용, 운용, 조작, 수술; (수학) 연산; (군사) 작전   **E** *operation*

> operator, operatoris, m. 운용자, 수술자, 작동유전자(作動遺傳子); (수학) 연산자   **E** *operator*

> cooperor, cooperatus sum, cooperari (< co- (< cum) *with, together*) 함께
일하다, 협동하다   **E** *cooperate*

> cooperatio, cooperationis, f. 협동   **E** *cooperation*

> opero, **operavi**, operatum, operare 일어나게 하다, 작용케 하다

> opifex, opificis, m., f. (< opus *work* + facĕre *to make*) 제조자, 수공업인

> opificina, opificinae, f. 제조소

> officina, officinae, f. 제조소

> officinalis, officinale 제조법의, 약전(藥典)에 따른, 약용(藥用)의   **E** *officinal*

> opificium, opificii, n. (< opus *work* + facĕre *to make*) 일, 활동, 제조

> officium, officii, n. 직무, 의무   **E** *office, officer*

> officialis, officiale 직무상의, 공무상의   **E** *official*

> officiosus, officiosa, officiosum 제구실하는   **E** *officious*

> officio, **officiavi**, officiatum, officiare 직무를 수행하다, 의무를 다하다   **E** *officiate*

< IE. op- *to work, to produce in abundance*

> L. ops, opis, f. 힘, 도움; (pl.) 세력, 병력, 재산

> L. opulentus, opulenta, opulentum (opulens, (gen.) opulentis) 힘 있는, 풍요한   **E** *opulent*

> L. Opis, Opis, f. 풍요와 수확의 여신   **E** *Opis*

> L. optimus, optima, optimum (< *wealthiest*) (bonus, bona, bonum의 최상급) 가장 좋은　　　　　　　　　　　　　　　　　　　　**E** *optimum, optimal, optimism, optimize*

> L. copia, copiae, f. (< co- (< cum) *with, together; intensive* + opes *wealth*) 풍부; (Copia) (로마 신화) 풍요의 여신　**E** *copy*, (cornu copiae *'horn of plenty'* >) *cornucopia*

　> L. copiosus, copiosa, copiosum 풍부한, 풍성한　　　　　　　**E** *copious*

> L. omnis, omne (< *abundant*) 모든 (Vide OMNIS; *See* E. *omni-*)

sidus, sideris, n. 성좌, 별

> sidereus, siderea, sidereum 성좌의, 별의　　　　　　　　　　**E** *sidereal*

> (*suggested*) considero, consideravi, consideratum, considerare (< *to observe the stars carefully* < con- (< cum) *with, together; intensive* + sidus *star*) 주의 깊게 관찰하다, 깊이 생각하다　　　　　　　　　　　　　　　　　　　**E** *consider*

> (*suggested*) desidero, desideravi, desideratum, desiderare (< *to await what the stars will bring* < de sidere *from the constellation*) 고대하다, 열망하다, 욕망 하다　　　　　　　　　　　　**E** *desiderate, desiderative, desire, undesired*

< IE. sweid- *to shine*

vulnus, vulneris, n. (volnus, volneris, n.) 상처

> vulnero, vulneravi, vulneratum, vulnerare 상처 입히다

　> vulnerarius, vulneraria, vulnerarium 상처에 관한, 외과의　**E** *vulnerary*

　> vulnerabilis, vulnerabile 상처 입을 수 있는, 범할 수 있는　**E** *vulnerable*

　> vulnificus, vulnifica, vulnificum (< vulnus *wound* + -ficus (< facĕre) *making*) 상처 입히는, 살해하는　　　　　　　　　　　　　**E** (*obsolete*) *vulnific*

< IE. welə- *to strike, to wound*

E ((*Old Norse*) valr *'those slain in battle'* + kyrja *'chooser'* >) *Valkyrie*, ((*Old Norse*) valr *'those slain in battle'* + hall *'hall'* >) *Valhalla*

> G. oulē, oulēs, f. *scar*　　　　　　　　　**E** *ul(o)- (ule-), ulectomy, ulegyria*

∞ (*probably*) IE. welə- *wool* (Vide VELLUS; *See* E. *vellus*)

∞ (*probably*) IE. wel- *to tear, to pull* (Vide VILLUS; *See* E. *villus*)

pectus, pectoris, n. 가슴, 흉부; 마음, 양심, 용기, 지혜　　　**E** *parapet*

[용례] pectus carinatum (< *pigeon chest*) 새가슴, 구흉(鳩胸), 돌출흉　**E** *pectus carinatum*

pectus excavatum (< *funnel chest*) 오목가슴, 누두흉(漏斗胸), 함몰흉　**E** *pectus excavatum*

[문법] pectus 가슴: 단수 주격

carinatum 용골(龍骨)을 댄: 과거분사, 중성형 단수 주격

< carinatus, carinata, carinatum

< carino, carinavi, carinatum, carinare 용골을 대다

excavatum 파인: 과거분사, 중성형 단수 주격

< excavatus, excavata, excavatum

< excavo, excavavi, excavatum, excavare 파내다

> pectoralis, pectorale 가슴의   **E** *pectoralis, pectoral*

> expectoro, **expectoravi**, expectoratum, expectorare (< ex- *out of, away from*) 가슴

밖으로 내보내다, 가슴속에서 (공포 등을) 몰아내다   **E** *expectorate*

> expectorans, expectorantis, n. (< *present participle*) 거담제(祛痰劑),

가래약   **E** *expectorant*

< IE. peg- *breast*

tempus, temporis, n. (< *span of time* < *span*) 때, 시간   **E** *tense,* It. *tempo*

[용례] ex tempore 그때그때, 즉석의, 즉흥적,

준비 없이   **E** *extempore, extemporary, extemporaneous, extemporize*

(문법) ex ~부터: 전치사, 탈격지배

tempore 때: 단수 탈격

> temporalis, temporale 때의, 시간의   **E** *temporal*

> temporarius, temporaria, temporarium 그때그때의, 일시적인   **E** *temporary*

> *contemporarius, *contemporaria, *contemporarium (< con- (< cum)

with, together) 동시대의   **E** *contemporary*

> tempestas, tempestatis, f. 계절, 기후, 나쁜 날씨, 폭풍우   **E** *tempest*

> tempero, **temperavi**, temperatum, temperare 때를 조절하다, 배합하다, 섞다,

균형 잡다, 절제하다, 상냥하게 대하다   **E** *temper, tamper, distemper,* It. *tempera*

> temperantia, temperantiae, f. (< *present participle*) 절제, 극기   **E** *temperance*

> temperatus, temperata, temperatum (*past participle*) 조절된, 잘 배치된,

절제 있는, 온후한   **E** *temperate*

> intemperatus, intemperata, intemperatum (< in- *not* + temperatus

temperate) 무절제한   **E** *intemperate*

> temperatura, temperaturae, f. 균형 잡힌 배합, 체질, 온도   **E** *temperature*

> temperamentum, temperamenti, n. 균형 잡힌 배합, 체질, 온도   **E** *temperament*

< IE. temp- *to stretch*

> L. templum, templi, n. (베틀에서 베를 팽팽하게 당겨 주는) 쳇발   **E** *temple, template*

> L. tempus, temporis, n. (< (*suggested*) *where the skin is stretched from*

behind the eye to the ear) (흔히 복수로 씀) 관자놀이   **E** *temple*

> L. temporalis, temporale 관자놀이의   **E** *temporal*

> (*Iranian*) *tap- *carpet*

> G. tapēs, tapētos, m. *carpet*

> G. tapētion, tapētiou, n. (< + -ion *diminutive suffix*) *tapestry*   **E** *tapestry*

> L. tapetum, tapeti, n. 양탄자, 융단, 요   **E** *tapetum*

< IE. ten- *to stretch* (Vide TENĒRE: *See* E. *tenet*)

ebur, eboris, n. 상아, 상아 제품

> eboreus, eborea, eboreum 상아의, 상아로 만든   **E** *ivory*

< (*probably*) *Via Phoenician from an African source*

femur, femoris, n. 윗다리, 넓적다리, 대퇴부(大腿部); 넓적다리뼈, 대퇴골(大腿骨)   **E** *femur*

> femoralis, femorale 넓적다리의, 대퇴부의; 넓적다리뼈의, 대퇴골의   **E** *femoral*

murmur, murmuris, n. 웅성거림, 중얼거림, 잡음   **E** *(noun) murmur*

> murmuro, **murmuravi**, murmuratum, murmurare 중얼거리다, 투덜거리다   **E** *(verb) murmur*

< IE. mormor–, murmur– *echoic root*

> G. mormyrein *to roar*

gutter, gutturis, n., m. 목구멍, 탐식   **E** *guttural*

> gutturosus, gutturosa, gutturosum 갑상샘종(腫)의   **E** *goiter (goitre), goitrous, goitrogen*

< IE. geu– *to bend, to arch*   **E** *cot, cottage*

맞대보기   –ma로 끝나는 그리스어 제3변화 중성명사는 라틴어 중성 명사가 되며 위의 변화 (제3변화 제1식 b)를 따른다. 결과의 명사 접미사 –ma (–sma)와 종양의 명사 접미사 –oma로 끝나는 그리스어 기원의 학술용어도 마찬가지이다. (단수 속격은 –matis, –omatis가 되고, 복수 주격은 –mata, –omata가 된다)

---

aroma, aromatis, n. 방향(芳香), 정취   **E** *aroma*

< G. arōma, arōmatos, n. *spice*

> G. arōmatikos, arōmatikē, arōmatikon *aromatic*

> L. aromaticus, aromatica, aromaticum 방향이 있는, 방향성의; (화학) 방향족(芳香族)의   **E** *aromatic, (aromatic polyamide >) aramid*

> G. arōmatizein *to spice*

> L. aromatizo, **aromatizavi**, aromatizatum, aromatizare 방향을 내다; (화학) 방향족화(芳香族化)하다   **E** *aromatize, aromatase*

bregma, bregmatis, n. 정수리점   **E** *bregma, bregmatic*

< G. bregma, bregmatos, n. *the front part of the head*

< IE. mregh–m(n)o– *brain*

   E *brain, forebrain (prosencephalon), midbrain (mesencephalon), hindbrain (rhombencephalon)*

chroma, chromatis, n. 치장, 피부색, 색채(色彩), 음색(音色)

E *chromat(o)- (chrom(o)-)*, *chromatography* (< 'originally, showing colored bands of the separated plant pigments'), *chromatophil (chromophil)* (< 'a cell or element that stains readily'), *chromophobe* (< 'a cell or element that does not stain readily'), *chromophore* (< 'color radical'), *chromatophore* (< 'pigment-bearing cell, pigment-bearing plastid'), *chromogen* (< 'coloring agent'); *chromatin* (< 'proposed to discriminate the denser element (nucleus) which eagerly takes the color (D. Chromatin) from the one (cytoplasm) which refuses it (D. Achromatin)'), *euchromatin* (< 'weakly staining chromatin'), *heterochromatin* (< 'densely staining chromatin'), *chromosome* (< 'chromatic bodies'), *chromatid* (< 'one-half of a replicated chromosome; when separated, it is called a daughter chromosome'); *cytochrome(s)* (< 'any electron transfer hemoprotein, originally described as cellular pigment'); *chromatic, -chromatic, achromatic, trichromat, dichromat*; *chromium (Cr)* (< 'brilliant colors, red, yellow, or green, of its compounds'), *chrome, chromic (Cr^{+++}), chromous (Cr^{++}), chromate, chromaffin* (< 'stained on exposure to chromates')

> L. -chromia, -chromiae, f. (< + -ia) *coloring*

> **E** *-chromia, -chromic, hyperchromic, orthochromic (normochromic), hypochromic; normochromic (orthochromic)*

> L. heterochromia, heterochromiae, f. (< G. heteros *different*)
이색증(異色症), 얼룩증　　　　　　　　　　　　　**E** *heterochromia*

> L. metachromasia, metachromasiae, f. (< G. met(a)- *between, along with, across, after* + chrōma, chrōmatos, n. *color* + -sia) 이염색성 (異染色性)　　　　　　　　　**E** *metachromasia, metachromatic*

> L. haemochromatosis, haemochromatosis, f. (< G. haima, haimatos, n. *blood* + chrōma, chrōmatos, n. *color* + -ōsis *condition*) (< *deposition of hemosiderin in the parenchymal cells with associated tissue damage*) 혈색소침착증　　　　**E** *haemochromatosis (hemochromatosis)*

< G. chrōma, chrōmatos, n. *embellishment, complexion, color*

< IE. ghreu- *to rub, to grind*

E *great* (< 'coarsely ground'), *grit* (< 'sand, gravel'), *grout* (< 'coarse meal'), *gruel* (< 'porridge'), (probably) *gravel*

> (*probably*) L. ruo, rui, rutum, ruĕre (< *gruĕre) 무너지다, 들이닥치다, 돌진하다

> L. congruo, congrui, −, congruĕre (< con- (< cum) *with, together* + ruĕre *to go ruin, to fall violently*) 맞아떨어지다, 일치하다, 조화 되다　　　　　　　　　　**E** *congruent, congruence (congruency)*

> L. congruus, congrua, congruum 맞는, 일치하는, 적절한　　**E** *congruous*

> L. congruitas, congruitatis, f. 일치, 적절　　**E** *congruity*

> L. inongruus, incongrua, incongruum (< in- *not*) 일치하지 않는, 부적절한　　　　　　　　　　**E** *incongruous*

> G. chrōs, chrōtos, m. *skin, complexion, color*　　**E** *dichroic* (< 'two-colored')

< IE. gher- *to scrape, to scratch*

> G. charassein *to sharpen, to notch, to carve, to cut*　　　　**E** *gash*

> G. charactēr, charactēros, m. *stamp, token, mark, character*

> L. character, characteris, m. (소유를 표시하기 위해 동물 등에 찍는)

낙인, 인호, 글자, 특성, 성격　　　　　　　　　　　　　　　　E *character*

　　　　> G. charaktēristikos, charaktēristikē, charaktēristikon

　　　　characteristic　　　　　　　　　　　　　　　　　　　E *characteristic*

　　　　> G. charaktērizein *characterize*　　　　　　　　　　E *characterize*

> IE. ghrendh- *to grind*　　　　　　　　　　　　　　　　　E *grind, gristle*

　　> (*suggested*) G. chondros, chondrou, m. *grain, lump, cartilage* (Vide CHONDROS: See E. *chondr(o)–*)

> (*reduplicated*) L. furfur, furfuris, m. 겨, 밀기울; 비듬

　　　E *furfur, furfural* (< '*an aldehyde*'), (*furfur* >) *furfuran (furan)*, (*furan* >) *furanose, furosemide (fursemide, frusemide)*

　　　> L. furfuraceus, furfuracea, furfuraceum 겨의, 밀기울의; 비듬이 많은　　E *furfuraceous*

pneuma, pneumatis, n. 숨, 공기, 바람, 영(靈), 정신

　　　E *pneumat(o)-, pneumatic, pneumatization, pneum(o)-, pneumothorax, pneumo-peritoneum, pneumopericardium*

　< G. pneuma, pneumatos, n. *breath, air, wind, spirit, mind*

< IE. pneu- (*imitative root*) *to breathe*　　　　　　　E *sneeze, snore, snort, sneer*

　> G. pnein (pneein) *to breathe, to blow*

　　> G. pnoē, pnoēs, f. *breath, breathing*

　　> G. –pnoia, –pnoias, f. *breath,*

　　breathing　　E *-pnoea (-pnea), tachypnoea (tachypnea), bradypnoea (bradypnea)*

　　> G. apnoia, apnoias, f. (< a- *not*) *breathlessness*

　　　> L. apnoea, apnoeae, f. 무호흡　　　　E *apnoea (apnea), apneic*

　　> G. dyspnoia, dyspnoias, f. (< dys- *bad*) *difficulty of breathing*

　　　> L. dyspnoea, dyspnoeae, f. 호흡곤란　　E *dyspnoea (dyspnea), dyspneic*

　　> G. orthopnoia, orthopnoias, f. (< orthos *upright, straight, correct*)

　　orthopnea

　　　> L. orthopnoea, orthopnoeae, f. 앉아숨쉬기, 좌위호흡

　　　　E *orthopnoea (orthopnea)* (< '*dyspnoea that is most severe in recumbency and that is alleviated by assuming an upright position*'), *orthopneic*

　　> L. hyperpnoea, hyperpnoeae, f. 과다호흡,

　　호흡항진　　　　　　　　　E *hyperpnoea (hyperpnea), hyperpneic*

aenigma, aenigmatis, n. 수수께끼, 모호한 비유, 은어　　　　E *enigma, enigmatic*

　　< G. ainigma, ainigmatos, n. (< + -ma *resultative noun suffix*) *riddle*

　　< G. ainissesthai *to speak in riddles, to hint*

　< G. ainos, ainou, m. *saying, story*

comma, commatis, n. 코머　　　　　　　　　　　　　　　E *comma*

< G. komma, kommatos, n. (< + -ma *resultative noun suffix*) *stamp, piece
cut off, short clause*

> L. osteocomma, osteocommatis, n. (< G. osteon *bone*) 낱뼈, 골편 **E** *osteocomma*

< G. koptein *to strike, to cut off*

> G. apokopē, apokopēs, f. (< ap(o)- *away from, from* + koptein) *apocope*

> L. apocope, apocopes, f. (음성) 어미음(語尾音) 소실 **E** *apocope*

> G. synkopē, synkopēs, f. (< syn- *with, together* + koptein) *syncope*

> L. syncope, syncopes, f. (syncopa, syncopae, f.) 결여, 실신(失神), 졸도
(卒倒); (음성) 어중음(語中音) 소실; (음악) 당김음법 **E** *syncope, syncopal*

> L. syncopo, **syncopavi**, syncopatum, syncopare 정신 잃다, 기절
하다; (음성) 어중음을 생략하다; (음악) 당김음을 쓰다 **E** *syncopate*

> L. Sarcoptes, Sarcoptis, f. (< G. sarx, sarkos, f. *flesh* + koptein) (진드기)
옴진드기속(屬) **E** *Sarcoptes, sarcoptic*

< IE. kop- *to beat, to strike* **E** *hoof, hatchet (< 'small ax')*

---

asthma, asthmatis, n. 천식(喘息) **E** *asthma*

< G. asthma, asthmatos, n. (< + -ma *resultative noun suffix*) *asthma*

> G. asthmatikos, asthmatikē, asthmatikon *asthmatic*

> L. asthmaticus, asthmatica, asthmaticum 천식의 **E** *asthmatic*

< G. azein *to breathe hard*

---

eczema, eczematis, n. 습진(濕疹), 아토피성 피부염 **E** *eczema, eczematous*

< G. ekzema, ekzematos, n. (< *something thrown out by boiling, by
heat* < + -ma *resultative noun suffix*) *eczema*

< G. ekzein (ekzeein) (< ek- *out of, away from*) *to boil over, to break out*

< G. zein (zeein) *to boil* **E** *zeolite (< 'swelling when heated')*

< IE. yes- *to boil, to foam, to bubble* **E** *yeast*

---

ependyma, ependymatis, n. 뇌실막(腦室膜), 수강막(髓腔膜) **E** *ependyma, ependymal; subependymal*

< G. ependyma, ependymatos, n. (< + -ma *resultative noun suffix*)
upper garment

[용례] ependyma ventriculorum 뇌실상피(腦室上皮)
(문법) ependyma 막: 단수 주격
ventriculorum 뇌실들의: 복수 속격
< ventriculus, ventriculi, m. 작은 배[腹], 실(室),
심실(心室), 뇌실(腦室)

< G. ependyein (< ep(i)- *upon* + en- *in* + dyein *to put on*) *to put on over*
< G. dyein *to sink, to enter, to put on*

oedema, oedematis, n. 부기, 부종(浮腫)　　　　　　　　　**E** *oedema (edema), edematous*

    < G. oidēma, oidēmatos, n. (< + -ma *resultative noun suffix*) *swelling, swollen*
        condition

   < G. oidein (oideein) *to swell*

     > G. Oidipous, Oidipodos, m. (< *swollen-footed* < pous, podos, m. *foot* + oidein)
       Oedipus

      > L. Oedipus, Oedipodis, m. (Oedipus, Oedipi, m.) 오이디푸스　　　**E** *Oedipus*

 < IE. oid- *to swell*　　　　　　　　　　　　　　　　　　　**E** *(perhaps) oat*

charisma, charismatis, n. 특별한 은혜, 특별한 능력　　　　　**E** *charisma, charismatic*

     < G. charisma, charismatos, n. (< + -ma *resultative noun suffix*) *favor*
       given, gift of grace, gift of God's grace

    < G. charizesthai *to show favor, to give free*

     > G. eucharistia, eucharistias, f. (< eu- *well*) *thanksgiving*　　**E** *Eucharist*

   < G. charis, charitos, f. *grace, favor*

 < IE. gher- *to like, to want*　　　　　　　　　　　　　**E** *yearn, greedy*

   > L. hortor, hortatus sum, hortari 격려하다, 권장하다　　　　**E** *hortative*

     > L. exhortor, exhortatus sum, exhortari (< ex- *out of, away from*) 열심히
      권하다, 훈계하다　　　　　　　　　　　　　　　　　**E** *exhort*

      > L. exhortatio, exhortationis, f. 권고, 훈계　　　　　　**E** *exhortation*

chiasma, chiasmatis, n. 교차(交叉),

  교차점　　　**E** *chiasma (chiasm), (pl.) chiasmata (chiasms), chiasmatic (chiasmal)*

     < G. chiasma, chiasmatos, n. (< + -ma *resultative noun suffix*) *two things*
      crossed

    < G. chiazein *to mark with a chi (X)*

     > G. chiasmos, chiasmou, m. (< + -mos *resultative noun suffix*) *crossing,*
      diagonal arrangement

      > L. chiasmus, chiasmi, m. X 모양의 기호; 교차배열법　　　**E** *chiasmus*

miasma, miasmatis, n. 장기(瘴氣, 대기 속에 있다는 전염성 독)　**E** *miasma (miasm), (pl.) miasmata*

    < G. miasma, miasmatos, n. (miasmos, miasmou, m.) (< + -sma *extended form*
      of -ma *resultative noun suffix*) *stain, defilement, pollution, abomination*

   < G. miainein *to stain, to soil, to pollute*

     > G. amiantos, amiantos, amianton (< a- *not* + miantos *defiled*) *undefiled*

      > L. amiantus, amianti, m. (amianthus, amianthi, m.) (< *free from all stains*
       by being thrown in the fire, it being itself incombustible) 석면(石綿),
       섬유 모양의 사문석(蛇紋石)　**E** *amiantus (amianthus), amiantoid (amianthoid)*

 < IE. mai- *to soil, to defile*　　　　　　　　　　　　**E** *mole (< 'spot, blemish')*

prisma, prismatis, n. 프리즘   **E** *prism, prismatic*

        < prisma, prismatos, n. (< + -ma *resultative noun suffix*) *thing sawn, prism*

      < prizein *to saw*

  < IE. pris- *to crush*

carcinoma, carcinomatis, n. 암(癌),

        암종(癌腫)   **E** *carcinoma, (pl.) carcinomata (carcinomas), carcinomatous*

       < G. karkinōma, karkinōmatos, n. (< (*suggested*) *the swollen veins surrounding*

         the part affected bear a resemblance to the limbs of a crab (Galen of Pergamon)

          < + -ōma *noun suffix denoting tumor*) *carcinoma*

      < G. karkinos, karkinou, m. *crab*

  < IE. kar-, ker- *hard* (Vide CANCER; *See* E. *cancer*)

sarcoma, sarcomatis, n. 육종(肉腫)   **E** *sarcoma, (pl.) sarcomata (sarcomas), sarcomatous*

       < G. sarkōma, sarkōmatos, n. (< + -ōma *noun suffix denoting tumor*) *sarcoma*

      < G. sarx, sarkos, f. (< *piece of meat*) *flesh*

  < IE. twerk- *to cut* (Vide SARX; *See* E. *sarcophagus*)

••• 제 3 변화 제 2 식 a

단수 속격의 음절수가 많아지며 어간 끝에 자음이 둘 이상 있는 남성, 여성 명사. 단수의 속격 어미는 -is; 복수의 주격 어미는 -es, 속격 어미는 -ium이 된다.

dens, dentis, m. 이, 치아

	단 수	복 수	
주격	dens	dent-es	~이, ~가, ~은, ~는, ~께서
속격	dent-is	dent-ium	~의
여격	dent-i	dent-ibus	~게, ~에게, ~께, ~한테
대격	dent-em	dent-es	~을, ~를
탈격	dent-e	dent-ibus	~에서, ~로부터, ~으로부터
호격	dens	dent-es	~여, ~이여

dens, dentis, m. 이, 치아(齒牙)

    E *dens, denture, dentist, (dentist >) dentistry, dentin, dentinal,* (dens leonis '*lion's tooth*'
    >) *dandelion*

돌기   **E** *denticle*

> denticulatus, denticulata, denticulatum 작은 이의, 작은 이 모양을 한   **E** *denticulate*

> dentalis, dentale 이의   **E** *dental, labiodental, interdental*

> dentatus, dentata, dentatum 이를 가진, 이 모양을 한   **E** *dentate*

> dentio, **dentivi**, dentitum, dentire 이가 나다

> dentitio, dentitionis, f. 치아 발생, 생치(生齒), 치열(齒列)   **E** *dentition*

> edento, **edentavi**, edentatum, edentare (< e- *out of, away from*) 이 뽑다,
이 빠지다   **E** *edentate*

> edentulus, edentula, edentulum (< e- *out of, away from*) 이 빠진, 이 없는   **E** *edentulous*

> indento, **indentavi**, indentatum, indentare (< in- *in, on, into, toward*) 톱니 모양을
내다, 톱니처럼 되다   **E** *indent, indenture, indentation*

> tridens, (**gen.**) tridentis (< tri- (< tres) *three*) 뾰족한 이가 셋 달린, 삼지창의, 세
갈래 난   **E** *trident*

< IE. dent- *biting* > *tooth*   **E** *tooth, tusk*

> G. odous, odontos, m. *tooth*

> **E** *odont(o)-, odontoid, odontology, odontoblast, periodontal (periodontic), -odontics,*
exodontics, orthodontics, periodontics, prosthodontics, gerodontics, -odont, -odon,
mastodon, -odus

> L. periodontium, periodontii, n. (< G. peri- *around, near, beyond, on ac-*
count of) 치아주위조직, 치주   **E** *periodontium*

> L. Tetrodon, Tetrodontis, m. (Tetraodon, Tetraodontis, m.) (< *four large*
teeth < G. tetr(a)- *four*) (참복과) 복어속(屬)   **E** *tetrodotoxin*

fons, fontis, m. 샘, 분천(噴泉), 원천   **E** *(fons baptismi 'fountain of baptism' >) font*

> fonticulus, fonticuli, m. (< + -culus *diminutive suffix*) 작은 샘, 작은 분수; 천문(泉門),
숫구멍   **E** *fonticulus (fontanelle)*

> fontanus, fontana, fontanum 샘의, 분수의

> fontana, fontanae, f. 샘, 분수   **E** *fountain*

> fontanella, fontanellae, f. (< + -ella *diminutive suffix*) 작은 샘, 작은 분수;
천문(泉門), 숫구멍   **E** *fontanelle (fontanel) (fonticulus), fontanellar*

< IE. dhen- *to run, to flow*

mons, montis, m. 산, 구(丘)

> **E** *(noun) mount, mountain, (ad montem 'uphill' >) amount, tantamount (< 'amount to as*
much'), paramount (< 'far above')

[용례] mons pubis (mons veneris) 치구(恥丘), 치골구(恥骨丘), 음부(陰阜),
불두덩   **E** *mons pubis (mons veneris)*

(문법) mons 구(丘): 단수 주격

pubis 두덩의: 단수 속격 < pubes, pubis, f. 음부, 두덩

veneris 사랑의: 단수 속격 < venus, veneris, f. 사랑;
(Venus) 비너스, 금성

> L. montanus, montana, montanum 산의, 산골의, 산골에
사는　　　　　　　　　　　　　　　　　　　**E** *montane, cismontane, tramontane*
　> L. verumontanum, verumontani, n. (< veru, verus, n. *spit, dart* + montanum
hilly) 둔덕, 과녁, 요도 둔덕(seminal colliculus)　　　**E** *verumontanum*
> L. *monto, *montavi, *montatum, *montare 오르다, 타다, 올라타다, 올려놓다, 설치
하다　　　　　　　　　　　　**E** *(verb)* *mount, surmount*, F. *montage* (< *'to mount'*)
< IE. men- *to project*　　　　　　　　　　　　　　　　　　　　　　**E** *mouth*
> L. mentum, menti, n. 턱
　> L. mentalis, mentale 턱의　　　　　　　　　　**E** *mental, (mental >) submental*
> L. minae, minarum, f. (pl.) 성의 흉벽, 첨탑, 총안; 위협
　> L. minor, minatus sum, minari 돌출하다, 임박하다, 위협하다
　　> L. minax, (gen.) minacis 돌출한, 위협적인　　　　　**E** *menace, minacious*
　　> L. minatorius, minatoria, minatorium 위협적인, 겁주는　　　**E** *minatory*
　　> L. mino, minavi, minatum, minare 가축을 소리 질러
몰다　　　　　　**E** *amenable* (< *'to lead to'*), *demean* (< *'to lead to'*)
　　　> L. promino, -, -, prominare (< pro- *before, forward, for, instead*
of + minare *to drive animals*) 가축을 몰고 가다　　　**E** *promenade*
> L. mineo, minui, -, minēre 돌출하다
　> L. emineo, eminui, -, eminēre (< e- *out of, away from* + minēre *to project*)
돌출하다, 융기하다, 출현하다　　　　　　　　　　**E** *eminent, eminence*
　> L. immineo, imminui, -, imminēre (< in- *in, on, into, toward* + minēre
to project) 임박하다, 절박하다　　　　　　　　　　　**E** *imminent*
　> L. promineo, prominui, -, prominēre (< pro *forth* + minēre *to project*)
융기(隆起)하다, 뛰어나다　　　　　　　　　　　　　　**E** *prominent*
　　> L. prominentia, prominentiae, f. 융기, 뛰어남, 현저, 탁월　　**E** *prominence*
　　> L. promontorium, promontorii, n. (< *influenced by* mons, montis, m.
mountain) 돌출부, 등성이, 갑(岬), 곶,
갑각융기(岬角隆起)　　　　　　　　　　**E** *promontorium, promontory*

pons, pontis, m. (< *earliest meaning of 'way, passage'*) 다리 [橋]; 뇌교(腦橋), 다리뇌, 교뇌

> **E** *pons, (pons >)* **pontine**, *(pons >)* **pontic** (<*'an artificial tooth that forms part of a dental bridge, being held in place by attachment to its neighbouring teeth, and not fixed directly to the jaw'*), **punt** (< *'flatbottom boat'*)

< IE. pent- *to tread, to go*　　　　　　　　　**E** *find, foundling, path, pathway, footpad*
> G. patein (pateein) *to tread, to walk*
　> G. patos, patou, m. *trodden way, beaten way, path*
　　> *(suggested)* G. apatē, apatēs, f. (< ap(o)- *away from, from* + patos)
cheating, deceit, fraud
　　　> **E** *apatite* (< *'diverse forms and colors of the mineral'*), **hydroxyapatite, fluoroapatite**
　> G. peripatein (peripateein) (< peri- *around, near, beyond, on account of*)

to walk about   **E** *Peripatetic*

> (*Russian*) sputnik (< put' *path, way*) *fellow traveler*   **E** *Sputnik*

Mars, Martis, m. (로마 신화) 군신(軍神); 화성(火星)   **E** *Mars*

> Martius, Martia, Martium 군신의; 화성의   **E** (Martius mensis *'month of Mars'* >) *March, Martian*

> martialis, martiale 전쟁의   **E** *martial*

< Mawort- (*Roman mythology*) *god of war and agriculture*

frons, frondis, f. (엽상체의) 잎   **E** *frond*

> frondosus, frondosa, frondosum 잎이 많은, 잎이 무성한   **E** *frondose*

frons, frontis, f. 이마,

얼굴   **E** *front, frontier,* (ad frontem *'to the face'* >) *affront, confront* (< *'with the face'*)

> frontalis, frontale 이마의, 앞의   **E** *frontal*

> effrons, (gen.) effrontis 뻔뻔스러운 (< ef- (< ex) *out of, away from* + frons *front*)   **E** *effrontery*

< (*possibly*) IE. ser- *base of prepositions and preverbs with the basic meaning 'above, over, up, upper'*

glans, glandis, f. 도토리, 도토리같이 생긴 것, 선(腺), 샘, 귀두(龜頭)   **E** *gland*

[용례] glans penis 음경귀두(陰莖龜頭)   **E** *glans penis*

glans clitoridis 음핵귀두(陰核龜頭)   **E** *glans clitoridis*

(문법) glans 귀두: 단수 주격

penis 음경의: 단수 속격 < penis, penis, m. 음경, 꼬리

clitoridis 음핵의: 단수 속격 < clitoris, clitoridis, f. 음핵

> glandula, glandulae, f. (< + -ula *diminutive suffix*) 선(腺), 편도선, 샘, 돼지멱

(목덜미)의 고기

   E *glandular, glanders* (< *'a contagious disease in horses, the chief symptoms of which are glandular swellings beneath the jaw and discharge of mucous matter from the nostrils'*)

< IE. gʷelə- *acorn*

> G. balanos, balanou, f. *acorn*

> L. balanus, balani, f. 도토리   **E** *balanic, balan(o)-, balanitis, balanoposthitis*

ars, artis, f. 기술, 솜씨, 예술, 미술

   E *art,* (arte factum *'something made by art'* >) *artefact (artifact), artefactual (artifactual),* (*artitianus* >) *artisan*

> artista, artistae, m. 예술인   **E** *artist*

> artifex, artificis, m. (ars *art* + facĕre *to make*) 예술인, 기능인

> artificium, artificii, n. 기술, 기교   **E** *artifice*

> artificialis, artificiale 인공적, 인위적   **E** *artificial*

> iners, inertis (< in- *not* + ars *skill, art*) 아무 기술도 없는, 굼뜬, 타성적인   **E** *inert*

> inertia, inertiae, f. 타성, 관성, 무기력, 무력증   **E** *inertia*

< IE. ar- *to fit together*   **E** *arm, forearm*

> L. artus, arta, artum 죈, 좁은, 긴밀한

   > L. arto, artavi, artatum, artare (arcto, arctavi, arctatum, arctare) 죄다, 좁히다

     > L. coarto, coarctavi, coarctatum, coarctare (coarcto, coarctavi, coarctatum, coarctare) (< co- (< cum) *with, together; intensive*) 죄다, 좁히다

       > L. coarctatio, coarctationis, f. 협착   **E** *coarctation*

> L. artus, artus, m. 맞물림, 관절, (pl.) 사지

   > L. articulus, articuli, m. (< + -culus *diminutive suffix*) (작은) 관절, 마디; (말이나 문장의) 부분, 관사, 조목, 논설, 논문   **E** *article*

     > L. articularis, articulare 관절의, 관절이 있는   **E** *articular*

     > L. articulo, articulavi, articulatum, articulare 맞물리다, 똑똑히 발음하다, 관절로 연결하다   **E** *articulate, (articulate >) disarticulate*

       > L. articulatio, articulationis, f. 명료한 발음, 조음(調音), (통화의) 명료도; 관절에 의한 연결, 관절; (치의학) 교합(咬合)   **E** *articulation*

> L. armus, armi, m. 위팔

   > L. armilla, armillae, f. (< + -illa *diminutive suffix*) 팔찌   **E** *armillary*

> L. arma, armorum, n. (pl.) 도구, 무기   **E** *arms,* (Ad illa arma! *'To the arms!'* >) *alarm*

   > L. armo, armavi, armatum, armare 무장하다

     E *arm,* (armata *(feminine past participle)* > *'armed'* >) *army, disarm, unarmed,* Sp. *Armada* (< *'armed'*), Sp. *armadillo* (< *'small armed one'*)

     > L. armatura, armaturae, f. 무장, 무기, 무장군인   **E** *armature, armor (armour)*

     > L. armamenta, armamentorum, n. (pl.) 장비, 병기   **E** *armament*

       > L. armamentarium, armamentarii, n. 의료장비, 의료기술   **E** *armamentarium,* (pl.) *armamentaria*

   > L. armistitium, armistitii, n. (< arma *arms* + -stitium *stopping* (< sistěre *to make to stand*) 휴전, 정전   **E** *armistice*

   > L. inermis, inerme (inermus, inerma, inermum) 무장하지 않은

> G. artios, artia, artion *fitting, (of numbers) even*   **E** *artiodactyl*

> G. arthron, arthrou, n. *joint, limb, article, articulation*   **E** *arthr(o)-, arthrology, arthralgia, arthrospore*

   > G. arthrosis, arthroseōs, f. (< + -ōsis *condition*) *articulation, connection by a joint*

     > L. arthrosis, arthrosis, f. 관절에 의한 연결

       > L. diarthrosis, diarthrosis, f. (< G. di(a)- *through, thoroughly, apart*) 가동(可動)관절   **E** *diarthrosis*

     > L. -arthrosis, -arthrosis, f. (< + G. -ōsis *condition*) 관절증   **E** *-arthrosis, hemarthrosis*

     > L. arthrodesis, arthrodesis, f. (< + G. desis *binding*) 관절유합술(癒合術), 관절고정술   **E** *arthrodesis*

> L. Arthropoda, Arthropodorum, n. (pl.) (< + G. pous, podos, m. *foot*) 절지
　　(節肢) 동물문(門)　　**E** Arthropoda, *arthropod*, *(arthropod-borne virus >)* **arbovirus**

　　> L. dysarthria, dysarthriae, f. (< + G. dys- *bad*) 조음(調音)곤란(증)　　**E** *dysarthria*

> G. aristos, aristē, ariston *best* (< *best fitting*), *noblest*　　**E** *aristocracy, Aristoteles*

> G. harmos, harmou, m. *fitting, joint*

　　> G. harmonia, harmonias, f. *harmony*　　**E** *harmony, dysharmony, harmonica*

pars, partis, f. 부분, 부(部)

> **E** (*noun*) **part**, *(part + taker >)* **partaker**, *(partaker >)* **partake**, (*partitianus >)* **partisan**,
> ((*probably*) pars orationis *'part of speech' >*) **parse**, (ad partem *'to the side' >*) **apart**,
> ((*Dutch*) apart *'separate'* + heid *'-hood' > 'separatedness' >*) **apartheid**

[용례] pars distalis (뇌하수체 전엽의) 먼쪽부분　　**E** *pars distalis*
　　　　pars tuberalis (뇌하수체 전엽의) 융기부분　　**E** *pars tuberalis*
　　　　pars intermedia (뇌하수체 전엽의) 중간부분　　**E** *pars intermedia*
　　　　pars nervosa (뇌하수체 후엽의) 신경부분　　**E** *pars nervosa*
　　　　(문법) pars 부분, 부: 단수 주격
　　　　　　distalis 먼쪽의: 형용사, 남·여성형 단수 주격 < distalis, distale
　　　　　　tuberalis 융기한: 형용사, 남·여성형 단수 주격 < tuberalis, tuberale
　　　　　　intermedia 중간의: 형용사, 여성형 단수 주격
　　　　　　　< intermedius, intermedia, intermedium
　　　　　　nervosa 신경의: 형용사, 여성형 단수 주격 < nervosus, nervosa, nervosum

[용례] pars plicata (안구 섬모체의) 주름부분　　**E** *pars plicata*
　　　　pars plana (안구 섬모체의) 납작부분　　**E** *pars plana*
　　　　(문법) pars 부분, 부: 단수 주격
　　　　　　plicata 주름잡힌: 과거분사, 여성형 단수 주격
　　　　　　　　< plicatus, plicata, plicatum
　　　　　　　< plico, plicavi (plicui), plicatum (plicitum), plicare 접다, 접어 겹치다
　　　　　　plana 납작한: 형용사, 여성형 단수 주격
　　　　　　　< planus, plana, planum 편평한, 평평한, 납작한, 평이한, 명확한

[용례] pars tensa (고막의) 긴장부　　**E** *pars tensa*
　　　　pars flaccida (고막의) 이완부　　**E** *pars flaccida*
　　　　(문법) pars 부분, 부: 단수 주격
　　　　　　tensa 긴장된: 과거분사, 여성형 단수 주격
　　　　　　　　< tensus, tensa, tensum 빳빳이 펴진, 팽팽한, 긴장된
　　　　　　　< tendo, tetendi, tentum (tensum), tendĕre 뻗치다, 향하다
　　　　　　flaccida 이완된: 형용사, 여성형 단수 주격
　　　　　　　< flaccidus, flaccida, flaccidum 축 늘어진, 처진, 무기력한

> partialis, partiale 부분적인, 부분에 치우친, 편파적인　　**E** *partial, (partial >)* **impartial**
> particula, particulae, f. (< + -cula *diminutive suffix*) 작은 부분; (물리) 입자(粒子);
　　(문법) 불변화사　　**E** *particle*

> particella, particellae, f. (< + -cella *diminutive suffix*) 작은 부분, 꾸러미　　E *parcel*

> particulatus, particulata, particulatum 작은 부분의, 작은 부분들로 이루어진　E *particulate*

> particularis, particulare 작은 부분에 관한, 개별적인, 특별한　E *particular, particularize*

> partio, partivi (partii), partitum, partire (partior, partitus sum, partiri) 나누다　E *(verb) part*

　> partitus, partita, partitum (*past participle*) 나누인

　　E *partite, bipartite, tripartite,* (partita (f.) *'divided into parts'* >) *party,* (jocus partitus *'divided game, game with even chances, alternative'* >) *jeopardy*

> partitio, partitionis, f. 나눔, 분할, 분리, 분배, 구획, 구분, 칸막이　　E *partition, partner*

> appartio, appartivi (appartii), appartitum, appartire (< ap- (< ad) *to, toward, at, according to* + partire *to part*) 할당하다, 분배하다　　E *apartment*

　> dispertio, dispertivi (dispertii), dispertitum, dispertire (< dis- *apart from, down, not* + partire *to part*) 여러 부분으로 나누다, 분류하다　　E *depart, department, departure*

> impartio, impartivi (impartii), impartitum, impartire (< im- (< in) *in, on, into, toward* + partire *to part*) 나누어 주다, 부여하다, 수여하다　　E *impart*

　> compartior, compartitus sum, compartiri (< com- (< cum) *with, together; intensive* + partiri *to part*) 나누다　　E *compart*

　　> compartmentum, compartmenti, n. 구획, 칸　　E *compartment*

> portio, portionis, f. (< pro portione *in respect of (its or a person's) share* < (*perhaps*) *pro partione) 부분, 몫, 비율　　E *portion*

　> proportio, proportionis, f. (< pro portione *in the degree proper to each, proportionately* < G. analogia *analogy*) 비례, 비, 균형, 조화

　　E *proportion, proportional, proportionate,* (proportion >) *disproportion, disproportional, disproportionate*

> particeps, (gen.) participis (< + -ceps *taking* < capĕre *to take*) 한몫 가지는, 참가하는

　> participo, participavi, participatum, participare 한몫 끼다, 참가하다　　E *participate, participant*

　　> participium, participii, n. 참여; (문법) 분사(分詞)　　E *participle*

　　　> participialis, participiale (문법) 분사의　　E *participial*

< IE. perə- *to grant, to allot; reciprocally to get in turn*

　> L. par, (gen.) paris 짝이 맞는, 같은

　　E *par,* ((*neuter* pl.) paria >) *pair, peer, apparel* (< *'to make equal or fit'*), *disparage* (< *'unequal inferior rank'*), (non *'not'* + par *'paired'* > *'not paired'* >) *umpire*

[용례] pari passu (< *with paired pace*) 같은 걸음으로, 보조를 맞추어　　E *pari passu*
　　(문법) pari 같은: 형용사, 남·여·중성형 단수 탈격
　　　　passu 걸음으로: 단수 탈격 < passus, passus, m. 걸음

> L. paritas, paritatis, f. 같음, 동등함　　E *parity*

　> L. disparitas, disparitatis, f. (< dis- *apart from, down, not* + paritas *parity*) 부등(不等), 부동(不同), 상이(相異)　　E *disparity*

> L. paro, paravi, paratum, parare 짝 지우다, 같게 하다

> L. compar, (gen.) comparis (< com- (< cum) *with, together* + par *paired*)

같은, 동등한

> L. comparo, **comparavi**, comparatum, comparare 대등하게 하다, 짝을

맞추다, 비교하다, 대조하다 **E** *compare*

> L. comparatio, comparationis, f. 비교, 대조 **E** *comparison*

>L. comparativus, comparativa, comparativum 비교의, 비교적;

(문법) 비교급의 **E** *comparative*

> L. impar, (gen.) imparis (< im- (< in-) *not* + par *paired*) 짝이 맞지 않는,

홀의, 틀린 **E** *impar, unpaired*

[용례] ganglion impar 홀신경절 **E** *ganglion impar*

(문법) ganglion 신경절: 단수 주격 < ganglion, ganglii, n.

impar: 형용사, 남·여·중성형 단수 주격

< IE. perə- *to grant, to allot; reciprocally to get in turn* (Vide PARS; *See* E. *part*)

urbs, urbis, f. 도시

> urbanus, urbana, urbanum 도시의 **E** *urban, urbanity*

> suburbium, suburbii, n. (< sub- *under, up from under* + urbs *city*) 성 밖,

교외 **E** *suburb, (suburb >) suburbia*

calx, calcis, f., m. 발꿈치

> calcaneus, calcanea, calcaneum 발꿈치의

> calcaneus, calcanei, m. 발꿈치, 배반자; 발꿈치뼈, 종골(踵骨) **E** *calcaneus, calcaneal*

> calcar, calcaris, n. 박차(拍車), 며느리발톱, 조거(鳥距); 자극 **E** *calcar*

> calcarinus, calcarina, calcarinum 며느리발톱의, 조거(鳥距)의, 며느리발톱

모양의 **E** *calcarine*

> calco, **calcavi**, calcatum, calcare 밟다, 밟아 다져넣다, 밟고 지나

가다 **E** *calque (< 'to copy by tracing'), decalcomania (< 'mania for copying by tracing')*

> inculco, **inculcavi**, inculcatum, inculcare (< in- *in, on, into, toward* + calcare

to tread) 짓밟다, 집어넣다, 심어주다 **E** *inculcate*

> calcitro, calcitravi, calcitratum, calcitrare 뒷발질하다, 날뛰다, 반항하다

> recalcitro, **recalcitravi**, –, recalcitrare (< re- *back, again; intensive* + calcitrare

to kick) 뒷발질하다, 날뛰다, 반항하다 **E** *recalcitrate, recalcitrant*

< IE. (s)kel- *crooked, with derivatives referring to a bent or curved part of the body, such*

as a heel or a leg

> G. skelos, skelous, n. *leg* **E** *triskelion (< 'three-legged'), skelalgia*

> G. isoskelēs, isoskelēs, isoskeles *with equal legs, isosceles* **E** *isosceles*

> G. skolios, skolia, skolion *crooked*

> G. skoliōsis, skoliōseōs, f. (< + -ōsis *condition*) *crookedness*

> L. scoliosis, scoliosis, f. 척추측만증, 척추옆굽음증 **E** *scoliosis, scoliotic*

> G. skōlēx, skōlēkos, m. *earthworm, grub (< that which twists and turns)*

> L. scolex, scolecis, m. (촌충의) 두절(頭節) **E** *scolex*

> G. kōlon, kōlou, n. *limb, member*

> L. colon, coli, n. 운문(韻文)의 단위　　　　　　　　E *colon, semicolon*

> (*suggested*) G. kylindein *to roll*

> G. kylindros, kylindrou, m. *roller*

> L. cylindrus, cylindri, m. (땅을 고르고 굳게 하는, 돌로 만든) 로울러,

원통(圓筒), 원주(圓柱)　　　　　　　　E *cylinder, cylindrical*

calx, calcis, f., m. 석회(石灰), 석회석(*calcium carbonate, CaCO₃*), 생석회(*calcium oxide,*

CaO), 소석회(*calcium hydroxide, Ca(OH)₂*)　　　E *chalk, calc(i)- (calco-), calcospherule*

> calcarea, calcareae, f. 생석회, 소석회　　　　　　　　E *calcarea*

> *calcifer, *calcifera, *calciferum (< calx *lime* + -fer (< ferre *to carry, to bear*)

carrying, bearing) 석회를 함유하는, 석회를 생성하는

E *calciferous, (calciferous >) calciferol(s), (ergot + calciferol >) ergocalciferol, (cholesterol + calciferol >) cholecalciferol*

> *calcifico, *calcificavi, *calcificatum, *calcificare (< calx *lime* + -ficare (< facĕre)

to make) 석회화(石灰化)하다　　　　　　　　E *calcify, calcification*

> calcinosis, calcinosis, f. (< + G. -ōsis *condition*) 석회증　　E *calcinosis*

> calcium, calcii, n. 칼슘

E *calcium (Ca), calcitonin (thyrocalcitonin) (< 'involved in the regulation of the normal tone of calcium in the body fluids'), calmodulin (< 'calcium-binding protein that modulates a variety of cellular responses to calcium')*

> calculus, calculi, m. (< + -ulus *diminutive suffix*) 조약돌, (로마) 고누의 말, 셈 돌,

투표용 조약돌 (흰 돌은 찬성 또는 사면의 표시였고 검은 돌은 반대 또는 단죄의

표시였음); 돌, 결석(結石)　　　　　　　　E *calculus, (pl.) calculi*

> calculosus, calculosa, calculosum 조약돌이 많은, 자갈투성이의;

결석에 걸린　　　　　　　　E *calculous; acalculous*

> calculo, calculavi, calculatum, calculare 셈하다, 계산하다　E *calculate; dyscalculia*

merx, mercis, f. 상품

> mercor, mercatus sum, mercari 매매하다

> mercatus, mercatus, m. 장사, 시장　　　　　　　　E *market, mart*

> *mercato, *mercatavi, *mercatatum, *mercatare (*frequentative*) 장사하다

> *mercatans, *mercatantis, m. (< *present participle*)

장사꾼　　　　　　　　E *merchant, merchandise*

> commercium, commercii, n. (< com- (< cum) *with, together* + merx *merchandise*)

거래, 교역　　　　　　　　E *commerce, commercial*

> merces, mercedis, f. 보수　　　　E *mercy (< 'heavenly reward, favor, pity')*

> mercenarius, mercenaria, mercenarium 보수를 받는, 고용된, 용병의　E *mercenary*

> (*probably*) Mercurius, Mercurii, m. (로마 신화) 상업의 신; 수성(水星); (mercurius)

(연금술) 수은(水銀)

< (*Italic root, possibly from Etruscan*) merk- *root referring to aspects of commerce*

맞대보기	어간 끝에 자음이 둘 이상 있는 증음절의 그리스어 제3변화 남성과 여성 명사는 위의 변화(제3변화 제2식 a)를 따르는 라틴어 명사가 되며 성은 그리스어의 성을 따르는 것을 원칙으로 한다.

---

larynx, laryngis, m. (< *the air passageway between the oropharynx and the trachea*)

후두(喉頭)　　　　　　　　　　　　　　　**E** *larynx, laryngeal, laryng(o)-*

< G. larynx, laryngos, m. *throat, gullet*

pharynx, pharyngis, m. (< *the chasm behind the nasal cavity, oral cavity, and larynx*)

인두(咽頭)　　　　　　　　　　　　　　　**E** *pharynx, pharyngeal, pharyng(o)-*

< G. pharynx, pharyngos, f. *chasm, throat*

< (*perhaps*) IE. bher-, bherə- *to cut, to pierce, to bore* (Vide FORARE: *See* E. *foramen*)

gaster, gastris, f. 배[腹], 위[胃]　**E** *gastr(o)-, gastrin* (< '*a hormone that stimulates gastric secretion*')

> gastrula, gastrulae, f. (< + -ula *diminutive suffix*) 장배(腸胚),

창자배　　　　　　　　　　　　**E** *gastrula, (gastrula >) gastrulation*

< G. gastēr, gastros, f. (< *grastēr) *belly, womb, sausage*

> L. gastricus, gastrica, gastricum 배[腹]의, 위[胃]의　　　　**E** *gastric*

> L. digastricus, digastrica, digastricum (< G. di- *two*) 배[腹]가

둘인, 이복(二腹)의　　　　　　　　　　　**E** *digastric*

> G. epigastrios, epigastrios, epigastrion (< ep(i)- *upon*) *epigastric*

> L. epigastrium, epigastrii, n. 명치, 상복부,

심와부(心窩部)　　　　　　　　　**E** *epigastrium, epigastric*

> G. hypogastrios, hypogastrios, hypogastrion (< hyp(o)- *under*)

hypogastric

> L. hypogastrium, hypogastrii, n. 아랫배,

하복부　　　　　　　　　　　**E** *hypogastrium, hypogastric*

> G. gastronomia, gastronomias, f. (< + nomos *usage*) *the art and science*

of delicate eating　　　　　　　　　　**E** *gastronomy*

< G. gran (graein) *to gnaw, to eat*

< IE. gras- *to devour*　　　　　　　　　　**E** *cress* (< '*fodder*')

> L. gramen, graminis, n. 목초, 꼴　　**E** *gramineous, graminivorous*

> G. gangraina, gangrainēs, f. *gangrene, cancer*

> L. gangraena, gangraenae, f. 괴저(壞疽)　　　　　　　**E** *gangrene*

> L. gangraenosus, gangraenosa, gangraenosum 괴저의　　**E** *gangrenous*

phalanx, phalangis, f. (창과 방패로 무장한) 밀집부대, 방진(方陣), 군집(群集), 손(발)가락뼈,

마디뼈   **E** *phalanx*, (pl.) *phalanges, phalangeal, phalang(o)-*

   < G. phalanx, phalangos, f. *beam, line of battle, finger bone*

< IE. bhelg-, bhelk- *plank, beam*

    E *balcony* (< 'scaffold'), *balk (baulk)* (< 'ridge'), *debauch* (< 'to trim wood to make a beam out of it')

salpinx, salpingis, f. 나팔, 나팔관, 관, 자궁관, 난관   **E** *salpinx*, (pl.) *salpinges, salpingian, salping(o)-*

   > L. mesosalpinx, mesosalpingis, f. (< G. mesos *middle*) 자궁관간막,

난관간막   **E** *mesosalpinx*

   < G. salpinx, salpingos, f. *trumpet*

● ● ●   ## 제 3 변화 제 2 식 b

단수 속격의 음절수가 많아지며 어간 끝에 자음이 둘 이상 있는 중성 명사. 단수의 속격 어미는 -is; 복수의 주격 어미는 -a, 속격 어미는 -ium이 된다. 단수 및 복수에서 주격, 대격, 호격이 똑같다.

cor, cordis, n. 심장, 마음

	단 수	복 수	
주격	cor	cord-a	~이, ~가, ~은, ~는, ~께서
속격	cord-is	cord-ium	~의
여격	cord-i	cord-ibus	~게, ~에게, ~께, ~한테
대격	cor	cord-a	~을, ~를
탈격	cord-e	cord-ibus	~에서, ~로부터, ~으로부터
호격	cor	cord-a	~여, ~이여

cor, cordis, n. 심장, 마음, 의지, 용기, 지혜   **E** *cord(i)-*, (suggested) *core, corrin* (< 'core of vitamin B$_{12}$')

  > cordatus, cordata, cordatum 심장 모양의, 현명한   **E** *cordate*

  > cordialis, cordiale 마음에서 우러나는   **E** *cordial*

  > *coraticum, *coratici, n. 용기, 열정, 욕망, 분노   **E** *courage, encourage*

  > praecordium, praecordii, n. (< prae- *before, beyond*) 전흉부(前胸部), 명치부위   **E** *precordium*

    > praecordialis, praecordiale 전흉부의, 명치부위의   **E** *precordial*

  > concors, (gen.) concordis (< con- (< cum) *with, together*) 한마음의, 합치하는,

일치하는, 화목하는   **E** *concord*

> discors, (gen.) discordis (< dis- *apart from, down, not*) 어긋나는, 상반되는, 불목
하는　　　　　　　　　　　　　　　　　　　　　　　　　　　　　E *discord*

> misericors, (gen.) misericordis (< miser *wretched*) 자비로운　　　E *misericord*

> accordo, **accordavi**, accordatum, accordare (< ac- (< ad) *to, toward, at, according
to*) 일치시키다, 조화시키다, 상응시키다　　　　　　　　　　　　　　E *accord*

> recordor, recordatus sum, recordari (< re- *back, again*) 기억하고 있다　E *record*

< IE. kerd- *heart*　　　　　　　　　　　E *heart, hearty, heartful, heartless, hearten*

　> G. kardia, kardias, f. *heart, mind, soul*

　　　　E *cardi(o)-, electrocardiogram (ECG),* (D. Elektrokardiogramm >) *EKG, cardiomegaly*

　　> G. kardiakos, kardiakē, kardiakon (< + -akos *adjective suffix*) *of heart*

　　　> L. cardiacus, cardiaca, cardiacum 심장의, 심장병의; (*on the heart side
of the body* >) 위(胃)의, 위병(胃病)의, (ostium cardiacum gastris,
pars cardiaca gastris >) 들문(~門)의　　　　　　　E *cardiac; cardia*

　　> G. kardioeidēs, kardioeidēs, kardioeides (< + eidos *shape*) *heart-shaped*　E *cardioid*

　　> G. perikardios, perikardia, perikardion (< peri- *around, near, beyond, on
account of*) *pericardial*

　　　> L. pericardium, pericardii, n. 심장막, 심낭(心囊)　E *pericardium, pericardial*

　　> L. endocardium, endocardii, n. (< G. end(o)- < endon *within*) 심내막, 심장
속막　　　　　　　　　　　　　　　　　E *endocardium, endocardial*

　　> L. myocardium, myocardii, n. (< G. my(o)- < mys, myos, m. *mouse, muscle*)
심근층, 심장근육층　　　　　　　　　　　E *myocardium, myocardial*

　　> L. epicardium, epicardii, n. (< G. ep(i)- *upon*) 심외막,
심장바깥막　　　　　　　　　　　　　　E *epicardium, epicardial*

　　> L. bradycardia, bradycardiae, f. (< G. bradys *slow*) 서맥(徐脈),
느린맥　　　　　　　　　　　　　　　　E *bradycardia, bradycardiac*

　　> L. tachycardia, tachycardiae, f. (< G. tachys *swift*) 빈맥(頻脈).
빠른맥　　　　　　　　　　　　　　　　E *tachycardia, tachycardiac*

　　> L. dextrocardia, dextrocardiae, f. (< L. dexter, dextra, dextrum *right*)
우심증　　　　　　　　　　　　　　　　　　　　E *dextrocardia*

> IE. kred-dhə- (< + IE. dhə- *to do, to place*) *to place trust*

　> L. credo, **credidi**, creditum, credĕre 믿다, 맡기다

　　　E (*first personal singular, present indicative, active 'I believe'* >) *credo,* (credo
>) *creed, grant* (< *'consent to support'*)

　　> L. creditum, crediti, n. 신용, 신뢰, 영예,
남에게 맡겨놓은 (빌려준) 것　　　　　　　　　　E *credit, accredit*

　　> L. credentia, credentiae, f. 신뢰, 신임　　　　　　E *credence*

　　　> L. credentialis, credentiale 신뢰의, 신임의　　　E *credential*

　　> L. credibilis, credibile 믿을 만한, 신용할 만한　　　E *credible*

　　　> L. credibilitas, credibilitatis, f. 신뢰성, 신용　　E *credibility*

　　　> L. incredibilis, incredibile (< in- *not*) 믿을 수 없는,
믿어지지 않는　　　　　　　　　　　　　　E *incredible*

> L. incredibilitas, incredibilitatis, f. 믿을 수 없음   **E** *incredibility*

> L. credulus, credula, credulum 쉽게 믿는   **E** *credulous*

> L. credulitas, credulitatis, f. 쉽게 믿음, 경신(輕信), 맹신(盲信)   **E** *credulity*

> L. incredulus, incredula, incredulum (< in- *not*) 의심 많은,
회의적인   **E** *incredulous*

> L. incredulitas, incredulitatis, f. 의심 많음, 회의   **E** *incredulity*

lac, lactis, n. 젖, 우유

E *lact(o)-, lactic, lactic acid, (lactic acid >) lactate, lactose (< 'milk sugar'), lactulose (< 'perhaps on the pattern of cellulose'), (lactic acid + -one (< ketone) >) lactone, (lactone + amide >) lactam, (lactone + imide >) lactim; lactotropin (prolactin)*

> lacteus, lactea, lacteum 젖의, 젖빛의   **E** *lacteal*

> lactifer, lactifera, lactiferum (< lact- *milk* + -i- + -fer (< ferre *to carry, to bear*)
carrying, bearing) 젖을 나르는, 유관(乳管)의; 젖을 내는   **E** *lactiferous*

> lactuca, lactucae, f. (< *milky juice of the plant*) 상치   **E** *lettuce*

> lacto, lactavi, lactatum, lactare 젖을 먹이다, 젖을 내다, 젖을 빨다   **E** *lactate, lactation*

> lactobacillus, lactobacilli, m. (< *a microorganism that produces lactic acid from
sugars* < lact- *milk* + -o- + bacillus *a rod-shaped bacterium*) 유산균   **E** *lactobacillus*

< IE. g(a)lag-, g(a)lakt- *milk*

> G. gala, galaktos, n. *milk*   **E** *galactic, galactose, galactorrhoea (galactorrhea)*

> G. galaxias, galaxiou, m. *galaxy*

> L. galaxias, galaxiae, m. 은하수, 유석(乳石)   **E** *galaxy*

mel, mellis, n. 꿀

> melleus, mellea, melleum 꿀의, 꿀이 들어 있는, 달콤한, 사랑스러운

> mellitus, mellita, mellitum 꿀의, 꿀이 들어 있는, 달콤한, 사랑스러운

> mellifer, mellifera, melliferum (< mel *honey* + -fer (< ferre *to carry, to bear*) *carrying,
bearing*) 꿀이 나는, 꿀을 내는   **E** *melliferous*

< IE. melit- *honey*   **E** *mildew*

> L. mulsus, mulsa, mulsum 꿀을 섞은   **E** *mousse*

> G. meli, melitos, n. *honey*

E *hydromel (< 'fermented honey and water'), (melimēlon 'honey and apple' >) marmalade*

> G. (*Attic*) melitta, melittēs, f., (*non-Attic*) melissa, melissēs, f. *honey,
bee*   **E** *melittin (< 'present in bee venom')*

os, ossis, n. 뼈

   E *os*

[용례] os hyoideum 목뿔뼈, 설골(舌骨)

os frontale 이마뼈, 전두골(前頭骨)

os coxae (< *hip bone*) 볼기뼈, 관골(臗骨)   **E** *os coxae*

(문법) os 뼈: 단수 주격

hyoideum ∪ 모양의: 형용사, 중성형 단수 주격

< hyoideus, hyoidea, hyoideum

frontale 이마의, 앞의: 형용사, 중성형 단수 주격 < frontalis, frontale

coxae 볼기의: 단수 속격 < coxa, coxae, f.

> ossiculum, ossiculi, n. (< + -culum *diminutive suffix*) 작은 뼈, 소골(小骨)　　**E** *ossicle*

> osseus, ossea, osseum

뼈의　　**E** *osseous, interosseous, intraosseous, ossein (< 'the collagen of bone')*

> ossuarium, ossuarii, n. 유골함, 납골당　　**E** *ossuary*

> *ossifico, *ossificavi, *ossificatum, *ossificare (< + -ficare (< facĕre) *to make*)

뼈가 되다, 골화하다　　**E** *ossify*

> ossificatio, ossificationis, f. 뼈되기, 골화(骨化) **E** *ossification, (ossification >) ossificated*

< IE. ost- *bone*

> G. osteon, osteou, n. *bone*

E *osteon (< 'the structural unit of bone'), oste(o)-, osteology, osteoblast, osteoblastic, osteocyte, osteoclast, osteoclastic, osteoid (< 'originally, bone-like; later, the initial unmineralized collagen matrix of bone'), osteoplastic, osteolytic, teleost*

> L. osteogenesis, osteogenesis, f. (< G. osteon + genesis *birth*) 뼈발생, 골발생　　**E** *osteogenesis*

> G. periosteon, periosteou, n. (< G. peri- *around, near, beyond, on account of* + osteon) *periosteum*

> L. periosteum, periostei, n. 뼈막, 골막, 뼈바깥막　　**E** *periosteum, periosteal*

> L. endosteum, endostei, n. (< end(o)- < endon *within* + osteon) 뼈속막, 골내막　　**E** *endosteum, endosteal*

> G. -ostōsis, -ostōseōs, f. (< + -ōsis *condition*) -ostosis　　**E** *-ostosis*

> G. exostōsis, exostōseōs, f. (< ex- *out of, away from*) *exostosis*

> L. exostosis, exostosis, f. 뼈연골종증　　**E** *exostosis*

> L. synostosis, synostosis, f. (< G. syn- *with, together*) 뼈융합, 골유합　　**E** *synostosis*

> L. dysostosis, dysostosis, f. (< G. dys- *bad*) 뼈발생이상　　**E** *dysostosis*

> G. ostreon, ostreou, n. *oyster*　　**E** *oyster*

> G. ostrakon, ostrakou, n. *fragment of pottery, potsherd, shell*　　**E** *ostracon, ostracize*

> G. astragalos, astragalou, m. *huckle-bone,* (pl.) *dice (< originally huckle bones); a moulding in the capital of a column; a leguminous plant*

> L. astragalus, astragali, m. (옛이름) 복사뼈, (옛이름) 목말뼈 (거골 距骨); 복사뼈처럼 생긴 기둥 장식, 쇠시리; 자운영(紫雲英) 속(屬)의 콩과 식물, 자운영　　**E** *astragal, astragalus*

∽ (*probably*) IE. kost- *bone*

> L. costa, costae, f. 갈비, 늑골(肋骨), 엽맥(葉脈), 옆구리　　**E** *(F. costelette 'little rib' > F. cotelette >) cutlet, coast, accost (< 'to the side')*

> L. costalis, costale 갈비의, 갈비뼈의, 늑골의　　**E** *costal*

> L. intercostalis, intercostale (< inter- *between, among*) 갈비 사이의,
늑골간의, 늑간의

> L. costatus, costata, costatum 늑골이 있는; (식물) 잎이 주맥이 있는

●●● 제3변화 제2식 c

단수 주격과 단수 속격의 음절수가 같은 남성, 여성 명사. 단수의 속격 어미는 -is; 복수의
주격 어미는 -es, 속격 어미는 -ium이 된다. 단수 주격의 어간과 단수 속격의 어간이 같다.

auris, auris, f. 귀

	단 수	복 수	
주격	aur-is	aur-es	~이, ~가, ~은, ~는, ~께서
속격	aur-is	aur-ium	~의
여격	aur-i	aur-ibus	~게, ~에게, ~께, ~한테
대격	aur-em	aur-es	~을, ~를
탈격	aur-e	aur-ibus	~에서, ~로부터, ~으로부터
호격	aur-is	aur-es	~여, ~이여

auris, auris, f. 귀

> auricula, auriculae, f. (< + -cula *diminutive suffix*) 귓바퀴, 심이(心耳)

> auricularis, auriculare 귓바퀴의, 심이(心耳)의

< IE. ous- *ear*

> L. ausculto, **auscultavi**, auscultatum, auscultare (< *aus- *ear* + *klito- *inclined*)
귀를 기울이다, 청진하다

> L. auscultatio, auscultationis, f. 경청, 청진

> G. ous, ōtos, n. *ear*

> G. ōtikos, ōtikē, ōtikon *of ear*

> L. oticus, otica, oticum 귀의

> G. myosōtis, myosōtidos, f. (< mys, myos, m. *mouse*) *a plant with leaves
like a mouse's ears*

> L. myosotis, myosotidis, f. 물망초, 물망초속(屬)의 식물

> G. parōtis, parōtidos, f. (< par(a)- *beside, along side of, beyond*) *parotid*

> L. parotis, parotidis, f. 귀밑샘, 이하선(耳下腺)

axis, axis, m. 굴대, 축(軸); 제2경추(頸椎), 중쇠뼈

> axilla, axillae, f. (< *axis point of the upper arm* < + -illa *diminutive suffix*) 겨드랑이, (준말) 겨드랑, 액와(腋窩)　　　　　　　　　　**E** *axilla; axil*

　　> axillaris, axillare 겨드랑이의, 겨드랑의　　　　　　　　**E** *axillary*

> neuraxis, neuraxis, f. (< *axis of the nervous system; the brain and spinal cord*) 중추신경계통　　　　　　　　　　　　　　　　　　**E** *neuraxis*

< IE. aks- *axis*　　　　　　　　　　　　　　　　　　　　　**E** *axle*

　　> L. ala, alae, f. (< *axla, *axlae, f.) 날개, 사람의 어깨, 겨드랑이, 기병대　**E** *ala, aisle*

　　　> L. alaris, alare 날개의, 날개깃의, 겨드랑이의　　　　　**E** *alar*

　　　> L. alarius, alaria, alarium 날개의, 날개깃의　　　　　**E** *alary*

　> G. axōn, axōnos, m. *axle*

　　> L. axon, axonis, m. 축삭(軸索)

> **E** *axon, axonal, axoplasm, mesaxon* (< 'the covering of an axon formed by invagination of the plasma membrane of a Schwann cell or oligodendrocyte, so named on account of the analogy with the mesentery in electron micrographs'), *axoneme*

civis, civis, m., f. (< *member of a household*) 시민

　> civicus, civica, civicum (공민으로서) 시민의　　　　　　　**E** *civic*

　> civilis, civile (민간인으로서) 시민의, 예의 바른　　　**E** *civil, (civil >) uncivil*

　　> civilitas, civilitatis, f. 예의　　　　　　　　　　　　**E** *civility*

　　> incivilis, incivile (< in- *not*) 비시민적인, 무례한　　　**E** *†incivil*

　　　> incivilitas, incivilitatis 무례　　　　　　　　　　**E** *incivility*

　　> civilizo, civilizavi, civilizatum, civilizare 문명화하다　**E** *civilize, (civilize >) uncivilize*

　> civitas, civitatis, f. 도시　　　　　**E** *city, citizen, citadel* (< 'little city')

< IE. kei- *to lie; bed, couch; beloved, dear*

　> L. cunae, cunarum, f. (pl.) 요람

　　> L. incunabula, incunabulorum, n. (pl.) (< in- *in, on, into, toward*) 배내옷, 기저귀, 요람기, 여명기, 발상(發祥)　　　**E** (sing.) *incunabulum*, (pl.) *incunabula*

　> (*possibly*) G. koiman (koimaein) *to put to sleep*

　　> G. kōma, kōmatos, n. *deep sleep, lethargy*

　　　> L. coma, comatis, n. 혼수(昏睡)　　　　　　　　**E** *coma, comatose*

　　> G. koimētērion, koimētēriou, n. *dormitory, (Christian writers) burial ground*

　　　> L. coemeterium, coemeterii, n. 묘지　　　　　　**E** *cemetery*

　> (*Sanskrit*) siva- *auspicious, dear*　　　　　　　　　　**E** *Shiva*

follis, follis, m. 가죽주머니, 가죽 공, 풀무　　　　　　**E** *folly, fool*, F. *folie*

　> folliculus, folliculi, m. (< + -culus *diminutive suffix*) (작은) 주머니, 소포(小胞), 난포(卵胞), 여포(濾胞), 낭(囊)　　　　　　**E** *follicle (follicule)*

　　> follicularis, folliculare (작은) 주머니의, 소포(小胞)의, 난포(卵胞)의　　　　　　　　　　　　　　**E** *follicular; parafollicular*

< IE. bhel- *to blow, to swell; with derivatives referring to various round objects and to the notion of tumescent masculinity*

> G. phallos, phallou, m. *penis, phallus*

> L. phallus, phalli, m. (Bacchus 축제 때에 메고 돌아다니던 나무·유리·가죽 등으로 만든 생식력 상징의) 남근상　**E** *phallus, phallic, phallicism (phallism), phalloplasty*

> L. phalloides, (gen.) phalloidis (< + G. eidos *shape*) 음경 모양의　**E** (Amanita phalloides >) *phalloidin (phalloidine), phallacidin*

> G. ithyphallos, ithyphallou, m. (< ithys *straight*) *the phallus carried in procession at the festivals of Bacchus*　**E** *ithyphallic*

> IE. bhel- *to thrive, to bloom*

> IE. bhle- *to thrive, to bloom* (Vide FLOS; See E. *floral*)

> IE. bhol-yo- *leaf* (Vide FOLIUM; See E. *folio*)

> IE. bhelgh- *to swell*　**E** *bellows, belly, billow* (< 'a wave')

> L. bulga, bulgae, f. 가죽부대　**E** *bulge, budget*

> IE. bhlei- *to blow, to swell*　**E** *blister, blain,* (chill + blain >) *chilblain*

> IE. bhleu- *to swell, to well up, to overflow* (Vide FLUÉRE; See E. *fluent*)

funis, funis, m. 띠, 줄, 탯줄, 제대(臍帶)　**E** *funis, funic, funiform, funambulism*

> funiculus, funiculi, m. (< + -culus *diminutive suffix*) 작은 띠, 삭(索), 속(束), 대(帶), 섬유단　**E** *funiculus, funicle, funicular*

orbis, orbis, m. 원(圓), 바퀴, 구(球)　**E** *orb*

> orbiculus, orbiculi, m. (< + -culus *diminutive suffix*) 작은 원(圓), 작은 바퀴

> orbicularis, orbiculare 둥근, 원형의, 둘레의　**E** *orbicular*

> orbita, orbitae, f. 수레바퀴 자국, 전철(前轍), (원형의) 궤도; 눈확, 안와(眼窩) (< *the bony cavity that contains the eyeball*)　**E** *orbit, orbital*

> exorbito, exorbitavi, exorbitatum, exorbitare (< ex- *out of, away from*) 궤도를 벗어나다, 이탈하다　**E** *exorbitant*

< (*perhaps*) IE. ergh- *to mount*

> G. orchis, orcheōs, m. (orchis, orchios, m.) *testis*

E *orchi(o)-, orchiopexy (orchiorrhaphy), orchid(o)-* (< 'mistaken stem'), *orchic (orchidic)*

> L. cryptorchismus, cryptorchismi, m. (cryptorchidismus, cryptorchidismi, m.) (< G. kryptos *hidden* + orchis *testis* + -ismos *noun suffix*) 잠복고환증　**E** *cryptorchism (cryptorchidism)*

> L. Clonorchis, Clonorchis, f. (< G. klōn, klōnos, m. *twig, shoot, sprout*) (흡충) 간흡충속(屬); 간디스토마　**E** *Clonorchis, clonorchiasis*

> L. Opisthorchis, Opisthorchis, f. (< G. opisth(o)- (< opisthen) *behind*) (흡충) 오피스토르키스속(屬), 후고(後睾)흡충, 간흡충　**E** *Opisthorchis, opisthorchiasis*

> L. orchis, orchis, f. (orchis, orchitis, f.) (< *the shape of the, frequently paired, tubers in many species*) 난초　**E** *orchis, orchid*

panis, panis, m. 빵

  > (*Portuguese*) pão 빵

    > (*Japanese*) パン

      > (*Korean*) 빵

  > panataria, panatariae, f. 주방　**E** *pantry*

  > compania, companiae, f. (< *a group sharing bread* < com- (< cum) *with, together* + panis *bread*) 일단(一團)　**E** *company (co., Co.)*

  > companio, companionis, m. (< *bread fellow, messmate* < com- (< cum) *with, together* + panis *bread*) 동료, 반려, 동반　**E** *companion,* (ac- (< ad) *to, toward, at, according to* + companio >) *accompany*

< IE. pa- *to protect, to feed*　**E** *fur, food, fodder, forage, foray* (< '*to forage*'), *feed, feedback, foster*

  > L. pabulum, pabuli, n. 사료, 양식　**E** *pabulum*

  > L. pasco, pavi, pastum, pascĕre 사료를 주다, 가축을 치다

    > L. pastura, pasturae, f. 꼴, 목초, 사료　**E** *pasture*

    > L. pastor, pastoris, m. 목자, 목동　**E** *pastor, pester* (< '*hobble of herdsman*')

      > L. pastoralis, pastorale 목자의, 전원의　**E** *pastoral, pastorale*

  > (*Persian*) pad *protecting against*

    > (*Persian*) padzahr (< pad + zahr *poison* (< IE. gwhen- *to strike, to kill*)) *counter-poison*

      E *bezoar* (< '*a small stony concretion found in the stomachs of ruminants, once used as an antidote for various ailments*'), *phytobezoar, trichobezoar*

penis, penis, m. 음경(陰莖), 꼬리　**E** *penis*

  > penilis, penile 음경의　**E** *penile*

  > peniculus, peniculi, m. (< + -culus *diminutive suffix*) 작은 꼬리, 꼬리 끝의 털 뭉치, 붓

    > penicillus, penicilli, m. (< + -illus *diminutive suffix*) 작은 붓　**E** *pencil, penicillar*

      > penicillium, penicillii, n. 작은 붓; 페니실륨, 푸른곰팡이

      E *penicilliary; penicillium, penicillin, penicillamine* (< '*an amine product of penicillin degradation*')

      [용례] Penicillium chrysogenum 푸른곰팡이　**E** *Penicillium chrysogenum*

        (문법) penicillium 페니실륨: 단수 주격

          chrysogenum 황금빛 색소를 만드는: 형용사, 중성형 단수 주격

            < chrysogenus, chrysogena, chrysogenum

              < G. chrysos, chrysou, m. *gold*

< IE. pes- *penis*

  > G. peos, peos, n. *penis*

unguis, unguis, m. 손톱, 발톱, 조(爪)　　　　　　　　　E *unguis*, (pl.) *ungues*, *ungual*, *subungual*

> ungula, ungulae, f. (< + -ula *diminutive suffix*) (동물의) 발톱, 발굽, 갈퀴　　E *ungulate*

< IE. nogh- *nail, claw*　　　　　　　　　　　　　　　　E *nail*

> G. onyx, onychos, m. *nail, claw, talon, hoof*　　　E *onych(o)-, onychomycosis, onycholysis*

> L. onyx, onychis, m. (< *from the resemblance in color between the stone and a finger-nail*) 마노(瑪瑙)　　　　　　E *onyx*

> L. eponychium, eponichii, n. (< G. ep(i)- *upon*) 손발톱위허물　　E *eponychium*

> L. hyponychium, hyponichii, n. (< G. hyp(o)- *under*) 손발톱아래허물　E *hyponychium*

> L. onychia, onychiae, f. (< + -ia) (< *on the pattern of* paronychia) 손발톱염, 조염(爪炎), 조상염(爪床炎), 손발톱증　　　　　　E *onychia*

> L. paronychia, paronychiae, f. (< G. par(a)- *beside, along side of, beyond*) 손발톱주위염, 조갑(爪甲)주위염　　　　　　E *paronychia (perionychia)*

> L. koilonychia, koilonychiae, f. (< *hollow nail* < G. koilos *hollow*) 숟가락 손발톱　　　　　　　　　　　E *koilonychia*

natis, natis, f. (주로 pl.) 궁둥이, 볼기, 꽁무니　　　　　　E *natal*

< IE. not- *buttock, back*

> G. nōton, nōtou, n. (nōtos, nōtou, m.) *back*　　　E *notochord, notomelia*

pestis, pestis, f. 전염병, 흑사병, 멸망, 불행　　　　　　E *pest, pesticide*

> pestilens, (gen.) pestilentis 전염병이 도는, 전염병의, 유해한　　E *pestilent*

> pestilentia, pestilentiae, f. 전염병, 흑사병, 해악　　E *pestilence*

syphilis, syphilis, f. (< *originally the title of a poem by Girolamo Fracastoro, but used also as the name of the disease; the subject is the story of a shepherd Syphilus, the sufferer from the disease*) 매독(梅毒)　　　　E *syphilis, syphilitic, syphilid*

triremis, triremis, f. (< *an ancient galley (originally Greek, afterwards also Roman) with three ranks of oars one above another, used chiefly as a ship of war* < tri- *three* + remus *oar*) 삼단 노가 달린 배　　　　　　　　E *trireme*

< remus, remi, m. (배 젓는) 노

< IE. erə- *to row*　　　　　　　　　　　　　　　E *row, rudder*

> G. triērēs, triērous, f. *trireme*

turris, turris, f. 탑, 요새　　　　　　　　　　　　E *tower, turret*

vestis, vestis, f. 옷　　　　　　　　　　　　　　E (noun) *vest*

> vestio, vestivi, vestitum, vestire 옷 입히다, 옷 입다, 덮다　　　E (verb) *vest* (< '*to dress*'), *divest* (< '*to undress*'), *transvestism*

240 • 의학어원론

> investio, **investivi**, investitum, investire (< in- *in, on, into, toward* + vestire *to dress, to clothe*) 입히다, 덮다, 장식하다, 둘러막다   **E** *invest, investment*

     < IE. wes- *to clothe*   **E** *wear*

         > G. hennynai *to clothe*

             > G. hima, himatos, n. (heima, heimatos, n.) *garment, cover*

                 > G. himation, himatiou, n. (< + -ion *diminutive suffix*) *small garment*   **E** *himation*

< IE. eu- *to put on*

     > L. omentum, omenti, n. (< o- (< eu-) + -mentum *noun suffix*) 그물막, 망(網)   **E** *omentum, omental*

     > L. exuo, **exui**, exutum, exuĕre (< ex- *out of, away from*) 벗다, 벗기다

         > L. exuviae, exuviarum, f. (pl.) (몸에 지닌 물건, 특히) 옷, 장신구; (동물의) 가죽, 껍질, 허물   **E** *exuviae*

     > (*suggested*) L. induo, **indui**, indutum, induĕre 입히다, 입다, 가지다, 취하다   **E** *endue (indue)*

         > L. indusium, indusii, n. 부인용 내복; 포막(包膜), 포피막(包皮膜)   **E** *indusium*

             [용례] indusium griseum 회색층   **E** *indusium griseum*

               (문법) indusium: 단수 주격

                   griseum 회색의: 형용사, 중성형 단수 주격

                     < griseus, grisea, griseum

---

fames, famis, f. 굶주림, 기아, 기근   **E** *famine, famish*

     ∞ fatigo, **fatigavi**, fatigatum, fatigare 지치게 하다, 피로하게 하다   **E** *fatigue*

         > fatigabilis, fatigabile 피로해지는, 지치는   **E** *fatigable, fatigability*

         > defatigo, **defatigavi**, defatigatum, defatigare (< de- *apart from, down, not; intensive* + fatigare *to fatigue*) 지치게 하다, 피로하게 하다

             > defatigabilis, defatigabile 피로해지는, 지치는

                 > indefatigabilis, indefatigabile (< in- *not*) 피로를 모르는, 지치지 않는   **E** *indefatigable*

     < IE. dhe- *to wither away*

---

nubes, nubis, f. 구름   **E** *nuance* (< *'shade of color'*)

     > nubilus, nubila, nubilum (nubilosus, nubilosa, nubilosum) 구름 낀, 오리무중의   **E** *nubilous*

     < IE. sneudh- *mist, cloud*

---

tabes, tabis, f. 와해, 소멸, 부패, 노(癆), 위축, 소모증, 타베스   **E** *tabes, tabetic*

     [용례] tabes dorsalis (< *slowly progressive degeneration of the posterior parts of the spinal cord in neurosyphilis*) 척수매독   **E** *tabes dorsalis*

         (문법) tabes 소모증: 단수 주격

             dorsalis (척수) 뒷부분의: 형용사, 남·여성형 단수 주격

< dorsalis, dorsale

    < IE. ta- *to melt, to dissolve*   **E** *thaw*

          > G. tēkein *to melt*   **E** *eutectic*

예외   단수 주격과 단수 속격의 음절수가 같은 명사 중 다음의 남성과 여성 명사는 복수 속격
어미를 –um으로 한다.

---

pater, patris, m. 아버지, 조상, 창시자   **E** *patrilineal*

    > paternus, paterna, paternum 아버지의

        > paternalis, paternale 아버지의   **E** *paternal*

        > paternitas, paternitatis, f. 부성(父性), 부계(父系)   **E** *paternity*

    > patronus, patroni, m. 평민 보호를 담당하던 귀족, 석방한 노예의 보호자로서의 옛 주인,

        보호자, 수호자, 후원자   **E** *patron, pattern* (< *'a patron giving an example to be copied'*)

    > patria, patriae, f. 조국

        > expatrio, **expatriavi**, expatriatum, expatriare 국외로 추방하다, 조국을 떠나다,

            국적을 이탈하다   **E** *expatriate*

    > patrimonium, patrimonii, n. 부모로부터 물려받은 것, 세습 재산   **E** *patrimony*

    > patro, **patravi**, patratum, patrare 이룩하다, 저지르다

        > perpetro, **perpetravi**, perpetratum, perpetrare (< per- *through, thoroughly* +

        patrare *to bring about*) 완성하다, 저지르다   **E** *perpetrate*

< IE. pə ter- *father*   **E** *father, forefather*

    > G. patēr, patros, m. *father, ancestor, founder*

        > G. patrios, patria, patrion *of one's father, native*

            > G. patriōtēs, patriōtou, m. *fellow-countryman*

                > L. patriota, patriotae, m. 동향인, 동포, 애국자   **E** *patriot, patriotism*

           > G. patria, patrias, f. *descent, lineage, tribe, family*

                > G. patriarchēs, patriarchou, m. (< + -archēs *ruling, ruler*)

                  patriarch   **E** *patriarch*

                  > G. patriarchia, patriarchias, f. *patriarchy*   **E** *patriarchy*

∽ IE. papa *a child's word for father, a linguistic near-universal found in many languages*

    > G. pappas, pappou, m. *papa; spiritual father*

        > L. papa, papae, m. 아버지; 교황   **E** *papal, papacy, pope*

    > G. pappos, pappou, m. *grandfather, first down on the chin, white down on certain*

        seeds

        > L. pappus, pappi, m. 할아버지, 노인; (민들레·엉겅퀴 등 씨의)

        관모(冠毛)   **E** *pappus,* (pl.) *pappi*

    > F. papa *father*   **E** *papa*

mater, matris, f. 어머니; (어머니의 역할을 하는) 모교(母校), 뇌막(腦膜),

척수막(脊髓膜)   **E** *matrilineal, matriarchy (< 'on the pattern of patriarchy')*

> maternus, materna, maternum 어머니의

     > maternalis, maternale 어머니의   **E** *maternal*

     > maternitas, maternitatis, f. 모성(母性), 모계(母系)   **E** *maternity*

> matrona, matronae, f. 기혼부인, 귀부인   **E** *matron*

> matrix, matricis, f. (번식을 위한 암컷, 자궁 >) 바탕질, 모질(母質); 명부;

(수학) 행렬   **E** *matrix, (pl.) matrices, matrical (matricial)*

     > matricula, matriculae, f. (< -ula diminutive suffix) 명부, 등록부,

       등록   **E** *matriculate*

> materia, materiae, f. (바탕 > 나무의 몸통 > 목재 > 재료 >) 물질(物質)   **E** *matter*

     > materialis, materiale 물질의   **E** *material, (hazardous material >) hazmat*

> matrimonium, matrimonii, n. 결혼, 결혼 생활   **E** *matrimony*

< IE. mater- *mother (based ultimately on the baby-talk form* ma-, *with the kinship*

term suffix -ter-)   **E** *mother*

> G. mētēr, mētros, f. *mother*   **E** *metropolis, metropolitan*

     > G. mētra, mētras, f. *womb*   **E** *metr(o)-, -metrium*

         > L. endometrium, endometrii, n. (< G. end(o)- < endon *within*)

            자궁내막, 자궁속막   **E** *endometrium, endometrial*

         > L. myometrium, myometrii, n. (< G. my(o)- < mys, myos, m.

            mouse, muscle) 자궁근층, 자궁근육층   **E** *myometrium, myometrial*

         > L. perimetrium, perimetrii, n. (< G. peri- *around, near, beyond,*

            on account of) 자궁외막, 자궁바깥막   **E** *perimetrium, perimetrial*

         > L. parametrium, parametrii, n. (< *the extension of the subserous*

            coat of the supracervical portion of the uterus laterally

            between the layers of the broad ligament < G. par(a)- *beside,*

            along side of, beyond) 자궁곁(조직)   **E** *parametrium, parametrial*

         > L. mesometrium, mesometrii, n. (< G. mesos *middle*)

            자궁간막   **E** *mesometrium*

         > L. metrorrhagia, metrorrhagiae, f. (< + G. -rrhagia < -rrhag-

            stem of rhēgnynai *to break, to burst*) 자궁출혈   **E** *metrorrhagia*

     > G. Dēmētēr, Dēmētros, f. (< de- *possibly meaning 'earth'* + mētēr) (*Greek*

       mythology) *Goddess of produce, especially cereal crops*   **E** *Demeter*

< IE. ma- *mother; a linguistic near-universal found in many of the world's languages, often*

in reduplicated form   **E** *mamma (mama)*

> L. mamma, mammae, f. 엄마, 젖, 유방(乳房)

     E *mamma, (pl.) mammae; mammotrope, mammoplasty (mammaplasty), mammogram,*
     Mammotome®

     > L. mammarius, mammaria, mammarium 유방의   **E** *mammary*

     > L. mammalis, mammale 유방의

         > L. Mammalia, Mammalium, n. (*neuter* pl.) (동물)

            포유강(哺乳綱)   **E** *Mammalia, (Mammalia >) mammal, mammalian*

     > L. mammilla, mammillae, f. (mamilla, mamillae, f.) (< + -illa *diminutive*

suffix) 유두(乳頭), 젖꼭지　　　　　　　**E** *mammilla (mamilla),* (pl.) *mammillae (mamillae)*

　　　> L. mammillaris, mammillare (mamillaris, mammillare) 유두의,

　　　　　젖꼭지의　　　　　　　　　　　　　　　　　**E** *mammillary (mamillary)*

　> G. maia, maias, f. *good mother, foster mother, midwife;* (Maia) (*Greek mythology*)

　　　the daughter of Atlas and mother of Hermes　　　　　**E** *Maia*

　　　> G. maieuesthai *to act as a midwife*

　　　　　> G. maieutikos, maieutikē, maieutikon *obstetric; of Socratic process*　**E** *maieutic*

frater, fratris, m. 형제

E *friar*

　　　> fraternus, fraterna, fraternum 형제의, 우애 있는　　　**E** *fraternal*

　　　　　> fraternitas, fraternitatis, f. 형제관계, 우애, 동포애　　　**E** *fraternity*

< IE. bhrater- *brother, male agnate*　　　　　　**E** *brother, bully* (< 'brother')

　　　> G. phratēr, phrateros, m. *member of a phratry*

　　　　　> G. phratria, phratrias, f. *tribe, clan; phratry (at Athens, a subdivision of*

　　　　　　phylē)　　　　　　　　　　　　　　**E** *phratry*

　　　> (*Sanskrit*) bhrata *brother*　　　　　　　　**E** *pal*

senex, senis, m., f. 노인, 어르신

< senex, m., senex, f., (gen.) senis 늙은, 나이 많은

　　> (*comparative*) senior, m., senior, f., (gen.) senioris

　　　　> senior, senioris, m., f. 연장자

　　　　　E *senior,* (senior >) *sire,* (sire >) *sir,* (sirly >) *surly;* (meus senior 'my senior' >)
　　　　　F. *monsieur,* (pl.) *messieurs*

　　> senilis, senile 노인의, 노쇠한　　　　　　　**E** *senile, senility*

　　> senesco, **senui**, –, senescĕre (< + -escĕre *suffix of inceptive (inchoative)*

　　　verb) 늙다　　　　　　　　　　　**E** *senescent, senescence*

　　> senecio, senecionis, m. 늙은이; (식물) (*white pappus* >) 솜방망이

　　> senatus, senatus, m. 원로원　　　　　　　**E** *senate*

< IE. sen- *old*

juvenis, juvenis, m., f. 젊은이

　　< juvenis, m., juvenis, f., (gen.) juvenis 젊은　　　　**E** *rejuvenate*

　　　　> (*comparative*) junior, m., junior, f., (gen.) junioris

　　　　　　> junior, junioris, m., f. 젊은이, 후배　　　　**E** *junior*

　　　　> juvenilis, juvenile 젊은　　　　　　　**E** *juvenile, juvenility*

　　　　> juvenesco, **juvenui**, –, juvenescĕre 늙다　　　**E** *juvenescent, juvenescence*

　　< IE. yeu- *vital force, youthful vigor*　　　　　**E** *young, youth*

　　　> Juno, Junonis, f. (로마 신화) 유노(주노) 여신　　　**E** *Juno*

　　　　> Junonius, Junonia, Junonium (Junius, Junia, Junium) 유노(주노)

　　　　　여신의　　　　　　　　　　**E** (Junius mensis 'month of Juno' >) *June*

< IE. aiw-, ayu- *vital force, life, long life, eternity; also endowed with the acme of vital force, young* **E** *ever, every* (<'*ever each*'); *no* (<'*not ever*'), *never* (<'*not ever*')

> L. aevum, aevi, n. 생애, 연령, 시대 **E** (medium aevum '*middle age*' >) *mediaeval (medieval)*

> L. aevitas, aevitatis, f. 나이

> L. aetas, aetatis, f. 나이 **E** *age*

> L. aeviternus, aeviterna, aeviternum 영원한

> L. aeternus, aeterna, aeternum 영원한

> L. aeternalis, aeternale 영원한 **E** *eternal*

> L. sempiternus, sempiterna, sempiternum (< semper *always*
+ aeternus *eternal*) 영원한

> L. sempiternalis, sempiternale 영원한 **E** *sempiternal*

> L. longaevus, longaeva, longaevum (< longus *long* + aevum *age*) 오래 사는

> L. longaevitas, longaevitatis, f. 장수 **E** *longevity*

> L. primaevus, primaeva, primaevum (< primus *first* + aevum *age*)
원시의 **E** *primaeval (primeval)*

> G. aiōn, aiōnos, m., f. *age, lifetime, period, eternity*

> L. aeon, aeonis, m., f. 영겁; (지질) 누대(累代, 연대 구분의 최대 단위,
100억 년) **E** *aeon (eon)*

> G. ouk, ou (< *not 'on your life*') (*adverb*) *not* **E** *Utopia*

> G. hygiēs, hygiēs, hygies (< + IE. gʷeiǝ-, gʷei- *to live*) *healthy*

> G. hygieia, hygieias, f. (hygeia, hygeias, f.) *health, soundness of body;*
(Hygieia) (*Greek mythology*) *goddess of health, daughter of*
Asclepius **E** *hygiology (hygieology)*

> L. Hygeia, Hygeiae, f. (Hygieia, Hygieiae, f.) (그리스 신화) 히게이아
(건강의 여신, 아스클레피우스의 딸) **E** *Hygeia (Hygieia)*

> G. hygieinos, hygieinē, hygieinon *healthful*

> L. hygieina, hygieinae, f. (< G. hygieinē technē *healthful art*) 건강법,
위생법 **E** *hygiene, hygienic, hygienics, hygienist*

> (*Sanskrit*) ayuh *life, health*

> (*Sanskrit*) Ayurveda (< + veda *knowledge, sacred knowledge, sacred book*)
the traditional Hindu system of medicine **E** *Ayurveda*

맞대보기 명사 접미사 -sis(행위·과정·상태), -osis(정상·비정상 상태), -(i)asis(질병 상태)로
끝나는 그리스어 기원의 학술용어는 위의 변화(제3변화 제2식 c)를 따르는 라틴어
여성 명사가 된다.

---

gnosis, gnosis, f. 앎, 신비적 직관 **E** *gnosis, -gnosis*

> diagnosis, diagnosis, f. (< G. di(a)- *through, thoroughly, apart*) 진단

E *diagnosis,* (pl.) *diagnoses, diagnostic, diagnostician,* (*diagnosis* >) *diagnose*

> prognosis, prognosis, f. (< G. pro- *before, in front*) 예후(豫後), 예측

    E *prognosis, (pl.) **prognoses, prognostic, prognosticate**, (prognosis >) **prognose***

< G. gnōsis, gnōseōs, f. (< + -sis *feminine noun suffix*) *knowledge, wisdom,*
judicial sentence, inquiry   **E** *-gnosia*

    > L. agnosia, agnosiae, f. (< G. a- *not*) 인식불능증   **E** *agnosia*

        > L. prosopagnosia, prosopagnosiae, f. (< G. prosōpon *face*)
        얼굴인식불능증   **E** *prosopagnosia*

< G. gignōskein (ginōskein) (gnō- *root of* gignōskein) *to know, to think, to judge*

    > G. gnōmōn, gnōmonos, m. *indicator, carpenter's square, rule, judge*

        > L. gnomon, gnomonis, m. 자[尺], (해시계의) 바늘   **E** *gnomon*

        > L. norma, normae, f. (*possibly from an Etruscan borrowing of* G. gnōmōn)
        (목수의) 직각자 > 기준, 규범, 정규   **E** *norm*

            > L. normalis, normale 직각자의, 직각의, 기준에 맞는, 규범적인,
            정규의, 정상의

                E *normal, (normal >) **normality**, (normal >) **normalcy**, (normal >) **normalize**, (normal >) **abnormal**, (abnormal >) **abnormality***

            > L. enormis, enorme (< e- *out of, away from*) 파격적인, 엄청난,
            어마어마하게 큰   **E** *enormous, enormity*

    > G. physiognōmia, physiognōmias, f. (< physiognōmonia < physis
    nature + gnōmōn) *judging a person's character by his or her*
    features

        > L. physiognomia, physiognomias, f. (< physiognomonia) 관상술,
        인상학, 용모, 외관   **E** *physiognomy, physiognomic (physiognomonic)*

    > G. pathognōmikos, pathognōmikos, pathognōmikon (< pathognōmonikos
    < pathos *suffering* + gnōmōn) *characteristic or indicative of a*
    particular disease or disorder

        > L. pathognomicus, pathognomica, pathognomicum (< pathognomon-
        icus) (어떤 질병에) 특징적인, 질병 특유의, 진단적인

            E *pathognomonic, (pathognomonic >) **pathognomic**, (pathognomic >) **pathognomy***

    > G. gnōtos, gnōtē, gnōton *known*   **E** *gnotobiotic*

< IE. gno- *to know* (Vide GNOSCĔRE: *See* E. *notorious*)

    > G. gnōrimos, gnōrimos, gnōrimon *well-known*

        > G. gnōrizein *to make known, to become acquainted*

            > G. anagnōrizein (< an(a)- *up, upward; again, throughout; back, backward;*
            against; according to, similar to + gnōrizein) *to recognize*

                > G. anagnōrisis, anagnōriseōs, f. (< + -sis *feminine noun suffix*)
                recognition

                    > L. anagnorisis, anagnorisis, f. 인지, 발견   **E** *anagnorisis*

lysis, lysis, f. 용해(溶解), 분해(分解), 박리(剝離), 환산(渙散)

E *lysis, (lysis + -ate ('on the pattern of filtrate, precipitate') >) lysate, lysin, lysine (Lys, K) (< 'obtained by decomposition of various proteins'), hydrolysis, hydrolysate, (hydrolysis >) hydrolase, karyolysis*

> autolysis, autolysis, f. (< G. autos *self* + lysis *loosening*) 자가용해　**E** *autolysis*

> electrolysis, electrolysis, f. (< G. elektr(o)- *electric* + lysis *loosening*)

　　전기분해　　　　　　　　　　　　　　　　　　　　　**E** *electrolysis*

> haemolysis, haemolysis, f. (< G. haima, haimatos, n. *blood* + lysis

　　loosening) 용혈(溶血)　　　**E** *haemolysis (hemolysis), hemolytic, hemolysin*

< G. lysis, lyseōs, f. (< + -sis *feminine noun suffix*) *loosening, release, dissolution*

< G. lyein *to loosen, to release, to dissolve*　　　　**E** *lyase, lyophilic, lyophilize*

> G. lytos, lytē, lyton *loosened*　　　　　　　　　　　　**E** *electrolyte*

> G. lytikos, lytikē, lytikon *able to loosen*

> L. lyticus, lytica, lyticum 용해성의　　　　　　　　**E** *lytic, -lytic*

> G. analyein (< an(a)- *up, upward; again, throughout; back, backward; against;*

according to, similar to + lyein) *to analyze*

> G. analysis, analyseōs, f. *dissolution, end, retirement, death*

> L. analysis, analysis, f. 분석(分析)

E *analysis, (pl.) analyses, analytic (analytical), analyze, (urine analysis >) urinalysis*

> G. katalyein (< kat(a)- *down, mis-, according to, along, thoroughly* + lyein)

to dissolve, to destroy; (middle) to cease

> G. katalysis, katalyseōs, f. *dissolving, destruction, expulsion, resting*

place

> L. catalysis, catalysis, f. 접촉,

촉매(觸媒)작용　　**E** *catalysis, catalytic, catalyst, catalyze, catalase*

> G. dialyein (< di(a)- *through, thoroughly, apart*) *to separate, to dissolve*

> G. dialysis, dialyseōs, f. *dialysis*

> L. dialysis, dialysis, f. 해리(解離),

투석(透析)　　　　**E** *dialysis, dialyze, dialysate, hemodialysis*

> G. paralyein (< par(a)- *beside, along side of, beyond*) *to loosen on one side,*

to be disabled

> G. paralysis, paralyseōs, f. *paralysis*

> L. paralysis, paralysis, f. 마비(痲痺)

E *paralysis, (pl.) paralyses, (paralysis >) palsy, paralytic, paralyze*

< IE. leu- *to loosen, to divide, to cut* (Vide SOLVĔRE: *See* E. *solve*)

phasis, phasis, f. 상(相), 위상(位相), (변화·발달의) 단계

E *phasis, (pl.) phases, phase, phasic, monophasic, diphasic, triphasic, interphase (< 'between' phase), prophase (< 'before' phase), metaphase (< 'after' phase), anaphase (< 'up' phase), telophase (< 'end' phase); biphasic*

< G. phasis, phaseōs, f. (< + -sis *feminine noun suffix*) *appearance*

< G. phainesthai (*passive*) *to be brought to light, to appear*

> G. phainomenon, phainomenou, n. (< phainomenon (*neuter present participle*)) *thing that appears, appearance, phenomenon*

> L. phaenomenon, phaenomeni, n. 현상(現象), 징후(徵候)

> **E** *phenomenon*, (pl.) *phenomena*, (*phenomenon* >) *epiphenomenon*, (pl.) *epiphenomena*

< G. phainein *to bring to light, to cause to appear, to show*

> **E** *phenotype, diaphanous, sycophant, phosphene* (< 'a subjective sensation of light produced by mechanical stimulation of the retina (as by pressure on the eyeball) or by electrical stimulation of various parts of the visual pathway'), *-phane, Cellophane®* (< 'transparent material made from regenerated cellulose'), *tryptophan (Trp, W)* (< 'appeared during pancreatic (tryptic) digestion of proteins'), *phen(o)-* (< 'the term first used to indicate derivatives from coal-tar, byproducts in manufacturing illuminating gas; now the term indicating benzene'), (*phen(o)- + -ol* >) *phenol*, (*phen(o)- + -yl* >) *phenyl*, (*diisoprophylphenol* >) *propofol*, (*trans + amine + oxy- + phenol* >) *tamoxifen*

> G. phaneros, phaneros (phanera), phaneron *visible, evident*　　**E** *phanerogam, phanerogenic* (< 'opposed to cryptogenic')

> G. phantazein *to make visible;* phantazesthai (*middle*) *to imagine*　　**E** *fantastic*

> G. phantasia, phantasias, f. *appearance, show, imagination*

> L. phantasia, phantasiae, f. 상상, 환상

> **E** *phantasy (fantasy)*, (fantasy >) *fancy*, ((probably) phantasia > 'to suffer from a nightmare' >) *pant*

> G. phantasma, phantasmatos, n. *appearance, fantom*

> L. phantasma, phantasmatis, n. 유령, 환영　　**E** *phantom (fantom)*

> G. emphainein (< em- (< en) *in* + phainein) *to show, to make visible or conspicuous*

> G. emphasis, emphaseōs, f. *reflection (in mirror etc.)*

> L. emphasis, emphasis, f. 강조　　**E** *emphasis, emphasize, emphatic*

> G. epiphainein (< ep(i)- *upon* + phainein) *to manifest*

> G. epiphaneia, epiphaneias, f. *manifestation, striking appearance, an appearance of a divinity*

> L. epiphania, epiphaniae, f. 출현, 현현(顯現), 직각(直覺), 통찰　　**E** *epiphany*

> G. theophaneia, theophaneias, f. *an appearance of a god to a human*　　**E** *theophany*

< IE. bha- *to shine*

> **E** *beacon, beckon, buoy, buoyant*, (buoyant >) *buoyancy (buoyance), banner;* (perhaps) *berry, -berry, frambesia (framboesia)* (< 'bramble berry')

> G. phōs, phōtos, n. *light*

> **E** *phot(o)-, photon, photograph (photo), photopia, photopsin(s)* (< 'cone opsin(s) for color vision'), *photochromogen, photophilia, photophobia*

> G. phōteinos, phōteinē, phōteinon *shining, bright*

> G. phōsphoros, phōsphoros, phōsphoron (< + -phoros, -phoros, -phoron *carrying, bearing*) *light-bearing*

> G. Phōsphoros, Phōsophorou, m. (< phōsphoros astēr) *the morning star*

    > L. Phosphorus, Phosphori, m. 금성, 샛별, 계명성, 명성, 개밥바라기;

       (phosphorus) 인(燐)   `E Phosphor, phosph(o)-`

> L. photosynthesis, photosynthesis, f. (< + G. syn- *with, together* + tithenai

   to put) 광합성   `E photosynthesis`

  > G. phaethein *to shine, to burn*   `E Phaeton`

physis, physis, f. 성장, 자연, 피조물; 성장판(*growth plate*),

   뼈끝연골(*epiphyseal plate*)   `E physis, (pl.) physes, physeal`

  > symphysis, symphysis, f. (< *a growing together, a natural junction*

     formed without a synovial membrane < G. sym- (< syn) *with,*

     together) 결합, 섬유연골 결합   `E symphysis, (pl.) symphyses, symphyseal`

     [용례] symphysis (ossium) pubis 치골결합, 두덩결합   `E symphysis pubis`

      (문법) symphysis: 단수 주격

             ossium 뼈들의: 복수 속격 < os, ossis, n.

             pubis 두덩의: 단수 속격 < pubes, pubis, f. 음부, 두덩

  > epiphysis, epiphysis, f. (< G. ep(i)- *upon*) 골단(骨端),

    뼈끝   `E epiphysis, (pl.) epiphyses, epiphyseal`

  > metaphysis, metaphysis, f. (< G. met(a)- *between, along with, across,*

    after) 골간단(骨幹端), 뼈몸통끝   `E metaphysis, (pl.) metaphyses, metaphyseal`

  > diaphysis, diaphysis, f. (< G. di(a)- *through, thoroughly, apart*)

    골간(骨幹), 뼈몸통   `E diaphysis, (pl.) diaphyses, diaphyseal`

  > apophysis, apophysis, f. (< *outgrowth, offshoot* < G. ap(o)- *away*

    from, from) 돌기, (뼈)곁돌기, 견인골단, 부푼홀씨

    > zygapophysis, zygapophysis, f. (< G. zyg(o)- < zygoun (zygoein)

      to yoke) 척추관절돌기   `E zygapophyseal`

  > hypophysis, hypophysis, f. (< G. hyp(o)- *under*) 뇌하수체(腦下垂體),

    하수체(下垂體)   `E hypophysis, hypophyseal`

    > adenohypophysis, adenohypophysis, f. (< G. adēn *acorn, gland*)

      샘뇌하수체, 선(腺)하수체   `E adenohypophysis, adenohypophyseal`

    > neurphypophysis, neurohypophysis, f. (< G. neuron *nerve*) 신경

      뇌하수체, 신경하수체   `E neurohypophysis, neurohypophyseal`

< G. physis, physeōs, f. (< + -sis *feminine noun suffix*) *growth, nature,*

   creature   `E physi(o)-`

  > G. physikos, physikē, physikon *natural*

    > L. physicus, physica, physicum 자연의, 물리적인, 물질의,

      신체의   `E physical, physician (< 'on the pattern of physicianus')`

      > L. physica, physicorum, n. (pl.) (< G. (*neuter* pl.) ta physica

        natural things) 자연과학; 물리학   `E physics, physicist`

        > L. metaphysica, metaphysicae, f. (< G. (*neuter* pl.) ta meta

ta physica *the things after the physics* < meta *between, along with, across, after*) 형이상학
    E *metaphysics*

> G. physiologia, physiologias, f. (< physis + -logia *study*) *natural philosophy*

> L. physiologia, physiologiae, f. 자연과학;
생리학
    E *physiology, physiologic, physiological*

> G. physiognōmia, physiognōmias, f. (< physiognōmonia < physis + gnōmōn *judge*) *judging a person's character by his or her features*

> L. physiognomia, physiognomiae f. (< physiognomonia) 관상술,
인상학, 용모, 외관
    E *physiognomy, physiognomic (physiognomonic)*

< G. phyein *to make grow, to bring forth*

> G. phyē, phyēs, f. *growth, stature, nature*

> G. heterophyēs, heterophyēs, heterophyes (< heteros *different*) *of different nature*

> L. Heterophyes, Heterophyis, f. (흡충) 이형(異形)흡충속(屬)
    E Heterophyes

> G. phyma, phymatos, n. *tumor*

> L. phyma, phymatis, n. 결절(結節), 종류(腫瘤)
    E *osteophyma*

> L. rhinophyma, rhinophymatis, n. (< G. rhis, rhinos, f. *nose* + G. phyma, phymatos, n. *tumor*) 딸기코종(~腫), 비류(鼻瘤),
주사비(酒皶鼻)
    E *rhinophyma*

> G. phyton, phytou, n. *plant, tree; creature, child*

E *phyt(o)-, -phyte, -phytic, neophyte, epiphyte, saprophyte, exophytic, endophytic, dermatophyte, osteophyte; phytocide (< 'agent lethal to plants'), phytoncide (< 'lethal agent from plants'); phytol (< 'a diterpenoid alcohol derived from chlorophyll'), phytanic acid (< 'a diterpenoid acid derived from phytol'), phytane (< 'a diterpenoid alkane')*

> L. trichophyton, trichophyti, n. (< *hair-plant which luxuriates on the beard* < G. thrix, trichos, f. *hair, wool, bristle*) 백선균(白癬菌)
    E *trichophyte*

< IE. bheuə-, bheu- *to be, to exist, to grow*

E *be, forebear (forbear) (< 'someone who exists before'), bondage, husband (< 'house holder'), husbandry (< 'management of a household'), neighbour (neighbor) (< 'near dweller'), bylaw (< 'local ordinance'), booth, build, boodle, (Dutch) Boer, D. Bauhaus, bound (< 'ready'); beam (< 'growing thing')*

> L. futurus, futura, futurum 장차 일어날, 미래의
    E *future (< 'that is to be')*

> L. fio, factus sum, fieri (변칙동사, 수동형) 되다,
이루어지다 **E** *(third personal singular, present subjunctive, passive 'let it be done' >) fiat*

> G. phylē, phylēs, f. *tribe (ten of these were formed at Athens by Cleisthenes), people, contingent of soldiers provided by a tribe*

> G. phyletēs, phyletou, m. *tribesman*

> G. phyletikos, phyletikē, phyletikon *pertaining to tribesman*
    E *phyletic, monophyletic*

> G. phylon, phylou, n. *race, stock, tribe*

> L. phylum, phyli, n. (생물 분류의) 문(門)　　**E** *phylum, phylogeny*

> IE. -bhw- *being*

> L. dubius, dubia, dubium (< du- (< duo) *two*) 이리 쏠리고 저리 쏠리고 하는,

의심스러운　　**E** *dubious*

> L. dubito, dubitavi, dubitatum, dubitare 의심하다,

서슴다　　**E** *doubt, dubitable, indubitable, redoubtable*

> L. probus, proba, probum (< *growing straightforward, growing well* < pro-

forward) 올곧은, (질적으로) 좋은, 정직한

> L. probo, probavi, probatum, probare 시험하다, 입증하다, 증명하다

E (probandus (*masculine gerundive*) 'one who must be proved' >) *proband, probate* (< 'something proved'), *prove, (prove >) proof, (prove >) disprove, (proof >) disproof*

> L. proba, probae, f. 시험, 입증, 증명　　**E** *probe*

> L. probatio, probationis, f. 시험, 입증, 증명　**E** *probation, probationary*

> L. probabilis, probabile 있음직한, 개연성(蓋然性)

있는　　**E** *probable, probabilism, probabilistic*

> L. probabilitas, probabilitatis, f. 있음직함, 개연성, 확률　**E** *probability*

> L. approbo, approbavi, approbatum, approbare (< ad- *to, toward, at, according to* + probare *to try, to test*) 승인

하다　　**E** *approve, (approve >) approval*

> L. superbus, superba, superbum (< *being above* < super- *above*) 뛰어난, 오만한　**E** *superb*

phylaxis, phylaxis, f. 감염에 대한 저항력　　**E** *-phylaxis*

> prophylaxis, prophylaxis, f. (< G. pro- *before, in front*)

예방　　**E** *prophylaxis, prophylactic*

> anaphylaxis, anaphylaxis, f. (< G. an(a)- *up, upward; again, throughout; back, backward; against; according to, similar to*) 과민증, 아나

필락시스　　**E** *anaphylaxis, anaphylactic*

< G. phylaxis, phylaxeōs, f. (< + -sis *feminine noun suffix*) *guarding*

< G. phylassein (phylact- *stem*) *to guard*

taxis, taxis, f. 배열, 순서, 배치,

주성(走性)　**E** *taxis, taxidermy, taxonomy, (taxonomy >) taxon, (taxon >) (pl.) taxa*

> L. chemotaxis, chemotaxis, f. (< G. chem(o)- *chemical*) 화학주성,

화학쏠림성　　**E** *chemotaxis, chemotactic*

> L. rheotaxis, rheotaxis, f. (< G. rheos *current*) 주류성(走流性), 흐름

쏠림성　　**E** *rheotaxis, rheotactic*

> L. stereotaxis, stereotaxis, f. (< G. stere(o)- *solid, three-dimensional*)

향착성(向着性), 접촉쏠림성, 정위술(定位術)　**E** *stereotaxis, stereotactic*

< G. taxis, taxeōs, f. (< + -sis *feminine noun suffix*) *arrangement, order, rank*

> G. ataxia, ataxias, f. (< a- *not* + taxis + -ia) *disorderliness*

> L. ataxia, ataxiae, f. 조화운동(調和運動)불능, 조화운동 못함증,

실조(失調), 운동실조(증)   **E** *ataxia, ataxic, diataxia*

< G. tassein ((*Attic*) tattein) *to arrange*

> G. taktos, taktē, takton *arranged*

> G. taktikos, taktikē, taktikon *of arrangement,*

of tactics   **E** *tactic, tactics, phonotactics, tactoid*

> G. syntassein (< syn- *with, together*) *to arrange together, to organize*   **E** *syntactic*

> G. syntaxis, syntaxeōs, f. *arranging, syntax, financial contribution to*

the alliance

> L. syntaxis, syntaxis, f. 문장 구성법, 구문론(構文論), 통사론(統辭論)   **E** *syntax*

> G. syntagma, syntagmatos, n. *arrangement*

> L. syntagma, syntagmatis, n. (언어) 신태그머 (발화 중 통합적 관

계를 갖는 어구)   **E** *syntagma*

< IE. tag- *to set in order*

thesis, thesis, f. 논제   **E** *thesis,* (pl.) *theses*

< G. thesis, theseōs, f. (< + -sis *feminine noun suffix*) *placing*

< G. tithenai (the- *root of* tithenai) *to put, to place*

> G. thema, thematos, n. (< the- + -ma *resultative noun suffix*) *what is*

placed down

> L. thema, thematis, n. 주제, 제목   **E** *theme, thematic*

> G. thetos, thetē, theton *placed, adopted*

> G. athetos, athetos, atheton (< a- *not*) *not placed, not fixed*

> L. athetosis, athetosis, f. (< + G. -ōsis *condition*) 무정위(無定位)

운동, 곰지락운동   **E** *athetosis*

> G. anatithenai (< an(a)- *up, upward; again, throughout; back, backward;*

against; according to, similar to) *to set up, to dedicate*

> G. anathema, anathematos, n. *something dedicated (to eternal*

damnation), accursed thing

> L. anathema, anathematis, n. 저주, 파문, 이단 배척   **E** *anathema*

> G. antitithenai (< ant(i)- *before, against, instead of*) *to oppose*

> G. antithesis, antitheseōs, f. *opposition*

> L. antithesis, antithesis, f. 대조,

상반   **E** *antithesis,* (pl.) *antitheses, antithetically*

> G. diatithenai (< di(a)- *through, thoroughly, apart*) *to arrange, to dispose*

> G. diathesis, diatheseōs, f. *disposition, state, condition*

> L. diathesis, diathesis, f. 특성, 체질, 소질,

경향   **E** *diathesis,* (pl.) *diatheses, diathetic*

> G. entithenai (< en- *in* + tithenai) *to put in*

> G. enthesis, entheseōs, f. *insertion*

> L. enthesis, enthesis, f. 삽입, 근육힘줄뼈부착부　　**E** *enthesis, enthetic*

> G. epentithenai (< ep(i)- *upon* + entithenai) *to insert additionally*

　　> G. epenthesis, epentheseōs, f. *additional insertion*

　　　　> L. epenthesis, epenthesis, f. 삽입음(挿入音),

　　　　삽입자(挿入字)　　**E** *epenthesis, epenthetic*

> G. parentithenai (< par(a)- *beside, along side of, beyond* + entithenai)

　　to put in beside

　　　　> G. parenthesis, parentheseōs, f. *rhetorical device by which an*

　　　　example or aside is inserted

　　　　　　> L. parenthesis, parenthesis, f. 삽입어구(挿入語句),

　　　　　　괄호(括弧)　　**E** *parenthesis,* (pl.) *parentheses, parenthetically*

> G. epitithenai (< ep(i)- *upon*) *to put on, to add*

　　> G. epithetos, epithetos, epitheton *added*

　　　　> L. epitheton, epitheti, n. (epithetum, epitheti, n.) 덧말, 부가어,

　　　　꾸밈말, 형용어, 뜻을 가진 이름, 별명　　**E** *epithet*

> G. hypotithenai (< hyp(o)- *under*) *to put under, to suppose*

　　> G. hypothesis, hypotheseōs, f. *disposition, state, condition*

　　　　> L. hypothesis, hypothesis, f. 가설, 가정, 전제

　　　　　　E *hypothesis,* (pl.) *hypotheses, hypothetic (hypothetical), hypothesize*

> G. metatithenai (< met(a)- *between, along with, across, after*) *to change the*

　　position of, to transpose

　　> G. metathesis, metatheseōs, f. *transposition*

　　　　> L. metathesis, metathesis, f. 전환(轉換)　　**E** *metathesis, metathetical*

> G. prostithenai (< pros- *towards, near, beside(s)*) *to put to, to add*

　　> G. prosthesis, prostheseōs, f. *addition*

　　　　> L. prosthesis, prosthesis, f. 첨가물, 보형물, 인공삽입물,

　　　　의지(義肢), 보철(補綴)

　　　　　　E *prosthesis,* (pl.) *prostheses, prosthetic, prosthetics, prosthetist,*
　　　　　　prosthodontics

> G. syntithenai (< syn- *with, together*) *to put together*

　　> G. synthesis, syntheseōs, f. *composition, logical or mathematical*

　　　　synthesis

　　　　> L. synthesis, synthesis, f. 합성

　　　　　　E *synthesis,* (pl.) *syntheses, synthetic (synthetical), synthesize,*
　　　　　　(synthesis + -ase > 'a synthesizing enzyme that does not require
　　　　　　nucleoside triphosphates as an energy source' >) **synthase,**
　　　　　　(synthetic + -ase > 'a synthesizing enzyme that requires
　　　　　　nucleoside triphosphates as an energy source' >) **synthetase,**
　　　　　　biosynthesis

　　　　> L. photosynthesis, photosynthesis, f. (< G. phōs, phōtos, n.

　　　　light) 광합성　　**E** *photosynthesis*

< IE. dhe- *to put, to set* (Vide FACÉRE: *See* E. *facsimile*)

stenosis, stenosis, f. 협착(狹窄), 협착증   **E** *stenosis, stenotic, stenosed, -stenosis; stenograph*

         < G. stenōsis, stenōseōs, f. (< + -sis *feminine noun suffix*) *narrowing*

       < G. stenoun (stenoein) *to make narrow*

     < G. stenos, stenē, stenon *narrow*

   < IE. sten- *narrow*

osmosis, osmosis, f. (< + G. -sis *feminine noun suffix*) 삼투(滲透)

       E *osmosis, endosmosis, exosmosis, (-osmosis >) osmose, osmotic, (osmotic + mole >) osmole, (osmotic + molar >) osmolar, (osmolar >) osmolarity, (osmotic + molal >) osmolal, (osmolal >) osmolality*

      < G. ōsmos, ōsmou, m. (< + -mos *resultative noun suffix*) *push, thrust*

     < G. ōthein *to push, to thrust*

   < IE. wedhə- *to strike, to kill*

myosis, myosis, f. (miosis, miosis, f.) 축동(縮瞳), 동공축소   **E** *myosis (miosis), myotic (miotic)*

      < G. myosis, myoseōs, f. (< + -ōsis *condition*) *constriction of the pupil of the eye*

     < G. myein *(to close the lips >) to close the eyes*

   < IE. meuə- *to be silent* (Vide MUTUS: *See* E. *mute*)

helminthiasis, helminthiasis, f. (< + G. -sis *feminine noun suffix*) 연충증(蠕蟲症),

     기생충증   **E** *helminthiasis*

      < G. helminthian (helminthiaein) *to suffer from worms*

     < G. helmins, helminthos, m. *parasitic worm*

      > L. helmins, helminthis, m. 연충(蠕蟲)   **E** *helminth*

   < IE. wel- *to turn, to roll; with derivatives referring to curved, enclosing objects*

     (Vide VOLVĒRE: *See* E. *volute*)

pityriasis, pityriasis, f. 잔비늘증, 비강진(粃糠疹)   **E** *pityriasis*

     < G. pityron, pityrou, n. *bran, scale*

      + -iasis (< *originally verbs in* -ian (-iaein), -iazein *or nouns in* -ia + -sis *feminine noun suffix, denoting state or process*) *suffering from*

mydriasis, mydriasis, f. 동공확대, 산동(散瞳), 동공산대   **E** *mydriasis, mydriatic*

      < G. mydriasis, mydriaseōs, f. (< *perhaps because the pupil is particularly bright or sparkling when dilated*) *dilatation of the pupil of the eye*

   < G. mydros, mydrou, m. *mass of red hot material in a forge or from a volcano*

      + -iasis (< *originally verbs in* -ian (-iaein), -iazein *or nouns in* -ia + -sis *feminine noun suffix, denoting state or process*) *suffering from*

••• 제 3 변화 제 3 식

단수 주격이 –al, –ar, –e로 끝나는 중성 명사. 복수 속격의 어미는 –ium이다. 단수 및 복수에서 주격, 대격, 호격이 똑같다.

mare, maris, n. 바다

	단 수	복 수	
주격	mar-e	mar-ia	~이, ~가, ~은, ~는, ~께서
속격	mar-is	mar-ium	~의
여격	mar-i	mar-ibus	~게, ~에게, ~께, ~한테
대격	mar-e	mar-ia	~을, ~를
탈격	mar-i	mar-ibus	~에서, ~로부터, ~으로부터
호격	mar-e	mar-ia	~여, ~이여

mare, maris, n. 바다   **E** *mare, mariculture*
> marinus, marina, marinum 바다의, 바다에 사는,

     해양의   **E** *marina, marine, submarine,* (ros marinus *'marine dew'* >) *rosemary*
> maritimus, maritima, maritimum 바다의, 바다에 사는, 바닷가의, 연해의   **E** *maritime*
< IE. mori– *body of water*   **E** *(mere + maid* >) *mermaid, marsh*

animal, animalis, n. 동물   **E** *animal*
< IE. anə– *to breathe* (Vide ʜᴀʟᴀʀᴇ: *See* E. *inhale*)

hepar, hepatis, n. 간(肝)

> **E** *hepat(o)–, hepatocyte, hepatocytic, hepatocellular, heparan sulfate (< 'a sulfated glycosaminoglycan isolated from the liver'), heparin (< 'a glycosaminoglycan isolated from the liver, similar to but more sulfated than heparan sulfate; present mainly in mast cells and basophils'), hepatomegaly*

[용례] porta hepatis 간문(肝門)   **E** *porta hepatis*
     (문법) porta 문(門): 단수 주격 < porta, portae, f.
       hepatis 간의: 단수 속격

< G. hēpar, hēpatos, n. *liver*
> G. hēpatikos, hēpatikē, hēpatikon *of the liver*
> L. hepaticus, hepatica, hepaticum 간의   **E** *hepatic*
< IE. yek^{w}r– *liver*

> L. jecur, jecoris, n. 간, 사랑, 격정, 용기, 슬기

> **E** †*jecorary* (< *'hepatic'*), *jecorin* (< *'lipoidal substance isolated from the liver'*), *jecorize* (< *'to impart to fats or oils some of the properties of cod-liver oil as by irradiation with ultraviolet light'*)

altare, altaris, n. (altar, altaris, n.) 제단　　　　　　　　　　　　　**E** *altar*

　< IE. al-, ol- *to burn*

　　> (*perhaps*) L. alacer, alacris, alacre 활기찬, 경쾌한, 재빠른, 즐거운　　**E** lt. *allegro*

　　　> L. alacritas, alacritatis, f. 활기, 경쾌, 재빠름, 즐거움　　　**E** *alacrity*

monile, monilis, n. 목걸이, (pl.) 보석　　　　　　　　　**E** *moniliform, monilethrix*

　　> monilia, moniliae, f. (< (pl.) monilia < *fungi having conidia arranged in chains like beads on a string*) 모닐리아 (*A genus of hyphomycetes chiefly comprising anamorphic forms of the ascomycetes* Neurospora *and* Monilinia, *but it has at various times included numerous other species, particularly in medical mycology, species of yeast now included in the genus* Candida.)　　　**E** *monilial; moniliosis (moniliasis) (candidiasis)*

　< IE. mon- *neck, nape of the neck*　　　　　　　　　　　**E** *mane*

rete, retis, n. 그물[網]　　　　　　　　　　　　　　　**E** *rete, retiform*

　　[용례] rete testis 고환그물　　　　　　　　　　　　**E** *rete testis*
　　　　rete ovarii 난소그물　　　　　　　　　　　　**E** *rete ovarii*
　　　(문법) rete 그물: 단수 주격
　　　　　testis 불알의: 단수 속격 < testis, testis, m.
　　　　　ovarii 난소의: 단수 속격 < ovarium, ovarii, n.

　　> reticulum, reticuli, n. (< + -culum *diminutive suffix*) 작은 그물, 세망(細網); 벌집위, 봉소상(蜂巢狀)위, 반추동물의 제2위　**E** *reticulum, reticule (reticle), reticulin; reticulocyte*
　　　> reticulatus, reticulata, reticulatum 그물 모양의, 망상(網狀)의　**E** *reticulate*
　　　> reticularis, reticulare 그물 모양의, 망상(網狀)의　　　　**E** *reticular*

　　> retina, retinae, f. (< *delicate structure or net-like vessels* < G. amphiblēstroeidēs chitōn *fishing net-like tunic*) 망막(網膜)

　　E *retina, (retina >) retinal; retinol, retinoic acid, (retinol + aldehyde >) retinal, retinoid(s)*

　　　[용례] macula lutea retinae 망막 황반　　　　　**E** *macula lutea (retinae)*
　　　　(문법) macula 반(斑): 단수 주격
　　　　　　lutea 노란: 형용사, 여성형 단수 주격 < luteus, lutea, luteum
　　　　　　retinae 망막의: 단수 속격

　< IE. erə- *to separate*

　　> L. rarus, rara, rarum 드문, 희박한　　　　　　　　　　**E** *rare*

> L. raritas, raritatis, f. 희박   **E** *rarity*

> L. rarefacio, **rarefeci**, rarefactum, rarefacĕre (< **rarifacĕre** < **rarus** + **facĕre**

  to make) 희박하게 하다   **E** *rarefy*

  > L. rarefactio, rarefactionis, f. 희박화   **E** *rarefaction*

> G. erēmos, erēmē, erēmon *solitary, desolate*

  > G. erēmitēs, erēmitou, m. *hermit*

    > L. eremita, eremitae, m. 은둔자   **E** *eremite, hermit, hermitage*

●●● 제4변화

단수 속격의 어미가 -us인 남성, 여성, 중성 명사. 단수 주격의 어간과 단수 속격의 어간이 같다.

●●● 제4변화 제1식

단수 주격 어미가 -us, 속격 어미가 -us; 복수의 주격 어미가 -us, 속격 어미가 -uum인 남성과 여성 명사. 성은 거의 남성이다.

manus, manus, f. 손

	단 수	복 수	
주격	man-us	man-us	~이, ~가, ~은, ~는, ~께서
속격	man-us	man-uum	~의
여격	man-ui	man-ibus	~게, ~에게, ~께, ~한테
대격	man-um	man-us	~을, ~를
탈격	man-u	man-ibus	~에서, ~로부터, ~으로부터
호격	man-us	man-us	~여, ~이여

manus, manus, f. 손

> **E** *manage* (< 'to handle (a horse)'), (manus + cura 'care' >) *manicure*, (manu facĕre 'to make by hand' >) *manufacture*, (manu operari 'to work by hand' >) *maneuver (manoeuvre)*, (manu operari 'to cultivate' >) *manure*, F. *manchette* (< 'ornamental sleeve')

> manubrium, manubrii, n. 손잡이, 자루, 병(柄)   **E** *manubrium*

> manualis, manuale 손의, 손에 들 만한, 소책자의, 교범(敎範)의   **E** *manual, bimanual*

> manuarius, manuaria, manuarium 손의, 손으로 하는   **E** *manner, mannerism*

> manicula, maniculae, f. (< + -cula *diminutive suffix*) 작은 손, 쟁깃자루; 수갑, 속박   **E** *manacle*

> manipulus, manipuli, m. (< *handful* < manus *hand* + plēre *to fill*) 한줌, 한 묶음,
중대(中隊) **E** (manipulus > *'skillful handling'* >) **manipulation,** *(manipulation >)* **manipulate**
> manceps, mancipis, m. (< manus *hand* + -ceps *taking* < capĕre *to take*) 소유자,
매입자
> mancipium, mancipii, n. (법적 절차를 밟은) 취득, 소유권, 노예
> emancipo, **emancipavi,** emancipatum, emancipare (< e- *out of, away*
from) (법적 소유권을) 해제하다, 해방하다 **E** *emancipate*
> mando, **mandavi,** mandatum, mandare (< manus *hand* + dare *to give*) 권한을 위임
하다, 명령하다 **E** *mandate*
> mandator, mandatoris, m. 위임자, 명령자
> mandatorius, mandatoria, mandatorium 위임의, 명령의, 의무적인 **E** *mandatory*
> commendo, **commendavi,** commendatum, commendare (< com- (< cum)
with, together; intensive + mandare *to entrust*) 위임하다, 추천하다, 명령
하다 **E** *commend, recommend*
> demando, **demandavi,** demandatum, demandare (< de- *apart from, down,*
not; intensive + mandare *to entrust*) (명령적으로) 요구하다 **E** *demand*
< IE. man- *hand*

anus, anus, f. 할머니
> anilis, anile 노파의, 노파 같은 **E** *anile*
> anilitas, anilitatis, f. 여자의 노년기 **E** *anility*
< IE. an- (*nursery word*) *old woman, ancestor*

metus, metus, m. 두려움, 경외심
> meticulosus, meticulosa, meticulosum 세심한, 꼼꼼한, 소심한 **E** *meticulous*

singultus, singultus, m. 흐느낌, 딸꾹질 **E** *singultus*

sinus, sinus, m. 굽이, 굽어 들어간 곳, 만(灣), 굴(窟), toga의 앞자락, 동(洞), 정맥동(靜脈洞),
도관(導管), 누(瘻), 농루(膿漏)

E *sinus,* (pl.) *sinuses, sinusal;* (sinus > *'translation error of (Arabic)* jiba *'chord of an arc'*
derived from (Sanskrit) jya *'bowstring'* >) *sine,* (complementi sinus *'sine of the*
complement of a given angle' >) *cosine, sinusoid* (< *'sine wave-shaped'), (sinusoid >)*
sinusoidal

> sinuosus, sinuosa, sinuosum 굽이치는, 꾸불꾸불한, 물결모양의 **E** *sinuous*
> *sinuositas, *sinuositatis, f. 만곡(彎曲) **E** *sinuosity*
> sinuo, sinuavi, sinuatum, sinuare 굽이지게 하다, 굽이지다 **E** *sinuate*
> insinuo, **insinuavi,** insinuatum, insinuare (< in- *in, on, into, toward* + sinuare
to curve) 들이밀다, 암시하다, 스며들다 **E** *insinuate*

situs, situs, m. 위치, 장소   **E** *situs, site*

    [용례] in situ (제)자리에서, 제자리, 정위치   **E** *in situ*

        (문법) in ~에서: 전치사, 탈격지배

          situ 위치: 단수 탈격

    [용례] situs inversus (viscerum) 내장역위증(逆位症), 내장자리바꿈증   **E** *situs inversus (viscerum)*

        (문법) situs 위치: 단수 주격

          inversus 뒤집힌, 바뀐: 과거분사, 남성형 단수 주격

            < inversus, inversa, inversum

            < inverto, inversi, inversum, invertĕre 안과 밖을 뒤집다, 바꾸다

          viscerum 내장들의: 복수 속격 < viscus, visceris, n.

    > situo, situavi, situatum, situare (*obsolete*) 위치를 정하다, 위치하다, 자리 잡다   **E** *situate*

      > situatio, situationis, f. 위치, 처지, 상황   **E** *situation*

< IE. tkei- *to settle, to dwell, to be home*   **E** *home, haunt (< 'to frequent', 'to go home', 'to bring home')*

    > L. sino, sivi (sii), situm, sinĕre 내버려두다, ~하도록 허락하다

        > L. desino, desivi (desii), desitum, desinĕre (< de- *apart from, down, not* +

           sinĕre *to leave*) 그만두다, 그치다, 끝나다

           > L. desinentia, desinentiae, f. (문법) 어미(語尾), 접미사(接尾辭)   **E** *desinence*

도움말   동사의 과거분사는 수동 또는 완료의 뜻을 가지며 -us (m.), -a (f.), -um (n.)으로 끝나는데, 남성형 -us를 위 변화(제4변화 제1식)의 남성 명사로 차용할 수 있다.

---

ductus, ductus, m. 잡아 늘임, 지휘, 도관(導管), 관(管)   **E** *ductus,* (pl.) *ductus, duct*

        < ductus, ducta, ductum (과거분사)

      < duco, duxi, ductum, ducĕre 이끌다, 잡아 늘이다

  < IE. deuk- *to lead* (Vide DUCĔRE: *See* E. *ductile*)

fremitus, fremitus, m. 으르렁거림, 포효(咆哮), 진동음, 진동감   **E** *fremitus*

        < fremitus, fremita, fremitum (과거분사)

      < fremo, fremui, fremitum, fremĕre 으르렁거리다, 포효하다

  < IE. bhrem- *to growl*

    > (*perhaps*) G. brontē, brontēs, f. *thunder*

      > L. Brontosaurus, Brontosauri, m. (< G. brontē + sauros *lizard*) 브론토사우루스

        속(屬), 뇌룡속(雷龍屬)   **E** *brontosaurus (brontosaur)*

fructus, fructus, m. 열매, 과실

      E *fruit, fruitful, fruitless, fruitarian* (< 'on the pattern of vegetarian'), *tructose* (< 'fruit sugar')

-ficare (< facĕre) *to make*) 열매를 맺다, 결실하다   **E** *fructification*

    < fructus, fructa, fructum (fruitus, fruita, fruitum) (과거분사)

        > fruitio, fruitionis, f. 누림, 향유   **E** *fruition*

    < fruor, fructus (fruitus) sum, frui 누리다, 향유하다

        > frumentum, frumenti, n. 곡식   **E** *frumentaceous*

< IE. bhrug- *agricultural produce; also to enjoy (results, produce)*

    > L. frux, frugis, f. 과실, 농산물, 소산, 건실함   **E** *frugivorous*

        > L. frugalis, frugale 농작물의, 건실한, 절약하는   **E** *frugal*

           > L. frugalitas, frugalitatis, f. 농작물, 건실함, 절약   **E** *frugality*

●●● 제 4 변화 제 2 식

> 단수 주격 어미가 -u, 속격 어미가 -us; 복수의 주격 어미가 -ua, 속격 어미가 -uum 인 중성 명사. 단수 및 복수에서 주격, 대격, 호격이 똑같다.

cornu, cornus, n. 뿔

	단 수	복 수	
주격	corn-u	corn-ua	~이, ~가, ~은, ~는, ~께서
속격	corn-us	corn-uum	~의
여격	corn-u	corn-ibus	~게, ~에게, ~께, ~한테
대격	corn-u	corn-ua	~을, ~를
탈격	corn-u	corn-ibus	~에서, ~로부터, ~으로부터
호격	corn-u	corn-ua	~여, ~이여

cornu, cornus, n. 뿔, 각(角)

E (*'horn'* >) (unicornis *'single-horned'* >) **unicorn**, (capricornus *'goat-horned'* >) **Capricorn**, (cornu copiae *'horn of plenty'* >) **cornucopia, corn, corner**; (*'horny substance'* >) **cornify**

> cornuatus, cornuata, cornuatum 뿔이 난, 뿔 모양의   **E** *cornuate, unicornuate, bicornuate*

> corniculum, corniculi, n. (< + -culum *diminutive suffix*) 작은 뿔, 소각(小角), 각상 (角狀)돌기   **E** *corniculate*

> corneus, cornea, corneum 뿔의, 뿔로 만든, 각질(角質)의

    > cornea, corneae, f. (< tunica cornea *horny tunic* < tela cornea *horny web* < *from its horny consistence*) 각막(角膜)   **E** *cornea, corneal*

< IE. ker- *horn, head; with derivatives referring to horned animals, horn-shaped objects, and projecting parts*   **E** *horn, horny, hart, reindeer* (< *'horned animal'*)

> L. cerebrum, cerebri, n. 대뇌(大腦)

> **E** *cerebrum*, (*cerebrum* >) *cerebration*, (*cerebration* >) *cerebrate*, *decerebrate*, *cerebr(i)- (cerebro-)*, *cerebroside(s)* (< 'found in the brain, with a sugar residue; hence, glucocerebroside and galactocerebroside')

> L. *cerebralis, *cerebrale 대뇌의   **E** *cerebral*

> L. cerebellum, cerebelli, n. (< + -ellum *diminutive suffix*) 소뇌(小腦)   **E** *cerebellum*

> L. *cerebellaris, *cerebellare 소뇌의   **E** *cerebellar, cerebell(i)- (cerebello-)*

> L. cervus, cervi; m. 숫사슴, 사슴   **E** *cervine*

> L. cervix, cervicis, f. 목, 경부(頸部)   **E** *cervix; ectocervix (exocervix), endocervix*

> L. *cervicalis, *cervicale 목의, 경부의   **E** *cervical*

> G. keras, keratos, n. *horn*

> **E** ('horn' >) *triceratops* (< 'three-horned face'); ('horny substance' >) *kerat(o)-, keratolysis*, (*noun*) *keratohyalin*, (*adjective*) *keratohyaline, keratin;* ('keratin' >) *keratin(o)-, keratinocyte* (< 'keratin-synthesizing cell'), *keratinize;* ('horny consistence' > 'cornea' >) *keratocyte* (< 'corneal connective tissue cell'), *keratitis, keratoplasty, keratotomy, keratan sulfate* (< 'a sulfated glycosaminoglycan isolated from the cornea')

> G. monokerōs, monokerōtos, m. (< monos *alone*) *one-horned creature*

> L. monoceros, monocerotis, m. 일각수(一角獸)   **E** *monoceros*

> G. rhinokerōs, rhinokerōtos, m. (< rhis, rhinos, f. *nose*) *rhinoceros*

> L. rhinoceros, rhinocerotis, m. 코뿔소   **E** *rhinoceros*

> G. keration, keratiou, n. (< + -ion *diminutive suffix*) *little horn, (little horn-shaped) carob pod; carob seed*   **E** *carat (karat)* (< 'a carob seed as a unit of weight')

> L. keratosis, keratosis, f. (< + G. -ōsis *condition*) 각화증(角化症)   **E** *keratosis*

> L. hyperkeratosis, hyperkeratosis, f. (< G. hyper- *over*) 각화과다증, 과(過)각화증, 각질증식증   **E** *hyperkeratosis*

> L. parakeratosis, parakeratosis, f. (< *originally, abnormal keratinization; later, retention of nuclei in the stratum corneum, as a normal or abnormal finding* < G. par(a)- *beside, along side of, beyond*) 부전(不全)각화증, 착(錯)각화증, 이상각화증   **E** *parakeratosis*

> L. dyskeratosis, dyskeratosis, f. (< *abnormal keratinization below the stratum granulosum* < G. dys- *bad*) 이상각화증   **E** *dyskeratosis*

> G. kara, karatos, n. *head, person, summit*   **E** *cheer* (< 'a good mood shown by the face')

> G. karoun (karoein) (< *to feel heavy headed*) *to stupefy, to be stupefied*

> G. karōtis, karōtidos, f. *one of the two great arteries of the neck (compression of these arteries was said to produce deep sleep or stupor)*   **E** *carotid*

> G. karōton, karōtou, n. *carrot*

> L. carotà, carotae, f. 당근(唐根), 홍당무(紅唐~)   **E** *carrot, carotene (carotin), carotenoid(s)*

> L. Toxocara, Toxocarae, f. (< *arrow-shaped* < G. toxon, toxou, n. *bow;* (pl.) toxa *bow and arrows*) (선충) 톡소카라속(屬)   **E** Toxocara

> G. kranos, kranou, n. *helmet*

    > G. kranion, kraniou, n. *skull, upper part of the head*

        > L. cranium, cranii, n. 머리뼈   **E** *cranium, cranial, intracranial*

            > L. neurocranium, neurocranii, n. (< G. neuron *nerve*) 뇌머리뼈,

                뇌두개(腦頭蓋)   **E** *neurocranium*

            > L. splanchnocranium, splanchnocranii, n. (< G. (pl.) splanchna

                internal organs) 내장머리뼈,

                얼굴머리뼈   **E** *splanchnocranium (viscerocranium)*

            > L. viscerocranium, viscerocranii, n. (< (pl.) viscera *internal parts*)

                내장머리뼈, 얼굴머리뼈   **E** *viscerocranium (splanchnocranium)*

        > G. ōlekranon, ōlekranou, n. (< ōlenē *elbow, forearm* + kranion) *point*

            of the elbow

            > L. olecranon, olecrani, n. 팔꿈치머리, 주두(肘頭)   **E** *olecranon*

        > G. hemikrania, hemikranias, f. (< hemi- *half*) *headache confined to*

            one side of the head, imperfect development or total defect of one

            side of the brain and its coverings

            > L. hemicrania, hemicraniae, f. 편두통, 반뇌증   **E** *migraine*

> G. korys, korythos, f. *helmet*

    > G. korydos, korydou, m. *crested lark, lark*

        > L. corydalis, corydalis, f. (식물) 현호색속(屬)   **E** *corydalis*

> G. korymbos, korymbou, m. *top, peak; cluster of fruit or flowers*

    > L. corymbus, corymbi, m. 꽃·열매의 송아리,

        산방화서(散房花序)   **E** *corymb, corymbiform, corymbose*

> G. korynē, korynēs, f. *club, mace*

    > L. Corynebacterium, Corynebacterii, n. (< *non-spore-forming, Gram-positive*

    rods that are often swollen at one end < + G. bakterion *bacterium*) (세균)

    코리네박테륨속(屬)   **E** Corynebacterium, *('corynebacterium-form'* >) *coryneform*

gelu, gelus, n. 얼음, 한냉

    > gelidus, gelida, gelidum 얼음같이 찬, 오싹하는   **E** *gelid*

    > gelo, gelavi, gelatum, gelare 얼리다, 굳히다

        E *jelly (< 'a semisolid substance from animal or vegetable material'), gelate, gelation, gelatin (< 'jelly of hydrolyzed collagen'), gelatinize, (gelatin >) gel*

        > congelo, congelavi, congelatum, congelare (< con- (< cum) *with, together;*

        intensive) + gelare *to freeze*) 얼리다, 딴딴하게 하다   **E** *congeal, congelation*

< IE. gel- *cold, to freeze*   **E** *cold, chill, (chill + blain >) chilblain, cool*

    > (*probably*) L. glacies, glaciei, f. 얼음   **E** *glacier*

        > L. glacialis, glaciale 얼음의, 얼음으로 덮인, 혹한의   **E** *glacial*

genu, genus, n. 무릎, 초본식물의 마디   **E** *genu, genuflect*

> geniculum, geniculi, n. (< + -culum *diminutive suffix*) 작은 무릎, 작은 마디

> geniculatus, geniculata, geniculatum 무릎 꿇은, 만곡(彎曲)한, 매듭이 많은   **E** *geniculate*

< IE. genu- *knee; also angle*   **E** *knee, kneel*

> G. gony, gonatos, n. *knee*   **E** *gonitis*

> G. gōnia, gōnias, f. *angle, corner*

> **E** *goniometer (< 'an instrument used for measuring angles'), gonioscope (< 'an instrument for observing the iridocorneal angle')*

> G. -gōnos, -gōnos, -gōnon -*angled, -cornered*

> **E** *-gon, -gonal, tetragon, tetragonal, pentagon, pentagonal, hexagon, hexagonal, heptagon, heptagonal, octagon, octagonal, polygon, polygonal*

> G. trigōnos, trigōnos, trigōnon (< tri- (< treis) *three*) *three-angled*

> G. trigōnon, trigōnou, n. *triangle*

> L. trigonum, trigoni, n. 삼각,

삼각형   **E** *trigon, trigonometry;* F. *trigone*

> L. trigonalis, trigonale 삼각형의   **E** *trigonal*

> G. diagōnios, diagōnia, diagōnion (< di(a)- *through, thoroughly, apart*) *from angle to angle*

> L. diagonalis, diagonale 대각선의   **E** *diagonal*

> G. orthogōnios, orthogōnia, orthogōnion (< orthos *upright, straight, correct*) *right-angled*

> L. orthogonalis, orthogonale 직교하는   **E** *orthogonal*

> L. gonion, gonii, n. 턱모서리점, 악각점(顎角點)   **E** *gonion*

pecu, pecus, n. 가축

> pecunia, pecuniae, f. 돈, 재산   **E** *pecuniary, impecunious*

> peculium, peculii, n. 사유재산; (로마법) 가족이 가장으로부터 받은 사유재산, 노예가

주인으로부터 받은 사유재산   **E** *peculium*

> peculiaris, peculiare 사유재산의, 특유한, 독특한, 유별난   **E** *peculiar*

> peculor, peculatus sum, peculari 공금을 횡령하다, 독직하다   **E** *peculate*

< IE. peku- *wealth, movable property, livestock*

> **E** *fee (< 'cattle, goods, money'), fellow (< 'business partner' < 'one laying down wealth for a joint undertaking' < IE. peku- + IE. legh- 'to lie, to lay'), fief*

> L. feudum, feudi, n. (봉건제도) 봉토(封土), 영지(領地)

> L. feudalis, feudale 봉토의, 영지의   **E** *feudal*

catechu, catechus, n. 아선약(阿仙藥)   **E** *catechu, catechin(s), catechol, catecholamine*

< (*Malayan*) kachu *catechu*

••• 제 5 변화

> 단수의 주격 어미가 -es이고 속격 어미가 -ei; 복수의 주격 어미가 -es, 속격 어미가 -erum인 남성 또는 여성 명사. 성은 거의 여성이다. 단수 주격의 어간과 단수 속격의 어간이 같다.

dies, diei, m. 날; f. 날짜

	단 수	복 수	
주격	di-es	di-es	~이, ~가, ~은, ~는, ~께서
속격	di-ei	di-erum	~의
여격	di-ei	di-ebus	~게, ~에게, ~께, ~한테
대격	di-em	di-es	~을, ~를
탈격	di-e	di-ebus	~에서, ~로부터, ~으로부터
호격	di-es	di-es	~여, ~이여

dies, diei, m. 날; f. 날짜

> **E** (circa *'about'* + dies *'day'* >) ***circadian,*** (ultra *'beyond'* + dies *'day'* >) ***ultradian,*** (dies mali *'bad days'* >) ***dismal***

> dialis, diale 하루의, 일일의　　　　　　　　　　　　　　　　　**E** *dial* (< *'clock dial'*)

> diurnus, diurna, diurnum 하루의, 나날의, 낮의

> **E** (diurnum *'a day's travel'* >) ***journey,*** (ad diurnum *'to an (appointed) day'* > *'to discontinue in order to reconstitute it at another time or place'* >) ***adjourn,*** (sub- *'under'* + diurnum > *'a temporary stay'* >) ***sojourn***

> diurnalis, diurnale 하루의, 나날의

> **E** ***diurnal, journal*** (< *'originally denoting a book containing the appointed times of daily prayers'*)

> diarium, diarii, n. 하루 급여 식량 또는 하루분 급여, 그 기록　　　　**E** *diary*

> meridies, meridiei, m. (< (*dissimilated form of older*) medidies *midday* < medius *middle* + dies *day*) 정오, 남쪽

> meridianus, meridiana, meridianum 정오의, 남쪽의, 자오선(子午線)의, 경선(經線)의, 날줄의　　　　　　　　　　　　　　**E** *meridian, antemeridian, postmeridian*

> meridionalis, meridionale 남쪽의, 자오선의　　　　　　　**E** *meridional*

< IE. dyeu- *to shine* (*and in many derivatives,* *'sky, heaven, god'*)

> **E** (G. hēmera Areios *'day of* Arēs', L. dies Martis *'day of* Mars' > *'Tiw's day'* >) ***Tuesday***

> L. divus, diva, divum 신의

> L. diva, divae, f. 여신　　　　　　　　　　　　　　　　**E** *diva*

> L. divinus, divina, divinum 신의, 신적인　　　　　　　　**E** *divine*

> L. divinitas, divinitatis, f. 신성　　　　　　　　　　　　　**E** *divinity*

> L. deus, dei, m. (*vocative singular* deus) 신; 하느님

　　E *deity, deific, Deus*, F. (a Dieu *'to God'* >) *adieu*, Sp. (a Dios *'to God'* >) *adios*

> L. Diana, Dianae, f. (로마 신화) 달의 여신 (그리스 신화의 Artemis에 해당)　　**E** *Diana*

> L. Jupiter (Juppiter), Jovis, m. (< Jovis pater *Father Jovis*) (로마 신화) 쥬피터
　　(그리스 신화의 Zeus), 하늘; 목성(木星)　　　　　　　　　　　　**E** *Jupiter, Jove*

　　> L. Jovialis, Joviale 쥬피터의; (점성술) 목성의 영향을 받고 태어난, 쾌활한　　**E** *jovial*

　　　> L. Julius, Julii, m. (< *descended from Jupiter*) 로마의 씨족 이름(가장 유명한
　　　　사람은 Gaius Julius Caesar (100~44 B.C.E.))　　　　　　　**E** *Julius*

　　　　> L. Julius, Julia, Julium 율리우스 씨족의, 율리우스의,
　　　　　7월의　　　**E** (Julius mensis *'month of Julius (Gaius Julius Caesar)'* >) *July*

　　> L. dives, (gen.) divitis (< *divine, blessed, fortunate*) 부유한　　　**E** *Dives*

> G. Zeus, Dios, m. (*Greek mythology*) Zeus, the supreme deity of the ancient Greeks　**E** *Zeus*

　　> L. Dianthus, Dianthi, m. (< G. Dios *of Zeus* + anthos *flower*) (식물) 패랭이꽃
　　속(屬)　　　　　　　　　　　　　　　　　　　　　　　　　　**E** Dianthus

> G. dēlos, dēlē, dēlon *visible, evident, plain, clear*

　　> G. dēloun (dēloein) *to make visible, to show, to reveal*　　**E** *psychedelic*

res, rei, f. 사물, 일, 실제, 재산

　　E (abl. sing.) *re*, (abl. pl.) *rebus, reify*, (de re *'away from the matter'* >) *dereism*, (dereism >)
　　dereistic

　　[용례] Nomina sunt consequentia rerum. 이름은 사물의 귀결이다
　　　(문법) nomina 이름들은: 복수 주격 < nomen, nominis, n.
　　　　　sunt 이다: esse 동사, 직설법 현재 복수 삼인칭
　　　　　consequentia 필연적 결과, 귀결: 단수 주격
　　　　　　< consequentia, consequentiae, f.
　　　　　rerum 사물들의: 복수 속격

> realis, reale 물적(物的)인, 실제적, 현실적

　　E *real*, (real > *'real estate'* >) *realty*, (in- *'not'* > ir- > + real >) *irreal*, (real >) *realism*,
　　(F. sur- (< L. super- *'above'*) + realism >) *surrealism*, (surrealism >) *surreal*

　　> realitas, realitatis, f. 실제, 사실, 실질, 현실성　　　　　　　**E** *reality*
> respublica, reipublicae, f. (< res *thing, affair* + publicus *public*) 공화국　**E** *republic*

　　[용례] Respublica Coreana 대한민국
　　　(문법) respublica 공화국: 단수 주격
　　　　　Coreana 한국의: 형용사, 여성형 단수 주격
　　　　　　< Coreanus, Coreana, Coreanum < Corea, Coreae, f.

< IE. re- *to bestow, to endow; goods, wealth, property*

caries, cariei, f. 부식(腐蝕), 우식(齲蝕), 카리에스　　　　　**E** *caries, cariogenic*
> cariosus, cariosa, cariosum 부식된, 우식의, 카리에스에 걸린　　　**E** *carious*

< IE. kerə- *to injure, to break apart*

> G. kēr, kēros, f. *destruction, death, goddess of death, fate*

scabies, scabiei, f. 옴, 개선(疥癬)

E *scabies*

[용례] Sarcoptes scabiei 옴진드기

E Sarcoptes scabiei

(문법) sarcoptes 옴진드기속(屬): 단수 주격

< Sarcoptes, Sarcoptis, f.

scabiei 옴의: 단수 속격

< scabo, scabi, −, scabĕre 긁다

> scaber, scabra, scabrum 껄껄한, 껄끄러운

E *scabrous* (< 'scratched')

< IE. (s)kep- *base of words with various technical meanings such as 'to cut with a sharp tool', 'to scrape', 'to hack'*

E *shape* (< 'cutting'), *-ship* (< 'state, condition'), *landscape, scoop* (< 'thing cut out'), *shaft, scab, shabby* (< 'cutting'), *shave*

> L. scapula, scapulae, f. (< *a tool for scraping*) 어깨뼈, 견갑골(肩胛骨), 어깨, 견갑(肩甲)

E *scapula, scapular*

> G. skaphē, skaphēs, f. (< *thing cut out*) *hollow vessel, boat*

> L. scapha, scaphae, f. 거룻배, 쪽배

E *scapha*

> G. skaphoeidēs, skaphoeidēs, skaphoeides (< + eidos *shape*) *boat-shaped*

> L. scaphoides, (gen.) scaphoidis 배 모양의, 주상(舟狀)의

E *scaphoid*

●●● 불변화 명사

수와 격에 따른 어미변화를 하지 않는 명사이다. 그러나 라틴어식 어미변화를 하는 경우도 있다. 차용한 명사가 많다.

cherub, m. (pl. cherubim) (불변화) 케루빔, 지천사(智天使); (미술) 케루빔의 그림 (아기 천사의 모습; *A rabbinic folk etymology, which explains the Hebrew singular form as representing Aramaic* ke-rabya *'like a child', led to the representation of the cherub as a child*)

E *cherubism*

< G. cheroub, (pl.) cheroubim

< (*Hebrew*) kerub, (pl.) kerubim

Adam, m. (불변화) (Adamus, Adami, m.) 아담

E *Adam*

< (*Hebrew*) adam *human being, man, humanity*

< (*Semitic root*) dm *human being*

manna, n. (불변화) (manna, mannae, f.) 만나, 만나 나무 (*manna ash* (Fraxinus ornus) <

manna sugar from the sap
compared to the Biblical manna)   **E** *mannitol* (< '*manna sugar*'), (*mannitol* >) ***mannose***
   < (*Aramaic*) manna *manna*
  < (*Hebrew*) man *manna*
< (*Semitic root*) mnn *to be kind, to show favor, to patronize; to disdain*

benzoin, f. (불변화) 안식향(安息香)   **E** *benzene*
  < (*Arabic*) luban jawi *incense of Java (probably confused with Sumatra) obtained from the*
    Styrax benzoin

지소사

영어에서는 명사에 축소 접미사를 붙여 지소사(指小辭, *diminutive*)를 만든다.

- *-en*   (예) *chicken* < **keuk-* (*echoic*)
      kitten < L. cattus *cat*

- *-ie*   (예) *birdie* < *bird*

- *-kin*   (예) *lambkin* < *lamb*
      napkin < L. mappa *tablecloth*

- *-ling* (< *-le* + *-ing*) (예) *duckling* < *duck*
      suckling < *suck*

- *-ock*   (예) *buttock* < *butt*
      hillock < *hill*

- *-let*   (예) *rootlet* < *root*
      leaflet < *leaf*
      piglet < *pig*
      hooklet < *hook*
      platelet < *plate* < G. platys *flat*

- *-et, -ette*   (예) *islet* < L. insula *island*
      lancet < L. lancea *lance*
      rosette < L. rosa *rose*

라틴어에서도 명사 어간에 축소 접미사를 붙여 지소사를 만든다. 지소사는 본
디 낱말의 성을 따라 남성(-us), 여성(-a), 중성(-um) 명사가 되는 것이 원칙이

며, 제1명사변화(-a) 또는 제2명사변화(-us, -um, -aster)를 따른다. 라틴어의
축소 접미사는 다음과 같다.

- -ulus, -ula, -ulum (-olus, -ola, -olum *after a bowel*)
- -culus, -cula, -culum
- -ellus, -ella, -ellum
- -illus, -illa, -illum
- -aster

-ulus (m.), -ula (f.), -ulum (n.)

-ulus, -uli, m.

flocculus, flocculi, m. 작은 양털 송아리, 솜털; 타래, 편엽(片葉); 면상침강물(綿狀沈降物)
> E *flocculus,* (pl.) *flocculi,* (flocculus >) *floccular,* (flocculus >) *flocculent,* (flocculus >) *flocculate, flocculation*

< floccus, flocci, m. 양털 송아리, 실 부스러기, 지푸라기, 사소한 것,
그까짓 것   E *floccus,* (pl.) *flocci, flock* (< *'lock of wool'*)
> floccosus, floccosa, floccosum 양털로 덮인, 솜털 모양의   E *floccose*
> *floccillus, *floccilli, m. (< + -illus *diminutive suffix*) 뜻은
flocculus와 같음   E *floccillation* (carphology)
< IE. bhlok- *flock of wool*

glomerulus, glomeruli, m. 토리, 구(球), 사구(絲毬), 사구체(絲毬體)
> E *glomerulus,* (pl.) *glomeruli,* (glomerulus >) *glomerular, juxtaglomerular, glomerulo-*
> glomerulosus, glomerulosa, glomerulosum 토리의, 토리 모양의 구상(毬狀)의
< glomus, glomeris, n. 실뭉치, 토리, 사구(絲毬), 소체(小體)   E *glomus*
> glomero, glomeravi, glomeratum, glomerare 둥글게 뭉치다
> conglomero, conglomeravi, conglomeratum, conglomerare (< con- (<
cum) *with, together*) 둥글게 뭉치다, 집괴(集塊) 모양으로 만들다,
복합체가 되다   E *conglomerate*

tubulus, tubuli, m. 세관(細管), 소관(小管),
관(管)   E *tubulus,* (pl.) *tubuli, tubule,* (tubulus >) *tubular, microtubule, tubulin*
< tubus, tubi, m. 관(管)
> E *tube,* (tubus >) *tubal,* (tubus >) *intubate,* (intubate >) *intubation, extubation* (< *'on the pattern of intubation'*), *tuba*

–ula, –ulae, f.

cellula, cellulae, f. 세포(細胞)   **E** *cell*

     < cella, cellae, f. 광

   < IE. kel- *to cover, to conceal, to save* (Vide CELLULA: *See* E. *cell*)

venula, venulae, f. 세정맥(細靜脈)   **E** *venule*
                                                   E *vein*

     < vena, venae, f. 맥, 혈관, 정맥(靜脈)

–ulum, –uli, n.

ovulum, ovuli, n. 작은 알, 난자   **E** *ovule*

       < ovum, ovi, n. 알, 난(卵), 난자(卵子), 난세포(卵細胞)

     < IE. owyo-, oyyo- *egg* (Vide OVUM: *See* E. *ovum*)

   < IE. awi- *bird* (Vide AVIS: *See* E. *avian*)

granulum, granuli, n. 작은 알맹이, 과립(顆粒)

> **E** *granule, granular, nongranular, granulation* (< *'the formation of grain-like prominences on sores when healing; (pl.) the grain-like bodies so formed'*); *granulocyte* (< *'granular leukocytes: neutrophil, eosinophil, basophil'*), *agranulocyte* (< *'nongranular leukocytes: lymphocyte, monocyte'*), *granulocytosis* (< *'increased number of granulocytes'*), *agranulocytosis* (< *'decreased number of granulocytes'*), *granulomere* (< *'granular part of platelet'*)

   > granulosus, granulosa, granulosum 작은 알맹이가 많은, 과립의   **E** *granulosa*

   > granuloma, granulomatis, n. (< *a term coined by Virchow to include certain 'neoplasms' which generally do not advance in structure beyond the stage of granulation tissue, and which usually proceed to ulceration* < + G. -ōma *noun suffix denoting tumor*) 육아종(肉芽腫)   **E** *granuloma, granulomatous*

     [용례] granuloma inguinale 샅고랑육아종   **E** *granuloma inguinale*

       (문법) granuloma 육아종: 단수 주격

          inguinale 샅고랑의: 형용사, 중성형 단수 주격

            < inguinalis, inguinale

     > lymphogranuloma, lymphogranulomatis, n. 림프육아종   **E** *lymphogranuloma*

       [용례] lymphogranuloma venereum 성병림프육아종   **E** *lymphogranuloma venereum*

         (문법) lymphogranuloma 림프육아종: 단수 주격

           venereum 사랑의, 색정의: 형용사, 중성형 단수 주격

< venereus, venerea, venereum

< granum, grani, n. 낟알, 알맹이, 과립, 입자

> **E** *granum,* (pl.) *grana, grain, granite,* (filum *'thread'* + granum *'grain'* > *'jewel work of a delicate kind made with threads and beads, usually of gold and silver'* >) *filigree, ingrain (engrain)* (< *'to dye with grain (cochineal)'*)

> granaria, granariorum, n. (pl.) 곡물 창고, 곡창, 곡창 지대, 저장고   **E** *granary, garner*

> granatus, granata, granatum 알맹이가 많은, 알곡이 풍성한

> **E** *garnet, grenade,* (pomum granatum *'apple with many seeds'* >) *pomegranate*

< IE. grəno- *grain*   **E** *corn* (< *'grain'*), *kernel,* D. *Kern* (< *'kernel'*), *kernicterus* (< *'nuclear jaundice'*)

–olus (m.), –ola (f.), –olum (n.)

–olus, –oli, m.

nucleolus, nucleoli, m. 핵소체(核小體)   **E** *nucleolus,* (pl.) *nucleoli*

     < nucleus, nuclei, m. 핵(核)

     < (*syncopated variant*) nuculeus, nuculea, nuculeum (< + –eus *adjective suffix*) 작은 견과의

     < nucula, nuculae, f. (< + –ula *diminutive suffix*) 작은 견과

     < nux, nucis, f. 견과(堅果)

   < IE. kneu– *nut* (Vide NUCLEUS; *See* E. *nucleus*)

–ola, –olae, f.

areola, areolae, f. 작은 뜰, 작은 틈; 윤(輪), 유륜(乳輪), 젖꽃판   **E** *areola*

   > areolaris, areolare 작은 틈이 있는, 그물코 모양의; 젖꽃판의   **E** *areolar, subareolar*

  < area, areae, f. 뜰, 영역, 구역, 역(域), 부위, 부(部), 야(野), 면(面)

> **E** *area, areal; are* (< *'a metric unit of 100 square meters'*), (G. hekaton *'a hundred'* > *'100 ares'* >) *hectare*

   > areatus, areata, areatum 구역 지어 생기는, 원형으로 생기는

arteriola, arteriolae, f. 세동맥(細動脈)   **E** *arteriole*

   < arteria, arteriae, f. 동맥(動脈)

  < G. artēria, artērias, f. *windpipe* > *artery, vein*

< IE. wer– *to raise, to lift, to hold suspended* (Vide ARTERIA; *See* E. *artery*)

-culus (m.), -cula (f.), -culum (n.)

-culus, -culi, m.

homunculus, homunculi, m. (< homun- (< homin-) + -culus *diminutive suffix*) 난쟁이,
축소인간, 변변치 못한 사람, 정자미인(精子微人)   **E** *homunculus*
< homo, hominis, m. 사람
< **IE.** dhghem- *earth, earthling* (Vide HOMO; *See* E. *homo*)

panniculus, panniculi, m. 천조각, 헝겊, 층(層)   **E** *panniculus*

[용례] panniculus adiposus 지방층   **E** *panniculus adiposus*
panniculus carnosus 근육층   **E** *panniculus carnosus*
(문법) panniculus 층: 단수 주격
adiposus 지방이 많은, 지방의: 형용사, 남성형 단수 주격
< adiposus, adiposa, adiposum
< adeps, adipis, m. 비계
carnosus 근육이 많은, 근육의: 형용사, 남성형 단수 주격
< carnosus, carnosa, carnosum
< caro, carnis, f. 근육

< pannus, panni, m. 천, 옷감,
판누스   **E** *pannus, pane, panel* (< 'piece of cloth, list on a piece of parchment')
< **IE.** pan- *fabric*   **E** *vane*

-cula, -culae, f.

buticula, buticulae, f. (butticula, butticulae, f.) 단지, 동이, 병   **E** *bottle, butler* (< 'cup-bearer')
< butis, butis, f. (buttis, buttis, f.) 통
< (*perhaps*) *Of* non-IE. *origin*

molecula, moleculae, f. 분자(分子)
E *molecule, molecular,* (molecule >) *mole,* (mole >) *molar* (< 'of a solution containing one mole of solute per liter of solvent'), (molar >) *molarity,* (mole >) *molal* (< 'of a solution containing one mole of solute per kilogram of solvent'), (molal >) *molality, macromolecule*

< moles, molis, f. 애씀, 어려움; 큰 축조물, 제방, 덩어리
> molestus, molesta, molestum 힘든, 귀찮은   **E** *molest*

> molesto, **molestavi**, molestatum, molestare 괴롭히다, 학대하다　　**E** *molestation*

> molior, molitus sum, moliri 애쓰다, 공사하다

> molimen, moliminis, n. 애씀, 어려움, 장애, 곤란　　**E** *molimen*

> demolior, demolitus sum, demoliri (< de- *apart from, down, not* + moliri

to construct) 헐다, 분쇄하다, 해체하다　　**E** *demolish, demolition*

< IE. mo- *to exert oneself*

-culum, -culi, n.

---

corniculum, corniculi, n. 작은 뿔, 소각(小角), 각상(角狀)돌기　　**E** *corniculate*

< cornu, cornus, n. 뿔

< IE. ker- *horn, head; with derivatives referring to horned animals, horn-shaped objects, and projecting parts* (Vide CORNU; *See* E. *unicorn*)

corpusculum, corpusculi, n. 인간의 (보잘 것 없는) 육체, 소체(小體), 미립자　**E** *corpuscle (corpuscule)*

< corpus, corporis, n. 몸, 체(體), 몸통, 전집(全集)

< IE. kʷrep- *body, form, appearance* (Vide CORPUS; *See* E. *corpus*)

-ellus (m.), -ella (f.), -ellum (n.)

-ellus, -elli, m.

---

pedicellus, pedicelli, m. 작은 발, 족돌기(足突起)　　**E** *pedicel*

< pediculus, pediculi, m. (< + -culus *diminutive suffix*) 작은 발, 꼭지, 족(足),

각(脚), 경(莖), 병(柄)

< pes, pedis, m. 발, 족(足)

< IE. ped- *foot* (Vide PES; *See* E. *pedal*)

-ella, -ellae, f.

---

umbella, umbellae, f. 우산, 양산, 해파리의 갓, 보호물

> umbellatus, umbellata, umbellatum 산형(繖形) 꽃차례의　　**E** *umbellate*

> umbellifer, umbellifera, umbelliferum (< umbella *parasol* + -fer (< ferre *to carry, to bear*) *carrying, bearing*) 산형의 꽃이 피는　　**E** *umbellifer, umbelliferous*

< umbra, umbrae, f. 그늘　**E** *umbra,* (sub umbra >) *sombre (somber),* (It. ombrella >) *umbrella*

> penumbra, penumbrae, f. (< paene (pene) *almost* + umbra *shadow*) 반음영
(半陰影), 반암부(半暗部), 명암이나 농담이 흐릿한 부분, 두 가지가 섞인
모호한 경계부　　　　　　　　　　　　　　　　　　　　　　　**E** *penumbra*

< IE. andho- *blind, dark*

–ellum, –elli, n.

rostellum, rostelli, n. 작은 부리, 작은 주둥이, 액취(額嘴)　　　**E** *rostellum*

< rostrum, rostri, n. 부리, 주둥이, 문(吻), 취(嘴), 뱃부리, (pl.) 연단

< IE. red- *to scrape, to scratch, to gnaw* (Vide RADĒRE; *See* E. *razor*)

–illus (m.), –illa (f.), –illum (n.)

–illus, –illi, m.

penicillus, penicilli, m. (penicillum, penicilli, n.) 붓　　　　　**E** *pencil*

< peniculus, peniculi, m. (< + –culus *diminutive suffix*) 작은 꼬리, 꼬리 끝의
털뭉치, 붓

< penis, penis, m. 음경(陰莖), 꼬리

< IE. pes- *penis* (Vide PENIS; *See* E. *penis*)

morbilli, morbillorum, m. (pl.) 홍역(紅疫)　　　　　　　　　**E** *morbilliform*

< morbus, morbi, m. 병(病)

< IE. mer- *to rub away, to harm* (Vide MORI; *See* E. *mortal*)

–illa, –illae, f.

papilla, papillae, f. (< papula + –illa *diminutive suffix*) 젖꼭지, 유두(乳頭), 유두상(乳頭狀)
구조, 시신경 원판(*optic disc, optic papilla*)　　　　　　**E** *papilla,* (pl.) *papillae*

> papillaris, papillare 유두(乳頭) 모양의, 유두상(乳頭狀)의　　**E** *papillary*

> papilloma, papillomatis, n. (< + G. –ōma *noun suffix denoting tumor*)
유두종(乳頭腫)　　　　　　　　　　　　　　　　　　　　**E** *papilloma*

> papilloedema, papilloedematis, n. (< *edema of the optic disc* (*optic papilla*)
< + G. oidēma *swelling*) 유두부종(乳頭浮腫),
시각신경유두부종　　　　　　　**E** *papilloedema (papilledema)*

< papula, papulae, f. 구진(丘疹), 솟음

    E *papule, papular*

   < IE. pap- *to swell*

       > (*suggested*) L. papaver, papaveris, n. 양귀비(楊貴妃), 앵속(罌粟)

    E *poppy, papaverine*

tonsillae, tonsillarum, f. (pl.) 편도(扁桃)

    E *tonsil*

       > tonsillaris, tonsillare 편도의

    E *tonsillar*

    < toles, tolium, m., f. (pl.) 편도염, 갑상샘 종양

-aster, -astri, m.　　　　E *-aster* (< *'a person or thing that is inferior or not genuine'*)

---

philosophaster, philosophastri, m. 철학자연하는 사람, 사이비 철학자

    E *philosophaster*

    < philosophus, philosophi, m. 철학자

   < G. philosophos, philosophou, m. (< philein (phileein) *to love* + sophia *wisdom*)
philosopher

명사를 만드는 방법

● ● ●　형용사의 차용

> 형용사를 명사처럼 쓸 수 있다. 형용사의 명사적 용법이다.

medicina, medicinae, f. 의학, 약

    E *medicine*

     < medicinus, medicina, medicinum 의사의, 의학의

    < medicus, medici, m. 의사

    E *medic, paramedics*

   , < medicus, medica, medicum 치료의, 의술의

   < medeor, −, mederi 치료하다

 < IE. med- *to take appropriate measures* (Vide MEDERI: *See* E. *medic*)

● ● ●　동사의 차용

> 형용사의 기능을 갖는 분사를 명사로 쓸 수 있다. 형용사의 명사적 용법과 같다.

현재분사　능동 또는 진행의 뜻을 가지는 현재분사를 명사로 차용한다.

pariens, parientis, f. 산모(産母)

< pariens, (gen.) parientis (현재분사) 낳는

  < pario, **peperi**, partum, par**ĕ**re 낳다, 해산하다

< IE. per**ə**- *to produce, to procure* (Vide PAR**Ĕ**RE; *See* E. *-parous*)

serpens, serpentis, m., f. 뱀   **E** *serpentine*

   < serpens, (gen.) serpentis (현재분사) 기는

    < serpo, **serpsi**, serptum, serp**ĕ**re 기다

 < IE. serp- *to crawl, to creep* (Vide SERPENS; *See* E. *serpentine*)

과거분사   수동 또는 완료의 뜻을 가지는 과거분사를 명사로 차용한다.

---

pruritus, pruritus, m. 가려움, 소양증(搔痒症), 색정   **E** *pruritus, pruritic, pruritogenic*

   < pruritus, prurita, pruritum (과거분사) 가려운

   < prurio, -, -, prurire 가렵다, 몹시 하고 싶어 하다, 색정이 일다   **E** *prurient*

    > prurigo, pruriginis, f. 양진(痒疹), 가려움발진   **E** *prurigo, pruriginous*

 < IE. preus- *to freeze, to burn*   **E** *freeze, frost, frostbite, (permanent frost >) permafrost*

   > L. pruina, pruinae, f. 서리

    > L. pruinosus, pruinosa, pruinosum 서리에 덮인   **E** *pruinose*

tinnitus, tinnitus, m. 귀울음, 이명(耳鳴)   **E** *tinnitus*

   < tinnitus, tinnita, tinnitum (과거분사) 울림소리가 나는

  < tinnio, **tinnivi (tinnii)**, tinnitum, tinnire (의성어) 땡그랑 소리 내다, 동전 소리를 내다,

  재잘대는 소리가 나다, 귀에 울리다

수동형 미래분사   당위의 뜻을 가지는 수동형 미래분사를 명사로 차용한다.

---

pudendum, pudendi, n. (여성의) 음부, 외음부   **E** *pudendum, (pl.) pudenda*

    > pudendalis, pudendale 음부의   **E** *pudendal*

   < pudendus, pudenda, pudendum (수동형 미래분사) 부끄러워해야 할   **E** *pudendous*

  < pudeo, **pudui**, puditum, pud**ĕ**re 부끄럽게 하다, 부끄러워하다

   > pudens, (gen.) pudentis (*present participle*) 부끄러워하는   **E** *(rare) pudent*

    > pudentia, pudentiae, f. 수줍음, 수줍어함, 단정함   **E** *pudency*

    > impudens, (gen.) impudentis (< im- (< in-) *not*) 부끄러워하지 않는   **E** *impudent*

     > impudentia, impudentiae, f. 뻔뻔스러움   **E** *impudence*

> pudicus, pudica, pudicum 부끄러워하는, 정숙한, 순결한

< IE. (s)peud- *to push, to repulse*

> L. repudium, repudii, n. 파혼, 이혼, 소박

E *repudiate*

●●● **명사 접미사의 이용**

접미사를 붙여 명사를 만든다.

–io, –ionis, f.	동사의 어간에 붙여 행위를 가리키는 추상명사 (–io) 또는 행위의	E *-ion*
–ura, –urae, f.	결과를 가리키는 구체명사 (–ura)를 만든다.	E *-ure*

fissio, fissionis, f. 쪼갬, 열개(裂開), 분열(分裂), 분할(分割)

E *fission*

fissura, fissurae, f. 틈새, 열(裂), 열창(裂創), 구(溝)

E *fissure*

    < findo, fidi, fissum, findĕre (fid- *stem*) 쪼개 벌리다

E *fissi-, -fid*

      > fissilis, fissile (쉽게) 쪼개지는

E *fissile*

      > bifidus, bifida, bifidum (< bi- *two*) 두 갈래의

E *bifid*

      > multifidus, multifida, multifidum (< multus *many*) 여러 갈래의

E *multifid*

  < IE. bheid- *to split; with Germanic derivatives referring to biting (hence also to eating and to hunting) and woodworking*

>   E *bit, bite, (bite > 'altered not to be misspelled as bit' >) byte, beetle (< 'to bite'), bait, bitter, abet (< 'to harrass with dogs'), boat (< 'dugout canoe, split planking')*

tinctio, tinctionis, f. 담그기, 세례, 염색

E *tinction*

tinctura, tincturae, f. 염료, 팅크제, 정기제(丁幾劑), 염색

E *tincture*

    < tingo (tinguo), tinxi, tinctum, tingĕre 적시다, 물들이다, 염색하다

E *tinge, taint, stain, destain*

      > tinctus, tinctus, m. 염색

E *tinct, tint*

      > tinctor, tinctoris, m. 염색업자

        > tinctorius, tinctoria, tinctorium 물이 드는, 색을 내는, 빛깔의

E *tinctorial*

      > *tingibilis, *tingibile 물들 수 있는

E *tingible*

  < IE. teng- *to soak*

E *dunk*

–or, –oris, m.	동사의 어간에 붙여 행위자나 상태를 가리키는 명사를 만든다.	E *-or*

actor, actoris, m. 움직이게 하는 자, 실행자; (법률) 원고, (남자) 배우

E *actor, actress*

    > actrix, actricis, f. (법률) 여자 원고, 여배우

  < ago, egi, actum, agĕre 하다, 움직이다, 몰다, 무게를 달다

< IE. ag- *to drive, to draw, to move* (Vide AGĔRE; *See* E. *act*)

terror, terroris, m. 공포   **E** *terror*

    < terreo, **terrui**, territum, terrēre 무섭게 하다

        > terribilis, terribile 무서운   **E** *terrible*

        > terrificus, terrifica, terrificum (< +-ficus (< facĕre) *making*) 무섭게 하는   **E** *terrific*

        > deterreo, **deterrui**, deterritum, deterrēre (< de- *apart from, down, not* + terrēre *to frighten*) 위협해서 못하게 하다   **E** *deter*

    < IE. tres- *to tremble*

< (*possibly*) IE. ter- *to tremble*

    > IE. trem- *to tremble*

        > L. tremo, **tremui**, –, tremĕre 떨다, 무서워하다   **E** (tremendus *'that is to be trembled at'* >) *tremendous*

        > L. tremor, tremoris, m. 떨림, 진전(震顫), 겁(怯)   **E** *tremor*

        > L. tremulus, tremula, tremulum 떠는   **E** *tremulous*

            > L. tremulo, **tremulavi**, tremulatum, tremulare 떨다   **E** *tremulate, tremble*

    > IE. trep- *to tremble*

        > L. trepidus, trepida, trepidum 동요하는, 겁내는   **E** *trepid*

        > L. trepido, **trepidavi**, trepidatum, trepidare 동요하다, 겁내다, 전율하다   **E** *trepidation*

        > L. intrepidus, intrepida, intrepidum (< in- *not* + trepidus *alarmed*) 두려움을 모르는   **E** *intrepid*

–men, –minis, n.
–mentum, –menti, n.   동사의 현재어간에 붙여 행위 또는 행위의 결과를 가리키는 명사를 만든다.   **E** *–men*   **E** *–ment*

---

carmen, carmimis, n. 빗, 얼레빗

    > carmino, **carminavi**, carminatum, carminare (양털을) 빗질하다

         E *carminative* (< *'a medical term from the old theory of humors; the object of carminatives is to expel wind, but the theory was that they dilute and relax the gross humors from whence the wind arises, combing them out like the knots in wool'*)

    < caro, –, –, carēre (양털을) 빗질하다

  < IE. kars- *to card*

    > (*perhaps*) L. carduus, cardui, m. 엉겅퀴, (엉거시과) 삽주   **E** *card*

ligamentum, ligamenti, n. 잡아매는 것 (노끈·줄·붕대·인대 등), 유대, 결연   **E** *ligamentum (ligament),* (pl.) *ligamenta (ligaments)*

    < ligo, **ligavi**, ligatum, ligare 매다, 결박하다

  < IE. leig- *to bind* (Vide LIGARE; *See* E. *ligate*)

-monia, -moniae, f.　　　(< *related by ablaut to the suffix* -men) 명사, 형용사, 분사의　　**E** *-mony*
-monium, -monii, n.　　어간에 붙여 상태, 조건, 행위를 가리키는 명사를 만든다.

testimonium, testimonii, n. 증언, 선언　　　　　　　　　　　　　　**E** *testimony*

　　　　　< testis, testis, m., f. 증인

　　　　< *tri-st-i- *third person standing by*

　　< IE. trei- *three* (Vide IE. trei-; *See* E. *three*)

　+ IE. sta- *to stand* (Vide STARE: *See* E. *stay*)

parsimonia, parsimoniae, f. 절약, 검소　　　　　　　　　　　　　**E** *parsimony*

　　　　　[용례] lex parsimoniae (< *law of parsimony*) 절약의 법칙

　　　　　　(문법) lex 법칙: 단수 주격 < lex, legis, f. 법(法), 법칙(法則)

　　　　　　　parsimoniae 절약의: 단수 속격

　　　　　< parco, peperci (parsi), parsum (parcitum), parcĕre 아끼다, 절약하다

　　　　< parcus, parca, parcum 아끼는, 절약하는, 인색한, 얼마 안 되는, 문체가 간결한

-ia (-tia), -iae (-tiae), f.　　　　　　　　　　　　　　　**E** *-ia (-tia, -ce)*
-itas, -itatis, f.　　　　형용사나 현재분사의 어간에 붙여 상태를　　　**E** *-ity*
-tudo, -tudinis, f.　　　가리키는 명사를 만든다.　　　　　　　　　**E** *-tude*

patientia, patientiae, f. 인내　　　　　　　　　　　　　　　　　**E** *patience*

　　　　　< patiens, (gen.) patientis (현재분사) 참는, 괴로움당하는, 병 앓는, 꿋꿋한

　　　　< patior, passus sum, pati 당하다, 견디다, 참다, 고통받다, 내버려 두다

　< IE. pe(i)- *to hurt* (Vide PATI: *See* E. *patient*)

caritas, caritatis, f. 사랑, 박애, 자선, 귀함　　　　　　　　　　　**E** *charity*

　　　　　< carus, cara, carum 사랑스러운, 귀한　　　　　**E** *caress, cherish*

　　< IE. ka- *to like, to desire*　　　　　　　　　　　　**E** *whore, whoredom*

　　　　> (*Sanskrit*) kamah *love, desire*　　　　　　　**E** *Kama, Kamasutra*

hebetudo, hebetudinis, f. 지둔(遲鈍), 우둔　　　　　　　　　　　**E** *hebetude*

　　　　　> hebeto, hebetavi, hebetatum, hebetare 무디게 하다　　**E** *hebetate*

　　　　< hebes, (gen.) hebetis 무딘, 둔한, 굼뜬

–arium, –arii, n. –orium, –orii, n. –ium, –ii, n.	동사의 어근이나 명사의 어간에 붙여 장소, 기간, 도구를 가리키는 명사를 만든다.	**E** *-ary* **E** *-ory* **E** *–ium*

vocabularium, vocabularii, n. 자전(字典)　　　　　　　　　　　　　　　　**E** *vocabulary*

   < vocabulum, vocabuli, n. 명칭, 용어

   < voco, **vocavi**, vocatum, vocare 부르다

  < vox, vocis, f. 목소리, 언어

 < IE. wek^w– *to speak* (Vide vox: *See* E. *voice*)

sensorium, sensorii, n. 감각력, 지각중추　　　　　　**E** *sensorium, sensorial, sensory*

   < sensus, sensus, m. 감각, 감각기관, 감정, 생각, 의미

  < sentio, **sensi**, sensum, sentire (< *to go mentally*) 느끼다, 생각하다, 깨닫다

 < IE. sent– *to head for, to go* (Vide sentire: *See* E. *sentient*)

tentorium, tentorii, n. 천막, 야영　　　　　　　　　**E** *tentorium, tentorial*

   < tendo, **tetendi**, tentum (tensum), tendĕre 뻗치다, 향하다

 < IE. ten– *to stretch* (Vide tenēre: *See* E. *tenet*)

silentium, silentii, n. 침묵　　　　　　　　　　　　　**E** *silence*

   < sileo, silui, –, silēre 잠잠하다, 침묵을 지키다, 고요하다, 멎다　　**E** *silent*

 < IE. si–lo– *silent*

–ulum (–ula) –bulum (–bula) –culum –brum (–bra), –crum, –trum	동사의 어근이나 명사의 어간에 붙여 도구, 수단, 장소를 가리키는 명사를 만든다.	**E** *-ulum (-ula)* **E** *-bulum (-bula, -ble)* **E** *-culum (-cle)* **E** *-brum (-bra), -crum, -trum*

cingulum, cinguli, n. 띠, 검대(劍帶), 견대(肩帶), 뱃대끈,

  지대(地帶)　　**E** *cingulum,* (pl.) *cingula, cingule, shingles,* (Sp. cincha >) *cinch*

   > cingulatus, cingulata, cingulatum 띠의, 띠 모양의, 대상(帶狀)의　　**E** *cingulate*

  < cingo, **cinxi**, cinctum, cingĕre 두르다, 띠다

   > praecingo, **praecinxi**, praecinctum, praecingĕre (< prae- *before, beyond* +

    cingĕre *to gird*) 띠를 두르다, 둘러싸다　　　　　　　**E** *precinct*

   > succingo, **succinxi**, succinctum, succingĕre (< suc- (< sub) *under* + cingĕre

    to gird) 띠를 허리에 두르다, 대비하다, 띠로 묶다, 간추리다　　**E** *succinct*

< IE. kenk- *to gird, to bind*

mandibulum, mandibuli, n. (mandibula, mandibulae, f.) 턱, 아래턱뼈, 하악골(下顎骨)   **E** *mandible*
> mandibularis, mandibulare 턱의, 아래턱뼈의, 하악골의   **E** *mandibular, submandibular*
< mando, **mandi**, mansum, mandĕre 씹다, 먹다
> manduco, **manducavi**, manducatum, manducare 먹다, 씹다   **E** *mange, manger*
< IE. mendh- *to chew*
> G. manasthai *to chew*
> G. masētēr, masētēros, m. *a chewer*
> L. masseter, masseteri, m. 깨물근, 교근(咬筋)   **E** *masseter*
> G. mastax, mastakos, f. *mouth, morsel*   **E** *moustache (mustache)*
> G. mastichan (mastichaein) *to grind the teeth*
> (*probably*) G. mastichē, mastichēs, f. *mastic*
> L. mastiche, mastiches, f. 유향수지(乳香樹脂)나무, 유향수지   **E** *mastic*
> L. mastico, **masticavi**, masticatum, masticare 씹다, 저작(咀嚼)하다   **E** *masticate*

vehiculum, vehiculi, n. (수레·배 등) 운반기구, 운반체   **E** *vehicle, vehicular*
< veho, **vexi**, vectum, vehĕre 나르다, 운반하다
< IE. wegh- *to go, to transport in a wheeled vehicle* (Vide VEHĔRE: *See* E. *vector*)

cribrum, cribri, n. 체[篩], 어레미   **E** *cribriform*
> cribrosus, cribrosa, cribrosum 체[篩] 모양의, 체처럼 작은 구멍이 많은
< cerno, **crevi**, cretum (certum), cernĕre 체로 치다, 분별하다, 이해하다
< IE. krei- *to sieve, to discriminate, to distinguish* (Vide CERNĔRE: *See* E. *crime*)

palpebra, palpebrae, f. (< *that which shakes or moves quickly*) 눈꺼풀,
안검(眼瞼)   **E** *palpebra*, (pl.) *palpebrae*
< palpo, **palpavi**, palpatum, palpare 어루만지다, 쓰다듬다, 다독거리다
< IE. pal- *to touch, to feel, to shake* (Vide PALPARE: *See* E. *palpate*)

sepulcrum, sepulcri, n. 무덤, 매장지   **E** *sepulchre (sepulcher), sepulchral*
< sepelio, **sepelivi** (sepelii), sepultum, sepelire (< *originally 'to perform ritual manual
operations on a corpse'*) 매장하다
> sepultura, sepulturae, f. 매장   **E** *sepulture*
< IE. sep- *to handle (skillfully), to hold (reverently)*

haustrum, haustri, n. 양수기, 팽대, 잘록창자팽대   **E** *haustrum*, (pl.) *haustra, haustral*
> haustellum, haustelli, n. (< + -ellum *diminutive suffix*) 문관(吻管),

흡관(吸管)　　　　　　　　　　　　　　　　　　　　**E** *haustellum*, (pl.) *haustella*

    < haurio, **hausi,** haustum, haurire 물을 긷다

       > haustor, haustoris, m. 물 긷는 사람, 마시는 사람

         > haustorium, haustorii, n. (기생식물의) 흡기(吸氣), 기생근(寄生根)　　**E** *haustorium*

        > exhaurio, **exhausi,** exhaustum, exhaurire (< *to draw out* < ex- *out of, away*

          from + haurire *to draw (water), to drain*) 물을 다 퍼내다, 바닥내다, 힘을

          다 빼다, 탈진(脫盡)하다　　　　　　**E** *exhaust, exhaustible, inexhaustible*

  < IE. aus- *to draw water*

      > (*probably*) G. arytein (< IE. we-r- (ur-) *water, liquid, milk* + IE. aus-) *to draw water*

        > G. arytaina, arytainas, f. *funnel, pitcher, ladle*　　**E** *arytenoid* (< '*pitcher-shaped*')

-ago, -aginis, f. -igo, -iginis, f. -ugo, -uginis, f.	동사의 어근이나 명사의 어간에 붙여 질환 또는 표면에 생기는 것을 가리키는 명사를 만든다.	**E** -ago, -age **E** -igo **E** -ugo

lumbago, lumbaginis, f. 요통　　　　　　　　　　　**E** *lumbago, lumbaginous*

     < lumbus, lumbi, n. 허리, 요부(腰部), (가축) 등심, 성욕의 자리

  < IE. lendh- *loin* (Vide LUMBUS; See E. *loin*)

lentigo, lentiginis, f. 렌즈콩 모양의 반점, 검정사마귀,

    흑색점(黑色點)　　　　　　　　　**E** *lentigo*, (pl.) *lentigines, lentiginous*

     < lens, lentis, f. 렌즈콩, 제비콩, 불콩[扁豆]; 렌즈, 수정체 (Vide LENS; See E. *lens*)

vitiligo, vitiliginis, f. (< *blemish*) 백반증(白斑症)　　　　　　　**E** *vitiligo*

     < vitium, vitii, n. 흠, 결점, 악습

  < IE. wei- *vice, fault, guilt* (Vide VITIUM; See E. *vitiate*)

impetigo, impetiginis, f. (< *contagious skin infection*) 고름딱지증,

    농가진(膿痂疹)　　　　　　　　　　　**E** *impetigo, impetiginous*

     < impeto, impetivi (impetii), impetitum, impetĕre (< im- (< in) *in, on, into,*

       toward + petĕre *to go toward, to seek*) 습격하다

     < peto, petivi (petii), petitum, petĕre 날아가다, (어느 방향으로) 가다, 찾아다니다, 청하다

  < IE. pet- *to fly, to rush* (Vide PETĔRE; See E. *petition*)

intertrigo, intertriginis, f. 피부스침증, 간찰진(間擦疹)　　　**E** *intertrigo, intertriginous*

     < *intertero, *intertrivi, *intertritum, *interterĕre (< inter- *between, among*

      + terĕre *to wipe*) 서로 비비다, 서로 분쇄하다

     < tero, trivi, tritum, terĕre 비비다, 분쇄하다

< IE. terə- *to rub, to turn* (Vide TERĔRE; *See* E. *trite*)

prurigo, pruriginis, f. 가려움발진, 양진(痒疹)　　　　　　　　　

    < prurio, −, −, prurire 가렵다, (몹시 하고 싶어 하다, 색정이 일다)

  < IE. preus- *to freeze, to burn* (Vide PRURITUS; *See* E. *pruritus*)

serpigo, serpiginis, f. 사행상(蛇行狀) 피부질환　　　　　　　　

    < serpo, **serpsi**, serptum, serpĕre 기다

  < IE. serp- *to crawl, to creep* (Vide SERPENS; *See* E. *serpentine*)

vertigo, vertiginis, f. 회전운동, 회전기구, 현기증, 어지러움, 현혹　　

    < verto, **versi**, versum, vertĕre 돌리다, 돌다, 바꾸다

  < IE. wer- *to turn, to bend, to wind* (Vide VERTĔRE; *See* E. *verse*)

aerugo, aeruginis, f. 동녹(銅綠), 돈 독

      > aeruginosus, aeruginosa, aeruginosum 녹청(綠靑)색의　

    < aes, aeris, n. 금속, 구리, 청동, 동전

  < IE. ayes- *metal, copper or bronze* (Vide AERUGINOSUS; *See* E. *era*)

albugo, albuginis, f. 백반(白斑)

      > albugineus, albuginea, albugineum 흰, 계란

      흰자위의　　　　　

    < albus, alba, album 흰

  < IE. albho- *white* (Vide ALBUS; *See* E. *albino*)

ferrugo, ferruginis, f. 쇠의 녹, 암갈색, 질투　　　　　　　　　

      > ferrugineus, ferruginea, ferrugineum 녹슨 쇳빛의, 암갈색의, 쇠비린내 나는,

      철분이 함유된

    < ferrum, ferri, n. 철, 쇠

  < (*possibly*) *Borrowed (via Etruscan) from the same obscure source as brass* (Vide FERRUM; *See* E. *ferrum*)

lanugo, lanuginis, f. (동식물의) 솜털, 배냇솜털　　　　　　　　

    < lana, lanae, f. 양털, (동물의) 털, 모직물, (식물의) 솜털, 새털구름

  < IE. welə- *wool* (Vide VELLUS; *See* E. *vellus*)

대명사

라틴어 대명사에는 여덟 가지가 있다. 인칭대명사(재귀대명사 포함), 소유대명사, 지시대명사, 관계대명사, 의문대명사, 부정대명사, 대명사적 형용사, 상관대명사이다. 학술용어를 이해하기 위해서는 몇 가지 대명사의 뜻과 관용어구 정도만 알면 된다.

인칭대명사

라틴어 인칭대명사의 속격은 '~에게 대한' '~을(를)'의 뜻을 갖는 객어적 속격이며 속격을 지배하는 동사나 형용사와만 함께 쓰인다. 제1인칭과 제2인칭의 복수 속격 nostrum, vestrum은 분할 속격으로서 '~ 중의', '~ 중에서'의 뜻을 갖는다. '~의'라는 소유의 뜻으로는 다음에 나오는 소유대명사를 사용한다.

●●● 제1인칭

	단 수			복 수	
주격	ego	나는, 내가	nos		우리는, 우리가
속격	mei	나에게 대한, 나를	nostri		우리에게 대한, 우리를
			nostrum		우리 중의
여격	mihi	나에게	nobis		우리에게
대격	me	나를	nos		우리를
탈격	me	나로	nobis		우리로

ego, mei, mihi, me, me (m., f.) 나, 자아(自我)

> **E** *ego, egocentric, superego* (< 'a censor on the wishes of the ego, the agent of self-criticism or self-observation')

> egoismus, egoismi, m. 이기주의   **E** *egoism, egotism* (< 'with intrusive -t-')

< IE. eg *nominative form of the personal pronoun of the first person singular*　　　　 E *I*
　　> G. egō *I, myself*

< IE. me- *oblique form of the personal pronoun of the first person singular*　 E *my, mine, me, myself*
　　> L. meus, mea, meum 나의

> E (mea domina *'my lady'* >) It. *Madonna,* (mea domina *'my lady'* >) F. *Madame,* (meus senior *'my senior'* >) F. *Monsieur*

nos, nostri (nostrum), nobis, nos, nobis (m., f.) 우리

　　> noster, nostra, nostrum 우리의
　　　　> nostrum, nostri, n. 비약(秘藥), 만병통치약　 E *nostrum (< '(something) of our own making')*
　　　> nostras, (gen.) nostratis 우리 조국의, 우리 민족의, 우리 종교의　 E *Nostratic*
< IE. nes- *oblique cases of the personal pronoun of the first person plural*　 E *our, ours, us*

● ● ●　**제 2 인칭**

	단 수		복 수	
주격	tu	너는, 네가	vos	너희는, 너희가
속격	tui	너에게 대한, 너를	vestri vestrum	너희에게 대한, 너희를 너희 중의
여격	tibi	너에게	vobis	너희에게
대격	te	너를	vos	너희를
탈격	te	너로	vobis	너희로

tu, tui, tibi, te, te (m., f.) 너

　　[용례] Et tu, Brute! (< *And you, Brutus!*) 브루투스, 너 마저!
　　　　(문법) et 그리고: 접속사
　　　　　　tu 너, 당신: 인칭대명사 (제2인칭), 단수 주격
　　　　　　Brute 브루투스여: 단수 호격 < Brutus, Bruti, m. 브루투스
　　　　　　(Marcus Junius Brutus, 85-42 B.C.E.)

vos, vestri (vestrum), vobis, vos, vobis (m., f.)
　　　　너희　　　　　　　　　　 E (F. rendez vous *'render yourselves'* >) *rendezvous*
< IE. wos (pl.) *you*

●●● 제 3 인칭 (재귀대명사)

문장 내의 주어 자신을 가리킨다. 목적어적 재귀대명사로 쓰이기 때문에 주격
은 없다. (일인칭과 이인칭에서는 인칭대명사의 각 격이 재귀대명사로 쓰인다.)

	단 수		복 수	
주격	—		—	
속격	sui	자신에게 대한, 자신을	sui	자신들에게 대한, 자신들을
여격	sibi	자신에게	sibi	자신들에게
대격	se	자신을	se	자신들을
탈격	se	자신으로	se	자신들로

—, sui, sibi, se, se (m., f.) (sing., pl.) 자신

> [용례] sui generis (< *of its own kind*) 그 종류 자신에게 대한, 그 자신에게 독특한,
> 그 자신만의　　　　　　　　　　　　　　　　　　　　　　　E *sui generis*
> 　(문법) sui 자신에게 대한: 인칭대명사, 제3인칭, 단수 속격
> 　　　　generis 종류의: 단수 속격 < genus, generis, n. 혈통, 족속, 종류, 속(屬)

> [용례] per se 자신을 통하여, 그 자체로서, 본질적으로　E *per se, (and per se and'* >) *ampersand*
> 　(문법) per 통하여: 전치사, 대격지배
> 　　　　se 자신을: 인칭대명사, 제3인칭, 단수 대격

> [용례] inter se 그들 사이에서, 그들끼리만, 동일종끼리 (교배하는)　　　E *inter se*
> 　(문법) inter 사이에: 전치사, 대격지배
> 　　　　se 자신을: 인칭대명사, 제3인칭, 복수 대격

> > suicidium, suicidii, n. (< sui *of oneself* + caedĕre *to cut, to kill*) 자살　E *suicide, suicidal*

< IE. s(w)e- *pronoun of the third person and reflexive (referring back to the subject of the sentence),*
one's own; further appearing in various forms referring to the social group as an entity,
'(we our-)selves'

> E *self, sib, sibling, gossip* (< *'idle talk'* < *'familiar acquaintance'* < *'godparent'*), *swain* (< *'one's own (man), attendant, servant'*), *boatswain*

> > L. se-, sed- (부사, 전치사) 자신만의 것으로 해 놓은 > (접두사) 분리, 이탈　E *se- (sed-)*
> > L. solus, sola, solum 홀로　　　　　　　　　　　　　E *sole*, It. *solo, sullen*
> > > L. solitarius, solitaria, solitarium 단독의, 고독한　　　　E *solitary*
> > > L. solitudo, solitudinis, f. 고독　　　　　　　　　　　E *solitude*
> > > L. desolo, desolavi, desolatum, desolare (< de- *apart from, down, not; intensive*)
> > > 　혼자 남겨놓다, 황폐케 하다　　　　　　　　　　　　E *desolate*

> L. desolatio, desolationis, f. 외로움, 황폐   **E** *desolation*

> L. suesco, **suevi**, suetum, suescĕre (< + -escĕre *suffix of inceptive (inchoative) verb*) 익숙해지다, 습관들이게 하다

  > L. consuesco, **consuevi**, consuetum, consuescĕre (< con- (< cum) *with, together* + suescĕre *to become accustomed*) 익숙해지다, 습관들이게 하다

    > L. consuetudo, consuetudinis, f. 습관, 관습, 생활양식

> **E** *consuetude, consuetudinary, custom, customary, accustom, customs* (< *'customary due paid to a ruler'*), *costume* (< *'dress'* < *'manner of dressing, wearing the hair, etc.'*)

  > L. mansuesco, **mansuevi**, mansuetum, mansuescĕre (< manus *hand* + suescĕre *to become accustomed*) 길들다, 길들이다   **E** *mastiff*

    > L. mansuetudo, mansuetudinis, f. 길들어 있음, 순치(馴致)된 상태, 온순, 유순   **E** *mansuetude*

> L. (*possibly*) soleo, solitus sum, solēre (반탈형 동사) 늘 (상습적으로) ~하다

  > L. solitus, solita, solitum (*past participle*) 평소의, 상례적인

    > L. insolens, (gen.) insolentis (< in- *not*) 서투른, 이례적인, 건방진   **E** *insolent*

      > L. insolentia, insolentiae, f. 건방짐, 오만   **E** *insolence*

  > L. obsolesco, **obsolevi**, obsoletum, obsolescĕre (< ob- *before, toward(s), over, against, away* + solēre *to become accustomed* + -escĕre *suffix of inceptive (inchoative) verb*) 못 쓰게 되어가다   **E** *obsolescent, obsolete (obs.), obsolescence, obsolesce*

> G. ēthos, ēthous, n. *disposition, trait, character, custom, morality*   **E** *ethos, ethology, ethics, ethical*

> G. ethnos, ethnous, n. *company, band, people, nation*   **E** *ethnos, ethnic, (ethnic >) ethnicity, ethnology, ethnocentric*

> G. hetaira, hetairas, f. *female companion, sweetheart, courtesan, prostitute*   **E** *hetaira, (pl.) hetairai*

  > L. hetaera, hetaerae, f. (고대 그리스의) 첩, 고급 매춘부   **E** *hetaera, (pl.) hetaerae*

> G. idios, idia, idion *own, private, peculiar*

> **E** *idio-, idiogram* (< *'a diagrammatic representation of a chromosome complement, based on measurement of the chromosomes of a number of cells'* < *'one's private mark'*), *idiograph* (< *'one's private mark or signature'*), *idiolect* (< *'the dialect of an individual'* < *'on the pattern of dialect'*)

  > G. idiōtēs, idiōtou, m. *private person, common man, plebeian, one without professional knowledge, 'layman; ignorant, ill-informed person*

    > L. idiota, idiotae, m. (idiotes, idiotae, m.) 못 배운 사람, 천치   **E** *idiot*

  > G. idioesthai *to make one's own, to make appropriate*

    > G. idiōma, idiōmatos, n. (< + -ma *resultative noun suffix*) *peculiarity, property, peculiar phraseology*

      > L. idioma, idiomatis, n. 특수한 어법, 관용어, 방언   **E** *idiom, idiomatic*

  > G. idiopatheia, idiopatheias, f. (< + -patheia -*pathy*) *idiopathy*

    > L. idiopathia, idiopathiae, f. 특발증, 자발증(自發症),

원인불명증   **E** *idiopathy, idiopathic*

> G. idiosynkrasia, idiosynkrasias, f. (< + synkrasis (< syn- *with, together* + krasis *mixing, tempering*) + -ia *noun suffix*) *peculiarity of constitution or temperament*

     > L. *idiosyncrasia, *idiosyncrasiae, f. 특이체질, 특이습관, 특이성   **E** *idiosyncrasy, idiosyncratic*

소유대명사

소유대명사는 항상 형용사적으로만 사용하며 형용사의 어미변화(제1·2변화)를 따른다.

	단 수		복 수	
일인칭	meus, mea, meum	나의	noster, nostra, nostrum	우리의
이인칭	tuus, tua, tuum	너의	vester, vestra, vestrum	너희의
삼인칭	suus, sua, suum	자기의	suus, sua, suum	자기들의

meus, mea, meum 나의

   < IE. me- *oblique form of the personal pronoun of the first person singular*

      (Vide EGO; *See* E. *ego*)

noster, nostra, nostrum 우리의

   < IE. nes- *oblique cases of the personal pronoun of the first person plural*

      (Vide NOS; *See* E. *nostrum*)

지시대명사

지시대명사는 명사적으로 사용하기도 하고 형용사적으로 사용하기도 하며, 성·수·격에 따라 변화한다.

is (m.), ea (f.), id (n.) 그 사람, 그 남자; 그 여자; 그것; 그, 저

	단 수			복 수		
	남성	여성	중성	남성	여성	중성
주격	is	ea	id	ii (ei)	eae	ea
속격	ejus	ejus	ejus	eorum	earum	eorum
여격	ei	ei	ei	iis (eis)	iis (eis)	iis (eis)
대격	eum	eam	id	eos	eas	ea
탈격	eo	ea	eo	iis (eis)	iis (eis)	iis (eis)

hic (m.), haec (f.), hoc (n.) 이 사람, 이 남자; 이 여자; 이것; 이

	단 수			복 수		
	남성	여성	중성	남성	여성	중성
주격	hic	haec	hoc	hi	hae	haec
속격	hujus	hujus	hujus	horum	harum	horum
여격	huic	huic	huic	his	his	his
대격	hunc	hanc	hoc	hos	has	haec
탈격	hoc	hac	hoc	his	his	his

is (m.), ea (f.), id (n.) 그 사람, 그 남자; 그 여자; 그것; 그, 저　　　　　　E (D. es 'if' >) id

　　[용례] id est (i.e.) (< that is) 그것이다, 즉　　　　　　　　　　E id est (i.e.)
　　　　　(문법) id 그것: 지시대명사, 중성 단수 주격
　　　　　　　　est 이다: esse 동사, 직설법 현재 단수 삼인칭

　　> idem (m.), eadem (f.), idem (n.) (< id it + -dem (demonstrative suffix)) 같은 사람,
　　　같은 것; 동일한

　　　　E (idem 'same' + gulose (< glucose) > 'epimeric with gulose'>) idose, iduronic acid
　　　> identitas, identitatis, f. 동일성, 일체성, 독자성, 정체성, 주체성　　E identity
　　　　> identicus, identica, identicum 동일한　　　　　　　　　　E identical
　　　　> identifico, identificavi, identificatum, identificare (< + -ficare (< facĕre
　　　　to make) 동일함을 확인하다, 동정(同定)하다, 식별하다　　　　E identify
　　　　　> identificatio, identificationis, f. 동일시, 동정, 식별, 확인　E identification

< IE. i- pronominal stem　　　E yea (< 'so'), yes (< 'so it be' < + IE. es- 'to be'), yet, if, beyond
　　>L. ita (부사) 이렇게, 이렇듯이, 그렇게

> L. item (부사) 마찬가지로, 역시, 다시

> **E** *item* (< *'used to introduce a new fact or statement, or, more frequently, each new article or particular in an enumeration, especially in a formal list or document'*), *itemize*

> L. iterum (부사) 다시

> L. itero, iteravi, iteratum, iterare 다시 하다, 되풀이하다,
반복하다　　　　　　　　　　　　　　　　　**E** *iterate, iterative, reiterate*

> L. ibi (부사) 거기에, 그곳에

> L. ibidem (< ibi *there* + -dem (*demonstrative suffix*)) (부사) 바로 그곳에,
같은 곳에　　　　　　　　　　　　　　　　　　**E** *ibidem (ibid., ib.)*

> L. alibi (< alius *other of more than two* + ibi *there*) (부사) 다른 곳에서　　**E** *alibi*

hic (m.), haec (f.), hoc (n.) 이 사람, 이 남자; 이 여자; 이것, 이

[용례] Hoc quoque transibit. 이 또한 지나가리라

(문법) hoc 이것, 이: 지시대명사, 중성 단수 주격

quoque 또한, 까지도: 부사

transibit 지나갈 것이다: 능동태 직설법 미래 단수 삼인칭

< transeo, transivi (transii), transitum, transire 지나가다

[용례] ad hoc (< *to this*) 이것까지, 특별히 이 경우에 한하여　　　　**E** *ad hoc*

(문법) ad 까지: 전치사, 대격지배

hoc 이것: 지시대명사, 중성 단수 대격

< IE. gho- *base of demonstrative pronouns and deictic pronouns*

+ IE. ke- (< IE. ko- *stem of demonstrative pronoun meaning 'this'*; Vide CIS; *See* E. *he*)
(*deictic particle*) *this, here*

iste (m.), ista (f.), istud (n.) 그 사람, 그 남자; 그 여자; 그것; 그

ille (m.), illa (f.), illud (n.) (< *that* < *yonder*) 저 사람, 저 남자; 저 여자; 저것; 저

> **E** (Ad illa arma! *'To the arms!'* >) *alarm*, (ad illam erectam *'to the watch tower'* >) *alert*; (ille lacertus *'the lizard'* > Sp. el lagarto >) *alligator*, (illa *reaptata (< re- *'again'* + aptare *'to fit'*) *'to tie again'* > Sp. la reata >) *lariat*, Sp. *El Niño* (< (masculine) *'the child'*), *La Niña* (< (feminine) *'the child'*)

< IE. al- *beyond*　　　　　　　　　　　　　　　　　　　**E** *else, other*

> L. ulter, ultra, ultrum 저쪽의, 너머의 [超], 지나친 [過] (부사형 ultra, ultro 외에는
쓰지 않음)

(비교급) ulterior, ulterior, ulterius ((gen.) ulterioris) 저 너머의　　**E** *ulterior*

(최상급) ultimus, ultima, ultimum 가장 멀리 있는, 마지막의　　　　**E** *ultima*

[용례] ultima ratio 최후 수단

(문법) ultima 마지막의: 형용사, 여성형 단수 주격

ratio 방법: 단수 주격

< ratio, rationis, f. 고려, 계산, 방법, 근거

> L. ultimo, −, −, ultimare 끝에 이르다

> L. ultimatus, ultimata, ultimatum (*past participle*) 맨 끝의, 최후의,

극한의　　　　　　　　　　　　　E *ultimate (ult), ultimatum, (ultimate >) ultimacy*

> L. paenultimus, paenultima, paenultimum (penultimus, penultima, penultimum)

(< paen *almost* + ultimus *last*) 끝에서 두 번째의　　　E *penultimate, penult*

> L. antepaenultimus, antepaenultima, antepaenultimum (< ante-

before + paenultimus *second last*) 끝에서

세 번째의　　　　　　　　E *antepenultimate, antepenult; preantepenult*

> L. ultra (전치사, 대격지배) 저쪽으로, 저 너머, 한도를

넘어　　　E *ultra, outrage (< 'meaning influenced by association with rage'), outre*

> L. ultra- *on the other side of, beyond*　　　E *ultra-, ultrasonic, ultrafiltrate*

> L. alter, altera, alterum (둘 중에) 다른 하나의　E *(alteri huic 'to this other' >) altruism, altruistic*

> L. altero, alteravi, alteratum, alterare 다른 것으로 바꾸다, 바뀌다,

변하다　　　　　　　　　　　　　　E *alter, alterative*

> L. alteratio, alterationis, f. 변경, (변경의 결과로서) 변화　　　E *alteration*

> L. alternus, alterna, alternum 교대로 하는, 서로 주고받는

> L. alterno, alternavi, alternatum, alternare 교대로 하다, 번갈아 하다, 교대로

일어나다　　　　　　　　　　　　E *alternate, alternative*

> L. alternatio, alternationis, f. 교대　　　　E *alternation*

> L. altercor, altercatus sum, altercari 언쟁하다　　　　E *altercate, altercation*

> L. adulter, adultera, adulterum (< ad alterum < ad *to, toward, at, according*

to + alter *another, other*) 변질된, 위조된, 행실이 나쁜, 간음의　　E *adultery*

> L. adultero, adulteravi, adulteratum, adulterare 변질시키다, 간음하다　E *adulterate*

> L. alius, alia, aliud 다른 사람, 다른 남자; 다른 여자; 다른 것

[용례] et alii (et al.) (< *and others*) 그리고 다른 사람들　　　E *et alii (et al.)*

(문법) et 그리고: 접속사

alii 다른 사람들: 남성형 복수 주격

> L. alienus, aliena, alienum 남의, 낯선　　　　　　　　　　　E *alien*

> L. alieno, alienavi, alienatum, alienare 남의 손에 넘기다, 양도하다, 소외

시키다, 멀리하다　　　　E *alienate, alienable, inalienable (unalienable)*

> L. alias (부사) 다른 때에, 다른 데로, 다른 방법으로, 달리　　　E *alias*

> L. alibi (< ali- *other of more than two* + ibi *there*) (부사) 다른 곳에서　　E *alibi*

[용례] et alibi (et al.) (< *and elsewhere*) 그리고 다른 곳에서　　E *et alibi (et al.)*

> L. aliquot (< ali- *other of more than two* + quot *how many*) (형용사, 불변화)

몇몇의, 약간의; (명사, 불변화) 몇몇, 약간　　　　　　　E *aliquot*

> G. allos, allē, allon *other (of the same kind)*　　　　　E *all(o)-*

ipse (m.), ipsa (f.), ipsum (n.) 자신, 자체; 바로 그　　E *ipsi-, (solus 'alone' + ipse 'self' >) solipsism* idem (m.), eadem (f.), idem (n.) 같은 사람, 같은 것; 동일한

　< IE. i- *pronominal stem* (Vide ɪs: *See* E. *id*)

관계대명사

　　　관계대명사는 성, 수, 격에 따라 변화한다. 성과 수는 선행사에 맞추며 격은 관계절에 맞춘다. 관계대명사가 전치사의 지배를 받을 때에는 전치사를 관계대명사 앞에 놓는다. 다만 전치사 cum 만은 관계대명사 뒤에 붙여 쓸 수 있다.

qui (m.), quae (f.), quod (n.)

	단 수			복 수		
	남성	여성	중성	남성	여성	중성
주격	qui	quae	quod	qui	quae	quae
속격	cujus	cujus	cujus	quorum	quarum	quorum
여격	cui	cui	cui	quibus	quibus	quibus
대격	quem	quam	quod	quos	quas	quae
탈격	quo	qua	quo	quibus	quibus	quibus

qui (m.), quae (f.), quod (n.) (관계대명사)

> **E** (quorum vos . . . unum (duos, *etc.*) esse volumus *'of whom we wish that you . . . be one (two, etc.)'* >) ***quorum***

[용례] Non caret is qui non desiderat. 욕망하지 않는 자는 아쉬움이 없다 (Marcus
　　　Tullius Cicero, 106-43 B.C.E.)
　　　(문법) non 아니: 부사
　　　　caret 없다, 모자라다, 아쉽다: 능동태 직설법 현재 단수 삼인칭
　　　　　< careo, carui, caritum, carēre
　　　　is 그 사람은: 지시대명사, 남성 단수 주격; caret의 주어, 관계대명사
　　　　　qui의 선행사 < is (m.), ea (f.), id (n.)
　　　　qui *who*: 관계대명사, 남성 단수 주격; 선행사는 is, desiderat의 주어
　　　　desiderat 욕망하다: 능동태 직설법 현재 단수 삼인칭
　　　　　< desidero, desideravi, desideratum, desiderare

[용례] status quo (< *status in which (the things are)*) 현 상태대로, 현상 유지　　**E** *status quo*

(문법) status 상태: 남성 단수 주격 < status, status, m.

quo *in which*: 관계대명사, 남성형 단수 탈격

[용례] (causa) sine qua non (< *(a cause) without which not (a thing can be done)*)

없으면 안 되는 원인, 필수조건

(문법) causa 까닭, 원인: 단수 주격 < causa, causae, f.

sine 없이: 전치사, 탈격지배

qua *which*: 관계대명사, 여성형 단수 탈격

non 아니: 부사

[용례] sine quo non (< *without whom not (a thing can be done)*)

없으면 안 되는 사람

(문법) sine 없이: 전치사, 탈격지배

quo *whom*: 관계대명사, 남성형 단수 탈격

non 아니: 부사

[용례] quod erat demonstrandum (< *what was to be demonstrated*) (이상이) 증명되어야

할 것이었다, 증명 끝

(문법) quod *what*: 관계대명사, 중성형 단수 주격

erat 이었다: esse 동사, 직설법 과거 단수 삼인칭

demonstrandum 증명되어야 할: 수동태 미래분사, 중성형 단수 주격

< demonstro, demonstravi, demonstratum, demonstrare

< IE. k^{w}o-, k^{w}i- *stem of interrogative and relative pronouns* (Vide infra)

의문대명사

의문대명사는 명사적으로 사용하는 것과 형용사적으로 사용하는 것 두 가지가 있다. 명사적 의문대명사는 관계대명사와 비슷하게 변화하며, 형용사적 의문대명사는 관계대명사와 똑같이 변화한다.

quis (m.), quis (f.), quid (n.) (명사적 의문대명사) 누구,

무엇　E (quid nunc? *'what now?'* > *'a person who constantly asks 'What now?' '* >) *quidnunc*

< IE. k^{w}o-, k^{w}i- *stem of interrogative and relative pronouns* (Vide infra)

qui (m.), quae (f.), quod (n.) (형용사적 의문대명사) 어떤, 어느

< IE. k^{w}o-, k^{w}i- *stem of interrogative and relative pronouns* (Vide infra)

quot (불변화) (의문형용사) 얼마나 많은

> quoties (quotiens) (부사) 몇 번, 몇 번이나

E *quotient* (< 'the number of times one number is contained in another as ascertained by division')

> quotidie (부사) 날마다

> quotidianus, quotidiana, quotidianum (형용사) 날마다의, 일상의   **E** *quotidian*

> aliquot (< alius *other* + quot *how many*) (불변화) (형용사) 몇, 몇몇, 약간의; (명사)
몇몇, 몇 사람   **E** *aliquot*

< IE. kʷo-, kʷi- *stem of interrogative and relative pronouns* (Vide infra)

quotus (m.), quota (f.), quotum (n.) (< quot *how many*) (의문형용사) 몇,

몇째   **E** (quota pars *'how great a part'* >) *quota*

> quoto, quotavi, quotatum, quotare (< *mark a book with numbers or marginal refer-
ences*) 번호를 매기다, 번호로 구분하다, 인용하다, 시세를 매기다, 견적하다   **E** *quote*

> quotatio, quotationis, f. 인용, 시세, 견적   **E** *quotation*

< IE. kʷo-, kʷi- *stem of interrogative and relative pronouns* (Vide infra)

qualis (m.), qualis (f.), quale (n.) (의문형용사) (성질·품질이) 어떤

> qualitas, qualitatis, f. 질(質)   **E** *quality*

> qualitativus, qualitativa, qualitativum 질적(質的)인   **E** *qualitative*

> qualifico, qualificavi, qualificatum, qualificare (< qualis *of what kind, of such a kind*
+ -ficare (< facĕre) *to make*) 성질을 부여하다, 성질을 나타내다   **E** *qualify, qualification*

< IE. kʷo-, kʷi- *stem of interrogative and relative pronouns* (Vide infra)

quantus (m.), quanta (f.), quantum (n.) (의문형용사) 얼마나 큰, 얼마나 많은   **E** *quantile*

> quantum, quanti, n. 얼마나 큰 것, 얼마 만큼의 것, ~ 만큼 큰 것, ~ 만큼의 것   **E** *quantum*

[용례] quantum satis (q.s.) (< *as much as is needed to achieve the desired
result, but not more*) 적당량   **E** *quantum satis (q.s.)*

(문법) quantum ~ 만큼의 양을: 단수 대격

satis 충분히, 필요한 만큼: 부사 < satis

> quantitas, quantitatis, f. 양(量)   **E** *quantity, (quantity >) quantitation*

> quantitativus, quantitativa, quantitativum 양적(量的)인   **E** *quantitative*

> quantifico, quantificavi, quantificatum, quantificare (< quantus *how great, how much*
+ -ficare (< facĕre) *to make*) 양을 정하다, 양을 나타내다,
정량화하다   **E** *quantify, quantification*

< IE. kʷo-, kʷi- *stem of interrogative and relative pronouns*

E *who, whose, whom, what, why, which, how, when, whence, whither, where, whether,
neither* (< *'no whether'*), *either*

> L. quando (의문부사) 언제   **E** (suggested) *cue*

> L. quam (접속사) 만큼, ~보다; (부사) 얼마나

> L. quasi (< quam *as, than, how* + si *if*) (접속사) ~(이)기나 한 듯이; (부사) 얼추,
준(準)   **E** *quasi, (quasi-stellar >) quasar, quasi-*

> L. ubi (의문부사) 어디에; (관계부사) ~ 곳에; (부정(不定)부사) 어디든지

> L. ubique (< ubi *where* + -que *and*) (부사) 어디든지

> L. ubiquitas, ubiquitatis, f. 널리 존재함, 두루 퍼져 있음, 편재(遍在)

> **E** *ubiquity, ubiquitous, ubiquitin, (ubiquitous + quinone(s) > 'its widespread distribution and properties' >)* ***ubiquinone(s)***

> L. uter, utra, utrum (대명사적 형용사) 둘 중 하나

> L. neuter, neutra, neutrum (< ne *not* + uter *either of two*) (대명사적 형용사)
둘 다 ~ 아니 (Vide NON; *See* E. *non-*)

부정(不定)대명사

nemo, neminis (nullius), m., f. 아무도 ~ 아니

nihil, n. (불변화) 아무것도 ~ 아니, 무(無) (Vide NON; *See* E. *non-*)

quisque (m.), quaeque (f.), quodque (n.) (< quis, quae, quod + -que *and* (전접 前接)
연계접속사, 일반화 접사) 각자, 각 (형용사적 부정대명사; 관계대명사의 변화를 따름)

[용례] quaque die (q.d.) 매일
quaque hora (q.h.) 매시간
(문법) quaque 각: 여성형 단수 탈격
die 날짜에: 단수 탈격 < dies, diei, m. 날; f. 날짜
hora 시간에: 단수 탈격 < hora, horae, f.

E *quaque die (q.d.)*
E *quaque hora (q.h.)*

대명사적 형용사

원래 형용사이나 명사적으로도 사용한다. 형용사와 비슷하게 변화한다.

alius (m.), alia (f.), aliud (n.) 다른 사람, 다른 남자; 다른 여자; 다른 것

	단 수			복 수		
	남성	여성	중성	남성	여성	중성
주격	alius	alia	aliud	alii	aliae	alia
속격	alterius (alius)	alterius (alius)	alterius (alius)	aliorum	aliarum	aliorum
여격	alii	alii	alii	aliis	aliis	aliis

대격	alium	aliam	aliud	alios	alias	alia
탈격	alio	alia	alio	aliis	aliis	aliis

unus, una, unum 하나의 (Vide IE. oi-no- *one; See* E. *one*)

solus, sola, solum 홀로 (Vide IE. s(w)e- *pronoun of the third person and reflexive; See* E. *suicide*)

totus, tota, totum 온, 전 (Vide ᴛᴏᴛᴜs; *See* E. *total*)

nullus, nulla, nullum (< ne *not* + ullus, ulla, ullum *any*) 아무 ~도 아니, 하나도 없는, 무효의 (Vide ɴᴏɴ; *See* E. *non-*)

neuter, neutra, neutrum (< ne *not* + uter, utra, utrum *either of two*) 둘 다 ~ 아니 (Vide ɴᴏɴ; *See* E. *non-*)

alter, altera, alterum (둘 중에) 다른 하나의 (Vide ɪʟʟᴇ; *See* E. *alarm*)

alius, alia, aliud 다른 사람, 다른 남자; 다른 여자; 다른 것 (Vide ɪʟʟᴇ; *See* E. *alarm*)

▌상관대명사

형용사적으로 사용하는 것과 부사적으로 사용하는 것 두 가지 종류가 있다.

talis …, qualis … (형용사적 상관대명사) ~같은

[용례] Qualis pater, talis filius. 그 아버지에 그 아들
(문법) qualis 어떠한: 형용사적 상관대명사, 남·여성 단수 주격 < qualis, quale
pater 아버지: 단수 주격 < pater, patris, m.
talis 이러한: 형용사적 상관대명사, 남·여성 단수 주격 < talis, tale
filius 아들: 단수 주격 < filius, filii, m.

toties …, quoties … (부사적 상관대명사) ~ 만큼 그 만큼 많이

형용사

　　라틴어 형용사는, 어간을 그대로 둔 채 어미를 바꿈으로써, 성과 수와 격을 드러낸다. 어간은 단수 속격에서 어미를 떼어내고 남은 부분이며, 형용사의 변화뿐 아니라 파생어나 합성어를 만들 때에도 축의 역할을 한다.

　　라틴어사전은 남·여·중성형의 단수 주격을 제시한다. 명사의 경우와 달리 단수 속격을 제시하지 않는 것은 남·여·중성형에 따라 바뀌는 단수 주격의 꼴만으로도 어간을 알 수 있기 때문이다. 남·여성형의 단수 주격이 같은 꼴이고 중성형의 단수 주격만 다른 꼴인 제3변화 제2식 형용사의 경우에는 남·여성형의 단수 주격과 중성형의 단수 주격을 제시하며, 남·여·중성형의 단수 주격이 같은 꼴이고 주격어간과 속격어간이 다른 제3변화 제3식 형용사의 경우에는 단수 주격과 함께 단수 속격을 제시한다.

　　형용사의 성, 수, 격은 수식하는 명사나 대명사의 성, 수, 격과 일치하여야 한다.

형용사변화

●●● 제1·2변화

남성형 변화는 명사의 제2변화 제1식 또는 제2식을 따르며, 여성형 변화는 명사의 제1변화를 따르고, 중성형 변화는 명사의 제2변화 제3식을 따른다.

●●● 제1·2변화 제1식

남성형의 변화가 명사 제2변화 제1식을 따른다.

bonus, bona, bonum 좋은

	단 수			복 수		
	남성	여성	중성	남성	여성	중성
주격	bon-us	bon-a	bon-um	bon-i	bon-ae	bon-a
속격	bon-i	bon-ae	bon-i	bon-orum	bon-arum	bon-orum

여격	bon-o	bon-ae	bon-o	bon-is	bon-is	bon-is
대격	bon-um	bon-am	bon-um	bon-os	bon-as	bon-a
탈격	bon-o	bon-a	bon-o	bon-is	bon-is	bon-is
호격	bon-e	bon-a	bon-um	bon-i	bon-ae	bon-a

---

bonus, bona, bonum (< *useful, efficient, working*) 좋은

> **E** *bonus, boon,* Fr. *bonbon* (< *'good-good:' a name originating in the nursery*), Sp. *bonanza* (< *'fair weather, prosperity'*)

> bonitas, bonitatis, f. 좋음 **E** *bounty*

> bene (부사) 좋게, 잘

>> bene- *well* **E** *bene-, benefaction, benevolent*

>> benignus, benigna, benignum (< + gignĕre *to beget*) 인자한, 어진

>>> **E** *benign, benignant* (< *'on the pattern of malignant'*), *benignancy* (< *'on the pattern of malignancy'*)

> bellus, bella, bellum (*diminutive form*)

예쁜 **E** *beau, belle,* It. *belvedere* (< *'fair sight'*), *embellish*

>> *bellitas, *bellitatis, f. 아름다움 **E** *beauty, beautiful*

>> belladonna, belladonnae, f. (< *perhaps from the use of its juice to add brilliance to the eyes by dilating the pupils* < It. bella donna < L. bella domina *fair lady*) 벨라도나(가지과의 유독 식물) **E** *belladonna*

> beo, **beavi**, beatum, beare 복되게 하다

>> beatus, beata, beatum (*past participle*) 복된

>>> beatitudo, beatitudinis, f. 복됨 **E** *beatitude*

< IE. deu- *to do, to perform, to show favor, to revere*

---

malus, mala, malum 나쁜 **E** (dies mali *'bad days'* >) *dismal,* (It. mala aria *'bad air'* > mal'aria >) *malaria*

> malitia, malitiae, f. (malities, malitiei, f.) 악의 **E** *malice*

>> malitiosus, malitiosa, malitiosum 악의 있는 **E** *malicious*

> male (부사) 나쁘게 **E** (male habitus *'badly had'* >) *malady*

>> male-, mal- *badly, bad*

>>> **E** *male- (mal-), malefaction, malevolent, malaise* (< *'bad ease'*), *malinger* (< *'badly weak'*), *malodorous, malformed, malformation, malnutrition, malabsorption, malposition, malpresentation, malrotation, malocclusion, malfunction, malpractice*

> malignus, maligna, malignum (< + gignĕre *to beget*) 간악한, 사악한 **E** *malign*

>> maligno, **malignavi**, malignatum, malignare 악의를 보이다 **E** *malignant, malignancy, premalignant*

> F. mal, m. (< L. (*neuter* sing.) malum)

sickness **E** F. *grand mal* (< *'grand sickness'*), F. *petit mal* (< *'little sickness'*)

< IE. mel- *false, bad, wrong*

> G. blasphēmein (blasphēmeein) (< (*perhaps*) blas- (< IE. mel-) + phēmē (< IE.
bha- *to speak*) *speech, saying*) to blaspheme, slander

E *blaspheme, blame*

magnus, magna, magnum 큰

E *magnum*

[용례] Magna Graecia 대(大) 그리스 (그리스의 이탈리아 식민도시들)
(문법) magna 큰: 형용사, 여성형 단수 주격
　　　 Graecia 그리스: 단수 주격 < Graecia, Graeciae, f.

> Maia, Maiae, f. (로마 신화) 마이아 여신(증산의 여신; 뒤에 그리스 신화의 Maia와 혼동됨)
　　 > Maius, Maia, Maium 마이아 여신의, 5월의 　E (Maius mensis *'month of Maia'* >) *May*
> magnas, magnatis, m. 거물, 요인 　E *magnate*
> magnitudo, magnitudinis, f. 크기, 위대 　E *magnitude*
> †magnificus, †magnifica, †magnificum (< magnus *great* + -ficus (< facĕre) *making*)
　 웅장한, 훌륭한, 화려한, 과장된 　E *magnificent*
　　 > magnifico, **magnificavi**, magnificatum, magnificare 찬양하다, 확대하다 　E *magnify*
　　　 > magnificatio, magnificationis, f. 찬양, 확대 　E *magnification*
> magister, magistri, m. 장(長), 교사
E *master*, It. *maestro*, (master > (unstressed form) >) *mister*, (master + -ess ,(< L.
-issa 'feminine suffix') >) *mistress*, (mistress > (shortened form) >) *miss*
　　 > magistralis, magistrale 장(長)의, 교사의 　E *magistral*
　　 > magisterius, magisteria, magisterium 권위 있는 　E *magisterial*
　　 > magistratus, magistratus, m. 관직, 관리 　E *magistrate*
> major, major, majus ((gen.) majoris) (비교급) 더 큰 　E *major, mayor*
　　 > majusculus, majuscula, majusculum (< + -culus *diminutive suffix*) 좀더 큰,
　　　 좀더 높은; (문법) 대문자의 　E *majuscule*
　　 > majoritas, majoritatis, f. (소수에 대한) 다수, 성년 　E *majority*
　　 > majestas, majestatis, f. 위엄 　E *majesty*
> maximus, maxima, maximum (최상급) 가장 큰
E *maximum, maximal*, (propositio maxima 'greatest proposition' >) *maxim, maximize*
< IE. meg- *great* 　E *much, mickle*
> G. megas, megalē, mega *large, great, big*
E *meg(a)-, megalith, omega, megal(o)-, megaloblast, cytomegalovirus (CMV), -megaly,
acromegaly, organomegaly*
　　 > G. megistos, megistē, megiston (최상급) *greatest* 　E *almagest*
> (*Sanskrit*) maha-, mahat- *great* 　E *maharajah, maharani, mahatma, Mahayana*

parvus, parva, parvum 작은; 적은 　E *parvovirus* (< 'small virus'); *parvicellular* (< 'of few cells')
< IE. pau-, pou- *little, few* (Vide PUER; *See* E. *puerile*)

multus, multa, multum 많은, *many, much* 　E *multi-, multicellular, multiarticular*
　　 > multitudo, multitudinis, f. 많음, 군중 　E *multitude*

< IE. mel- *strong, great*

> L. melior, melior, melius ((gen.) melioris) (bonus, bona, bonum의 비교급)
더 좋은　　　　　　　　　　　　　　　　　　　　　　　E *meliorism*

> L. melioro, **melioravi**, melioratum, meliorare 더 좋아지게 하다, 나아지게 하다,
개선하다　　　E *meliorate,* (ad *'to'* + meliorare *'to make better'* >) *ameliorate*

paucus, pauca, paucum 적은, 소수의, 드문　　　E *pauci-, paucicellular, pauciarticular*

> paucitas, paucitatis, f. 소수　　　　　　　　　　　　　E *paucity*

< IE. pau-, pou- *little, few* (Vide PUER: *See* E. *puerile*)

densus, densa, densum 빽빽한, 조밀(稠密)한　　　　　　　　E *dense*

> densitas, densitatis, f. 밀도　　　　　　　　E *density, radiodensity*

> condensus, condensa, condensum (< con- (< cum) *with, together*) 몹시 빽빽한,
몹시 조밀한

> condenso, **condensavi**, condensatum, condensare 농축시키다,
응축시키다　　　　　　　　　　E *condense, condensation*

< IE. dens- *dense, thick*

> G. dasys, daseia, dasy *hairy, bushy, rough*　　　　　E *dasyure*

rarus, rara, rarum 성긴, 드문, 희소(稀少)한, 희박(稀薄)한, 희귀(稀貴)한　　　E *rare*

> raritas, raritatis, f. 희소　　　　　　　　　　　　　　　E *rarity*

> rarefacio, **rarefeci**, rarefactum, rarefacĕre (< rarus *rare* + facĕre *to make*)
희박하게 하다　　　　　　　　　　　　　E *rarefy, rarefaction*

< IE. erə- *to separate* (Vide RETE: *See* E. *rete*)

femininus, feminina, femininum 여성의,
암컷의　　　　　E *feminine (f.), femininity, (feminine condom* >) *Femidom*®

< femina, feminae, f. (< *she who suckles*) 여성　E *feminism, feminize, defeminize,* F. *femme (fem)*

> femineus, feminea, femineum 여성의, 여성다운, 여성 같은

> femella, femellae, f. (< + -ella *diminutive suffix*) 젊은 여자　　E *female*

> effemino, **effeminavi**, effeminatum, effeminare (< ef- (< ex) *out of, away
from*) 여자같이 만들다, 여성화하다, 나약해지다　　　E *effeminate*

< IE. dhe(i)- *to suck*

> L. fetus, feta, fetum 비옥한, 새끼 밴

> L. fetus, fetus, m. ((*incorrectly written*) foetus, foetus, m.)
태아(胎兒)　　　　　　　　　E *fetus, fetiparous, feticide; fawn*

[용례] fetus in fetu 태아내태아(胎兒內胎兒)　　　　E *fetus in fetu*
(문법) fetus 태아: 단수 주격
in ~에서: 전치사, 탈격지배
fetu 태아(내): 단수 탈격

> L. fetalis, fetale 태아의 ‖ E *fetal*

> L. feto, −, −, fetare 새끼 치다 ‖ E *fetation*

　　> L. superfeto, −, −, superfetare (< super- *above* + fetare *to produce*
　　offspring) 다시 임신하다

　　　　> L. superfetatio, superfetationis, f. 임신중임신, 과다수태

　　　　　E **superfetation** (< *'fertilization of ova during different ovulatory
　　　　　cycles'*)

　　> L. effetus, effeta, effetum (< ef- (< ex) *out of, away from* + fetus *breeding*)
　　새끼를 낳아 버린, 산고에 지친, 쇠퇴한, 생산력이 없어진 ‖ E *effete*

> L. fecundus, fecunda, fecundum 다산의, 비옥한 ‖ E *fecund, fecundity, fecundability*

　　> L. fecundo, **fecundavi**, fecundatum, fecundare 비옥하게 하다, 수정(受精)
　　시키다

　　　　> L. fecundatio, fecundationis, f. 수정(受精)

　　　　　E **fecundation, superfecundation** (< *'fertilization of ova during the
　　　　　same ovulatory cycle by separate coital acts'*)

> L. felix, (gen.) felicis 풍요한, 행복한

　　> L. felicitas, felicitatis, f. 풍요, 행복 ‖ E *felicity, (felicity >) felicitous*

> L. fello, **fellavi**, fellatum, fellare (젖을) 빨다 ‖ E *fellate, fellator, fellatorism*

　　> L. fellatio, fellationis, f. 구강성교 ‖ E *fellatio*

> L. filius, filii, m. 아들; filia, filiae, f. 딸 ‖ E *filicide,* F. *fils*

　　> L. filialis, filiale 아들의, 자식으로서의, 자식의 위치에
　　있는 E **filial**, *(the first filial generation >)* F_1, *(the second filial generation >)* F_2

　　> L. affilio, **affiliavi**, affiliatum, affiliare (< af- (< ad) *to, toward, at, according
　　to* + filius *son*) 양자를 들이다, 양자로 들어가다 ‖ E *affiliate*

> G. thēlys, thēleia, thēly *female, feminine* ‖ E *thely-*

> G. thēlē, thēlēs, f. *nipple, mammilla, papilla* ‖ E *thel(o)- (thele-)*

　　> L. thelium, thelii, n. 젖꼭지, 유두(乳頭) ‖ E *thelium,* (pl.) *thelia*

　　> L. thelarche, thelarchae, f. (< G. thēlē + archē *beginning*) 유방발육 개시 ‖ E *thelarche*

　　> L. *thelalgia, *thelalgiae, f. (< G. thēlē + algos *pain* + -ia) 유두통 ‖ E *thelalgia*

　　> L. *thelorrhagia, *thelorrhagiae, f. (< G. thēlē + -rrhagia < -rrhag- *stem of*
　　rhēgnynai *to break, to burst*) 유두출혈 ‖ E *thelorrhagia*

　　> L. polythelia, polytheliae, f. (< G. polys *many* + thēlē + -ia) 다유두증, 유두
　　과다증 ‖ E *polythelia*

　　> L. epithelium, epithelii, n. (< *a layer upon the dermal papillae* < G. ep(i)-
　　upon + thēlē + -ium) 상피(上皮); (식물) 신피(新皮), 피막조직

　　　　E **epithelium**, (pl.) *epithelia, epithelial, epithelialize, epithelioid; intraepithelial,
　　　　subepithelial*

　　> L. endothelium, endothelii, n. (< *on the pattern of* epithelium < G. end(o)-
　　< endon *within*) 내피(內皮) ‖ E *endothelium, endothelial*

　　> L. mesothelium, mesothelii, n. (< *on the pattern of* epithelium < G. mes(o)-
　　< mesos *middle*) 중피(中皮) ‖ E *mesothelium, mesothelial*

> L. urothelium, urothelii, n. (< *on the pattern of* epithelium < G. ur(o)-
< ouron *urine*) 요로상피(尿路上皮)　　　　　　　　　　　**E** *urothelium, urothelial*

> G. thēlazein *to suckle, to suck*

> L. Thelazia, Thelaziae, f. (선충) 텔라지아속(屬); 안충(眼蟲)　　**E** *Thelazia*

masculinus, masculina, masculinum 남성의, 수컷의,

남자다운　　　　　　　　　**E** *masculine (m.), masculinity, masculinize, demasculinize*

< masculus, mascula, masculum (< + -culus *diminutive suffix*) 남성의,

수컷의　　　　　　　　　　　　　　　**E** *male*, Sp. *macho*

< mas, maris, m. 남성, 수컷

> (*suggested*) maritus, marita, maritum 결혼의

> maritalis, maritale 결혼의　　　　　**E** *marital, extramarital*

> marito, **maritavi**, maritatum, maritare 결혼시키다, 장가들이다, 시집

보내다　　　　　　　　　　　　　　　**E** *marry, marriage*

< IE. mari- *young woman;* marito- *provided with a bride*

> G. meirakion, meirakiou, m. *boy, lad*

> G. meirakidion, meirakidiou, n. (< + -idion *diminutive suffix*) *little boy*

> L. miracidium, miracidii, n. 흡충섬모유충　　　　**E** *miracidium*

internus, interna, internum 안의　　　　**E** *intern, internment, internal, internalize*

< inter (전치사, 대격지배) 가운데에서, 사이에서

< IE. en *in* (Vide IN: *See* E. *in-*)

externus, externa, externum 바깥의, 외부의, 외래의　　　**E** *extern, external, externalize*

[용례] lamina densa 치밀판(緻密板)　　　　　　　　**E** *lamina densa*

lamina rara interna 내희박판(內稀薄板)　　　　**E** *lamina rara interna*

lamina rara externa 외희박판(外稀薄板)　　　　**E** *lamina rara externa*

(문법) lamina 판: 단수 주격 < lamina, laminae, f. 판, 층

densa 조밀한: 형용사, 여성형 단수 주격 < densus, densa, densum

rara 희박한: 형용사, 여성형 단수 주격 < rarus, rara, rarum

interna 안의: 형용사, 여성형 단수 주격

externa 바깥의: 형용사, 여성형 단수 주격

< exter (exterus), extera, exterum 바깥의

< ex, e (전치사, 탈격지배) 에서, 부터

< IE. eghs *out* (Vide EX. E: *See* E. *ex-*)

aequus, aequa, aequum 같은, 평등한, 평탄한　　　　　　　　　**E** *equi-*

> aequalis, aequale 같은, 평등한, 평탄한　　**E** *equal, (equal >) unequal, equalize*

> aequalitas, aequalitatis, f. 동등, 평등, 균등　　**E** *equality, equalitarian (egalitarian)*

> inaequalis, inaequale (< in- *not* + aequalis *equal*) 같지 않은, 불평등한, 평탄
하지 않은

> inaequalitas, inaequalitatis, f. 부동(不同), 불평등, 불균등   **E** *inequality*

> aequitas, aequitatis, f. 공평, 불편부당(不偏不黨), 형평(衡平), 평면,
평정(平靜)   **E** *equity, (equity >) inequity*

> iniquus, iniqua, iniquum (< in- *not* + aequuus *equal*) 같지 않은, 불평등한, 평탄하지
않은, 부당한, 불의한

> iniquitas, iniquitatis, f. 불평등, 불의, 불법, 죄악   **E** *iniquity*

> aequo, **aequavi**, aequatum, aequare 같게 하다   **E** *equate*

> aequatio, aequationis, f. 같게 함, 등식, 방정식, 반응식   **E** *equation*

> aequator, aequatoris, m. (< (circulus) aequator diei et noctis *the equalizer
of day and night*) 적도(赤道)   **E** *equator, equatorial*

> aequabilis, aequabile 한결 같은, 평등한, 안정된   **E** *equable*

> adaequo, adaequavi, adaequatum, adaequare (< ad- *to, toward, at, according
to* + aequare *to make or to become equal or level*) 같게 하다, 다다르다,
적절하다   **E** *adequate, (adequate >) adequacy, inadequate, inadequacy*

amplus, ampla, amplum 여유 있게 충분히 큰, 널찍한, 커다란, 훌륭한   **E** *ample*

> amplitudo, amplitudinis, f. 넓이, 폭, 진폭, 크기   **E** *amplitude*

> amplifico, **amplificavi**, amplificatum, amplificare (< amplus *large* + -ficare (< facĕre)
to make) 크게 하다, 증폭하다   **E** *amplify, amplifier (amp)*

arduus, ardua, arduum 가파른, 험한, 힘드는   **E** *arduous*

< IE. erədh- *high*

> G. orthos, orthē, orthon *upright, straight,
correct*   **E** *orth(o)-, orthodox, orthopaedics (orthopedics), orthodontics*

bassus, bassa, bassum 낮은   **E** *base, abase, debase, bass, contrabass, bassoon*

< (*possibly*) (*Oscan*) bassus *low*

broccus, brocca, broccum 불쑥 내민, 돌출한, 뻐드렁니의   **E** It. *broccoli (< 'little protruding shots')*

> brocca, broccae, f. 꼬챙이

E *broach, brooch, brochure (< 'pages stitched together'), broker (< 'wine dealer' < 'to
broach, to tap')*

< *Of Celtic origin*

cavus, cava, cavum 우묵한, 파인, 빈

> cavum, cavi, n. 구멍, 굴, 강(腔), 동(洞), 공동(空洞), 와(窩)   **E** *cave*

> cavitas, cavitatis, f. 구멍, 굴, 강(腔), 동(洞), 공동(空洞),
와(窩)   **E** *cavity, (cavity >) cavitary, (cavity >) cavitation*

> cavea, caveae, f. 새장, 우리, 움집, 실(室)   **E** *cage*, ((Dutch) de kooi 'the cage' >) *decoy*

    > caveola, caveolae, f. (< + -ola *diminutive suffix*)

       소포(小胞)   **E** *caveola*, (pl.) *caveolae, caveolar, caveolin, jail (gaol)*

> caverna, cavernae, f. 굴, 바위굴   **E** *cavern*

    > cavernosus, cavernosa, cavernosum 굴이 많은, 움푹하게 파인   **E** *cavernous*

> concavus, concava, concavum (< con- (< cum) *with, together; intensive*)

       오목한   **E** *concave, concavity, biconcave, biconcavity*

> cavo, **cavavi**, cavatum, cavare 움푹하게 하다; 파내다

    > excavo, excavavi, excavatum, excavare (< ex- *out of, away from* + cavare

       to hollow) 움푹하게 하다, 파내다   **E** *excavate*

< IE. keuə- *to swell; vault, hole*

  > L. cumulus, cumuli, m. 더미, 퇴적, 구(丘)   **E** *cumulus*

    > L. cumulo, **cumulavi**, cumulatum, cumulare 쌓다, 축적하다   **E** *cumulate, cumulative*

      > L. accumulo, **accumulavi**, accumulatum, accumulare (< ac- (< ad) *to,*

        toward, at, according to + cumulare *to heap up, to amass*) 쌓아

        올리다, 축적하다   **E** *accumulate, accumulative*

  > G. koilos, koilē, koilon *hollow*   **E** *coel(o)- (cel(o)-), koilocyte*

    > G. koilia, koilias, f. *hollow of the belly, belly, womb,*

      body cavity   **E** *-coele (-cele, -coel), blastocoele*

      > G. koiliakos, koiliakē, koiliakon *of body cavity, belonging to the belly,*

        suffering in the bowels

        > L. coeliacus, coeliaca, coeliacum 복강(腹腔)의   **E** *coeliac (celiac)*

    > G. koilōma, koilōmatos, n. *cavity*

      > L. coeloma, coelomatis, n. 체강(體腔)   **E** *coelom (celom), coelomic (celomic)*

    > L. Coelenterata, Coelenteratorum, n. (< *hollow intestine* < + G. enteron *gut*

      + L. -ata *neuter plural of* -atus -ate) 강장(腔腸)동물   **E** *coelenterate*

    > L. coelacanthus, coelacanthi, m. (< *hollow spines* < + G. akantha *thorn, thistle*)

      실러캔스   **E** *coelacanth*

    > L. koilonychia, koilonychiae, f. (< *spoon nail* < *hollow nail* < + G. onyx *nail*)

      숟가락손발톱   **E** *koilonychia*

  > G. kōos, kōou, m. *hollow, den*

    > G. kōdōn, kōdōnos, m., f. *bell, patrol*

    > G. kōdeia, kōdeias, f. *poppy head*   **E** *codeine*

  > G. kyein *to swell, to be pregnant*

    > G. kyma, kymatos, n. (< *anything swollen*) *wave, billow, surge,*

       sprout   **E** *cymography (kymography)* (< 'drawing in curves')

      > L. cyma, cymatis, n. (cyma, cymae, f.) (식물) 새싹, 취산(聚繖)꽃차례;

       (건축) 반곡선 쇠시리   **E** *cyma (cyme), cymose*

    > G. kyēsis, kyēseōs, f. *pregnancy, conception*

      > L. cyesis, cyesis, f. 임신(姙娠)   **E** *cyesis*

       > L. pseudocyesis, pseudocyesis, f. (< G. pseudēs *false*) 거짓임신,

       가임신(假姙娠)   **E** *pseudocyesis*

> G. kyrios, kyriou, m. (< *strong, powerful* < *swollen*) *lord, master, ruler, owner*　**E** *Kyrie*

> G. kyriakos, kyriakē, kyriakon *of lord*　**E** (kyriakon (dōma) *'lord's (house)'* >) *church*

crudus, cruda, crudum 날 것 그대로의, 거친

E *crude*

> crudelis, crudele 잔인한

E *cruel*

> crudesco, **crudui**, –, crudescĕre (< + –escĕre *suffix of inceptive* (*inchoative*) *verb*)
거칠어지다, 사나워지다

> recrudesco, **recrudui**, –, recrudescĕre (< re– *back, again*) 더치다,
재발하다

E *recrudesce*

< IE. kreuə– *raw flesh*

E *raw*

> G. kreas, kreōs, n. *flesh,*
meat　**E** *creatine* (< *'discovered first in the juice of flesh'*), (creatine >) *creatinine*

> G. pankreas, pankreatos, n. (< pan– (< pas, pasa, pan) *all* + kreas) *pancreas*

> L. pancreas, pancreatis, n. 췌장(膵臟),
이자　**E** *pancreas* (< *'all fleshy, sweetbread'*), *pancreat(o)–, pancreatin*

> L. pancreaticus, pancreatica, pancreaticum 췌장의,
이자의　**E** *pancreatic, pancreatic(o)–*

> G. kallikreas, kallikreatos, f. (< *sweetbread* < *pancreas or thymus of an*
animal, especially as used for food; esteemed a delicacy < kallos *beauty*
+ kreas) *pancreas*　**E** *kallikrein* (< *'found in the human pancreas'*), *prekallikrein*

∽ IE. kreus– *to form a crust, to begin to freeze*

> L. crusta, crustae, f. 더껑이, 버캐, 딱지, 껍질, 살얼음

E *crust, encrust, custard* (< *'compound of eggs and milk'* < *'something covered*
with crust')

> L. crustaceus, crustacea, crustaceum 갑각(甲殼)의,
갑각류(甲殼類)의　**E** *crustaceous, crustacean*

> G. kryos, kryou, n. *frost, ice*

E *cry(o)–, cryosurgery, cryopexy; cryopreservation, cryoprecipitation, cryoglobulin*

> G. krystallos, krystallou, m. *ice, rock crystal* (< *supposed to be a modified or*
permanent form of ice)

> L. crystallum, crystalli, n. 얼음, 수정(水晶), 결정체

E *crystal, crystallize, crystalloid, crystallin(s)* (< *'protein(s) isolated from*
crystalline lens')

> G. krystallinos, krystallinē, krystallinon *of ice, of crystal*

> L. crystallinus, crystallina, crystallinum 수정의, 수정 같은,
결정체의　**E** *crystalline, paracrystalline*

curvus, curva, curvum 굽은

E *curve, curvilinear (curvilineal)*

> curvo, **curvavi**, curvatum, curvare (곡선으로) 구부리다, 휘다,
(뜻·마음을) 굽히게 하다　**E** *curb* (< *'strap fastened to the bit'*)

> curvatura, curvaturae, f. 굽이, 만곡(灣曲), 곡률(曲率)　**E** *curvature*

< IE. (s)ker– *to turn, to bend*

> L. crispus, crispa, crispum 곱슬곱슬한, (양배추 잎이 싱싱하여) 똘똘 말린, (음식물이)

바삭바삭한, 부서지기 쉬운, (공기·날씨가) 상쾌한, (의미가) 명쾌한   **E** *crisp (crispy)*

> L. crispo, **crispavi**, crispatum, crispare 곱슬곱슬하게 하다   **E** *crispate*

> L. crista, cristae, f. (닭의) 볏, 도가머리, 맨드라미, 투구의 깃털;

능(稜), 능선(稜線)   **E** *crista, (pl.) cristae, crest, (perhaps) crease*

[용례] crista galli 계관(鷄冠), 볏돌기   **E** *crista galli*

crista ampullaris 팽대부 능선   **E** *crista ampullaris*

(문법) crista 볏, 능선: 단수 주격

ampullaris 팽대부의: 형용사, 남·여성형 단격 주격

< ampullaris, ampullare < ampulla, ampullae, f. 단지; 팽대부

> L. cristatus, cristata, cristatum 볏을 가진, 도가머리 있는, 장식 깃털 달린   **E** *cristate*

> (*suggested*) L. cortina, cortina, f. 가마솥, 장막, 휘장   **E** *curtain*

> G. kyrtos, kyrtē, kyrton *curved, arched, bulging, convex*   **E** *kurtosis*

> G. korōnē, korōnēs, f. *curved object, handle of a door, tip of a bow (on which the bowstring was hooked), wreath*

> L. corona, coronae, f. 관(冠), 화관, 왕관, 영예

> L. coronalis, coronale 관의, 화관의, 관 모양의; 관상봉합의, 관상면의   **E** *coronal*

> L. coronarius, coronaria, coronarium 관의, 화관의, 관 모양[冠狀]의; 관상

동맥의, 관상정맥의, 심장의   **E** *coronary*

> L. corolla, corollae, f. (< + -ola *diminutive suffix*) 작은 화관; 꽃부리,

화관   **E** *corolla*

> L. corollarium, corollarii, n. (< *money paid for a small garland, gratuity*) 선물, 덤으로 주는 물건; 부가 결론   **E** *corollary*

> L. corono, **coronavi**, coronatum, coronare 관을 씌워주다, 장식하다

> L. coronatio, coronationis, f. 대관식   **E** *coronation*

> G. kirkos, kirkou, m. *ring, circle, bracelet*

> L. circus, circi, m. 원, (원형의) 경기장   **E** *circus*

> L. circulus, circuli, m. (< + -ulus *diminutive suffix*) 원, 고리, 순환,

회전, 원형의 물건, 모임

> L. circularis, circulare 둥근, 원형의, 회람의   **E** *circular*

> L. circulor, circulatus sum, circulari 원형을 이루다,

순환하다   **E** *circulate, circulatory*

> L. circulatio, circulationis, f. 순환(循環)   **E** *circulation*

> L. semicirculus, semicirculi, m. (< semi- *half*) 반원   **E** *semicircle*

> L. semicircularis, semicirculare 반원의, 반고리의   **E** *semicircular*

> L. circinus, circini, m. 콤파스

>L. circino, **circinavi**, circinatum, circinare 원을 그리다   **E** *circinate*

> L. circo, **circavi**, circatum, circare (걸어서) 한 바퀴 돌아오다   **E** *search, research*

> L. circa (부사; 전치사, 대격지배) 주위에, 무렵에, 경에   **E** *circa (ca., c.)*

> L. circa- *about*   **E** *circa-,* (circa *'about'* + dies *'day'* >) *circadian*

> L. circum (부사; 전치사, 대격지배) 둘러싸고, 두루

> L. circum- *around*   **E** *circum-*

> G. krikos, krikou, m. *ring, circle, bracelet*   **E** *cricoid*

> IE. (s)kerb- *to turn, to bend*   **E** *scorch, rimple, ramp, rampant, shrimp*

> IE. kreuk- *to turn, to bend*

> L. crux, crucis, f. 십자가, 십자가형(刑)

> **E** ***cross, across, cruise*** *(< 'to sail crossing to and fro'),* (instantia crucis *'crucial instance, a metaphor from a crux or finger-post at bifurcation of a road'* >) ***crucial, cruciform, crusade***

> L. cruciatus, cruciata, cruciatum 십자형(型)의   **E** *cruciate*

> L. crucio, **cruciavi**, cruciatum, cruciare 십자가형(刑)에 처하다, 고문하다

> L. excrucio, **excruciavi**, excruciatum, excruciare (< ex- *out of, away from; intensive* + cruciare *to torment*) 큰 고통을 주다   **E** *excruciate*

deliciosus, deliciosa, deliciosum 쾌감을 주는, 맛있는   **E** *delicious*

< delicia, deliciae, f. 쾌락, 귀여움

> delicatus, delicata, delicatum 쾌감을 주는, 맛 좋은, 풍미 있는, 부드러운, 섬세한, 미묘한   **E** *delicate, delicacy, delicatessen*

< delicio, -, -, delicĕre (< de- *apart from, down, not; intensive* + lacĕre *to entice*) 마음을 끌다, 유혹하다

> (*frequentative*) delecto, **delectavi**, delectatum, delectare 즐겁게 하다, 기쁨을 주다   **E** *delectable, delight, dilettante (< 'a lover of arts')*

< lacio, -, -, lacĕre 속이다

> elicio, **elicui**, elicitum, elicĕre (< e- *out of, away from* + lacĕre *to entice*) 끌어 내다, 일으키다   **E** *elicit*

< IE. lek- *twig, snare*

> L. laqueus, laquei, m. 고를 낸 매듭, 올가미, 그물, 음모, 계략   **E** *lace, lasso*

ebrius, ebria, ebrium 술 취한, 도취한

> ebrietas, ebrietatis, f. 술 취함, 명정(酩酊)   **E** *ebriety, (ebriety >) inebriety*

> ebrio, **ebriavi**, ebriatum, ebriare 취하게 하다

> inebrio, **inebriavi**, inebriatum, inebriare (< in- *in, on, into, toward* + ebriare *to intoxicate*) 만취시키다   **E** *inebriate, inebriation*

> sobrius, sobria, sobrium (< se- *apart, without* + ebrius *drunk*) 술을 삼가는, 술

기운 없는, 제정신의, 절제하는

> sobrietas, sobrietatis, f. 금주, 절제

< IE. egʷh- *to drink*

E *sober*

E *sobriety*

---

facetus, faceta, facetum 멋진, 재치 있는, 익살스러운

> facetia, facetiae, f. 재치, 익살

< IE. ghwokw- *to twinkle, to shine*

E (pl.) *facetiae, facetious*

---

ferus, fera, ferum 사나운

> ferox, (gen.) ferocis 사나운

> ferocitas, ferocitatis, f. 사나움, 흉포함

< IE. ghwer- *wild beast*

> G. thēr, thēros, m. *wild beast*

> G. thērion, thēriou, n. (< + -ion *diminutive suffix*) *little wild beast*

> G. thēriakos, thēriakē, thēriakon *of little wild beast*

E *feral, ferine, fierce*

E *ferocious*

E *ferocity*

E *theroid, theropod*

E *theri(o)-, theriogenology, dinothere*

E *treacle* (< 'antidote against venom')

---

flaccidus, flaccida, flaccidum 축 늘어진, 처진, 무기력한

< flaccus, flacca, flaccum 축 늘어진, 처진

E *flaccid, (flaccid >) flaccidity*

---

francus, franca, francum 프랑크인의, (*only Franks had full freedom in Frankish Gaul* >) 자유로운

E *frank*, It. *lingua franca* (< 'common hybrid language' < 'European (Frankish) language used in the eastern Mediterranean'), *franchise* (< 'freedom from restriction'), *frankincense* (< 'high-quality incense')

< Francus, Franci, m. 프랑크 사람

< (*of Germanic root*) Frankon- (< *javelin*) *Frank*

> L. Francia, Franciae, f. (< *land of Franks*) 프랑스

E *Frank, French*

E *France, francium (Fr)*

---

geminus, gemina, geminum 쌍둥이의, 짝지은, 같이 생긴

> gemini, geminorum, m. (pl.) 쌍둥이 형제; (천문) (Gemini) 쌍둥이좌

E *Gemini*

> gemellus, gemella, gemellum (< + -ellus *diminutive suffix*) 작은 쌍둥이의, 짝지은

[용례] musculus gemellus 쌍자근

E *gemellus (muscle)*, (pl.) *gemelli (muscles)*

(문법) musculus 근육, 근: 단수 주격 < musculus, musculi, m.

gemellus: 형용사, 남성형 단수 주격

> bigeminus, bigemina, bigeminum (< bis *twice*) 두 쌍의, 둘이 짝지은

E (*neuter* sing. 'one of the bigemina' >) *bigeminum*, (pl.) *bigemina, bigeminal, bigeminy*

> tergeminus, tergemina, tergeminum (< ter *thrice*) 세 쌍의, 셋이 짝지은

trigeminus, trigemina, trigeminum (< tri- *three*) 세 쌍의, 셋이 짝지은   E *trigeminal, trigeminy*

> quadrigeminus, quadrigemina, quadrigeminum (< quadri- *four*) 네 쌍의,

넷이 짝지은   E *quadrigeminal, quadrigeminy*

[용례] corpora quadrigemina (< *the superior and inferior colliculi*

considered together) 네둔덕   E *corpora quadrigemina*

(문법) corpora 몸, 체(體): 복수 주격 < corpus, corporis, n.

quadrigemina: 형용사, 중성형 복수 주격

< IE. yem- *to pair*

gratus, grata, gratum 마음에 드는, 고마운   E *grateful*

> gratia, gratiae, f. 호의, 우호, 우아, 은혜,

감사   E *grace, gracious, graceful,* (gratiis (abl. pl.) *'out of favor'* > (*contracted*) >) *gratis*

> gratitudo, gratitudinis, f. 사의(謝意)   E *gratitude*

> gratuitus, gratuita, gratuitum 무상(無償)의   E *gratuitous*

> gratuitas, gratuitatis, f. 은전(恩典), 축의금, 팁   E *gratuity*

> gratulor, gratulatus sum, gratulari (남의 경사를) 기뻐하다

> congratulor, congratulatus sum, congratulari (< con- (< cum) *with, together* +

gratulari *to manifest or express one's joy*) 축하하다   E *congratulate*

> gratifico, gratificavi, gratificatum, gratificare (< gratus *pleasing* + -ficare (< facĕre)

to make) 만족시키다   E *gratify*

> *adgrato, *adgratavi, *adgratatum, *adgratare (< ad- *to, toward, at, according to* +

gratus *pleasing*) 동의하다   E *agree, disagree*

< IE. gʷerə- *to favor*   E (*probably*) *bard* (< *'he who makes praises'*)

grossus, grossa, grossum 굵은, 두꺼운; 총계의, 눈으로 보이는

E *gross, grossly, engross, grocery* (< *'selling food and household goods in the gross, in large
quantities'*)

< IE. gʷres- *thick, fat*

largus, larga, largum 크고 널찍한, 풍부한, 마음이 넓은, 헤픈   E *large, enlarge,* lt. *largo*

< (*possibly*) IE. lai- *fat*

> L. lardum, lardi, n. (laridum, laridi, n.) (돼지) 비계, 라드   E *lard*

> L. lardaceus, lardacea, lardaceum (돼지) 비계의, 라드의   E *lardaceous*

> G. larinos, larinē, larinon *fattened*

latus, lata, latum 넓은   E *latifundium*

> latitudo, latitudinis, f. (지리·천문) 씨줄, 위도; (사진) 관용도   E *latitude*

> dilato, dilatavi, dilatatum, dilatare (< dis- *apart from, down, not* + latus *broad, wide*)

넓히다, 확장(擴張)시키다   E *dilatate (dilate), vasodilate*

> dilatatio, dilatationis, f. (dilatio, dilationis, f. (*etymologically incorrect*)) 확장,

팽창(膨脹)   **E** *dilatation (dilation)*

> dilatator, dilatatoris, m. (dilator, dilatoris, m. (*etymologically incorrect*)) 보급자,

확장근, 확장기   **E** *dilatator (dilator)*

[용례] musculus dilatator pupillae (musculus dilator pupillae) 동공확대근,

산동근(散瞳筋)   **E** *dilator pupillae (muscle)*

(문법) musculus 근육, 근: 단수 주격 < musculus, musculi, m.

dilatator (dilator) 확장근: 단수 주격 (musculus와 동격)

pupillae 동공의: 명사, 단수 속격 < pupilla, pupillae, f.

< IE. stelə- *to extend*

> (*suggested*) L. latus, lateris, n. 옆구리, 곁, 옆   **E** *laterad (< + -ad 'toward')*

> L. lateralis, laterale 옆구리의, 옆의

E *lateral, laterality, lateralize, -lateral, unilateral, bilateral, equilateral, ipsilateral, contralateral*

> L. collateralis, collaterale (< *side by side with one another* < col- (< cum) *with, together*) 옆으로 늘어선, 나란히 나아가는, 곁의, 부수적, 방계(傍系)의   **E** *collateral*

> L. quadrilaterus, quadrilatera, quadrilaterum (< quadri- *four* + latus *side*) 사변형의   **E** *quadrilateral*

> (*suggested*) L. later, lateris, m. 벽돌   **E** *laterite*

> L. lateritius, lateritia, lateritium 벽돌의, 벽돌로 된, 붉은 벽돌 색깔의

lascivus, lasciva, lascivum 흥겨워하는, 자유분방한, 외설적인, 색을 좋아하는   **E** *lascivious*

< IE. las- *to be eager, to be wanton, to be unruly*   **E** *list (< 'to please'), listless, lust, wanderlust*

maturus, matura, maturum 때가 다된, 익은, 성숙한   **E** *mature, demure*

> maturitas, maturitatis, f. 성숙, 성숙도   **E** *maturity*

> maturo, **maturavi**, maturatum, maturare 익히다, 성숙하게 하다, 익다, 성숙하다   **E** *maturate*

> maturatio, maturationis, f. 성숙시킴, 성숙해짐, 성숙   **E** *maturation*

> immaturus, immatura, immaturum (< im- (< in-) *not* + maturus *ripe*) 때가 아닌, 익지 않은, 미숙한   **E** *immature, immaturity*

> praematurus, praematura, praematurum (< prae- *before, beyond* + maturus *ripe*) 너무 이른, 일찍 익은, 조숙한   **E** *premature, prematurity*

< IE. ma- *good; with derivatives meaning 'occurring at a good moment, timely, seasonable, early'*

> L. mane (불변화 명사) 아침; (부사) 아침에

> L. Matuta, Matutae, f. (고대 이탈리아) 새벽의 여신

> L. matutinus, matutina, matutinum 이른 아침의, 아침의   **E** *matin, matinee*

mirus, mira, mirum 기묘한, 경탄할 만한

> miror, miratus sum, mirari 기묘히 여기다, 경탄하다, 경탄하는 눈으로 바라보다   **E** *mirage, mirror*

> miraculum, miraculi, n. 경이, 기적   **E** *miracle*

> miraculuosus, miraculuosa, miraculuosum 경이로운, 기적의   **E** *miraculous*

> mirabilis, mirabile 기묘한, 경이로운, 불가사의한   **E** *marvel, marvelous*

> admiror, admiratus sum, admirari (< ad- *to, toward, at, according to* + mirari

to wonder) 경탄하다, 경탄하는 눈으로 바라보다   **E** *admire*

< IE. smei- *to laugh, to smile*   **E** *smirk, smile*

novus, nova, novum 새로운   **E** (nova stella *'new star'* >) *nova*

> novicius, novicia, novicium (novitius, novitia, novitium) 풋내기의, 신참의   **E** *novice*

> novo, **novavi**, novatum, novare 새롭게 하다   **E** *novation*

> innovo, **innovavi**, innovatum, innovare (< in- *in, on, into, toward* + novare

to make new) 쇄신하다   **E** *innovate*

> renovo, renovavi, renovatum, renovare (< re- *back, again* + novare *to make*

new) 쇄신하다   **E** *renovate*

> novellus, novella, novellum (< + -ellus *diminutive suffix*) 갓난, 햇, 풋   **E** *novel, novelty*

< IE. newo- *new* (*related to* IE. nu- *now*)   **E** *new, renew, renewal*

> G. neos, nea, neon *new, early, young*   **E** *neon (Ne)* (< *'new element'*), *neo-, misoneism*

> (*comparative*) G. neōteros, neōtera, neōteron   **E** *neoteric*

> G. neanias, neaniou, m. *young man, youth*

> G. nearos, neara, nearon *fresh, youthful*

> G. nēros, nēra, nēron *fresh* (*used of fish and of water*), *wet, damp*

E *Nereus, Nereid, aneroid* (< *'a barometer, in which the pressure of the air is measured, not by the height of a column of mercury or other fluid which it sustains, but by its action on the elastic lid of a box exhausted of air'*)

nudus, nuda, nudum 벗은   **E** *nude*

> nudo, **nudavi**, nudatum, nudare 벗기다

> denudo, **denudavi**, denudatum, denudare (< de- *apart from, down, not; intensive*

+ nudare *to make naked*) 발가벗기다   **E** *denude, denudate*

< IE. nog^w- *naked*   **E** *naked*

> G. gymnos, gymnē, gymnon (< *with metathesis due to taboo deformation*) *naked*   **E** *gymn(o)-*

> G. gymnazein *to train naked, to train, to exercise*   **E** *gymnastics*

> G. gymnasion, gymnasiou, n. *exercise, place of exercise*

> L. gymnasium, gymnasii, n. (그리스 남자들이 옷을 벗고 신체를

단련하던) 체육장   **E** *gymnasium*

planus, plana, planum 편평한, 평평한, 납작한, 평이한, 명확한

E *plain, plane, plan* (< *'drawing, sketch, or diagram made by projection on a horizontal plane showing the layout of a building, city, area, etc'*), It. (piano et forte *'soft and loud'* >) *pianoforte (piano), plan(i)- (plano-)*

> planaris, planare 평평한, 평면의   **E** *planar*

> planula, planulae, f. (< *flattened form* < + -ula *diminutive suffix*) 플라눌라 (*a larval*

coelenterate)   **E** *planula*

> explano, **explanavi**, explanatum, explanare (< ex- *out of, away from*) 평평하게 만들다,

펴다, 설명하다 ☐**E** *explain, explanation, explanatory*

> applano, **applanavi**, applanatum, applanare (< ap- (< ad) *to, toward, at, according*

to) 누르는 힘을 가해 평평하게 만들다 ☐**E** *applanation*

< **IE.** pelə- *flat, to spread* ☐**E** *field, floor*

> **L.** palma, palmae, f. 손바닥, 수장(手掌), 종려잎, 종려, 종려열매, 승리

☐**E** *palm, palmistry, palmitic acid* (< '*found in palm oil*'), (*naphthenate + palmitate* >) *napalm*

> **L.** palmaris, palmare 손바닥의, (동물) 앞발바닥의, 종려의, 승리의 ☐**E** *palmar*

> **L.** palmatus, palmata, palmatum 손바닥 모양을 한, (동물) 물갈퀴가 있는, 종려

잎 무늬가 있는 ☐**E** *palmate*

> **G.** plassein (< *to shape, to spread out*) *to mold, to form*

> **G.** plasis, plaseōs, f. *molding, formation*

> **L.** -plasia, -plasiae, f. ~형성(形成)

☐**E** *-plasia, -plastic, symplastic* (< '*multinucleated or interconnected*')

> **L.** aplasia, aplasiae, f. (< **G.** a- *not*) 무형성(증)(無形成(症)), 형성

부전(形成不全), 발육부전, 재생불량 ☐**E** *aplasia*

> **L.** hypoplasia, hypoplasiae, f. (< **G.** hyp(o)- *under*)

형성저하(증) ☐**E** *hypoplasia*

> **L.** hyperplasia, hyperplasiae, f. (< **G.** hyper- *over*) 과다 형성,

과형성, 증식(증) ☐**E** *hyperplasia*

> **L.** metaplasia, metaplasiae, f. (< **G.** met(a)- *between, along with,*

across, after) 화생(化生) ☐**E** *metaplasia*

> **L.** dysplasia, dysplasiae, f. (< **G.** dys- *bad*) 형성이상 (< *abnormal*

development), 이형성(異形成) (< *precancerous formation*) ☐**E** *dysplasia*

> **L.** anaplasia, anaplasiae, f. (< *backward formation to the primitive,*

embryonic, or undifferentiated form < **G.** an(a)- *up, upward;*

again, throughout; back, backward; against; according to, similar

to) 역형성(逆形成) ☐**E** *anaplasia*

> **L.** neoplasia, neoplasiae, f. (< **G.** neos *new*) 신생(新生), 신생물

(新生物), 종양(腫瘍) ☐**E** *neoplasia, neoplastic, paraneoplastic*

> **G.** plasma, plasmatos, n. *something molded, something formed, figure, image,*

fiction, forgery

> **L.** plasma, plasmatis, n. 형질(形質), 원형질, 세포질, 장(漿), 혈장(血漿)

☐**E** *plasma* (< '*from which blood is molded or made*'), *plasmin*
(< '*fibrinolytic enzyme in plasma*'), *plasmid* (< '*a genetic structure in a*
cell that replicates independently of the chromosomes; specially any of
the small circular strands of DNA occurring in the cytoplasm of many
bacteria and protozoans' <+ -*id*); *plasm(o)- (plasma-), plasmalemma,*
plasmocyte (plasmacyte, plasma cell) (< '*abundant cytoplasm*'),
-plasma (-plasm), -plasmic, (D. Zytoplasma >) *cytoplasm, ectoplasm,*
endoplasm; nucleoplasm; heteroplasmy (< '*a mixture of more than one*
type of an organellar genome within a cell or individual')

> L. protoplasma, protoplasmatis, n. (< G. prōtos *first*) 최초의
피조물, 최초의 인간; 원형질(原形質)　　　**E** *protoplasm, protoplasmic*

> L. neoplasma, neoplasmatis, n. (< G. neos *new*) 신생물(新生物),
종양(腫瘍)　　　**E** *neoplasm*

> L. cataplasma, cataplasmatis, n. (< G. kat(a)- *down, mis-, according
to, along, thoroughly*) 찜질, 찜질약, 습포(濕布)　　　**E** *cataplasm*

> L. Histoplasma, Histoplasmatis, n. (< G. histos *tissue*) (불완전
곰팡이) 히스토플라스마속(屬)　　　**E** Histoplasma

> L. plasmodium, plasmodii, n. (< G. plasm(o)- + G. -ōdēs *like, resembling*
+ L. -ium *noun suffix*) (1) (*a multinucleate mass of cytoplasm
formed by the aggregation of a number of amoeboid cells, as
that characteristic of the vegetative phase of the slime molds* >)
변형체(變形體), 합포체(合胞體), (2) (*a protozoan of the genus*
Plasmodium, *which includes the parasites that cause malaria* >)
말라리아원충속(原蟲屬), 열원충속(熱原蟲屬)　　　**E** *plasmodium*

> G. plastos, plastē, plaston *molded, formed*

> **E** *plastid* (< '*an organelle in the cytoplasm of a plant cell, usually containing
pigment or food substances*' < + -id < G. -idion '*diminutive suffix*'), -plast,
chloroplast, chromoplast, amyloplast, proteinoplast, elaioplast; blepharoplast
(< '*basal body*')

> G. plastikos, plastikē, plastikon *being molded, belonging to molding,
plastic*

> L. plasticus, plastica, plasticum 틀에 넣어 만드는, 모양을 만드는,
형성력 있는, 가소성(可塑性)의, 소성(塑性)의, 인공적인, 성형의,
조직을 형성하는　　　**E** *plastic, plasticity, plasticizer*

> G. -plastia, -plastias, f. *molding, forming*　　　**E** *-plasty*

> G. emplassein (< em- (< en) *in* + plassein) *to plaster up*

> G. emplastron, emplastrou, n. *plaster, salve*

> L. emplastrum, emplastri, n. 고약, 연고; (식물) 접붙이기　　　**E** *plaster*

> G. planan (planaein) (< *to spread out*) *to lead astray*　　　**E** *aplanatic*
planasthai (*passive*) *to wander*

> G. planētēs, planētou, m. *wanderer*

> L. planeta, planetae, m. 행성(行星), 혹성(惑星)　　　**E** *planet*

> IE. plat-, pletə- *to be flat, to spread*　　　**E** *flat, flatter* (< '*to smooth, to caress with flat hand*')

> L. planta, plantae, f. 발바닥

> L. plantaris, plantare 발바닥의　　　**E** *plantar, plantarflexion*

> L. planto, plantavi, plantatum, plantare 발바닥으로 땅을 고르다, 식물을
심다, 세우다　　　**E** *(verb) plant, plantation*

> L. planta, plantae, f. 식물　　　**E** *(noun) plant, clan* (< '*plant, sprout*')

> L. implanto, implantavi, implantatum, implantare (< im- (< in)
in, on, into, toward + plantare *to plant*) 심다, 단단히 박아
넣다　　　**E** *implant, implantation*

> L. transplanto, **transplantavi**, transplantatum, transplantare (< *trans-*
over, across, through, beyond + plantare *to plant*) 옮겨 심다,
이식(移植)하다

> **E** *transplant, transplantation, autotransplantation* (< *'self'*), *isotransplantation*
> (< *'equal'*), *allotransplantation* (< *'other'*), *xenotransplantation* (< *'foreign'*)

> L. supplanto, **supplantavi**, supplantatum, supplantare (< *sub- under,*
up from under + planta *sole*) 걸어 넘어뜨리다, 딴죽 걸다, 뒤엎다,
대신 들어앉다 **E** *supplant*

> L. plantago, plantaginis, f. 질경이 **E** *plantain*

> G. platys, plateia, platy *flat, broad* **E** *platy-, platybasia*

 > G. Platōn, Platōnos, m. (< *broad-shouldered*) *Plato*

  > L. Plato, Platonis, m. (Platon, Platonis, m.) 플라톤 **E** *Plato (Platon)*

  > G. Platōnikos, Platōnikē, Platōnikon *of Plato*

   > L. Platonicus, Platonica, Platonicum 플라톤의 **E** *Platonic*

 > G. plateia, plateias, f. *broad street*

  > L. platea, plateae, f. 한길, 저자거리,

   안뜰 **E** *place,* Sp. *plaza,* It. *piazza, displace, misplace, replace*

 > G. platanos, platanou, f. *plane-tree*

  > L. platanus, platani, f. 플라타너스 **E** *platanus, plane-tree*

 > G. platynein *to widen*

  > G. platysma, platysmatos, n. (< + -sma *extended form of* -ma
   resultative noun suffix) *a plate*

   > L. platysma, platysmatis, n. 넓은 목근, 활경근(闊頸筋) **E** *platysma*

 > L. plata, platae, f. (편평한) 금속판

> **E** *plate,* (*diminutive*) *platelet, platter, platform* (< *'flat form'*), *platitude* (<
> *'on the pattern of latitude'*), *electroplate,* F. *plateau,* (Sp. plata *'silver*
> *plate'* > Sp. (*diminutive*) *platina* >) *platinum (Pt)*

 > L. Platyhelminthes, Platyhelminthium, m. (pl.) (< + G. helmins, helminthos,
  m. *parasitic worm*) (기생충) 편형동물문(扁形動物門) **E** *platyhelminth*

> (*suggested*) G. pleura, pleuras, f. *rib, side, flank*

> **E** *somatopleure* (< *'embryonic body wall'*), *splanchnopleure* (< *'embryonic gut wall'*)

 > L. pleura, pleurae, f. 가슴막, 흉막(胸膜), 늑막(肋膜)

> **E** *pleura, pleur(o)-,* (*pleuritis* >) *pleurisy,* (*pleuritis* >) *pleuritic*

  > L. pleuralis, pleurale 가슴막의, 흉막의, 늑막의 **E** *pleural*

  > L. pleurodesis, pleurodesis, f. (< + G. desis *binding*) 가슴막유착,
   흉막유착, 늑막유착 **E** *pleurodesis*

> IE. plak- *to be flat* **E** *flake, fluke, flaw, flawless*

> L. planca, plancae, f. 널빤지, 널판대기 **E** *plank*

> L. plaga, plagae, f. (< *something flat and extended*) 그물, 올가미

 > L. plagium, plagii, n. 그물, 유괴, 표절

  > L. plagiarius, plagiarii, m. 유괴자, 표절자 **E** *plagiarism*

> L. placeo, **placui**, placitum, placēre (여격지배) 마음에

들다　　　　　　　　　　　　　　　　　　　　　　　　　**E** *please, pleasure, pleasant*

[용례] placebo 나는 (주님의) 마음에 들 것이다 (주님께서 나를 받아주실
　　　　것이다)　　　　　　　　　　　　　　　　　　　　　　**E** *placebo*
　　　　(문법) 능동태 직설법 미래 단수 일인칭; (1) 죽은 자를 위해 부르는
　　　　　　기도 (placebo로 시작한다: Placebo Domino in regione
　　　　　　vivorum (*Psalm*). *I shall please the Lord in the land of
　　　　　　the living.*), (2) 가약(假藥), 위약(僞藥), 플라시보

> L. placitum, placiti, n. 마음의 흡족, 뜻, 결정, 의견, 학설　　　**E** *plea, plead*
> L. placidus, placida, placidum 평온한　　　　　　　　　　　**E** *placid*
> L. placo, **placavi**, placatum, placare (*causative*) 평온하게 하다, 진정
　　시키다, 화해시키다　　　　　　　　　　　　　　　　　　**E** *placate*
　　> L. placabilis, placabile 달래기 쉬운, 화해될 수 있는, 온화한　**E** *placable*
　　　　> L. implacabilis, implacabile (< im- (< in-) *not*) 달래기
　　　　　　어려운, 화해될 수 없는, 용서 없는　　　　　　　　**E** *implacable*
> L. complaceo, **complacui**, complacitum, complacēre (< com- (< cum)
　　with, together; intensive + placēre *to please*) 마음에 들게 하다,
　　마음에 들다　　　　　　　　　　　　　　　　　　　　　**E** *complacent*
> G. plax, plakos, f. *plaque, slab*

E (plakoeidēs (< + eidos *'shape'*) > *'plaquelike'* >) *placoid*, (plakōdēs (< +
eidos *'shape'*) > *'a plaquelike structure of ectoderm in the early embryo, from
which a sense organ develops'* >) *placode*

　　> G. plakous, plakountos, m. *cake, pan-cake*
　　　　> L. placenta, placentae, f. 케이크,
　　　　　　태반　**E** *placenta*, (pl.) *placentae (placentas), (placenta >) placentation*
　　　　　　> L. placentalis, placentale 태반의　　　　　　　　**E** *placental*
　　> L. electroplax, electroplacis, f. (< G. electr(o)- *electric*) 전기판　**E** *electroplax*
　　> L. erythroplakia, erythroplakiae, f. (< G. erythros *red*) 홍색판　**E** *erythroplakia*
　　> L. leukoplakia, leukoplakiae, f. (< G. leukos *bright, white*)
　　　　백색판증　　　　　　　　　　　　　　　　　　　　　**E** *leukoplakia*
　　> L. malacoplakia, malacoplakiae, f. (< G. malakos *soft*)
　　　　연화판증　　　　　　　　　　　　　　　　　　　　　**E** *malacoplakia*
> G. plagos, plagou, n. *side*
　　> G. plagios, plagia, plagion *sideways, slanting, oblique*　**E** *plagi(o)-*
> G. (*possibly*) pelagos, pelagous, n. *open sea*

E *pelagic, archipelago* (< *'an extensive group of islands'* < *'sea studded with
islands'* < *'the Aegean Sea'* < *'the chief sea'*)

pravus, prava, pravum 꾸부러진, 비틀린, 못된, 나쁜
　　> pravitas, pravitatis, f. 기형, 타락, 부패　　　**E** *pravity, (pravity >) depravity*
　　> depravo, **depravavi**, depravatum, depravare (< de- *apart from, down, not; intensive*
　　　　+ pravus *crooked*) 비틀리게 하다, 나빠지게 하다, 타락시키다　**E** *deprave*

> depravatio, depravationis, f. 변질, 악화, 타락　　　　　　　　　　　E *depravation*

< IE. pra- *to bend*

> (*probably*) L. pratum, prati, n. 풀밭, 초원　　　　　　　　　　　E *prairie*

purus, pura, purum 깨끗한, 맑은, 순수한　　　　　　　　　　　　E *pure*

> puritas, puritatis, f. 깨끗함, 순수, 순결　　　　　　　　E *purity, Puritan*

> purgo, **purgavi**, purgatum, purgare (< *purigare < *puragare < purus *pure* + agĕre
to drive, to do) 깨끗이 하다, 정화하다　　　　　　E *purge, purgative, purgatory*

> purifico, purificavi, purificatum, purificare (< purus *pure* + -ficare (< facĕre) *to make*)
깨끗이 하다, 정화하다　　　　　　　　　　　　　　　　　E *purify*

> purificatio, purificationis, f. 정화　　　　　　　　　　E *purification*

< IE. peuə- *to purify, to cleanse*

> (*probably*) L. pius, pia, pium 효성스러운, 애정이 두터운, 나라를 사랑하는, 경건한,
자애로운, 상냥한

E *pious;* (pia mater *'tender mother'* >) **pia, pial, subpial, pia-arachnoid (piarachnoid)**

> L. pietas, pietatis, f. 효성, 애정, 조국애, 경건, 자애　　E *piety, pity,* It. *Pieta*

> L. pio, **piavi**, piatum, piare 종교적으로 정화하다, 속죄하다

> L. expio, expiavi, expiatum, expiare (< ex- *out of, away from; intensive*
+ piare *to seek to appease*) 속죄하다, 보상하다　　　E *expiate*

serus, sera, serum 늦은, 저문, 뒤늦은　　　　　　　　　　　　E *soiree*

> serotinus, serotina, serotinum 늦되는, 저녁의　　　　　E *serotine (serotinous)*

< IE. se- *long,*

late E *side* (< *'long surface, long part'*), **aside, since, syne,** (men *'stone'* + hir *'long'* >) *menhir*

spurius, spuria, spurium 사생(私生)의, 가짜의, 거짓의　　　　　E *spurious*

< *Of Etruscan origin*

vagus, vaga, vagum 이리저리 다니는, 정처 없는, 방랑하는　　　　E *vague*

[용례] nervus vagus 미주(迷走)신경

(문법) nervus 신경: 단수 주격 < nervus, nervi, m.

vagus 이리저리 다니는: 형용사, 남성형 단수 주격

> vagus, vagi, m. 방랑자, 편력자, 무적자, 음유시인; (nervus vagus >)
미주(迷走)신경　　　　　　　　　　　　E *vagus,* (pl.) *vagi, vagal, vag(o)-*

> vagor, vagatus sum, vagari 떠돌아다니다, 방황하다

E *vagarious, vagary,* (extra vagari *'to wander outside'* >) **stray,** (extra vagari *'to
wander outside'* >) **astray,** (extra vagari *'to wander outside'* >) **extravagant**

> vagabundus, vagabunda, vagabundum 떠돌아다니는, 방황하는　　E *vagabond*

< IE. wag- *to be bent*

< (*probably*) IE. wa- *to bend apart, to turn*

> L. vacillo, **vacillavi**, vacillatum, vacillare 흔들거리다, 동요하다   **E** *vacillate*

> L. varus, vara, varum 안쪽 들린, 안으로 구부러진, 내번(內翻)의

varus, vara, varum 안쪽 들린, 안으로 구부러진, 내번(內翻)의   **E** *varus*

   < (*probably*) IE. wa- *to bend apart, to turn* (Vide supra)

valgus, valga, valgum 가쪽 들린, 밖으로 구부러진, 외번(外翻)의   **E** *valgus*

   < IE. wel- *to turn, to roll; with derivatives referring to curved, enclosing objects* (Vide
     VOLVĒRE: *See* E. *volute*)

varius, varia, varium 잡다한, 여러 가지의, 다른, 변하는   **E** *various*

   > varietas, varietatis, f. 잡다함, 변화   **E** *variety*

   > vario, **variavi**, variatum, variare 여러 가지로 변화시키다, 다르게 하다,

     다르다   **E** *vary, variant, invariant, univariate, multivariate*

     > variabilis, variabile 변할 수 있는, 변할 만한   **E** *variable*

     > variatio, variationis, f. 변이   **E** *variation*

     > variantia, variantiae, f. 변동, 변이, 분산   **E** *variance*

   > variego, **variegavi**, variegatum, variegare (< varius *various* + agĕre *to drive, to do*)

     여러 가지로 변화시키다   **E** *variegate*

   > variola, variolae, f. (< *speckled, variegated* < + -ola *diminutive suffix*) 천연두

     (天然痘), 두창(痘瘡), 마마(媽媽)   **E** *variola (smallpox), (variola >) variolation*

     > varicella, varicellae, f. (< + -cella *diminutive suffix*) 수두(水痘), 물마마   **E** *varicella*

  < IE. wer- *high raised spot or other bodily infirmity*   **E** *wart*

   > L. varus, vari, m. 소농포, 작은 부스럼

     > L. (*possibly*) varix, varicis, m., f. 정맥류(靜脈瘤),

      맥관류   **E** *varix, (pl.) varices, (varix >) variceal*

      > L. varicosus, varicosa, varicosum 정맥류의   **E** *varicose, varicosity*

   > L. verruca, verrucae, f. 불쑥 나온 것, 사마귀, 결점, 티   **E** *verruca, (pl.) verrucae, verruciform*

     [용례] verruca vulgaris 보통 사마귀   **E** *verruca vulgaris*

     verruca plana 편평 사마귀   **E** *verruca plana*

     (문법) verruca 사마귀: 단수 주격

      vulgaris 보통의: 형용사, 남·여성형 단수 주격

       < vulgaris, vulgare 서민적, 일반적, 보통의, 통속적, 저속한

      plana 편평한: 형용사, 여성형 단수 주격

       < planus, plana, planum 편평한, 평평한, 납작한, 평이한, 명확한

     > L. verrucosus, verrucosa, verrucosum 사마귀가 많은, 사마귀의, 사마귀

     모양의   **E** *verrucose (verrucous), verrucosity*

vernaculus, vernacula, vernaculum 주인집 태생노예의, 그 고장의, 자기 나라의, 풍토적,

   통속적   **E** *vernacular*

   < verna, vernae, m., f. 태생노예(버릇없는 자로 통하였음), 토착민, 자기 나라에서 태어

난 사람

< (*probably*) *Of Etruscan origin*

verus, vera, verum 참된   **E** *very*

      > veritas, veritatis, f. 진리   **E** *verity, veritable*

      > verifico, **verificavi**, verificatum, verificare (< verus *true* + -ficare (< facĕre) *to make*)

          진실성을 증명하다, 검증하다   **E** *verify*

        > verax, (gen.) veracis 참된, 진실한   **E** *veracious*

          > veracitas, veracitatis, f. 진실성, 정확성   **E** *veracity*

   < IE. werə-o- *true, trustworthy*

맞대보기 1   어미 -os, -ē(-a), -on으로 끝나는 그리스어 제1·2변화 형용사는 -us, -a, -um 으로 끝나는 라틴어 형용사가 되어 위의 변화(제1·2변화)를 따른다.

---

austerus, austera, austerum 시큼한, 딱딱한, 준엄한   **E** *austere*

         > austeritas, austeritatis, f. 시큼한 맛, 준엄, 긴축   **E** *austerity*

      < G. austēros, austēra, austēron (< *making the tongue dry and rough*) *sour,*

         harsh, severe

     < G. auein (hauein) *to dry, to kindle, to singe*

   < IE. saus- *dry*   **E** *sear (sere)*

cardiacus, cardiaca, cardiacum 심장의; (*on the heart side of the body* >) 위(胃)의,

      (위의) 들문(~門)의   **E** *cardiac,* (ostium cardiacum gastris, pars cardiaca gastris >) *cardia*

       [용례] ostium cardiacum gastris (위의) 들문(~門), 분문(噴門)

           pars cardiaca gastris (위의) 들문부(~門部), 분문부(噴門部)

        (문법) ostium 입구: 중성 단수 주격 < ostium, ostii, n.

           cardiacum 심장의: 형용사, 중성형 단수 주격

           gastris 위의: 단수 속격 < gaster, gastris, f. 위, 배

           pars 부: 단수 주격 < pars, partis, f. 부분, 부(部)

           cardiaca 심장의: 형용사, 여성형 단수 주격

      < G. kardiakos, kardiakē, kardiakon (< + -akos *adjective suffix*) *of heart*

     < G. kardia, kardias, f. *heart, mind, soul*

   < IE. kerd- *heart* (Vide COR: *See* E. *courage*)

gastricus, gastrica, gastricum 위의   **E** *gastric*

       [용례] ulcus gastricum (< *gastric ulcer*) 위궤양

          (문법) ulcus 궤양: 단수 주격 < ulcus, ulceris, n.

gastricum 위의: 형용사, 중성형 단수 주격

< G. gastrikos, gastrikē, gastrikon *gastric*

< G. gastēr, gastros, f. *belly, womb, sausage* + -ikos *adjective suffix*

< IE. gras- *to devour* (Vide GASTER: *See* E. *gastrin*)

histolyticus, histolytica, histolyticum (< G. histos *tissue*) 조직을 녹이는

E *histolytic*

[용례] Entamoeba histolytica 이질(痢疾) 아메바

E Entamoeba histolytica

(문법) Entamoeba (체내 기생성) 아메바속(屬): 단수 주격

< Entamoeba, Entamoebae, f.

histolytica 조직을 녹이는: 형용사, 여성형 단수 주격

< G. lytikos, lytikē, lytikon (< + -tikos *adjective suffix*) *histolytic*

< G. lyein *to loosen, to release, to dissolve*

< IE. leu- *to loosen, to divide, to cut* (Vide SOLVĔRE: *See* E. *solve*)

맞대보기 2 어미 -ēs(-es)로 끝나는 그리스어 제3변화 형용사도 -us, -a, -um으로 끝나는 라틴어 형용사가 되어 위의 변화(제1·2변화)를 따른다.

---

thyroideus, thyroidea, thyroideum 방패 모양의, 갑상(甲狀)의, 갑상연골(甲狀軟骨)의, 갑상샘의, 갑상선(甲狀腺)의

E *thyr(o)- (thyre(o)-)*, **thyroid, thyrotropin,** *(thyroid + -n- + -ine > 'the amino acid of thyroid hormones' >)* **thyronine, tetraiodothyronine** *(thyroxine, T₄), (thyr(o)- + ox(y)- + indole > 'after the original erroneous description of its chemical composition' >)* **thyroxine** (T_4)**, triiodothyronine** (T_3)**, hyperthyroidism, hypothyroidism**

> parathyroideus, parathyroidea, parathyroideum (< G. par(a)- *beside, along side of, beyond*) 부갑상샘의, 부갑상선(副甲狀腺)의

E *parathyroid, (parathyroid + hormone >)* **parathormone, hyperparathyroidism, hypoparathyroidism**

[용례] glandula thyroidea (< *thyroid gland, thyroid*) 갑상샘, 갑상선

glandula parathyroidea (< *parathyroid gland, parathyroid*) 부갑상샘, 부갑상선

(문법) glandula 샘, 선(腺): 단수 주격 < glandula, glandulae, f.

< glans, glandis, f. 도토리, 샘, 선(腺)

thyroidea: 형용사, 여성형 단수 주격

parathyroidea: 형용사, 여성형 단수 주격

< G. thyreoeidēs, thyreoeidēs, thyreoeides (< + -o- + eidos, eidous, n. *act of seeing, appearance, shape*) *shield-shaped*

E *thyre(o)- (thyr(o)-)*

< G. thyreos, thyreou, m. *door-stone, large shield*

< IE. dhwer- *door, doorway* (Vide FORENSIS: *See* E. *forensic*)

sigmoideus, sigmoidea, sigmoideum Σ (sigma) 문자 모양의, S 문자 모양의　**E** *sigmoid, sigmoidal*

> [용례] colon sigmoideum (< *sigmoid colon, sigmoid*) S상(狀)결장, 구불결장,
> 　　　구불잘록창자
> 　　　(문법) colon 결장, 잘록창자: 단수 주격 < colon, coli, n.
> 　　　　　sigmoideum S 문자 모양의: 형용사, 중성형 단수 주격
>
> 　< G. sigmoeidēs, sigmoeidēs, sigmoeides (< + -o- + eidos, eidous, n. *act of*
> 　　　*seeing, appearance, shape*) *sigmoid*
> 　< G. sigma *sigma (Σ)*

●●● 제 1 · 2 변화 제 2 식

> 남성형의 변화가 명사 제2변화 제2식을 따른다.

niger, nigra, nigrum 검은

	단 수			복 수		
	남성	여성	중성	남성	여성	중성
주격	niger	nigr-a	nigr-um	nigr-i	nigr-ae	nigr-a
속격	nigr-i	nigr-ae	nigr-i	nigr-orum	nigr-arum	nigr-orum
여격	nigr-o	nigr-ae	nigr-o	nigr-is	nigr-is	nigr-is
대격	nigr-um	nigr-am	nigr-um	nigr-os	nigr-as	nigr-a
탈격	nigr-o	nigr-a	nigr-o	nigr-is	nigr-is	nigr-is
호격	niger	nigr-a	nigr-um	nigr-i	nigr-ae	nigr-a

niger, nigra, nigrum 검은　　　　　　　　　**E** (Sp., *Portuguese*) *negro*

> > nigro, nigravi, nigratum, nigrare 검다, 어둡다, 검게 하다, 어둡게 하다
> > 　> denigro, denigravi, denigratum, denigrare (< de- *apart from, down, not;*
> > 　　*intensive* + nigrare *to blacken*) 검게 하다, 먹칠하다, 중상하다　**E** *denigrate*
> > > nigrico, -, -, nigricare 거무스름하다, 검다
> < IE. nekʷt- *night* (Vide NOX: *See* E. *nocturn*)

ruber, rubra, rubrum 붉은　　　　　　　**E** *bilirubin* (< 'a reddish pigment occurring in bile')

> [용례] nucleus ruber (< *red nucleus* < *brain nucleus, pink in fresh specimens because*
> 　*of iron-containing pigments*) 적색핵(赤色核)　　　**E** *nucleus ruber, rubral*

(문법) nucleus 핵(核): 단수 주격 < nucleus, nuclei, m.

　　　　　ruber 붉은: 형용사, 남성형 단수 주격

> rubricus, rubrica, rubricum 붉게 물들여진　　　　　　　　　**E** *rubric*

　　> rubrico, −, rubricatum, rubricare 붉게 물들이다　　　　**E** *rubricate*

> rubeus, rubea, rubeum 붉은, 적갈색의　　　　　**E** *rubefacient, ruby, rouge*

　　> *rubeolus, *rubeola, *rubeolum (< + -olus *diminutive suffix*)

　　　　> rubeola, rubeolae, f. (< *neuter* pl. *of* *rubeolum) 홍역(紅疫, *measles*)　　**E** *rubeola*

> rubellus, rubella, rubellum (< + -ellus *diminutive suffix*) 붉은 빛 도는

　　> rubella, rubellorum, n. (*neuter* pl. *of* rubellum) 풍진(風疹, *German measles*)　　**E** *rubella*

> rubeo, rubui, −, rubēre 붉다, 붉어지다

　　> rubor, ruboris, m. 적색, 홍안, 부끄러움, 발적(發赤)　　　**E** *rubor*

　　> rubidus, rubida, rubidum 불그레한　　**E** *rubidium (Rb)* (< *'two red lines in its spectrum'*)

　　> rubeosis, rubeosis, f. (< + G. -ōsis *condition*) 피부홍조　　　**E** *rubeosis*

　　> rubesco, rubui, −, rubescĕre (< + -escĕre *suffix of inceptive (inchoative) verb*)

　　　　붉어지다　　　　　　　　　　　　　　　　**E** *rubescent*

< IE. reudh- *red, ruddy*　　　　**E** *red, reddish, infrared (IR), ruddy, rust, rowan*

> L. russus, russa, russum 붉은, 불그스름한　　　　　**E** *russet*

> L. rubus, rubi, m. 나무딸기, 가시덤불

> L. robus, roboris, n. (robur, roboris, n.) *red oak* (붉은 떡갈나무 등의 참나무) > 견고, 힘

　　> L. robustus, robusta, robustum 참나무로 만든 > 견고한　　　**E** *robust*

　　> L. roboro, roboravi, roboratum, roborare 튼튼하게 하다, 강장케 하다　　**E** *roborant*

　　　　> L. corroboro, corroboravi, corroboratum, corroborare (< cor- (< cum)

　　　　with, together; intensive + roborare *to make strong*) 튼튼하게 하다,

　　　　입증하다, 확증하다　　　　　　　　　　　　**E** *corroborate*

> G. erythros, erythra, erythron *red*

E *erythr(o)-, erythroblast, erythrocyte, erythroplakia; erythropoietin, erythremia;*
(erythrocyte >) **erythrose**, *(erythrose >)* **threose**, *(threose >)* **threonine (Thr, T)**
(< 'spatial configuration analogous to that of D-threose')

[용례] erythroblastosis fetalis 태아 적혈모구증(赤血母球症),

　　　　태아 적아구증(赤芽球症)　　　　　　　**E** *erythroblastosis fetalis*

(문법) erythroblastosis 적혈모구증, 적아구증: 단수 주격

　　　　< erythroblastosis, erythroblastosis, f.

　　　　< erythroblast + G. -ōsis *condition*

　　fetalis 태아의: 형용사, 남·여성형 단수 주격 < fetalis, fetale

> G. erythainein *to redden*

　　> G. erythēma, erythēmatos, n. *redness*

　　　　> L. erythema, erythematis, n. 홍반(紅斑)　　**E** *erythema, (pl.) erythemata*

　　　　　　> L. erythematosus, erythematosa, erythematosum 홍반

　　　　　　(紅斑)의　　　　　　　　　　　　**E** *erythematous*

> (*suggested*) G. erysipelas, erysipelatos, n. (< *erysis *reddening* + pella *skin*)

　　> L. erysipelas, erysipelatis, n. 단독(丹毒), 얕은연조직염(~軟組織炎)　　**E** *erysipelas*

sacer, sacra, sacrum 거룩한

　　[용례] os sacrum (< G. hieron osteon *strong ('sacred') bone*) 엉치뼈,

　　　　천골(薦骨)　　　　　　　　　　　　　　　　　　　　　E *sacrum, sacr(o)-*

　　　　[문법] os 뼈: 단수 주격 < os, ossis, n.

　　　　　　sacrum 거룩한: 중성형 단수 주격

　　　> sacralis, sacrale 엉치뼈의, 천골(薦骨)의　　　　　　　E *sacral*

　　> sacro, sacravi, sacratum, sacrare 신에게 바치다　　　　E *sacred*

　　　> consecro, consecravi, consecratum, consecrare (< con- (< cum) *with, together;*

　　　　intensive + sacrare *to dedicate*) 신에게 바치다, 신성하게 하다, 바치다,

　　　　전념하다　　　　　　　　　　　　　　　　　　　　E *consecrate*

　　　> exsecror, exsecratus sum, exsecrari (< ex- *out of, away from* + sacrare *to*

　　　　dedicate) 저주하다, 악담하다, 증오하다　　　　　　E *execrate, execrable*

　　> sacrificus, sacrifica, sacrificum (< sacer *holy* + -ficus (< facĕre) *making*) 제사의

　　　> sacrificium, sacrifii, n. 제사, 제물, 희생물, 희생　　　E *sacrifice*

　　> sacrilegus, sacrilega, sacrilegum (< sacer *holy* + legĕre *to choose*) 성물(聖物)을 훔

　　　치는, 신전을 터는, 신성모독의

　　　> sacrilegus, sacrilega, sacrilegum 성물절도, 신성모독　E *sacrilege*

　< IE. sak- *to sanctify*

　　> L. sancio, sanxi (sancii), sanctum (sancitum), sancire (종교 예식으로) 신성하게 만들다,

　　　(법을) 제정하다

　　　> L. sanctus, sancta, sanctum 거룩한　　　　　　　　　E *saint, sanctify*

　　　　> L. sanctitas, sanctitatis, f. 거룩함　　　　　　　　E *sanctity*

　　　　> L. sanctuarium, sanctuarii, n. 성역　　　　　　　　E *sanctuary*

　　　> L. sanctio, sanctionis, f. (구속력을 가진) 법률, 제재　E *sanction*

liber, libera, liberum 자유로운

　　> liberalis, liberale 자유로운, 너그러운　　　　　　　　E *liberal*

　　> libertas, libertatis, f. 자유　　　　　　　　　　　　　E *liberty*

　　> libero, liberavi, liberatum, liberare 자유롭게 하다, ~에서 벗어나게

　　　하다　　E *liberate, livery* (< *'the dispensing of food, provisions, or clothing to servants'*)

　　　[용례] Lingua liberabit vos. 언어가 너희를 자유롭게 하리라

　　　　　(문법) lingua 언어가: 단수 주격 < lingua, linguae, f. 혀, 소리, 언어

　　　　　　liberabit 자유롭게 하리라: 능동태 직설법 미래 단수 삼인칭

　　　　　　vos 너희를: 인칭대명사, 제2인칭, 복수 대격

　　　> delibero, deliberavi, deliberatum, deliberare (< de- *apart from, down, not;*

　　　　intensive) ~에서 벗어나게 하다, 배달하다, (견해를) 표명하다, (판결을) 내리다,

　　　　분만하다　　　　　　　　　　　　　　　　　　　　E *deliver, delivery*

　　> libertus, liberti, m. (노예신분에서 해방된) 자유인　　E *libertine*

　< IE. leudh- *to mount up, to grow*

　　> G. eleutheros, eleuthera, eleutheron *free*　　　　　　E *eleuther(o)-*

제3변화

> 명사 제3변화에서처럼 단수 속격의 어미가 –is로 끝나며 남·여·중성형에서 단수 속격이 모두 같다. 단수 주격의 꼴에 따라 세 가지로 나눈다.

제3변화 제1식

> 단수 주격이 남성형은 –er, 여성형은 –is, 중성형은 –e로 끝난다.

acer, acris, acre 신, 날카로운, 혹독한

	단 수			복 수		
	남성	여성	중성	남성	여성	중성
주격	acer	acr-is	acr-e	acr-es	acr-es	acr-ia
속격	acr-is	acr-is	acr-is	acr-ium	acr-ium	acr-ium
여격	acr-i	acr-i	acr-i	acr-ibus	acr-ibus	acr-ibus
대격	acr-em	acr-em	acr-e	acr-es	acr-es	acr-ia
탈격	acr-i	acr-i	acr-i	acr-ibus	acr-ibus	acr-ibus
호격	acer	acr-is	acr-e	acr-es	acr-es	acr-ia

acer, acris, acre 신, 날카로운, 혹독한　**E** *acrid, eager* (< 'keen'), (vinum acre 'acrid wine' >) *vinegar*
　< IE. ak- *sharp* (Vide ACUTUS; *See* E. *acute*)

celer, celeris, celere 빠른
　　　　> celeritas, celeritatis, f. 신속, 민첩　　　　　　　　　　　　**E** *celerity*
　　　　> accelero, **acceleravi**, acceleratum, accelerare (< ac- (< ad) *to, toward, at,*
　　　　　　according to + celer *swift*) 가속하다, 촉진하다　**E** *accelerate, (accelerate >) decelerate*
　　< IE. kel- *to drive, to set in*
　　　　swift motion　　　　**E** *hold* (< 'to possess' < 'to tend' < 'to drive (cattle, etc.)'), *halt*
　　　　> L. celeber, celebris, celebre 사람이 많이 모여드는, 붐비는, 경축하는, 유명한
　　　　　　> L. celebritas, celebritatis, f. 번화, 축제, 유명　　**E** *celebrity, (celebrity >) celeb*
　　　　　　> L. celebro, **celebravi**, celebratum, celebrare 붐비다, 경축하다　　**E** *celebrate*
　　　　　　　　> L. celebratio, celebrationis, f. 붐빔, 경축, 축전　　　　**E** *celebration*
　　　　> G. klonos, klonou, m. *turmoil, agitation*
　　　　　　> L. clonus, cloni, m. (< *alternate muscular contraction and relaxation in rapid*
　　　　　　　　succession) 간대성경련(間代性痙攣), 클로누스　　　　**E** *clonus, clonic*
　　　　　　　　> L. myoclonus, myocloni, m. (< *shocklike contractions of muscle(s)* <

G. my(o)- < mys, myos, m. *mouse, muscle*) 간대성근경련(間代性筋痙攣),
근간대(筋間代)   **E** *myoclonus*

> L. paramyoclonus, paramyocloni, m. (< *myoclonus in several*
unrelated muscles < G. par(a)- *beside, alongside of, beyond*)
근간대경련(筋間代痙攣)   **E** *paramyoclonus*

● ● ● 제 3 변화 제 2 식

단수 주격이 남·여성형은 -is, 중성형은 -e로 끝난다. 남성형과 여성형의 어미변화가
같으므로 사전은 남·여성형과 중성형 두 가지만의 단수 주격을 제시한다.

omnis, omne 모든

	단 수			복 수		
	남성	여성	중성	남성	여성	중성
주격	omn-is	omn-is	omn-e	omn-es	omn-es	omn-ia
속격	omn-is	omn-is	omn-is	omn-ium	omn-ium	omn-ium
여격	omn-i	omn-i	omn-i	omn-ibus	omn-ibus	omn-ibus
대격	omn-em	omn-em	omn-e	omn-es	omn-es	omn-ia
탈격	omn-i	omn-i	omn-i	omn-ibus	omn-ibus	omn-ibus
호격	omn-is	omn-is	omn-e	omn-es	omn-es	omn-ia

omnis, omne (< *abundant*) 모든   **E** (dat. pl.) *omnibus (bus), omnium-gatherum, omni-*
< IE. op- *to work, to produce in abundance* (Vide opus; *See* E. *opus*)

dulcis, dulce 감미로운   **E** *dulcin, Dulcinea,* It. *dolce*
< IE. dlku- *sweet*
> G. glykys, glykeia, glyky *sweet*

> **E** *glyc(o)-;* ('sugar' >) ***glycoside(s)*** (< 'on the pattern of glucoside'), ***glycosamine(s)*** (< 'on
the pattern of glucosamine'), ***glycolipid(s)***, ***glycoprotein(s)***, ***glycocalyx***, (glyc(o)- + -an (<
L. -anus 'adjective suffix') >) ***glycan(s)*** (polysaccharide(s)), ***glycosaminoglycan(s)*** (***GAGs***)
(formerly, mucopolysaccharide(s)), ***peptidoglycan(s)*** (< 'peptide chain-linked glycan(s)';
murein(s)), ***proteoglycan(s)*** (< 'protein-linked glycan(s)'), ***glycation*** (< 'nonenzymatic
attachment of a sugar'), ***glycosylation*** (< 'enzymatic attachment of a sugar'); ('glucose' >)
glycogen, ***hyperglycaemia*** (***hyperglycemia***), ***hypoglycaemia*** (***hypoglycemia***), ***glycosuria***
(***glucosuria***); ('sweet' >) (glykyrrhiza 'sweet root' >) ***liquorice*** (***licorice***), ***glycine*** (***Gly, G***) (<
'sweet tasting')

> L. glycolysis, glycolysis, f. (< G. glykys *sweet, 'glucose'* + lysis *loosening*)
해당작용(解糖作用)
E *glycolysis, glycolytic*

> L. glycogenolysis, glycogenolysis, f. (< *glycogen* + G. lysis *loosening*)
당원분해
E *glycogenolysis*

> L. glycogenosis, glycogenosis, f. (< *glycogen* + G. -ōsis *condition*)
당원축적병
E *glycogenosis*

> G. glykeros, glykera, glykeron *sweet*

E *glycerol (glycerin), nitroglycerin, glyceride(s), triglyceride(s); glycol (< 'intermediate in composition between glycerol and alcohol')*

> G. gleukos, gleukous, n. *sweet wine*

E *glucose, (glucose > 'carbohydrate' >) -ose, glucoside(s), glucosamine, glucan(s) (< 'polysaccharide(s) of glucose'), glucagon (< 'hyperglycemic substance, driving glucose'), glucocorticoid(s), glucuronic acid, glucuronide(s)*

> L. gluconeogenesis, gluconeogenesis, f. (< G. gleukos *sweet wine, 'glucose'* + neos *new* + genesis *birth*) 글루코스신생성, 포도당신생성, 당신생, 포도당신생
E *gluconeogenesis*

grandis, grande (*replacing* magnus *in Late Latin and Romance languages*) 거대한, 나이 많은
E *grand, grandeur, grandiose, (grandiose >) grandiosity, grandiloquence*

gravis, grave 무거운, 중(重)한, 중대한, 임신한, 억눌린, 혹독한, 중증(重症)의
E *grave*

> gravitas, gravitatis, f. 무거움, 병세의 중태, 중력
E *gravity (g)*

> gravito, **gravitavi**, gravitatum, gravitare 중력에 끌리다, 침하하다, 끌리다
E *gravitate*

> gravitatio, gravitationis, f. 중력, 침하, 인력

E *gravitation, (gravitation + -on 'a termination of Greek neuter nouns and adjectives' >) graviton*

> gravidus, gravida, gravidum 가득한, 임신한

E *gravid, progravid, (feminine sing. >) gravida (G.), primigravida, secundigravida, tertigravida, multigravida*

[용례] striae gravidarum (pl.) 임신선(姙娠線)
E *(pl.) striae gravidarum*
(문법) striae 선(線): 복수 주격
< stria, striae, f. 도랑, 밭이랑, 폭이 좁은 띠, 조(條), 선(線)
gravidarum 임신부들의: 형용사의 명사적 용법, 여성 복수 속격

> graviditas, graviditatis, f. 임신
E *gravidity*

> gravo, **gravavi**, gravatum, gravare 무겁게 하다, 악화시키다, 괴롭히다
E *grieve, grief*

> aggravo, **aggravavi**, aggravatum, aggravare (< ag- (< ad) *to, toward, at, according to* + gravare *to make heavy*) 더 무겁게 하다, 악화시키다
E *aggrieve, aggravate*

< IE. gʷerə- *heavy*
E *brigade, brigand,* D. *Krieg,* D. *Blitzkrieg,* D. *Sitzkrieg*

> G. barys, bareia, bary *heavy, mighty, burdensome*

> **E** *barytone (baritone), barycenter,* (baryta 'an alkaline earth distinguished by its great weight' >) *barium (Ba), baryon*

> G. baros, barous, n. *weight, burden, plenty, grief*

> **E** *bar, isobar, hyperbaric, bar(o)–, barometer, barotrauma* (< 'injury caused by pressure changes'), *bariatrics* (< 'treatment of weight')

> L. brutus, bruta, brutum 묵직한, 굼뜬, 이성이 없는   **E** *brute*

> L. brutalis, brutale 짐승의   **E** *brutal,* (brutal >) *brutalism*

levis, leve 가벼운

E *levitate* (< 'on the pattern of gravitate'), (levitate >) *levitation*

> levitas, levitatis, f. 가벼움, 경솔   **E** *levity*

> levo, levavi, levatum, levare 가볍게 하다, 위로하다, 들어 올리다

E *lever, levy,* (*carnem levare *'putting away or removal of flesh as food'* >) *carnival*

> levator, levatoris, m. 쉽게 해주는 자, 잠, 도둑, 올림근, 거근(擧筋)   **E** *levator*

    (용례) levator ani 항문거근, 항문올림근

    (문법) levator 거근: 단수 주격

      ani 항문의: 단수 속격 < anus, ani, m. 가락지, 항문

> levamen, levaminis, n. (< *means of raising*) 경감, 완화, 위로   **E** *leaven, unleavened*

> allevo, allevavi, allevatum, allevare (< al- (< ad) *to, toward, at, according to* + *levare to raise*) 치켜세우다, 거들어주다, 완화하다, 경감하다   **E** *alleviate*

> elevo, elevavi, elevatum, elevare (< ex- *out of, away from*) 들어 올리다   **E** *elevate*

   > elevatio, elevationis, f. 올림, 높임, 융기   **E** *elevation*

   > elevator, elevatoris, m. 들어 올리는 사람(물건), 지렛대, 올림근   **E** *elevator*

> relevo, relevavi, relevatum, relevare (< re- *back, again*) (다시) 일으키다, 경감하다, 완화하다, 위로하다   **E** *relieve, relief, relevant* (< 'to bear upon' < 'to lift up'), *irrelevant*

   > *relevantia, *relevantiae, f. (< *to bear upon* < *to lift up*) (당면 문제와의) 관련성, 적합성, 타당성   **E** *relevance*

< IE. leg^wh- *light, having little weight*   **E** *light, lung*

mitis, mite 양순한

> immitis, immite (< im- (< in-) *not* + mitis *mild*) 양순하지 않은

[용례] Coccidioides immitis 콕시디오이데스 이미티스   **E** Coccidioides immitis

   (문법) coccidioides 콕시디오이데스속(屬): 단수 주격

     < coccidioides, coccidioidis, f. (병원성 불완전 진균) 콕시디오이데스속(屬)

    immitis 양순하지 않은: 형용사, 남·여성형 단수 주격

> mitigo, mitigavi, mitigatum, mitigare (< mitis *mild* + agĕre *to drive, to do*) 완화시키다   **E** *mitigate, mitigable, immitigable*

< IE. mei- *mild*

fertilis, fertile 산출하는, 비옥한, 다산의, 임신 가능한,

　　　　가임의　　　**E** *fertile, (fertile >) fertilize, (fertilize >) fertilization, fertilizer, unfertilized*

　　　　　> fertilitas, fertilitatis, f. 생식능력, 출산력　　　　　　　　　　　　**E** *fertility*

　　　　　> infertilis, infertile (< in- *not* + fertilis *productive*) 불모의, 불임의　　**E** *infertile*

　　　　　　　　> infertilitas, infertilitatis, f. 불임증　　　　　　　　　　　　**E** *infertility*

　　　　< fero, tuli, latum, ferre 옮기다, 가져가다, 가져오다, 지니다, 견디다

　　< IE. bher- *to carry, also to bear children* (Vide FERRE; *See* E. *-ferous*)

sterilis, sterile 불모의, 불임의, 무균의　　　　　　　**E** *sterile, sterilize, (sterilize >) sterilant*

　　　　> sterilitas, sterilitatis, f. 불모, 불임, 불임증　　　　　　　　　　**E** *sterility*

　　< IE. ster- *barren*

medialis, mediale 가운데의, 안쪽의

　　　　E *medial,* (medialia (*neuter* pl.) *'coins worth half a denarius'* >) *medal, medallion*

　　< medius, media, medium 가운데의

　　　　E (medidies *'midday'* >) *meridian,* (medium aevum *'middle age'* >) *mediaeval*
　　　　(medieval), Mediterranean, (medius *'middle'* >) It. *mezzo* (< *'half'*), (medius
　　　　locus *'middle place'* >) F. *milieu*

　　> medium, medii, n. 매체(媒體), 배지(培地)　　　　　　　　**E** *medium,* (pl.) *media*

　　> media, mediae, f. (< tunica media *middle tunic*) 중간막(中間膜)　**E** *media, medial*

　　> medianus, mediana, medianum 한가운데의,

　　　　정중(正中)의　　　　　　　**E** *median, mean* (< *'middle'*); *paramedian*

　　> medietas, mediatatis, f. 가운데, 절반, 부분; 중용　　　　　　**E** *moiety*

　　> mediastinus, mediastina, mediastinum 가운데의

　　　　> mediastinum, mediastini, n. 세로칸, 종격(縱隔)　**E** *mediastinum, mediastinal*

　　> medio, mediavi, mediatum, mediare 가운데를 나누다, 중간에 있다, 중개

　　　　하다, 매개하다　　　　　　　　　**E** (verb) *mediate*

　　　　> mediatus, mediata, mediatum (*past participle*) 중개에 의한,

　　　　　　간접의　　　　　　　　　**E** (adjective) *mediate*

　　　　　　> immediatus, immediata, immediatum (< im- (< in-) *not*)

　　　　　　　　직접의, 바로, 즉각　　**E** *immediate, (immediate >) immediacy*

　　> mediocris, mediocre (< *halfway up a mountain* < medius *middle* +

　　　　ocris *rugged mountain*) 중간의, 평범한, 이류의　　　　**E** *mediocre*

　　> dimidius, dimidia, dimidium (< di- (< dis-) *apart from, down, not* +

　　　　medius *mid*) 절반의

　　　　E (F. demi *'half'* >) *demi-,* (L. semideus >) *demigod, demilune, demi-*
　　　　mondaine (< *'half-world woman'*), *demifacet*

　　> intermedius, intermedia, intermedium (< inter- *between, among* + medius

　　　　mid) 중간의, 사이에 있는　　　　　　　**E** *intermediate, intermediary*

< IE. medhyo- *middle*

> **E** *middle, mid, mid-, midst, amid, Midgard (< 'middle garden'), ((Gallo-Roman) Mediolanum (< + -lanum 'plain' < IE. pelə- 'flat', 'to spread') 'in the middle of the plain' >) Milan*

> G. mesos, mesē, meson *middle*

> **E** *mes(o)-, meson, mesenchyma, mesoderm, mesentery, mesocolon, mesoappendix, mesometrium, mesosalpinx, mesovarium, mesaxon, mesangium, Mesopotamia; mesial, mesiad (<+ -ad 'toward')*

< IE. me- *in the middle of*   **E** *midwife (< 'woman who is with the mother at childbirth')*

> G. meta > met(a)-, meth- (*before* aspirate) *between, along with, across, after*

> **E** *met(a)- (meth-), metamorphosis, meteor, method; metalanguage (< 'a language or set of terms used for the description or analysis of another language'), metanalysis (< 'different analysis of words or word-groups'), meta-analysis (< 'analysis of data from a number of independent studies of the same subject, especially in order to determine overall trends and significance')*

---

lateralis, laterale 옆구리의, 옆의   **E** *lateral, -lateral*

> < latus, lateris, n. 옆구리, 곁, 옆

< (*probably*) IE. stelə- *to extend* (Vide LATUS; See E. *latitude*)

---

inanis, inane 비어 있는, 헛된, 어리석은   **E** *inane*

> inanitas, inanitatis, f. 비어 있음, 헛됨, 어리석음   **E** *inanity*

> inanio, **inanivi**, inanitum, inanire 비우다, 공허하게 하다, 헛되게 하다

> inanitio, inanitionis, f. 비움, 공허함, (사회적, 도덕적) 무기력, 기아, 영양실조, 기아성 쇠약   **E** *inanition*

---

satis (형용사, 무변화) 충분한, 필요한 만큼의; (부사) 충분히, 필요한 만큼   **E** *(ad- 'to, toward, at, according to' + satis 'enough' >) asset*

> satur, satura, saturum 포만한, 풍부한

> satira, satirae, f. (< lanx satura *full dish*) (여러 가지 운율과 내용의) 혼합시, 풍자시, 풍자   **E** *satire*

> saturo, **saturavi**, saturatum, saturare 배불리 먹이다, 충족시키다, 포화시키다   **E** *saturate, supersaturate, unsaturated*

> saturatio, saturationis, f. 배불리 먹임, 충족, 포화   **E** *saturation, supersaturation*

> satietas, satietatis, f. 풍부, 포만, 물림   **E** *satiety*

> satio, **satiavi**, satiatum, satiare 배불리 먹이다, 물리게 하다   **E** *satiate*

> satisfacio, **satisfeci**, satisfactum, satisfacĕre (< satis *enough* + facĕre *to make*) 만족시키다   **E** *satisfy, unsatisfied*

< IE. sa- *to satisfy*   **E** *sate, sad (< 'sorrowful' < 'serious, sober' < 'steadfast, firm')*

> G. hadros, hadra, hadron *bulky, thick*   **E** *hadron*

●●● 제3변화 제3식

> 남·여·중성형에서 단수 주격은 주격끼리, 단수 속격은 속격끼리 같으며 단수 속격의 음절 수가 많아진다. 단수 주격의 끝음절이 -ns, -s, -x, -l, -r로 끝나는 형용사이다. 사전은 단수 주격과 단수 속격을 제시한다.

potens, (gen.) potentis 힘 있는, 능력 있는

	단 수			복 수		
	남성	여성	중성	남성	여성	중성
주격	potens	potens	potens	potent-es	potent-es	potent-ia
속격	potent-is	potent-is	potent-is	potent-ium	potent-ium	potent-ium
여격	potent-i	potent-i	potent-i	potent-ibus	potent-ibus	potent-ibus
대격	potent-em	potent-em	potens	potent-es	potent-es	potent-ia
탈격	potent-i	potent-i	potent-i	potent-ibus	potent-ibus	potent-ibus
호격	potens	potens	potens	potent-es	potent-es	potent-ia

potens, (gen.) potentis 힘 있는, 능력 있는   **E** *potent*

     < possum, potui, −, posse (< potis *able, possible* + esse *to be*) 할 수 있다, 가능성 있다, 힘이 있다, 능력이 있다

     < potis (pote) (불변화) 할 수 있는, 능력이 있는

   < IE. poti- *powerful, lord* (Vide POSSE: *See* E. *posse*)

recens, (gen.) recentis (< re- *back, again* + IE. ken-) 싱싱한, 새로운, 최근의   **E** *recent*

   < IE. ken- *fresh, new, young*

     > G. kainos, kainē, kainon *new, strange*

> **E** *caen(o)- (cen(o)-, cain(o)-), Caenozoic (Cenozoic, Cainozoic), -cene, kainite (< 'the mineral's recent formation')*

sagax, (gen.) sagacis 감각이 예민한, 명민한, 총명한   **E** *sagacious*

     > sagacitas, sagacitatis, f. 명민, 총명   **E** *sagacity*

   < IE. sag- *to seek out*

> **E** *seek, beseech, sake, forsake (< for- 'prefix denoting exclusion or rejection' < IE. per basic meanings of 'forward', 'through'), (perhaps) seize (< 'to take possession of' < 'to lay claim to one's rights'), (seize >) seizure*

     > L. sagio, −, −, sagire 냄새를 잘 맡다, 예민하게 감지하다, 직감적으로 알다

> L. praesagio, praesagivi (praesagii), praesagitum, praesagire (< prae- *before, beyond* + sagire *to perceive keenly*) 예감하다
>> L. praesagium, praesagii, n. 예감, 전조, 예언 `E` *presage*
> G. hēgeisthai (< *to track down*) *to lead, to guide*
>> G. hēgemōn, hēgemonos, m., f. *leader*
>>> G. hēgemonia, hēgemonias, f. *leadership* `E` *hegemony*
>> G. exēgeisthai (< ex- *out of, away from*) *to interpret*
>>> G. exēgēsis, exēgēseōs, f. *interpretation*
>>>> L. exegesis, exegesis, f. 해석, 주석 `E` *exegesis*

memor, (gen.) memoris 기억하고 있는

> memoria, memoriae, f. 기억 `E` *memory, memorial*
> memoror, memoratus sum, memorari 기억하다
>> rememoror, rememoratus sum, rememorari (< re- *back, again*) 기억하고 있다 `E` *remember*
> memoro, memoravi, memoratum, memorare 생각나게 하다, 언급하다

`E` ((*neuter gerundive*) '*something to be remembered*' >) *memorandum,* (pl.) *memoranda,* (*memorandum* >) *memo,* (pl.) *memos, memorable*

>> commemoro, commemoravi, commemoratum, commemorare (< com- (< cum) *with, together*) 기념하다 `E` *commemorate*

< IE. (s)mer- *to remember* `E` *mourn* (< '*to remember sorrowfully*')

맞대보기 어미 -ēs (-es)로 끝나는 그리스어 제3변화 형용사꼴로서 관례상 그대로 라틴어 형용사로 쓰이는 낱말은 위의 변화(제3변화 제3식)를 따른다.

---

botryoides, (gen.) botryoidis 포도송이 모양의 `E` *botryoid (botryoidal)*

[용례] sarcoma botryoides 포도육종 `E` *sarcoma botryoides*
　　(문법) sarcoma 육종: 단수 주격 < sarcoma, sarcomatis, n.
　　　　botryoides 포도송이 모양의: 형용사, 남·여·중성형 단격 주격

< G. botryoeidēs, botryoeidēs, botryoeides (< + -o- + eidos, eidous, n. *act of seeing, appearance, shape*)
< G. botrys, botryos, m. *bunch of grapes* `E` *botry(o)-; botryose*

lumbricoides, (gen.) lumbricoidis (< + G. -oeidēs, -oeidēs, -oeides < -o- + eidos, eidous, n. *act of seeing, appearance, shape*) 지렁이 모양의 `E` *lumbricoid*

[용례] Ascaris lumbricoides 회충(蛔蟲) `E` *Ascaris lumbricoides*
　　(문법) ascaris, ascaridis, f. 회충(蛔蟲)

lumbricoides: 형용사, 남·여·중성형 단수 주격

< lumbricus, lumbrici, m. 지렁이, 회충

> lumbricalis, lumbricale 지렁이 모양의; 벌레근의, 충양근(蟲樣筋)의

E *lumbrical*

< (*possibly*) IE. sleng^wh- *to slide, to make slide, to sling, to throw*

E *sling, slink*

pyogenes, (gen.) pyogenis (< + G. -genēs, -genēs, -genes *producing*) 고름을 만드는, 화농(化膿)의

[용례] Streptococcus pyogenes 고름 사슬알균, 화농 연쇄구균

E Streptococcus pyogenes

(문법) streptococcus 사슬알균, 연쇄구균: 단수 주격

< streptococcus, streptococci, m.

pyogenes: 형용사, 남·여·중성형 단수 주격

< G. pyon, pyou, n. *pus* (Vide PUS: *See* E. *pus*)

●●● 제3변화 제3식 예외

제3변화 제1식의 명사변화를 따라 단수 탈격이 –e, 복수 속격이 –um; 중성 복수 주격, 호격, 대격이 –a로 끝난다.

vetus, (gen.) veteris 나이든, 늙은, 묵은, 옛, 낡은

	단 수			복 수		
	남성	여성	중성	남성	여성	중성
주격	vetus	vetus	vetus	veter-es	veter-es	veter-a
속격	veter-is	veter-is	veter-is	veter-um	veter-um	veter-um
여격	veter-i	veter-i	veter-i	veter-ibus	veter-ibus	veter-ibus
대격	veter-em	veter-em	vetus	veter-es	veter-es	veter-a
탈격	veter-e	veter-e	veter-e	veter-ibus	veter-ibus	veter-ibus
호격	vetus	vetus	vetus	veter-es	veter-es	veter-a

vetus, (gen.) veteris 나이든, 늙은, 묵은, 옛, 낡은

E *veteran*

> veterinus, veterina, veterinum (일할 수 있을 만큼) 나이가 든, 짐바리 짐승의

(용례) veterina bestia (일할 수 있을 만큼) 나이가 든 짐승, 역축(役畜)

(문법) veterina: 형용사, 여성형 단수 주격

bestia 짐승: 단수 주격 < bestia, bestiae, f.

> veterinarius, veterinaria, veterinarium 짐바리 짐승의, 수의사의 E *veterinary, veterinarian*

< IE. wet- *year* (Vide VITULUS; *See* E. *veal*)

●●● 불변화 형용사

성·수·격에 따른 어미변화를 하지 않는 형용사이다.

semis 반(半)　　　　　　　　　　　　　　　　　　　　　　　　　　　　　**E** *semi-*
　　　> sesqui (sesque) (< semis *half* + -que *and*) (부사) 반이 더 많게, 1.5배로　　**E** *sesqui-*
　　　> sestertius, sestertia, sestertium (< semis *half* + tertius *third*) (형용사) 한 배 반이
　　　　　　더 많은, 2.5배의　　　　　　　　　　　　　　　　　　　　　　　　　**E** *sester-*
　　< IE. semi- *half, as first member of a compound*
　　　　> G. hēmisys, hēmiseia, hēmisy *half*　　　　　　　　　　　　　　　　**E** *hemi-*

뜻의 비교

변화의 양식은 다르나 뜻이 대조되기 때문에 사용상 무리를 이루는 형용사들
을 함께 모아 놓았다.

omnis, omne (< *abundant*) 모든　　　　　　　　　　　　　　　　　　　　**E** *omni-*
　　< IE. op- *to work, to produce in abundance* (Vide OPUS; *See* E. *opus*)

totus, tota, totum ((gen.) totius, (dat.) toti) 전체의, 온전한
　　　> totum, toti, n. 전체, 핵심　　　　　　　　　　**E** (Fac totum! *Do everything!* >) *factotum*
　　　　[용례] in toto 전체적으로, 고스란히　　　　　　　　　　　　　　**E** *in toto*
　　　　　　(문법) in ~ 안에서, ~ 안의: 전치사, 탈격지배
　　　　　　　　toto 전체: 단수 탈격
　　　> totalis, totale 전체의,
　　　　　전액의　　　　　**E** *total, subtotal, totalism,* (total > (emphatic extension) >) *teetotal*
　　　　　　> totalitas, totalitatis, f. 전체, 전액, 전체성, 완전성　　**E** *totality, totalitarian*

dexter, dextra, dextrum (dexter, dextera, dexterum) 오른쪽의, 길조의, 오른손잡이의,
　　　솜씨 좋은
　　　E *dexter, dextrous (dexterous), dextr(o)-, dextrorotatory* (D-), *(dextrorotatory glucose >)*
　　　dextrose, dextrin (< *'the property of turning the plane of polarization 138.68° to the*
　　　right'), dextran

> dextra, dextrae, f. (dextera, dexterae, f.) 오른손, 오른편　**E** *dextrad* (< + -ad 'toward')

　　> dextralis, dextrale 오른손의, 오른편의, 오른편에 있는　**E** *dextral*

　> dextrorsum (< dextrovorsum < dexter + vortĕre (vertĕre) *to turn*) (부사)
　　오른쪽으로　**E** *dextrorse*

　> dexteritas, dexteritatis, f. 능숙, 다행　**E** *dexterity*

　> ambidexter, ambidextra, ambidextrum (< amb(i)- *on both sides, around*) 양손잡이의,
　　솜씨가 비상한, 언행이 다른, 표리부동한　**E** *ambidexter, ambidexterity*

< IE. deks- *right*

　> G. dexios, dexia, dexion (dexiteros, dexitera, dexiteron) *right*　**E** *dexiocardia, dexiotropic*

laevus, laeva, laevum 왼쪽의, 서투른, 흉조의

> **E** *laev(o)- (lev(o)-), levorotatory (L-), levulose* (< 'formerly, levorotatory glucose; now, the naturally occurring (levorotatory) form of fructose'), (levulose >) *levulinic acid*

< IE. laiwo- *left*

　> G. laios, laia, laion *left*

sinister, sinistra, sinistrum 왼쪽의, 서투른, 흉조의 (< *Early Roman augurs faced south, with the east (lucky side) to the left, but the Greeks (followed by later Romans) faced the north.*)　**E** *sinister, sinistr(o)-*

　> sinistra, sinistrae, f. 왼손, 왼편, (훔친 것을) 슬쩍 감추는 손　**E** *sinistrad* (< + -ad 'toward')

　　> *sinistralis, *sinistrale 왼손의, 왼편의　**E** *sinistral*

　> sinistrorsum (< sinistrovorsum < sinister + vortĕre (vertĕre) *to turn*) (부사)
　　왼쪽으로　**E** *sinistrorse*

< IE. sene- *to prepare, to achieve; related to (Sanskrit)* saniyan *'more winning', 'more favorable', a euphemistic expression for taboo replacement*

superficialis, superficiale 표면의, 피상적인　**E** *superficial*

　　　< superficies, superficiei, f. (< super- *above* + facies *face*) 겉, 허울, 표면,
　　　　(법률) 지상권　**E** *superficies, surface*

　　　< (*probably*) facies, faciei, f. 얼굴, 면(面)

　　< facio, feci, factum, facĕre 만들다

< IE. dhe- *to put, to set* (Vide FACĔRE: *See* E. *facsimile*)

intermedius, intermedia, intermedium (< inter- *between, among*) 중간의,
　　사이에 있는　**E** *intermediate, intermediary*

　　< medius, media, medium 가운데의

< IE. medhyo- *middle* (Vide MEDIĄLIS: *See* E. *medial*)

basalis, basale 바닥의, 기저의, 기초의, 기본적인　**E** *basal*

< basis, basis, f. 바닥, 기저, 바탕, 기초, 기본
　< G. basis, baseōs, f. *stepping, tread, base*
　　< G. bainein *to go, to walk, to step*
< IE. gʷa-, gʷem- *to go, to come* (Vide VENIRE: *See* E. *venue*)

profundus, profunda, profundum (< pro- *before, forward, for, instead of* + fundus *bottom*)
깊은　　　　　　　　　　　　　　　　　　　　　　**E** *profound, profundity*
　< fundus, fundi, m. 바닥, 토지, 토대, 기저(基底)
< IE. bhudh-, budh- *bottom, base* (Vide FUNDUS: *See* E. *fundus*)

patens, (gen.) **patentis** (*present participle*) 열려 있는　　　　　**E** *patent*
　< pateo, patui, –, patēre 열리다, 열려 있다
< IE. petə- *to spread* (Vide PANDĒRE: *See* E. *pass*)

caecus, caeca, caecum (cecus, ceca, cacum) 눈먼, 막힌

[용례] foramen caecum 막구멍, 맹공(盲孔)　　　　**E** *foramen caecum (foramen cecum)*
　　　 intestinum caecum 막창자, 맹장(盲腸)　　　**E** *caecum (cecum), cecal*
　　　 (문법) foramen 구멍, 공(孔): 단수 주격 < foramen, foraminis, n.
　　　　　　 intestinum 창자, 장(腸): 단수 주격 < intestinum, intestini, n.
　　　　　　 caecum 막힌: 형용사, 중성형 단수 주격

　< IE. kaiko- *one-eyed*

mutus, muta, mutum 벙어리의, 소리 안 나는　　　　　　　　**E** *mute, mutism*
　< IE. meuə- *to be*
silent **E** *mum (< 'imitative of a sound made with closed lips'), (mum (frequentative) >) mumble*
　　> G. myein (*to close the lips* >) *to close the eyes*
　　　　> G. myosis, myoseōs, f. (< + G. –ōsis *condition*) *constriction of the pupil of*
　　　　　　the eye
　　　　　　> L. myosis, myosis, f. (miosis, miosis, f.) 축동(縮瞳),
　　　　　　　 동공축소　　　　　　　　　**E** *myosis (miosis), myotic (miotic)*
　　　　> G. myōps, myōpos, f. (< myein + ōps, ōpos, f. *eye*)
　　　　　　> L. myopia, myopiae, f. 근시(近視)　　　　**E** *myopia*
　　　　> G. mystēs, mystou, m. (< (*probably*) *person vowed to keep silence*) *one initiated*
　　　　　　> G. mystikos, mystikē, mystikon *belonging to secret rites*
　　　　　　　　> L. mysticus, mystica, mysticum 비교(秘敎)의, 신비한　　**E** *mystic, mystical*
　　　　　　> G. mystērion, mystēriou, n. *secret rites*
　　　　　　　　> L. mysterium, mysterii, n. 비교(秘敎), 신비　　　　**E** *mystery*

surdus, surda, surdum 참고 들을 수 없는, 귀먹은, 소리 안 나는; (음성) 무성음의; (수학) 무리
　　수(無理數)의 (< G. alogos *irrational, speechless*)　　　　　　　　　**E** *surd*
　　　　> absurdus, absurda, absurdum (< *away from the right sound* < ab- *off, away from;*
　　　　　　intensive + surdus *insufferable to the ear*) 어처구니없는, 불합리한, 부조리한　**E** *absurd*
　　　　　　　　> absurditas, absurditatis, f. 어처구니없는 짓, 불합리, 부조리　　**E** *absurdity*
　< IE. swer- *to buzz, to whisper*　　　　　　　　　　　　　　　　　**E** *swirl, swarm*
　　　　> L. susurrus, susurri, m. 윙윙거림, 중얼거림, 수군거림, 속삭임　**E** *susurrous, susurration*

durus, dura, durum 단단한, 굳은, 투박한, 엄한, 잘 견디어내는
　　　　E (dura mater *'hard mother'* >) *dura, dural, epidural, subdural, extradural, intradural*
　　　　> induro, induravi, induratum, indurare (< in- *in, on, into, toward* + durus *hard*) 굳히다,
　　　　　　무감각하게 만들다, 단련하다　　　　　　　　　　　　　　　**E** *indurate, endure*
　　　　　　　> induratio, indurationis, f. 경화(硬化)　　　　　　　　**E** *induration*
　　　　> obduro, obduravi, obduratum, obdurare (< ob- *before, toward(s), over, against, away*
　　　　　　+ durus *hard*) 굳어지게 하다, 완고해지다　　　　　　　　**E** *obdurate*
　< IE. deru-, dreu- *to be firm, solid, steadfast; hence specialized senses 'tree', 'wood', and*
　　　derivatives referring to objects made of wood
　　　　E *tree, tray* (< *'wooden board'*), *trough* (< *'wooden vessel'*), *trim* (< *'to make firm'*), *tar*
　　　　(< *'obtained from the pine tree'*), *true, truth, trust, truce* (< *'pledge'*), *troth, betroth*
　　　　> L. Druidae, Druidarum, m. (Druides, Druidum, m.) (pl.) (< (*probably*) (*Celtic*) *dru-wid-
　　　　　　(< *strong seer* < IE. deru-, dreu- + IE. weid- *to see*) 고대 Celt족의 제관들　**E** *Druid*
　　　　> G. drys, dryos, f. *oak, wood,*
　　　　　　tree　　　**E** *dryad,* (drys + pepon > drypepes *'tree-ripened'* > *'a stone-fruit'* >) *drupe*
　　　　> G. dendron, dendrou, n. *tree*
　　　　　　　E *dendr(o)-, dendroid, dendrocyte, oligodendroglia (oligodendrocyte), -dendron;*
　　　　　　　dendriform
　　　　　　> G. dendritēs, dendritēs, dendrites *of a tree*　　**E** *dendrite,* (*dendrite* >) *dendritic*
　　　　　　> G. rhododendron, rhododendrou, n. (< rhodon *rose* + dendron) *rhododendron*
　　　　　　　　>L. rhododendron, rhododendri, n. 진달래속(屬)의 식물　　**E** *rhododendron*
　　　　> (*Sanskrit*) daru *wood, timber*　　　　　　　　　　　　　　**E** *deodar*

mollis, molle 부드러운, 무른
　　　　> mollio, mollivi (mollii), mollitum, mollire 부드럽게 하다, 무르게 하다, 완화(緩化)시키다,
　　　　연화(軟化)시키다
　　　　　　> emollio, emollivi (emollii), emollitum, emollire (< e- *out of, away from; intensive*
　　　　　　　　+ mollire *to make soft*) 부드럽게 하다, 무르게 하다, 완화(緩化)시키다, 연화
　　　　　　　　(軟化)시키다　　　　　　　　　　　　　　　　　　　　**E** *emollient*
　　　　> mollifico, −, −, mollificare (< mollis *soft* + -ficare (< facĕre) *to make*) 무르게
　　　　하다, 완화시키다　　　　　　　　　　　　　　　　　　**E** *mollify, mollification*
　　　　> molluscus, mollusca, molluscum 부드러운, 무른　　　　　**E** *mollusc (mollusk)*
　　　　　　> molluscum, mollusci, n. 물렁종, 연속종(軟屬腫), 연우(軟疣)　　**E** *molluscum*

< IE. mel- *soft; with derivatives referring to soft or softened materials of various kinds*

> **E** melt, smelt, malt *(< 'grain softened by steeping in water, allowed to germinate in order to develop the saccharifying enzyme diastase, dried, and ground'), (malt sugar formed by the action of diastase on starch >)* **maltose, mild, mulch,** *(en- 'on' + amel 'enamel' >)* **enamel** *(< 'a vitreous composition inlaid or encrusted to the (metal) surface by fusion'), (enamel >)* **ameloblast**

> (*possibly*) L. blandus, blanda, blandum 부드러운, 순한, 평범한   **E** *bland*

> G. malakos, malakē, malakon soft   **E** *malac(o)-, malacology*

     > G. malakia, malakias, f. *softness, homosexual desire, sickness*

         > L. malacia, malaciae, f. 바다의 고요함, 무풍 상태; 무기력, 구역질, 입덧; 연화(軟化), 연화증(軟化症)   **E** *malacia, -malacia*

           > L. encephalomalacia, encephalomalaciae, f. (< G. enkephalos, enkephalou, m. *brain*) 뇌연화증   **E** *encephalomalacia*

           > L. keratomalacia, keratomalaciae, f. (< G. keras, keratos, n. *horn*) 각막연화증, 각질연화증   **E** *keratomalacia*

           > L. osteomalacia, osteomalaciae, f. (< G. osteon, osteou, n. *bone*) 뼈연화증, 골연화증   **E** *osteomalacia*

     > G. malassein *to soften*

         > G. malagma, malagmatos, n. *softening substance*

         E (*probably*) **amalgam** *(< 'mixture' < 'originally, a soft mass formed by chemical manipulation, especially a soft or plastic condition of gold, silver, etc. produced by combination of mercury'),* **amalgamate**

     > L. malacoplakia, malacoplakiae, f. (< + G. plax, plakos, f. *plaque*) 연화판증   **E** *malacoplakia*

> G. blenna, blennas, f. *slime, mucus*   **E** *blenny (< 'mucous coating of its scales')*

     > L. blennorrhoea, blennorrhoeae, f. (< + G. rhoia, rhoias, f. *flow*) 농루(膿漏)   **E** *blennorrhoea (blennorrhea)*

> G. amblys, ambleia, ambly *blunt, dull, dim*

     > G. amblyōpia, amblyōpias, f. (< amblys + ōps, ōpos, f. *eye* + -ia *noun suffix*) *dimsightedness*

         > L. amblyopia, amblyopiae, f. 약시(弱視)   **E** *amblyopia*

firmus, firma, firmum (< *firm, strong*) 튼튼한, 확고한   **E** *(adjective) firm*

> firmo, firmavi, firmatum, firmare 튼튼하게 하다, 확실하게 하다, 증명하다, 보증하다, 계약을 맺다

     E *(noun)* **firm** *(< 'one's signature under which the business of a firm was contracted'),* **farm** *(< 'rent or tax contracted'),* **farmer**

> firmamentum, firmamenti, n. 버티는 수단, 확고성, 창공(蒼空)   **E** *firmament*

> affirmo, affirmavi, affirmatum, affirmare (< af- (< ad) *to, toward, at, according to*) 확언하다   **E** *affirm*

> confirmo, **confirmavi**, confirmatum, confirmare (< con- (< cum) *with, together*) 확인하다   **E** *confirm*

     > confirmatio, confirmationis, f. 확인   **E** *confirmation*

> *confirmatorius, *confirmatoria, *confirmatorium 확인해주는   **E** *confirmatory*

> infirmus, infirma, infirmum (< in- *not* + firmus *firm*) 약한, 병든, 설득력 없는   **E** *infirm*

> infirmaria, infirmariae, f. 요양소, 의무실, 부속진료소   **E** *infirmary*

< IE. dher- *to hold firmly, to support*

> L. frenum, freni, n. 재갈, 소대(小帶), 주름띠   **E** *frenum*

> L. frenulum, frenuli, n. (< + -ulum *diminutive suffix*) 소대(小帶), 계대(繫帶), 작은 주름띠   **E** *frenulum*

> L. refreno, **refrenavi**, refrenatum, refrenare (< re- *back, again*) (재갈을 당겨 말을) 세우다, 못하게 하다, 막다   **E** *refrain*

> G. thronos, thronou, m. (< *support*) *throne*

> L. thronus, throni, m. 왕좌, 주교좌, 교황좌   **E** *throne, dethrone*

> (*suggested*) G. thōrax, thōrakos, m. *breastplate, cuirass; breast, chest*

> L. thorax, thoracis, m. 가슴받이 갑옷, 가슴, 흉부(胸部), 흉곽(胸廓)

E *thorax, thorac(o)-, thoracocentesis (thoracentesis), pneumothorax, hydrothorax, hemothorax, pyothorax*

> G. thōrakikos, thōrakikē, thōrakikon *thoracic*

> L. thoracicus, thoracica, thoracicum 가슴의, 흉부의, 흉곽의   **E** *thoracic*

> L. thoracopagus, thoracopagi, m. (< *Siamese twins joined at the thorax* < + G. pagos *that which is fastened*) 가슴 붙은 쌍둥이   **E** *thoracopagus*

> L. thoracodelphus, thoracodelphi, m. (< *a double monster with one head, two arms, and four legs, the bodies being joined above the navel* < + G. adelphos *brother*) 가슴결합체   **E** *thoracodelphus*

> (*Old Persian*) Darius (< *holding firm the good*)   **E** *Darius*

> (*Sanskrit*) dharma (< *that which is established firmly*) *law*   **E** *dharma*

fragilis, fragile (섬세하게 만들어져) 깨지기 쉬운   **E** *fragile, frail*

> fragilitas, fragilitatis, f. 깨지기 쉬움, 여림, 취약성   **E** *fragility, frailty*

< frango, **fregi**, fractum, frangĕre 분지르다, 깨트리다

< IE. bhreg- *to break* (Vide FRANGĔRE; *See* E. *fractal*)

rigidus, rigida, rigidum (< *stiff*) 뻣뻣한, 꼿꼿한, 꿋꿋한   **E** *rigid*

> rigiditas, rigiditatis, f. 경직   **E** *rigidity*

< rigeo, **rigui**, −, rigēre 뻣뻣해지다, 뻣뻣하다

> rigor, rigoris, m. 경직, 엄격, 혹독   **E** *rigor*

[용례] rigor mortis 사후경직   **E** *rigor mortis*

(문법) rigor 경직: 단수 주격

mortis 주검의: 단수 속격 < mors, mortis, f. 죽음, 주검

> rigorosus, rigorosa, rigorosum 엄격한, 혹독한   **E** *rigorous*

< IE. reig- *to reach, to stretch out*   **E** *reach*

> G. rhigos, rhigous, n. *frost, cold*

> L. *rhigosis, *rhigosis, f. (< + G. -ōsis *condition*) 냉각(冷覺)　　　**E** *rhigosis*

lenis, lene 부드러운, 온화한, 평정한; 연음(軟音)의　　　**E** *lenis,* (pl.) *lenes*

　　> lenitas, lenitatis, f. 부드러움, 온화　　　**E** *lenity*

　　> lenio, lenivi (lenii), lenitum, lenire 달래다, 진정시키다, 완화하다　　　**E** *lenient, lenitive, lenition*

< IE. le- *to let go, to slacken*

　　E *let, inlet, outlet, late,* (comparative) *later,* (comparative) *latter,* (superlative) *last*

　　> L. lassus, lassa, lassum 지친, 처진, 내키지 않은　　**E** (ah lassus *'ah (I am) miserable'* >) *alas*

　　　　> L. lassitudo, lassitudinis, f. 나른함, 권태, 무기력　　　**E** *lassitude*

fortis, forte (< *strong*) 용맹한, 힘센, 강한; 경음(硬音)의

　　E *fortis,* (pl.) *fortes, force,* It. (piano et forte *'soft and loud'* >) *pianoforte (piano), fort, fortress*

　　> fortitudo, fortitudinis, f. 역경 속의 용기, 불굴의 용기　　　**E** *fortitude*

　　> fortifico, −, −, fortificare (< fortis *strong* + -ficare (< facĕre) *to make*)

　　　　강화하다　　　**E** *fortify, fortification*

　　> conforto, confortavi, confortatum, confortare (< con- (< cum) *with, together; intensive*

　　　　+ fortis *strong*) 용맹하게 하다, 튼튼하게 하다, 격려하다,

　　　　편하게 하다　　　**E** *comfort, comfortable, discomfort*

　　> *effortio, *effortiavi, *effortiatum, *effortiare (< ef- (< ex) *out of, away from* + fortis

　　　　strong) 노력하다　　　**E** *effort*

　　> infortio, infortiavi, infortiatum, infortiare (< in- *in, on, into, toward* + fortis *strong*)

　　　　노력하다, 강화하다, 집행하다　　　**E** *enforce, reinforce*

< IE. bhergh- *high; with derivatives referring to hills and hill-forts*

　　E *iceberg, borough, -burg, -bury, harbor* (< *'army hill, hill-fort'* < IE. koro- *'war, war-band,*
　　host, army'), *harbinger* (< *'army hill, hill-fort'* < IE. koro- *'war, war-band, host, army'*)

　　> L. burgus, burgi, m. 성곽이 있는

　　　　도시　　**E** *bourg, bourgeois,* (suggested) *burglar* (< *'fortress thief'*), (burglar >) *burgle*

debilis, debile (< de- *apart from, down, not*) 쇠약한, 불구의

　　> debilitas, debilitatis, f. 쇠약　　　**E** *debility*

　　> debilito, debilitavi, debilitatum, debilitare (< de- *apart from, down, not; intensive*)

　　　　쇠약하게 하다, 불구로 만들다　　　**E** *debilitate*

< IE. bel- *strong*

　　> (*Russian*) bolshoi *large, great*　　**E** ((Russian) bolshe (comparative) *'greater'* >) *Bolshevik*

solidus, solida, solidum 완전한, (비어 있지 않고 같은 종류의 것으로 가득 차) 충실한, 견실한,

　　진짜의, 견고한, 고체의, 입체의　　　**E** *solid, solidify*

　　[용례] (nummus) solidus (콘스탄틴 황제가 발행한 순금의) 금화　　　**E** *soldier*

　　　　(문법) nummus 주화(鑄貨): 단수 주격 < nummus, nummi, m.

　　　　solidus 충실한: 형용사, 남성형 단수 주격

> soliditas, soliditatis, f. 충실, 견실, 견고, 고체, 입체   **E** *solidity*

> solidaris, solidare 연대의, 연대 책임의   **E** *solidarity*

> solido, **solidavi**, solidatum, solidare 굳게 하다, (땜질 등으로) 붙게 하다   **E** *solder*

>> consolido, **consolidavi**, consolidatum, consolidare (< con- *with, together;*
intensive + solidare *to make firm or solid*) 굳게 하다   **E** *consolidate*

< sollus, solla, sollum 온통의, 통짜의   **E** *solicit*

> (*suggested*) sollemnis, sollemne (solemnis, solemne) (< sollus *whole* + annus
year) 일년에 한 번 지내는, 장엄한, 성대한   **E** *solemn, solemnity*

< IE. sol-, solə- *whole*

> L. salvus, salva, salvum 고스란한, 무사한, 안전한, 구제된   **E** *safe*

> L. salvitas, salvitatis, f. 안전   **E** *safety*

> L. salvo, **salvavi**, salvatum, salvare 낫게 하다, 구하다, 구원하다

> **E** *save, salvage, salvation,* (salvare + arsenic + -an > 'arsenic compound to save'
>) *Salvarsan®, salver,* Sp. *El Salvador*

> L. salus, salutis, f. 건강, 안녕, 문안 인사; (Salus) (로마 신화) 안녕의 여신

> L. salutaris, salutare 건강에 좋은   **E** *salutary*

> L. saluto, **salutavi**, salutatum, salutare 인사하다   **E** *salute, salutation*

> L. salutatorius, salutatoria, salutatorium 인사의   **E** *salutatory*

> L. salvia, salviae, f. 샐비어, 세이지   **E** *salvia, sage*

> G. holos, holē, holon *whole, complete, entire,*
all   **E** *hol(o)-, holism* (< 'whole making'), *holistic, hologram* (< 'wholly written')

> G. holokaustos, holokaustos, holokauston (< + kaustos *burnt*) *burnt in whole,*
of burnt-offering

> L. holocaustum, holocausti, n. 번제(燔祭, 희생동물을 통째로 태워 바치던
유대교의 제사)   **E** *holocaust*

> G. katholou (< kath- (< kata) *down, mis-, according to, along, thoroughly*)
(*adverb*) *on the whole, generally, universally*

> G. katholikos, katholikē, katholikon *general, universal*

> L. catholicus, catholica, catholicum 일반적, 보편적   **E** *catholic*

asper, aspera, asperum 거칠거칠한, 거친

> asperitas, asperitatis, f. 거칢, 어려움, 매서움   **E** *asperity*

> aspero, **asperavi**, asperatum, asperare 거칠게 만들다, 더 어렵게 만들다   **E** *asperate*

> exaspero, **exasperavi**, exasperatum, exasperare (< ex- *out of, away from;*
intensive + asperare *to roughen*) 거칠게 만들다, 악화시키다   **E** *exasperate*

> G. aspros, aspra, aspron (< *rough silver coin* < *carved silver coin*) *white*

> G. diaspros, diaspra, diaspron (< di(a)- *through, thoroughly, apart*) *pure
white, white interspersed with other color*

> L. diasprus, diaspra, diasprum 흰   **E** *diaper*

glaber, glabra, glabrum 매끈한, 털이 없는

> glabella, glabellae, f (< + -ella *diminutive suffix*) 미간(眉間),
눈썹활사이　　　　　　　　　　　　　　　　　　　　　　E *glabella, glabellar*

> glabrosus, glabrosa, glabrosum 매끈한, 털이 없는, 몸의　　　　E *glabrous*

< IE. gladh- *smooth*

laevis, laeve (levis, leve) 매끈한, 평활(平滑)한, 갈고닦은, 유창한

> laevigo, **laevigavi**, laevigatum, laevigare (levigo, **levigavi**, levigatum, levigare)
(< laevis, laeve (levis, leve) *smooth* + agĕre *to drive, to do*) 매끈하게 하다,
갈고닦다　　　　　　　　　　　　　　　　　　　　　　　E *levigate*

< IE. (s)lei- *slimy*

E *slime, slimy, slip, slippery, slippage, slipper, slick* (< 'smooth'), (slick >) *sleek, slight*
(< 'slender' < 'smooth'), *lime* (< 'birdlime, quicklime')

> G. leios, leia, leion *smooth, polished, bald*　　　　E *leio- (lio-), leiomy(o)-*

> G. litos, litē, liton *plain, simple*

> G. litotēs, litotētos, f. *plainness, simplicity*

> L. litotes, litotis, f. 곡언법(曲言法), 완서법(緩敍法)　　　E *litotes*

> (*suggested*) G. leimax, leimakos, f. *slug*

> L. limax, limacis, m., f. 괄태충(括胎蟲), 민달팽이, 창녀

> L. Endolimax, Endolimacis, f. (아메바) 엔도리막스속(屬)　E *Endolimax*

> L. lino, livi (levi, lini), litum, linĕre (기름·약·도료 등을) 바르다, 씌우다, 지우다

> L. linimentum, linimenti, n. 바르는 약　　　　　E *liniment*

> L. deleo, **delevi**, deletum, delēre (< de- *apart from, down, not*)
지워버리다　　　　　　　　　　　　　　E *delete, (delete >) undelete*

> L. deletio, deletionis, f. 지워버림, 삭제, 결손　　E *deletion*

> L. delebilis, delebile 지울 수 있는　　　　　　E *delible*

> L. indelebilis, indelebile (< im- < in- *not*) 지울 수 없는　E *indelible*

> L. obliviscor, oblitus sum, oblivisci (< *to let slip from the mind* < ob- *before, toward(s),
over, against, away*) 잊어버리다

> L. oblivium, oblivii, n. 망각　　　　　　　　E *oblivion*

> L. obliviosus, obliviosa, obliviosum 잊어버리는, 염두에 없는　E *oblivious*

> (*Sanskrit*) alayah *abode*

> (*Sanskrit*) Himalaya (< himah *snow* < IE. ghei- *winter*) *Himalaya*　E *Himalayas*

> IE. sleidh- *to slip, to slide*　　　　　E *slide, sled, sledge, sleigh*

> (*probably*) G. olisthein (olisthanein) *to slip, to glide*　E *olisthe (olisthy)*

> G. olisthēsis, olisthēseōs, f. *dislocation*

> L. -olisthesis, -olisthesis, f. 전위(轉位)　　　E *-olisthesis*

> L. spondylolisthesis, spondylolisthesis, f. (< *dislocation of
the vertebra* < G. spondylos *vertebra*) 척추탈위증(脫位
症), 척추일출증(逸出症)　　　　　E *spondylolisthesis*

moderatus, moderata, moderatum 절도 있는, 중등도(中等度)의　　　E *moderate*

> immoderatus, immoderata, immoderatum (< im- < in- *not*) 절제 없는,

지나친, 터무니없는　　　　　　　　　　　　　　　　　　　　　　**E** *immoderate*

　　　< moderor, moderatus sum, moderari 절도를 지키다, 조정하다

　　　　　> moderator, moderatoris, m. 조정자, 중재자, 조절기, 사회자　　**E** *moderator*

　　　< modus, modi, m. 절도, 양식, 척도, 기준

< IE. med- *to take appropriate measures* (Vide MEDICINA; *See* E. *medicine*)

severus, severa, severum 엄격한, 심한　　　　　　　　　　　　**E** *severe*

　　　　> severitas, severitatis, f. 엄격, 가차없음, 중증도(重症度)　　**E** *severity*

< IE. segh- *to hold* (Vide SCHOLA; *See* E. *scholar*)

celer, celeris, celere 빠른

　　　　> celeritas, celeritatis, f. 신속, 민첩　　　　　　　　　**E** *celerity*

< IE. kel- *to drive, to set in swift motion* (Vide CELER; *See* E. *celerity*)

lentus, lenta, lentum 잘 휘는, 나긋나긋한, 질질 끄는, 느린, 둔감한, 온순한

　　E *relent* (< '*to become less harsh'*)*, relentless, lentivirus* (< '*responsible for slow virus diseases'*)

< IE. len-to- *flexible*　　　　　　　　　**E** *lithe, linden* (< '*pliable bast'*)

tardus, tarda, tardum 더딘, 지체되는, 지연되는　　　　　**E** *tardive, tardy, tardyon*

　　　　> retardo, **retardavi**, retardatum, retardare (< re- *back, again* + tardus *slow*) 지체
　　　　하다, 지연시키다　　　　　　　　　　　　**E** *retard, retardant, retardation*

acutus, acuta, acutum 날카로운, 매운, 급성의　　　　　　**E** *acute, subacute*

　　　< acuo, **acui**, acutum, acuĕre 뾰족하게 만들다

　　　　　> acumen, acuminis, m. 뾰족한 끝, 정점, 예민　　　　**E** *acumen*

　　　　　　　> acumino, **acuminavi**, acuminatum, acuminare 뾰족하게 하다
　　　　　　　　> acuminatus, acuminata, acuminatum (*past participle*)
　　　　　　　뾰족한, 첨형(尖形)의
　　　　　　　> acuitas, acuitatis, f. (첨단의) 날카로움, 총명, 명료도　　**E** *acuity*

　　　< acus, acus, f. 바늘

　　　E (acu (abl.) '*with a needle'* + *puncture* >) *acupuncture, (acupuncture point* >) *acupoint*

< IE. ak- *sharp*　　**E** *edge, ear* (< '*spike of a cereal plant'*)*, hammer* (< '*stone hammer'* < '*sharp stone'*)

　　> L. acer, acris, acre 신, 날카로운, 혹독한　　**E** *acrid, eager,* (vinum acre '*acrid wine'* >) *vinegar*

　　　　> L. acrimonia, acrimoniae, f. 신랄함, 통렬함　　　　　**E** *acrimony*

　　　　> L. acerbus, acerba, acerbum 떫은, 덜된, 신랄한, 혹독한　　**E** *acerbic*

　　　　　　> L. exacerbo, **exacerbavi**, exacerbatum, exacerbare (< ex- *out of, away*
　　　　　　from + acerbus *harsh, bitter*) 격분시키다, 악화시키다　　**E** *exacerbate*

　　　　> L. aceo, **acui**, −, acēre 시어지다, 시큰둥하다

　　　　　　> L. acidus, acida, acidum 신, 신랄한

> **E** *acid, acidic,* (D. Essigaether *'vinegar ether (ethyl acetate)'* > (*contracted*) > *'a compound formed by an acid joined to an alcohol'* >) *ester, esterase; acidophil, acidophilic, antacid*

> L. aciditas, aciditatis, f. 산성, 산성도 **E** *acidity*

> L. acidifico, acidificavi, acidificatum, acidificare (< acidus *acid* + -ficare (< facĕre) *to make*) 산성화하다 **E** *acidify*

> L. acidosis, acidosis, f. (< *acid* + G. -ōsis *condition*) 산증(酸症) **E** *acidosis*

> L. acetum, aceti, n. 식초, 신랄한 비판

> **E** *acet(o)-, acetic acid, acetate* (< *'a salt or ester of acetic acid'), acetyl (< 'the acyl group of acetic acid'), (acet(o)- + -one (< G. -ōnē 'feminine patronymic suffix') >) acetone, (acetone >) ketone, (ketone >) ket(o)-, (ket(o)- >) keto, (ket(o)- >) ketosis, (ketone >) -one, (acetic acid + alcohol > 'arisen from alcohol during the formation of acetic acid' >) acetal, ('acetal derived from ketone' >) ketal, (hemi- 'half' + acetal > 'an intermediate in the preparation of acetal' >) hemiacetal, ('half ketal' >) hemiketal*

> L. acetabulum, acetabuli, n. 식초 종지, 비구(髀臼), 관골구(膻骨臼), 절구, 흡반, 빨판 **E** *acetabulum, acetabular*

> L. acetobacter, acetobacteris, m. (< *a microorganism that produces acetic acid from ethanol* < acetum *vinegar* + -bacter *bacteria*) (세균) 초산균 **E** *acetobacter*

> G. akē, akēs, f. *point*

> G. akantha, akanthēs, f. *thorn, thistle* **E** *acanthocyte, coelacanth, tragacanth*

> L. acanthosis, acanthosis, f. (< + G. -ōsis *condition*) 가시세포증, 극세포증(棘細胞症) **E** *acanthosis, acanthotic*

[용례] acanthosis nigricans 흑색가시세포증 **E** *acanthosis nigricans*
(문법) acanthosis 가시세포증: 단수 주격
nigricans 거무스름한, 검은: 현재분사,
남·여·중성형 단수 주격
< nigricans, (gen.) nigricantis
< nigrico, -, -, nigricare 거무스름하다, 검다

> L. acantholysis, acantholysis, f. (< + G. lysis *loosening*) 가시세포분리(증), 극세포분리(증) **E** *acantholysis, acantholytic*

> G. akanthos, akanthou, m. *acanthus*

> L. acanthus, acanthi, m. (식물) 어캔서스(Acanthus spinosus); (건축) 어캔서스 잎 모양 장식 **E** *acanthus*

> (*probably*) G. akakia, akakias, f. (< *in reference to its thorns*) *acacia*

> L. acacia, acaciae, f. 아카시아 **E** *acacia*

[용례] Acacia farnesiana *Farnese acacia tree*

> **E** *farnesol (< 'a sesquiterpenoid alcohol obtained from Farnese acacia flowers'), (farnesol >) farnesyl, farnesylate*

(문법) acacia 아카시아: 단수 주격

farnesiana (사람 이름): 형용사, 여성형 단수 주격

< Odoardo Farnese (1573-1626), *Italian cardinal*

> L. Anisakis, Anisakis, f. (< *two unequal spicules* < G. anisos *unequal* + akē)

(선충) 아니사키스

E *Anisakis, anisakiasis*

> G. akmē, akmēs, f. *point, highest point*

E *acme*

> (*supposed to be corrupted*) L. acne, acnes, f. 여드름,

좌창(痤瘡)

E *acne, acneic, acneiform (acneform)*

> G. akonē, akonēs, f. *whetstone*

> G. parakonan (parakonaein) (< par(a)- *beside, along side of, beyond* + akonē)

to sharpen

> It. paragone *touchstone to test gold*

E *paragon* (< *'a model'*)

> G. akros, akra, akron *extreme, topmost,*

terminal

E *acr(o)-, acropolis, acrophobia, acrosome, acral*

> G. oxys, oxeia, oxy *sharp, quick, sour*

E (oxys *'sharp'* >) **oxycephaly;** (oxys *'quick'* >) **oxytocin;** (oxys *'sour'* > *'acid'* >) **oxyphil, oxyphilic;** (oxys *'sour'* > *'acidifying principle'* >) **oxygen (O),** (oxygen >) **oxygenate, deoxygenate, oxygenation, oxygenator, oxyhemoglobin, oxymeter (oximeter), dioxin(s);** (oxygen + acid >) **oxide(s), hydroxide(s), peroxide(s), superoxide(s),** (epi *'upon'* + oxide > *'oxygen atom upon two carbon atoms'* >) **epoxide(s),** (epoxide >) **epoxy;** (oxide >) **oxidation,** (reduction + oxidation >) **redox, oxidative, oxidant, antioxidant, oxidize, oxidase;** (oxide >) **-ide;** (oxygen + -yl >) **carboxyl, hydroxyl**

> G. oxynein *to sharpen, to make acid*

E *oxyntic*

> G. paroxynein (< par(a)- *beside, along side of, beyond*) *to incite*

> G. paroxysmos, paroxysmou, m. *inciting, provoking*

> L. paroxysmus, paroxysmi, m. (감정·행동의) 폭발,

(주기적) 발작

E *paroxysm, paroxysmal*

> G. oxalis, oxalidos, f. (< *sour foliage*) *sorrel*

> L. oxalis, oxalidis, f. 괭이밥

E *oxalis, oxalic acid, oxalate*

> L. anoxia, anoxiae, f. (< G. an- *not* + *oxygen* + -ia)

무산소증(無酸素症)

E *anoxia, anoxic*

> L. hypoxia, hypoxiae, f. (< G. hyp(o)- *under* + *oxygen* + -ia)

저산소증(低酸素症)

E *hypoxia, hypoxic*

> L. hyperoxia, hyperoxiae, f. (< G. hyper- *over* + *oxygen* + -ia)

고산소증(高酸素症)

E *hyperoxia, hyperoxic*

chronicus, chronica, chronicum 연대(年代)에 관한, 만성의

E *chronic, chronicity, chronicle*

< G. chronikos, chronikē, chronikon *of time*

< G. chronos, chronou, m. *time*

E *chron(o)-, chronometry, chronotropic* (< *'affecting the time or rate of muscle contractions'*)

> L. chronologia, chronologiae, f. (< + G. -logia *study*) 연대기(年代記),

연표(年表)   **E** *chronology, chronological*

> G. -chronos, -chronos, -chronon *of a period of time*

> **E** *-chronous, diachronic (< 'through the course of time, historical' < 'on the pattern of synchronic')*

> G. synchronos, synchronos, synchronon (< syn- *with, together*)

    synchronous

> L. synchronus, synchrona, synchronum 동시대(同時代)의, 동시(同時)의, 동기(同期)의

> **E** *synchronous, (synchronous >) synchrony, (synchronous >) asynchronous, (asynchronous >) asynchrony, (synchronus >) synchronic, synchronicity*

> G. synchronismos, synchronismou, m. *being synchronous*

> L. synchronismus, synchronismi, m. 동시성(同時性)

> **E** *synchronism, (synchronism >) synchronize, synchronization, asynchronism*

> G. metachronos, metachronos, metachronon (< met(a)- *between, along with, across, after*) *occurring at different times, occurring at later times*

    E *metachronous, metachronism*

> G. isochronos, isochronos, isochronon (< is(o)- *equal*) *equal in age, equal in time*

    E *isochronous, isochronism, isochrony*

> G. anachronizein (< an(a)- *up, upward; again, throughout; back, backward; against; according to, similar to* + chronos) *to refer to a wrong time*

> G. anachronismos, anachronismou, m. *referring to a wrong time*   **E** *anachronism*

---

tropicus, tropica, tropicum 방향을 돌리는, 향하는, 회귀선(回歸線)의, 열대의

E *tropic, -tropic, heliotropic, geotropic, hydrotropic, (tropic >) tropical, subtropical, isotropic (< 'of an object or substance having a physical property which has the same value when measured in different directions'), anisotropic (< 'of an object or substance having a physical property which has a different value when measured in different directions')*

영향을 미치는

E *-tropic, psychotropic, neurotropic, pleiotropic, pleiotropism (pleiotropy), (chaos > 'disorder-making' >) chaotropic, (kosmos > 'order-making' >) kosmotropic*

조절하는

E *-tropic, -tropin, -trope; somatotropic (somatotrophic), somatotropin (somatotrophin), somatotrope (somatotroph); lactotropic (lactotrophic), lactotropin (lactotrophin), lactotrope (lactotroph); adrenocorticotropic (corticotropic) (adrenocorticotrophic, corticotrophic), adrenocorticotropin (corticotropin) (adrenocorticotrophin, corticotrophin), corticotrope (corticotroph); thyrotropic (thyrotrophic), thyrotropin (thyrotrophin), thyrotrope (thyrotroph); gonadotropic (gonadotrophic), gonadotropin(s) (gonadotrophin(s)), gonadotrope (gonadotroph); ionotropic (< 'modulating ion channels'), metabotropic (< 'modulating metabolic steps')*

< G. tropikos, tropikē, tropikon *of turning, tropic*

< G. tropē, tropēs, f. *turning, turn, solstice (< the turning of the sun at the solstice), flight, defeat, victory, change* **E** *entropy (< 'turning (transformational) contents, after the analogy of energy')*

> G. tropaion, tropaiou, n. *sign of victory, trophy*

> L. tropaeum, tropaei, n. (trophaeum, trophaei, n.) 전승 기념물 (나무기둥 위에 전리품을 걸었음), 전리품, 승리 **E** *trophy*

> L. tropia, tropiae, f. 사시(斜視) **E** *-tropia*

> L. esotropia, esotropiae, f. (< G. esō- *inwards*) 내사시(內斜視) **E** *esotropia*

> L. exotropia, exotropiae, f. (< G. exō- *outwards*) 외사시(外斜視) **E** *exotropia*

> L. *hypertropia, *hypertropiae, f. (< G. hyper- *over*) 상사시 (上斜視) **E** *hypertropia*

> L. *hypotropia, *hypotropiae, f. (< G. hyp(o)- *under*) 하사시 (下斜視) **E** *hypotropia*

G. tropos, tropou, m. *turn, direction, manner, way, fashion, custom, mode of life, character, temper*

E *tropism, chemotropism, dromotropism, trop(o)-, tropomyosin, (tropomyosin >) troponin, contrive (< 'to find out'), contrivance, retrieve (< 'to find again'), retrieval*

G. tropos, tropē, tropon *of manner, flexible, changeable*

> G. allotropos, allotropos, allotropon (< allos *other*) *of other manner*

> G. allotropia, allotropias, f. *variation, changeableness*

E *allotropy (< 'the variation of physical properties without change of substance, first noted in the case of charcoal and the diamond), (allotropy >) **allotrope***

> G. atropos, atropos, atropon (< a- *not*) *inflexible, unchangeable, inexorable*

> G. Atropos, Atropou, f. *(Greek mythology) one of the three Fates who severs the thread of life* **E** *Atropos*

> L. Atropa, Atropae, f. (가지과의 유독성 식물) 아트로파속(屬) **E** Atropa, *atropine*

< G. trepein *to turn, to turn away*

> G. treponema, treponematos, n. (< trep(o)- *turning* + nēma, nēmatos, n. *thread*) *treponema*

> L. treponema, treponematis, n. 트레포네마균 **E** *treponema, treponemal*

[용례] Treponema pallidum (< *a pale turning thread*) 매독균 **E** Treponema pallidum

(문법) treponema 트레포네마균: 단수 주격

pallidum 창백한: 형용사, 중성형 단수 주격

< pallidus, pallida, pallidum

> G. apotrepein (< ap(o)- *away from, from*) *to turn away, to avert* **E** *apotropaic*

> G. ektrepein (< ek- *out of, away from*) *to turn outwards*

> G. ektropion, ektropiou, n. *eversion*

> L. ectropium, ectropii, n. 겉말림, 외번(外飜) **E** *ectropion (ectropium)*

> G. entrepein (< en- *in*) *to turn inwards*

> G. entropion, entropiou, n. *inversion*

> L. entropium, entropii, n. 속말림, 내번(內飜) **E** *entropion (entropium)*

< IE. trep- *to turn*

***trophicus, *trophica, *trophicum** 영양물질을 만드는, 영양물질을 찾는

E *trophic, autotrophic, heterotrophic, phototroph, chemotroph, lecithotrophic, psychrotrophic*

유지하는, 조절하는 **E** *neurotrophic*

< G. trophikos, trophikē, trophikon

< G. trophē, trophēs, f. *food, nourishment*

> G. -trophia, -trophias, f. *nourishment* **E** *-trophy, -trophic*

> L. atrophia, atrophiae, f. (< G. a- *not*) 위축(萎縮) **E** *atrophy, hemiatrophy*

> L. atrophicus, atrophica, atrophicum 위축의 **E** *atrophic*

> L. hypertrophia, hypertrophiae, f. (< G. hyper- *over*) 비대(肥大) **E** *hypertrophy, hemihypertrophy*

> L. eutrophia, eutrophiae, f. (< G. eu- *well*) 영양 양호, 정상 발육, 부(富)영양상태 **E** *eutrophy, eutrophication*

> L. dystrophia, dystrophiae, f. (< G. dys- *bad*) 영양장애, 퇴행 위축, 이상증(異常症), 이영양(증)(異營養(症)) **E** *dystrophy, dystrophin*

> L. dystrophicus, dystrophica, dystrophicum 영양장애의, 퇴행위축의, 이상증의, 이영양(증)의 **E** *dystrophic*

> L. leukodystrophia, leukodystrophiae, f. (< G. leukos *bright, white*) 백색질(白色質)장애, 백질이영양증, 대뇌 백질위축증 **E** *leukodystrophy, adrenoleukodystrophy*

> L. amyotrophia, amyotrophiae, f. (< G. a- *not* + my(o)- *muscle*) 근육위축, 근위축 **E** *amyotrophy*

< G. trephein *to feed, to nourish*

E *trophology, trophoblast* (< 'a layer which supplies nutrition to the embryo'), *cytotrophoblast* (< 'the inner cellular trophoblast'), *syncytiotrophoblast* (< 'the outer syncytial trophoblast'), *trophozoite* (< 'a protozoon in the feeding stage')

< IE. dherebh- *to coagulate*

> G. thrombos, thrombou, m. *lump, piece, curd of milk, blood clot*

> L. thrombus, thrombi, m. 혈전(血栓)

E *thrombus,* (pl.) *thrombi, thromb(o)-, thrombin, prothrombin, antithrombin(s), thromboplastin, thrombosthenin, thrombogenic, thrombolytic, thromboembolism, thrombocyte, thrombasthenia*

> G. thrombōsis, thrombōseōs, f. (< + -ōsis *condition*) *thrombosis*

> L. thrombosis, thrombosis, f. 혈전증(血栓症)

E *thrombosis, thrombotic, antithrombotic, prothrombotic,* (thrombosis >) *thrombose*

longus, longa, longum 긴, 먼, 오랜   E *lunge*

  [용례] Ars (est) longa. 예술은 길다, (배워야 할) 의술은 길다

    (문법) ars 예술, 기술: 단수 주격 < ars, artis, f.

        est 이다: esse 동사, 직설법 현재 단수 삼인칭

        longa: 형용사, 여성형 단수 주격

  > longitudo, longitudinis, f. 길이, 거리, 기간, 날줄, 경도(經度)   E *longitude*

    > longitudinalis, longitudinale 세로의, 종적(縱的)인, 날줄의, 경도의   E *longitudinal*

  > longaevus, longaeva, longaevum (< longus *long* + aevum, aevi, n. *age*) 오래 사는   E *longevous*

    > longaevitas, longaevitatis, f. 장수, 수명   E *longevity*

  > oblongus, oblonga, oblongum (< ob- *before, toward(s), over, against, away* + longus *long*) 옆으로 긴, 장방형의   E *oblong*

    > oblongatus, oblongata, oblongatum 길쭉한, 장방형의, 연(延)

  > elongo, elongavi, elongatum, elongare (< e- *out of, away from* + longus *long*) (모양을) 길게 끌다, 늘어나서 가늘게 되다   E *elongate*

  > prolongo, prolongavi, –, prolongare (< pro- *before, forward, for, instead of* + longus *long*) (시간을) 길게 끌다   E *prolong, prolongate, purloin (< 'to put at a distance')*

< IE. del- *long*

  E *long, length, along, belong, linger (< 'to continue alive, though oppressed by sickness or other distress' < 'to make long'), malinger (< 'badly weak'), Lent (< 'lengthening of the days in the spring')*

  > (*possibly*) G. dolichos, dolichē, dolichon *long, far*

    E *dolich(o)-, dolichol (< 'long-chain isoprenoid alcohols'), dolichocephalic (< 'long-headed'), dolichocranial (< 'of long skull')*

brevis, breve 짧은, 간결한   E *(neuter sing.) breve, brief*

  [용례] Vita (est) brevis. 인생은 짧다

    (문법) vita 생명은: 단수 주격 < vita, vitae, f.

        est 이다: esse 동사, 직설법 현재 단수 삼인칭

        brevis: 형용사, 남·여성형 단수 주격

  > brevitas, brevitatis, f. 짧음, 간결   E *brevity*

  > brevio, breviavi, breviatum, breviare 줄이다, 단축하다

    > abbrevio, abbreviavi, abbreviatum, abbreviare (< ab- (< ad) *to, toward, at, according to* + breviare *to shorten*) 줄이다, 단축하다   E *abbreviate, abridge, unabridged*

< IE. mregh-u- *short*   E *merry (< 'to shorten time'), mirth*

  > G. brachys, bracheia, brachy *short, not far off, little, shallow*

    E *brachy-, brachycephalic (< 'short-headed'), brachycranial (< 'of short-skull'); brachytherapy (< 'short distance therapy')*

    > G. brachiōn, brachionos, m. *arm; especially upper arm (as opposed to the longer forearm)*

      > L. brachium, brachii, n. 팔; 위팔, 상완(上腕);

팔짓, 포옹   **E** *brace, bracelet, embrace, brassiere*

    > L. brachialis, brachiale 위팔의   **E** *brachial*

    > L. antebrachium, antebrachii, n. (antibrachium, antibrachii, n.)

      (< ante- *before* + brachium *upper arm*) 아래팔,

      전완(前腕)   **E** *antebrachium (antibrachium)*

      > L. *antebrachialis, *antebrachiale (*antibrachialis, *anti-

      brachiale) 아래팔의   **E** *antebrachial (antibrachial)*

    > L. brachiocephalicus, brachiocephalica, brachiocephalicum (< *of both*

      arm and head < + G. kephalē *head*) 팔과 머리의   **E** *brachiocephalic*

    > L. Brachiosaurus, Brachiosauri, m. (< *long humerus* < G. brachiōn +

      saurus *lizard*) 브라키오사우루스속(屬)   **E** *brachiosaurus (brachiosaur)*

    > G. tribrachys, tribrachýos, m. *a metrical foot consisting of three short syllables*

      > L. tribrachys, tribrachyos, m. 삼단격(三短格), 삼약격(三弱格)   **E** *tribrach*

rotundus, rotunda, rotundum 둥근   **E** *round, rotund, rotunda, (probably) prune (< 'to round off')*

    < rota, rotae, f. 바퀴   **E** *rotavirus (< 'wheel-shaped virus'), roulette (< 'small wheel')*

    > rotarius, rotaria, rotarium 회전하는, 윤번제의, 환상(環狀)의   **E** *rotary*

    > rotula, rotulae, f. (< + -ula *diminutive suffix*) 작은 바퀴   **E** *(verb) roll*

      > rotulus, rotuli, m. 두루마리

      E *(noun) roll, role (< 'the roll of paper on which the actor's part was written'),* (contrarotulus *'copy of a roll to check accounts'* >) *control;* F. *rouleau,* (pl.) *rouleaux*

    > roto, **rotavi,** rotatum, rotare

      돌리다   **E** *rotate, rotatory,* Sp. *rodeo (< 'going-round, cattle-ring')*

      > rotatio, rotationis, f. 돌림, 회전, 자전, 교대   **E** *rotation, malrotation*

      > rotator, rotatoris, m. 회전자(回轉子); 돌림근(筋),

      회전근(回轉筋)   **E** *rotator, (rotator >) rotor*

  < IE. ret- *to run, to roll*

ovalis, ovale 난형의, 난원형의   **E** *oval*

    < IE. owyo-, oyyo- *egg* (Vide OVUM: *See* E. *ovum*)

  < IE. awi- *bird* (Vide AVIS: *See* E. *avian*)

spinosus, spinosa, spinosum 가시 많은, 가시의, 뾰족한, 까다로운   **E** *spinous*

    < spina, spinae, f. 가시; 등마루, 척추(脊椎), 척주(脊柱)   **E** *spine, spiny*

    > spinalis, spinale 등마루의, 척추의; 척수(脊髓)의   **E** *spinal*

  < IE. spei- *sharp point* (Vide SPINA: *See* E. *spine*)

lacer, lacera, lacerum 찢어진

    > lacero, **laceravi,** laceratum, lacerare 찢다, 찢어발기다   **E** *lacerate*

> laceratio, lacerationis, f. 찢김, 찢긴 상처, 열창(裂創)　　　　　　　**E** *laceration*

< IE. lek- *to tear*

> L. lacinia, laciniae, f. 옷자락　　　　　　　　　　　　　　　　　**E** *laciniate*

> L. lancino, lancinavi, lancinatum, lancinare 찢어발기다　　　　　　**E** *lancinate*

[용례] foramen rotundum 원형구멍, 정원공(正圓孔)　　　　　**E** *foramen rotundum*

foramen ovale 타원구멍, 난원공(卵圓孔)　　　　　　**E** *foramen ovale*

foramen spinosum 뇌막동맥구멍, 극공(棘孔)　　　　**E** *foramen spinosum*

foramen lacerum 파열구멍, 열공(裂孔)　　　　　　　**E** *foramen lacerum*

(문법) foramen 구멍, 공(孔): 단수 주격 < foramen, foraminis, n.

rotundum 둥근: 형용사, 중성형 단수 주격

ovale 난형의, 난원형의: 형용사, 중성형 단수 주격

spinosum 뾰족한: 형용사, 중성형 단수 주격

lacerum 찢어진: 형용사, 중성형 단수 주격

crassus, crassa, crassum 두터운, 투박한, 살찐, 우둔한　　　　　**E** *crass, grease*

< IE. kert- *to turn, to entwine* (Vide CARTILAGO; *See* E. *cartilage*)

tenuis, tenue 가는, 엷은　　　　　　　　　　　　　　　　　　　**E** *tenuous*

< IE. ten- *to stretch* (Vide TENĒRE; *See* E. *tenet*)

gracilis, gracile 가늘고 긴　　　　　　　　　　　**E** *gracile, gracilis (muscle)*

> gracilitas, gracilitatis, f. 가느다라함, 날씬함, 가냘픔, (문체의) 간결함　**E** *gracility*

albus, alba, album 흰　　　　　　　　　　　　**E** *albino, albinism, albatross*

> album, albi, n. 흰색, 흰 부분, 흰 도료, 흰 게시판　　　　　　**E** *album*

> albumen, albuminis, n. 계란 흰자위, 단백질　　**E** *albumen, (albumen >) albumin*

> albugo, albuginis, f. 백반(白斑)

> albugineus, albuginea, albugineum 계란 흰자위의, 흰

[용례] tunica albuginea 백색막　　　　　**E** *tunica albuginea (albuginea)*

(문법) tunica 막: 단수 주격 < tunica, tunicae, f. 층, 막

albuginea 흰: 형용사, 여성형 단수 주격

> albedo, albedinis, f. 흰색, 흰빛　　　　　　　　　　　　　**E** *albedo*

> albo, albavi, albatum, albare 희게 하다

> dealbo, dealbavi, dealbatum, dealbare (< de- *apart from, down, not; intensive*

+ albicare *to whiten*) 희게 하다, 흰 칠하다, 석회를 바르다　　**E** *daub*

> albico, albicavi, albicatum, albicare 하얗다, 하얗게 되다

[용례] Candida albicans 칸디다 알비칸스　　　　　　**E** Candida albicans

corpus albicans, (pl.) corpora albicantia 백체,

백색체   **E** *corpus albicans,* (pl.) *corpora albicantia*

(문법) Candida 칸디다속(屬): 단수 주격

    < Candida, Candidae, f. (불완전 진균) 칸디다속(屬)

corpus 몸, 체(體): 단수 주격 < corpus, corporis, n.

corpora: corpus의 복수 주격

albicans 하얀: 현재분사, 남·여·중성형 단수 주격

    < albicans, (gen.) albicantis

albicantia 하얀: 현재분사, 중성형 복수 주격

< IE. albho- *white*   **E** *elf* (< (possibly) 'white ghostly apparition')

ruber, rubra, rubrum 붉은

< IE. reudh- *red, ruddy* (Vide RUBER; *See* E. *rubric*)

fulvus, fulva, fulvum 적황색의   **E** *fulvous*

[용례] Penicillium griseofulvum 페니실륨 그리세오풀붐   **E** *griseofulvin*

(문법) penicillium 페니실륨: 단수 주격 < penicillium, penicillii, n.

    < penicillum, penicilli, n. 붓

griseofulvum 회색을 띤 황갈색의: 형용사, 중성형 단수 주격

    < griseus *grayish* + fulvus *reddish yellow*

< IE. ghel- *to shine; with derivatives referring to colors, bright materials, gold* (*probably* '*yellow metal*'), *and bile or gall*

E *yellow, yolk; gold, gild; gall, gallbladder, gallstone; glad* (< 'shining'), *glee, glass, glassy, glance, gleam, glimpse, glare, glitter, gloss, glow, aglow,* (possibly) *glide*

> (*probably*) L. galbus, galba, galbum 노란

> L. galbinus, galbina, galbinum (galbanus, galbana, galbanum) 노란, 연두빛의, 초록빛의, 초록빛 의복의, 여성적인   **E** *jaundice*

> G. chlōros, chlōra, chlōron *yellowish green, green*

E *chlor(o)-, chlorine (Cl)* (< 'yellowish green gas'), *chlorinate, chloride, hydrochloric acid (HCl, chlorhydric acid),* (chlorhydric acid >) *achlorhydria, chloroplast, chlorophyll (chlorophyl)* (< 'the coloring matter of the green leaves')

> L. chlorosis, chlorosis, f. (< *making green* < + G. -ōsis *condition*) 위황병(萎黃病)   **E** *chlorosis, chlorotic*

> L. chloroma, chloromatis, n. (< *greenish tumor* < + G. -ōma *noun suffix denoting tumor*) 녹색종(綠色腫)   **E** *chloroma*

> L. chlorella, chlorellae, f. (< *green alga* < + -ella *diminutive suffix*) 단세포 녹조류(綠藻類)   **E** *chlorella*

> G. chloos, chloē, chloon *light green*

> G. chloazein *to be green*

> L. chloasma, chloasmatis, n. 기미   **E** *chloasma* (melasma)

> G. cholē, cholēs, f. *bile, gall*

E cholic, chol(o)- (chole-), cholagogue, cholecyst(o)-, choledoch(o)-, choline (< 'obtained from bile'), **acetylcholine** (< 'acetyl ester of choline'), **cholesterol** (< 'first found in gallstones'), (cholesterol + calciferol >) **cholecalciferol**, **cholesteatoma** (< 'fatty tumor principally composed of cholesterol crystals'), **cholic acid**, (tauros 'bull' >) **taurocholic acid**, (chēn 'goose' >) **chenodeoxycholic acid**, (L. ursus 'bear' >) **ursodeoxycholic acid**

> G. cholera, choleras, f. *a disorder, attended with bilious diarrhea, vomiting, stomach-ache, and cramps*

> L. cholera, cholerae, f. 콜레라, 호열자(虎列刺)　　　　**E** *cholera, choleraic*

> G. melancholē, melancholēs, f. (< melan(o)- *black*) *black bile*

> G. melancholia, melancholias, f. *condition of having black bile*

> L. melancholia, melancholiae, f. 검은 담즙, 우울, 우울증　　**E** *melancholy*

> G. acholos, acholos, acholon (< a- *not*) *lacking bile*　**E** *acholous, acholia, acholic*

> L. cholesterolosis, cholesterolosis, f. (cholesterosis, cholesterosis, f.) (< *cholesterol deposition in tissue* < *cholesterol* + G. -ōsis *condition*)

콜레스테롤증　　　　　　　　　　　**E** *cholesterolosis (cholesterosis)*

> (*Persian*) zar *gold*

> (*Arabic*) al-zarnik *the (yellow) orpiment (arsenic trisulphide, As₂S₃, a bright yellow mineral which was formerly used as a dye or artist's pigment)*

> G. arsenikon, arsenikou, n. *(yellow) orpiment*

> L. arsenicum, arsenici, n. 비소(砒素)　　　　**E** *arsenic (As), arsenical*

flavus, flava, flavum 노란

E flavin(s), riboflavin, flavoprotein(s); (flavone >) flavonoid(s), flavivirus (< 'type species yellow fever virus')

< IE. bhel- *to shine, to flash, to burn; shining white, various bright colors*

E blank, blanket, blanch, bleach, bleak, blemish (< 'to injure, to make pale'), **blind** (< 'cloudy'), **blunder** (< 'to do blindly') (pitch + blende 'to blind, to deceive; because it resembles lead ore' >) **pitchblende**, **blend** (< 'to make cloudy'), **blink** (< 'to open one's eyes'), **blush**, **blond**, **blue**, **black** (< 'burned'), **blaze**, D. **Blitzkrieg**

> L. fulgeo, fulsi, -, fulgēre 번쩍이다, 번개 치다

> L. fulgur, fulguris, n. 번개, 전광(電光)

> L. fulguro, fulguravi, fulguratum, fulgurare 전광처럼 번쩍이다, 번개 치다, 전기불꽃으로 처치하다　　　　　　　**E** *fulgurate*

> L. fulguratio, fulgurationis, f. 전광, 방전요법　**E** *fulguration*

> L. fulmen, fulminis, n. (< *fulgmen) 벼락, 낙뢰

> L. fulmino, fulminavi, fulminatum, fulminare 벼락 치다, 낙뢰 치다　　　　　　　　　**E** *fulminate, fulminant*

> L. flagro, flagravi, flagratum, flagrare 불타다, 타오르다　　**E** *flagrant*

> L. flamma, flammae, f. (< *flagma) 불꽃, 화염　**E** *flame,* (suggested) *flamingo*

> L. flammo, flammavi, flammatum, flammare 불붙이다　**E** *flammable, flamboyant*

> L. inflammo, inflammavi, inflammatum, inflammare (< in- *in, on, into, toward* + flammare *to set on fire*) 불붙이다, 염증(炎症)을

일으키다   **E** *inflame, inflammable, inflammatory*

> L. inflammatio, inflammationis, f. 점화, 방화, 염증,

자극   **E** *inflammation*

> L. conflagro, **conflagravi**, conflagratum, conflagrare (< con- *with, together:*

intensive + flagrare *to blaze*) 불길에 싸이다   **E** *conflagrant*

> L. conflagratio, conflagrationis, f. 대화재   **E** *conflagration*

> G. phlegein *to burn*

> G. phlegethein *to flame, to blaze*

> G. Phlegethōn, Phlegethontos, m. (< *present participle*) (*Greek mythology*)

the river of fire, one of the five rivers of Hades   **E** *Phlegethon*

> G. phlegma, phlegmatos, n. *flame, fire, heat; morbid humor, phlegm*

> L. phlegma, phlegmatis, n. (체액설에서 네 가지 체액 중의 하나)

점액질   **E** *phlegm, phlegmatic*

> G. phlegmasia, phelgmasias, f. (< + -sia) *inflammation, swelling*

> L. phlegmasia, phlegmasiae, f. 염증(*rare or disused*), 급성 결합

조직염(*rare or disused*), 하지 종창   **E** *phlegmasia*

> G. phlegmonē, phlegmonēs, f. *heat, inflammation, inflammation beneath*

the skin

> L. phlegmone, phlegmones, f. (phlegmon, phlegmonis, f.)

결합조직염   **E** *phlegmon, phlegmonous*

> G. phlox, phlogos, f. *fire, flame*   **E** *phloxine*

> L. phlox, phlogis, f. 플록스   **E** *phlox*

> G. phlogizein *to burn up*

> G. phlogistos, phlogistē, phlogiston *burnt*

> G. phlogiston, phlogistou, n. *phlogiston*   **E** *phlogiston*

---

luteus, lutea, luteum 루툼 염색 색깔의, 누런   **E** *luteous*

[용례] corpus luteum 황체(黃體)

> **E** *corpus luteum, luteal, lutein, luteinize (<'to cause the corpus luteum to form lutein'), luteotropic (<'affecting the corpus luteum'), luteotropin, luteolysis*

(문법) corpus 몸, 체(體): 단수 주격 < corpus, corporis, n.

luteum 누런: 형용사, 중성형 단수 주격

< lutum, luti, n. 진흙탕, 진펄, 루툼(진펄에서 자라는 풀 이름, 누런 물감의 원료로 쓰였음)   **E** *lute*

> polluo, pollui, pollutum, polluĕre (< pol- (< pro) *forth*) 더럽히다,

오염시키다   **E** *pollute, (pollute >) pollutant*

> pollutio, pollutionis, f. 오염, 유정(遺精), 몽정(夢精)   **E** *pollution*

---

aureus, aurea, aureum 금으로 만든, 도금한, 금빛의, 싯누런

[용례] Staphylococcus aureus (< *grape-like clusters when viewed through a microscope* and golden-yellow colonies when cultured on agar plates) 포도알균,

황색포도상구균　　　　　　　　　　　　　　**E** Staphylococcus aureus

(문법) staphylococcus 포도알균, 포도상구균: 단수 주격

< staphylococcus, staphylococci, m.

aureus 금빛의: 형용사, 남성형 단수 주격

< aurum, auri, n. 금, 금화

< IE. aus- *to shine (said especially of the dawn), gold* (Vide AURUM; *See* E. *aurum*)

viridis, viride 초록의, 푸른, 싱싱한

E (F. verd- '*green*'>) **verdure, verdant, biliverdin** (< '*a green pigment occurring in bile*')

> viriditas, viriditatis, f. 초록색, 신록, 신선, 미숙　　　　**E** *viridity*

> virido, **viridavi**, viridatum, viridare 푸르게 하다, 푸르다

[용례] Streptococcus viridans (< *green coloration on blood agar plates*)

스트렙토코쿠스 비리단스　　　　　　　　**E** Streptococcus viridans

(문법) streptococcus 사슬알균, 연쇄구균: 단수 주격

< streptococcus, streptococci, m.

viridans 초록색의: 현재분사, 남·여·중성형 단수 주격

< viridans, (gen.) viridantis

> viridesco, −, −, viridescĕre 푸르게 되다　　　　**E** *viridescent*

∞ vireo, virui, −, virēre 푸르러지다, 번창하다

> viresco, −, −, virescĕre 푸르러지다, 번창하다　　　　**E** *virescent*

∞ virga, virgae, f. 연한 가지, 회초리, 막대기, 권장(權杖); 권장의 힘이 미치는 범위, 그

경계　　　　　　　　　　　　　　　　　**E** *verge, virgate*

> virgula, virgulae, f. 작은 가지, 작은 막대기, 신장(神杖); (인쇄) 문장부호, 빗금　**E** *virgule*

∞ virgo, virginis, f. 처녀　　　　**E** *virgin, Virginia* (< '*in honor of Queen Elizabeth*')

> virginalis, virginale 처녀의　　　　　　　　　　　　　**E** *virginal*

aeruginosus, aeruginosa, aeruginosum 동녹(銅綠)색의, 녹청(綠靑)색의　**E** *aeruginous*

[용례] Pseudomonas aeruginosa 녹농균(綠膿菌),

슈도모나스 에루지노사　　　　　　　　**E** Pseudomonas aeruginosa

(문법) Pseudomonas (세균) 슈도모나스속(屬): 단수 주격

< Pseudomonas, Pseudomonadis, f.

aeruginosa 동녹(銅綠)색의: 형용사, 여성형 단수 주격

< aerugo, aeruginis, f. (< + -ugo 표면에 생기는 것) 동녹(銅綠), 돈 독

< aes, aeris, n. 금속, 구리, 청동, 동전　　　　**E** *era* (< '*counters used in calculation*')

< IE. ayes- *metal, copper or bronze*　　　　**E** *ore*

caeruleus, caerulea, caeruleum (coeruleus, coerulea, coeruleum)

짙푸른　　　　**E** *cerulean, ceruloplasmin* (< '*deep blue colored protein in blood plasma*')

[용례] locus caeruleus (locus coeruleus) (< *the spot deep blue colored, due to light scattering from melanin in noradrenergic nerve cell bodies*) 청색반점,

청반　　　　　　　　　　　　　　　　　　　**E** *locus caeruleus (locus coeruleus, locus ceruleus)*

(문법) locus 장소, 지방, 자리: 단수 주격 < locus, loci, m.

caeruleus (coeruleus) 짙푸른: 형용사, 남성형 단수 주격

< caelum, caeli, n. (coelum, coeli, n.) 하늘, 천국

> caelestis, caeleste 하늘의, 천상의

> caelestialis, caelestiale 하늘의, 천상의　　　　　　　　　**E** *celestial*

∞ caesius, caesia, caesium

청회색의　　　　　　　**E** *caesium (cesium, Cs)* (< *'two distinctive blue lines in the spectrum'*)

violaceus, violacea, violaceum 자줏빛의, 자주색의　　　　　　　**E** *violaceous*

< viola, violae, f. 제비꽃, 오랑캐꽃, 자줏빛꽃, 자줏빛　　　　**E** *viola, violet, ultraviolet (UV)*

< *Of Mediterranean origin*

> G. ion, iou, n. *violet*

> G. iōdēs, iōdēs, iōdes (< ion *violet* + eidos *shape*) *violet-colored*

E *iodopsin(s)* (< *'visual violet(s), photopsin(s) with retinal'*; *iodine (I)* (< *'violet-colored vapor'*), *iodide, iod(o)-, periodic acid, iodinate*

brunus, bruna, brunum 갈색의, 밤색의　　　　　　　　　　**E** *brunescent*

< IE. bher- *bright, brown*　　　　　**E** *brown, bear* (< *'brown animal'*), *beaver* (< *'brown animal'*)

canus, cana, canum 흰 잿빛의, 희끄무레한, (동물·열매 등의) 털이 흰, 연로한, 존경할 만한,

엄숙한　　　　　　　　　　　　　　　　　　　　　　　**E** *canescent*

> incanus, incana, incanum (< in- *in, on, into, toward* + canus *white, hoary*) 회백

색의, 백발의

< IE. kas- *gray*　　　　　　　　　　　　　　　　　　　**E** *hare*

cinereus, cinerea, cinereum 재[灰]의, 잿빛의　　　　　　　　**E** *cinereous*

< cinis, cineris, m., f. 재[灰]

< IE. keni- *dust, ashes* (Vide CINIS: *See* E. *incinerate*)

griseus, grisea, griseum 회색의, 푸르스름한 회색의　　　　　**E** *griseous, griseofulvin*

< (*Germanic root*) gh(e)r- *to shine, to glow, gray*　　　　**E** *gray (grey), greyhound, grizzle, grizzly*

lividus, livida, lividum 검푸른, 납빛의, 멍든, 질투하는　　　　**E** *livid,* (*suggested*) *lavender*

> livor, livoris, m. 검푸름, 납빛, 질투

[용례] livor mortis 시반(屍斑)　　　　　　　　　　　　　　**E** *livor mortis*

(문법) livor 검푸름: 단수 주격

mortis 주검의: 단수 속격 < mors, mortis, f. 죽음, 주검

> lividitas, lividitatis, f. 검푸름, 흑청색화　　　　　　　　　**E** *lividity*

< liveo, −, −, livēre 검푸르다, 멍들다

> livedo, livedinis, f. 울혈반(鬱血斑), 청색피반(靑色皮斑)　　**E** *livedo*

< IE. sleiə- *bluish*　　**E** *sloe* (< 'bluish fruit')

niger, nigra, nigrum 검은

< IE. nekʷt- *night* (Vide NIGER; *See* E. *negro*)

lucidus, lucida, lucidum 빛나는, 밝은, 투명한, 또렷한　　**E** *lucid*

< IE. leuk- *light, brightness* (Vide LUX; *See* E. *lux*)

opacus, opaca, opacum 그늘진, 어두운, 빽빽한, 불투명한,
혼탁한　　**E** *opaque, radiopaque,* (opacus >) *opacification*

> opacitas, opacitatis, f. 그늘짐, 어두움, 불투명, 혼탁　　**E** *opacity*

fuscus, fusca, fuscum 어둠침침한, 가무잡잡하게 그을린, 갈색의　　**E** *fuscous*

< IE. dheu-, dheuə- *the base of a wide variety of derivatives meaning 'to rise in a cloud', as dust, vapor, or smoke, and related to semantic notions of breath, various color adjectives, and forms denoting defective perception or wits.* (Vide FUMUS; *See* E. *fume*)

pallidus, pallida, pallidum 창백한　　**E** *pallid, pale, appall (appal)* (< 'to make pale')

[용례] globus pallidus 창백핵, 담창구(淡蒼球)　　**E** *globus pallidus (pallidum)*

(문법) globus 구: 단수 주격 < globus, globi, m.

pallidus 창백한: 형용사, 남성형 단수 주격

> pallidum, pallidi, n. 창백핵, 담창구(淡蒼球)　　**E** *pallidum (globus pallidus)*

< palleo, pallui, −, pallēre 창백해지다, 겁에 질리다

> pallor, palloris, m. 창백, 공포　　**E** *pallor*

< IE. pel- *pale*　　**E** (F. tauve 'reddish yellow', 'wild animal' >) *fauvism*

> G. polios, polia, polion *grayish white*

E *poliomyelitis* (< 'involvement of the grey matter of the spinal cord'), (poliomyelitis >) *polio, poliovirus*

> G. pelios, pelia, pelion *dark, livid*

> G. Pelōps, Pelōpos, m. (< *dark-faced* < + ōps *face, eye*) (*Greek mythology*) *Pelops, king of Olympia and eponymous hero of the Peloponnesus, the land of Pelops*　　**E** *Pelops, Peloponnesus*

> L. peliosis, peliosis, f. (< + G. -ōsis *condition*) 자반병(紫斑病)　　**E** *peliosis*

비교급과 최상급

형용사에는 원급·비교급·최상급이 있으며, 어미만 규칙적으로 바뀌는 규칙 형용사와 어간까지 바뀌는 불규칙 형용사 두 가지가 있다.

●●● 규칙 형용사

비교급은 원급의 형용사 어간에 –ior(남성형과 여성형)와 –ius(중성형)를 붙여 만든다. 비교급 형용사는 제3변화 제1식의 명사변화를 따르므로 단수 탈격의 어미는 –e, 복수 속격의 어미는 –um 이 된다. 중성형의 경우, 복수 주격, 호격, 대격의 어미는 –a 가 된다. a priori 나 a posteriori 에서처럼 관용구에서는 단수 탈격의 어미 –e 대신 –i 를 쓰기도 한다.

최상급은 원급의 형용사 어간에 –issimus (남성형), –issima (여성형), –issimum (중성형)을 붙여 만든다. 남성형 단수 주격이 –er 로 끝나는 형용사는 남성 단수 주격에다 –rimus (남성형), –rima (여성형) –rimum (중성형)을 붙여 만든다. 최상급 형용사는 제1·2변화 제1식의 형용사변화를 따른다.

원 급 lat–us, lat–a, lat–um 넓은

비교급 lat–ior, lat–ior, lat–ius ((gen.) latior–is) 더 넓은

최상급 lat–issimus, lat–issima, lat–issimum 가장 넓은

    [용례] musculus latissimus dorsi 넓은 등근, 광배근(廣背筋)   **E** *latissimus dorsi (muscle)*

      (문법) musculus 근육, 근: 단수 주격 < musculus, musculi, m.

        latissimus 가장 넓은: 형용사 최상급, 남성형 단수 주격

        dorsi 등의: 단수 속격 < dorsum, dorsi, n.

  < IE. stelə– ***to extend*** (Vide LATUS; *See* E. *latitude*)

원 급 fort–is, fort–is, fort–e 강한   **E** It. *forte*

비교급 fort–ior, fort–ior, fort–ius ((gen.) fortior–is) 더 강한

최상급 fort–issimus, fort–issima, fort–issimum 가장 강한   **E** It. *fortissimo*

  < IE. bhergh– ***high; with derivatives referring to hills and hill-forts*** (Vide FORTIS; *See* E. *force*)

원 급 niger, nigra, nigrum 검은

비교급 nigr–ior, nigr–ior, nigr–ius ((gen.) nigrior–is) 더 검은

최상급 niger–rimus, niger–rima, niger–rimum 가장 검은

  < IE. nekʷt– ***night*** (Vide NIGER; *See* E. *negro*)

원 급 acer, acr–is, acr–e 신, 날카로운, 혹독한

비교급 acr–ior, acr–ior, acr–ius ((gen.) acrior–is) 더 신, 더 날카로운, 더 혹독한

최상급 acer–rimus, acer–rima, acer–rimum 가장 신, 가장 날카로운, 가장 혹독한

  < IE. ak– *sharp* (Vide ACUTUS: *See* E. *acute*)

●●● 불규칙 형용사

원 급 bonus, bona, bonum 좋은

     < IE. deu– *to do, to perform, to show favor, to revere* (Vide BONUS: *See* E. *bonus*)

비교급 melior, melior, melius ((gen.) melioris) 더 좋은   **E** *meliorism*

     < IE. mel– *strong, great* (Vide MULTUS: *See* E. *multi–*)

최상급 optimus, optima, optimum (< *wealthiest*) 가장 좋은   **E** *optimum, optimism*

     < IE. op– *to work, to produce in abundance* (Vide OPUS: *See* E. *opus*)

원 급 malus, mala, malum 나쁜

     < IE. mel– *false, bad, wrong* (Vide MALUS: *See* E. *male–*)

비교급 pejor, pejor, pejus ((gen.) pejoris) 더 나쁜   **E** *pejorate*

     < (*verbal root*) IE. ped– *to walk, to stumble, to fall*

    < IE. ped– *foot* (Vide PES: *See* E. *pedal*)

최상급 pessimus, pessima, pessimum 가장 나쁜   **E** *pessimism*

     < (*verbal root*) IE. ped– *to walk, to stumble, to fall*

    < IE. ped– *foot* (Vide PES: *See* E. *pedal*)

원 급 magnus, magna, magnum 큰

비교급 major, major, majus ((gen.) majoris) 더 큰   **E** *major*

최상급 maximus, maxima, maximum 가장 큰   **E** *maximum*

  < IE. meg– *great* (Vide MAGNUS: *See* E. *magnum*)

원 급 multus, multa, multum 많은

     < IE. mel– *strong, great* (Vide MULTUS: *See* E. *multi–*)

비교급 단수 –, –, plus ((gen.) pluris) 더 많은   **E** *plus, plural*

   복수 plures, plures, plura ((gen.) plurium)

     < IE. pelə– *to fill; with derivatives referring to abundance and multitude*

       (Vide PLĒRE: *See* E. *complete*)

최상급 plurimus, plurima, plurimum 가장 많은

< IE. pelə- *to fill; with derivatives referring to abundance and multitude*

(Vide PLĒRE: *See* E. *complete*)

원 급 **parvus, parva, parvum** 작은, 적은　　E *parvovirus (< 'small virus'); parvicellular (< 'of few cells')*

　　< IE. pau-, pou- *little, few* (Vide PUER: *See* E. *puerile*)

비교급 **minor, minor, minus** ((gen.) **minoris**) 더 작은, 더 적은　　E *minor, minus*

　　　[용례] musculus pectoralis major 큰가슴근, 대흉근(大胸筋)　　E *pectoralis major (muscle)*

　　　　　 musculus pectoralis minor 작은가슴근, 소흉근(小胸筋)　　E *pectoralis minor (muscle)*

　　　　　(문법) musculus 근육, 근: 단수 주격 < musculus, musculi, m.

　　　　　　　 pectoralis, pectorale 가슴의: 형용사, 남·여성형 단수 주격

　　　　　　　　 < pectus, pectoris, n.

　　　　　　　 major: 형용사 비교급, 남·여성형 단수 주격

　　　　　　　 minor: 형용사 비교급, 남·여성형 단수 주격

　　　[용례] labium majus, (pl.) labia majora 대음순　　E *labium majus, (pl.) labia majora*

　　　　　 labium minus, (pl.) labia minora 소음순　　E *labium minus, (pl.) labia minora*

　　　　　(문법) labium 입술: 단수 주격 < labium, labii, n.

　　　　　　　 labia 입술들: 복수 주격 < labium, labii, n.

　　　　　　　 majus: 형용사 비교급, 중성형 단수 주격

　　　　　　　 majora: 형용사 비교급, 중성형 복수 주격

　　　　　　　 minus: 형용사 비교급, 중성형 단수 주격

　　　　　　　 minora: 형용사 비교급, 중성형 복수 주격

　　　> minusculus, minuscula, minusculum (< + -culus *diminutive suffix*) 꽤 작은,

　　　　 왜소한; (문법) 소문자의　　E *minuscule (miniscule)*

　　　> minoritas, minoritatis, f. (다수에 대한) 소수, 미성년　　E *minority*

　　　> minuo, minui, minutum, minuĕre 줄이다

　　　　　> minutus, minuta, minutum (*past participle*) 작은, 세분된, 짧은

　　　　　　　E *minute,* (pars minuta prima *'first minute part'* >) *minute,* (F. menu
　　　　　　　'small, detailed' > *'detailed list'* >) *menu,* (F. menu *'small, detailed'* >
　　　　　　　'fine, delicate' >) *minuet*

　　　　　　　> minutia, minutiae, f. 부스러기; (pl.) 사소한 것,

　　　　　　　　 사소한 일　　E *(pl.) minutiae, mince*

　　　　　> comminuo, comminui, comminutum, comminuĕre (< com- (< cum) *with,*

　　　　　　 together; intensive + minuĕre *to make smaller*) 산산조각을 내다,

　　　　　　 분쇄하다　　E *comminute*

　　　　　> diminuo, diminui, diminutum, diminuĕre (< di- (< dis-) *apart from, down,*

　　　　　　 not + minuĕre *to lessen*) 줄이다　　E *diminish*

　　　　　　　> diminutivus, diminutiva, diminutivum 작은, 축소형의;

　　　　　　　　 (문법) 지소사(指小辭)의　　E *diminutive*

　　　> minister, ministri, m. 시종, 봉사자　　E *minister*

　　　　　> ministerium, ministerii, m. 시중, 봉사, 직무　　E *ministry*

> ministerialis, ministeriale 시중드는, 봉사의, 직무의   **E** *ministerial, minstrel*

> ministro, **ministravi**, ministratum, ministrare 시중들다, 섬기다, (먹을 것을)

내놓다, 보살피다, 관리하다

> administro, **administravi**, administratum, administrare (< ad- *to,*

toward, at, according to + ministrare *to serve*) 시중들다, 섬기다,

(먹을 것을) 내놓다, 보살피다, 관리하다   **E** *administrate, administrative*

< IE. mei- *small*

> G. meiōn, meiōn, meion (mikros, mikra, mikron *small, little, short*의 비교급)

lesser   **E** *mei(o)- (mio-, mi-), Miocene*

> G. meioun (meioein) *to lessen*

> G. meiōsis, meiōseōs, f. (< + G. -sis *feminine noun suffix*) *lessening*

> L. meiosis, meiosis, f. (miosis, miosis, f.) 완서법(緩敍法),

경감기(輕減期), 감수(減數)분열   **E** *meiosis (miosis), meiotic (miotic)*

> (*Russian*) men'she *less*   **E** *Menshevik*

최상급 minimus, minima, minimum 가장 작은, 가장 적은   **E** *minimum, minimal, minim, minimize*

< IE. mei- *small* (Vide supra)

원 급 senex, senex, – ((gen.) senis) 늙은   **E** *senile*

비교급 senior, senior, – ((gen.) senioris) 더 늙은   **E** *senior*

최상급 (없음)

< IE. sen- *old* (Vide SENEX; *See* E. *senile*)

원 급 juvenis, juvenis, – ((gen.) juvenis) 젊은   **E** *juvenile*

비교급 junior, junior, – ((gen.) junioris) 더 젊은   **E** *junior*

최상급 (없음)

< IE. yeu- *vital force, youthful vigor* (Vide JUVENIS; *See* E. *juvenile*)

●●● 불규칙 형용사

두 가지 최상급을 가지는 장소의 형용사

원 급 exter (exterus), extera, exterum 바깥의

비교급 exterior, exterior, exterius ((gen.) exterioris) 더 바깥의   **E** *exterior*

최상급 extremus, extrema, extremum 맨 바깥의   **E** *extreme*

extimus, extima, extimum

< IE. eghs *out* (Vide EX; *See* E. *ex-*)

원 급 superus, supera, superum 위쪽의, 상부(上部)의

비교급 superior, superior, superius ((gen.) superioris) 더 위쪽의, 더 상부의   **E** *superior*

최상급 supremus, suprema, supremum 맨 위쪽의, 가장 상부의   **E** *supreme*

       summus, summa, summum   **E** *summa, (pl.) summae*

> [용례] Summum jus, summa injuria. 최고의 공정(公正)은 최고의 불의(이다) (극단적으로
> 엄격한 법규정은 극단의 불의이다) (Marcus Tullius Cicero, 106-43 B.C.E.)
> (문법) summum 정상의, 지대한, 마지막의: 형용사 최상급, 중성형 단수 주격
>   jus 법: 단수 주격 < jus, juris, n.
>   summa 정상의, 지대한, 마지막의: 형용사 최상급, 여성형 단수 주격
>   injuria 불법, 불의, 모욕, 침해, 손상: 단수 주격 < injuria, injuriae, f.

  < IE. uper *over* (Vide SUPER: *See* E. *super-*)

원 급 inferus, infera, inferum 아래쪽의, 하부(下部)의

비교급 inferior, inferior, inferius ((gen.) inferioris) 더 아래쪽의, 더 하부의   **E** *inferior*

최상급 infimus, infima, infimum 맨 아래쪽의, 가장 하부의

       imus, ima, imum   **E** *ima*

> [용례] arteria thyroidea ima (< *lowest thyroid artery*, *thyroid ima artery*)
>   맨아래갑상샘동맥
> (문법) arteria 동맥: 단수 주격 < arteria, arteriae, f.
>   thyroidea 갑상샘의: 형용사, 여성형 단수 주격
>   < thyroideus, thyroidea, thyroideum
>   ima 맨 아래의: 형용사 최상급, 여성형 단수 주격

  < IE. ndher- *under* (Vide INFRA: *See* E. *infra-*)

원 급 posterus, postera, posterum 뒤의

비교급 posterior, posterior, posterius ((gen.) posterioris) 더 뒤의   **E** *posterior*

최상급 postremus, postrema, postremum 맨 뒤의

       postumus, postuma, postumum   **E** *posthumous*

  < (*probably*) IE. apo-, ap- *off, away* (Vide AB: *See* E. *ab-*)

● ● ● **불규칙 형용사**

원급 없이 비교급과 최상급만을 가지는 형용사. 대부분 전치사로부터 파생한 형용사이다.

(전치사) ante 앞에

비교급 anterior, anterior, anterius ((gen.) anterioris) 앞의, 이전의

최상급 (없음)

　< IE. ant- *front, forehead* (Vide ANTE: *See* E. *ante-*)

E *anterior*

(전치사) inter 가운데에서, 사이에서

비교급 interior, interior, interius ((gen.) interioris) 안쪽의

최상급 intimus, intima, intimum 맨 안쪽의

　< IE. en *in* (Vide IN: *See* E. *in-*)

E *interior*

E *intima*

(전치사) prope 가까이

비교급 propior, propior, propius ((gen.) propioris) 더 가까운

최상급 proximus, proxima, proximum 가장 가까운

　< IE. per *basic meanings of 'forward', 'through'* (Vide PER: *See* E. *per-*)

E *proximal*

형용사의 위치

　　형용사는 명사를 한정적 또는 서술적으로 꾸민다. 학술용어에서는 한정적 용법의 형용사가 대부분이다. 한정적 용법의 형용사 위치는, 딱히 정해져 있지 않으나, 일반적으로 다음과 같다.

속성을 나타내는 형용사와 형용사적으로 쓰이는 소유대명사는 명사의 뒤에 놓는다. 그러나 뜻을 강조하기 위해 형용사나 소유대명사를 명사 앞에 놓을 수 있다.

　　[용례] Terminologia Anatomica (TA) 해부학 용어
　　　　(문법) terminologia 용어론, (총칭) 용어: 단수 주격
　　　　　　　< terminologia, terminologiae, f.
　　　　　　anatomica 해부학의: 형용사, 여성형 단수 주격
　　　　　　　< anatomicus, anatomica, anatomicum

　　[용례] Nomina Anatomica (NA) 해부학 용어
　　　　(문법) nomina 이름들: 복수 주격 < nomen, nominis, n.
　　　　　　anatomica 해부학의: 형용사, 중성형 복수 주격

　　[용례] Veritas (est) lux mea. 진리는 나의 빛(이다)
　　　　(문법) veritas 진리: 단수 주격 < veritas, veritatis, f.
　　　　　　est 이다: esse 동사, 직설법 현재 단수 삼인칭
　　　　　　lux 빛: 단수 주격 < lux, lucis, f.

mea 나의: 형용사적 소유대명사, 여성형 단수 주격

[용례] mea culpa 내 탓으로, 내 잘못으로
(문법) mea 나의: 형용사적 소유대명사, 여성형 단수 탈격
culpa 탓으로, 잘못으로: 단수 탈격 < culpa, culpae, f.

수량을 나타내는 형용사나 지시형용사, 의문형용사는 명사의 앞에 놓는다.

[용례] Omnis cellula e cellula 모든 세포는 세포로부터 (Rudolf Ludwig Carl Virchow, 1821-1902)
(문법) omnis 모든: 형용사, 남·여성형 단수 주격 < omnis, omne
cellula 세포는: 단수 주격 < cellula, cellulae, f.
e ~로부터: 전치사, 탈격지배
cellula 세포: 단수 탈격 < cellula, cellulae, f.

관례상 명사의 앞에 놓는 경우에는 관례를 따른다.

[용례] dura mater (< *hard mother*) 경막(硬膜), 경질막(硬質膜)

arachnoidea mater (< *cobweb-like mother*) 거미막, 지주막(蜘蛛膜)

pia mater (< *tender mother*) 연막(軟膜), 연질막(軟質膜)

(문법) dura 단단한, 엄한: 형용사, 여성형 단수 주격
< durus, dura, durum 단단한, 굳은, 투박한, 엄한, 잘 견디어내는
arachnoidea 거미줄 같은: 형용사, 여성형 단수 주격
< arachnoideus, arachnoidea, arachnoideum 거미줄 같은
pia 자애로운: 형용사, 여성형 단수 주격
< pius, pia, pium 효성스러운, 애정이 두터운, 나라를 사랑하는, 경건한,
자애로운, 상냥한
mater 뇌척수막(腦脊髓膜): 단수 주격
< mater, matris, f. 어머니; (어머니의 역할을 하는) 뇌막(腦膜), 척수막(脊髓膜)

E *dura mater*

E *arachnoidea mater*

E *pia mater*

형용사의 명사적 용법

형용사를 명사처럼 사용할 수 있다. 형용사 남성형은 '~ 남자' 또는 '~ 사람', 여성형은 '~ 여자' 또는 추상명사, 중성형은 '~ 것' 또는 추상명사로 사용할 수 있는 것이다.

---

novus, nova, novum 새로운

[용례] de novo (< *from new*) 처음부터, 새로이   **E** *de novo*

    (문법) de ~로부터, ~에 대하여: 전치사, 탈격지배

       novo 새로움으로: 형용사의 명사적 용법, 중성 단수 탈격

< IE. newo- *new* (*related to* IE. nu- *now*) (Vide NOVUS; *See* E. *nova*)

omnis, omne (< *abundant*) 모든

[용례] omnibus (모든 사람에게 > 모든 사람을 위한) 합승마차, 버스, 총괄,

  일괄   **E** (dat. pl.) *omnibus (bus)*

    (문법) 형용사의 명사적 용법, 남·여·중성 복수 여격 (여기서는 남성으로 사용)

< IE. op- *to work, to produce in abundance* (Vide OMNIS; *See* E. *omni-*)

similis, simile 비슷한

[용례] Fac simile! 비슷한 것을 만들어라!   **E** *facsimile,* (facsimile >) *fax*

    (문법) fac 너는 만들어라: facĕre (*to make*)의 능동태 명령법 현재 단수 이인칭

      simile 비슷한 것을: 형용사의 명사적 용법, 중성 단수 대격

< IE. sem- *one; also adverbially 'as one', together with* (Vide IE. sem-; *See* E. *same*)

형용사를 아예 명사로 전용하기도 한다.

---

membrana, membranae, f. 가죽, 껍질, 양피지, 막(膜),

        피막(皮膜)   **E** *membrane, membranous (membraneous), pseudomembranous*

         > membranaceus, membranacea, membranaceum 막으로 덮인,

      막 모양의   **E** *membranaceous*

            [용례] placenta membranacea 막태반(膜胎盤)   **E** *placenta membranacea*

             (문법) placenta 태반: 단수 주격 < placenta, placentae, f.

               membranacea 막 모양의: 형용사, 여성형 단수 주격

           > semimembranosus, semimembranosa, semimembranosum (< semi- *half*)

             반막 모양의 **E** *semimembranosus (muscle)* (< '*fascial in half*'), *semimembranous*

        < *membranus, *membrana, *membranum 몸을 구성하는

     < membrum, membri, n. 사지(四肢), 지체(肢體), 구성원   **E** *member*

       > dismembro, **dismembravi**, dismembratum, dismembrare (< dis- *apart from,*

       down, not) 사지를 절단하다, 분할하다, 축소하다   **E** *dismember*

  < IE. mems- *flesh, meat*

     > (*possibly*) L. mensa, mensae, f. (< *food on a table*) 식탁, 상   **E** Sp. *mesa*

       > L. mensalis, mensale 식탁의   **E** *mensal*

         > L. commensalis, commensale (< com- (< cum) *with, together*) 함께 식사

하는; 공생의, 기거생활의, 편리공생의 　　　　　E *commensal, commensalism*

> G. mēninx, mēningos, f. *membrane (of the brain)*

　　> L. meninx, meningis, f. 수막(髓膜),

　　　　뇌막(腦膜) 　　　　　　　E *meninx,* (pl.) *meninges, meningeal, mening(o)-*

　　　　> L. leptomeninx, leptomeningis, f. (< *the pia-arachnoid* < G. leptos *thin*)

　　　　　　연질뇌척수막, 연수막(軟髓膜) 　　E *leptomeninx,* (pl.) *leptomeninges*

　　　　> L. pachymeninx, pachymeningis, f. (< G. pachys *thick*)

　　　　　　경수막(硬髓膜) 　　　　　　　E *pachymeninx*

　　　　> L. meningismus, meningismi, m. (< + -ismus *noun suffix*)

　　　　　　수막자극증 　　　　　　　　　E *meningismus (meningism)*

　　　　> L. meningitis, meningitidis, f. (< + -itis *noun suffix denoting inflammation*)

　　　　　　수막염(髓膜炎) 　　　　　E *meningitis,* (pl.) *meningitides, meningitic*

　　> L. myrinx, myringis, f. (< myringa < meninga) 고막(鼓膜) 　E *myring(o)-, myringoplasty*

intestinum, intestini, n. 내장, 창자 　　　　　　　　　　　　E *intestine*

　　　　　> intestinalis, intestinale 내장의, 창자의 　　　　　E *intestinal*

　　　　< intestinus, intestina, intestinum 안의, 안에 있는

　　< intus (부사) 안에서, 안으로

< IE. en *in* (Vide IN: *See* E. *in-*)

mediastinum, mediastini, n. 세로칸, 종격(縱隔) 　　　　E *mediastinum, mediastinal*

　　　　< mediastinus, mediastina, mediastinum 가운데의

　　　　< medius, media, medium 가운데의

< IE. medhyo- *middle* (Vide MEDIALIS: *See* E. *medial*)

sericum, serici, n. 명주, 비단　E *sericulture, sericin* (< *'silk protein'*), (*'sericin'* >) *serine (Ser, S), silk*

　　　　　　< sericus, serica, sericum 명주의,

　　　　　　비단의 　　　　　　　　E (serica lana *'Seric wool'* >) *serge*

　　　　< Sericus, Serica, Sericum 동방의, 중국의

　　　　< Ser, Seris, m. ((pl.) Seres, Serum, m.) (명주로 유명하던) 동방 아시아

　　　　　　주민, 중국 서북부의 민족, 중국인

　　< G. Sērikos, Sērikē, Sērikon *of Sēres*

< G. Sēres *the oriental people, perhaps the Chinese, from whom silk was first obtained*

vivum, vivi, n. 생체, 생살, 원금(原金)

　　　　[용례] in vivo 생체 안에서, 생체 안의, 생체내 　　　　E *in vivo*

　　　　　　ex vivo 생체 밖에서, 생체 밖의, 생체외 　　　　E *ex vivo*

　　　　(문법) in ~ 안에서, ~ 안의: 전치사, 탈격지배

　　　　　　ex ~ 밖으로, ~ 밖의: 전치사, 탈격지배

　　　　　　vivo 생체: 단수 탈격

< vivus, viva, vivum 살아 있는

< IE. gʷeiə-, gʷei- *to live* (Vide VIVĒRE: *See* E. *vivarium*)

bacteroides, bacteroidis, m. 박테로이드

< L. *bacteroides, (gen.) *bacteroidis (< *bacterium-like* < + G. eidos *shape*)

박테로이드의

< G. baktērion, baktēriou, n. (< + -ion *diminutive suffix*) *small staff, bacterium*

< G. baktēria, baktērias, f. (baktron, baktrou, n.) *staff, stick*

< IE. bak- *staff used for support* (Vide BACTERIUM: *See* E. *bacterium*)

원래는 명사를 수식하는 형용사였으나 명사를 생략하여도 뜻이 분명하기 때문에 형용사 단독으로 사용되다가 명사로 전용되기도 한다.

---

cornea, corneae, f. 각막(角膜)

< corneus, cornea, corneum 뿔의, 뿔로 만든, 각질(角質)의

[용례] tunica cornea (tela cornea) (< *from its horny consistence*) 각질막, 각질 조직

(문법) tunica 막: 단수 주격 < tunica, tunicae, f. 층, 막

tela 조직: 단수 주격

< tela, telae, f. 베, 직물, 거미줄, 날실, 막, 조직

cornea 각질(角質)의: 형용사, 여성형 단수 주격

< cornu, cornus, n. 뿔

< IE. ker- *horn, head; with derivatives referring to horned animals, horn-shaped objects, and projecting parts* (Vide CORNU: *See* E. *unicorn*)

conjunctiva, conjunctivae, f. 결막(結膜), 이음막

< conjunctivus, conjunctiva, conjunctivum 연결시키는, 잇는; 접속어의

[용례] tunica conjunctiva (< *conjoining the eyeball with the eyelid*) 결막(結膜), 이음막

(문법) tunica 막: 단수 주격 < tunica, tunicae, f. 층, 막

conjunctiva 연결시키는: 형용사, 여성형 단수 주격

< conjungo, conjunxi, conjunctum, conjungĕre (< con- (< cum) *with, together* + jungĕre *to yoke*) 짝지어 멍에 메우다, 연결시키다, 잇다

< IE. yeug- *to yoke* (Vide JUNGĔRE: *See* E. *join*)

choroidea, choroideae, f. (chorioidea, chorioideae, f.)

맥락막(脈絡膜)

< choroideus, choroidea, choroideum (chorioideus, chorioidea, chorioideum)

(< + G. eidos *shape*) 융모막 모양의, 혈관이 얼기설기한, 맥락(脈絡)의

[용례] tela choroidea (tela chorioidea) (< *the choroid coat (of the eye)*

< G. chorioeidēs chitōn) 맥락막(脈絡膜)

(문법) tela 조직: 단수 주격 < tela, telae, f.

choroidea (chorioidea) 혈관이 얼기설기한: 형용사, 여성형 단수 주격

< G. chorion, choriou, n. *intestinal membrane, fetal membrane, afterbirth*

< IE. gherə- *gut, entrail* (Vide CHORDA: *See* E. *chord*)

intima, intimae, f. 내막(內膜), 속막   **E** *intima, intimal*

< intimus, intima, intimum (형용사 최상급) 맨 안쪽의

[용례] tunica intima 맨 안쪽 막

(문법) tunica 막: 단수 주격 < tunica, tunicae, f. 층, 막

intima 맨 안쪽의: 형용사 최상급, 여성형 단수 주격

< IE. en *in* (Vide IN: *See* E. *in-*)

media, mediae, f. 중간막(中間膜)   **E** *media, medial*

< medius, media, medium 가운데의

[용례] tunica media 가운데 막

(문법) tunica 막: 단수 주격 < tunica, tunicae, f. 층, 막

media 가운데의: 형용사, 여성형 단수 주격

< IE. medhyo- *middle* (Vide MEDIALIS: *See* E. *medial*)

adventitia, adventitiae, f. 외막(外膜), 바깥막   **E** *adventitia, adventitial*

< adventitius, adventitia, adventitium (< ad- *to, toward, at, according to* + venire

to come) (바깥에서부터) 다가오는, 외래의, 우발적인

[용례] tunica adventitia 바깥막

(문법) tunica 막: 단수 주격 < tunica, tunicae, f. 층, 막

adventitia 외래의: 형용사, 여성형 단수 주격

< IE. gʷa-, gʷem- *to go, to come* (Vide VENIRE: *See* E. *venue*)

mucosa, mucosae, f. 점막(粘膜)   **E** *mucosa, mucosal*

< mucosus, mucosa, mucosum 점액이 많은, 점액을 분비하는, 점액의, 점액성의

[용례] tunica mucosa (< *mucous membrane*) 점액성 막

(문법) tunica 막: 단수 주격 < tunica, tunicae, f. 층, 막

mucosa 점액성의: 형용사, 여성형 단수 주격

< mucus, muci, m. 콧물, 점액

< IE. meug- *slimy, slippery* (Vide MUCUS: *See* E. *mucus*)

submucosa, submucosae, f. 점막하조직   **E** *submucosa, submucosal (submucous)*

    < submucosus, submucosa, submucosum (< sub- *under, up from under* + mucosa

    mucous membrane) 점막 아래의

       [용례] tela submucosa 점막 아래 조직

        (문법) tela 조직: 단수 주격 < tela, telae, f.

          submucosa 점막 아래의: 형용사, 여성형 단수 주격

  < IE. upo *up from under, over, under* (Vide SUB; *See* E. *sub-*)

muscularis, muscularis, f. 근육층 **E** *muscularis (muscularis externa, muscular tunic, muscular coat)*

    < muscularis, musculare 근육의

      [용례] tunica muscularis (externa) (바깥) 근육층

       (문법) tunica 막: 단수 주격 < tunica, tunicae, f. 층, 막

        muscularis 근육의: 형용사, 남·여성형 단수 주격

        externa 바깥의: 형용사, 여성형 단수 주격

         < externus, externa, externum

    < musculus, musculi, m. 근육, 근

  < IE. mus- *mouse* (Vide MUSCULUS; *See* E. *muscle*)

subserosa, subserosae, f. 장막하조직   **E** *subserosa, subserosal*

    < subserosus, subserosa, subserosum (< sub- *under, up from under*) 장막 아래의

      [용례] tela subserosa 장막 아래 조직

       (문법) tela 조직: 단수 주격 < tela, telae, f.

        subserosa 장막 아래의: 형용사, 여성형 단수 주격

serosa, serosae, f. 장막(漿膜)   **E** *serosa, serosal*

    < serosus, serosa, serosum 장액성(漿液性)의, 혈청의

      [용례] tunica serosa (< *serous membrane*) 장액성 막

       (문법) tunica 막: 단수 주격 < tunica, tunicae, f. 층, 막

        serosa 장액성의: 형용사, 여성형 단수 주격

    < serum, seri, n. 장액, 혈청

  < IE. ser- *to stream*

duodenum, duodeni, n. 십이지장(十二指腸), 샘창자   **E** *duodenum*

    > duodenalis, duodenale 십이지장의   **E** *duodenal*

    < duodeni, duodenae, duodena *twelve each*, 열둘씩

      [용례] intestinum duodenum digitorum (< *intestine of twelve fingerbreadths*

      (in length)) (길이에 있어서) 열두 손가락(폭)의 창자

(문법) intestinum 내장, 창자: 단수 주격

　　　　　　　　duodenum: 배분수사, 남성형 복수 속격; digitorum을 수식

　　　　　　　　digitorum 손가락들의: 복수 속격 < digitus, digiti, m.

　< IE. dwo- **two** (Vide IE. dwo-; *See* E. *two*)

　+ IE. dekm **ten** (Vide IE. dekm; *See* E. *ten*)

jejunum, jejuni, n. 빈창자, 공장(空腸)　　　　　　　　　　　**E** *jejunum, jejunal*

　　　< jejunus, jejuna, jejunum 굶주린,

　　　　속이 빈　　　　　　　　**E** *jejune,* (*disjejunare *'to break one's fast'* >) *dine, dinner*

　　　　[용례] intestinum jejunum (< *empty intestine, usually found so after death*)

　　　　　　　　빈 창자

　　　　　　(문법) intestinum 내장, 창자: 단수 주격

　　　　　　　　jejunum 빈: 형용사, 중성형 단수 주격

ileum, ilei, n. 돌창자, 회장(回腸)　　　　　　　　　　　　　　**E** *ileum, ileal*

　　　< ileus, ilea, ileum 아랫배 옆구리의, 샅의

　　　　[용례] intestinum ileum (< *intestine in flanks, intestine in groins*) 아랫배 창자

　　　　　　(문법) intestinum 내장, 창자: 단수 주격

　　　　　　　　ileum 아랫배 옆구리의: 형용사, 중성형 단수 주격

　　< ilia, ilium, n. (pl.) (< (sing.) ile, ilis, n.) 아랫배 옆구리; 샅, 사타구니,

　　　서혜부(鼠蹊部)　　　　**E** *jade* (< Sp. piedra de ijada *'stone of the flank (stone for colic)'*)

　　　> ilium, ilii, n. 엉덩뼈, 장골(腸骨)　　　　　　　　　　　　**E** *ilium*

　　　　> iliacus, iliaca, iliacum 엉덩뼈의, 장골의　　　　　　　　**E** *iliac*

　　　　　[용례] musculus iliacus 엉덩근, 장근　　　　　　　**E** *iliacus (muscle)*

　　　　　　　(문법) musculus 근육, 근: 단수 주격 < musculus, musculi, m.

　　　　　　　　iliacus 엉덩뼈의, 장골의: 형용사, 남성형 단수 주격

caecum, caeci, n. 막창자, 맹장(盲腸)　　　　　　　　　**E** *caecum (cecum), cecal*

　　　< caecus, caeca, caecum 눈먼, 막힌

　　　　[용례] intestinum caecum (< *blind intestine*) 막힌 창자

　　　　　　(문법) intestinum 내장, 창자: 단수 주격

　　　　　　　　caecum 막힌: 형용사, 중성형 단수 주격

　< IE. kaiko- **one-eyed**

rectum, recti, n. 곧창자, 직장(直腸)　　　　　　　　　　　**E** *rectum, rectal*

　　　< rectus, recta, rectum 곧은

　　　　[용례] intestinum rectum (< *straight intestine*) 곧은 창자

　　　　　　(문법) intestinum 내장, 창자: 단수 주격

rectum 곧은: 형용사(과거분사), 중성형 단수 주격

< IE. reg- *to move in a straight line* (Vide REGÉRE; *See* E. *regent*)

형용사를 만드는 방법

●●● 동사의 차용

동사와 형용사의 기능을 함께 갖는 분사를 형용사로 쓸 수 있다.

현재분사 동사의 현재분사를 형용사로 차용한다. 능동 또는 진행의 뜻을 가진다. 남·여·중
성형의 단수 주격이 –ns, 단수 속격이 –ntis가 되며 제3변화 제3식의 형용사변화를
따른다.

communicans, (gen.) communicantis 교통(交通)하는

< communico, communicavi, communicatum, communicare (< com- (< cum) *with, together*
+ munis *of duty*) 함께 참여시키다, 교류하다, 교통하다, 소통하다

[용례] ramus communicans, (pl.) rami communicantes 교통가지,

교통지　　　　　　　　　　　**E** *ramus communicans,* (pl.) *rami communicantes*

(문법) ramus 가지[枝]: 단수 주격 < ramus, rami, m.

communicans 교통하는: 현재분사, 남·여·중성형 단수 주격

< communicans, (gen.) communicantis

rami 가지[枝]들: 복수 주격

communicantes 교통하는: 현재분사, 남·여성형 복수 주격

< IE. mei- *to change, to go, to move* (Vide MUTARE; *See* E. *mutate*)

occludens, (gen.) occludentis 가두는, 막는

< occludo, occlusi, occlusum, occludĕre (< oc- (< ob-) *before, toward(s), over, against,*
away + claudĕre *to shut*) 가두다, 막다

[용례] zonula occludens, (pl.) zonulae occludentes 폐쇄띠,

폐쇄소대(小帶)　　　　　　　**E** *zonula occludens,* (pl.) *zonulae occludentes*

(문법) zonula 작은 띠, 소대(小帶): 단수 주격 < zonula, zonulae, f.

occludens 가두고 있는: 현재분사, 남·여·중성형 단수 주격

< occludens, (gen.) occludentis

zonulae 작은 띠들, 소대(小帶)들: 복수 주격

occludentes 가두고 있는: 현재분사, 남·여성형 복수 주격

< IE. klau- (*possibly*) *hook, peg* (Vide CLAUDĔRE: *See* E. *close*)

과거분사 동사의 과거분사를 형용사로 차용한다. 수동 또는 완료의 뜻을 가진다. 남·여·중
성형의 단수 주격이 –us, –a, –um으로 끝나며 형용사 제1·2변화를 따른다.

---

falsus, falsa, falsum 거짓의 **E** *false, falsehood,* (*probably*) *faucet* (< '*to make a breach in*')

> falsificus, falsifica, falsificum (< falsus *false* + –ficus (< facĕre) *making*)

속이는, 조작의

> falsifico, **falsificavi**, falsificatum, falsificare 속이다, 조작하다 **E** *falsify*

> falsificatio, falsificationis, f. 착오, 조작, 변조 **E** *falsification*

< falsus, falsa, falsum (과거분사) 속은

< fallo, **fefelli**, falsum, fallĕre 속이다 **E** *fail, failure*

> fallax, (**gen.**) fallacis 속이는

> fallacia, fallaciae, f. 속임수 **E** *fallacy*

> fallaciosus, fallaciosa, fallaciosum 속임수의 **E** *fallacious*

> *fallita, *fallitae, f. 잘못, 결함;

(지질) 단층 **E** *fault, default* (< '*due to failure to fulfil an obligation*')

< IE. ghwel– *to bend, to deviate*

hamatus, hamata, hamatum 낚시 달린, 갈고리 모양의, 걸려들게 하는 **E** *hamate*

< hamatus, hamata, hamatum (과거분사) 낚인

< hamo, **hamavi**, hamatum, hamare 낚시하다, 낚다

< hamus, hami, m. 낚시, 갈고리, 속임수

> hamulus, hamuli, m. (< + –ulus *diminutive suffix*) 작은 낚시, 작은 갈고리 **E** *hamulus*

● ● ● **형용사 접미사의 이용**

접미사를 붙여 형용사를 만든다.

–ivus, –iva, –ivum 동사의 어근이나 어간에 붙여 관계나 성격을 가리키는 형용사를 **E** *-ive*
만든다.

---

activus, activa, activum 활동적인, 능동의; (문법) 능동태의 **E** *active*

> activitas, activitatis, f. 활동, 활성도 **E** *activity*

< ago, **egi**, actum, agĕre 하다, 움직이다, 몰다, 무게를 달다

< IE. ag– *to drive, to draw, to move* (Vide AGĔRE: See E. *act*)

passivus, passiva, passivum 당하는, 수동적인, 피동의, 소극적인;

　　(문법) 수동태의　　　　　　　　E *passive, passivity* (< (probably) on the pattern of activity)

　　　　< patior, passus sum, pati 당하다, 견디다, 참다, 고통받다, 내버려 두다

　< IE. pe(i)- *to hurt* (Vide PATI: *See* E. *patient*)

nativus, nativa, nativum 태어난 그대로의, 천부(天賦)의, 토박이의　　　　　E *native*

　　　　　　> nativitas, nativitatis, f. 출생, 탄생　　　　　　　　　E *nativity*

　　　　< L. nascor, natus sum, nasci (자동사) 태어나다, 출생하다, 생기다

　< IE. genə-, gen- *to give birth, to beget; with derivatives referring to aspects and results of procreation and to familial and tribal groups* (Vide GIGNĔRE: *See* E. *genital*)

-idus, -ida, -idum　　동사의 어근이나 어간 또는 명사의 어간에 붙여 상태를 가리키는　　E *-id*
　　　　　　　　　　형용사를 만든다.

---

frigidus, frigida, frigidum 추운, 찬, 냉담한　　　　　　　　　　　E *frigid*

　　　　　　> frigiditas, frigiditatis, f. 추위, 한랭, 냉감증, 불감증　　E *frigidity*

　　　　< frigeo, frigui (frixi), -, frigēre 차게 되다, 냉대받다

　　　< frigus, frigoris, n. 추위

　　　　　　> frigero, frigeravi, frigeratum, frigerare 차게 하다　　E *refrigerator*

　< IE. srig- *cold*

rancidus, rancida, rancidum 썩은 냄새가 나는, 쉰, 악취 나는;

　　역겨운　　　　　　　　E *rancid*, (rancid >) *rancidity*, (rancid >) *rancidify; rancor (rancour)*

　　　　< ranceo, -, -, rancēre (*obsolete*) 썩다, 쉬다, 악취 나다

sordidus, sordida, sordidum 더러운, 때 묻은, 비천한　　　　　E *sordid*

　　　　< sordeo, sordui, -, sordēre 더럽다, 때 묻다, 비천하다

　< IE. swordo- *black, dirty*　　　　　　　　　　　　　　E *swart (swarthy)*

tepidus, tepida, tepidum 따뜻한, 미지근한, 식은　　　　　　E *tepid*

　　　　< tepeo, -, -, tepēre 따뜻하다, 미지근하다

　< IE. tep- *to be hot*

timidus, timida, timidum 무서워하는　　　　　　　　　　　E *timid*

　　　　　> timiditas, timiditatis, f. 겁, 소심　　　　　　　E *timidity*

　　　　　> intimido, intimidavi, intimidatum, intimidare (< in- *in, on, into, toward*)

　　　　　　겁주다　　　　　　　　　　　　　　E *intimidate, intimidation*

　　　< timeo, timui, -, timēre 무서워하다

morbidus, morbida, morbidum 병의, 병든, 병에 잘 걸리는 ⟦E⟧ *morbid*

         > morbiditas, morbiditatis, f. 병적 상태, 이환(罹患), 이환율 ⟦E⟧ *morbidity*

     < morbus, morbi, m. 병(病)

   < IE. mer– *to rub away, to harm* (Vide MORI: *See* E. *mortal*)

–ilis, –ile   동사의 어근이나 어간에 붙여 가능성을 뜻하는 ⟦E⟧ *–ile*
–bilis, –bile   형용사를 만든다. ⟦E⟧ *–ble (–able, –ible)*

---

reptilis, reptile 기어 다니는, 파행(爬行)의, 파충류(爬蟲類)의 ⟦E⟧ *reptile*

     < repo, repsi, reptum, repĕre 기다, 기어 다니다

   < IE. rep– *to creep, to slink*

miserabilis, miserabile 불쌍한 ⟦E⟧ *miserable*

       < miseror, miseratus sum, miserari 불쌍히 여기다

     < miser, misera, miserum 불쌍한 ⟦E⟧ *miser, miserly*

       > miseria, miseriae, f. 비참, 고통 ⟦E⟧ *misery*

   < IE. mais–, mis– *wretched*

–bundus, –bunda, –bundum   동사의 어근이나 어간에 붙여 진행을 뜻하는 ⟦E⟧ *–bund, –bond*
                                      형용사를 만든다.

---

moribundus, moribunda, moribundum 죽어 가는, 빈사 상태의, 치명적인 ⟦E⟧ *moribund*

     < morior, mortuus sum, mori 죽다

   < IE. mer– *to rub away, to harm* (Vide MORI: *See* E. *mortal*)

vagabundus, vagabunda, vagabundum 떠돌아다니는, 방황하는 ⟦E⟧ *vagabond*

       < vagor, vagatus sum, vagari 떠돌아다니다, 방황하다

     < vagus, vaga, vagum 이리저리 다니는, 정처 없는, 방랑하는

    < IE. wag– *to be bent*

  < (*probably*) IE. wa– (Vide VAGUS: *See* E. *vague*)

–us, –a, –um   (제1·2변화 제1식)
–is, –e   (제3변화 제2식)   명사 어간에 붙여 속성을 가리키는 형용사를 만든다.
–or, (gen.) –oris   (제3변화 제3식)

–florus, –flora, –florum 꽃의, 꽃을 피우는, 꽃피는

> densiflorus, densiflora, densiflorum (< densus, densa, densum *dense*) 빽빽
하게 꽃피는

[용례] Pinus densiflora 소나무

E Pinus densiflora

(문법) pinus 소나무: 단수 주격 < pinus, pinus, f.

densiflora 빽빽하게 꽃피는: 형용사, 여성형 단수 주격

< flos, floris, m. 꽃

< IE. bhle- *to thrive, to bloom* (Vide FLOS; See E. *floral*)

-formis, -forme ~ 모양의, ~형(形)의

E -form

> multiformis, multiforme (< multus, multa, multum *many, much*) 여러 모양의,
다형(多形)의

E multiform

[용례] erythema multiforme 다형 홍반(紅斑)

E erythema multiforme

(문법) erythema 홍반: 단수 주격 < erythema, erythematis, n.

multiforme 다형의: 형용사, 중성형 단수 주격

< forma, formae, f. 모양, 형식, 방식

< G. morphē, morphēs, f. *form, shape, appearance, beauty* (Vide FORMA; See E. *form*)

-color, (gen.) -coloris ~색의

> multicolor, (gen.) multicoloris (< multus, multa, multum *many, much*)
여러 가지 색의, 다색(多色)의

E multicolored

> varicolor, (gen.) varicoloris (< varius, varia, varium *various*) 여러 가지
색의, 잡색의, 색색의

E varicolored

> versicolor, (gen.) versicoloris (< vers- < versare *to turn often* < vertĕre
to turn) 변색하는, 얼룩덜룩한

E versicolored (versicolor)

< color, coloris, m. 색, 외모, 가식(假飾)

< celo, celavi, celatum, celare 숨기다

< IE. kel- *to cover, to conceal, to save* (Vide CELLULA; See E. *cell*)

-inus, -ina, -inum 명사 어간에 붙여 성격을 뜻하는 형용사를 만든다. **E** -ine (-in), (-ine >) -yne

---

bovinus, bovina, bovinum 소의

E bovine

< bos, bovis, m., f. 소, 황소

< IE. gʷou- *ox, bull, cow* (Vide BOS; See E. *beef*)

salinus, salina, salinum 소금의

E saline

< sal, salis, m., n. 소금

< IE. sal- *salt* (Vide SAL; See E. *sal*)

-eus, -ea, -eum	**E** -eous
-ius, -ia, -ium	**E** -ious
-aceus, -acea, -aceum	**E** -aceous
-aneus, -anea, -aneum	**E** -aneous

명사의 어간에 붙여 출처, 성격, 비슷함을 뜻하는 형용사를 만든다.

---

carneus, carnea, carneum 고기의, 살의, 육신의   **E** carneous

[용례] trabecula carnea, (pl.) trabeculae carneae

근소주(筋小柱)   **E** trabecula carnea, (pl.) trabeculae carneae

(문법) trabecula 소주(小柱): 단수 주격 < trabecula, trabeculae, f.

carnea 살의: 형용사, 여성형 단수 주격

trabeculae 소주(小柱)들: 복수 주격

carneae 살의: 형용사, 여성형 복수 주격

< caro, carnis, f. 고기, 살, 육신

< IE. (s)ker- *to cut* (Vide CORTEX: *See* E. *cortex*)

tendineus, tendinea, tendineum 힘줄의, 건(腱)의

[용례] chorda tendinea, (pl.) chordae tendineae 힘줄끈,

건삭(腱索)   **E** chorda tendinea, (pl.) chordae tendineae

(문법) chorda 현(弦), 줄, 끈, 삭(索): 단수 주격

< chorda, chordae, f. (corda, cordae, f.)

tendinea 힘줄의, 건의: 형용사, 여성형 단수 주격

chordae 끈들, 삭(索)들: 복수 주격

tendineae 힘줄의, 건의: 형용사, 여성형 복수 주격

< L. tendo, tendinis, m. (*form influenced by* L. tendĕre *to stretch*) 힘줄, 건(腱)

< G. tenōn, tenontos, m. *sinew, tendon*

< G. teinein *to stretch*

< IE. ten- *to stretch* (Vide TENĒRE: *See* E. *tenet*)

sartorius, sartoria, sartorium 수선공의, 재봉사의

[용례] musculus sartorius (< *tailor's muscle* < *involved for cross-legged sitting*

position used by tailors) 넙다리빗근, 봉공근(縫工筋)   **E** sartorius (muscle)

(문법) musculus 근육, 근: 단수 주격 < musculus, musculi, m.

sartorius 재봉사의: 형용사, 남성형 단수 주격

< sartor, sartoris, m. 수선공, 옷 깁는 사람, 재봉사   **E** sartorial

< sarcio, sarsi, sartum, sarcire 보상하다, 수선하다, 깁다

< IE. serk- *to make whole*

> L. sarcina, sarcinae, f. 짐짝, 봇짐, (로마) 군인 각자의 분담화물, 부담, 걱정, 뱃속의 새끼;

팔련구균(八聯球菌)   **E** *sarcina*

> (*suggested*) G. horkos, horkou, m. *oath*

     > G. exorkizein (< *ex- out of, away from*) *to bind by oath, to swear a person to banish an evil spirit, to exorcize*

         > L. exorcizo, **exorcizavi**, exorcizatum, exorcizare 악마를 쫓아내다, 구마 (驅魔)하다   **E** *exorcize (exorcise)*

         > G. exorkismos, exorkismou, m. *exorcism*

             > L. exorcismus, exorcismi, m. 악마를 쫓아냄, 구마(驅魔), 주술(呪術), 액막이, 주문(呪文)   **E** *exorcism*

         > G. exorkistēs, exorkistou, m. *exorcist*

             > L. exorcista, exorcistae, m. 주술사(呪術師)   **E** *exorcist*

venerius, veneria, venerium ((*misspelled*) **venereus, venerea, venereum**) 비너스 여신의, 색정(色情)의   **E** *venereal*

     < venus, veneris, f. 사랑; (Venus) (로마 신화) 비너스, 금성   **E** *Venus*

         > veneror, veneratus sum, venerari 존경하다   **E** *venerate, venerable*

   < IE. wen- *to desire, to strive for*

> **E** *win* (< '*to seek to gain*'), *winsome* (< '*pleasure, joy*'), *wont* (< '*to become accustomed to, to dwell*'), *wean* (< '*to accustom*'), *ween* (< '*to expect, to imagine, to think*'), *wish*, (Vanadis '*a name of the Scandinavian goddess Freya*' >) *vanadium* (V)

     > L. venenum, veneni, n. (< *love potion*) 미약(媚藥), 독(毒), 독물(毒物, 뱀·곤충 등에서 정상적으로 분비되는 유독물질)   **E** *venom, (venom + -in >) venin, antivenin*

         > L. venenosus, venenosa, venenosum 유독한, 악의에 찬   **E** *venomous*

     > L. venia, veniae, f. 친절, 호의, 용서   **E** *venial*

     > L. venior, venatus sum, venari 사냥하다

         > L. venatio, venationis, f. 사냥, 사냥감   **E** *venison*

papyraceus, papyracea, papyraceum 파피루스의, 종이의   **E** *papyraceous*

     < papyrus, papyri, m., f. (papyrum, papyri, n.) 파피루스(이집트·시리아 등의 물가에서 자라는 방동사니과 다년초 Cyperus papyrus), 파피루스 종이, 종이; 파피루스 사본; (파피루스 섬유로 엮어 만든) 밧줄, 짚신, 옷

> **E** *papyrus, (pl.) papyri (papyruses), paper, papery,* (*probably, dissimilated*) *taper* (< '*use of papyrus pith as wick*')

     < G. papyros, papyrou, m. *papyrus-reed; papers, textiles, etc., made from papyrus-reed*

   < (*suggested*) (*Egyptian*) p-n-pr- *that of the pharaoh*

cutaneus, cutanea, cutaneum 피부의   **E** *cutaneous*

     < cutis, cutis, f. 껍질, 가죽, 살갗, 피부

   < IE. (s)keu- *to cover, to conceal* (Vide CUTIS: *See* E. *cutin*)

-arius, -aria, -arium -orius, -oria, -orium -ius, -ia, -ium	명사의 어간에 붙여 속성을 가리키는 형용사를 만든다.	**E** -ary **E** -ory **E** -ium

arbitrarius, arbitraria, arbitrarium 중재하는, 재량의, 임의의, 인위적인   **E** *arbitrary*

     < arbiter, arbitri, m. (< ad- *to, toward, at, according to* + bito (beto), -, -, bitĕre (betĕre)

         to go) 중재인, 재판관   **E** *arbiter*

exploratorius, exploratoria, exploratorium 답사의, 탐색의, 탐험의   **E** *exploratory*

         < explorator, exploratoris, m. 답사자, 탐색자, 탐험가

       < exploro, exploravi, exploratum, explorare (< *to set up a loud cry to scare an*

            animal from its hiding place, to beat the bushes < ex- *out of, away from*

            + plorare *to cry out, to wail*) 살피다, 탐색하다, 검사하다   **E** *explore, exploration*

     < ploro, ploravi, ploratum, plorare 소리 지르다, 통곡하다

       > deploro, deploravi, deploratum, deplorare (< de- *apart from, down, not; intensive*

         + plorare *to cry out, to wail*) 한탄하다, 통곡하다, 애통해 하다   **E** *deplore*

       > imploro, imploravi, imploratum, implorare (< im- (< in) *in, on, into, toward*

         + plorare *to cry out, to wail*) 애원하다, 간청하다   **E** *implore*

regius, regia, regium 왕의

         < rex, regis, m. 왕

      < rego, rexi, rectum, regĕre 올바로 이끌다, 다스리다

   < IE. reg- *to move in a straight line, with derivatives meaning 'to direct in a straight line,*

     to lead, to rule' (Vide REGĔRE: *See* E. *regent*)

-alis, -ale -aris, -are -ilis, -ile	명사의 어간에 붙여 관계 또는 속성을 가리키는 형용사를 만든다.	**E** -al **E** -ar **E** -ile

mineralis, minerale 광산의, 채석장의, 광석의, 금속의   **E** *mineral, mineralocorticoid(s)*

        < minera, minerae, f. 광석

      < mina, minae, f. 광산   **E** *mine*

   < *Of Celtic origin*

saecularis, saeculare (secularis, seculare) 세기의, 현세의, 세속의   **E** *secular*, F. *siecle*

       < saeculum, saeculi, n. (seculum, seculi, n.) (< *successive human generations as the*

         links that 'bind' the chain of human life) 세대, 시대, 세기, 현세, 세속

   < IE. sai- *to bind, to tie*   **E** *sinew*

> L. saeta, saetae, f. (seta, setae, f.) 짐승의 빳빳한 털, 강모(剛毛)　　**E** *seta*, (pl.) *setae*

> L. saetiger, saetigera, saetigerum (setiger, setigera, setigerum) (< saeta (seta)
bristle + -ger *bearing*) 강모를 가진, 강모가 나 있는　　**E** *setigerous*

> L. equisaetum, equisaeti, n. (equisetum, equiseti, n.) (< equus *horse* + saeta
(seta) *bristle*) (속새 · 쇠뜨기 등) 속새속(屬)의 식물　　**E** *equisetum*

militaris, militare 군인의, 군사(軍事)의　**E** *military, militarize, demilitarize, militarism, (military >) militaria*

< miles, militis, m. 군인

> militia, militiae, f. 병역　　**E** *militia*

> milito, **militavi**, militatum, militare 군에 복무하다, 싸우다　**E** *militate, militant, militancy*

virilis, virile 어른의, 성인 남자의, 남성의; 용감한　　**E** *virile*

< vir, viri, m. 어른, 남자 어른, 장부

< IE. wi-ro- **man** (Vide VIR: *See* E. *vir*)

-anus, -ana, -anum
-enus, -ena, -enum
-aneus, -anea, -aneum
-(i)ensis, -(i)ense
-(e)stris, -(e)stre

명사의 어간에 붙여 장소, 기원, 소속을 가리키는
형용사를 만든다.

E *-an, -ane*
E *-ene*
E *-anean*
E *-ese*
E *-strial*

---

mundanus, mundana, mundanum 세상의, 세속의　**E** *mundane, demimondaine (< 'half-world woman')*

< mundus, mundi, m. 세상, 세속

terrenus, terrena, terrenum 땅의, 현세의　　**E** *terrene, (terrenum >) terrain*

< terra, terrae, f. (< *dry land*) 땅, 지구; (Terra) (로마 신화) 땅의 여신

< IE. ters- *to dry* (Vide TERRA: *See* E. *terrace*)

mediterraneus, mediterranea, mediterraneum (< medius *middle* + terra *land*) 내륙의,
육지로 둘러싸인; (Mediterraneus) 지중해(地中海)의　　**E** *Mediterranean*

< terra, terrae, f. (< *dry land*) 땅, 지구

< IE. ters- *to dry* (Vide TERRA: *See* E. *terrace*)

forensis, forense 시장의, 광장의, 법정의, 공공장소의　　**E** *forensic*

< forum, fori, n. 시장, 광장, 법정　　**E** *forum*

< foras (부사: fora의 복수 대격) 문 밖으로

> foraneus, foranea, foraneum 집 밖의　　**E** *foreign*

< foris (부사: fora의 복수 탈격) 문 밖에
있는   **E** (foris facĕre *'to do outside'* > *'to transgress'* >) *forfeit*
> forestis, forestis, f. 숲   **E** *forest*
< *fora, *forae, f. 문
< IE. dhwer- *door, doorway*   **E** *door*
> G. thyra, thyras, f. *fold of a door, door, gate*
> G. thyreos, thyreou, m. *door-stone, large shield*   **E** *thyroid, parathyroid*

terrestris, terrestre 땅의, 지구의, 지상의, 현세의   **E** *terrestrial, extraterrestrial*
< terra, terrae, f. (< *dry land*) 땅, 지구
< IE. ters- *to dry* (Vide TERRA: *See* E. *terrace*)

−osus, −osa, −osum   명사의 어간에 붙여 가득 참, 많음을 가리키는   **E** *-ose, -ous*
−lentus, −lenta, −lentum   형용사를 만든다.   **E** *-lent*

fastidiosus, fastidiosa, fastidiosum 넌더리 나는, 까다로운   **E** *fastidious*
< fastidium, fastidii, n. 오만불손, 넌더리, 까다로움
< fastus, fastus, m. (< *prickliness*) 오만불손
< IE. bhars-, bhors- *projection, bristle, point*   **E** *bristle*
> L. fastigium, fastigii, n. 꼭대기, 절정; (병의) 최고점, 극기   **E** *fastigium, fastigial*
> L. fastigiatus, fastigiata, fastigiatum (뾰족하게) 높이 솟은, 절정에 이른,
경사진   **E** *fastigiate*
> IE. (*probably*) bhars- *barley*   **E** *barley, barn* (< *'barley house'*)
> L. far, farris, n. 곡물, 곡물가루
> L. farina, farinae, f. 곡물가루, 밀가루, 가루   **E** *farina*
> L. farinaceus, farinacea, farinaceum 가루의   **E** *farinaceous*

fibrosus, fibrosa, fibrosum 섬유가 많은, 섬유 모양의, 섬유성의   **E** *fibrous*
< fibra, fibrae, f. 가는 줄, 섬유
< IE. (*possibly*) gʷhi- *thread, tendon* (Vide FIBRA: *See* E. *fiber*)

somnolentus, somnolenta, somnolentum 몹시 졸리는   **E** *somnolent*
< somnus, somni, m. 잠
< IE. swep- *to sleep* (Vide SOMNUS: *See* E. *Somnus*)

succulentus, succulenta, succulentum (suculentus, suculenta, suculentum) 즙이 많은   **E** *succulent*
< succus, succi, m. (sucus, suci, m.) 즙, 맛, 활력소
< IE. seuə- *to take liquid* (Vide SUGĔRE: *See* E. *suction*)

-atus, -ata, -atum -itus, -ita, -itum	동사의 과거분사 어미로서 명사의 어간에 붙여 속성을 가리키는 형용사를 만든다.	E *-ate, -ade, -ee* E *-ite*

guttatus, guttata, guttatum 물방울 모양의 얼룩이 있는, 반점 있는

E *guttate*

< gutta, guttae, f. (액체의) 방울, 물방울, 반점(斑點), 얼룩점

E *gutta*

mellitus, mellita, mellitum 꿀의, 꿀이 들어 있는, 달콤한, 사랑스러운

< mel, mellis, n. 꿀

< IE. melit- *honey* (Vide MEL; *See* E. *melliferous*)

수사

라틴어 수사에는 기본수사, 순서수사, 배분수사의 세 가지가 있다. 모두 형용사이므로 어미변화를 하는 경우에는 어미를 수식하는 명사의 성, 수, 격에 맞춰 주어야 한다. 학술용어를 이해하기 위해 알아야 할 수사는 많지 않다.

●●● **기 수**

다음 중 unus, duo, tres, quingenti, milia가 어미변화를 한다. (mille는 단수에서는 어미변화를 하지 않고 복수에서만 중성 명사 제3변화 제3식에 따른 어미변화를 한다.) 어원론에서는 어미변화까지 알아둘 필요는 없다.

unus (m.)	una (f.)	unum (n.)	하나	1 (I)
duo (m.)	duae (f.)	duo (n.)	둘	2 (II)
tres (m.)	tres (f.)	tria (n.)	셋	3 (III)
quattuor			넷	4 (IV)
quinque			다섯	5 (V)
sex			여섯	6 (VI)
septem			일곱	7 (VII)
octo			여덟	8 (VIII)
novem			아홉	9 (IX)
decem			열	10 (X)

undecim			열하나	11 (XI)
duodecim			열둘	12 (XII)
viginti			스물	20 (XX)
quadraginta			마흔	40 (XL)
quinquaginta			쉰	50 (L)
centum			백	100 (C)
quingenti	quingentae (f.)	quingenta (n.)	오백	500 (D)
mille, (pl.) millia (milia)			천	1000 (M)

[용례] E pluribus unum. (< *Out of many, one.*) 다수로부터 하나
    (문법) e ~로부터: 전치사, 탈격지배
        pluribus 다수: 형용사의 명사적 용법, 중성 복수 탈격
          < (sing.) −, −, plus ((gen.) pluris)
            (pl.) plures, plures, plura ((gen.) plurium) 더 많은
        unum 하나: 형용사의 명사적 용법, 중성 단수 주격

●●● 서수

서수는 형용사 제1·2변화 제1식의 어미변화를 따른다.

primus (m.)	prima (f.)	primum (n.)	첫째	1 (I)
secundus (m.)	secunda (f.)	secundum (n.)	둘째	2 (II)
tertius (m.)	tertia (f.)	tertium (n.)	셋째	3 (III)
quartus (m.)	quarta (f.)	quartum (n.)	넷째	4 (IV)
quintus (m.)	quinta (f.)	quintum (n.)	다섯째	5 (V)
sextus (m.)	sexta (f.)	sextum (n.)	여섯째	6 (VI)
septimus (m.)	septima (f.)	septimum (n.)	일곱째	7 (VII)
octavus (m.)	octava (f.)	octavum (n.)	여덟째	8 (VIII)
nonus (m.)	nona (f.)	nonum (n.)	아홉째	9 (IX)
decimus (m.)	decima (f.)	decimum (n.)	열째	10 (X)
undecimus (m.)	undecima (f.)	undecimum (n.)	열한째	11 (XI)
duodecimus (m.)	duodecima (f.)	duodecimum (n.)	열두째	12 (XII)
centesimus (m.)	centesima (f.)	centesimum (n.)	백째	100 (C)

millesimus (m.)　　　millesima (f.)　　　millesimum (n.)　　　천째　1000 (M)

[용례] ostium primum 일차구멍, 일차공

E *ostium primum*

　　　ostium secundum 이차구멍, 이차공

E *ostium secundum*

　　　(문법) ostium 입구, 구(口), 구멍: 중성 단수 주격 < ostium, ostii, n.

　　　　　primum 첫째: 수사, 중성형 단수 주격

　　　　　secundum 둘째: 수사, 중성형 단수 주격

[용례] quaque hora (q.h.) 시간마다 < 각 시간에

E *quaque hora (q.h.)*

　　　quaque secunda hora (q. 2h.) 두 시간마다 < 각 두 번째 시간에

　　　quaque tertia hora (q. 3h.) 세 시간마다

　　　quaque quarta hora (q. 4h., q.q.h.) 네 시간마다

　　　quaque sexta hora (q. 6h., q.s.h.) 여섯 시간마다

　　　(문법) quaque 각자, 각: 형용사적 부정대명사, 여성형 단수 탈격

　　　　　secunda, tertia, quarta, sexta: 서수, 여성형 단수 탈격

　　　　　hora 시간에: 단수 탈격 < hora, horae, f.

● ● ●　**배분수사**

배분수사는 복수로만 쓰이며 형용사 제1·2변화 제1식의 어미변화를 따르므로 주격의 남성형이 -i, 여성형이 -ae, 중성형이 -a가 된다. 남성형과 중성형 속격에서 -orum 대신 -um이 되기도 한다.

singuli, singulae, singlula	하나씩	E *single*
bini, binae, bina	둘씩	E *binary*
terni, ternae, terna (trini, trinae, trina)	셋씩	E *ternary, trinity*
quaterni, quaternae, quaterna	넷씩	E *quaternary, quaternity*
deni, denae, dena	열씩	E *denary*
duodeni, duodenae, duodena	열둘씩	E *duodenum*

● ● ●　**수사에서 파생한 형용사**

simplus, simpla, simplum 한 배의, 단순한

E *simple, simpleton*

simplex, (gen.) simplicis 홑겹의, 단순한

E *simplex*

singulus, singula, singulum 단일의

E *single, singleton, singlet*

duplus, dupla, duplum 두 배의, 갑절의

E *duple, double, doublet, (double >) dub*

duplex, (gen.) duplicis 두 겹의, 이중의, 복식의   `E duplex, duplicate`

triplus, tripla, triplum 세 배의   `E triple, triplet`

triplex, (gen.) triplicis 세 겹의, 삼중의   `E triplex, triplicate`

quadruplus, quadrupla, quadruplum 네 배의   `E quadruple, quadruplet`

quadruplex, (gen.) quadruplicis 네 겹의, 사중의   `E quadruplex, quadruplicate`

multiplus, multipla, multiplum 여러 배의   `E multiple`

multiplex, (gen.) multiplicis 여러 겹의, 여러 곱절의, 복합된   `E multiplex, multiplicate, multiply`

••• 수사에서 파생한 횟수의 부사

semel   한 번 > semel in die (s.i.d.) *once a day*   `E s.i.d.`

bis   두 번 > bis in die (b.i.d.) *twice a day*   `E b.i.d.`

ter   세 번 > ter in die (t.i.d.) *three times a day*   `E t.i.d.`

quater   네 번 > quater in die (q.i.d.) *four times a day*   `E q.i.d.`

unus, una, unum 하나   `E uni-, unary (< 'on the pattern of binary'), triune (< 'three in one')`

> unio, unionis, f. 합일, 결합, (골절·손상의) 치유;
  구근(球根)   `E union, nonunion, malunion, onion (< 'no shoots, a single entity')`

> unitas, unitatis, f. 유일성, 단일성, 일(一), 단위   `E unity, unit, subunit`

> unitarius, unitaria, unitarium 단일의, 일원론의   `E unitary, unitarian`

> unicus, unica, unicum 하나뿐인   `E unique`

> unio, univi, unitum, unire 하나로 묶다   `E unite`

> uncia, unciae, f. 12분의 1, 1인치, 1온스   `E inch, ounce, uncial`

< IE. oi-no- *one, unique*

`E one, an, a, eleven (< 'one left (beyond ten)'), once, nonce (< 'the one'); none (< 'not one'); alone, lone, lonely; any`

> L. ullus, ulla, ullum 어느

> L. nullus, nulla, nullum (< ne *not* + ullus *any*) 아무 ~도 아니, 하나도 없는,
  무효의   `E null, nullify, annul`

singulus, singula, singulum (형용사) 단일의   `E single, singleton, singlet`

> singularis, singulare 단일의, 뛰어난, 특이한; (문법) 단수의   `E singular`

singuli, singulae, singlula (배분수사) 하나씩   `E single`

< IE. sem- *one; also adverbially 'as one',*
together with　　　　　　　　　　 **E** *same; seem, seemingly; some* (< *'a certain one'*), *-some* (< *'-like'*)
　　> L. semel (부사) 한번
　　　　> L. semper (< *once for all* < semel *once* + per *through*) (부사) 늘, 언제나
　　　　> L. simplus, simpla, simplum (< semel *once* + -plus (< IE. pel- *to fold*)) 한
　　　　　　배의, 단순한　　　　　　　　　　　　　　　　　**E** *simple, simpleton*
　　　　　　> L. simplifico, **simplificavi**, simplificatum, simplificare (< + -ficare (< facĕre)
　　　　　　　　to make) 하나로 되게 하다, 단순하게 하다　　　**E** *simplify*
　　　　> L. simplex, (gen.) simplicis (< semel *once* + -plex (< IE. plek- *to plait* <
　　　　　　IE. pel- *to fold*)) 홑겹의, 단순한　　　　　　　　**E** *simplex*
　　　　　　> L. simplicitas, simplicitatis, f. 단순　　　　　　**E** *simplicity*
　　　　　　> L. simpliciter (부사) 단순히　　　　　　　　　　**E** *simpliciter*
　　> L. simul (부사) 함께, 동시에　　　　　　　**E** (in + simul >) *ensemble, simulcast*
　　　　> L. *simultaneus, *simultanea, *simultaneum (형용사) 동시의 **E** *simultaneous, simultaneity*
　　　　> L. assimulo, **assimulavi**, assimulatum, assimulare (< as- (< ad) *to, toward, at,*
　　　　　　according to + simul *together*) 모으다　　**E** *assemble, assembly, assemblage*
　　> L. similis, simile 비슷한
　　　　> L. simile, similis, n. 비슷한 것, 유사; 직유
　　　　　　(直喩) **E** (Fac simile! *'Make a similar thing!'* >) *facsimile, (facsimile >) fax; simile*
　　　　> L. *similaris, *similare 비슷한　　　　　　　　　　**E** *similar, similarity*
　　　　> L. similitudo, similitudinis, f. 비슷함　　　　　　**E** *similitude*
　　　　> L. similo, **similavi**, similatum, similare 비슷해지다,
　　　　　　닮다　　　　　　　　　　　**E** *semblance, resemble, resemblance*
　　　　　　> L. assimilo, **assimilavi**, assimilatum, assimilare (< as- (< ad) *to, toward,*
　　　　　　　　at, according to + similare *to seem, to be like*) 비슷하게 만들다,
　　　　　　　　같게 하다　　**E** *assimilate, dissimilate* (< *'on the pattern of assimilate'*)
　　　　　　　　> L. assimilatio, assimilationis, f. 비슷하게 만듦, 같게 함, 동화(同化),
　　　　　　　　　　동화작용, 융합　　**E** *assimilation, dissimilation* (< *'assimilation'*)
　　　　> L. simulo, **simulavi**, simulatum, simulare 비슷하게 만들다, 모방하다, ~ 체하다,
　　　　　　가장하다　　　　　　　　　　**E** *simulate, simulant, simulator*
　　　　　　> L. simulatio, simulationis, f. 가상, 모의, 꾀병　　**E** *simulation*
　　　　　　> L. simulacrum, simulacri, n. 모형, 환영(幻影), 가짜 **E** *simulacrum, (pl.) simulacra*
　　　　　　> L. dissimulo, **dissimulavi**, dissimulatum, dissimulare (< dis- *apart from,*
　　　　　　　　down, not + simulare *to feign*) 위장하다, 숨기다　**E** *dissimulate, dissemble*
　　　　> L. dissimilis, dissimile (< dis- *apart from, down, not*) 다른　**E** *dissimilar*
　　　　> L. verisimilis, verisimile (< verus *true*) 정말 같은　　**E** *verisimilar*
　　　　　　> L. verisimilitudo, verisimilitudinis, f. 정말 같음, 박진감(迫進感) **E** *verisimilitude*
　　> L. sincerus, sincera, sincerum (< *of one growth* < IE. sem- *one* + IE. ker- *to grow*)
　　　　자연 그대로의, 순수한, 성실한　　　　　　　　　　　　**E** *sincere*
　　> G. heis, mia, hen *one*　　**E** *henotheism,* (hen dia dyoin *'one by means of two'* >) *hendiadys*
　　　　> G. hyphen (< hyp(o)- *under* + hen *one*) (adverb) *together*　　**E** *hyphen*

> G. hekaton *one hundred*

> G. hekatombē, hekatombēs, f. (< hekaton + bous *ox*) *an offering of a hundred oxen, a great public sacrifice*　　　　　　　　　　　`E hecatomb`

> G. haploos, haploē, haploon (< ha- *one* + -ploos (< IE. pel- *to fold*)) *onefold, simple, single*　　　　　　　　　`E haplotype (< 'haploid genotype')`

> G. homos, homē, homon *common, of the same* (Vide HOMOS: *See* E. *hom(o)–*)

> G. heteros, hetera, heteron ((*earlier*) hateros) *another, different (of different kinds)*
(Vide HETEROS: *See* E. *heter(o)–*)

> (*Sanskrit*) sam *together*

　　`E ((IE. sem- >) sam 'together' + krta > 'made together' > 'perfected' >) Sanskrit, (sam + sr 'to run, to glide, to move' >) samsara`

duo, duae, duo 둘　　　　　　`E duo, (It. duetto 'diminutive of duo' >) duet, deuce, du-`

> bis (*adverb, multiplicative*) 두 번

　　`E bis- (< 'used in the names of compounds to signify two identical groups substituted in the same way'), (L. *biscoctus panis 'twice baked bread' >) biscuit`

> bi-, bin- (*before* vowel) *twice, two*　　　　　　　　`E bi- (bin-)`

> bilanx, (gen.) bilancis (< libra bilanx < bi- *twice, two* + lanx, lancis, f. *flat plate, scale*) 두 개의 저울판을 가진　`E balance, unbalanced, imbalance`

> bini, binae, bina 둘씩　　　　`E binocular, pinochle (< 'binocular')`

> binarius, binaria, binarium 둘로 이루어진　　`E binary, (binary digit >) bit`

> combino, **combinavi**, combinatum, combinare (< com- (< cum) *with, together* + bini *two together*) 짝 지우다, 결합시키다, 조합(組合)시키다

　　`E combine, combinatorial, (combine >) recombine, (recombine >) recombinant`

> combinatio, combinationis, f. 짝맞춤, 결합, 조합　　`E combination, (combination >) recombination`

> dualis, duale 둘의　　　　　　　　　　　　　　`E dual`

> duplus, dupla, duplum (< duo *two* + -plus (< IE. pel- *to fold*)) 두 배의, 갑절의　　　　　　　　`E duple, double, doublet, (double >) dub`

> duplex, (gen.) duplicis (< duo *two* + -plex (< IE. plek- *to plait* < IE. pel- *to fold*)) 두 겹의, 이중의, 복식의　　　　　　　　　　　`E duplex`

> duplicitas, duplicitatis, f. 이중, 중복, 표리부동　　`E duplicity`

> duplico, **duplicavi**, duplicatum, duplicare 중복하다, 갑절하다, 구부리다　`E duplicate`

> dubius, dubia, dubium 이리저리 양쪽으로 흔들리는, 의심하는, 의심스러운　`E dubious`

> dubito, **dubitavi**, dubitatum, dubitare 의심하다　　`E doubt`

> duodecim (< duo *two* + decem *ten*) 열둘　　`E dozen, duodecimal`

> duodeni, duodenae, duodena 열둘씩　　　　`E duodenum`

> dis-, dif- (*before* f), di- (*before* b, d, g, l, m, n, r, v) *apart from, down, not; intensive*　　　　　`E dis- (dif-, di-), disinfect, difficult, direct`

< IE. dwo- *two*

E *two, twain, twin, twelve* (< 'two left (beyond ten)'), *twice, twenty* (< 'twice ten'), *twilight, twist* (< 'divided objects, fork, rope'), *twine* (< 'double thread, twisted thread'), *entwine, intertwine, between* (< 'at the middle point of two' < *bi- 'at, by' < IE. ambhi 'around'), *twig* (< 'fork'), (D. zwei 'two' > Zwitter 'hybrid' + ion >) *zwitterion*

> G. dyo, dyo, dyo *two*   **E** (hen dia dyoin 'one by means of two' >) *hendiadys*

> G. dis (*adverb, multiplicative*) *twice, double*

> G. di– *twice, two*   **E** *di-*

> G. dicha *in two*

> G. dichotomos, dichotomos, dichotomon (< + tomos *cutting, cut*) *cut in half, equally divided*

> L. dichotomus, dichotoma, dichotomum 양분(兩分)하는, 두 갈래로 갈라지는   **E** *dichotomous*

> G. dichotomia, dichotomias, f. *cutting in two*

> L. dichotomia, dichotomiae, f. 양분(兩分), 이분법 (二分法)   **E** *dichotomy*

> G. dissos, dissē, disson ((*Attic*) dittos, dittē, ditton) *twice, double*   **E** *diss(o)- (ditt(o)-)*

> G. dyas, dyados, f. *the number two, pair, dyad*   **E** *dyad*

> G. (*reduplicated*) didymos, didymē, didymon *double, twofold, twin*

> G. didymoi, didymōn, m. (pl.) *testicles*

> L. epididymis, epididymidis, f. (< G. ep(i)– *upon*) 부고환(副睾丸)   **E** *epididymis*, (pl.) *epididymides, epididym(o)-*

> G. dia (전치사, 속격·대격지배; 부사) *through, thorough, apart*

> G. di(a)– *through, thoroughly, apart*   **E** *di(a)-*

> IE. dwei– *to fear* (*original meaning* 'to be in doubt, to be of two minds')

> L. dirus, dira, dirum 무시무시한, 끔찍스런, 모진   **E** *dire*

> L. Dirofilaria, Dirofilariae, f. (< filaria < filum *thread*) (사상충 絲狀蟲) 디로필라리아속(屬), 개사상충속(屬)   **E** *Dirofilaria*

> G. deinos, deinē, deinon *fearful, terrible, powerful, venerable*

> L. dinosaurus, dinosauri, m. (< G. deinos + sauros *lizard*) 공룡(恐龍)   **E** *dinosaur, dinosaurian*

> L. dinotherium, dinotherii, n. (< G. deinos + thērion, thēriou, n. (< thēr, thēros, m. *wild beast* + –ion *diminutive suffix*)) 공수(恐獸)   **E** *dinothere*

tres, tres, tria 셋

E *tri-;* (trifolium 'three-leaved' >) *trefoil,* (tres fines 'three ends' >) *trephine,* (trephine >) *trephination, trocar* (< 'three-sided'), It. *trio*

> ter (부사) 세 번

> terni, ternae, terna 셋씩

> ternarius, ternaria, ternarium 셋으로 이루어진   **E** *ternary*

> trini, trinae, trina 셋씩

> trinitas, trinitatis, f. 세 개 한 벌, 3인조, 삼위일체   **E** *trinity*

> triplus, tripla, triplum (< tri- *three* + –plus (< IE. pel- *to fold*)) 세 배의   **E** *triple, triplet*

> triplex, (gen.) triplicis (< tri- *three* + –plex (< IE. plek- *to plait* < IE. pel- *to fold*))

　세 겹의, 삼중의   **E** *triplex*

　> triplico, **triplicavi**, triplicatum, triplicare 세 겹 하다, 세 곱 하다   **E** *triplicate*

> triquetrus, triquetra, triquetrum (< tri- *three* + IE. kʷed- *to sharpen*) 세모난, 삼각의,

　뿌리가 셋 있는   **E** *triquetrous, (os triquetrum >) triquetrum*

> tribus, tribus, f. (로마 세 부족 중 하나의) 부족   **E** *tribe, tribal, tribalism*

　> tribunus, tribuni, m. ((gen. pl.) tribunum) 로마의 세 부족의 부족장 중 한 명,

　　세 명의 호민관 중 한 명   **E** *tribune*

　> tribuo, **tribui**, tributum, tribuĕre 로마의 세 부족 간에 세금을 분배하다, 분할하다,

　　주다, ~의 공으로 돌리다

　　> tributum, tributi, n. 세공(稅貢), 공물(貢物), 증정품   **E** *tribute*

　　　> tributarius, tributaria, tributarium 세공의, 공물의, 세공을 바치는;

　　　　(강의) 지류(支流)의   **E** *tributary*

　　> attribuo, **attribui**, attributum, attribuĕre (< at- (< ad) *to, toward, at,*

　　　according to + tribuĕre *to allot, to pay*) 지정해주다, 속성(屬性)을

　　　부여하다   **E** *attribute*

　　> contribuo, **contribui**, contributum, contribuĕre (< con- (< cum) *with,*

　　　together + tribuĕre *to allot, to pay*) 할당하다, 분담하다, 기여하다,

　　　공헌하다   **E** *contribute*

　　> distribuo, **distribui**, distributum, distribuĕre (< dis- *apart from, down, not*

　　　+ tribuĕre *to allot, to pay*) 분배하다, 분포시키다   **E** *distribute*

　　> retribuo, **retribui**, retributum, retribuĕre (< re- *back, again* + tribuĕre

　　　to allot, to pay) 돌려주다, 보답하다, 보복하다   **E** *retribute*

> trivium, trivii, n. (< tri- *three* + via *way*) 삼거리, 광장; (역사) 삼학(三學) (문법, 수사,

　논리)

　> trivialis, triviale 보통 있는, 하찮은, 저속한, 야비한; 삼학의   **E** *trivial*

< IE. trei- *three*   **E** *three, thirteen, thirty, trillium; third; thrice*

> L. tertius, tertia, tertium 셋째

　> L. tertiarius, tertiaria, tertiarium 삼분의 일의   **E** *tertiary*

　> L. tertianus, tertiana, tertianum (당일까지 합쳐) 사흘마다 일어나는,

　　사흘거리의   **E** *(febris tertiana 'tertian fever' >) tertian*

> L. testis, testis, m., f. (< *tri-st-i- *third person standing by* < IE. trei- *three* +

　*-st- *standing* (< IE. sta- *to stand*; Vide STARE; See E. *stay*)) 증인

　> L. testimonium, testimonii, n. 증언, 선언   **E** *testimony*

　> L. testor, testatus sum, testari 증언하다, 유언하다   **E** *testate*

　　> L. testamentum, testamenti, n. 입증, 유언, 계약; (Testamentum) 성서   **E** *testament*

　　> L. attestor, attestatus sum, attestari (< ad- (< ad) *to, toward, at,*

　　　according to + testari *to witness*) 입증하다, 증거가 되다   **E** *attest*

　　> L. contestor, contestatus sum, contestari (< con- (< cum) *with, together;*

　　　intensive + testari *to witness*) 증인으로 삼다, 호소하다   **E** *contest*

> L. detestor, detestatus sum, detestari (< de- *apart from, down, not* + testari *to witness*) 저주하다, 몹시 싫어하다   **E** *detest*

> L. protestor, protestatus sum, protestari (< pro- *before, forward, for, instead of* + testari *to witness*) 증언하다, 공언하다, 항의하다   **E** *protest*

> L. testificor, testificatus sum, testificari (< testis *witness* + -ficari (< facĕre) *to make*) 증언하다   **E** *testify*

> L. testis, testis, m. (< *two glands side by side, as by-standers* < G. parastatēs *by-stander, legal supporter*) 불알, 고환(睾丸)   **E** *testis,* (pl.) *testes*

> L. testiculus, testiculi, m. (< + -culus *diminutive suffix*) 불알, 고환   **E** *testicle, testicular*

> G. treis, treis, tria *three*   **E** *tri-*

> G. tris (*adverb, multiplicative*) *three times, thrice*

E *tris-* (< '*used prefixed to the names of complex radicals or compounds, signifying that the whole complex is present thrice over, and not merely the single element or radical immediately following the prefix*'), *trisoctahedron*

> G. tri- *three*   **E** *tri-*

> G. triploos, triploē, triploon (< tri- *thrice* + -ploos (< IE. pel- *to fold*)) *threefold, triple*   **E** *triploid, triploidy, triploblastic*

> G. trias, triados, f. *the number three, triad*   **E** *triad*

> G. tritos, tritē, triton *third*

> L. tritium, tritii, n. (< *the third of the naturally occurring hydrogen isotopes (protium, deuterium, and tritium)*) 삼중수소 (三重水素)   **E** *tritium (^3H, T), tritiated,* (tritium > '*on the pattern of proton*' >) *triton*

> (*Russian*) troe *three*   **E** *troika* (< '*group of three*')

> (*Persian*) si *three*   **E** *sitar, teapoy*

quattuor 넷   **E** *quadr(i)- (quadru-)*

> quater (부사) 네 번, 네 곱

> quaterni, quaternae, quaterna 넷씩

> quaternarius, quaternaria, quaternarium 넷으로 이루어진

E *quaternary, paraquat* (< '*the bond between the two pyridyl groups is in the para position with respect to their quaternary nitrogen atoms*')

> quaternitas, quaternitatis, f. 네 개 한 벌, 4인조   **E** *quaternity*

> quadruplus, quadrupla, quadruplum (< quadru- *four* + -plus (< IE. pel- *to fold*)) 네 배의   **E** *quadruple, quadruplet*

> quadruplex, (gen.) quadruplicis (< quadru- *four* + -plex (< IE. plek- *to plait* < IE. pel- *to fold*)) 네 겹의, 사중의   **E** *quadruplex*

> quadruplico, quadruplicavi, quadruplicatum, quadruplicare 네 겹 하다, 네 곱 하다   **E** *quadruplicate*

> quadrus, quadra, quadrum 네모난   **E** *cadre* (< '*four-sided frame*')

> quadro, quadravi, quadratum, quadrare 네모지게 하다, 꼭 맞게 하다   **E** *quadrate, quarry, square,* (square >) *squarish, squad*

> quadrans, quadrantis, m. (< *present participle*) 4분의 1　　　**E** *quadrant*

< IE. kʷetwer- *four*　　　**E** *four, fourteen, fortnight, forty; fourth*

> L. quartus, quarta, quartum 넷째　　　**E** *quart, quartet*

> L. quartanus, quartana, quartanum (당일까지 합쳐) 나흘마다 일어나는,

제4군단의　　　**E** *(febris quartana 'quartan fever' >) quartan*

> L. quartarius, quartarii, m. (용량) sextarius의 4분의 1, (이익금의 4분의 1을

받던) 노새몰이 품꾼, 측정값의 4분의 1　　　**E** *quarter*

> L. quartilis, quartile 네 번째의, 4분의 1의, 4분위(分位)의　　　**E** *quartile*

> G. tessares, tessares, tessara ((*Ionic*) tesseres, tesseres, tessera) *four*　　　**E** *tetr(a)- (tra-)*

> G. tetrakis (*adverb, multiplicative*) *four-times*

E *tetrakis-* (< 'used in the names of compounds to signify four identical groups all substituted in the same way')

> G. tetras, tetrados, f. *the number four, tetrad*　　　**E** *tetrad*

> G. tessera, tesseras, f. *a small tablet of wood or bone used as a token*

> L. tessera, tesserae, f. 네모난 돌, 주사위 돌, 네모 명패, 배급표, 증표　　　**E** *tessera*

> L. tessella, tessellae, f. (< + -ella *diminutive suffix*) 네모난 돌,

주사위 돌, 모자이크 돌, 네모난 판　　　**E** *tessellate*

> G. tetraploos, tetraploē, tetraploon (< tetr(a)- *four* + -ploos (< IE. pel- *to*

fold)) *fourfold, quadruple*　　　**E** *tetraploid, tetraploidy*

> G. tetratos, tetratē, tetraton *third*

quinque 다섯　　　**E** *quinqu(e)-,* (quinquefolium *five leaves* >) *cinquefoil*

> quini, quinae, quina 다섯씩

> quindecim (< quinque *five* + decem *ten*) 열다섯　　　**E** *quindecennial*

> quinquaginta (< quinque *five* + -ginta *ten times*) 쉰　　　**E** *quinquagenarian*

> quinquagesimus, quinquagesima, quinquagesimum 쉰 번째의

> quingenti, quingentae, quingenta (< quinque *five* + centum *hundred*) 오백　**E** *quincentenary*

< IE. penkʷe *five*　　　**E** *five, fifteen, fifty; fifth; femto-* (< 'fifteen'); *finger* (< 'one of five'), *fist*

> L. quintus, quinta, quintum 다섯째　　　**E** *quintet*

> L. quintanus, quintana, quintanum (당일까지 합쳐) 닷새마다

일어나는　　　**E** *(febris quintana 'quintan fever' >) quintan*

> L. quintilis, quintile 다섯 번째의, 5분의 1의, 5분위(分位)의　　　**E** *quintile*

> L. quintuplex (< quintus *fifth* + -plex (< IE. plek- *to plait* < IE. pel- *to fold*))

다섯 배의　　　**E** *quintuple, quintuplicate*

> L. quintessentia, quintessentiae, f. (< quinta essentia < G. pemptē ousia

the fifth essence) 제5원(元) (물·불·흙·공기 4원 외의 원), (물질의) 가장

순수한 본질　　　**E** *quintessence*

> G. pente *five*　　　**E** *pent(a)-*

> G. pentakis (*adverb, multiplicative*) *five-times*

> G. pentas, pentados, f. *the number five, pentad*　　　**E** *pentad*

> G. pemptos, pemptē, pempton *fifth*

> (*Sanskrit*) panca *five*　　　**E** *punch* (< 'originally prepared from five ingredients')

sex 여섯　　　　　　　　　　　　　　　　　　　　　　　　　　　　　　　　　　　　　E *sex(i)-*

> semestris, semestre (semenstris, semenstre) (< se- (< sex) *six* + mensis *month*)
　　6개월의　　　　　　　　　　　　　　　　　　　　　　　　　　　　　　　　　E *semester, semestral*

< IE. s(w)eks *six*　　　　　　　　　　　　　　　　　　　　　　　　E *six, sixteen, sixty; sixth*

> L. sextus, sexta, sextum 여섯째

　　E (sexta hora *'sixth hour, noon; counting from dawn'* >) *siesta*, (Pope Sixtus IV >) *Sistine*

> L. sextans, sextantis, m. 6분의 1　　　　　　　　　　　　　　　　　　　　E *sextant*

> L. sextilis, sextile 여섯 번째의, 6분의 1의, 6분위(分位)의　　　　　　　　　E *sextile*

> G. hex *six*　　　　　　　　　　　　　　　　　　　　　　　　　　　　　E *hex(a)-*

　　> G. hexakis (*adverb, multiplicative*) *six-times*

　　> G. hexas, hexados, f. *the number six, hexad*　　　　　　　　　　　　E *hexad*

> G. hektos, hektē, hekton *sixth*

septem 일곱　　　　　　　　　　　　　　　　　　　　　　　　　　E *sept(i)-, septennial*

> septuaginta (< septem *seven* + -ginta *ten times*) 일흔　　　　　　　　　E *Septuagint*

> September, Septembris, Septembre (고대 로마력의) 제7월의,
　　(개정 로마력의) 9월의　　　　　　　E (September mensis *'the seventh month'* >) *September*

< IE. septm *seven*　　　　　　　　　　　E *seven, seventeen, seventy; seventh*

> L. septimus, septima, septimum 일곱째

> G. hepta *seven*　　　　　　　　　　　　　　　　　　　　　　　　　　E *hept(a)-*

　　> G. heptakis (*adverb, multiplicative*) *seven-times*

　　> G. heptas, heptados, f. *the number seven, heptad*　　　　　　　　　E *heptad*

　　> G. hebdomas, hebdomados, f. *the number seven, a period of seven days*　E *hebdomad*

> G. hebdomos, hebdomē, hebdomon *seventh*

octo 여덟　　　　　　　　　　　　　　　　　　　E *oct(o)-, octet (< 'a group of eight')*

> octoginta (< octo *eight* + -ginta *ten times*) 여든　　　　　　　　　E *octogenarian*

> October, Octobris, Octobre (고대 로마력의) 제8월의,
　　(개정 로마력의) 10월의　　　　　　　E (October mensis *'the eighth month'* >) *October*

< IE. okto(u) *eight*　　　　　　E *eight, eighteen, eighty; eighth; atto- (< 'eighteen')*

> L. octavus, octava, octavum 여덟째　　　　　　　　　　　　　　　　　E *octave*

> G. oktō *eight*　　　　　　　　　　　　　　　　　　　　　　　　　E *oct(o)- (octa-)*

　　> G. oktakis (*adverb, multiplicative*) *eight-times*

　　> G. oktas, oktados, f. *the number eight, octad*　　　　　　　　　　　E *octad*

> G. ogdoos, ogdoē, ogdoon *eighth*

novem 아홉

> nonaginta (< novem *nine* + -ginta *ten times*) 아흔　　　　　　　　　E *nonagenarian*

> November, Novembris, Novembre (고대 로마력의) 제9월의,
　　(개정 로마력의) 11월의　　　　　　　E (November mensis *'the ninth month'* >) *November*

< IE. newn *nine*　　　　　　　　　　　　　　　　　　　　**E** *nine, nineteen, ninety; ninth*

　　> L. nonus, nona, nonum 아홉째

　　　　E (nona hora *'ninth hour'* >) ***noon, nonan*** *(< 'recurring every ninth day or at intervals of eight days'),* ***non(a)-***

　　> G. ennea *nine*

　　　　> G. enakis (*adverb, multiplicative*) *nine-times*

　　　　> G. enneas, enneados, f. *the number nine, ennead*　　　　　**E** *ennead*

　　> G. enatos, enatē, enaton *ninth*

decem 열

　　> December, Decembris, Decembre (고대 로마력의) 제10월의,

　　　　(개정 로마력의) 12월의　　　**E** (December mensis *'the tenth month'* >) *December*

　　> deni, denae, dena 열씩

　　　　> denarius, denaria, denarium

　　　　　　열씩의　　　**E** *denary,* (denarius nummus *'coin containing ten asses'* >) *denarius*

　　> decussis, decussis, m. 열, X자형

　　　　> decusso, **decussavi**, decussatum, decussare X자형으로 만들다, X자형으로

　　　　　　나누다, X자형으로 교차시키다　　　　　　　　　　　**E** *decussate*

　　> decanus, decani, m. 열 명 단위 조직의 장, 십장　　　　　　**E** *dean*

　　> decimus, decima, decimum 열째　　　　　　　**E** *decimal, deci-, dime*

　　　　> decimo, **decimavi**, decimatum, decimare 열 번째를 골라내다, 열 명에 하나씩

　　　　　　사형시키다, 10분의 1의 조세를 물리다　　　　　　　**E** *decimate*

< IE. dekm *ten*　　　　　　　　　　　　　　　　**E** *ten, -teen, -ty; tenth*

　　> G. deka *ten*

　　　　E *dec(a)-,* (hoi deka logoi *'the ten sayings'* >) *Decalogue,* (G. **dekaēmeron* (*dechēmeron) *'ten days'* >) *Decameron*

　　　　> G. dekakis (*adverb, multiplicative*) *ten-times*

　　　　> G. dekas, dekados, f. *the number ten (the perfect number of the Pythagoreans), decade*

　　　　　　> L. decas, decadis, f. 열, 열을 한 묶음으로 한 단위　　　**E** *decad, decade*

　　　　> G. hendeka *eleven*　　　　　　　　　　　　　　　　**E** *hendec(a)-*

　　　　> G. dōdeka *twelve*　　　　　　　　　　　　　　　　**E** *dodec(a)-*

　　> G. dekatos, dekatē, dekaton *tenth*

　　> IE. dkm-ta *ten times*

　　　　> L. -ginta 열 배

　　　　　　> L. quadraginta (quadra- *four* + -ginta) 마흔

　　　　　　　　E (It. quaranta *'forty'* > *'a period of forty days set aside or used for a specific purpose'*) >) *quarantine*

　　　　> G. -konta *ten times*

　　　　　　> G. triakonta (< tria *three* + -konta) *thirty*　　　　**E** *triacontanol*

　　　　　　> G. pentēkonta (< pente *five* + -konta) *fifty*

　　　　　　　　> G. pentēkostos, pentēkostē, pentēkoston *fiftieth*　　**E** *Pentecost*

> IE. wikmti- *twenty* (< IE. wi- *in half, hence two*)

> L. viginti 스물

> G. eikosi *twenty*

> **E** *eicos(a)- (icos(a)-), eicosanoic acid (icosanoic acid)* (< *'a saturated fatty acid with a 20-carbon chain, arachidic acid'*), *eicosanoid(s)* (< *'biologically active molecules that are, similar to arachidonic acid, around 20 carbon units in length'*), *eicosapentaenoic acid (EPA)* (< *'a fatty acid with a 20-carbon chain and five double bonds'*), *icosahedron*

> G. dōkosi (< dyo kai eikosi *two and twenty*) *twenty-two*

> **E** *docosahexaenoic acid (DHA)* (< *'a fatty acid with a 22-carbon chain and six double bonds'*)

> IE. dkm-tom, km-tom *hundred* **E** *hundred; thousand* (< *'swollen hundred'* < IE. teuə- *'to swell'*)

> L. centum (불변화) 백(百)

> **E** *centum, cent,* (per centum >) *percent,* (percent >) *percentage,* (percent > *'on the pattern of quartile'* > *'each of the 99 intermediate values of a variate which divide a frequency distribution into 100 groups each containing one percent of the total population; each of the 100 groups so formed'* >) *percentile, cent(i)-*

> L. centesimus, centesima, centesimum 백 번째   **E** *centesimal*

> L. centenarius, centenaria, centenarium 백의,

백 되는 수의   **E** *centenary, centenarian*

> L. centuria, centuriae, f. **Servius Tullius**가 193등급으로 나눈 로마 시민의

단위, 백인조(百人組), 백인대(百人隊),

백 개의 묶음   **E** *(a century of years >) century*

> L. centurio, centuriavi, centuriatum, centuriare 백인대로 편성하다

> L. succenturio, succenturiavi, succenturiatum, succenturiare

(< L. suc- (< sub) *under, up from under*) 백인대를 보충

하다, 보충대를 편성하다   **E** *succenturiate*

> G. hekaton (< IE. sem- *one* + IE. dkm-tom, km-tom *hundred*)

hundred   **E** *(hekaton > (contracted) >) hect(o)-*

> G. hekatombē, hekatombēs, f. (< hekaton + bous *ox*) *an offering of a*

hundred oxen, a great public sacrifice   **E** *hecatomb*

> (*Avestan*) satem *hundred*   **E** *satem*

mille, (pl.) millia (milia) 천

> **E** *milli-,* (milia passuum *'thousand of paces'* >) *mile, milestone* (< *'a stone set up beside a road indicating the distance in miles'*), ((probably) It. mille *'thousand'* + -one *'augmentative suffix'* > millione >) *million,* (bi- *'two'* > *'the second power of a million'* >) *billion,* (tri- *'three'* > *'the third power of a million'* >) *trillion,* (quadri- *'four'* > *'the fourth power of a million'* >) *quadrillion*

> L. millesimus, millesima, millesimum 천 번째   **E** *millesimal*

> L. millennium, millennii, n. (< mille *thousand* + annus *year*) 천년   **E** *millennium*

< IE. (*suggested*) gheslo- *thousand*

> G. chilioi (m.), chiliai (f.), chilia (n.) (pl.) *thousand*

E *kilo-*

동사

라틴어 동사에는 정형(定形)동사와 탈형(脫形)동사가 있다. 정형동사란 능동태와 수동태의 구분이 분명한 동사를 가리킨다. 탈형동사란 꼴은 수동태이지만 뜻은 능동태인 동사를 가리킨다. 탈형동사를 이태(異態)동사라고 하기도 한다. 그 외에 정형과 탈형이 섞인 반탈형동사, 불규칙 변화를 하는 불규칙동사, 법·시제·인칭 등이 결여되어 있는 불비(不備)동사가 있다. 동사라고 하면 정형동사를 가리킬 정도로 대부분의 동사가 정형동사이다.

정형동사

정형동사의 변화

정형동사는 태(능동태·수동태), 법(직설법·가정법·명령법·부정법), 시제(현재·과거·미래·완료·과거완료·미래완료), 수(단수·복수), 인칭(일인칭·이인칭·삼인칭), 분사(현재분사·미래분사·과거분사·목적분사) 등에 따라 꼴이 달라지므로 동사의 변화는 명사나 형용사의 변화보다도 훨씬 더 복잡하다. 그러나 변화에 필요한 네 가지 기본꼴만 알고 있으면 모든 변화를 시킬 수 있으며, 라틴어사전도 네 가지 기본꼴만을 제시한다.

- 능동태 직설법 현재 단수 일인칭: 현재어간과 동사변화의 종류를 보여준다.

- 능동태 직설법 완료 단수 일인칭: 완료어간을 보여준다.

- 능동태 목적분사: 능동태 목적분사 어간(수동태 과거분사 어간)을 보여준다.

- 능동태 현재부정법: 현재어간과 동사변화의 종류를 보여준다.

(보기) am-o, amav-i, amat-um, am-are 사랑하다

- am-o 나는 사랑한다

  능동태 직설법 현재 단수 일인칭 (영어에서와 같음)

- amav-i 나는 사랑하였다

  능동태 직설법 완료 단수 일인칭 (영어의 현재완료에 해당함)

- amat-um 사랑하러

  능동태 목적분사 ('오다', '가다' 등의 목적을 제시해주는 부사어)

- am-are 사랑하기는(를)

  능동태 현재부정법 (영어의 부정법 '*to* + 동사원형'에 해당함)

네 가지 기본꼴 중 능동태 현재부정법과 능동태 직설법 현재 단수 일인칭 두 가지를 보면 현재어간과 동사변화의 종류를 알 수 있고, 네 가지를 모두 보면 나머지 두 어간과 동사변화 전체를 알 수 있다.

수동태는 수동태 직설법 현재 단수 일인칭, 수동태 직설법 완료 단수 일인칭, 수동태 현재부정법의 세 가지를 알면 변화시킬 수 있는데, 이 셋은 각각 능동태 직설법 현재 단수 일인칭, 능동태 목적분사, 그리고 능동태 현재부정법의 어미를 살짝 바꾸어줌으로써 쉽게 만든다.

정형동사의 변화에는 네 가지가 있다.

제1변화   능동태 현재부정법이 -are로 끝나는 동사. 능동태 직설법 현재 단수 일인칭은 -o로 끝난다. 이에 해당하는 수동태 어미는 -ari, -or이다.

(능동태) am-o, amav-i, amat-um, am-are 사랑하다
(수동태) am-or, amat-us (amat-a, amat-um) sum, am-ari 사랑받다

제2변화   능동태 현재부정법이 -ēre로 끝나는 동사. 어미 -ēre의 첫 음절이 장음이며 거기에 강세가 있다. 능동태 직설법 현재 단수 일인칭은 -eo로 끝난다. 해당하는 수동태 어미는 -eri, -eor이다.

(능동태) hab-eo, habu-i, habit-um, hab-ēre 가지다
(수동태) hab-eor, habit-us (habit-a, habit-um) sum, hab-eri 가지게 되다

제3변화   능동태 현재부정법이 -ĕre로 끝나는 동사. 어미 -ĕre의 바로 앞 음절이 장음이며 거기에 강세가 있다. 능동태 직설법 현재 단수 일인칭은 -o (A식) 또는 -io (B식)로 끝난다. 해당하는 수동태 어미는 -i 와 -or (A식) 또는 -ior (B식)이다.

(능동태) leg-o, leg-i, lect-um, leg-ĕre 모으다, 뽑다, 읽다

(수동태) leg-or, lect-us (lect-a, lect-um) sum, leg-i 모아지다, 뽑히다, 읽히다

(능동태) cap-io, cep-i, capt-um, cap-ĕre 붙잡다

(수동태) cap-ior, capt-us (capt-a, capt-um) sum, cap-i 붙잡히다

제4변화 능동태 현재부정법이 –ire로 끝나는 동사. 능동태 직설법 현재 단수 일인칭은 –io로 끝난다. 해당하는 수동태 어미는 -iri, -ior이다.

(능동태) aud-io, audiv-i, audit-um, aud-ire 듣다

(수동태) aud-ior, audit-us (audit-a, audit-um) sum, aud-iri 들리다

제2변화와 제3변화 동사의 능동태 현재부정법 어미는 철자가 같으나 첫 음절의 장단과 강세가 다르다. 이를 라틴어사전은 장단과 강세 표시로 구분한다. 어원론에서는, 강세 표시를 생략하므로, –ēre와 –ĕre처럼 장단으로 구분한다. 제3변화 A식과 B식 동사는 능동태 직설법 현재 단수 일인칭이 다르다. 동사가 어느 변화에 속하는지 알려면 능동태 현재부정법과 능동태 직설법 현재 단수 일인칭 두 가지를 같이 보아야 하는 것이다.

능동태 직설법 현재 단수 일인칭 (*first personal singular, present indicative, active*)

라틴어사전의 표제어이다. 일부 어원론에서 제시하는 형이기도 하다. 'ego(나는)'라는 인칭대명사 없이도 '나는 ~한다'의 뜻을 갖는다. 'ego'라는 인칭대명사를 사용하면 특별히 '나'를 강조하는 뜻을 가지나 그런 문장은 매우 드물다.

[용례] Cogito, ergo sum. 나는 생각한다, 그러므로 나는 존재한다 (René Descartes, 1596–1650)
　　　(문법) cogito 나는 생각한다: 능동태 직설법 현재 단수 일인칭
　　　　　　＜ cogito, cogitavi, cogitatum, cogitare 생각하다 (제1변화)
　　　　　ergo 그러므로: 접속사
　　　　　sum 나는 있다: esse 동사의 직설법 현재 단수 일인칭
　　　　　　＜ sum, fui, –, esse ~이다, 있다 (불규칙 변화)

능동태 직설법 완료 단수 일인칭 (*first personal singular, perfect indicative, active*)

라틴어 동사는 결과가 현재까지 미치는 지난 일 또는 딱 한번 일어난 지난 일을 완료(*perfect*)라고 하여, 지속적 또는 반복적으로 일어난 일인 미완료 과거(*imperfect*)와 구분한다.

> [용례] Veni, vidi, vici. 나는 왔다, 보았다, 이겼다 (Gaius Julius Caesar, 100–44 B.C.E.)
> (문법) veni 나는 왔다: 능동태 직설법 완료 단수 일인칭
>   < venio, veni, ventum, venire 오다 (제4변화)
> vidi 나는 보았다: 능동태 직설법 완료 단수 일인칭
>   < video, vidi, visum, vidēre 보다 (제2변화)
> vici 나는 이겼다: 능동태 직설법 완료 단수 일인칭
>   < vinco, vici, victum, vincěre 이기다 (제3변화 A식)

능동태 목적분사 (*supine*)

'오다', '가다' 등의 목적을 제시해 주는 목적부사어이다. 대격(–um)과 탈격(–u)만 있어 서 있지 못하고 누워버린 꼴이다. 영어 *supine*도 누워 있는 낱말(supinum verbum)임을 뜻한다.

> [용례] Venisti dictum, veni actum. 너는 말하기 위해 왔고, 나는 행동하기 위해 왔다
> (문법) venisti 너는 왔다: 능동태 직설법 완료 단수 이인칭
>   < venio, veni, ventum, venire 오다 (제4변화)
> dictum 말하기 위해: 능동태 목적분사
>   < dico, dixi, dictum, dicěre 말하다 (제3변화 A식)
> veni 나는 왔다: 능동태 직설법 완료 단수 일인칭
>   < venio, veni, ventum, venire 오다 (제4변화)
> actum 행동하기 위해: 능동태 목적분사
>   < ago, egi, actum, agěre 하다 (제3변화 A식)

능동태 목적분사의 용례는 위와 같으나 위 문장은 자주 보는 문장이 아니다. 능동태 목적분사의 실제적 기능은 과거분사의 어간을 보여준다는 점이다. 그래서 능동태 목적분사 어간을 과거분사 어간이라고도 한다.

> [용례] Vox audita perit, litera scripta manet. (< *The heard voice perishes, the written letter remains.*) 들린 목소리는 사라지나, 쓰인 글자는 남는다
> (문법) vox 목소리는: 단수 주격 < vox, vocis, f.

audita 들린: 과거분사, 여성형 단수 주격

    < auditus, audita, auditum

   < audio, audivi (audii), auditum, audire 듣다 (제4변화)

perit 사라진다: 능동태 직설법 현재 단수 삼인칭

   < pereo, perivi (perii), peritum, perire (< per- *through, thoroughly* +
     ire *to go*) 사라지다, 죽다, 망하다 (불규칙변화)

litera 글자는: 단수 주격 < litera, literae, f. (littera, litterae, f.)

scripta 쓰인: 과거분사, 여성형 단수 주격

    < scriptus, scripta, scriptum

   < scribo, scripsi, scriptum, scribĕre 새기다, 글을 쓰다 (제3변화 A식)

manet 남는다: 능동태 직설법 현재 단수 삼인칭

   < maneo, mansi, mansum, manēre 머물다, 거주하다, 남다 (제2변화)

능동태 현재부정법 (*present infinitive, active*)

능동태 현재부정법은 '~하기', '~한다는 것'의 뜻을 가지며 수동태 현재부정법은 '~받기', '~되기', '~받는다는 것', '~된다는 것'의 뜻을 가진다. 부정법은 동사 겸 명사로 사용되기도 하고 그냥 명사로만 사용되기도 하는데 중성의 단수 명사로 취급하고 주격 또는 대격만 허용한다. 어미변화는 없다. (어원론에서는 능동태 현재부정법을 동사의 기본꼴로 간주하기 때문에 '~하기', '~한다는 것'이라기보다는 편의상 '~하다'라고 옮긴다. 같은 맥락에서 수동태 현재부정법을 '~받기', '~되기'라기보다는 '~받다', '~되다'라고 옮긴다.)

[용례] Errare humanum est. (< *To err is human.*) 실수하는 것은 인간적이다, 실수하는
     것은 인간이기 때문이다
    (문법) errare 실수하는 것은: 능동태 현재부정법, 중성 단수 주격
       < erro, erravi, erratum, errare 실수하다 (제1변화)
     humanum 사람의, 인간적인: 형용사, 중성형 단수 주격
       < humanus, humana, humanum
     est 이다: esse 동사의 직설법 현재 단수 삼인칭
       < sum, fui, -, esse ~이다, 있다 (불규칙변화)

[용례] Primum (est) non nocēre. (< *Not to do harm is first.*) 안 해치는 것이 첫째이다
    (문법) primum 첫째: 수사, 중성형 단수 주격 < primus, prima, primum
     non 아니: 부사
     nocēre 해치는 것이: 능동태 현재부정법, 중성 단수 주격
       < noceo, nocui, nocitum, nocēre 해치다 (제2변화)

어원론에 필요한 정형동사의 변화

동사변화가 복잡하다고 하나 어원을 이해하고 학술용어를 구사하기 위해 필요한 꼴은 다음 넷이다.

- 능동태 현재부정법 (*present infinitive*)
- 능동태 현재분사 (*present participle*)
- 수동태 미래분사 (*gerundive*)
- 수동태 과거분사 (*past participle*)

'모으다', '뽑다', '읽다'라는 정형동사 'lego, legi, lectum, legĕre'에서 어원론에 필요한 꼴과 그로부터 비롯한 영어 낱말은 다음과 같다.

- 능동태 현재부정법

  leg‑ĕre 모으다, 뽑다, 읽다   E *legible, …*

- 능동태 현재분사

  legens, (gen.) legent‑is ~하는, ~하고 있는   E *diligent, …*

- 수동태 미래분사

  legend‑us, legend‑a, legend‑um ~받아야 할   E *legend, …*

- 수동태 과거분사

  lect‑us, lect‑a, lect‑um ~받은, ~받고서   E *lecture, …*

이 외의 몇몇 동사변화 꼴이 영어 속에 들어오기도 한다. 미래형 *placebo*, 명령형 *recipe* 등 관용어처럼 쓰이는 낱말들이다.

[용례] placebo 나는 (주님의) 마음에 들 것이다 (주님께서 나를 받아주실 것이다)   E *placebo*
　　　　(문법) 능동태 직설법 미래 단수 일인칭; (1) 죽은 자를 위해 드리는 기도
　　　　　　　(placebo로 시작한다: Placebo Domino in regione vivorum
　　　　　　　(Psalm). *I shall please the Lord in the land of the living.*),
　　　　　　　(2) 가약(假藥), 위약(僞藥), 플라시보
　　　　< placeo, placui, placitum, placēre (여격지배) 마음에 들다   E *please*

[용례] Recipe! 받으십시오!   E *recipe*

(문법) recipe 당신께서는 받으십시오: 능동태 명령법 현재 단수 이인칭
< recipio, recepi, receptum, recipĕre 받다

E *receive*

이들 낱말까지 이해하기 위해서는 어원에 필요한 네 가지 꼴 외에 몇 가지를 추가할 필요가 있다. 정형동사 legĕre를 예로 들면 다음 표와 같다. 이 책의 부록 〈변화표〉에 수록되어 있는 형식이다.

능동태					
부정법	현재			leg-ĕre	모으다, 뽑다, 읽다
직설법	현재	단수	일인칭	leg-o	나는 ~한다
			이인칭	leg-is	너는 ~한다
			삼인칭	leg-it	그는 ~한다
		복수	일인칭	leg-imus	우리는 ~한다
			이인칭	leg-itis	너희는 ~한다
			삼인칭	leg-unt	그들은 ~한다
	과거	단수	일인칭	leg-ebam	나는 ~하였다
	미래	단수	일인칭	leg-am	나는 ~하겠다
	완료	단수	일인칭	leg-i	나는 ~하였다
가정법	현재	단수	일인칭	leg-am	나는 ~하리라
명령법	현재	단수	이인칭	leg-e	너는 ~하라
		복수	이인칭	leg-ite	너희는 ~하라
분 사	현재			legens, (gen.) legent-is	~하는, ~하고 있는
목적분사				lect-um	~하러, ~하기 위하여
수동태					
부정법	현재			leg-i	모아지다, 읽히다
분 사	미래			legend-us, legend-a, legend-um	~받아야 할
	과거			lect-us, lect-a, lect-um	~받은, ~받고서

위 표처럼 능동태 현재부정법, 능동태 현재분사, 수동태 미래분사, 수동태 과거분사 넷을 필요할 때마다 제시해 준다면 보는 사람은 마음에 든다고 할 것이다. 그러나 그렇게 해주지 않는다. 라틴어사전에서처럼 동사변화에 필요한 기본 꼴만을 제시하거나, 기껏해야, 그중 일부만을 제시해줄 따름이다. 어원론은 그 정도만 가지고도 나머지는 보는 사람이 알아서 해석할 수 있을 것이라고 전제하

기 때문이다.

동사에서 만들어진 파생어나 합성어는 명사나 형용사에서 만들어진 파생어나 합성어보다 훨씬 많다. 또한 학술용어에서는 능동태 현재분사와 수동태 과거분사를 라틴어 형용사처럼 라틴어 문법에 맞춰 사용하는 경우가 많다. Caenorhabditis elegans의 elegans도 라틴어 동사의 능동태 현재분사를 형용사처럼 라틴어 문법에 맞춰 사용한 예이다. 따라서, 생명과학을 공부하는 사람이라면, 라틴어사전에서 제시하는 기본꼴이나 어원론에서 제시하는 일부 기본꼴을 보고서 어원과 관련된 꼴을 찾아낼 줄 알아야 한다. 그것은, 일단 규칙을 알고 나면, 쉽다.

어원론에 필요한 동사꼴을 찾아내는 방법과 꼴의 뜻

라틴어사전이 정형동사에 대해 보여주는 내용은 다음이 전부이다.

am-o	amav-i	amat-um	am-are	사랑하다	(제1변화)
hab-eo	habu-i	habit-um	hab-ēre	가지다	(제2변화)
leg-o	leg-i	lect-um	leg-ĕre	모으다, 뽑다, 읽다	(제3변화 A식)
cap-io	cep-i	capt-um	cap-ĕre	붙잡다	(제3변화 B식)
aud-io	audiv-i	audit-um	aud-ire	듣다	(제4변화)

여기서부터 어원론에 필요한 꼴을 찾아내는 방법과 찾아낸 꼴의 뜻은 다음과 같다.

능동태 현재부정법 (*present infinitive*)

라틴어사전은 능동태 직설법 현재 단수 일인칭을 표제어로 제시하고 능동태 현재부정법을 뒤에 제시하나 대부분의 어원론에서는 능동태 현재부정법만 제시한다.

능동태 현재부정법을 보면 동사의 현재어간을 알 수 있으며, 능동태 현재부정법과 능동태 직설법 현재 단수 일인칭을 같이 보면 동사변화의 종류를 알 수 있다.

능동태 현재분사 (*present participle*)

am–o	⋯	amat–um	am–are	>	amans	(gen.)	amant–is	(제1변화)
hab–eo	⋯	habit–um	hab–ēre	>	habens	(gen.)	habent–is	(제2변화)
leg–o	⋯	lect–um	leg–ĕre	>	legens	(gen.)	legent–is	(제3변화 A식)
cap–io	⋯	capt–um	cap–ĕre	>	capiens	(gen.)	capient–is	(제3변화 B식)
aud–io	⋯	audit–um	aud–ire	>	audiens	(gen.)	audient–is	(제4변화)

능동태 현재분사는 동사의 현재어간에 –ans(제1변화), –ens(제2변화), –ens (제3변화 A식), –iens(제3변화 B식), –iens(제4변화)를 붙여 만든다. 형용사 제3변화 제3식에 따른 어미변화를 한다. 따라서 능동태 현재분사의 단수 주격 은 남·여·중성에서 모두 같은 꼴을 가지며, 단수 속격은 –ntis로 끝나고, 어간 은 –nt–까지이다.

능동태 현재분사는 능동 또는 진행의 뜻을 가진다. 수동태에는 현재분사가 없 다. 따라서 현재분사라고만 하여도 능동태이다. 능동태 현재분사의 영어 표기가 *present participle*인 것은 이 때문이다.

라틴어에서 능동태 현재분사는 동사와 형용사의 기능을 함께 가지나 학술용어 에서는 형용사적으로만 쓰인다. 형용사와 마찬가지로, 수식하는 명사의 성·수· 격을 따른다.

[용례] luna crescens 상현달
　　　(문법) luna 달: 단수 주격 < luna, lunae, f.
　　　　　　crescens 커지는: 능동태 현재분사, 남·여·중성형 단수 주격
　　　　　　　　< crescens, (gen.) crescentis
　　　　　　　　< cresco, crevi, cretum, crescĕre 커지다 (제3변화)

[용례] res moventes (pl.) 동산(動産)
　　　(문법) res 재산: 복수 주격 < res, rei, f. 사물, 일, 재산
　　　　　　moventes 움직이는: 능동태 현재분사, 남·여성형 복수 주격
　　　　　　　　< movens, (gen.) moventis
　　　　　　　　< moveo, movi, motum, movēre 움직이다, 움직이게 하다 (제2변화)

[용례] corpus albicans, (pl.) corpora albicantia 백체, 백색체
　　　(문법) corpus 몸, 체(體): 단수 주격 < corpus, corporis, n.

albicans 하얀, 하얗게 되는: 능동태 현재분사, 남·여·중성형 단수 주격

    < albicans, (gen.) albicantis

    < albico, albicavi, albicatum, albicare 하얗다, 하얗게 되다 (제1변화)

corpora: corpus의 복수 주격

albicantia: albicare의 능동태 현재분사, 중성형 복수 주격

수동태 미래분사 (*gerundive*)

am-o	⋯	am-are	>	amans	(gen.) amant-is	> amand-us, -a, -um (제1변화)
hab-eo	⋯	hab-ēre	>	habens	(gen.) habent-is	> habend-us, -a, -um (제2변화)
leg-o	⋯	leg-ĕre	>	legens	(gen.) legent-is	> legend-us, -a, -um (제3변화 A식)
cap-io	⋯	cap-ĕre	>	capiens	(gen.) capient-is	> capiend-us, -a, -um (제3변화 B식)
aud-io	⋯	aud-ire	>	audiens	(gen.) audient-is	> audiend-us, -a, -um (제4변화)

수동태 미래분사는 동사의 현재어간에 -andus (제1변화), -endus (제2변화), -endus (제3변화 A식), -iendus (제3변화 B식), -iendus (제4변화)를 붙여 만든다. 형용사 제1·2변화의 어미변화를 한다.

수동태 미래분사는 '~되어져야 할', '~받아야 할'이라는 뜻을 가지는 동사적 형용사이며 수동태 당위분사라고도 한다. 몇 가지 일반 영어나 학술용어의 어원을 이해하는데 필요한 정도이다.

[용례] Memorandum est. (그것은) 기억되어야 할 것이다

    (문법) memorandum 기억되어야 할: 수동태 미래분사, 중성형 단수 주격

        < memorandus, memoranda, memorandum

        < memoro, memoravi, memoratum, memorare 생각나게 하다, 언급하다

        est (그것은) 이다: esse 동사 직설법 현재 단수 삼인칭

        < sum, fui, -, esse ~이다, 있다 (불규칙동사)

수동태 과거분사 (*past participle*)

am-o	amav-i	amat-um	am-are >	amat-us, -a, -um (제1변화)
hab-eo	habu-i	habit-um	hab-ēre >	habit-us, -a, -um (제2변화)
leg-o	leg-i	lect-um	leg-ĕre >	lect-us, -a, -um (제3변화 A식)
cap-io	cep-i	capt-um	cap-ĕre >	capt-us, -a, -um (제3변화 B식)
aud-io	audiv-i	audit-um	aud-ire >	audit-us, -a, -um (제4변화)

수동태 과거분사는 능동태 목적분사 어간에 -us(m.), -a(f.), -um(n.)을 붙여 만든다. 형용사 제1·2변화에 따른 어미변화를 한다.

수동태 과거분사는 수동 또는 완료의 뜻을 가진다. 능동태에는 과거분사가 없다. 따라서 과거분사라고만 하여도 수동태이다. 수동태 과거분사의 영어 표기가 *past participle*인 것은 이 때문이다.

라틴어에서는, 능동태 현재분사와 마찬가지로, 동사와 형용사의 기능을 함께 하나 학술용어에서는 형용사적으로만 쓰인다. 형용사와 마찬가지로, 수식하는 명사의 성·수·격을 따른다.

[용례] placenta accreta 유착(癒着)태반   **E** *placenta accreta*
      placenta increta 함입(陷入)태반, 감입(嵌入)태반   **E** *placenta increta*
      placenta percreta 천공(穿孔)태반, 전감입(全嵌入)태반   **E** *placenta percreta*
    (문법) placenta 태반: 단수 주격 < placenta, placentae, f.
        accreta 자란: 수동태 과거분사, 여성형 단수 주격
            < accretus, accreta, accretum
          < accresco, accrevi, accretum, accrescĕre (< ac- (< ad) *to, toward,*
            at, according to + crescĕre *to grow*) (부착에 의해) 자라다, 더해가다
        increta 더 자란: 수동태 과거분사, 여성형 단수 주격
            < incretus, increta, incretum
          < incresco, increvi, incretum, increscĕre (< in- *in, on, into, toward*
            + crescĕre *to grow*) (점점) 자라나다
      percreta 많이 자란: 수동태 과거분사, 여성형 단수 주격
            < percretus, percreta, percretum
          < percresco, percrevi, percretum, percrescĕre (< per- *through, thoroughly*
            + crescĕre *to grow*) 많이 자라다

탈형동사

탈형동사는 꼴은 수동태이나 뜻이 능동태인 동사이다. 그러나 탈형동사라고 하더라도 현재분사와 수동형 미래분사는 능동태의 꼴을 갖는다.

탈형동사의 변화

탈형동사의 경우에는 변화에 필요한 세 가지 기본꼴만 알고 있으면 모든 변화를 시킬 수 있으며, 라틴어사전도 세 가지 기본꼴만을 제시한다.

- 직설법 현재 단수 일인칭: 현재어간과 동사변화의 종류를 보여준다.

- 직설법 완료 단수 일인칭(남성형): 완료어간을 보여준다.

- 현재부정법: 현재어간과 동사변화의 종류를 보여준다.

(보기) imit-or, imitat-us sum, imit-ari 모방하다

- imit-or 나는 모방한다

    직설법 현재 단수 일인칭

- imitat-us sum 나는 모방하였다

    직설법 완료 단수 일인칭(남성형)

- imit-ari 모방하기는(를)

    현재부정법

탈형동사의 변화에도 네 가지가 있다.

제1변화 현재부정법이 -ari로, 직설법 현재 단수 일인칭이 -or로 끝나는 동사.

imit-or, imitat-us sum, imit-ari 모방하다, 본받다

제2변화 현재부정법이 -eri로, 직설법 현재 단수 일인칭이 -eor로 끝나는 동사.

tue-or, tuit-us (tut-us) sum, tu-eri 지켜보다, 주시하다, 보살피다

제3변화 현재부정법이 -i로, 직설법 현재 단수 일인칭이 -or(A식) 또는 -ior(B식)로 끝나는 동사.

loqu-or, locut-us sum, loqu-i 말하다
pat-ior, pass-us sum, pat-i 참다, 고통받다

제4변화 현재부정법이 -iri로, 직설법 현재 단수 일인칭이 -ior로 끝나는 동사.

or-ior, ort-us sum, or-iri 돋다, 나다, 출현하다

직설법 현재 단수 일인칭 (*first personal singular, present indicative*)

라틴어사전의 표제어이며 일부 어원론에서 제시하는 형이다. 정형동사의 능동태 직설법 현재 단수 일인칭이 의미하는 것과 같다.

> [용례] Cura pecuniam crescentem sequitur. 걱정은 불어나는 돈을 따라다닌다
>   (Quintus Horatius Flaccus, 65-8 B.C.E.)
> (문법) cura 걱정은: 단수 주격 < cura, curae, f.
>   pecuniam 돈을: 단수 대격 < pecunia, pecuniae, f.
>   crescentem 커지는: 능동태 현재분사, 남·여성형 단수 대격
>   < crescens, (gen.) crescentis
>   < cresco, crevi, cretum, crescĕre 커지다 (정형 제3변화)
>   sequitur 뒤따른다: 직설법 현재 단수 삼인칭
>   < sequor, secutus sum, sequi (탈형 제3변화 A식)

직설법 완료 단수 일인칭 (남성형) (*first personal singular, perfect indicative*)

정형동사의 직설법 완료 단수 일인칭이 의미하는 것과 같다. -us (m.), -a (f.), -um (n.)뿐 아니라 esse 동사인 sum도 주어를 따라서 변화한다.

> [용례] Cicero locutus est, "Homo stultus." 치체로가 말하였다, "사람은 어리석다."
> (문법) Cicero 치체로(키케로)가: 단수 주격 < Cicero, Ciceronis, m.
>   < Marcus Tullius Cicero (106-43 B.C.E.)
>   locutus est 말하였다: 직설법 완료 단수 삼인칭, 남성형
>   < loquor, locutus sum, loqui 말하다 (탈형 제3변화 A식)
>   homo 사람은: 단수 주격 < homo, hominis, m.
>   stultus 어리석은: 형용사, 남성형 단수 주격 < stultus, stulta, stultum

현재부정법 (*present infinitive*)

정형동사의 능동태 현재부정법이 의미하는 것과 같다. 능동태 현재부정법과 마찬가지로 명사로 사용할 때에는 중성 단수 명사로 취급하고 주격 또는 대격으로만 사용한다. 어미변화는 없다.

> [용례] Memento mori. 죽는다는 것을 너는 기억하고 있으라
> (문법) memento 너는 기억하고 있으라: 명령법 현재 단수 이인칭
>   < -, memini, -, meminisse (과거부정법, 뜻은 현재) (불비동사) 기억하고 있다
>   mori 죽는다는 것을: 현재부정법, 중성 명사 단수 대격으로 사용
>   < morior, mortuus sum, mori 죽다 (탈형 제3변화 B식)

어원론에 필요한 탈형동사의 변화

탈형동사의 꼴은 법(직설법·가정법·명령법·부정법), 시제(현재·과거·미래·완료·과거완료·미래완료), 수(단수·복수), 인칭(일인칭·이인칭·삼인칭), 분사(현재분사·미래분사·과거분사) 등에 따라 달라진다. 어원을 이해하고 학술용어를 구사하기 위해 필요한 내용은 다음 넷이다. 탈형동사의 경우에는 태를 구분할 수 없기 때문에 능동태나 수동태라는 표현을 쓰지 않아서 그렇지 내용과 영어 표기는 정형동사의 경우와 똑같다.

- 현재부정법 (*present infinitive*)
- 현재분사 (*present participle*)
- 수동형 미래분사 (*gerundive*)
- 과거분사 (*past participle*)

'참다', '고통받다'라는 탈형동사 'patior, passus sum, pati'에서 어원론에 필요한 꼴과 그로부터 비롯한 영어 낱말은 다음과 같다.

- 현재부정법

  pat-i 참다, 고통받다   Ｅ *compatible, ⋯*

- 현재분사

  patiens, (gen.) patient-is ~하는, ~하고 있는   Ｅ *patient, ⋯*

- 수동형 미래분사

  patiend-us, patiend-a, patiend-um ~받아야 할

- 과거분사

  pass-us, pass-a, pass-um ~받은, ~받고서   Ｅ *passion, ⋯*

탈형동사 pati의 변화는 다음 표와 같다. 이 책의 부록 〈변화표〉에 수록되어 있는 형식이다.

부정법	현재			pat-i	참다, 고통받다
직설법	현재	단수	일인칭	pat-ior	나는 ~한다
			이인칭	pat-eris	너는 ~한다
			삼인칭	pat-itur	그는 ~한다
		복수	일인칭	pat-imur	우리는 ~한다
			이인칭	pat-imini	너희는 ~한다
			삼인칭	pat-iuntur	그들은 ~한다
	과거	단수	일인칭	pat-iebar	나는 ~하였다
	미래	단수	일인칭	pat-iar	나는 ~하겠다
	완료	단수	일인칭	pass-us, -a, -um sum	나는 ~하였다
가정법	현재	단수	일인칭	pat-iar	나는 ~하리라
명령법	현재	단수	이인칭	pat-ĕre	너는 ~하라
		복수	이인칭	pat-imini	너희는 ~하라
분　사	현재			patiens, (gen.) patient-is	~하는, ~하고 있는
	과거			pass-us, pass-a, pass-um	~한
수동형	미래분사			patiend-us, patiend-a, patiend-um	~받아야 할

어원론에 필요한 동사꼴을 찾아내는 방법과 꼴의 뜻

라틴어사전이 탈형동사에 대해 보여주는 내용은 다음이 전부이다.

imit-or	imitat-us sum	imit-ari	모방하다, 본받다	(제 1 변화)
tu-eor	tuit-us sum	tu-eri	지켜보다, 보살피다	(제 2 변화)
loqu-or	locut-us sum	loqu-i	말하다	(제 3 변화 A 식)
pat-ior	pass-us sum	pat-i	참다, 고통받다	(제 3 변화 B 식)
or-ior	ort-us sum	or-iri	돈다, 나다, 출현하다	(제 4 변화)

여기서부터 어원론에 필요한 꼴을 찾아내는 방법, 찾아낸 꼴의 뜻은 정형동사의 경우와 똑같다.

현재부정법 (*present infinitive*)

라틴어사전은 직설법 현재 단수 일인칭을 표제어로 제시하고 현재부정법을 뒤에 제시하나 대부분의 어원론에서는 현재부정법만 제시한다. 정형동사의 능동태 현재부정법이 의미하는 것과 같다.

현재분사 (*present participle*)

imit-or	imitat-us sum	imit-ari	>	imitans	(gen.)	imitant-is	(제1변화)
tu-eor	tuit-us sum	tu-eri	>	tuens	(gen.)	tuent-is	(제2변화)
loqu-or	locut-us sum	loqu-i	>	loquens	(gen.)	loquent-is	(제3변화 A식)
pat-ior	pass-us sum	pat-i	>	patiens	(gen.)	patient-is	(제3변화 B식)
or-ior	ort-us sum	or-iri	>	oriens	(gen.)	orient-is	(제4변화)

현재분사는 만드는 방법, 뜻, 어미변화에 있어서 정형동사의 능동태 현재분사와 똑같다.

수동형 미래분사 (*gerundive*)

imit-or	⋯	imit-ari	>	imitans	(gen.)	imitant-is	>	imitand-us, -a, -um	(제1변화)
tu-eor	⋯	tu-eri	>	tuens	(gen.)	tuent-is	>	tuend-us, -a, -um	(제2변화)
loqu-or	⋯	loqu-i	>	loquens	(gen.)	loquent-is	>	loquend-us, -a, -um	(제3변화 A식)
pat-ior	⋯	pat-i	>	patiens	(gen.)	patient-is	>	patiend-us, -a, -um	(제3변화 B식)
or-ior	⋯	or-iri	>	oriens	(gen.)	orient-is	>	oriend-us, -a, -um	(제4변화)

수동형 미래분사도 만드는 방법, 뜻, 어미변화에 있어서 정형동사의 수동태 미래분사와 똑같다.

과거분사 (*past participle*)

imit-or	imitat-us sum	imit-ari	>	imitat-us, -a, -um	(제1변화)
tu-eor	tuit-us sum	tu-eri	>	tuit-us, -a, -um	(제2변화)
loqu-or	locut-us sum	loqu-i	>	locut-us, -a, -um	(제3변화 A식)
pat-ior	pass-us sum	pat-i	>	pass-us, -a, -um	(제3변화 B식)
or-ior	ort-us sum	or-iri	>	ort-us, -a, -um	(제4변화)

과거분사는 완료어간에 -us(m.), -a(f.), -um(n.)을 붙여 만든다. 형용사 제1·2 변화에 따르는 어미변화를 한다. 뜻은 정형동사의 수동태 과거분사와 똑같다.

동사변화

정형동사의 변화

●●● 정형 제1변화

능동태 현재부정법이 -are로, 능동태 직설법 현재 단수 일인칭이 -o로 끝나는 동사.

amo, amavi, amatum, amare 사랑하다

능동태	부정법	현재			am-are	사랑하다
	직설법	현재	단수	일인칭	am-o	나는 ~한다
				이인칭	am-as	너는 ~한다
				삼인칭	am-at	그는 ~한다
			복수	일인칭	am-amus	우리는 ~한다
				이인칭	am-atis	너희는 ~한다
				삼인칭	am-ant	그들은 ~한다
		과거	단수	일인칭	am-abam	나는 ~하였다
		미래	단수	일인칭	am-abo	나는 ~하겠다
		완료	단수	일인칭	amav-i	나는 ~하였다
	가정법	현재	단수	일인칭	am-em	나는 ~하리라
	명령법	현재	단수	이인칭	am-a	너는 ~하라

			복수	이인칭	am-ate	너희는 ～하라
수동태	분 사 목적분사	현재			amans, (gen.) amant-is	～하는, ～하고 있는
					amat-um	～하러, ～하기 위하여
	부정법 분 사	현재 미래 과거			am-ari	사랑받다
					amand-us, amand-a, amand-um	～받아야 할
					amat-us, amat-a, amat-um	～받은, ～받고서

amo, amavi, amatum, amare 사랑하다

> amor, amoris, m. 사랑　　　　　　　　　　　　　　　　　　**E** F. *amour*

[용례] amor fati 운명애(運命愛)
(문법) amor 사랑: 단수 주격
fati 운명의: 단수 속격 < fatum, fati, n.

[용례] vena amoris 사랑의 혈관
(문법) vena 혈관: 단수 주격 < vena, venae, f. 혈관, 맥, 정맥
amoris: 단수 속격

> amator, amatoris, m. 연모자, 애호가, 호색가　　　　　　**E** *amateur*
　> amatorius, amatoria, amatorium 사랑하는, 연애의, 호색적인　**E** *amatory*
> amoenus, amoena, amoenum 기분 좋은, 즐거운, 쾌적한
　> amoenitas, amoenitatis, f. 기분 좋음, 즐거움, 쾌적　　　　**E** *amenity*
< IE. am- (*Latin and Celtic root*) '*various nursery words*'
　> L. amita, amitae, f. 고모　　　　　　　　　　　　　　**E** *aunt*
　> L. amicus, amica, amicum 친구의, 우호적인
　　　> L. amicus, amici, m. (amica, amicae, f.) (여자) 친구　**E** Sp. *amigo*
　　　　> L. amicabilis, amicabile 우호적인, 호감을 주는　**E** *amicable, amiable*
　　　　> L. *amicitas, *amicitatis, f. 우호관계, 친선　　　**E** *amity*
　　　> L. inimicus, inimica, inimicum (< in- *not* + amicus *friendly*) 비우호적인,
　　　원수의　　　　　　　　　　　　　　　　　　**E** *enemy, inimical*
　　　　> L. *inimicitas, *inimicitatis, f. 적의, 증오, 앙심　**E** *enmity*

aestimo, aestimavi, aestimatum, aestimare 값을 매기다,
평가하다　　　　　　　　**E** *estimate, esteem,* (ad '*to*' + aestimare '*to estimate*' >) *aim*

ambulo, ambulavi, ambulatum, ambulare (< amb(i)- *on both sides, around*) 거닐다,
산책하다, 왕래하다
　E *ambulate,* (ambulans (*present participle*) '*walking hospital*' >) *ambulance, ambulation, funambulism, somnambulism, alley,* It. *andante*

> ambulator, ambulatoris, m. 산책하는 사람, 빈둥빈둥 거니는 사람, 도부 장사, 행상인

　　> ambulatorius, ambulatoria, ambulatorium 보행의, 이동성의, 움직일 수 있는　**E** *ambulatory*

> perambulo, **perambulavi**, perambulatum, perambulare (< per- *through, thoroughly*

　　+ ambulare *to walk*) 배회하다, 순회하다　**E** *perambulate*

> praeambulo, **praeambulavi**, praeambulatum, praeambulare (< prae- *before, beyond*

　　+ ambulare *to walk*) 앞서가다

　　> praeambulum, praeambuli, n. 머리말, 전문(前文)　**E** *preamble*

< IE. al- *to wander, to be confused*

> L. hallucinor, hallucinatus sum, hallucinari 꿈과 같은 생각 속에서 헤매다, 횡설수설

　　하다, 환각에 사로잡히게 하다　**E** *hallucinant; hallucinogen*

　　> L. hallucinatio, hallucinationis, f. 환각　**E** *hallucination, (hallucination >) hallucinosis*

> L. exul, exulis, m., f. (< ex- *out of, away from* + IE. al-) 유배자, 추방자

　　> L. exilium, exilii, n. 유배, 망명　**E** *exile*

aro, **aravi**, **aratum**, **arare** 밭을 갈다, 경작하다

> arabilis, arabile 경작할 만한　**E** *arable*

< IE. arə- *to plow*

> L. aravus, arava, aravum 경작할 만한, 갈아 놓은

　　> L. arvum, arvi, n. 밭, 경작지

　　　> L. arvensis, arvense 밭의, 경작지의

bato, **batavi**, **batatum**, **batare** 입을 크게 벌리다, 크게 벌어지다　**E** *bevel, abash, abeyance*

< IE. bat- *yawning; Latin root of unknown origin, probably imitative*

calo, **calavi**, **calatum**, **calare** 부르다, 초대하다

> Calendae, Calendarum, f. (Kalendae, Kalendarum, f.) (pl.) (*the first day of the
month, when it was publicly announced on which days the nones and ides of
that month would fall*) 초하루, (시간의) 달　**E** *calends*

　　> calendarium, calendarii, n. 책력　**E** *calendar*

> concilium, concilii, n. (< *calling together* < con- (< cum) *with, together* + calare
to call) 연결, 회의, 협의회, 평의회, (고대 로마의) 국민회의　**E** *council*

　　> concilio, **conciliavi**, conciliatum, conciliare (보기에 모순된 것을) 조화시키다,
　　조정하다, 회유하다　**E** *conciliate*

　　　> reconcilio, **reconciliavi**, reconciliatum, reconciliare (< re- *back, again*)
　　　조정하다, 화해시키다　**E** *reconcile*

　　　　> reconciliatio, reconciliationis, f. 조정, 화해, 복귀　**E** *reconciliation*

> intercalo, **intercalavi**, intercalatum, intercalare (< *to insert an additional day, days,
or month in the calendar in order to bring the current reckoning of time into
harmony with the natural solar year* < inter- *between, among* + calare *to call*)

윤달이나 윤일(閏日)을 끼워 넣다, 끼워 넣다, 삽입하다, 개재(介在)시키다   **E** *intercalate*

> intercalaris, intercalare (intercalarius, intercalaria, intercalarium) 윤(閏)의,

끼워 넣은   **E** *intercalary*

> nomenclatura, nomenclaturae, f. (< nomen *name* + calatus (*past participle*) *called*)

명명법, 학명, 학술용어   **E** *nomenclature*

< IE. kelə- *to shout, to call hither*

> **E** *haul* (< '*to draw*' < '*to call hither*'), **overhaul** (< '*to haul over, as for examination*'), **low** (< '*to cry*')

> L. clamo, clamavi, clamatum, clamare 소리 지르다   **E** *claim, (claim >) claimant*

   > L. clamor, clamoris, m. 외침, 함성   **E** *clamor (clamour), clamorous*

   > L. acclamo, acclamavi, acclamatum, acclamare (< ac- (< ad) *to, toward, at,*

     according to + clamare *to shout*) 향하여 소리 지르다, 환호하다   **E** *acclaim*

   > L. declamo, declamavi, declamatum, declamare (< de- *apart from, down, not;*

     intensive + clamare *to shout*) 큰 소리로 말하다,

     웅변하다   **E** *declaim, declamation, declamatory*

   > L. disclamo, disclamavi, disclamatum, disclamare (< dis- *apart from, down,*

     not + clamare *to shout*) 부인하다   **E** *disclaim*

   > L. exclamo, exclamavi, exclamatum, exclamare (< ex- *out of, away from* +

     clamare *to shout*) 탄성을 지르다   **E** *exclaim, exclamation, exclamatory*

   > L. proclamo, proclamavi, proclamatum, proclamare (< pro- *before, forward, for,*

     instead of + clamare *to shout*) 소리쳐 알리다, 선언하다   **E** *proclaim, proclamation*

   > L. reclamo, reclamavi, reclamatum, reclamare (< re- *back, again* + clamare

     to shout) 소리 질러 항의하다, 요구하다   **E** *reclaim, reclamation*

> L. clarus, clara, clarum (< *clear* < *clear-sounding*) 낭랑한, 맑은, 밝은, 분명한, 유명한

> **E** *clear, clearance,* (clarus + videns (< vidēre '*to see*') > '*clear seeing*' >) F. *clairvoyant,* D. *Aufklärung* (< '*enlightenment*')

   > L. claritas, claritatis, f. 맑음, 밝음, 명백   **E** *clarity*

   > L. claro, claravi, claratum, clarare 분명히 하다

     > L. declaro, declaravi, declaratum, declarare (< de- *apart from, down,*

       not; intensive + clarare *to make clear*) 분명하게 드러내다, 선언하다   **E** *declare*

   > L. clarifico, clarificavi, clarificatum, clarificare (< clarus *clear* + -ficare (<

     facĕre) *to make*) 맑게 하다, 밝게 하다, 명백히 하다   **E** *clarify*

> L. classis, classis, f. (< *summons, division of citizens for military draft, hence*

army, fleet, also class in general) (고대 로마의 제6대 왕 Servius Tullius가

구분한 로마인의 여섯 가지) 신분계급, 무장한 육군, 함대, 등급, 계급, 계층   **E** *class*

   > L. classicus, classica, classicum 제1계급의, (권위의 인정을 받은) 제1류의,

     고전적   **E** *classic, classicism, classical*

   > L. *classifico, *classificavi, *classificatum, *classificare (< classis *division* +

     -ficare (< facĕre) *to make*) 분류하다   **E** *classify, classifier, classification*

> G. kalein (kaleein) *to shout*

   > G. ekkalein (ekkaleein) (< ek- *out of, away from*) *to shout out, to summon*

> G. ekklēsia, ekklēsias, f. *convoked general assembly of Athenian citizens, the Jewish congregation, the Christian church*
> > L. ecclesia, ecclesiae, f. (고대 아테네의) 민회; (유대) 회중, 교회
> > > E *ecclesia, ecclesiastical, Ecclesiastes (< 'one who addresses a public assembly')*

castro, castravi, castratum, castrare 자르다, 전정(剪定)하다, 거세(去勢)하다   E *castrate*
> castratio, castrationis, f. 거세   E *castration*

< IE. kes- *to cut*
> L. castrum, castri, n. (< *(perhaps) separated place*) 요새, 성채, 병영
> > L. castellum, castelli, n. (< + -ellum *diminutive suffix*) 요새, 성채, 부락, 은신처   E *castle, -chester, Lancaster (< 'fort on the Lune River'),* F. *chateau*
> > > L. castellatus, castellata, castellatum 성 모양의, 성같이 지은, 성이 많은   E *castellated*
> > > L. castellanus, castellani, m. 성주   E *castellan*
> L. castus, casta, castum (< *cut off from or free of faults*) 순결한   E *chaste, caste (< 'pure or unmixed (stock or breed)')*
> > L. castitas, castitatis, f. 순결   E *chastity*
> > L. castigo, castigavi, castigatum, castigare (< castus *pure* + agĕre *to drive, to do*) (잘 되게 하기 위해) 징벌하다   E *chasten, chastise, castigate*
> > L. incestus, incesta, incestum (< in- *not* + castus *chaste*) 불결한, 난륜의, 근친상간의   E *incest*
> L. careo, carui, caritum, carēre 없다, 결여되어 있다, 모자라다, 아쉽다   E *(third personal singular, present indicative, active 'it is lacking' >) caret*
> L. cassus, cassa, cassum 빈, 결여된, 헛된
> > L. casso, cassavi, cassatum, cassare 무효가 되게 하다, 파기하다   E *cashier (< 'to dismiss, to revoke'), cassation, quash*

clino, clinavi, clinatum, clinare 기울어지다
> declino, declinavi, declinatum, declinare (< de- *apart from, down, not* + clinare *to lean*) 벗어나게 하다, 구부리다, 저물다, 쇠퇴하다, 거절하다; (문법) (명사·대명사·형용사의) 어미변화를 하다   E *decline*
> > declinatio, declinationis, f. 구부림, 거절; (문법) (명사·대명사·형용사의) 어미변화, 곡용(曲用)   E *declination, declension (< 'bending aside from the nominative')*
> > declinabilis, declinabile (< + habilis *able* < habēre *to have*) 구부리는; (문법) 어미변화를 하는   E *declinable*
> > > indeclinabilis, indeclinabile (< in- *not*) 구부리지 않는, 의연한; (문법) 어미변화를 하지 않는   E *indeclinable*
> inclino, inclinavi, inclinatum, inclinare (< in- *in, on, into, toward* + clinare *to lean*) 기울어지게 하다, 쏠리게 하다, 기울어지다, 쏠리다   E *incline*

> reclino, **reclinavi**, reclinatum, reclinare (< re- *back, again* + clinare *to lean*) 뒤로
젖히다, 몸을 눕히다, 의지하다 　　　　　　　　　　　　　　　　　　　**E** *recline*

> (*suggested*) clemens, (gen.) clementis 온후한, 온화한 　　　**E** *clement, inclement*

< IE. klei- *to lean* 　　　　　　　　　　**E** *lean, lid (< 'that which bends over'), eyelid, ladder*

　　> L. clivus, clivi, m. 비탈, 비스듬틀, 경사대(傾斜臺) 　　　　　　　　　　**E** *clivus*

　　　　> L. acclivis, acclive (< ac- (< ad) *to, toward, at, according to* + clivus *slope*)
　　　　오르막의, 치받이의 　　　　　　　　　　　　　　　　　　　　　　**E** *acclivity*

　　　　> L. declivis, declive (< de- *apart from, down, not* + clivus *slope*) 내리막의　**E** *declivity*

　　　　> L. proclivis, proclive (< pro- *before, forward, for, instead of* + clivus *slope*)
　　　　앞으로 기울어진, 성향이 있는 　　　　　　　　　　　　　　　　　**E** *proclivity*

　　> L. cliens, clientis, m. (< *one leaning on another for protection*) (고대 로마 귀족에
　　예속되어 있는) 피보호 평민, 의뢰인 　　　　　　　　　　　　　　　　**E** *client*

　　> G. klinein *to lean, to slope* 　　　　　　　　　　　　　　**E** *cline, clinal*

　　　　> G. klitikos, klitikē, klitikon *leaning* 　　**E** *synclitic, syncliticism (synclitism), asynclitism*

　　　　> G. klinē, klinēs, f. (< *that on which one reclines*) *bed*

　　　　　　E *clinoid (< 'resembling a bed: applied to the four processes or apophyses of*
　　　　　　the sphenoid bone, from their resemblance to the knobs of a bedstead, or
　　　　　　from enclosing a quadrilateral space')

　　　　　　> G. klinikos, klinikē, klinikon *bed-ridden or sick*

　　　　　　　　> L. clinicus, clinici, m. 병상에 누워 있는 환자,
　　　　　　　　임상의(臨床醫) 　　　　**E** *clinic, polyclinic, clinical, clinician*

　　> G. klima, klimatos, n. *sloping surface of the earth, region, district, climate*

　　　　> L. clima, climatis, n. 풍토, 기후; 풍조

　　　　　　E *climate (< 'collection of atmospheric conditions' < 'region considered with*
　　　　　　regard to its prevailing weather conditions' < 'part of the earth determined
　　　　　　by its position relative to celestial objects'), **acclimate (acclimatize)** *(< 'to*
　　　　　　habituate or inure to a new climate, or to one not natural'), **acclimation**
　　　　　　(acclimatation, acclimatization)

　　> G. klimax, klimakos, f. *ladder, staircase*

　　　　> L. climax, climacis, f. 사다리, 계단, 단계; (수사) 점층법(漸層法), (점층
　　　　법의 마지막 단계인) 절정(絕頂) 　　　　　　　　**E** *climax, anticlimax*

　　　　> G. klimaktēr, klimaktēros, m. *rung of a ladder, definite or critical period*
　　　　of a man's life

　　　　　　> L. climacter, climacteris, m. 액년(厄年, 7과 9의 기수배가 되는 해),
　　　　　　대액년(大厄年, 7×9=63세가 되는 해), 갱년기(更年期)

　　　　　　　　> L. climacterium, climacterii, n. 갱년기　**E** *climacterium, climacteric*

　　> G. enklinein (< en- *in*) *to lean on* 　　　　　　　　　　**E** *enclitic*

　　　　> G. enklisis, enkliseōs, f. (*grammar*) *the transference of accentuation*
　　　　to a previous word

　　　　　　> L. enclisis, enclisis, f. (문법) 전접(前接) 　　　　**E** *enclisis*

　　> G. proklinein (< pro- *before, in front*) *to lean forward* 　　　　**E** *proclitic*

　　　　> G. proklisis, prokliseōs, f. (*grammar*) *the transference of accentuation*

to a following word

> L. proclisis, proclisis, f. (문법) 후접(後接)   **E** *proclisis*

> G. klitys *hill*

> G. kleitoris, kleitoridos, f. *clitoris* (<(*also suggested*) kleiein *to close, to hide*

< IE. klau- (*possibly*) *hook, peg* (Vide CLAUDĔRE; *See* E. *close*))

> L. clitoris, clitoridis, f. 음핵(陰核)   **E** *clitoris, clitorimegaly, clitoridectomy*

cubo, cubui, cubitum, cubare 침대에 눕다, 누워 자다, 병상에 눕다, 식탁에 다가가서 눕다

(로마인들은 왼팔로 머리를 괴고 반쯤 누워서 먹었음)

> cubitus, cubiti, m. (cubitum, cubiti, n.) 팔꿈치, 팔꿉, 완척(腕尺, 팔꿈치에서 가운데
손가락 끝까지의 거리, 약 44 cm)   **E** *cubitus, cubit, cubital, antecubital*

> incubo, incubui, incubitum, incubare (< in- *in, on, into, toward* + cubare *to lie down*)
위에 눕다, 엎디다, 기대다, (새·닭이) 알을 품다, 부화(孵化)시키다   **E** *incubate*

> incubatio, incubationis, f. 알을 품음, 부화   **E** *incubation*

> incubus, incubi, m. 잠자는 사람 위에 걸터앉아 괴롭힌다는 몽마(夢魔), 잠자는
여자를 범한다는 몽마   **E** *incubus*

> succubo, succubui, succubitum, succubare (< suc- (< sub) *under, up from under*
+ cubare *to lie down*) 밑에 눕다

> succuba, succubae, f. 첩(妾)   **E** *succubus (< 'on the pattern of incubus')*

> accumbo, accubui, accubitum, accumbĕre (< ac- (< ad) *to, toward, at, according to*
+ cubare *to lie down*) 눕다, 옆에 눕다, 식탁에 자리 잡다, 둘러앉다   **E** *accumbent*

[용례] nucleus accumbens septi (< *nucleus leaning against the septum pellucidum*)
중격기댐핵, 중격의지핵,
중격측좌핵, 중격측위핵   **E** *nucleus accumbens septi (nucleus accumbens)*

(문법) nucleus 핵: 단수 주격 < nucleus, nuclei, m.

accumbens 옆에 자리 잡는: 현재분사, 남·여·중성형 단수 주격
< accumbens, (gen.) accumbentis

septi 중격의: 단수 속격 < septum, septi, n.

> concumbo, concubui, concubitum, concumbĕre (< con- (< cum) *with, together* +
cubare *to lie down*) 함께 눕다, 동침하다

> concubina, concubinae, f. 첩(妾), 창녀   **E** *concubine*

> decumbo, decubui, decubitum, decumbĕre (< de- *apart from, down, not* + cubare
to lie down) 눕다, 엎드리다, 식탁에 다가가서 눕다, 쓰러지다   **E** *decumbent*

> decubitus, decubitus, m. 누움, 누운 자세, 욕창(褥瘡)   **E** *decubitus, decubital*

> incumbo, incubui, incubitum, incumbĕre (< in- *in, on, into, toward* + cubare *to lie
down*) 기대다, 힘쓰다, 몰두하다   **E** *incumbent*

> recumbo, recubui, recubitum, recumbĕre (< re- *back, again* + cubare *to lie down*)
눕다, 식탁에 다가가서 눕다, 기대다   **E** *recumbent*

> succumbo, succubui, succubitum, succumbĕre (< suc- (< sub) *under, up from under*
+ cubare *to lie down*) 밑에 눕다, 성교하다, 굴복하다   **E** *succumb*

< IE. keu–, keu(b)–, keu(p)–, kumb– *to bend, to curve, to arch*

　　　E *hip (< 'curved'), hop (< 'to bend forward'), (suggested) hope (< 'to leap up in expectation')*

　　> L. cupa, cupae, f. (cuppa, cuppae, f.) 큰 나무 통　　　　　**E** *cup, cupel, cupellation*

　　　　> L. cupula, cupulae, f. (< + –ula *diminutive suffix*) 작은 통　　**E** *cupula, cupule, cupola*

　　> G. kymbē, kymbēs, f. *bowl, boat*

　　　　> L. cymba, cymbae, f. 쪽배　　　　　　　　　　　　　　**E** *cymba*

　　　　　> L. cymbidium, cymbidii, n. (< *a hollow recess in the lip of the flower*

　　　　　　　< + –idium < G. –idion *diminutive suffix*) 심비듐(열대산 난)　**E** *cymbidium*

　　　　> G. kymbalon, kymbalou, n. *cymbal*

　　　　　> L. cymbalum, cymbali, n. (흔히) 심벌즈(청동이나 놋쇠로 만든 악기),

　　　　　　바라　　　　　　　　　　　　　　　　　　　　　**E** *cymbal, chime*

　　> G. kybos, kybou, m. *cube, die*

　　　　> L. cubus, cubi, m. 입방체, 정육면체　　　　　　**E** *cube (hexahedron), cubism*

　　　　> G. kybikos, kybikē, kybikon *cubic*

　　　　　> L. cubicus, cubica, cubicum 입방체의, 정육면체의　　　　**E** *cubic*

　　　　> G. kyboeidēs, kyboeidēs, kyboeides (< + eidos *shape*) *cuboid*

　　　　　> L. cuboides, (gen.) cuboidis 입방형의　　**E** *cuboid, (cuboid >) cuboidal*

　　> G. kyphos, kyphē, kyphon *bent, curved, stooping, hunchbacked*

　　　　> G. kyphōsis, kyphōseōs, f. (< + –ōsis *condition*) *hunchback*

　　　　　> L. kyphosis, kyphosis, f. 척추후만증, 척추뒤굽음증　　**E** *kyphosis*

> IE. kemb– *to bend, to turn, to change, to exchange*　　**E** *hump, Cambridge (< 'crooked')*

　　> L. cambio, campsi, –, cambiare (cambire) 바꾸다,

　　　교환하다　　　　　　　　　　　　　　**E** *change, exchange, interchange*

　　　　> L. cambium, cambii, n. 교환 장소; (식물) 형성층

　　　　　　　E *cambium (< 'sap that becomes or exchanges form with vegetative form')*

　　> G. kanthos, kanthou, m. *corner of the eye*

　　　　> L. canthus, canthi, m. 쇠바퀴, (쇠로 만든) 바퀴 테; 눈구석, 안각(眼角),

　　　　　눈초리　　　　　　　　　　　　　　**E** *canthus, cant, decant*

　　　　　> L. epicanthus, epicanthi, m. (< + G. ep(i)– *upon*) 눈구석주름,

　　　　　　내안각췌피(內眼角贅皮), 몽고주름　　　**E** *epicanthus, epicanthic*

> IE. kamp– *to bend*

　　> L. campus, campi, m. (< *corner, cove < bended*) 들, 연병장, 분야(分野)

　　　　　E *campus, camp, (F. Champagne 'field' >) champagne; campimetry*
　　　　　(< 'measuring of the central visual field')

　　　> L. campanius, campania, campanium 들의, 평야의

　　　　　E *campaign (< 'an army's practice of 'taking the field', i.e., moving from a*
　　　　　fortress or town to open country, at the onset of summer')

　　　　> L. Campania, Campaniae, f. (< *field*) (이탈리아 중부) 깜빠니아 지방

　　　　　(청동 제품으로 유명함)

　　　　　> L. campana, campanae, f. 종(鐘)

　　　　　　> L. campanula, campanulae, f. (< + –ula *diminutive*

suffix) 작은 종, 종 모양의 구조, 초롱꽃　　　　**E** *campanula*

> L. campio, campionis, m. 격투, 권투사　　　　**E** *champion (champ)*

> G. kampylos, kampylē, kampylon *bent, curved*　　　**E** *campyl(o)-*

> L. Campylobacter, Campylobacteris, m. (< *curved and spiral form*

< G. kampylos *bent, curved* + -bacter *bacterium*) (세균) 캄필로

박터속(屬)　　　　**E** *Campylobacter*

---

dissipo, dissipavi, dissipatum, dissipare (< dis- *apart from, down, not* + (*archaic*) sipare

(supare, suppare) *to throw about*) 흩어지게 하다　　　**E** *dissipate*

< IE. swep- *to throw, to sling, to cast*　　　**E** *swab*

---

do, dedi, datum, dare 주다

E (data (*feminine past participle*) *'the first word in Roman letters or documents, giving the place and time of writing' > 'given' >*) *date, update, die* (< *'something given or played'*), *dice* (< *'something given or played'*)

[용례] Data Romae pridie Kalendas Februarias 로마에서 2월 초하루 하루 전에 주어진

(편지나 문서에 쓴 관용어, 날짜는 기준일을 중심으로 역산하였음)

(문법) data 주어진 (편지·문서): 과거분사, 여성형 단수 주격

< datus, data, datum

Romae 로마에서: 단수 속격 (장소의 속격) < Roma, Romae, f.

pridie 전날: 불변화 명사

Kalendas 초하루: 복수 대격 < Kalendae, Kalendarum, f.

Februarias 2월의: 형용사, 여성형 복수 대격

< Februarius, Februaria, Februarium

[용례] Bis das, si cito das. 네가 빨리 주면 너는 두 번 준다 (주려거든 빨리 주라)

(문법) bis 두 번: 부사

das 너는 준다: 능동태 직설법 현재 단수 이인칭

si 만일 ~면: 종속 접속사

cito 빨리: 부사

> datum, dati, n. 준 것, 선물　　　　**E** *datum, data*

> dativus, dativa, dativum 주어지는; (문법) 여격(與格)의　　**E** *dative (dat.)*

> donum, doni, n. 선물

> dono, **donavi**, donatum, donare 선물로 주다, 기증하다,

바치다　　**E** (per- + donare > perdonare *'to present thoroughly'* >) *pardon*

> donatio, donationis, f. 기증　　**E** *donation, (donation >) donate*

> donator, donatoris, m. 기증자　　**E** *donator, (donator >) donor*

> condono, **condonavi**, condonatum, condonare (< con- (< cum) *with,*

together; intensive + donare *to present*) 용서하다　**E** *condone*

> mando, **mandavi**, mandatum, mandare (< *to give into any one's hand or charge* <

manus *hand* + dare *to give*) 권한을 위임하다, 명령하다   **E** *mandate*

> mandator, mandatoris, m. 위임자, 명령자

> mandatorius, mandatoria, mandatorium 위임의, 명령의, 의무적인   **E** *mandatory*

> commendo, **commendavi**, commendatum, commendare (< com- (< cum) *with, together; intensive* + mandare *to entrust*) 위임하다, 추천하다   **E** *commend*

> recommendo, **recommendavi**, recommendatum, recommendare (< re- *back, again; intensive* + commendare *to commend*) 추천하다   **E** *recommend*

> commando, **commandavi**, commandatum, commandare (< com- (< cum) *with, together; intensive* + mandare *to entrust*) 명령하다   **E** *command*

> demando, **demandavi**, demandatum, demandare (< de- *apart from, down, not; intensive* + dare *to give*) (명령적으로) 요구하다   **E** *demand*

> addo, **addidi**, additum, addĕre (< ad- *to, toward, at, according to* + dare *to give*) 더해주다   **E** *add, additive*

> addendum, addendi, n. (< (*neuter gerundive*) *something to be added*) 첨가물   **E** *addendum*

> additio, additionis, f. 첨가   **E** *addition, additional*

> addicamentum, addicamenti, n. 첨가물   **E** *addicament*

> edo, **edidi**, editum, edĕre (< e- *out of, away from* + dare *to give*) 내보내다, 출판하다   **E** *edition, editor, (editor >) editorial, (editor >) edit*

> perdo, **perdidi**, perditum, perdĕre (< per- *through, thoroughly* + dare *to give*) 파멸시키다

E *perdition,* (pro- *'for'* + perdĕre *'to destroy'* > *'for destruction'* > *'a positive regulator of the alternate pathway of the complement system'* >) *properdin*

> reddo, **reddidi**, redditum, reddĕre (< red- *back, again* + dare *to give*) 돌려주다, 되게 하다, 넘겨주다, 인도(引渡)하다

E *render, rendition, rent, surrender,* (F. rendez vous *'render yourselves'* >) *rendezvous*

> trado, **tradidi**, traditum, tradĕre (< tra- (< trans) *over, across, through, beyond* + dare *to give*) 건네주다, 물려주다, 적의 손에 넘기다, 반역하다   **E** *betray*

> traditio, traditionis, f. 전승, 전통, 배신, 반역

E *tradition, treason,* (ex *'out of, away from'* + traditio *'delivery'* >) *extradition,* (extradition >) *extradite*

> traditor, traditoris, f. 배신자, 반역자   **E** *traditor, traitor*

> vendo, **vendidi**, venditum, vendĕre (< venum *sale* + dare *to give*) 팔다   **E** *vend*

< IE. do- *to give*

> L. dos, dotis, f. 지참금

> L. doto, **dotavi**, dotatum, dotare 지참금을 주다; (능력·자질을) 부여하다   **E** *endow, dowager*

> L. dotarium, dotarii, n. 지참금; (천부의) 능력, 자질   **E** *dowry, dower*

> G. didonai (do- *root of* didonai) *to give*

> G. dōron, dōrou, n. *gift*

> G. Pandōra, Pandōras, f. (< *all-gifted* < pan- *all* + dōron) (*Greek*

*mythology) the first human female on whom all the Olympian gods
bestowed gifts*

> L. Pandora, Pandorae, f. 판도라   **E** *Pandora*

> G. dosis, doseōs, f. *act of giving, gift, portion*

    > L. dosis, dosis, f. 용량(用量)   **E** *dose, (dose >) dosage*

> G. ekdidonai (< ek- *out of, away from*) *to surrender, to marry, to publish*

    > G. ekdotos, ekdotos, ekdoton *surrendered, married, published*

       > G. anekdotos, anekdotos, anekdoton (< an- *not*) *unsurrendered,
unmarried, unpublished*

          > G. anekdota, anekdotōn, n. (< *neuter* pl.) *things unpublished*

            > L. anecdota, anecdotorum, n. (pl.) 일화(逸話)   **E** *anecdote*

> G. antididonai (< ant(i)- *before, against, instead of*) *to give in return*

    > G. antidotos, antidotos, antidoton *given against, given as a remedy*

       > G. antidoton, antidotou, n. (< *neuter* sing.) *remedy*

          > L. antidotum, antidoti, n. 해독제   **E** *antidote*

duro, duravi, duratum, durare 오래가다, 지속하다   **E** *during*

    > duratio, durationis, f. 지속, 지속 기간, 내구(耐久)   **E** *duration*

    > durabilis, durabile 오래가는, 내구성 있는   **E** *durable*

    > perduro, **perduravi**, perduratum, perdurare (< per- *through, thoroughly*) 지속하다,
영속하다   **E** *perdure, perdurable*

  < IE. deuə- *long in duration*

erro, erravi, erratum, errare 길을 잃다, 헤매다, 그르치다, 실수하다   **E** *err*

    > erratum, errati, n. 실수, 오류, 오자(誤字), ((pl.) errata) 정오표   **E** *erratum, (pl.) errata*

    > error, erroris, m. 방황, 실수, 오류, 오차, 이상   **E** *error*

    > erro, erronis, m. 떠돌이, 방랑자, 헤매는 사람

       > erroneus, erronea, erroneum 떠도는, 틀린   **E** *erroneous*

    > erraticus, erratica, erraticum 떠도는, 방랑하는, (나뭇가지 등) 제멋대로 뻗는, 상궤를
벗어난   **E** *erratic*

    > aberro, **aberravi**, aberratum, aberrare (< ab- *off, away from* + errare *to wander*)
길을 잃다, 벗어나다, 빗나가다   **E** *aberrant*

       > aberratio, aberrationis, f. 일탈(逸脫), 탈선, 이상(異常); (광학) 수차(收差)   **E** *aberration*

  < IE. ers- *to be in motion*   **E** *race (< 'rushing')*

festino, festinavi, festinatum, festinare 서두르다   **E** *festinate*

   [용례] Festina lente! (< *Make haste slowly!*) 천천히 서둘러라!, 급할수록 천천히!

     (문법) festina 너는 서둘러라: 능동태 명령법 현재 단수 이인칭

       lente 천천히: 부사 < lentus, lenta, lentum 느린

< IE. bhers- *quick*

flo, flavi, flatum, flare 불다

> flatus, flatus, m. (바람이) 붊, 바람, 숨결, (피리의) 음향, (pl.) 건방짐; 위창자내 공기,
방귀
> **E** *flatus, flavor (flavour)*
>> flatulentus, flatulenta, flatulentum 허풍의; 위창자내 공기가 찬,
고창(鼓脹)의
>> **E** *flatulent, flatulence*
> deflo, **deflavi**, **deflatum**, deflare (< de- *apart from, down, not* + flare *to blow*) 불어
날리다
> **E** *deflate, deflation*
> inflo, **inflavi**, **inflatum**, inflare (< in- *in, on, into, toward* + flare *to blow*) 불어넣다,
부풀리다
> **E** *inflate, inflation*
> sufflo, **sufflavi**, sufflatum, sufflare (< sub- *under, up from under* + flare *to blow*)
숨을 내불다, 불다
> **E** *souffle*
>> insufflo, **insufflavi**, insufflatum, insufflare (< in- *in, on, into, toward* + sufflare
to blow upon) 불어 넣다, 흡입시키다
>> **E** *insufflate*
> flabellum, flabelli, n. 부채, (의식용) 큰 부채
> **E** *flabellum, flabellate*
< IE. bhle- *to blow*
E *blow, blast, bladder (< 'something blown up'), gallbladder*
> G. phleps, phlebos, f. *vein*

E *phleb(o)-, phlebitis, phlebectasis, phlebothrombosis, thrombophlebitis, phlebotomy*

foro, foravi, foratum, forare 구멍 뚫다

> foramen, foraminis, n. 구멍, 공(孔)
> **E** *foramen, (pl.) foramina*

[용례] foramen magnum 큰 구멍, 대공(大孔)
> **E** *foramen magnum*
(문법) foramen: 단수 주격
magnum: 형용사, 중성 단수 주격
< magnus, magna, magnum 큰

> perforo, **perforavi**, perforatum, perforare (< per- *through, thoroughly*) 꿰뚫다,
관통하다
> **E** *perforate, (perforate >) imperforate*
>> perforatio, perforationis, f. 뚫림, 관통, 천공(穿孔)
>> **E** *perforation*
< IE. bher-, bhera- *to cut, to pierce, to bore*
> **E** *bore*
> L. ferio, -, -, ferire 때리다, 치다, (짐승을) 잡다

E *interfere (< 'to strike each other'), (interfere >) interference, interferon (<
interfering agent, inhibiting viral replication')*

> (*suggested*) L. barra, barrae, f. (< *cut wood*) 가로장, 빗장,
장해
> **E** *bar, unbar,* It. *barista, barrier, barricade, embarrass*
>> L. *imbarrico, *imbarricavi, *imbarricatum, *imbarricare (< im- (< in) *in, on,
into, toward* + barra *bar*) 금하다
>> **E** *embargo*
> (*perhaps*) G. pharynx, pharyngos, f. *chasm, throat*
>> L. pharynx, pharyngis, m. (< *the chasm behind the nasal cavity, oral cavity,*

and *larynx*) 인두(咽頭)

> **E** *pharynx, pharyngeal, glossopharyngeal, pharyng(o)–; nasopharynx, oropharynx, laryngopharynx (hypopharynx)*

> IE. bhreu-, bhreuə- *to cut,*
to break up   **E** *brittle, bruise, debris, brothel (< 'deteriorated' < 'broken up')*
> L. frustum, frusti, n. 조각, 단편(斷片), 절두체(截頭體)   **E** *frustum*

fragro, fragravi, fragratum, fragrare 향기 나다, 방향(芳香)을 풍기다   **E** *fragrant, flair*
> fragrantia, fragrantiae, f. 향기, 방향(芳香)   **E** *fragrance*
< IE. bhrag- *to smell*

frico, fricui, fricatum (frictum), fricare 쓰다듬다, 문지르다, 마찰하다   **E** *fray, fricative*
> frictio, frictionis, f. 마찰   **E** *friction, frictional*
> dentifricium, dentifricii, n. (< dens, dentis, m. *tooth* + fricare *to rub*) 치약   **E** *dentifrice*
> affrico, affricui, affricatum (affrictum), affricare (< af- (< ad) *to, toward, at,*
according to + fricare *to rub*) 비비다, 문지르다   **E** *affricate, affricative*
< IE. bhreiə- *to cut, to break*
> L. frivolus, frivola, frivolum 사소한, 경박한   **E** *frivolous*
> L. frio, friavi, friatum, friare 부수다, 빻다, 찧다, 갈다
> L. friabilis, friabile 부서지기 쉬운   **E** *friable, friability*

*frido, *fridavi, *fridatum, *fridare 평화롭게 하다
> *exfrido, *exfridavi, *exfridatum, *exfridare (< ex- *out of, away from* + *fridare
to make peace) 평화를 깨다   **E** *afraid, affray*
< IE. pri- *to love*

> **E** *free (< 'to love, to set free'), freebooter, filibuster, friend,* D. *Siegfried (< 'victorious peace'), Frigg (< 'goddess of the heavens, wife of Odin' < 'beloved, wife'),* (G. hēmera Aphroditēs 'day of Aphroditē', L. dies Veneris 'day of Venus' > 'Frigg day' >) *Friday*

*futo, *futavi, *futatum, *futare 치다
> confuto, confutavi, confutatum, confutare (< con- (< cum) *with, together* + futare
to beat, to strike) 가라앉히다, 반박하다, 논박하다   **E** *confute*
> refuto, refutavi, refutatum, refutare (< re- *back, again* + futare *to beat, to strike*)
물리치다, 반박하다, 논박하다   **E** *refute*
< IE. bhau- *to beat, to strike*

> **E** *beat, butt (< 'to strike or push with the head or horns', 'to thrust'), buttress, (butt 'to thrust' >) button,* F. *bouton,* F. *boutonniere (< 'buttonhole'), abut, butt (< 'thick end'), (butt 'thick end' + -ock 'diminutive suffix' >) buttock, (butt 'thick end' > 'target' >) debut (< 'to make the first stroke at a target')*

glenn, glennavi, glennatum, glennare 수확하고 남은 것을 모으다, 주워 모으다   `E glean`

gusto, gustavi, gustatum, gustare 맛보다   `E gust, gustatory, disgust`
     > gustatio, gustationis, f. 맛보기, 맛, 미각   `E gustation`
   < gustus, gustus, m. 맛봄, 맛, 미각, 풍미, 취향   `E gusto`
  < IE. geus- to taste, to choose   `E choose, choice`
     > G. geuein to give to taste; geuesthai (middle) to taste
       > G. geusis, geuseōs, f. taste   `E hypogeusia (hypogeusesthesia), dysgeusia`

halo, halavi, halatum, halare 입김을 내다, 증발하다, 숨 쉬다
     > halitus, halitus, m. 입김, 숨
       > halitosis, halitosis, f. (< + G. -ōsis condition) 입냄새, 구취(口臭)   `E halitosis`
    > exhalo, exhalavi, exhalatum, exhalare (< ex- out of, away from + halare to breathe)
    폐 밖으로 내뿜다   `E exhale`
      > exhalatio, exhalationis, f. 내쉼, 호기(呼氣)   `E exhalation`
    > inhalo, inhalavi, inhalatum, inhalare (< in- in, on, into, toward + halare to breathe)
    폐 안으로 빨아들이다   `E inhale, inhalant`
      > inhalatio, inhalationis, f. 흡입   `E inhalation`
  < IE. anə- to breathe
    > L. anima, animae, f. 숨, 바람, 생기, 목숨, 혼, 영혼   `E anima, animism`
      > L. animo, animavi, animatum, animare 생기를 불어넣다   `E animate, inanimate`
        > L. animatio, animationis, f. 생기를 불어넣음, 생기; (영화) 애니메이션   `E animation`
      > L. animal, animalis, n. 동물   `E animal`
        > L. animalculum, animalculi, n. (< + -culum diminutive suffix) 소(小)동물,
        극미(極微)동물   `E animalcule`
    > L. animus, animi, m. 생각, 정신, 의견, 의지, 용기, 원한
      > L. animosus, animosa, animosum 용기 있는, 원한 있는
        > L. animositas, animositatis, f. 용기, 원한   `E animosity`
      > L. aequanimus, aequanima, aequanimum (< aequus animus equal mind) 침
      착한, 태연한, 유장한
        > L. aequanimitas, aequanimitatis, f. 침착, 태연, 유장   `E equanimity`
      > L. magnanimus, magnanima, magnanimum (magnanimis, magnanime) (<
      magnus animus great soul) 관대한, 도량이 큰, 아량 있는   `E magnanimous`
        > L. magnanimitas, magnanimitatis, f. 관대, 도량, 아량   `E magnanimity`
      > L. unanimus, unanima, unanimum (unanimis, unanime) (< unus animus one
      mind) 한 생각의, 만장일치의   `E unanimous`
        > L. unanimitas, unanimitatis, f. (생각의) 일치, 만장일치   `E unanimity`
    > G. anemos, anemou, m. wind   `E anemometer`
      > G. anemōnē, anemōnēs, f. (< daughter of the wind (the flower was thought
      to open when the wind blows < anemos + -ōnē feminine patronymic suffix)

wind-flower

> L. anemone, anemones, f. 아네모네　　　　　　　　　　　E *anemone*

hio, hiavi, hiatum, hiare 벌어지다, 틈이 생기다, 입이 벌어지다, 낭독하다, 노래하다, 모음이

겹쳐 발음이 단절되다, (말의 내용이) 단절되다

> hiatus, hiatus, m. 틈새, 구멍, 간극(間隙), 열(裂), 열공(裂孔), 모음충돌, 모음단절　　E *hiatus, hiatal*

> dehisco, dehivi, –, dehiscĕre (< de- *apart from, down, not* + hiare *to gape* + -escĕre

　suffix of inceptive (inchoative) verb) 벌어지다, 틈이 생기다, 터지다　E *dehisce, dehiscent*

　　> dehiscentia, dehiscentiae, f. 벌어짐, 열개(裂開), 분리, 결손　　　　E *dehiscence*

< IE. ghai- *to gape, to yawn*　　　　　　　　　　　　　E *gape, agape, gap, gasp, yawn*

> G. chainein *to gape, to yawn, to gasp for, to utter*

　　> G. chasma, chasmatos, n. *cleft, chasm*

　　　　> L. chasma, chasmatis, n. 깊이 갈라진 틈, 간극, 균열　　　　　E *chasm*

> G. chēlē, chēlēs, f. *claw*

　　> L. chele, cheles, f. (게·가재 등의)

집게발　　　E *chelate, (cheloid > 'appearance like the claws of a crab' >) keloid*

∞ IE. gheu- *to gape, to yawn*　　　　　　　　　　　　　　E *gum*

> G. chaos, chaous, n. *vast gulf or chasm, empty space, the nether abyss, the first*

　state of the universe; (Chaos) (Greek mythology) the first created being, from

　which came the primeval deities Gaia, Tartarus, Erebus, and Nyx

　　> L. chaos, chai, n. 무한하고 공허한 암흑 공간(cosmos의 반대), 혼돈세계, 지하

　　세계, 대혼란; (Chaos) (그리스 신화) 원시혼돈의 신

E *chaos, chaotic, gas* (< *'occult principle'*), (*gas* >) *gaseous*, (*gas* + -ol *'oil'* +
-ine *'chemical suffix'* >) *gasoline*

irrigo, irrigavi, irrigatum, irrigare (< ir- (< in) *in, on, into, toward* + rigare *to wet,*

　to water) 적시다, 물을 대다, 관개(灌漑)하다, 관류(灌流)하다, 세척하다　　E *irrigate*

　> irrigatio, irrigationis, f. 관개, 관류, 세척　　　　　　　　　　E *irrigation*

< rigo, rigavi, rigatum, rigare 적시다, 물을 대다

< IE. reg- *moist*　　　　　　　　　　　　　　　　　　　　　E *rain*

juvo, juvi, jutum, juvare 돕다, 도움이 되다, 이롭다

　> juvans, (gen.) juvantis (*present participle*) 도움이 되는

　　> juvantia, juvantium, n. (*neuter* pl.) 보조제　　　　　　　　E *juvantia*

　> adjuvo, adjuvi, adjutum, adjuvare (< ad- *to, toward, at, according to* + juvare

　to help) 돕다　　　　　　　　　　　　　　　　　　　　　E *adjuvant*

　　> adjuto, adjutavi, adjutatum, adjutare (*frequentative*) 돕다　　E *aid*

lavo, lavavi (lavi), lavatum (lautum, lotum), lavare 씻다

E *lava* (<*'originally a stream or gutter suddenly caused by rain, applied in the Neapolitan dialect to a lava-stream from Vesuvius'*), *lavage, lavish,* (lavanda (pl. *neuter gerundive*) *'things to be washed'* >) *launder, laundry*

> lavatorium, lavatorii, n. 세숫대야, 세면장, 목욕탕 　　　　　　　　　　　　　　**E** *lavatory*
> lavatrina, lavatrinae, f. ((*contracted*) latrina, latrinae, f.) 욕실, 화장실, 변소 　　**E** *latrine*
> lotio, lotionis, f. 씻음, 세탁 　　　　　　　　　　　　　　　　　　　　　　**E** *lotion*
> luo, lui, lutum, luĕre 씻다
　　> abluo, ablui, ablutum, abluĕre (< ab- *off, away from* + luĕre *to wash*) 깨끗이
　　　씻다 　　　　　　　　　　　　　　　　　　　　　　　　　　　　　**E** *ablute*
　　　　> ablutio, ablutionis, f. 씻음, 세척, 목욕, 세정(洗淨) 　　　　　　　　**E** *ablution*
　　> colluo, collui, collutum, colluĕre (< col- (< cum) *with, together; intensive* +
　　　luĕre *to wash*) 씻어내다
　　　　> collutorium, collutorii, n. 양칫물, 구강 세척제, 양치질약 　　　　　**E** *collutory*
　　> diluo, dilui, dilutum, diluĕre (< dis- *apart from, down, not* + luĕre *to wash*)
　　　씻어 지우다, 묽게 하다, 약하게 하다, 희석하다 　　　　　　　　　　**E** *dilute, diluent*
　　　　> dilutio, dilutionis, f. 희석, 묽힘 　　　　　　　　　　　　　　　　**E** *dilution*
　　　　> diluvium, diluvii, n. (diluvio, diluvionis, f.) 홍수, 홍적물, 홍적층 　　**E** *deluge*
　　> eluo, elui, elutum, eluĕre (< e- *out of, away from* + luĕre *to wash*) 씻어서
　　　깨끗이 하다, 녹여서 분리하다 　　　　　　　　　　　　　　　　　　**E** *elute, eluent, eluate*
　　　　> elutio, elutionis, f. 용출(溶出), 용리(溶離) 　　　　　　　　　　　**E** *elution*
< IE. leu(ə)- *to wash* 　　　　　　　　　　　　　　　　　　　　　　　　　　**E** *lye, lather*

libo, libavi, libatum, libare 맛보다, 덜어내다; (제사 때) 제주(祭酒)를 제단·공중·바다 등에
　　　뿌리다
　　> libatio, libationis, f. 헌주(獻酒), 제주 　　　　　　　　　　　　　　　**E** *libation*
　　> praelibo, praelibavi, praelibatum, praelibare 미리 맛보다
　　　　> praelibatio, praelibationis, f. 시식(試食), (독을 확인하기 위해) 먼저 맛보기 　**E** *prelibation*
< IE. leig- *to bind*
　　> (*probably*) L. litus, litoris, n. 바닷가, 강가
　　　　> L. litoralis, litorale (littoralis, littorale) 바닷가의, 강가의 　　　　**E** *littoral*

ligo, ligavi, ligatum, ligare 매다,
　　결박하다　　**E** *ligate,* (ligandum (*neuter gerundive*) *'that to be tied'* >) *ligand, ligase, league*
　　> ligatio, ligationis, f. 잡아맴, 묶기, 결찰(結紮) 　　　　　　　　　　**E** *ligation, liaison*
　　> ligatura, ligaturae, f. 잡아매는 것, 결찰사(結紮絲) 　　　　　　　　　**E** *ligature*
　　> ligamentum, ligamenti, n. (노끈·줄·붕대·인대 등) 잡아매는 것, 유대, 결연

　　　E *ligamentum (ligament),* (pl.) *ligamenta (ligaments), ligamental (ligamentary, ligamentous)*

　　　[용례] ligamentum flavum, (pl.) ligamenta flava
　　　　　황색인대 　　　　　　　　　　　**E** *ligamentum flavum,* (pl.) *ligamenta flava*
　　　　(문법) ligamentum 인대: 단수 주격
　　　　　flavum 노란: 형용사, 중성형 단수 주격 < flavus, flava, flavum
　　　　　ligamenta 인대들: 복수 주격

flava 노란: 형용사, 중성형 복수 주격

> *ligabilis, *ligabile 책임져야 할, 의무가 있는, (병 등에) 걸리기 쉬운, 하기 쉬운　E *liable, liability*

> alligo, alligavi, alligatum, alligare (< ad- *to, toward, at, according to* + ligare *to bind*) 동여매다, 매이게 하다　E *ally, rally (< 're-ally'), alliance, alloy*

> colligo, colligavi, colligatum, colligare (< col- (< cum) *with, together* + ligare *to bind*) 한데 묶다, 결합하다, 총괄하다　E *colligate, colligative*

> obligo, obligavi, obligatum, obligare (< ob- *before, toward(s), over, against, away* + ligare *to bind*) 결박하다, 강제하다, 의무를 지우다　E *obligate, oblige*
>> obligatio, obligationis, f. 의무　E *obligation*
>> obligatorius, obligatoria, obligatorium 의무적인, 편성(偏性)의　E *obligatory*

> religo, religavi, religatum, religare (< re- *back, again* + ligare *to bind*) 매이게 하다　E *rely; (rely >) reliance, reliant, reliable, reliability*
>> religio, religionis, f. 종교(宗敎)　E *religion, religious*

< IE. leig- *to bind*

mano, manavi, manatum, manare 흘러나오다

> emano, emanavi, emanatum, emanare (< e- *out of, away from* + manare *to flow*) 흘러나오다, 내뿜다, 발산하다　E *emanate*

< IE. ma- *damp*　E *moor (< 'marsh, wilderness')*

muto, mutavi, mutatum, mutare 바꾸다, 바뀌다

E *mutate, mutant, molt (moult) (< 'with intrusive -l-'); mutagen, mutagenic, mutagenicity*

> mutatio, mutationis, f. 바꿈, 바뀜, 변이(變異), 돌연변이

E *mutation, (mutation >) dismutation (< 'disproportionation involving the simultaneous oxidation and reduction of a compound in a biological context'), (dismutation >) dismutase*

> mutabilis, mutabile 변하는, 변하기 쉬운　E *mutable*
>> immutabilis, immutabile (< im- (< in-) *not* + mutabilis *mutable*) 변하지 않는, 불변의　E *immutable*

> mutuus, mutua, mutuum 서로의, 상호적인　E *mutual*

> commuto, commutavi, commutatum, commutare (< com- (< cum) *with, together* + mutare *to change*) 서로 바꾸다, 교환하다, 대체하다; (정기권을 구입하여) 통근하다　E *commute*

> permuto, permutavi, permutatum, permutare (< per- *through, thoroughly* + mutare *to change*) 교환하다, 갈아 넣다; (수학) 순열을 바꾸다　E *permute*

> transmuto, transmutavi, transmutatum, transmutare (< trans- *over, across, through, beyond* + mutare *to change*) 자리를 바꾸다, (물질·모양·상태 등) 성질을 바꾸다　E *transmute*

< IE. mei- *to change, to go, to move; with derivatives referring to the exchange of goods and services within a society as regulated by custom or law*

E *mad (< 'changed for the worse'), mis- (< 'in a changed manner'), mistake, miss (< 'in a changed manner'), amiss, mean (< 'common'), demean (< 'to degrade')*

> L. meo, **meavi**, meatum, meare 통행하다

> L. meatus, meatus, m. 통행, 통로, 길, 도(道)　　　　　　　　　**E** *meatus*

> L. permeo, **permeavi**, permeatum, permeare (< per- *through, thoroughly* + meare *to pass*) 통과하다, 침투하다, 퍼지다, 투과하다　　**E** *permeate, permeant, impermeant*

> L. permeabilis, permeabile 침투할 수 있는, 투과할 수 있는

E *permeable, permeability, semipermeable, semipermeability, impermeable, impermeability*

> L. migro, **migravi**, migratum, migrare (< *to change one's place of living*) 옮기다, 이동하다　　　　　　　　　　　　　　　**E** *migrate, migrant, migratory*

[용례] larva migrans 유충이행증　　　　　　　　**E** *larva migrans*

(문법) larva 유충: 단수 주격

< larva, larvae, f. 유령, 탈, 가면; 애벌레, 유생(幼生)

migrans 이행하는, 이행하고 있는: 현재분사, 남·여·중성형 단수 주격

< migrans, (gen.) migrantis

> L. migratio, migrationis, f. 이동　　　　　　　　　**E** *migration*

> L. emigro, **emigravi**, emigratum, emigrare (< e- *out of, away from* + migrare *to migrate*) 나가 살다, 이민 가다　　　　　**E** *emigrate, emigrant*

> L. immigro, **immigravi**, immigratum, immigrare (< im- (< in) *in, on, into, toward* + migrare *to migrate*) 들어와 살다, 이민 오다　　**E** *immigrate, immigrant*

> L. transmigro, **transmigravi**, transmigratum, transmigrare (< trans- *over, across, through, beyond* + migrare *to migrate*) 옮겨 살다, 이주하다　　**E** *transmigrate*

> L. munus, muneris, n. 직무, 예물　　　　　　　　　**E** *municipal*

> L. munis, mune 직무를 다하는, 잘 돌보는, 고마워할 줄 아는

> L. communis, commune (< com- (< cum) *with, together* + munis *of duty*) 공공의, 공통의, 통상적인　　　　**E** *common, commune, communism*

> L. communitas, communitatis, f. 공공성, 공통성, 공동체, 공동사회, 지역사회　　　　　　　　　　　　　　　**E** *community*

> L. communico, **communicavi**, communicatum, communicare (< communis *common*) 함께 참여시키다, 교류하다, 소통하다, 의사를 소통하다, 통신하다　　　　　**E** *communicate, communicative*

> L. communicatio, communicationis, f. 교류, 소통, 의사소통, 통신　　　　　　　　　　　　　　　　**E** *communication*

> L. excommunico, **excommunicavi**, excommunicatum, excommunicare (< ex- *out of, away from* + communis *common*) 파문하다, 제명처분하다　　　　　　　　　　　　　**E** *excommunicate*

> L. immunis, immune (< im- (< in-) *not* + munis *of duty*) 직무에서 면제된, 벗어난; 면역(免疫)이 된

E *immune, immunize, immuno-, immunocompetent, immunocompetence, immunodeficiency, immunocompromised, immunoglobulin (Ig); autoimmune (< 'immune against autoantigens'), isoimmune (< 'immune against isoantigens')*

> L. immunitas, immunitatis, f. (의무·부담·부채 등의) 면제;
면역(免疫) **E** *immunity*

> L. muneror, muneratus sum, munerari 사례하다, 보답하다

> L. remuneror, remuneratus sum, remunerari (< re- *back, again;* *intensive*
+ munerari *to give*) 사례하다, 보답하다 **E** *remunerate*

> L. munificus, munifica, munificum (< munus *gift* + -ficus (< facĕre) *making*)
푸짐한, 후한, 인심 좋은 **E** *munificent*

> G. ameibein *to change*

> G. amoibē, amoibēs, f. *change*

> L. amoeba, amoebae, f. (단세포 원생동물)
아메바 **E** *amoeba (ameba),* (pl.) *amoebae (amebae), amebic, ameboid*

> L. Acanthamoeba, Acanthamoebae, f. (< *short filose extensions
from the margins of the body, giving a spiny appearance* <
G. akantha *thorn, thistle*) (원충) 가시아메바속(屬) **E** Acanthamoeba

> L. Entamoeba, Entamoebae, f. (< G. entos *within, inside*) (원충)
(체내 기생성) 아메바속(屬) **E** Entamoeba

opto, optavi, optatum, optare (*frequentative of* *opĕre) 선택하다, 원하다 **E** *opt, co-opt*

> optio, optionis, f. 선택 **E** *option*

> adopto, **adoptavi,** adoptatum, adoptare (< ad- *to, toward, at, according to* + optare
to choose) 채택하다, 양자로 삼다 **E** *adopt*

> adoptio, adoptionis, f. 채택, 양자 결연 **E** *adoption*

< IE. op- *to choose*

> L. opinor, opinatus sum, opinari 여기다, 추측하다

> L. opinio, opinionis, f. 의견, 견해, 추측 **E** *opinion,* (opinion >) *opinionated*

oro, oravi, oratum, orare 기도하다, 청하다, 말하다, 연설하다

> oratio, orationis, f. 기도, 연설; (문법) 화법 **E** *oration*

> orator, oratoris, m. 기도하는 사람, 청원인, 연설가, 웅변가 **E** *orator*

> oratorius, oratoria, oratorium 기도의, 연설의, 웅변의 **E** *oratory*

> oratorium, oratorii, n. 작은 예배당, 기도실, 성담곡(聖譚曲) **E** *oratorio*

> oraculum, oraculi, n. (< + -culum *diminutive suffix*) 신탁 **E** *oracle, oracular*

> adoro, **adoravi,** adoratum, adorare (< ad- *to, toward, at, according to* + orare *to pray,
to speak*) 간청하다, 숭배하다 **E** *adore*

> exoro, **exoravi,** exoratum, exorare (< ex- *out of, away from;* *intensive* + orare *to
pray, to speak*) 간청하다, 마음을 돌리게 하다

> exorabilis, exorabile 간청에 마음이 움직이는

> inexorabilis, inexorabile (< in- *not*) 간청에도 굽히지 않는, 용서 없는,
냉혹한 **E** *inexorable*

> peroro, **peroravi,** peroratum, perorare (< per- *through, thoroughly* + orare *to pray,*

to speak) 빼지 않고 다 말하다, 열변을 토하다, 말을 맺다　　　　　　　　**E** *perorate*

< IE. or- *to pronounce a ritual formula*

palpo, palpavi, palpatum, palpare 어루만지다, 쓰다듬다, 다독거리다　　　**E** *palpate*
> palpatio, palpationis, f. 어루만짐, 쓰다듬음, 다독거림, 아부, 촉진(觸診)　　**E** *palpation*
> palpabilis, palpabile 만져볼 수 있는, 만져서 알 수 있는　　　　　　　**E** *palpable*
　　> impalpabilis, impalpabile (< im- (< in-) *not*) 만져볼 수 없는, 만져서 알 수
　　　　없는　　　　　　　　　　　　　　　　　　　　　　　　**E** *impalpable*
> palpus, palpi, m. 쓰다듬음, 애무; (곤충의) 촉수(觸鬚)　　　**E** *palpus (palp)*, (pl.) *palpi*
> palpebra, palpebrae, f. (< *that which shakes or moves quickly*) 눈꺼풀,
　　안검(眼瞼)　　　　　　　　　　　　　　　　**E** *palpebra*, (pl.) *palpebrae*
　　> palpebralis, palpebrale 눈꺼풀의, 안검의　　　　　　　　　**E** *palpebral*
> (*probably*) papilio, papilionis, m. 나비;
　　천막, 군막　　**E** *papilionaceous, pavilion* (< *'a tent resembling a butterfly's wings'*)
> palpito, palpitavi, palpitatum, palpitare (*frequentative*) 팔딱이다, 두근거리다, 심장이
　　뛰다　　　　　　　　　　　　　　　　　　　　**E** *palpitate, palpitant*
　　> palpitatio, palpitationis, f. (심장의) 고동(鼓動), 두근거림, 심계항진(心悸亢進)　**E** *palpitation*
< IE. pal- *to touch, to feel, to shake*　　　　　　　　　　　　　　**E** *feel*
> G. polemos, polemou, m. *war, battle, fight*　　　　　　　　　　**E** *polemic*
> G. pallein *to shake, to swing, to toss*　　　　　　　　　　　**E** *pallesthesia*
　　> G. katapeltēs, katapeltou, f. (< kat(a)- *down, mis-, according to, along,*
　　　　thoroughly + pallein) *catapult*
　　　　> L. catapulta, catapultae, f. 투석기, 투창기　　　　　　　**E** *catapult*
> (*suggested*) G. psallein *to pull, to pluck, to play the lyre with the fingers, to sing,*
　　to praise
　　> G. psalmos, psalmou, m. *playing on the lyre, song, psalm*
　　　　> L. psalmus, psalmi, n. 성가, (구약 성서) 시편의 한 편　　　**E** *psalm*
　　> G. psaltērion, psaltēriou, n. *stringed instrument, psaltery, psalm*
　　　　> L. psalterium, psalterii, n. 수금(竪琴) 비슷하게 생긴 현악기의 일종, 현악기,
　　　　　　현악기 반주에 맞추어 부르는 노래, 시편(詩篇); 뇌궁교련(腦弓交聯),
　　　　　　뇌금(腦琴); (*now rare*) 겹주름위(중판위 重瓣胃, 반추동물의
　　　　　　제3위)　　　　　　　　　　　　　　　**E** *psalterium, psaltery*

paro, paravi, paratum, parare 준비하다

> **E** *pare, parry, parade,* (parare *'to make ready'* + F. chute *'fall'* > *'making ready against the*
> *fall'* >) *parachute,* (parare *'to make ready'* + sol *'sun'* > *'making ready against the sun'* >)
> *parasol,* (re- *'again'* + *anteparare *'to prepare'* >) *rampart*

> apparo, **apparavi**, apparatum, apparare (< ap- (< ad) *to, toward, at, according to*
　　+ parare *to make ready*) 계획적으로 준비하다
　　> apparatus, apparatus, m. 준비물, 장치, 기구, 기관　　**E** *apparatus*, (pl.) *apparatus*
> disparo, disparavi, disparatum, disparare (< dis- *apart from, down, not* + parare)

to make ready) 가르다, 분리하다　　　　　　　　　　　　　　　　　**E** *disparate*

> praeparo, **praeparavi**, praeparatum, praeparare (< prae- *before, beyond* + parare

　　to make ready) 미리 준비하다　　　　　　　　　　**E** *prepare, preparative*

　　> praeparatio, praeparationis, f. 준비; (약제·제제·표본 등) 준비물　**E** *preparation*

　　> praeparator, praeparatoris, m. 준비하는 사람　　　　　　　**E** *preparator*

　　　　> praeparatorius, praeparatoria, praeparatorium 준비의, 준비하는,

　　　　　　선행하는　　　　　　　　　　　　　　　　　　　**E** *preparatory*

> reparo, **reparavi**, reparatum, reparare (< re- *back, again* + parare *to make ready*)

　　보수하다, 회복하다, 수복(修復)하다　**E** *repair, reparation, reparative, reparable (repairable)*

> separo, **separavi**, separatum, separare (< se- *apart, without* + parare *to make ready*)

　　분리하다　　　　　**E** *separate,* (separare >) *sever, severance, separative, separable*

　　> separatio, separationis, f. 분리　　　　　　　　　　　　**E** *separation*

　　> separ, (gen.) separis 분리된, 별개의

　　　　> separalis, separale 따로따로의, 몇몇의　　　　　　　**E** *several*

　　> disseparo, **disseparavi**, disseparatum, disseparare (< dis- *apart from, down,*

　　　　not; intensive + separare *to separate*) 분리하다, 분할하다　　**E** *dissever*

> impero, **imperavi**, imperatum, imperare (< im- (< in) *in, on, into, toward* + -perare

　　(< parare) *to make ready*) (자금·군대·무기·선박·양곡의) 준비를 명령하다, 명령하다

　　> imperium, imperii, n. 명령, 통수권, 제국　　　　　　　　**E** *empire*

　　　　> imperialis, imperiale 제국의　　　　　　　　　　　　**E** *imperial*

　　　　> imperiosus, imperiosa, imperiosum 명령권을 쥐고 있는, 독단적인　**E** *imperious*

　　> imperator, imperatoris, m. 명령자, 통수권자, 황제　　　　**E** *emperor, empress*

　　> imperativus, imperativa, imperativum 명령적인; (문법) 명령법의　**E** *imperative*

< IE. pere- *to produce, to procure*

> L. pario, **peperi**, partum, parĕre 낳다, 해산하다

　　> L. pariens, parientis, f. (< *present participle*) 산모(産母)

　　> L. parens, parentis, m., f. (< *present participle (archaic form)*) 어버이;

　　　　(pl.) parentes, parentum, m. 양친　**E** *parent,* (pl.) *parents, parental, parentage*

　　> L. partus, partus, m. 분만, 출산　　**E** *peripartum* (< *'on the pattern of -partum'*)

　　　　[용례] ante partum 분만 전의, 산전의　　　　　**E** *antepartum, antepartal*

　　　　　　　intra partum 분만 중의, 산중의　　　　　**E** *intrapartum, intrapartal*

　　　　　　　post partum 분만 후의, 산후의　　　　　　**E** *postpartum, postpartal*

　　　　　　(문법) ante 전에: 전치사, 대격지배

　　　　　　　　 intra 안에: 전치사, 대격지배

　　　　　　　　 post 후에: 전치사, 대격지배

　　　　　　　　 partum: 단수 대격

　　> L. -parus, -para, -parum 낳는, 산부(産婦)의

　　　　E *-parous* (< *'bearing'*)*, oviparous, viviparous, fetiparous, sudoriparous, viper*
　　　　(< *'ovo-viviparous snake'*)*, (-parous >) parous*

　　　　> L. -para, -parae, f. 출산(出産), 산부(産婦), 분만부(分娩婦)　**E** *-para, para*

　　　　　> L. nullipara, nulliparae, f. (< nullus *none*)

미분만부(未分娩婦)　　　　　　　　　　　　**E** *nullipara, nulliparous*

> L. primipara, primiparae, f. (< primus *first*) 초산녀　**E** *primipara, primiparous*

> L. multipara, multiparae, f. (< multus *many*) 다분만부,

다분만녀　　　　　　　　　　　　　　　**E** *multipara, multiparous*

> L. puerpera, puerperae, f. (< puer *boy* + -pera (< -para)) 산후부

(産後婦), 산후녀, 산욕부(産褥婦)　　　　**E** *puerpera, puerperal*

> L. puerperium, puerperii, n. 산욕기(産褥期),

산후(産後)　　　　　　　　　　**E** *puerperium, puerperial*

> L. paritas, paritatis, f. 출산수, 임신분만력,

출산력　　　　　　**E** *parity, -parity, nulliparity, primiparity, multiparity*

> L. parturio, parturivi (parturii), -, parturire

분만하다　　　　　　**E** *parturient, parturition, parturifacient (< 'oxytocic')*

> L. pario, peperi, paritum, parire (*Early Latin, uncommon*) 낳다, 해산하다

> L. reperio, repperi, repertum, reperire (< re- *back, again* + parire *to produce,*

to bring forth) 획득하다, 발견하다

> L. repertorium, repertorii, n. 목록, 재산목록　　**E** *repertory, repertoire*

> L. Parcae, Parcarum, f. (pl.) 운명의 세 여신 (Nona (*the Roman goddess of pregnancy.*

She was called upon by pregnant women in their ninth month when the child

was due to be born.), Decima, Morta)

> L. pauper, (gen.) pauperis (< IE. pau-, pou- *little, few* + IE. perə-)

가난한　　　　　　　　　　　　　　　　**E** *pauper, poor, impoverish*

> L. paupertas, paupertatis, f. 가난　　　　　　　**E** *poverty*

pipio, pipiavi, pipiatum, pipiare (pipare, pipire) 삐삐거리며 울다,

지저귀다　　　　　　　　　　**E** *pipe, (pipe (diminutive) >) pipette*

> pipio, pipionis, m. 새끼 새, 비둘기 새끼　　　　**E** *pigeon*

< IE. pip(p)- (*imitative root*) *to peep*

plico, plicavi (plicui), plicatum (plicitum), plicare 접다,

접어 겹치다　　**E** *plait, pleat, ply, (ply >) pliers, pliant, pliable, pliability*

> plicatus, plicata, plicatum (*past participle*) 접힌, 주름잡힌,

주름이 있는　　　　　　　　　　　**E** *plicate, plight (< 'folded')*

> plicatio, plicationis, f. (접어 만드는) 주름잡음, 주름　　**E** *plication*

> plica, plicae, f. (접어 만든, 접힌) 주름, 습벽(褶襞), 추벽(皺襞)　**E** *plica, (pl.) plicae*

[용례] plica circularis, (pl.) plicae circulares 원형

주름　　　　　　　　**E** *plica circularis, (pl.) plicae circulares*

(문법) plica 주름: 단수 주격

circularis 둥근: 형용사, 남·여성형 단수 주격

< circularis, circulare 둥근, 원형의, 회람의

plicae 주름들: 복수 주격

circulares 둥근: 형용사, 남·여성형 복수 주격

> -plex, (gen.) -plicis ~배의　　　　　　　　　　　**E** *-plex, duplex, triplex, quadruplex*

　> simplex, (gen.) simplicis (< semel *once* + -plex *-fold*) 홑겹의,

　　단순한　　　　　　　　　　　　　　　　　　**E** *simplex, simplicity*

　> multiplex, (gen.) multiplicis (< multus *many* + -plex *-fold*) 여러 겹의,

　　여러 곱절의, 복합된　　　　　　　　　　　　**E** *multiplex, multiplicity*

　　> multiplico, **multiplicavi**, multiplicatum, multiplicare 많아지게 하다,

　　　곱하다, 증식시키다, 번식시키다　　　　　　**E** *multiplicate, multiply*

> supplex, (gen.) supplicis (< sup- (< sub) *under, up from under* + plicare

　to fold) 굽히는, 애원하는, 유연한　　　　　　**E** *supple*

> applico, **applicavi** (applicui), applicatum (applicitum), applicare (< ap- (< ad)

　to, toward, at, according to + plicare *to fold*) 갖다대다,

　적용하다　　　　　　　　　**E** *apply, applicant, applicable, (apply >) appliance*

　> applicatio, applicationis, f. 적용, 응용, 외용(外用), 지원　　**E** *application*

> complico, **complicavi** (complicui), complicatum (complicitum), complicare (< com-

　(< cum) *with, together* + plicare *to fold*) 접다; (*passive*) 뒤얽히다, 복잡해

　지다　　　　　　　　　　　　　　　　　　　　**E** *complicate*

　> complicatio, complicationis, f. 합병증　　　　**E** *complication*

> displico, **displicavi**, displicatum, displicare (< dis- *apart from, down, not* +

　plicare *to fold*) 펴다　　　　　　　**E** *display, (display >) splay, deploy*

> explico, **explicavi** (explicui), explicatum (explicitum), explicare (< ex-*out of,*

　away from + plicare *to fold*) 펼치다, 설명하다　　**E** *explicate, explicit, exploit*

> implico, **implicavi** (implicui), implicatum (implicitum), implicare (< im- (< in)

　in, on, into, toward + plicare *to fold*) 얽히게 하다, 끌어넣다, 내포하다,

　함축하다　　　　　　　　　　　　　**E** *implicate, implicit, imply, employ*

> replico, **replicavi**, replicatum, replicare (< re- *back, again* + plicare *to fold*)

　뒤로 접다, 되풀이하다　　**E** *replicate, reply,* It. *replica, (replicate >) replicase*

　> replicatio, replicationis, f. 반복, 회전　**E** *replication, (replication unit >) replicon*

> supplico, **supplicavi**, supplicatum, supplicare (< sup- (< sub) *under, up from*

　under + plicare *to fold*) 굽히다, 애원하다　　　**E** *supplicate, suppliant*

< IE. plek- *to plait*　　　　　　　　　　　　　　　　　　　　　**E** *flax*

　> L. plecto, **plexi** (plexui), plexum, plectĕre 엮다, 짜다　**E** *plectin*

　　> L. plexus, plexus, m. 얼기, 총(叢)　　　　　　　　**E** *plexus*

　　　> L. plexiformis, plexiforme 얼기 모양의　　　　　**E** *plexiform*

　　> L. perplexus, perplexa, perplexum (< per- *through, thoroughly*

　　　+ plectĕre *to weave, to braid*) 뒤얽힌　　　　　　**E** *perplex*

　　　> L. perplexitas, perplexitatis, f. 뒤얽힘, 까다로움, 당혹, 모호　**E** *perplexity*

　　> L. complector, complexus sum, complecti (< com- (< cum) *with, together*

　　　+ plectĕre *to weave, to braid*) 얽히다, 껴안다, 둘러싸다, 파악하다

　　　> L. complex, (gen.) complicis 얽혀 있는, 연루된, 복잡한,

　　　　복합된　　**E** *complex, complicity, accomplice, (complex >) complexity*

> L. complexio, complexionis, f. 결합, 연루, 체액의 결합, 기질, 외관,

안색 **E** *complexion*

> G. plekein *to plait, to twine* **E** *plecopteran*

> G. plektos, plektē, plekton *plaited, twisted* **E** *plect(o)-, plectognath, plectonemic*

< IE. pel- *to fold* **E** *fold, -fold, (suggested) falter*

> L. -plus, -pla, -plum ~배의 **E** *-ple*

> L. simplus, simpla, simplum (< semel *once* + -plus *-fold*) 한 배의,

단순한 **E** *simple, simpleton*

> L. simplifico, **simplificavi**, simplificatum, simplificare (< + -ficare (< facĕre)

to make) 하나로 되게 하다, 단순하게 하다 **E** *simplify*

> L. multiplus, multipla, multiplum (< multus *many, much* + -plus *-fold*) 여러

배의 **E** *multiple*

> G. -ploos, -ploē, -ploon *-fold*

E *(adjective)* **-ploid**, *(noun)* **-ploidy**, *(-ploidy > 'the number of homologous sets of chromosomes in a cell' >)* **ploidy, euploid, euploidy, aneuploid, aneuploidy**

> G. haploos, haploē, haploon (< ha- *one*) *onefold, simple,*

single **E** *(adjective)* **haploid**, *(noun)* **haploidy**

> G. diploos, diploē, diploon (diplous, diploē, diploun) (< di- *two*) *twofold,*

double **E** *(adjective)* **diploid**, *(noun)* **diploidy, dipl(o)-, diplotene**

> G. diploē, diploēs, f. *fold, doubling*

> L. diploē, diploēs, f. 판사이층, 판간층(板間層) **E** *diploë, diploic (diploetic)*

> G. diploun (diploein) *to double*

> G. diplōma, diplōmatos, n. (< -ma *resultative noun suffix*)

folded letter, letter of licence or privilege

> L. diploma, diplomatis, n. 인가서, 통과증, 공문서, 증서,

여권 **E** *diploma, diplomatic*

> L. diplococcus, diplococci, m. (< + G. kokkos *grain, berry*) 쌍알균,

쌍구균(雙球菌) **E** *diplococcus, (pl.) diplococci*

> G. polyploos, polyploē, polyploon (< polys *many*)

manyfold **E** *(adjective)* **polyploid**, *(noun)* **polyploidy**

> G. epiploos, epiploou, m. (< ep(i)- *upon*) *membrane enclosing the entrails*

> G. epiploon, epiploou, n. (< ep(i)- *upon*) *omentum, greater omentum*

> L. epiploön, epiploi, n. 망막(網膜, *omentum*) **E** *epiploon, epiploic*

porto, portavi, portatum, portare 나르다, 지니다

E *(folium 'leaf' > 'briefcase for carrying loose papers' >)* **portfolio**, *(mantellum 'manteau' > 'traveling bag' >)* **portmanteau, disport** *(< 'to carry away'), (disport >)* **sport**

> portator, portatoris, m. 운반인, 휴대자, 짐꾼 **E** *porter*

> portabilis, portabile 지닐 수 있는, 휴대용의, 간편한 **E** *portable*

> apporto, **apportavi**, apportatum, apportare (< ap- (< ad) *to, toward, at, according to*

+ portare *to carry*) 가지고 가다, 가져오다 **E** *apport, (re- + apport > 'bring back' >)* **rapport**

> deporto, **deportavi**, deportatum, deportare (< de- *apart from, down, not* + portare *to carry*) 운반하다, 추방하다   **E** *deport*

> exporto, **exportavi**, exportatum, exportare (< ex- *out of, away from* + portare *to carry*) 가져나가다, 수출하다   **E** *export*

> importo, **importavi**, importatum, importare (< im- (< in) *in, on, into, toward* + portare *to carry*) 들여오다, 의미하다, 수입하다   **E** *import, important, importance*

> proporto, **proportavi**, proportatum, proportare (< pro- *before, forward, for, instead of* + portare *to carry*) 주장하다, 의도하다, 의미하다   **E** *purport*

> reporto, **reportavi**, reportatum, reportare (< re- *back, again* + portare *to carry*) 가지고 돌아가다(오다), (소식·답을) 가지고 오다, 보고하다   **E** *report*

> supporto, **supportavi**, supportatum, supportare (< sup- (< sub) *under, up from under* + portare *to carry*) 메다, 지지하다   **E** *support, supportive*

> transporto, **transportavi**, transportatum, transportare (< trans- *over, across, through, beyond* + portare *to carry*) 옮겨 놓다, 운반하다, 운송하다   **E** *transport, transportation*

< IE. per- *to lead, to pass-over; a verbal root belonging to the group of* IE. per *forward, through*

   E *fare, farewell, welfare, warfare, ferry, ford, fjord (fiord), fern* (< *'having feathery fronds'* < *'feather which carries a bird in flight'*)

> L. portus, portus, m. (< *passage*)

항구   **E** *port, airport, passport* (< *'to pass seaport'*), (Portus Cale >) *Portugal*

> L. importunus, importuna, importunum (< im- < in- *not* + portus *haven*) 부적당한, 성가신, 끈질긴   **E** *importune, importunate*

> L. opportunus, opportuna, opportunum (< *originally a nautical term, qualifying a wind that blows towards harbor* < ob- *before, toward(s), over, against, away* + portus *haven*) (장소·시기가) 알맞은, 공격받기 쉬운, (위험 등을) 당하기 쉬운, (병에) 걸리기 쉬운   **E** *opportune, opportunism, opportunistic*

> L. opportunitas, opportunitatis, f. 기회   **E** *opportunity*

> L. porta, portae, f. 배의 하역구, 성문, 대문, 현관문, 문(門)   **E** *port, portcullis* (< *'straining door'*)

[용례] porta hepatis 간문(肝門)   **E** *porta hepatis*
(문법) porta 문: 단수 주격
hepatis 간의: 단수 속격 < hepar, hepatis, n.

> L. portalis, portale 문(門)의   **E** *portal*
> L. porticus, porticus, f. (지붕 있는) 주랑(柱廊), 회랑(回廊)   **E** *porch, portico*
> L. portarius, portarii, m. 문지기   **E** *porter*

> G. poros, porou, m. *passage, ford, means of achieving*   **E** *neuropore*, (G. poros + *polymeric* >) *poromeric*

> G. aporos, aporos, aporon (< a- *not* + poros) *impassable, difficult, helpless*

> G. aporia, aporias, f. *embarrassment, difficulty, helplessness, doubt*

> L. aporia, aporiae, f. 난처, 곤경, 무력, 의문, 아포리아   **E** *aporia*

> G. emporos, emporou, m. (< em- (< en) *in*) *passenger, merchant*

> G. emporion, emporiou, n. *trading place*

> L. emporium, emporii, n. 시장

E *emporium, (pl.) emporia*

> L. porus, pori, m. 도관(導管), 작은 구멍, 흡수공, 기공(氣孔)

E *pore, porin, aquaporin, nucleopore*

> L. porosus, porosa, porosum 구멍이 많은, (물·공기 등이) 스며드는

E *porous*

> L. porositas, porositatis, f. 다공성(多孔性)

E *porosity*

> L. osteoporosis, osteoporosis, f. (< G. osteon *bone* + poros + -ōsis *condition*) 골다공증(骨多孔症)

E *osteoporosis, osteoporotic*

> L. porosis, porosis, f. 다공증

E *porosis, porotic*

> G. peirein *to pierce, to run through*

> G. peronē, peronēs, f. (< *that which pierces through*) brooch, buckle, fibula

E *peroneal*

> L. peroneus, peronei, m. 종아리근, 비골근(腓骨筋)

E *peroneus (muscle)*

> G. petra, petras, f. (petros, petrou, m.) (< *what one comes through to*) bedrock, rock

E *Petra*

> G. petroselinon, petroselinou, n. (< *rock parsley* < petra + selinon *parsley*) parsley

> L. petroselinum, petroselini, n. 파슬리

E *parsley*

> L. petra, petrae, f. 반석, 바위

E *petrify, saltpetre (saltpeter)*

> L. petrosus, petrosa, petrosum 바위로 된, 바위처럼 딱딱한; (해부) (측두골) 추체(錐體)의

E *petrous, (petrous >) petrosal*

> L. petroleum, petrolei, n. (< petra *rock* + oleum *oil*) 석유(石油)

E *petroleum, petrol (< 'a light fuel oil made by distilling petroleum'), petrolatum (< 'petroleum jelly such as Vaseline®)*

> L. Petrus, Petri, m. 피터

E *Peter, F. Pierre, (diminutive of F. Pierre >) Pierrot, ((probably) diminutive of F. Pierre >) parrot*

> L. osteopetrosis, osteopetrosis, f. (< G. osteon *bone* + petra + -ōsis *condition*) 뼈화석증, 골화석증

E *osteopetrosis*

postulo, postulavi, postulatum, postulare 요구하다

E *postulate*

> expostulo, expostulavi, expostulatum, expostulare (< ex- *out of, away from* + postulare *to demand*) 요구하다

E *expostulate*

< posco, poposci, -, poscĕre 요구하다

< IE. prek- *to ask, to entreat*

> L. prex, precis, f. 간청, 기원, 기도

> L. precor, precatus sum, precari 간청하다, 기원하다, 기도하다

E *pray*

> L. precarius, precaria, precarium 간청해서 얻는(얻은), 주는 사람이 허락하는 동안만의, 가점유(假占有)의, 일시적인, 언제 어떻게 될지 모르는, 확실하지 않는

E *precarious*

> L. deprecor, deprecatus sum, deprecari (< *to pray against* < de- *apart from, down, not* + precari *to pray*) 않게 되기를 빌다

E *deprecate*

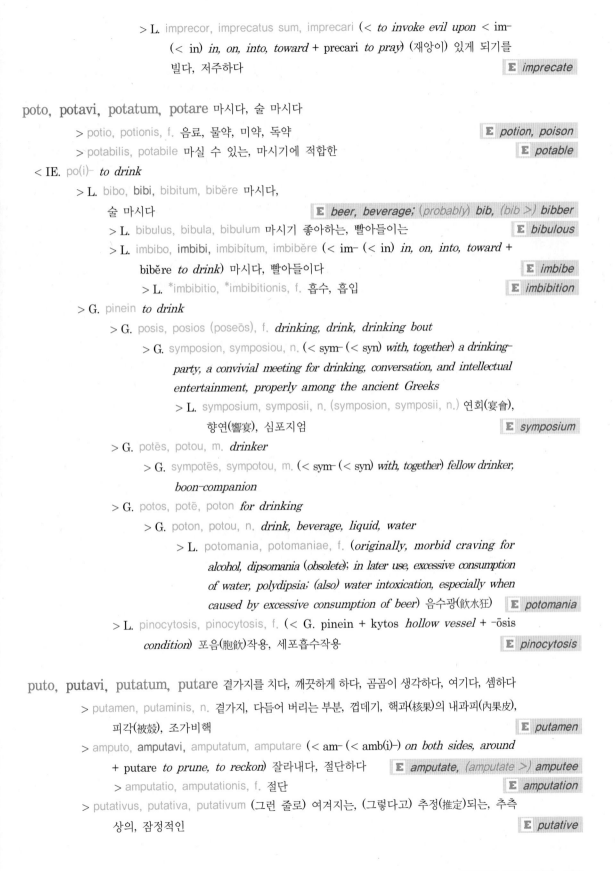

> L. imprecor, imprecatus sum, imprecari (< *to invoke evil upon* < im-
(< in) *in, on, into, toward* + precari *to pray*) (재앙이) 있게 되기를
빌다, 저주하다   **E** *imprecate*

poto, potavi, potatum, potare 마시다, 술 마시다

> potio, potionis, f. 음료, 물약, 미약, 독약   **E** *potion, poison*

> potabilis, potabile 마실 수 있는, 마시기에 적합한   **E** *potable*

   < IE. po(i)- *to drink*

     > L. bibo, **bibi**, bibitum, biběre 마시다,
술 마시다   **E** *beer, beverage;* (probably) *bib,* (bib >) *bibber*

       > L. bibulus, bibula, bibulum 마시기 좋아하는, 빨아들이는   **E** *bibulous*

       > L. imbibo, **imbibi**, imbibitum, imbiběre (< im- (< in) *in, on, into, toward* +
biběre *to drink*) 마시다, 빨아들이다   **E** *imbibe*

         > L. *imbibitio, *imbibitionis, f. 흡수, 흡입   **E** *imbibition*

    > G. pinein *to drink*

      > G. posis, posios (poseōs), f. *drinking, drink, drinking bout*

        > G. symposion, symposiou, n. (< sym- (< syn) *with, together*) *a drinking-
party, a convivial meeting for drinking, conversation, and intellectual
entertainment, properly among the ancient Greeks*

         > L. symposium, symposii, n. (symposion, symposii, n.) 연회(宴會),
향연(饗宴), 심포지엄   **E** *symposium*

       > G. potēs, potou, m. *drinker*

         > G. sympotēs, sympotou, m. (< sym- (< syn) *with, together*) *fellow drinker,
boon-companion*

       > G. potos, potē, poton *for drinking*

         > G. poton, potou, n. *drink, beverage, liquid, water*

          > L. potomania, potomaniae, f. (*originally, morbid craving for
alcohol, dipsomania* (obsolete); *in later use, excessive consumption
of water, polydipsia;* (also) *water intoxication, especially when
caused by excessive consumption of beer*) 음수광(飮水狂)   **E** *potomania*

      > L. pinocytosis, pinocytosis, f. (< G. pinein + kytos *hollow vessel* + -ōsis
condition) 포음(胞飲)작용, 세포흡수작용   **E** *pinocytosis*

puto, putavi, putatum, putare 곁가지를 치다, 깨끗하게 하다, 곰곰이 생각하다, 여기다, 셈하다

> putamen, putaminis, n. 곁가지, 다듬어 버리는 부분, 껍데기, 핵과(核果)의 내과피(內果皮),
피각(被殼), 조가비핵   **E** *putamen*

> amputo, amputavi, amputatum, amputare (< am- (< amb(i)-) *on both sides, around*
+ putare *to prune, to reckon*) 잘라내다, 절단하다   **E** *amputate,* (amputate >) *amputee*

   > amputatio, amputationis, f. 절단   **E** *amputation*

> putativus, putativa, putativum (그런 줄로) 여겨지는, (그렇다고) 추정(推定)되는, 추측
상의, 잠정적인   **E** *putative*

> computo, **computavi**, computatum, computare (< com- (< cum) *with, together* + putare *to prune, to reckon*) 헤아리다, 셈하다 **E** *compute, count, computer, counter, computation, computerize, account, discount*

> deputo, **deputavi**, deputatum, deputare (< de- *apart from, down, not* + putare *to prune, to reckon*) (대리인에게) 맡기다, 임명하다, 위임하다 **E** *depute, deputation, deputy*

> disputo, **disputavi**, disputatum, disputare (< dis- *apart from, down, not; intensive* + putare *to prune, to reckon*) 셈을 따지다, 논의하다, 토론하다 **E** *dispute, disputation*

> imputo, **imputavi**, imputatum, imputare (< im- (< in) *in, on, into, toward* + putare *to prune, to reckon*) 계산에 넣다, 탓으로 돌리다, 전가하다 **E** *impute, imputation*

> reputo, **reputavi**, reputatum, reputare (< re- *back, again* + putare *to prune, to reckon*) 계산하다, 평가하다, 숙고하다, 음미하다 **E** *repute, reputation*

< IE. pau- *to cut, to strike, to chop, to stamp*

> L. puteus, putei, m. 우물, 움, (노예를 가두어 벌주는 우물같이 생긴) 땅굴 **E** *pit*

> L. paveo, **pavi**, –, pavēre (< *to be struck*) 무서워 떨다, 무서워하다 **E** *pavid*

> L. pavor, pavoris, m. 공포, 경악; (Pavor) (로마 신화) 공포의 신 **E** *pavor*

> L. pavio, **pavivi**, pavitum, pavire 두드려 편편하게 하다, 다져서 굳게 하다 **E** *pave, pavement*

> G. paiein *to beat*

> G. anapaistos, anapaistos, anapaiston (< an(a)- *up, upward; again, through -out; back, backward; against; according to, similar to*) *struck back, reversed*

> L. anapaestum, anapaesti, n. (< *reversed dactyl*) 단단장격(短短長格), 약약강격(弱弱强格) **E** *anapaest (anapest)*

*redo, *redavi, *redatum, *redare 정돈하다

> *arredo, *arredavi, *arredatum, *arredare (< ar- (< ad) *to, toward, at, according to* + *redare *to arrange*) 배열하다 **E** *array, arrayal*

< IE. reidh- *to ride* **E** *ride, road, raid, ready* (< *'prepared for a journey'*), *already*

ructo, ructavi, ructatum, ructare 트림하다, 내뿜다, 풍기다

> eructo, **eructavi**, eructatum, eructare (< e- *out of, away from* + ructare *to belch, to emit*) 트림하다, 내뿜다

> eructatio, eructationis, f. 트림 **E** *eructation*

< IE. reug- *to vomit, to belch; smoke, cloud* **E** *reek*

seco, secui, sectum, secare 자르다, 베다, 나누다

E *secant,* (sectus *(past participle)* >) *transect,* (transect >) *transection,* (sectus *(past participle)* >) *bisect; hemisect*

> sectio, sectionis, f. 자름, 잘라낸 부분, 부서, 구역, 절단, 단면, 절편, 절개 **E** *section, sectional, sectionalism*

> sector, sectoris, m. 자르는 사람, 분야, 구역, 분야 **E** *sector, sectorial*

> sectilis, sectile 잘라진, 자를 수 있는 **E** *sectile*

> securis, securis, f. 도끼   **E** *securi-, securiform*

> segmentum, segmenti, n. 조각, 마디, 분절(分節), 체절(體節),

   구역(區域)   **E** *segment, segmental, (segment >) segmentate, (segment >) segmentation*

> disseco, dissecui, dissectum, dissecare (< dis- *apart from, down, not* + secare *to*

   cut) 잘게 자르다, 베다, 해부하다, 박리(剝離)하다   **E** *dissect*

    > dissectio, dissectionis, f. 해부, 박리, 절개, 절제   **E** *dissection*

> inseco, insecui, insectum, insecare (< in- *in, on, into, toward* + secare *to cut*) 안을

   자르다, 가르다, 끊다   **E** *(G. zöion entomon > L. animal insectum >) insect, insecticide*

> interseco, intersecui, intersectum, intersecare (< inter- *between, among* + secare

   to cut) 사이를 자르다, 교차하다   **E** *intersect*

> reseco, resecui, resectum, resecare (< re- *back, again; intensive* + secare *to cut*)

   베다, 절제(切除)하다   **E** *resect*

    > resectio, resectionis, f. 절제(切除)   **E** *resection, resectional*

> (*probably*) sexus, sexus, m. 성(性)   **E** *sex, intersex*

    > sexualis, sexuale 성의, 성에 관한, 성적인, 성욕의

       E *sexual, unisexual, bisexual, transsexual, transsexualism; asexual, heterosexual (hetero), homosexual (homo)*

      > *sexualitas, *sexualitatis, f. 성별, 성욕   **E** *sexuality*

< IE. sek- *to cut*

   E *scythe, saw, hacksaw, skin (< 'to peel off, to flay'), Saxon (< (traditionally but doubtfully) 'knife-bearer')*

> L. secula, seculae, f. (Campania 지방의 낱말) 낫   **E** *sickle*

> L. saxum, saxi, n. (< (*perhaps*) *broken-off piece*) 바위, 돌산   **E** *saxicolous (< 'rock-inhabiting')*

   > L. saxatilis, saxatile 바위의, 바위에 붙어 나는, 바위 틈에서 나는   **E** *saxatile*

   > L. Saxidomus, Saxidomi, m. (< saxum *rock* + domus *home*) *name of a genus*

     of clams

       E *saxitoxin (< 'a toxic alkaloid synthesized by dinoflagellates of the genus Gonyaulax and accumulated by molluscs (e.g., saxidomus) which feed on these')*

   > L. saxifragus, saxifraga, saxifragum (< saxum *rock* + frangĕre *to break*) 바위를

     깨는

     > L. saxifraga, saxifragae, f. (< saxifraga herba *rock-breaking herb*) 범의

      귀속(屬)의 식물   **E** *saxifrage*

> IE. sked- *to split, to scatter*   **E** *scatter, shatter*

   > L. scandula, scandulae, f. (scindula, scindulae, f.) (< *split piece*) 지붕널,

     너와   **E** *shingle*

> IE. skei- *to cut, to split*

   E *ski (< 'log, stick, snowshoe'), shin (< 'piece cut off'), shiver (< 'splinter'), sheath (< 'split stick'), (perhaps) skid (< 'stick of wood'), shed (< 'to separate'), watershed, shit*

   > L. scio, scivi (scii), scitum, scire (< *to separate one thing from another, to*

     discern) 알다   **E** *(scire licet 'it is permitted to know' >) scilicet (scil., sc.); sciology*

     > L. omnisciens, (gen.) omniscientis (< omnis *all* + sciens (*present*

participle) *knowing*) 전지의, 박식한　　　　　　　　　　　　　　**E** *omniscient*

> L. scientia, scientiae, f. (< sciens (*present participle*) *knowing*) 지식,
학문, 과학　　　　　　　　　　**E** *science, (science fiction >) sci-fi; Scientology*

　　> L. scientificus, scientifica, scientificum (< + -ficus (< facĕre)
making) 학문의, 과학의　　　　　　　　　　　　　　**E** *scientific*

> L. conscio, conscivi (conscii), conscitum, conscire (< consciens (*present
participle*) *knowing along with others* < con- (< cum) *with, together*
+ scire *to know*) 인식하다,
의식하다　　　　　**E** *conscious, consciousness, subconscious, unconscious*

　　> L. conscientia, conscientiae, f. 공동인식, 의식,
양심　　　　　　　　**E** *conscience, (conscience >) unconscionable*

　　　> L. conscientiosus, conscientiosa, conscientiosum 양심적인,
성실한　　　　　　　　　　　　　　　**E** *conscientious*

> L. nescio, nescivi (nescii), nescitum, nescire (< ne *not* + scire *to know*)
모르다　　　　　　　　　　　　　　　　**E** *nescient*

　　> L. nescius, nescia, nescium 모르는,
하지 못하는　　　　　　**E** *nice (< 'unclear sense development')*

> L. praescio, praescivi (praescii), praescitum, praescire (< prae- *before,
beyond* + scire *to know*) 미리 알다, 예지하다　　　　**E** *prescient*

> L. scisco, scivi, scitum, sciscĕre (*inchoative*) 알아보다, 조사하다, 재가
하다, 결정하다

　　> L. plebiscitum, plebisciti, n. (< plebis scitum *an ordinance of
the plebs* < plebs, plebis, f. *common people* + sciscĕre *to vote
for*) (원로원 의원·귀족을 제외한) 로마 시민의 의결, 국민투표　**E** *plebiscite*

> L. scindo, scidi, scissum, scindĕre 찢다, 갈래로 나누다

　　> L. scissio, scissionis, f. 분할, 분열　　　　　　　　　**E** *scission*

　　> L. scissilis, scissile 찢어지기 쉬운, 갈라지는　　　　　**E** *scissile*

　　> L. abscindo, abscidi, abscissum, abscindĕre (< ab- *off, away from* +
scindĕre *to cut*) 찢어내다,
갈라놓다　　　　　**E** *abscind, (abscissa linea 'cut-off line' >) abscissa*

　　　> L. abscissio, abscissionis, f. 절단, 분리, 이탈　**E** *abscission, abscisic acid*

　　> L. discindo, discidi, discissum, discindĕre (< di- (< dis-) *apart from,
down, not* + scindĕre *to cut*) 가르다, 절개하다　　　　**E** *discission*

　　> L. exscindo, exscidi, exscissum, exscindĕre (< ex- *out of, away from*
+ scindĕre *to cut*) 잘라내다, 근절시키다　　　　　　**E** *exscind*

　　> L. praescindo, praescidi, praescissum, praescindĕre (< prae- *before,
beyond* + scindĕre *to cut*) 갈라놓다　　　　　　　**E** *prescind*

　　> L. rescindo, rescidi, rescissum, rescindĕre (< re- *back, again* + scindĕre
to cut) 폐기하다, 무효로 하다　　　　　　　　　　**E** *rescind*

> L. scutum, scuti, n. (< *board*) (장방형의) 방패; (동물) 인갑(鱗甲);
(곤충) 순판(楯板)　　　　　　　**E** *scutum, (pl.) scuta, escutcheon*

> L. scutarius, scutaria, scutarium 장방형 방패의, 장방형 방패로 무장한

    > L. scutarius, scutarii, m. 방패 제조인,

        방패로 무장한 근위병   <u>E</u> *esquire, (esquire >) squire*

    > L. scutatus, scutata, scutatum 장방형 방패의, 장방형 방패로 무장한 <u>E</u> *scutate*

> (*perhaps*) L. scutra, scutrae, f. 접시, 쟁반, 대접

    > L. scutella, scutellae, f. (< + -ella *diminutive suffix*) 우묵한 접시, 받침

        접시, 운두가 얕은 사발   <u>E</u> *scuttle*

> G. schizein *to split, to cleave, to separate*   <u>E</u> *schiz(o)-, schism*

    > G. schizōn, (gen.) schizontos (*masculine present participle*) *splitting* <u>E</u> *schizont*

    > G. schiza, schizēs, f. (schidē, schidēs, f.) *cleft piece of wood, splinter*

        > L. scheda, schedae, f. 파피루스의 인피(靭皮), 종잇장, 책장

            > L. schedula, schedulae, f. (< + -ula *diminutive suffix*)

            쪽지, 일람표   <u>E</u> *schedule*

    > G. schisis, schiseōs, f. *division, by-road* <u>E</u> *-schisis, gastroschisis, rachischisis*

    > G. schistos, schistē, schiston *split, cleft* <u>E</u> *schist(o)-*

        > L. schistosoma, schistosomatis, n. (< + soma *body*) (흡충) 주혈

        흡충속(住血吸蟲屬)   <u>E</u> *Schistosoma*

    > L. schizophrenia, schizophreniae, f. (< + G. phrēn, phrenos, f. *mind*)

    정신분열증   <u>E</u> *schizophrenia, schizophrenic*

> IE. (s)ker- *to cut*

> <u>E</u> *shear, share, shore, sharp, short, shirt, skirt, score* (< '*to make an incision*'), *underscore, skirmish* (< '*to fight with a sword*'), (*skirmish* >) *scrimmage (scrummage), (scrummage* >) *scrum, screen* (< '*shield*' < '*to fence*' < '*to fight with a sword*'), *scrap* (< '*piece*'), *scrape, scrabble* (< '*to scrape*'), *scrub* (< '*to clean by rubbing*' < '*to scrape*'), *shrub* (< '*rough plant*'), *scurf, (scurf* >) *scurvy, (scurvy* > L. scorbutus > L. scorbuticus >) *scorbutic, (a-scorbutic* '*not scorbutic*' >) *ascorbic acid*

> L. caro, carnis, f. 고기, 살, 육신

> <u>E</u> (**carnem levare* >) *carnival, carnitine* (< '*first isolated in meat extract*'), *carrion* (< '*a piece of flesh*')

    > L. caruncula, carunculae, f. (< + -cula *diminutive suffix*) 작은 고깃

    덩어리, 살점   <u>E</u> *caruncle*

    > L. carneus, carnea, carneum 고기의, 살의, 육신의   <u>E</u> *carneous*

    > L. carnosus, carnosa, carnosum 근육이 많은, 근육의

    > L. carnalis, carnale 육신의, 육체적, 육욕의, 속세적   <u>E</u> *carnal; charnel*

    > L. carnivorus, carnivora, carnivorum (< + -vorus *devouring*) 육식의 <u>E</u> *carnivorous*

    > L. incarno, incarnavi, incarnatum, incarnare (< in- *in, on, into, toward*)

    육체화하다, 인간화하다   <u>E</u> *incarnate, incarnation, incarnadine*

> L. corium, corii, n. (< *piece of hide*) (짐승의) 가죽, 가죽 갑옷, 모피, 껍질,

진피(眞皮)   <u>E</u> *corium (dermis)*

    > L. coriaceus, coriacea, coriaceum

    가죽으로 만든   <u>E</u> (*vestis coriacea* '*leathern garment*' >) *cuirass*

    > L. excorio, excoriavi, excoriatum, excoriare (< ex- *out of, away from*)

가죽을 벗기다, 껍질을 벗기다　　　**E** *excoriate, (excoriate >) excoriation*

> L. cortex, corticis, m., f. (< *that which can be cut off*) 나무껍질, 수피(樹皮),
　피질(皮質), 겉질

> **E** *cortex, corticosteroid(s) (corticoid(s)), glucocorticoid(s), mineralocorticoid(s), gonadocorticoid(s); cortisol (hydrocortisone); paracortex*

　> L. corticalis, corticale 피질의, 겉질의　　　**E** *cortical*

　> L. corticatus, corticata, corticatum 피질이 있는　　　**E** *corticate*

　> L. decortico, decorticavi, decorticatum, decorticare (< de- *apart from,
　　down, not*) 껍질을 벗기다, 피질을 박리하다　　　**E** *decorticate*

　> L. isocortex, isocorticis, m., f. (< *six-layered neocortex* < G. isos *equal*
　　+ L. cortex *bark*) 동종피질　　　**E** *isocortex (homotypical cortex)*

　> L. allocortex, allocorticis, m., f. (< *three-, four-, five-layered archicortex
　　and paleocortex* < G. allos *other* + L. cortex *bark*)
　　이종피질　　　**E** *allocortex (heterotypical cortex)*

　> L. neocortex, neocorticis, m., f. (< G. neos *new* + L. cortex *bark*)
　　신(新)피질　　　**E** *neocortex (neopallium)*

　> L. archicortex, archicorticis, m., f. (< G. archē *beginning* + L. cortex
　　bark); archaeocortex, archaeocorticis, m., f. (< G. archaios *primitive*
　　+ L. cortex *bark*)
　　원시(原始)피질　　　**E** *archicortex (archaeocortex, archeocortex) (archipallium)*

　> L. palaeocortex, palaeocorticis, m., f. (< G. palaios *antient* + L. cortex
　　bark) 고(古)피질　　　**E** *palaeocortex (paleocortex) (paleopallium)*

> L. curtus, curta, curtum 절단된, 자른, 잘린, 짧은　　　**E** *curt, curtail*

> L. scrobis, scrobis, m., f. 구덩이, 우묵한 구멍

　> L. scrobiculus, scrobiculi, m. (< + -culus *diminutive suffix*) 작은 오목,
　　소와(小窩)　　　**E** *scrobiculus, scrobiculate*

> L. scrofa, scrofae, f. (scropha, scrophae, f.) (< *rooter, digger*) 씨암퇘지　　**E** *screw*

　> L. scrofulae, scrofularum, f. (scrophulae, scrophularum, f.) (pl.) (<
　　supposed to be subject to the disease < + -ula *diminutive suffix*)
　　결핵성 경부 림프절염, 피부샘병　　　**E** *scrofula*

> G. keirein (*ablaut stem* ker-, kor-) *to cut, to poll, to lop*

　> kormos, kormou, m. *tree trunk*

　　> L. cormus, cormi, m. (식물) 알줄기, 구경(球莖)　　　**E** *corm*

> G. epikarsios, epikarsios, epikarsion (< ep(i)- *upon*) *at an angle, oblique, sideways,
　crosswise, head foremost*　　　**E** *(perhaps) bias*

> IE. skreu- *to cut, cutting
　tool*　　　**E** *shred, shroud (< 'piece of garment'), scroll (< 'scrap of parchment')*

　> L. scrotum, scroti, n. (< *leather quiver for arrows*) 음낭(陰囊)　**E** *scrotum, scrotal*

　> L. scruta, scrutorum, n. (pl.) 헌 옷가지, 넝마

　　> L. scrutor, scrutatus sum, scrutari (< *to search even to the rags*)
　　　샅샅이 뒤지다

> L. scrutinium, scrutinii, n. 정밀 조사　　**E** *scrutiny, scrutinize*

> L. inscrutabilis, inscrutabile (< in- *not*) 헤아릴 수 없는,

　　꿰뚫어볼 수 없는　　**E** *inscrutable*

> IE. skribh- *to cut, to separate, to sift*

　> L. scribo, **scripsi,** scriptum, scribĕre 새기다, 글을

　　쓰다　　**E** *scribe,* (scriptum (*neuter past participle*) '*written*' >) *script, shrive*

　　> L. scriptura, scripturae, f. 글; (Scriptura) 성서　　**E** *scripture*

　　> L. scriptorium, scriptorii, n. 필사실, 문서실　　**E** *scriptorium*

　　> L. manuscriptus, manuscripta, manuscriptum (< manu (abl. sing.

　　　of manus) *with a hand* + scriptus (*past participle*) *written*)

　　　손으로 쓴　　**E** *manuscript*

　　> L. ascribo, **ascripsi,** ascriptum, ascribĕre (< a- (< ad) *to, toward,*

　　　at, according to + scribĕre *to write*) 덧붙여 쓰다, 명단에 기입

　　　하다, 가입시키다, (원인·동기·기원을 ~에게) 돌리다, (결과 등을

　　　~의) 탓으로 하다, 귀속시키다　　**E** *ascribe*

　　> L. circumscribo, **circumscripsi,** circumscriptum, circumscribĕre

　　　(< circum- *around* + scribĕre *to write*) 둘레에 경계선을 긋다,

　　　경계선으로 주위를 둘러싸다, 한계를 정하다　　**E** *circumscribe*

　　　> L. circumscriptio, circumscriptionis, f. 윤곽, 한계선,

　　　　한정　　**E** *circumscription*

　　> L. conscribo, **conscripsi,** conscriptum, conscribĕre (< con- (<

　　　cum) *with, together* + scribĕre *to write*) 기입하다, 등록하다,

　　　(병적에 등록하여) 징집하다　　**E** *conscript*

　　　> L. conscriptio, conscriptionis, f. 기입, 등록, 징집　　**E** *conscription*

　　> L. describo, **descripsi,** descriptum, describĕre (< de- *apart from,*

　　　down, not; intensive + scribĕre *to write*) 베끼다, 윤곽을 그리다,

　　　기술하다, 묘사하다　　**E** *describe, descriptive, nondescript*

　　　> L. descriptio, descriptionis, f. 기술, 묘사　　**E** *description*

　　> L. inscribo, **inscripsi,** inscriptum, inscribĕre (< in- *in, on, into,*

　　　toward + scribĕre *to write*) 써넣다, 새기다　　**E** *inscribe*

　　　> L. inscriptio, inscriptionis, f. 기입, 새김　　**E** *inscription*

　　> L. postscribo, **postscripsi,** postscriptum, postscribĕre (< post-

　　　after + scribĕre *to write*) 뒤에 쓰다, 뒤에 이어 쓰다

　　　E (postscriptum (*neuter past participle*) '*after-written*' >) *postscript*
　　　(P.S.)

　　> L. praescribo, **praescripsi,** praescriptum, praescribĕre (< prae-

　　　before, beyond + scribĕre *to write*) 앞에 기록하다, 규정하다,

　　　지시하다　　**E** *prescribe, prescript*

　　　> L. praescriptio, praescriptionis, f. 규정, 지시, 처방　　**E** *prescription*

　　> L. proscribo, **proscripsi,** proscriptum, proscribĕre (< pro- *before,*

　　　forward; for; instead of + scribĕre *to write*) 게시하다, 공고하다,

(고대 로마에서) 처벌자의 이름을 공포하다, 금지하다　　　**E** *proscribe*

> L. subscribo, **subscripsi**, subscriptum, subscriběre (< sub- *under,
up from under* + scriběre *to write*) 밑에 쓰다, 서명하다, 등록
하다, 응모하다, 구독하다　　　**E** *subscribe, subscript*

> L. superscribo, **superscripsi**, superscriptum, superscriběre (< super-
above + scriběre *to write*) 위에 쓰다　　　**E** *superscribe, superscript*

> L. transcribo, **transcripsi**, transcriptum, transcriběre (< trans- *over,
across, through, beyond* + scriběre *to write*) 옮겨 쓰다,
베끼다　　　**E** *transcribe, transcript*

> L. transcriptio, transcriptionis, f. 필사(筆寫),
전사(轉寫)　　　**E** *transcription, (transcription >) transcriptase*

> G. skariphos, skariphou, m. *pencil, stylus*

> G. skariphasthai *to scratch an outline, to sketch lightly, to do
anything slightly or slovenly*

> L. scarifo, **scarifavi**, scarifatum, scarifare 살짝 째다, 살짝
터트리다, 난절법(난자법)으로 치료하다　　　**E** *scarify, scarification*

> IE. skreup- *to cut*

> L. scrupus, scrupi, m. 거칠고 모난 돌, (신 안의 굵은 모래알 >) 걱정,
(병적인) 세심

> L. scrupulus, scrupuli, m. (< + -ulus *diminutive suffix*) 모난 작은
자갈, 미량, (신 안의) 굵은 모래알, (신 안의 굵은 모래알 >)
걱정, (병적인) 세심　　　**E** *scruple*

> L. scrupulosus, scrupulosa, scrupulosum 모난 작은 돌의,
세심한, 면밀한　　　**E** *scrupulous*

servo, servavi, servatum, servare 지키다, 주의하다

> conservo, **conservavi**, conservatum, conservare (< con- (< cum) *with, together*) 지키다,
보호하다, 보존하다　　　**E** *conserve, conservative, conservation*

> conservatorius, conservatoria, conservatorium 보호하는,
보존하는　　　**E** *conservatory, conservatoire*

> observo, **observavi**, observatum, observare (< ob- *before, toward(s), over, against,
away*) 지키다, 지켜보다, 관찰하다　　　**E** *observe, observation*

> observatorium, observatorii, n. 관측소, 전망대　　　**E** *observatory*

> praeservo, **praeservavi**, praeservatum, praeservare (< prae- *before, beyond*) 지키다,
보존하다　　　**E** *preserve, preservative, preservation*

> reservo, **reservavi**, reservatum, reservare (< re- *back, again*) (뒷일을 위해) 남겨 두다,
유보하다, 마련해 두다, 저장하다, 보유하다,
예약하다　　　**E** *reserve, reservation, reservatory, reservoir*

< IE. ser- *to protect*

> (*perhaps*) G. hērōs, hērōos, m. (< *protector*) *hero, demigod*

> L. heros, herois, m. 영웅

E *hero*, D. *heroin* (< *'inflation of the personality consequent upon taking the drug')*

> G. hērōinē, hērōinēs, f. *heroine*

    > L. heroina, heroinae, f. (heroine, heroines, f.) 여걸, 여주인공   **E** *heroine*

> G. hērōikos, hērōikē, hērōikon *heroic*

    > L. heroicus, heroica, heroicum 영웅의, 영웅다운   **E** *heroic*

sibilo, sibilavi, sibilatum, sibilare 식식 소리 나다, 식식 소리 내다, 휘파람 불다, 야유하다, 마찰음을 내다, 치찰음(齒擦音)을 내다   **E** *sibilate, sibilant*

  < IE. swei- (*imitative root*) *to whistle, to hiss*

spiro, spiravi, spiratum, spirare 입김을 내불다, 숨 쉬다, 발산하다, 생각하다, 갈망하다   **E** *spirograph, spirometer*

> spiritus, spiritus, m. 숨, 정신, 신, 정령   **E** *spirit*, F. *esprit*

    > spiritualis, spirituale 정신적인, 혼의, 정령의   **E** *spiritual, spiritualism*

> spiraculum, spiraculi, n. 바람구멍, 환기창, 영감, 호흡구멍, 기문(氣門)   **E** *spiracle*

> aspiro, **aspiravi**, aspiratum, aspirare (adspiro, **adspiravi**, adspiratum, adspirare) (< a-

    (< ad) *to, toward, at, according to* + spirare *to breathe*) 숨 쉬다, 흡인(吸引)하다, 갈망하다   **E** *aspirate, aspirator, aspire, aspirant*

    > aspiratio, aspirationis, f. 흡인, 갈망   **E** *aspiration*

> conspiro, **conspiravi**, conspiratum, conspirare (< con- (< cum) *with, together* + spirare

    to breathe) 호흡이 맞다, 뜻을 같이하다, 모의하다   **E** *conspire, conspiracy*

> exspiro, **exspiravi**, exspiratum, exspirare (expiro, **expiravi**, expiratum, expirare)

    (< ex- *out of, away from* + spirare *to breathe*) 숨을 내쉬다, 만기가 되다, 숨이 끊어지다   **E** *expire, expiratory, expiry*

    > expiratio, expirationis, f. 날숨, 호기(呼氣), 종료, (고어) 사망   **E** *expiration*

> inspiro, **inspiravi**, inspiratum, inspirare (< in- *in, on, into, toward* + spirare *to breathe*)

    숨을 들이쉬다, 흡입(吸入)하다, (사상·감정을) 불어넣다, 영감을 주다   **E** *inspire, inspiratory*

    > inspiratio, inspirationis, f. 들숨, 흡기(吸氣), 영감   **E** *inspiration*

> respiro, **respiravi**, respiratum, respirare (< re- *back, again* + spirare *to breathe*)

    숨 쉬다, 호흡하다   **E** *respire, respiratory*

    > respiratio, respirationis, f. 호흡   **E** *respiration*

> perspiro, **perspiravi**, perspiratum, perspirare (< per- *through, thoroughly* + spirare

    to breathe) 사방으로 불다, 땀 흘리다   **E** *perspire, perspiratory*

    > perspiratio, perspirationis, f. 발한(發汗), 분투   **E** *perspiration*

> suspiro, **suspiravi**, suspiratum, suspirare (< su- (< sub) *under, up from under* +

    spirare *to breathe*) 한숨 쉬다, 탄식하다   **E** *suspire*

    > suspiratio, suspirationis, f. 한숨, 탄식   **E** *suspiration*

> transpiro, **transpiravi**, transpiratum, transpirare (< trans- *over, across, through,

    beyond* + spirare *to breathe*) 증발하다, 땀 흘리다   **E** *transpire*

    > transpiratio, transpirationis, f. 증발, 발한(發汗), 불감수분손실, 증산(蒸散)   **E** *transpiration*

  < IE. (s)peis- *to blow*

sto, steti, statum, stare 서다, 서 있다, 오래가다

> **E** *stay, stage, staging,* (stans (*present participle*) *'standing'* >) It. *stanza,* (It. stanza >) *stance*

[용례] In medio stat virtus. 덕은 중용에 있다, 德在中庸

  (문법) in 안에: 전치사, 탈격지배

    medio 중용: 형용사의 명사적 용법, 중성 단수 탈격

      < medius, media, medium 가운데

    stat 서 있다: 능동태 직설법 현재 단수 삼인칭

    virtus 덕은: 단수 주격 < virtus, virtutis, f.

> status, status, m. 상태, 현상, 체질, 신분, 지위

> **E** *status, estate, state,* F. *etat, nystatin* (< *'acronym of New York State, where it was developed'*)

[용례] status asthmaticus 천식지속상태　　　　　　　　　　　**E** *status asthmaticus*

　　　status epilepticus 뇌전증지속상태　　　　　　　　　　**E** *status epilepticus*

　　　status praesens 현재상태 (현재소견)

　　　(문법) status 상태: 단수 주격

　　　　　asthmaticus 천식의: 형용사, 남성형 단수 주격

　　　　　　< asthmaticus, asthmatica, asthmaticum

　　　　　epilepticus 뇌전증의: 형용사, 남성형 단수 주격

　　　　　　< epilepticus, epileptica, epilepticum

　　　　　praesens 앞에 있는, 출석한, 현재의: 현재분사, 남·여·중성형 단수 주격

　　　　　　< praesens, (gen.) praesentis

　　　　　　< praeesse (< prae- *before, beyond* + esse *to be*) 앞에 있다

　> statista, statistae, m. 정치인

　　> statisticus, statistica, statisticum 정치의, 정치에 필요한 자료의,

　　　통계의　　　　　　　　　　　　　　　**E** *statistic, statistics, statistical*

> statio, stationis, f. 체류, 정지, 정박소　　　　　　　　　　**E** *station*

　> stationarius, stationaria, stationarium 움직이지 않는, 고정된, 정박소가 있는

> **E** *stationary, stationer* (< *'a tradesman (chiefly, a bookseller) who has a station or shop, as distinguished from an itinerant vendor'*), *stationery* (< *'the articles sold by a stationer; writing materials, writing-table belongings'*)

> statura, staturae, f. 키, 신장, 높이　　　　　　　　　　　**E** *stature*

> statua, statuae, f. (사람의) 상(像), 조상(彫像)　　　　　　　**E** *statue*

> stator, statoris, m. 지키는 사람; (Stator) (로마 신화) Jupiter의 별칭; (물리·전기)

　　고정자(固定子)　　　　　　　　　　　　　　　　　　**E** *stator*

> stamen, staminis, n. 베틀의 날실, 꽃의 수술, 운명의 실　**E** *stamen,* (pl.) *stamina (stamens)*

> stabulum, stabuli, n. 거처, 여인숙,

　　사육장, 마구간　　　　　　**E** *stable,* (comes stabuli *'count of the stable'* >) *constable*

> stabilis, stabile 견고한, 안정된　　　　　**E** *stable,* (stable >) *unstable, stabilize*

　> stabilitas, stabilitatis, f. 안정　　　　　　　　　　　　　**E** *stability*

　> instabilis, instabile (< in- *not*) 불안정한

　　　　　　　　　　　　　　　　　　　　　E (*now rare*) *instable*

> instabilitas, instabilitatis, f. 불안정　　　　　　　　**E** *instability*

　　　> stabilio, **stabilivi**, **stabilitum**, stabilire 견고히 하다, 안정되게 하다　　**E** *establish*

> statim (부사) 선 채로, 즉시　　　　　　　　　　　　　　**E** *stat*

> postis, postis, m. (< por- (< pro) *before, forward, for, instead of* + *stem of* stare)

　　　문설주, 문짝

　　　　E *post* (< *'piece of timber, etc., set upright'*), *poster* (< *'a notice fastened to a post'*)

> sisto, **stiti** (steti), **statum**, sistĕre 세우다, 멈추게 하다, 공고히 하다

　　　> armistitium, armistitii, n. 휴전, 정전 (< arma, armorum, n. *arms* + sistĕre

　　　　　to make to stand)　　　　　　　　　　　　　　**E** *armistice*

　　　> solstitium, solstitii, n. (< sol, solis, m. *sun* + sistĕre *to make to stand*)

　　　　　(하지·동지의) 지점(至點), 전환점　　　　　　　　**E** *solstice*

　　　> assisto, **astiti**, −, assistĕre (< as- (< ad) *to, toward, at, according to* + sistĕre

　　　　　to make to stand) 옆에 서다, 옆에서 거들다, 보조하다

　　　　E *assist,* (assistens (*present participle*) *'assisting'* + -ant (*Latin present participle*
　　　　suffix) >) *assistant,* (assistentia >) *assistance*

　　　> consisto, **constiti**, **constitum**, consistĕre (< con- (< cum) *with, together* + sistĕre

　　　　　to make to stand) 멈춰서다, 이루어지다, 성립하다　　**E** *consist, consistent*

　　　　　> consistentia, consistentiae, f. 성립　　　　　**E** *consistence (consistency)*

　　　> desisto, **destiti**, **destitum**, desistĕre (< de- *apart from, down, not* + sistĕre

　　　　　to make to stand) 그만두다, 단념하다　　　　　　**E** *desist*

　　　> exsisto, **exstiti**, **exstitum**, exsistĕre (existo, **existiti**, **existitum**, existĕre) (< ex-

　　　　　out of, away from + sistĕre *to make to stand*) 생겨나다, 존재하다　**E** *exist, existent*

　　　　　> existentia, existentiae, f. 존재, 실존　　　　　**E** *existence*

　　　　　　　> existentialis, existentiale 존재의, 실존의　**E** *existential, existentialism*

　　　> insisto, **institi**, −, insistĕre (< in- *in, on, into, toward* + sistĕre *to make to*

　　　　　stand) 위에 서다, 버티고 서다, 노력하다, 주장하다　**E** *insist, insistent*

　　　> intersisto, **interstiti**, **interstitum**, intersistĕre (< inter- *between, among* + sistĕre

　　　　　to make to stand) 사이에 서다

　　　　　> interstitium, interstitii, n. 간극(間隙),

　　　　　　　사이질　　　　**E** *interstitium,* (pl.) *interstitia, interstitial, interstice*

　　　> persisto, **perstiti**, −, persistĕre (< per- *through, thoroughly* + sistĕre *to make*

　　　　　to stand) 항구하게 머무르다, 지속하다　　　**E** *persist, persistent, persistence*

　　　> resisto, **restiti**, **restitum**, resistĕre (< re- *against* + sistĕre *to make to stand*)

　　　　　저항하다

　　　　E *resist,* (resistens (*present participle*) *'resisting'* + -ant (*Latin present participle*
　　　　suffix) >) *resistant,* (resistentia >) *resistance, resistible, irresistible, resistor*

　　　> subsisto, **substiti**, **substitum**, subsistĕre (< sub- *under, up from under* +

　　　　　sistĕre *to make to stand*) 머물다, 존속하다, 존재하다　**E** *subsist, subsistent*

　　　　　> subsistentia, subsistentiae, f. 존속, 존재, 생존　　**E** *subsistence*

> statuo, **statui**, **statutum**, statuĕre 세우다, 정하다, 결정하다, 제정하다,

　　　명령하다　　　　　　　**E** (statutum (*neuter past participle*) *'set up, placed'* >) *statute*

> constituo, **constitui**, constitutum, constituĕre (< con- (< cum) *with, together* + statuĕre *to set up, to place*) 세우다, 구성하다,
제정하다 **E** *constitute, constituent, (constituent >) constituency, reconstitute*
　　> constitutio, constitutionis, f. 구성, 체질, 제정, 헌법 **E** *constitution*
> destituo, **destitui**, destitutum, destituĕre (< de- *apart from, down, not* + statuĕre *to set up, to place*) 내버려두다 **E** *destitute*
　　> destitutio, destitutionis, f. 내버려둠 **E** *destitution*
> instituo, **institui**, institutum, instituĕre (< in- *in, on, into, toward* + statuĕre *to set up, to place*) 설립하다, 지정하다, 양성하다 **E** *(verb) institute*
　　> institutum, instituti, n. 계획, 제도, 연구기관, 교육기관 **E** *(noun) institute*
　　> institutio, institutionis, f. 체계, 제도, 양성 **E** *institution*
> prostituo, **prostitui**, prostitutum, prostituĕre (< *offered for sale* < *exposed publicly* < pro- *before, forward, for, instead of* + statuĕre *to set up, to place*) 몸을 팔게 하다, 몸을 팔다 **E** *prostitute, prostitution*
> restituo, **restitui**, restitutum, restituĕre (< re- *back, again* + statuĕre *to set up, to place*) 제자리에 도로 세워놓다, 복구하다, 복원하다 **E** *restitute, restitution*
> substituo, **substitui**, substitutum, substituĕre (< sub- *under, up from under* + statuĕre *to set up, to place*) 대신 세우다, 대체하다,
치환하다 **E** *substitute, substituent*
　　> substitutio, substitutionis, f. 대체, 치환 **E** *substitution*
> circumsto, **circumsteti**, −, circumstare (< circum- *around* + stare *to stand*) 둘러 서 있다, 둘러서다, 에워싸다
　> circumstantia, circumstantiae, f. 환경, 상황, 형편 **E** *circumstance*
> consto, **constiti**, constaturus, constare (< con- (< cum) *with, together* + stare *to stand*) 그대로 서 있다, 지속하다, 가치가 있다, 값이 ~이다 **E** *constant, cost*
　> constantia, constantiae, f. 지속성, 항상성(恒常性), 항존성(恒存性) **E** *constancy*
> contrasto, **contrastiti**, contrastatum, contrastare (< contra- *against* + stare *to stand*) 앞을 막다, 버티다, 대조를 이루다, 대비하다, 대비해서 뚜렷한 차이를 보이다 **E** *contrast*
> disto, −, −, distare (< dis- *apart from, down, not* + stare *to stand*) (공간적·시간적으로) 떨어져 있다 **E** *distant, equidistant*
　> distantia, distantiae, f. 거리, 간격 **E** *distance, equidistance*
　> distalis, distale (< *in contrast to proximal*) 기점(基點)에서 떨어져 있는, 먼쪽의, 원위(遠位)의, 말단의 **E** *distal*
> exsto, **exstiti**, exstatum, exstare (exto, **extiti**, extatum, extare) (< ex- *out of, away from* + stare *to stand*) 밖에 드러나 있다, (아직도) 남아 있다, 존재하다 **E** *extant*
> insto, **institi**, instaturus, instare (< in- *in, on, into, toward* + stare *to stand*) ~에 서 있다, (공간적·시간적으로) 가까이 있다, 임박하다 **E** *instant*
　> instantia, instantiae, f. 현재, 순간, 절박; (법률) 소송 **E** *instance*
> obsto, **obstiti**, obstatum, obstare (< ob- *before, toward(s), over, against, away* + stare *to stand*) 앞에 서다, 앞을 막다, 못 하게 하다 **E** *oust*
　> obstaculum, obstaculi, n. 장애, 장애물 **E** *obstacle*

> obstino, **obstinavi**, obstinatum, obstinare 끝까지 버티다, 고집하다   **E** *obstinate*

     > obstinatia, obstinatiae, f. 고집, 완고, 끈질김   **E** *obstinacy*

> obstetrix, obstetricis, f. (< *(midwife) being present*)

     조산원   **E** *obstetric, obstetrician, obstetrics*

> resto, **restiti**, −, restare (< re- *back, again* + stare *to stand*) 뒤에 남다, 남아 있다,

     멈추다

     E *rest,* (ad *'to'* + restare *'to remain, to stop'* >) *arrest, restive* (< *'inclined to remain still'*)

> supersto, **supersteti**, −, superstare (< super- *above* + stare *to stand*) 위에 서 있다,

     우위에 있다

     > superstitio, superstitionis, f. (< *(perhaps) standing over a thing in amazement*

         or awe, a state of religious exaltation) 미신(迷信)   **E** *superstition*

         > superstitiosus, superstitiosa, superstitiosum 미신에 사로잡힌, 미신의 **E** *superstitious*

> substo, −, −, substare (< sub- *under, up from under* + stare *to stand*) 밑에 서

     있다, 버티다, 존재하다

     > substantia, substantiae, f. 물질(物質), 질(質), 실체(實體)   **E** *substance, substantive*

         [용례] substantia nigra (< *black substance*) 흑색질(黑色質),

             흑질(黑質)   **E** *substantia nigra*

           substantia grisea (< *gray matter*) 회색질(灰色質)

           substantia alba (< *white matter*) 백색질(白色質)

           (문법) substantia: 단수 주격

              nigra 검은: 형용사, 여성형 단수 주격 < niger, nigra, nigrum

              grisea 회색의: 형용사, 여성형 단수 주격

                < griseus, grisea, griseum

              alba 흰: 형용사, 여성형 단수 주격 < albus, alba, album

         > substantialis, substantiale 물질적인, 실체가 있는, 본질적인   **E** *substantial*

         > substantio, **substantiavi**, substantiatum, substantiare 실체화하다, 실증

            하다, 입증하다   **E** *substantiate*

> destino, **destinavi**, destinatum, destinare (< de- *apart from, down, not; intensive* +

     stare *to stand*) 붙잡아 매다, 정하다,

     목표로 정하다   **E** *destine,* (destinata *(feminine past participle) 'determined'* >) *destiny*

     > destinatio, destinationis, f. 지정, 목표, 목적지   **E** *destination*

     > praedestino, **praedestinavi**, praedestinatum, praedestinare (< prae- *before,*

         beyond + destinare *to establish*) 미리 정하다   **E** *predestinate*

         > praedestinatio, praedestinationis, f. 예정, 숙명   **E** *predestination*

< IE. sta- *to stand, with derivatives meaning 'place or thing that is standing'*

   E *stand,* (*to stand still* >) *standstill, understand, withstand, bystander, stem, steady, stud,* *steed, stool* (< *'a wooden seat, the place of evacuation, the matter evacuated'*), *steer,* *stern* (< *'steering'*), *steel* (< *'that which stands firm'*), *stow* (< *'place'*), *bestow* (< *'to place'*)

> L. -stauro, -stauravi, -stauratum, -staurare 놓다, 세우다

     > L. instauro, **instauravi**, instauratum, instaurare (< in- *in, on, into, toward* +

         -staurare *to place, to erect*) 준비하다   **E** *store, storage, instauration*

> L. restauro, **restauravi**, restauratum, restaurare (< re- *back, again* + -staurare *to place, to erect*) 복원하다, 복구하다

> **E** **restore, restoration, restorative, restaurant** *(< 'where refreshments or meals are obtained')*

> G. histanai (sta- *root of* histanai) *to make stand, to set, to place*

> G. stasis, staseōs, f. (< sta- + -sis *feminine noun suffix*) *standing, standstill*

> **E** *dysstasia*

> L. stasis, stasis, f. 정지, 정체, 저류(貯溜), 울체(鬱滯), 울혈(鬱血)

> **E** *stasis, -stasis, bacteriostasis, bacteriostatic*

> L. homoeostasis, homoeostasis, f. (< G. homoios *like, similar, resembling, of the same*) 항상성(恒常性)

> **E** *homoeostasis (homeostasis), homeostatic*

> L. haemostasis, haemostasis, f. (< G. haima, haimatos, n. *blood*) 지혈(止血)

> **E** *haemostasis (hemostasis), hemostatic, hemostat*

> L. cholestasis, cholestasis, f. (< G. cholē, cholēs, f. *bile*) 쓸개즙 정체

> **E** *cholestasis, cholestatic*

> L. metastasis, metastasis, f. (< G. met(a)- *between, along with, across, after* + stasis *standing*) 전이(轉移), 전이종양, 전이병원체

> **E** *metastasis, (pl.) metastases, metastatic, metastasize*

> G. apostasis, apostaseōs, f. (< ap(o)- *away from, from*) *standing off, desertion of one's faith*

> L. apostasia, apostasiae, f. 배교(背敎)

> **E** *apostasy*

> G. ekstasis, ekstaseōs, f. (< ek- *out of, away from*) *standing outside oneself*

> L. ecstasis, ecstasis, f. 무아의 경지, 황홀경, 황홀감

> **E** *ecstasy*

> G. epistasis, epistaseōs, f. (< ep(i)- *upon*) *stopping, checking, halt; assembly; inspection; attention*

> L. epistasis, epistasis, f. 상위, 억제

> **E** *epistasis*

> G. statos, statē, staton *standing, stationary, placed*

> **E** **stat(o)-, -stat, -statin, statin(s)** *(< 'drugs which reduce cholesterol levels in the blood by inhibiting the rate-limiting enzyme, HMG-CoA reductase, for biosynthesis of cholesterol')*

> G. astatos, astatos, astaton *unstable* **E** *astatic, astatine (At)* *(< 'short half-life')*

> G. statikos, statikē, statikon *causing to stand*

> L. staticus, statica, staticum 정지시키는, 정지하고 있는, 정적인 **E** *static, -static*

> G. diistanai (< di(a)- *through, thoroughly, apart* + histanai) *to separate*

> G. diastasis, diastaseōs, f. (< di(a)- *through, thoroughly, apart* + stasis) *separation*

> L. diastasis, diastasis, f. 분리, 이개(離開), (심박) 정지(靜止)

> **E** *diastasis,* F. *diastase* *(< 'separating starch into simple sugars: amylase'), (diastase >) -ase*

> G. diastēma, diastēmatos, n. (< di(a)- *through, thoroughly, apart* +

-stēma) *space between, interval*

> L. diastema, diastematis, n. 틈, 이 틈새,

치아 틈새　　　　　　　　E *diastema (diastem),* (pl.) *diastemata*

> G. proistanai (< pro- *before, in front* + histanai) *to set before*

> G. prostatēs, prostatou, m. *front-rank man, protector, leader*

> L. prostata, prostatae, f. 전립선(前立腺)

E *prostate, prostatic, prostaglandin(s)* (< 'monocyclic structure');
prostacyclin (prostagladin I₂) (< 'bicyclic structure')

> G. synistanai (< syn- *with, together* + histanai) *to place together*

> G. systēma, systēmatos, n. (< sy- (< syn-) *with, together* + -stēma)
composition, organized government, constitution

> L. systema, systematis, n. 체계, 계통, 조직

E *system,* (system >) *systemic* (< 'used for differentiation of meaning
instead of the regular 'systematic'')

> G. systēmatikos, systēmatikē, systēmatikon *according to a system*

> L. systematicus, systematica, systematicum 체계적인, 잘

정돈된　　　　　　　　E *systematic*

> G. epistasthai (< ep(i)- *above* + histasthai (*passive of* histanai) *to know
how to do, to understand*

> G. epitēmē, epitēmēs, f. *knowledge, intelligence, insight; skill; science,
art*　　　　　　　　E *episteme*

> G. histos, histou, m. (< *that which is set up*) *ship's mast, loom, warp, web, tissue*

E *histogram* (< 'graphical representation by columns which are set upright'), *hist(o)-,
histology, histone, histidine (His, H), histamine* (< 'an amine formed from histidine
by decarboxylation')

> G. histion, histiou, n. (< histos *tissue* + -ion, -iou, n. *diminutive suffix*) *sail,
web, tissue*　　　　　　　　E *histi(o)-, histiocyte, histiocytic*

> G. stoa, stoas, f. *portico, roofed colonnade; specifically the great hall at Athens
(adorned with frescoes of the battle of Marathon), in which Zeno lectured, and
from which his disciples were called Stoics*　　　　　　E *stoa, Stoic*

> G. stylos, stylou, m. *pillar, prop*　　　　　　E *stylite, sarcostyle*

> G. styloeidēs, styloeidēs, styloeides (< + eidos *shape*) *pillar-like*

> L. styloideus, styloidea, styloideum 기둥 모양의, 경상(莖狀)의; (*meaning
influenced by unrelated* L. stilus (stylus) *pointed instrument*) 첨필(尖筆)
모양의, 붓 모양의　　　　　　　　E *styloid*

> (*Persian*) -stan (< *where one stands*) *country*　　E *-stan, Afghanistan* (< 'Land of Afghans')

> IE. tauro- *bull*

> G. tauros, taurou, m. *bull*　　E *taurine, taurocholic acid* (< 'obtained from ox-bile')

> L. taurus, tauri, m. 황소; (Taurus) (천문) 황소자리　　E *Taurus, toreador, torero*

> G. Minōtauros, Minōtaurou, m. (< Minōs *Minos*) (*Greek mythology*)
Minotaur

> L. Minotaurus, Minotauri, m. (그리스 신화) 미노타우루스　　　E *Minotaur*

sudo, sudavi, sudatum, sudare 땀 흘리다, 적시다, 방울방울 떨어뜨리다

E *sudation*

> sudor, sudoris, m. 땀, 발한(發汗)　　　　**E** *sudomotor* (< 'on the pattern of vasomotor')

　　> sudorificus, sudorifica, sudorificum (< sudor *sweat* + -ficus (< facĕre) *making*)

　　　　땀을 만드는, 발한(성)의　　　　　　　　　　　　**E** *sudorific*

　　> sudoriparus, sudoripara, sudoriparum (< sudor *sweat* + -parus (< parĕre *to bring*

　　　　forth, to bear) *bearing*) 땀을 낳는, 발한(성)의　　　**E** *sudoriparous*

　　> sudorifer, sudorifera, sudoriferum (< sudor *sweat* + -fer (< ferre *to carry,*

　　　　to bear) *carrying, bearing*) 땀을 흐르게 하는, 발한(성)의　**E** *sudoriferous*

　　> sudarium, sudarii, n. 수건, 손수건　　　　　　　　　**E** *sudarium*

> sudatorius, sudatoria, sudatorium 땀나게 하는, 발한성(發汗性)의

　　> sudatorium, sudatorii, n. 한증막, 증기 목욕　　　　**E** *sudatorium*

> exsudo, exsudavi, exsudatum, exsudare (exudo, exudavi, exudatum, exudare) (< ex-

　　out of, away from + sudare *to sweat*) 땀으로 나오다, 스며 나오다,

　　삼출(滲出)하다　　　　　　　　　　　　　　　　**E** *exude, exudate*

　　> exudatio, exudationis, f. 삼출(滲出)　　　　　　　**E** *exudation*

> insudo, insudavi, insudatum, insudare (< in- *in, on, into, toward* + sudare *to sweat*)

　　몹시 땀 흘리다

　　> insudatio, insudationis, f. (< *seepage of plasma or other constituents of*

　　　　blood through arterial wall) 벽내삼출(壁內滲出)　　**E** *insudation*

> transsudo, transsudavi, transsudatum, transsudare (transudo, transudavi, transudatum,

　　transudare) (< trans- *over, across, through, beyond* + sudare *to sweat*) 누출(漏出)

　　하다　　　　　　　　　　　　　　　　　　　**E** *transude, transudate*

　　> transudatio, transudationis, f. 누출(漏出)　　　**E** *transudation*

< IE. sweid- *sweat, to sweat*　　　　　　　　　　　**E** *sweat*

> G. hidrōs, hidrōtos, m. *sweat, perspiration*　　　**E** *hidr(o)-*

　　> G. hidrōsis, hidrōseōs, f. (< + -sis *feminine noun suffix*) *sweating*

　　　　> L. hidrosis, hidrosis, f. 발한(發汗)　　　　**E** *hidrosis, -hidrosis*

　　　　> L. osmidrosis, osmidrosis, f. (< G. osmē *smell*)

　　　　　　땀악취증　　　　　　　　　　　　**E** *osmidrosis (bromidrosis)*

　　　　> L. anidrosis, anidrosis, f. (< G. an- *not*)

　　　　　　땀없음증　　　　　　　　　　　　**E** *anidrosis (anhidrosis)*

　　　　> L. dysidrosis, dysidrosis, f. (< G. dys- *bad*)

　　　　　　땀흘림이상　　　　　　　　　　　**E** *dysidrosis (dyshidrosis)*

　　　　> L. bromidrosis, bromidrosis, f. (< G. brōmos *bad smell*)

　　　　　　땀악취증　　　　　　　　**E** *bromidrosis (bromhidrosis) (osmidrosis)*

　　　　> L. hyperidrosis, hyperidrosis, f. (< G. hyper- *over*) 땀과다증,

　　　　　　다한증(多汗症)　　　　　　　　**E** *hyperidrosis (hyperhidrosis)*

titubo, titubavi, titubatum, titubare 비틀거리다　　　　**E** *titubate*

tolero, toleravi, toleratum, tolerare 견디다, 용인하다, 내성이 있다

E *tolerate, tolerant*

> tolerantia, tolerantiae, f. 견딤, 용인, 관용, 허용 오차, 내성(耐性)　　　　**E** *tolerance*

　　> intolerantia, intolerantiae, f. (< in- *not*) 못 견딤, 불관용, 편협　　**E** *intolerance*

> tolerabilis, tolerabile 견딜 수 있는　　　　　　　　　　　　　　　**E** *tolerable*

　　> intolerabilis, intolerabile (< in- *not*) 견딜 수 없는　　　　　**E** *intolerable*

< IE. telə- *to lift, to support, to weigh; with derivatives referring to measured weights and*
　　thence to money and payment

　　> L. tollo, **sustuli**, sublatum, tollĕre 들어올리다, 들어내 버리다　　　**E** *extol*

　　> L. talio, talionis, f. 동태복수　　　　　　　　　　　　　　　　**E** *talion*

　　　　[용례] lex talionis (< *law of retaliation*) 동태복수법
　　　　　　(문법) lex 법: 단수 주격 < lex, legis, f.
　　　　　　　　talionis 동태복수의: 단수 속격

　　　　> L. retalio, **retaliavi**, retaliatum, retaliare (< re- *back, again*) (상대방과 같은
　　　　　　수단으로) 앙갚음하다, 보복하다, 동태복수법을 적용하다　　　**E** *retaliate*

　　> L. latus, lata, latum (**ferre**의 과거분사) 가져다준, 지닌 (Vide FERRE: *See* E. *-ferous*)

　　> G. telos, telous, n. *toll, tax, duty*　　　　　　　　　　　　　**E** *toll*

　　　　> G. atelēs, atelēs, ateles (< a- *not*) *free from tax or charge*

　　　　　　> G. ateleia, ateleias, f. *exemption from payment*

　　　　　　　　E *philately* (< '*a postage stamp, already paid as a result of the purchase*
　　　　　　　　and exempting the recipient from payment')

　　> G. tlēnai *to suffer, to bear, to endure, to resist*

　　　　> G. talas, talaina, talan *suffering, enduring, patient,*
　　　　　　wretched　　　　　　　　　　　　　**E** *oxytalan* (< '*acid-resistant*')

　　> G. talanton, talantou, n. *weight, specific weight of gold or silver, the sum of money*
　　　　represented by such a weight, weight of inclination

　　　　> L. talentum, talenti, n. 그리스의 무게 및 화폐 단위; 재능, 재주　　**E** *talent*

　　> G. telamōn, telamōnos, m. *bearer, supporter*

　　　　> L. telamon, telamonis, m. 남자 모양의 기둥,
　　　　　　남상주(男像柱)　　　　　　　**E** *telamon*, (pl.) *telamones* (*atlantes*)

　　> (*suggested*) G. Atlas, Atlantos, m. (< a- *prothetic* + tlan *bearing*) (*Greek mythology*)
　　　　Atlas (*one of the Titans, who was punished for this part in their revolt against*
　　　　Zeus by being made to support the heavens)

　　　　> L. Atlas, Atlantis, m. (그리스 신화)
　　　　　　아틀라스　　　　　　**E** *Atlas, Atlantic*, (pl.) (Atlantes >) *atlantes* (*telamones*)

　　　　　　> L. atlas, atlantis, m. (*a representation of Atlas supporting the heavens*
　　　　　　　　placed as a frontispiece to early maps >) 지도(地圖), 도해서(圖解書);
　　　　　　　　제1경추(頸椎), 고리뼈, 환추(環椎)　**E** *atlas*, (pl.) *atlases, atlantal, atlantoaxial*

tono, tonui, -, tonare 천둥치다, 폭음이 나다

　　E (Sp. tronada '*thunderstorm*' >) *tornado*, (ex- '*out of, away from*' + tonare '*to thunder*' >)
　　astonish, astound, (astonish >) *stun*

　　> detono, detonui, -, detonare (< de- *apart from, down, not; intensive* + tonare *to*

thunder) 천둥소리 내다, 요란하게 울리다, 폭발하다; 요란한 소리가 그치다, 멎다   **E** detonate

< IE. (s)tenə- *to thunder*

> **E** *Thor* ((*Scandinavian mythology*) *God of Thunder, son of Odin and Freya (Frigga)*), (G. hēmera Dios *'day of Zeus'*, L. dies Jovis *'day of Jupiter'* > '*Thor's day*' >) ***Thursday,*** *thunder, thunderbolt, thunderstorm*

ululo, ululavi, ululatum, ululare 소리 지르다   **E** *ululate*

> ulula, ululae, f. 올빼미소리, 올빼미

< IE. u(wa)l- (*imitative root*) *to howl*   **E** *owl, howl*

vaco, vacavi, vacatum, vacare 비어 있다, 쉬다   **E** *vacant, vacancy*

> vacuus, vacua, vacuum 비어 있는, 공허한, 진공의,

한가한   **E** *vacuous;* F. *vacuole, vacuolar, vacuolate, vacuolization; void, avoid, devoid*

> vacuum, vacui, n. 공간, 공허, 진공   **E** *vacuum*

> vacuitas, vacuitatis, f. 공간   **E** *vacuity*

> evacuo, evacuavi, evacuatum, evacuare (< e- *out of, away from* + vacuus *empty*)

비우다, 벗어나게 하다   **E** *evacuate*

> vacatio, vacationis, f. 면제, 휴가   **E** *vacation*

< IE. euə- *to leave, to abandon, to give out*   **E** *wane, want,* (wan + ton > '*badly led*' >) *wanton*

> L. vanus, vana, vanum 공허한, 헛된, 허영의   **E** *vain*

> L. vanitas, vanitatis, f. 공허, 헛됨, 허영   **E** *vanity*

> L. vanito, −, −, vanitare 자랑하다, 과시하다, 허풍 치다   **E** *vaunt*

> L. vanesco, −, −, vanescĕre (< vanus *empty* + -escĕre *suffix of inceptive* (*inchoative*) *verb*) 사라지다

> L. evanesco, evanui, −, evanescĕre (< e- *out of, away from* + vanescĕre *to vanish*) 사라지다   **E** *evanesce, evanescent, evanish,* (evanish >) *vanish*

> L. vastus, vasta, vastum 황폐한, 빈, 광대한   **E** *waste, vast*

> L. devasto, devastavi, devastatum, devastare (< de- *apart from, down, not; intensive*) 황폐케 하다, 유린하다   **E** *devastate*

veto, vetui, vetitum, vetare 금지하다,

반대하다   **E** (*first personal singular, present indicative, active 'I forbid'* >) *veto*

< *Of unknown origin*

vibro, vibravi, vibratum, vibrare 흔들다, 진동시키다, 흔들리다,

진동하다   **E** *vibrate, vibrant,* (vibrate >) *vibratory*

> vibratio, vibrationis, f. 진동   **E** *vibration*

> vibrio, vibrionis, m., f. (< *organisms characterized by vibratory motion*) 비브리오균   **E** *vibrio*

> vibrissae, vibrissarum, f. (pl.) 코털, (동물) 입 언저리의 진모(震毛)   **E** (pl.) *vibrissae*

< IE. weip- *to turn, to vacillate, to tremble ecstatically*

> **E** *waif, waive, wipe* (< '*to move back and forth*'), *whip* (< '*to move back and forth*')

vito, vitavi, vitatum, vitare 피하다

> evito, evitavi, evitatum, evitare (< e- *out of, away from* + vitare *to shun*) 피하다

> evitabilis, evitabile 피할 수 있는　　　　　　　　　　**E** *evitable, inevitable*

volo, volavi, volatum, volare 날다　　　　　　　　　　　**E** *volant, volley, volleyball*

[용례] Rumor volat. 소문은 날아다닌다
　　　(문법) rumor 소문은: 단수 주격 < rumor, rumoris, m.
　　　　　volat: 능동태 직설법 현재 단수 삼인칭

> volatilis, volatile 나는, 날개 달린; 일시적인; 휘발성의　　　**E** *volatile*
> volito, volitavi, volitatum, volitare (*frequentative*) 자주 날다, 여기저기 날아다니다

[용례] muscae volitantes 날파리증, 비문증(飛蚊症)　　　　**E** *muscae volitantes*
　　　(문법) muscae 파리들: 복수 주격 < musca, muscae, f.
　　　　　volitantes 여기저기 날아다니는: 현재분사, 남·여·중성형 복수 주격

< IE. gʷel- *to fly, a wing*
∞ IE. gʷelə- *to throw, to reach, with further meaning to pierce* (Vide EMBOLUS: *See* E. *embolus*)

●●● 정형 제 2 변화

능동태 현재부정법이 -ēre로, 능동태 직설법 현재 단수 일인칭이 -eo로 끝나는 동사.

habeo, habui, habitum, habēre 가지다

능동태	부정법	현재			hab-ēre	가지다
	직설법	현재	단수	일인칭	hab-eo	나는 ~한다
				이인칭	hab-es	너는 ~한다
				삼인칭	hab-et	그는 ~한다
			복수	일인칭	hab-emus	우리는 ~한다
				이인칭	hab-etis	너희는 ~한다
				삼인칭	hab-ent	그들은 ~한다
		과거	단수	일인칭	hab-ebam	나는 ~하였다
		미래	단수	일인칭	hab-ebo	나는 ~하겠다
		완료	단수	일인칭	habu-i	나는 ~하였다
	가정법	현재	단수	일인칭	hab-eam	나는 ~하리라
	명령법	현재	단수	이인칭	hab-e	너는 ~하라
			복수	이인칭	hab-ete	너희는 ~하라
분 사		현재			habens, (gen.) habent-is	~하는, ~하고 있는

수동태	목적분사				habit-um	~하러, ~하기 위하여
	부정법	현재			hab-eri	가지게 되다
	분 사	미래			habend-us, habend-a, habend-um ~받아야 할	
		과거			habit-us, habit-a, habit-um ~받은, ~받고서	

habeo, habui, habitum, habēre 가지다

[용례] habeas corpus 인신 보호 영장
　　(문법) habeas 너는 가지리라: 능동태 가정법 현재 단수 이인칭
　　　　corpus 몸을: 단수 대격 < corpus, corporis, n. 몸

> habitus, habita, habitum (*past participle*) 가진, 잘 보살핀, 돌본

　　[용례] male habitus 나쁘게 돌본　　　　　E (male habitus *'badly had'* >) *malady*
　　　(문법) male 나쁘게: 부사
　　　　habitus 돌본: 과거분사, 남성형 단수 주격

> habitus, habitus, m. 습관, 버릇, 벽(癖), 소질, 본성, 체형, 체질　　E *habitus, habit*
　　> habitualis, habituale 습관적인　　　　　　　　　　　　　　　E *habitual*
　　> habituo, habituavi, habituatum, habituare 길들이다, 익숙하게 하다,
　　　　습관이 되다　　　　　　　　　　　　　　　　　　　　　E *habituate*
> habitudo, habitudinis, f. 습성, 기질　　　　　　　　　　　　E *habitude*
> habena, habenae, f. 고삐, 끈, 굴레, 제어　　　　　　　E *habena, habenar*
　　> habenula, habenulae, f. (< + -ula *diminutive suffix*) 고삐,
　　　　작은 끈　　　　　　　　　　　　　　　　　E *habenula, habenular*
> habilis, habile 재주 있는, 숙달된

　　E *able, ableism, ably,* (*able* >) (*adjective*) *unable,* (*able* >) (*verb*) *enable,* (*able* >)
　　(*verb*) *disable*

　　> habilitas, habilitatis, f. 재주, 숙달

　　　E *ability,* (*ability* >) *inability* (< *'not being able'*), (*ability* >) *disability* (< *'being
　　　disabled'*)

　　　> habilito, habilitavi, habilitatum, habilitare 능력을 갖추게 하다　E *habilitate*
　　　　> habilitatio, habilitationis, f. 자격 획득　　　　　　E *habilitation*
　　　　> rehabilito, rehabilitavi, rehabilitatum, rehabilitare (< re- *back,
　　　　　again* + habilitare *to make fit, to enable*) (원래의 능력으로)
　　　　　되돌리다, 사회에 복귀시키다, 재활(再活)시키다　　　E *rehabilitate*
　　　　　> rehabilitatio, rehabilitationis, f. 복구, 복귀, 재활　E *rehabilitation*
> habito, habitavi, habitatum, habitare (*frequentative*) (어디에) 살다, 거주하다, 고집하다

　　E (*third personal singular, present indicative, active 'it dwells'* >) *habitat, habitant,
　　habitation, habitable*

　　> cohabito, cohabitavi, cohabitatum, cohabitare (< co- (< cum) *with, together*
　　　+ habitare *to dwell*) 함께 살다, 동거하다　　　　　E *cohabit, cohabitant*

> inhabito, **inhabitavi**, inhabitatum, inhabitare (< in- *in, on, into, toward* + habitare
 to dwell) (어디에) 살다, 거주하다   **E** *inhabit, inhabitant, inhabitation, inhabitable*
> debeo, **debui**, debitum, debēre (< de- *apart from, down, not* + habēre *to have*) 빚지다,
 의무가 있다

> **E** (debitum (*past participle*) *'something owed'* >) **debit**, (debitum *'something owed'* >)
> **debt**, (debitum *'something owed, as an enforceable obligation or debt'* >) **due**,
> (due >) **duty**, (due >) **undue, devoir, endeavour (endeavor)** (< *'to make it one's*
> *duty to do something')*

> exhibeo, **exhibui**, exhibitum, exhibēre (< ex- *out of, away from* + habēre *to have*)
 드러내다, 전시하다   **E** *exhibit*
  > exhibitio, exhibitionis, f. 표출, 제출, 전시   **E** *exhibition*
> inhibeo, **inhibui**, inhibitum, inhibēre (< in- *in, on, into, toward* + habēre *to have*)
 걷잡다, 억제하다, 저지하다   **E** *inhibit*
  > inhibitio, inhibitionis, f. 억제   **E** *inhibition*
  > inhibitor, inhibitoris, m. 억제제   **E** *inhibitor*
  > inhibitorius, inhibitoria, inhibitorium 억제하는   **E** *inhibitory*
> prohibeo, **prohibui**, prohibitum, prohibēre (< pro- *before, forward, for, instead of*
 + habēre *to have*) 보호하다, 말리다, 금하다   **E** *prohibit*
  > prohibitio, prohibitionis, f. 금지   **E** *prohibition*
< IE. ghabh-, ghebh- *to give, to receive*   **E** *give, gift, forgive* (< *'give away'*)

arceo, arcui, –, arcēre 가두다, 보호하다

> arca, arcae, f. 궤, 상자   **E** *ark*
  > arcanus, arcana, arcanum 비밀의, 신비로운   **E** *arcane*
> coerceo, **coercui**, coercitum, coercēre (< co- (< cum) *with, together* + arcēre *to keep
 in or away*) 제지하다, 억압하다   **E** *coerce*
> exerceo, **exercui**, exercitum, exercēre (< *to keep busy, to practice* < ex- *out of,
 away from* + arcēre *to keep in or away*) 움직이게 하다, 연습시키다
  > exercitium, exercitii, n. 연습, 훈련   **E** *exercise*
  > exercito, **exercitavi**, exercitatum, exercitare (*frequentative*) 줄곧 연습시키다
    > exercitatio, exercitationis, f. 연습, 실습, 실천   **E** *exercitation*
< IE. ark- *to hold, to contain, to guard*
  > G. arkein (arkeein) *to ward off, to suffice*
    > G. autarkeia, autarkeias, f. (< autos *self* + arkein) *self-sufficiency*   **E** *autarky*

areo, arui, –, arēre 마르다, 시들다, 목마르다

> aridus, arida, aridum 메마른, 무미건조한   **E** *arid*
  > ardeo, **arsi**, arsum, ardēre 타오르다, 뜨겁다   **E** *ardent*
    > ardor, ardoris, m. 화염, 정열   **E** *ardor (ardour)*
    > arsio, arsionis, f. 방화   **E** *arson, arsonist*
< IE. as- *to burn, to glow*

E ash, (pot ash 'obtained by leaching wood ashes and evaporating the leach in a pot' >) potash, (potash >) potassium, ashen

> G. azaleos, azalea, azaleon *parched, dry*

> L. azalea, azaleae, f. (< *from the dry soil in which it flourishes, or from its dry brittle wood*) 진달래　　　　　　　　　　　　　　　**E** azalea

augeo, auxi, auctum, augēre 증가시키다

> augmentum, augmenti, n. 증가, 증대, 확대　　　　　　　**E** (noun) augment

　> augmento, **augmentavi**, augmentatum, augmentare 증가시키다, 증대시키다, 확대시키다　　　　　　　　　　　　　　　　　　**E** (verb) augment

　　> augmentatio, augmentationis, f. 증가, 증대, 확대　　**E** augmentation

> augur, auguris, m. (< *he who obtains favorable presage* < *increase, divine favor*) (새의 나는 모양·먹는 모양·울음소리, 짐승의 창자, 천체의 현상 등으로 점을 치던) 복점관(卜占官), 신탁관(神託官)　　　　　　　　　　　**E** augur

　> augurium, augurii, n. 복점(卜占)　　　　　　　　　　**E** augury

　> auguro, **auguravi**, auguratum, augurare (새로써) 점치다

　　> inauguro, **inauguravi**, inauguratum, inaugurare (< in- *in, on, into, toward* + augurare *to take augurs*) 점치다, 점을 쳐서 터를 잡다, 점을 쳐서 제관으로 임명하다, 개막식을 거행하다, 즉위식을 올리다, 시작하다　　　　　　　　　　　**E** inaugurate, inaugural

> augustus, augusta, augustum 존엄한　　　　　　　　　**E** august

　> Augustus, Augusti, m. 로마 초대 황제의 별호(別號) (그 후 모든 로마 황제의 별호가 됨)　　　　　　　　　　　　　　　　　　**E** Augustus

　　> Augustus, Augusta, Augustum 아우구스투스 초대 황제의, 로마 황제의

　　　E (Augustus mensis 'month of Augustus Caesar, the first Roman Emperor' >) August

> auctor, auctoris, m., f. 창건자, 권위자, 저자　　　　　**E** author

　> auctoritas, auctoritatis, f. 권위　　　　　　　　　　**E** authority

　> auctorizo, **auctorizavi**, auctorizatum, auctorizare 권한을 주다, 위임하다, 인정하다　　　　　　　　　　　　　　　　　**E** authorize

> auctio, auctionis, f. (< *a sale by increase of bids*) 경매, 공매　**E** auction

> auxilium, auxilii, n. 도움, 보조

　> auxiliarius, auxiliaria, auxiliarium 도움의, 보조의; (문법) 조동사(助動詞)의　**E** auxiliary

< IE. aug- *to increase*　　**E** (an eke name >) nickname, wax (< 'to grow'), waist (< 'to grow')

　> G. auxein *to increase*　　　　　**E** auxin (< 'a plant grow hormone')

aveo, -, -, avēre 무슨 일에 호기심을 가지다, 하고 싶어 못 견디다

> avidus, avida, avidum 몹시 하고 싶어 하는, 갈망하는　**E** avid, avidin (< 'its avidity for biotin')

　> aviditas, aviditatis, f. 갈망, 욕망, 탐욕　　　　　　**E** avidity

> avarus, avara, avarum 탐욕스러운

　> avaritia, avaritiae, f. 탐욕　　　　　　　　　　　　**E** avarice

　　> *avaritiosus, *avaritiosa, *avaritiosum 탐욕 많은　**E** avaricious

∞ (*suggested*) audeo, ausus sum, audēre (반탈형동사) 감히 하다, 감행하다

> audax, (gen.) audacis 대담한　　　　　　　　　　　　　　　E *audacious*
>> audacitas, audacitatis, f. 대담, 대담성　　　　　　　　　E *audacity*

candeo, candui, –, candēre 불에 달궈져 빛을 내다, 백열(白熱)을 내다, 하얗다　E *candent*

> candor, candoris, m. 눈부신 흰빛, 순결, 솔직, 성실　　　E *candor (candour)*
> candidus, candida, candidum 흰, 순결한, 꾸밈없는　　　　E *candid*
>> candida, candidae, f. 백의(白衣, 선거나 경기의 후보자가 입는 흰 toga); (Candida)
>> (불완전 진균) 칸디다속(屬)

> E Candida (< 'white or creamy colonies'), *candidiasis (moniliasis, moniliosis)*
>> candidatus, candidata, candidatum 흰옷의, 흰옷 입은, 후보자의　E *candidate*
> candela, candelae, f. 양초, 칸델라(광도의 국제단위)　　　　E *candle, candela (cd)*
>> candelabrum, candelabri, n. 촛대　　　　　　　　　E *candelabrum*, F. *chandelier*
> candesco, candui, –, candescĕre (< candēre *to glow, to be white* + –escĕre *suffix*
> *of inceptive (inchoative) verb*) 백열을 내다, 하얗게 되다　E *candescent*
>> incandesco, incandui, –, incandescĕre (< in- *in, on, into, toward* + candescĕre
>> *to become white*) 백열을 내다, 하얗게 되다　E *incandescent, incandescence*
> incendo, incendi, incensum, incendĕre (< in- *in, on, into, toward* + candēre *to*
> *shine, to glow, to burn*) 불 피우다, 흥분시키다　　　　E *(verb) incense*
>> incensum, incensi, n. (< *neuter past participle*)
>> 향　　　　　E *(noun) incense, frankincense (< 'high-quality incense')*
>> incendium, incendii, n. 화재, 연소, 불길
>>> incendiarius, incendiaria, incendiarium 불내는, 방화의, 선동하는　E *incendiary*
< IE. kand-, kend- *to shine*

caveo, cavi, cautum, cavēre 조심하다, 주의하다, 삼가다, 돌보다　　　E *caveat*

[용례] Caveat emptor. (< *Let the buyer beware.*) 구매자가 주의해야 할 것이다,
매수자 위험 부담
(문법) caveat 주의해야 할 것이다: 능동태 가정법 현재 단수 삼인칭
emptor 구매자가: 단수 주격 < emptor, emptoris, m.

> cautio, cautionis, f. 조심, 주의　　　　　　　　　　　E *caution*
>> *cautiosus, *cautiosa, *cautiosum 조심성 있는, 주의 깊은　E *cautious*
> praecaveo, praecavi, praecautum, praecavēre (< prae- *before, beyond*) 사전에 조심
> 하다, 예방 조치를 취하다
>> praecautio, praecautionis, f. 예방 조치, 예방책　　　　E *precaution, precautious*
< IE. (s)keuə- *to pay attention, to perceive*
E *show* (< 'to look at'), *scavenger* (< 'to look at'), *sheen* (< 'conspicuous, attractive')

censeo, censui, censum, censēre 국세조사를 하다, 평가하다, 여기다

> census, census, m. 국세조사　　　　　　　　　　　　　E *census*

> censor, censoris, m. (고대 로마의 호구조사·재산조사·풍기감찰 등을 임무로 한) 감찰관, 검열관, 비평가　　　　　　　　　　　　　　　　　　　　　E *censor*

> censura, censurae, f. 감찰관직, 검열, 징계　　　　　　　E *censure*

< IE. kens- *to proclaim, to speak solemnly*

cieo, civi, citum, ciēre 움직이게 하다, 일으키다, 부르다

> citus, cita, citum (*past participle*) 움직이는, 빠른

> sollicitus, sollicita, sollicitum (< sollus *whole* + citus *set in motion*) 끊임없이
움직이게 하는 > 염려하는　　　　　　　　　　　　E *solicitous*

> sollicitudo, sollicitudinis, f. 근심, 걱정, 갈망　　　　E *solicitude*

> sollicito, sollicitavi, sollicitatum, sollicitare 부추기다, 유혹하다,
간청하다　　　　　　　　　　　　　　E *solicit, unsolicited*

> cito, citavi, citatum, citare (*frequentative*) 일이 일어나게 하다, 재촉하다, 불러내다,
인용하다　　　　　　　　　　　　　　　　　　　E *cite*

> citatio, citationis, f. 인용　　　　　　　　　　　E *citation*

> excito, excitavi, excitatum, excitare (< ex- *out of, away from* + citare *to rouse*)
나오게 하다, 흥분시키다　　　　　E *excite, excitatory, excitable, excitability*

> excitatio, excitationis, f. 자극, 흥분; (물리) 여기(勵起)　　E *excitation*

> incito, incitavi, incitatum, incitare (< in- *in, on, into, toward* + citare *to rouse*)
충동하다, 격려하다　　　　　　　　　　　　　　　E *incite*

> recito, recitavi, recitatum, recitare (< re- *back, again* + citare *to rouse*) 암송
하다　　　　　　　　E *recite, (recite >) recital, recitative*

> resuscito, resuscitavi, resuscitatum, resuscitare (< re- *back, again* + sus-
(< sub) *under, up from under* + citare *to rouse*) 되살아나게 하다, 소생
시키다　　　　　　　　　　　　　E *resuscitate, resuscitator*

< IE. keiə- *to set in motion*

> G. kinein (kineein) *to set in motion, to move*

E *kin(o)- (kine-), kinin, bradykinin* (< 'slow kinin' < 'slow contraction produced in isolated guinea pig ileum'), *cytokinin* (< 'a plant hormone promoting cell division'), *kinase, -kine, cytokine, chemokine*

> G. kinētos, kinētē, kinēton *moving, movable*　　E *kinetophore, kinetoplast, kinetochore*

> L. acinetobacter, acinetobacteris, m. (< G. a- *not* + kinētos + -bacter
bacterium) 아시네토박터　　　　　　　　　　　E *acinetobacter*

> G. kinētikos, kinētikē, kinētikon *moving, movable*　　E *kinetic, kinetics*

> G. kinēsis, kinēseōs, f. (< + -sis *feminine noun suffix*) *movement, tumult,
disturbance*

> L. kinesis, kinesis, f. 운동성,
운동　　　　　E *kinesis, kinesics, kinesiology, -kinesis, kinesin*

> L. hyperkinesis, hyperkinesis, f. (hyperkinesia, hyperkinesiae, f.) (< G.
hyper- *over*) 운동과다증　　　　　E *hyperkinesis (hyperkinesia)*

> L. hypokinesis, hypokinesis, f. (hypokinesia, hypokinesiae, f.) (< G.

hyp(o)- *under*) 운동감소증, 과소운동증   **E** *hypokinesis (hypokinesia)*

> L. autokinesis, autokinesis, f. (< G. autos *self*) (생리) 자동(自動)운동,

수의(隨意)운동   **E** *autokinesis*

> L. telekinesis, telekinesis, f. (< G. tēle *afar, far off*) (심령) 염동(念動)

작용   **E** *telekinesis*

> L. karyokinesis, karyokinesis, f. (< G. karyon *nut*)

유사(有絲)핵분열   **E** *karyokinesis*

> L. cytokinesis, cytokinesis, f. (< G. kytos *hollow vessel*)

세포질분열   **E** *cytokinesis*

> L. diakinesis, diakinesis, f. (< G. di(a)- *through, thoroughly, apart*)

이동기(移動期)   **E** *diakinesis*

> G. -kinēsia, -kinēsias, f. (< + -ia) *movement,*

motion   **E** *-kinesia, diadochokinesia, dysdiadochokinesia*

> G. akinēsia, akinēsias, f. (< a- *not*) *quiescence*

> L. akinesia, akinesiae, f. 운동불능증   **E** *akinesia*

> G. dyskinēsia, dyskinēsias, f. (< dys- *bad*) *difficulty of moving*

> L. dyskinesia, dyskinesiae, f. 운동이상증   **E** *dyskinesia*

> G. kinēma, kinēmatos, n. (< -ma *resultative noun suffix*) *motion*

E *kinematics, cinematograph (cinema, cine), cinematography, (cinematography*
>) cine-, cinemicrography

doceo, docui, doctum, docēre (< *to cause to accept*) 가르치다   **E** *docent*

> doctor, doctoris, m. 스승, 박사, 의사   **E** *doctor*

> doctrina, doctrinae, f. 가르침, 학과, 학설, 교의   **E** *doctrine*

> doctrino, **doctrinavi**, doctrinatum, doctrinare 가르치다   **E** *indoctrinate*

> doctrix, doctricis, f. 여교사

> docilis, docile 가르치기 쉬운, 다루기 쉬운, 유순한   **E** *docile*

> indocilis, indocile (< in- *not*) 가르치기 어려운, 다루기 어려운, 고분고분하지 않는   **E** *indocile*

> documentum, documenti, n. 교훈, 귀감, 기록문서   **E** *document, documentary, documentation*

< IE. dek- *to take, to accept*

> L. decet, decuit, -, decēre (비인칭 동사) 어울리다, 적합하다

> L. decens, (gen.) decentis (*present participle*) 어울리는, 적합한, 품위 있는   **E** *decent*

> L. decentia, decentiae, f. 어울림, 적합, 품위   **E** *decency*

> L. indecens, (gen.) indecentis (< in- *not*) 어울리지 않는, 꼴사나운,

야비한   **E** *indecent*

> L. indecentia, indecentiae, f. 어울리지 않음, 꼴사나움, 야비함   **E** *indecency*

> L. decus, decoris, n. 어울림, 장식   **E** *decor*

> L. decorus, decora, decorum 어울리는, 품위 있는,

예의 있는   **E** *decorum, decorous*

> L. decoro, **decoravi**, decoratum, decorare 장식하다   **E** *decorate*

> L. dignus, digna, dignum 어울리는, 자격 있는

> L. dignitas, dignitatis, f. 자격, 품위, 존엄성, 고상함 　E *dignity, dainty, (dignity >) dignitary*

> L. dignor, dignatus sum, dignari 자격 있다고 인정하다, 좋게 생각하다, 해주다 　E *deign*

    > L. dedignor, dedignatus sum, dedignari (< de- *apart from, down, not* +

      dignari *to consider worthy*) 부당하게 여기다, 멸시하다 　E *disdain*

      > L. indignor, indignatus sum, indignari (< in- *not* + dignari *to consider*

      worthy) 부당하게 여기다, 멸시하다 　E *indignant*

        > L. indignatio, indignationis, f. 분개 　E *indignation*

        > L. indignitas, indignitatis, f. 분개, 모욕 　E *indignity*

> L. disco, **didici**, discitum, discĕre 배우다

    > L. discipulus, discipuli, m. 학생, 제자 　E *disciple*

      > L. disciplina, disciplinae, f. 배움, 교육, 훈련,

      학과목 　E *discipline, disciplinary, multidisciplinary*

> G. dechesthai *to accept, to receive*

    > G. dektos, dektē, dekton *acceptable, to be accepted, to be re-*

    ceived 　E *chemodectoma (< 'a tumor (paraganglioma) of the chemoreceptor system')*

    > G. dektēs, dektou, m. *receiver*

      > G. pandektēs, pandektou, m. (< G. pan- *all*) *all-receiver*

        > L. pandectae, pandectarum, m. (pl.) 총람, 전집, 법전, 유스티니아누스

        (Justinianus) 법전 　E *pandect*

    > G. dochē, dochēs, f. *receptacle, banquet*

      > L. choledochus, choledocha, choledochum (< G. cholē *bile* + dochē

      receptacle) 담즙을 받아들이는 　E *choledoch(o)-, choledochal*

        [용례] ductus choledochus 총담관, 온쓸개관 　E *ductus choledochus*

        (문법) ductus 관: 단수 주격 < ductus, ductus, m.

          choledochus: 형용사, 남성형 단수 주격

    > G. diadechesthai (< di(a)- *through, thoroughly, apart* + dechesthai) *to receive*

    in turn, to succeed

      > G. diadochos, diadochos, diadochon *receiving in turn, successive*

        > G. diadochos, diadochou, m. *successor* 　E *((pl.) Diadochoi >) Diadochi*

        > L. diadochokinesia, diadochokinesiae, m. (< G. + -kinēsia) 되풀이

        운동, 반복운동 　E *diadochokinesia, dysdiadochokinesia*

> G. ekdechesthai (< ek- *out of, away from* + dechesthai) *to take, to take up*

    > G. synekdechesthai (< syn- *with, together* + dechesthai) *to take with*

    something else

      > G. synekdochē, synekdochēs, f. *synecdoche*

        > L. synecdoche, synecdoches, f. 제유법(提喩法),

        대유법(代喩法) 　E *synecdoche*

> G. dokein *to appear, to seem, to think, to believe* (< *to cause to accept or be accepted*)

    > G. doxa, doxēs, f. *opinion, glory*

      > G. -doxos, -doxos, -doxon *of opinion*

> L. orthodoxus, orthodoxa, orthodoxum (< G. orthos *upright, straight, correct*) 정통의   **E** *orthodox*

> L. heterodoxus, heterodoxa, heterodoxum (< G. heteros *different*) 비정통적인, 이단의   **E** *heterodox*

> L. paradoxus, paradoxa, paradoxum (< G. par(a)- *beside, along side of, beyond*) 예기치 않은, 역설의   **E** *paradox, paradoxical*

> G. dogma, dogmatos, n. *opinion, doctrine*

> L. dogma, dogmatis, n. 정설, 교의(敎義)   **E** *dogma, dogmatic*

faveo, favi, fautum, favēre (종교 예식에) 경건하게 참석하다, 호의를 보이다

> favor, favoris, m. 종교적 엄숙, 호의   **E** *favor (favour), favorite*

> favorabilis, favorabile 호의적   **E** *favorable*

< IE. ghow-e- *to honor, to revere, to worship*

ferveo, fervui, –, fervēre (fervo, fervi, –, fervĕre) 끓다, 뜨거워지다, 북받치다   **E** *fervent*

> fervor, fervoris, m. 백열, 혹서, 열정   **E** *fervor (fervour)*

> fervidus, fervida, fervidum 백열의, 혹서의, 열정적인   **E** *fervid*

> fermentum, fermenti, n. 누룩, 발효소, 울화   **E** *(noun) ferment*

> fermento, **fermentavi**, fermentatum, fermentare 발효시키다, 발효하다   **E** *(verb) ferment*

> fermentatio, fermentationis, f. 발효   **E** *fermentation*

> defervesco, **defervi (deferbui)**, –, defervescĕre (< de- *apart from, down, not* + fervēre *to boil* + -escĕre *suffix of inceptive (inchoative) verb*) (끓다가) 식기 시작하다, 차분해지다   **E** *defervescence*

> effervesco, **effervi (efferbui)**, –, effervescĕre (< ef- (< ex) *out of, away from* + fervēre *to boil* + -escĕre *suffix of inceptive (inchoative) verb*) 끓기 시작하다, 격노해지다   **E** *effervesce, effervescent, effervescence*

< IE. bhreuə-, bhreu- *to boil, to bubble, to effervesce, to burn; with derivatives referring to cooking and brewing*

E *bread (< 'leavened bread'), brew, brewery, brawn, brawny, broth, braise, brood, breed*

fleo, flevi, fletum, flēre 울다, 슬퍼하다

> flebilis, flebile 울게 하는, 눈물겨운, 슬픈   **E** *feeble, foible*

< IE. bhle- *to howl*   **E** *bleat, blare*

< IE. bhel- *to cry out, to yell*   **E** *bell, bellow, bawl, belch*

gaudeo, gavisus sum, gaudēre (반탈형동사) 기뻐하다   **E** *enjoy, rejoice, gaud, gaudy*

> gaudium, gaudii, n. 기쁨, 기쁘게 해주는 것, 관능적 쾌락   **E** *joy*

< IE. gau- *to rejoice; also to have religious fear or awe*

haereo, haesi, haesum, haerēre (hereo, hesi, hesum, herēre) 달라붙다

> h(a)esito, h(a)esitavi, h(a)esitatum, h(a)esitare (*frequentative*) 주저하다　　**E** *hesitate, hesitant*

　　> h(a)esitantia, h(a)esitantiae, f. 주저　　**E** *hesitance (hesitancy)*

> adh(a)ereo, adh(a)esi, adh(a)esum, adh(a)erēre (< ad- *to, toward, at, according to*
　+ h(a)erēre *to stick, to cling*) 달라붙다, 부착하다, 유착하다　　**E** *adhere, adherent, adhesive*

　　[용례] zonula adherens, (pl.) zonulae adherentes 부착띠,
　　　　　　부착소대(小帶)　　**E** *zonula adherens,* (pl.) *zonulae adherentes*
　　　　　macula adherens, (pl.) maculae adherentes 부착반점(斑點),
　　　　　　유착반(斑)　　**E** *macula adherens,* (pl.) *maculae adherentes*
　　　　(문법) zonula 작은 띠, 소대(小帶): 단수 주격 < zonula, zonulae, f.
　　　　　　zonulae 작은 띠들, 소대(小帶)들: 복수 주격
　　　　　macula 반점(斑點), 반(斑): 단수 주격 < macula, maculae, f.
　　　　　maculae 반점들: 복수 주격
　　　　　adherens 부착하고 있는: 현재분사, 남·여·중성형 단수 주격
　　　　　　< adherens, (gen.) adherentis
　　　　　adherentes 부착하고 있는: 현재분사, 남·여성형 복수 주격

　　　　> adh(a)esio, adh(a)esionis, f. 부착, 유착, 붙음, 부속　　**E** *adhesion*
> coh(a)ereo, coh(a)esi, coh(a)esum, coh(a)erēre (< co- (< cum) *with, together* +
　h(a)erēre *to stick, to cling*) 서로 달라붙다, 응집하다,
　결집하다　　**E** *cohere, coherent, cohesive, discohesive*
　　> coh(a)erentia, coh(a)erentiae, f. 밀착, 상호관련성, 응집, 결집　　**E** *coherence*
　　> *coh(a)esio, *coh(a)esionis, f. 결합, 응집　　**E** *cohesion*
> inh(a)ereo, inh(a)esi, inh(a)esum, inh(a)erēre (< in- *in, on, into, toward* + h(a)erēre
　to stick, to cling) 달라붙어 있다, 내재하다　　**E** *inhere, inherent, inherence*
< IE. ghais- *to adhere, to sting*

horreo, horrui, –, horrēre 빳빳이 일어서다, 삐죽삐죽 서 있다, 털이 곤두서다, 소름 끼치다,
　겁내다　　**E** (horrendus (*gerundive*) '*to be shuddered at*' >) *horrendous*
　> horror, horroris, m. 털이 곤두섬, 소름 끼침, 공포　　**E** *horror*
　> horridus, horrida, horridum 무서운, 아주 싫은　　**E** *horrid*
　> horribilis, horribile 무서운, 지긋지긋하게 싫은　　**E** *horrible*
　> abhorreo, abhorrui, –, abhorrēre (< ab- *off, away from* + horrēre *to bristle*) 몹시
　　싫어하다, 혐오하다　　**E** *abhor, abhorrent,* (abhorrent >) *abhorrence*
< IE. ghers- *to bristle*
　　> L. (h)ericius, (h)ericii, m. 고슴도치　　**E** *urchin*
　　> L. hircus, hirci, m. 염소, 산양, 노린내, 호색한
　　　　> L. hircinus, hircina, hircinum 염소의, 산양의, 노린내 나는　　**E** *hircine*
　　> L. hirsutus, hirsuta, hirsutum 털이 곤두선, 털로 덮인　　**E** *hirsute, hirsutism*
　　> L. (*probably*) hordeum, hordei, n. 보리
　　　　> L. hordeolum, hordeoli, n. (< + -olum *diminutive suffix*) 다래끼,
　　　　　　맥립종(麥粒腫)　　**E** *hordeolum*

> (*Oscan*) hirpus *wolf*

> L. hirpex, hirpicis, m. (irpex, irpicis, m.) (< *resemblance of harrow's teeth to those of a wolf*) 쇠스랑

> **E** *rehearse* (< *'to harrow again'*), (*rehearse* >) ***rehearsal, hearse*** (< *'a vehicle for conveying the coffin at a funeral' < 'harrow-shaped triangular frame for carrying candles at certain services'*)

indulgeo, indulsi, indultum, indulgēre 너그럽다, 전념하다, 탐닉하다   **E** *indulge*

> indulgentia, indulgentiae, f. 관용, 면죄, 탐닉   **E** *indulgence (indulgency)*

< IE. dlegh– *to engage oneself*   **E** *play* (< *'to exercise oneself'*), ***pledge, plight***

lateo, latui, –, latēre 잠복해 있다, 잠재해 있다, 은거하다, 알려져 있지 않다   **E** *latent*, (*latent* >) *latency*

> latebra, latebrae, f. 잠복처, 은신처, 빠져나가는 구멍   **E** *latebra*

< IE. ladh– *to be hidden*

> G. lanthanein *to escape notice*   **E** *lanthanum (La)* (< *'concealed in cerium oxide'*)

> G. lanthanesthai (*middle*) *to forget*

> G. lēthē, lēthēs, f. *forgetting;* (Lēthē) (*Greek mythology*) *a river in Hades, the water of which produced, in those who drank it, forgetfulness of the past*

> L. Lethe, Lethes, f. (그리스 신화) 망각의 강   **E** *Lethe*

> (*suggested*) G. alēthēs, alēthēs, alēthes (< a– *not*) *true*

> G. alētheia, alētheias, f. *truth*   **E** *alethic*

> G. lēthargia, lēthargias, f. (< lēthē + argos *idle*) *forgetfulness*

> L. lethargia, lethargiae, f. 졸음증, 기면(嗜眠)   **E** *lethargy, lethargic*

libet, libuit (libitum est), –, libēre (비인칭동사) 마음에 든다, 하고 싶다

> libitus, libitus, m. 마음에 든 것, 마음 내킴

[용례] ad libitum (ad libit., ad lib.) 임의로   **E** *ad libitum (ad libit., ad lib.)*
(문법) ad 따라: 전치사, 대격지배
libitum: 단수 대격

> libido, libidinis, f. 욕구, 욕망, 육욕, 리비도, 활력, 성욕   **E** *libido*

< IE. leubh– *to care, to desire; love*

> **E** *believe* (< *'to hold dear, to esteem, to trust'*), ***belief, leave*** (< *'permission' < 'approval' < 'pleasure'*), ***furlough, love***

licet, licuit (licitum est), –, licēre (비인칭동사) 허락되다,

~해도 좋다   **E** (licēre *'to be permitted'* >) *leisure*

> licitus, licita, licitum (*past participle*) 허락된, 정당한, 합법적인   **E** *licit*

> illicitus, illicita, illicitum (< il– (< in–) *not*) 허락되지 않은, 불법적인   **E** *illicit*

> licentia, licentiae, f. 허락, 인가, 자격, 면허, 자유, 방종   **E** *licence (license)*

     > licentiosus, licentiosa, licentiosum 방종한, 파격의   **E** *licentious*

     > scilicet (< scire licet *it is permitted to know*) (부사) 분명히, 즉   **E** *scilicet (scil., sc.)*

     > videlicet (< vidēre licet *it is permitted to see*) (부사) 분명히, 즉   **E** *videlicet (viz.)*

< IE. leik– *to offer for sale, to bargain*

liqueo, liqui (licui), –, liquēre 녹은 (액체) 상태에 있다, 맑다

> liquor, liquoris, m. 액체, 물, 알코올 음료   **E** *liquor*

> liquidus, liquida, liquidum 액체의   **E** *liquid*

     > liquido, liquidavi, liquidatum, liquidare 액체가 되다, 녹다, 정리하다   **E** *liquidate*

> liquesco, (licui), –, liquescĕre (< liquēre *to be liquid* + -escĕre *suffix of inceptive (inchoative) verb*) 액체가 되다   **E** *liquescent*

     > deliquesco, delicui, –, deliquescĕre (< de- *apart from, down, not; intensive* + liquescĕre *to melt*) 액체가 되다, 녹아 없어지다   **E** *deliquescent*

> liquefacio, liquefeci, liquefactum, liquefacĕre (< liquēre *to be liquid* + facĕre *to make*) 액체가 되게 하다   **E** *liquefy, liquefacient, liquefaction*

> prolixus, prolixa, prolixum (< pro- *before, forward, for, instead of*) 길게 늘어진, 장황한   **E** *prolix*

     > prolixitas, prolixitatis, f. 길게 늘어짐, 장황   **E** *prolixity*

< IE. wleik– *to flow, to run*

lugeo, luxi, luctum, lugēre (< *to be broken*) 슬퍼하다

     > lugubris, lugubre 슬픈   **E** *lugubrious*

< IE. leug– *to break*

maneo, mansi, mansum, manēre 머물다, 거주하다, 남다   **E** *manor*

> mansio, mansionis, f. 머무름, 숙소, 거처, 주택   **E** *mansion, menage, menagerie*

> immaneo, immansi, immansum, immanēre (< im- (< in) *in, on, into, toward* + manēre *to stay*) 안에 남다, 내재(內在)하다   **E** *immanent*

> permaneo, permansi, permansum, permanēre (< per- *through, thoroughly* + manēre *to stay*) 끝까지 머물다, 지속하다   **E** *permanent, (permanent frost >) permafrost*

> remaneo, remansi, remansum, remanēre (< re- *back, again* + manēre *to stay*) (빼고) 남다, 잔존하다   **E** *remain, remainder, remanent, (remanent >) remnant*

< IE. men– *to remain*

mereo, merui, meritum, merēre (mereor, meritus sum, mereri) 받을 만하다, 마땅히 받다   **E** *merit, (terra merita 'deserved earth' >) turmeric*

> meritum, meriti, n. 공적   **E** *merit; meritocracy*

> demereo, demerui, demeritum, demerēre (demereor, demeritus sum, demereri)

(< de- *apart from, down, not; intensive* + merēre *to deserve*) 마땅히 받을 만한
일을 하다

> demeritum, demeriti, n. (< *neuter past participle*) 죄과, 과실   **E** *demerit*

> emereo, **emerui**, emeritum, emerēre (emereor, emeritus sum, emereri) (< e- *out of,*
away from + merēre *to deserve*) 직책을 다하다, 공을 세우다

> emeritus, emerita, emeritum (*past participle*) 직책을 마친, 명예의   **E** *emeritus, emerita*

< IE. (s)mer- *to get a share of something*

> G. meros, merous, n. *part, share, lot*

> **E** *mer(o)-, merozoite (schizozoite) (< 'a protozoon resulted from merogony or schizogony'), (merozoite > 'producing merozoites' >) meront (< 'on the pattern of schizont'), (D. -mer >) -mer, isomer, enantiomer, epimer, anomer, metamer, monomer, dimer, oligomer, polymer, polymeric, polymerize, polymerase, protomer, (excited dimer >) excimer, (F. -mere >) -mere, centromere (< 'central part'), telomere (< 'end part'), sarcomere (< 'the contractile unit of myofibrils in striated muscle'), capsomere (< 'morphological unit of the viral capsid'), granulomere (< 'granular part of platelet'), hyalomere (< 'glassy part of platelet')*

> G. merizein *to divide*

> G. meristos, meristē, meriston *divided, divisible*   **E** *meristem, meristematic*

> G. moros, morou, m. *part, lot, fate*

> G. morion, moriou, n. (< + -ion *diminutive suffix*) *part, portion, division,*
limb   **E** *monomorium (< 'a single median hair on the clypeus')*

> G. moira, moiras, f. *part, portion, share, lot, fate;* ((pl.) Moirai) (*Greek mythology*)
the Fates (Clotho, Lachesis, Atropos)   **E** *(pl.) Moirai*

misceo, miscui, mixtum (mistum), miscēre 섞다

> **E** *mix, miscegenation, (mixtus 'mixed' >) Sp. mestizo, (animalia mixta 'mixed animals' >) mustang*

> mixtura, mixturae, f. 섞인 물건, 혼합물   **E** *mixture*

> miscellus, miscella, miscellum 섞어 놓은, 혼합된

> miscellaneus, miscellanea, miscellaneum 뒤섞어 놓은,
혼합된   **E** *miscellaneous, (miscellanea (neuter pl.) >) miscellany*

> miscibilis, miscibile 섞을 수 있는, 섞이는   **E** *miscible*

> misculo, **misculavi**, misculatum, misculare 섞다   **E** *meddle, medley*

> admisceo, **admiscui**, admixtum (admistum), admiscēre (< ad- *to, toward, at, according*
to + miscēre *to mix*) 섞다   **E** *admix, admixture*

> commisceo, **commiscui**, commixtum (commistum), commiscēre (< com- (< cum)
with, together + miscēre *to mix*) 섞다, 합치다   **E** *commixture*

> promiscuus, promiscua, promiscuum (< pro- *before, forward, for, instead of* + miscēre
to mix) 뒤섞인, 구별 없는, 통상적인, 문란한   **E** *promiscuous*

< IE. meik-, meig- *to mix*   **E** *mash*

> G. mignynai *to mix*

> G. mixis, mixeōs, f. *mixing, mingling*   **E** *amphimixis, apomixis, panmixis (panmixia)*

moveo, movi, motum, movēre 움직이다,

움직이게 하다　　　　　E *move, motile, motility, immotile, nonmotile, movable (moveable)*

> motus, motus, m. 움직임, 운동

> motio, motionis, f. 움직임, 운동　　　　　　　　　　　E *motion*

> motor, motoris, m. 움직이게 하는 사람, 원동력, 발동기　　　E *motor, -motor*

> motivus, motiva, motivum 원동력이 되는, 동기가 되는,

　　결정하는　　　　　E *motive, motif, (motive >) motivate, motivation*

> movimentum, movimenti, n. (*obsolete*) 움직임　　　　E *movement*

　　> momentum, momenti, n. 움직임, 계기, 순간,

　　　　중요성　　　　　E *momentum, moment, momentous (< 'of great importance')*

　　　　> momentarius, momentaria, momentarium 순간의　　E *momentary*

> *movita, *movitae, f. 반란　　　　　　　　　　E *mutiny, mutineer*

> mobilis, mobile 움직일 수 있는, 움직이기

　　쉬운 E *mobile, (mobile vulgus 'excitable crowd' >) mob, mobilize, demobilize; automobile*

　　> mobilitas, mobilitatis, f. 가동성, 기동성, 이동성, 유동성　　E *mobility*

　　> immobilis, immobile (< im- (< in-) *not*) 움직일 수 없는,

　　　　움직이기 어려운　　　　　　　　　　　E *immobile, immobilize*

　　　　> immobilitas, immobilitatis, f. 부동(不動) 상태　　E *immobility*

> commoveo, commovi, commotum, commovēre (< com- (< cum) *with, together; intensive*

　　+ movēre *to move*) 뒤흔들다, 충격을 주다, 격동시키다, 감동시키다

　　> commotio, commotionis, f. 진탕, 격동, 감동　　　　E *commotion*

> emoveo, emovi, emotum, emovēre (< e- *out of, away from* + movēre *to move*) 자리를

　　뜨게 하다, 일으키다

　　> emotio, emotionis, f. 감동, 감정, 정서　　　E *emotion, (emotion >) emotional*

> promoveo, promovi, promotum, promovēre (< pro- *before, forward, for, instead of*

　　+ movēre *to move*) 전진시키다, 승진시키다,

　　촉진하다　　　　　E *promote, (promote >) demote, (demote >) demotion*

　　> promotio, promotionis, f. 전진, 승진, 촉진　　　E *promotion*

　　> promotor, promotoris, m. 발기인, 승진자, 촉진제, 조촉매(助觸媒),

　　　　촉진유전자(促進遺傳子)　　　　　　　　E *promotor*

> removeo, removi, remotum, removēre (< re- *back, again* + movēre *to move*) 치우다,

　　물러가게 하다, 떨어지게 하다

　　E *remove, (remove >) removal, removable, (remotus (past participle) 'removed' >) remote*

< IE. meuə- *to push away*

mulgeo, mulsi (mulxi), mulsum (mulctum), mulgēre 젖을 짜다

> emulgeo, emulsi, emulsum, emulgēre (< e- *out of, away from* + mulgēre *to milk*)

　　(젖 등을) 짜내다　　　　　E *emulsify, emulsification, phacoemulsification*

　　> emulsio, emulsionis, f. 젖 같은 액체, 유제(乳劑), 유탁액(乳濁液)　　E *emulsion*

< IE. melg- *to rub off, to milk*　　　　　　　　　　　　　　　E *milk*

niteo, nitui, –, nitēre 빛나다, 찬란하다, 윤이 나다, 잘 가꾸어져 있다, 말쑥하다, 번창하다

> nitidus, nitida, nitidum 빛나는, 찬란한, 말쑥한, 세련된, 푸둥푸둥한   **E** *neat, net*

< IE. nei– *to be excited, to shine*

> (*possibly*) (*Sanskrit*) nila– *dark blue*

> **E** ((*Arabic*) an-nil >) **anil**, (*anil* >) **aniline**, ((*Persian*) nilak 'bluish' >) **lilac**, (*rose* + *aniline* >) **rosaniline**

noceo, nocui, nocitum, nocēre 해치다, 해롭다

E (nocēre 'to harm' + *receptive* >) **nociceptive**, (nocēre 'to harm' + *receptor* >) **nociceptor**, **nuisance**

[용례] nocebo (< *I shall cause harm.*, *I shall be harmful.*) 나는 해로울 것이다   **E** *nocebo*
(문법) nocebo: 능동태 직설법 미래 단수 일인칭

> nocens, (gen.) nocentis (*present participle*) 해를 끼치는, 유해한, 죄가 있는   **E** *nocent*

> innocens, (gen.) innocentis (< in– *not* + nocens *harming*) 무죄한, 무고한   **E** *innocent*

> noxa, noxae, f. 해(害)

> noxius, noxia, noxium 해로운   **E** *noxious*

> innoxius, innoxia, innoxium (< in– *not*) 해롭지 않는   **E** *innoxious*

> obnoxius, obnoxia, obnoxium (< ob– *before, toward(s), over, against, away*) (해를) 당할 수 있는

> obnoxiosus, obnoxiosa, obnoxiosum (해를) 당할 수 있는   **E** *obnoxious*

> innocuus, innocua, innocuum (< in– *not*) 해치지 않는   **E** *innocuous*

< IE. nek– *death*

> L. nex, necis, f. 죽임, 살육, 죽음, 위해(危害)

> L. neco, necavi, necatum, necare 죽이다, 멸하다

> L. necator, necatoris, m. 살해자; 구충(鉤蟲)   **E** *necator*

> L. interneco, internecavi, internecatum, internecare (< inter– *between, among* + necare *to kill*) 서로 죽이다, 몰살하다   **E** *internecine*

> L. pernicies, perniciei, f. (< per– *through, thoroughly* + nex *death*) 파멸, 해독

> L. perniciosus, perniciosa, perniciosum 파멸을 가져오는, 해독을 끼치는   **E** *pernicious*

> G. nekros, nekra, nekron *dead*

E **necr(o)–**, **necropsy** (*autopsy*) (< 'examination of a dead body'), **necromancy**, **necrophagous**, **necropolis**

> G. nekroun (nekroein) *to kill, to make dead*

> G. nekrōsis, nekrōseōs, f. (< +–ōsis *condition*) *making dead, deadness*

> L. necrosis, necrosis, f. 괴사(壞死)   **E** *necrosis, necrotic, necrotize*

> G. nektar, nektaros, n. (< *overcoming death* < IE. nek– + IE. terə– *to cross over, to pass through, to overcome*) *the drink of the gods, wine or other sweet drink*

> L. nectar, nectaris, n. 신들의 음료, 감로주   **E** *nectar, nectarine*

pareo, parui, paritum, parēre 나타나다, 뻗하다; (여격지배) 순종하다

> appareo, **apparui**, apparitum, apparēre (< ap- (< ad) *to, toward, at, according to* + parēre *to appear*) 나타나다,

드러나다　**E** *appear, apparent, (apparent >) inapparent, ((suggested) appear >) peer*

　　　> apparentia, apparentiae, f. 나타남, 출현, 겉보기, 외견　**E** *appearance*

　　　> apparitio, apparitionis, f. 시중들기; (갑작스러운) 출현, 출현물, 기묘한 현상,

유령　**E** *apparition*

> transpareo, **transparui**, transparitum, transparēre (< trans- *over, across, through, beyond* + parēre *to appear*) 투명하다　**E** *transparent*

　　　> transparentia, transparentiae, f. 투명, 투명도　**E** *transparency*

pleo, plevi, pletum, plēre (*obsolete*) 채우다

> manipulus, manipuli, m. (< manus, manus, f. *hand* + plēre *to fill*) 한줌; (고대 로마) 중대 (60명 또는 120명으로 구성됨)　**E** *manipulate*

> compleo, **complevi**, completum, complēre (< com- (< cum) *with, together; intensive* + plēre *to fill*) 채우다, 충만케 하다, 보완하다, 완성하다

E *complete, comply (< 'to be agreeable, to oblige, to obey' < 'to fulfil the requirements of courtesy'), (comply >) compliance*

　　　> completio, completionis, f. 완성, 완료, 종료　**E** *completion*

　　　> complementum, complementi, n. 보완물, 보완; (문법) 보어; (면역학) 보체(補體)

E *complement, complementary; ('a polite expression for fulfillment of the requirements of courtesy' >) compliment, complimentary*

　　　> accompleo, **accomplevi**, accompletum, accomplēre (< ac- (< ad) *to, toward, at, according to* + complēre *to fill up, to complete*) 완수하다　**E** *accomplish*

> depleo, **deplevi**, depletum, deplēre (< de- *apart from, down, not* + plēre *to fill*) 비우다, 없애다, 고갈시키다　**E** *deplete*

　　　> *depletio, *depletionis, f. 감소, 상실, 고갈　**E** *depletion*

> expleo, **explevi**, expletum, explēre (< ex- *out of, away from; intensive* + plēre *to fill*) 채우다

　　　> expletivus, expletiva, expletivum 채우는, 보완하는, 부가적인　**E** *expletive*

> impleo, **implevi**, impletum, implēre (< im- (< in) *in, on, into, toward* + plēre *to fill*) 채우다

　　　> implementum, implementi, n. 채움, 완성; 도구,

이행　**E** *implement, (implement >) implementation*

> repleo, **replevi**, repletum, replēre (< re- *back, again* + plēre *to fill*) 채우다　**E** *replete*

　　　> repletio, repletionis, f. 충만　**E** *repletion*

> suppleo, **supplevi**, suppletum, supplēre (< sup- (< sub) *under, up from under* + plēre *to fill*) 보충하다, 추가하다　**E** *supply*

　　　> suppletio, suppletionis, f. 보충, 추가; (문법) 보충법　**E** *suppletion*

　　　> supplementum, supplementi, n. 보충물, 추가물　**E** *supplement, supplementary*

　　　> suppletivus, suppletiva, suppletivum 보충하는, 추가적인　**E** *suppletive*

< IE. pelə- *to fill: with derivatives referring to abundance*
and multitude   **E** *fill, full, fulfil (fulfill), fulfilment (fulfillment), folk, folklore,* D. *Volkslied*

> L. pelvis, pelvis, f. 세숫대야, 반(盤), 골반(骨盤), 신우(腎盂)   **E** *pelvis, (pelvis >) pelvic*

> L. plebs, plebis, f. 평민, 서민, 민중   **E** *plebs, (pl.) plebes*

> L. plebeius, plebeia, plebeium 평민의, 서민의, 민중의   **E** *plebeian*

> L. plebiscitum, plebisciti, n. (< plebis scitum < plebs *common people* + sciscĕre
vote for) (원로원 의원·귀족을 제외한) 로마 시민의 의결, 국민투표   **E** *plebiscite*

> L. plenus, plena, plenum 가득한, 꽉 찬   **E** *deplenish, replenish*

> L. plenarius, plenaria, plenarium 전체의, 전원 출석의, 완전한   **E** *plenary*

> L. plenitas, plenitatis, f. 많음, 풍부   **E** *plenty*

> L. plenitudo, plenitudinis, f. 충분, 충만   **E** *plenitude*

> L. −, −, plus ((gen.) pluris) (multus, multa, multum의 비교급) 더 많은

E *plus, pluripotent, nonplus (< 'a state in which no more can be said or done'),*
(superplus >) *surplus*

> L. pluralis, plurale 여러; (문법) 복수의   **E** *plural*

> L. plusquamperfectum, plusquamperfecti, n. (< plus quam perfectum *more
than perfect*) (문법) 과거완료   **E** *pluperfect*

> G. plērēs, plērēs, plēres *full, filled with, complete*   **E** *plerocercoid (< 'completed cercoid')*

> G. plēroun (plēroein) *to make full, to fill*

> G. anaplēroun (anaplēroein) (< an(a)- *up, upward; again, throughout; back,
backward; against; according to, similar to) to fill up, to complete*

> G. anaplērōsis, anaplērōseōs, f. (< + -ōsis *condition*) *filling up of a
deficiency*

> L. anaplerosis, anaplerosis, f. 보충, 보전(補塡)   **E** *anaplerosis, anaplerotic*

> G. plēthein *to be full*

> G. plēthōra, plēthōras, f. *fullness, overabundance of one or more humors,
especially blood*

> L. plethora, plethorae, f. 충만, 과다, 다혈색, 다혈증   **E** *plethora, plethoric*

> G. plēthos, plēthous, n. *mass, throng, crowd, great number*

> G. plēthynein *to make full, to increase*

> G. plēthysmos, plēthysmou, m. *making full, increase*

E *plethysmograph (< 'an instrument for recording and measuring variation
in the volume of a part of the body, or of the whole body, especially as
caused by changes in blood pressure')*

> G. polys, pollē, poly *many, much, frequent*

E *poly-, polymorphism (< 'two or more forms in one species, as the castes of social
insects'), polycyte (< 'hypersegmented polymorphonuclear leukocyte of normal size,
appearing multinucleated')*

pleiōn, pleiōn, pleion (pleōn, pleōn, pleon) (비교급) *more*

E *pleio-, pleiotropism (pleiotropy), pleiotropic, pleo-, pleomorphism (< 'two or more
forms in one life cycle'), pleocytosis (< 'more cells in the cerebrospinal fluid'),
plio-, Pliocene*

E *Pleistocene*

rideo, risi, risum, ridēre 웃다, 비웃다

> risor, risoris, m. 웃는 사람, 비웃는 사람

> risorius, risoria, risorium 웃는, 잘 웃는

E *risorius (muscle)*

> ridiculus, ridicula, ridiculum 웃기는, 우스운

E *ridiculous*

> ridiculum, ridiculi, n. 웃음거리, 익살

E *ridicule*

> derideo, **derisi**, derisum, deridere (< de- *apart from, down, not; intensive* + ridēre *to laugh*) 비웃다, 조롱하다

E *deride, derisive*

> derisio, derisionis, f. 비웃음, 조롱

E *derision*

< IE. wrizd- *to avert the face*

sedeo, sedi, sessum, sedēre 앉다

E *siege*

> sedes, sedis, f. 자리, 지위, 왕좌, (주교・교황)좌, 거처, 본거지, 터전, 궁둥이, 항문

> sedentarius, sedentaria, sedentarium 앉아서 일하는, 정착성의

E *sedentary*

> sedimentum, sedimenti, n. 앙금, 침몰, 침전물

E *sediment, (sediment >) sedimentation*

> sessio, sessionis, f. 앉음, 착석, 개회, 회의, 회기

E *session*

> sessilis, sessile 앉을 만한, (술잔 등) 밑바닥이 넓어 안정성 있는; (식물) 옆으로 퍼진; 무경(無莖)의, 무병(無柄)의

E *sessile*

> sella, sellae, f. 안장

E *sella, sellar, suprasellar, infrasellar*

[용례] sella turcica 터키안(鞍), 안장

E *sella turcica*

(문법) sella: 단수 주격

turcica 터키식의: 형용사, 여성형 단수 주격

< turcicus, turcica, turcicum

[용례] tuberculum sellae 안장결절

E *tuberculum sellae*

dorsum sellae 안장등

E *dorsum sellae*

diaphragma sellae 안장가로막

E *diaphragma sellae*

(문법) tuberculum 결절: 단수 주격 < tuberculum, tuberculi, n.

dorsum 등: 단수 주격 < dorsum, dorsi, n.

diaphragma 가로막: 단수 주격 < diaphragma, diaphragmatis, n.

sellae: 단수 속격

> assideo, **assedi**, assessum, assidēre (< as- (< ad) *to, toward, at, according to* + sedēre *to sit*) 옆에 앉아 있다, (법정에) 배석하다, 보살피다, 힘쓰다

E *assize, (assize (aphetic) > 'an ordinance regulating weights and measures') >) size*

> assiduus, assidua, assiduum 늘 옆에 있는, 꾸준히 힘쓰는

E *assiduous*

> assesso, **assessavi**, assessatum, assessare (*frequentative*) 평가하다, 부과하다

E *assess*

> dissideo, **dissedi**, dissessum, dissidēre (< dis- *apart from, down, not* + sedēre *to sit*) 떨어져 앉다, 의견을 달리하다, 반대하다

E *dissident*

> dissidentia, dissidentiae, f. 상이, 반대   **E** *dissidence*

> insideo, **insedi**, insessum, insidēre (< in- *in, on, into, toward* + sedēre *to sit*) 자리
잡고 있다

    > insidiae, insidiarum, f. (pl.) 매복, 암계

       > insidiosus, insidiosa, insidiosum 암계를 꾸미는, 잠행성(潛行性)의, 서서히
진행하는   **E** *insidious*

    > *insessorius, *insessoria, *insessorium (새의 다리가) 나뭇가지에 앉기 적합한,
(새가) 나뭇가지에 앉는   **E** *insessorial*

> obsideo, **obsedi**, obsessum, obsidēre (< ob- *before, toward(s), over, against, away*
+ sedēre *to sit*) 자리 잡다, 포위하다, 점유하다,
(마음·정신 등을) 사로잡다   **E** *obsess, obsessive*

    > obsessio, obsessionis, f. 포위, 점유, 강박, 강박관념, 망상   **E** *obsession*

    > obses, obsidis, m., f. 볼모, 인질, 보증, 저당

       > obsidatus, obsidatus, m. 볼모로 넘겨줌(잡혀감), 볼모 신세   **E** *hostage*

> possideo, **possedi**, possessum, possidēre (< potis (pote) *able, possible* + sedēre
to sit) 차지하다, 소유하다   **E** *possess*

    > possessio, possessionis, f. 소유, 점유, 소유물   **E** *possession*

    > possessivus, possessiva, possessivum 소유의; (문법) 소유격(所有格)의   **E** *possessive*

> praesideo, **praesedi**, praesessum, praesidēre (< prae- *before, beyond* + sedēre *to sit*)
앞자리에 앉다, 지키다, 통할하다   **E** *preside*

    > praesidens, praesidentis, m. (< *present participle*) 주관자, 의장,
통치자   **E** *president, presidential*

       > praesidentia, praesidentiae, f. 주관자의 지위(직책, 임기)   **E** *presidency*

> resideo, **resedi**, resessum, residēre (< re- *back, again* + sedēre *to sit*) 앉아 있다,
거주하다, 남아 있다   **E** *reside, resident*

    > residentia, residentiae, f. 거주지, 임지, 거주,
(임지에서의) 정주(定住)   **E** *residence, residency, residential*

    > residuus, residua, residuum 남은, 나머지의, 잔존하는, 잔류하는

       > residuum, residui, n. 나머지, 잔존,
잔류   **E** *residuum,* (pl.) *residua, residue, residual*

> supersedeo, **supersedi**, supersessum, supersedēre (< super- *above* + sedēre *to sit*)
위에 앉다, 주재하다, 그치다   **E** *supersede*

< IE. sed- *to sit*

    E *sit, seat, saddle, settle, set, setup, onset, offset, beset, nest* (< '*bird's place of sitting
down*'), *nestle, nestling, soot* (< '*that which settles*'), (D. Sitzbad >) *sitz bath*, D. *Sitzkrieg*

> L. sido, **sidi** (sedi), sessum, sidēre 내려앉다, 가라앉다

    > L. subsido, **subsidi** (subsedi), subsessum, subsidēre (< sub- *under, up from
under* + sidēre *to sit down*) 엎드리다, 머물다, 망보다, 잠잠해지다   **E** *subside*

       > L. subsidium, subsidii, n. 예비군, 보조   **E** *subsidy,* (subsidy >) *subsidize*

          > L. subsidiarius, subsidiaria, subsidiarium 예비의, 보조의   **E** *subsidiary*

> L. sedo, **sedavi**, sedatum, sedare 진정시키다   **E** *sedate, sedative*

> L. sedatio, sedationis, f. 진정작용, 진정상태   **E** *sedation*

> L. solium, solii, n. 의자, 왕좌, 왕위, 물통, 목욕통,

　석관   **E** *soil (< 'in association with* L. solum *ground')*

> L. nidus, nidi, m. (*ni- *down* + *zd- (<*sed-) *to sit*) 새집, 둥지, 병터, 병소(病巢),

　핵   **E** *nidus, (nidus >) nidation, niche*

> G. hezesthai *to sit*

　　> G. hedra, hedras, f. *seat, base, side of a solid figure*

　　　　E *-hedron, -hedral, tetrahedron, hexahedron (cube), octahedron, dodecahedron, icosahedron, icosahedral, trisoctahedron, polyhedron, polyhedral*

　　　> G. ephedra, ephedras, f. (< eph- (< epi) *upon* + hedra) *shrubby horsetails*

　　　　> L. ephedra, ephedrae, f. 마황(麻黃)   **E** *ephedrine*

　　　> G. kathedra, kathedras, f. (< kath- (< kata) *down, mis-, according to,*

　　　　along, thoroughly + hedra) *seat*

　　　　> L. cathedra, cathedrae, f. 좌석, 팔걸이의자, 교수의 강좌,

　　　　　주교좌   **E** *cathedra, cathedral, chair*

> G. piezein (< *to sit upon* < IE. epi *upon* + IE. sed-) *to press*

　tight   **E** *piez(o)-, piezoelectricity, isopiestic*

> (*Sanskrit*) upanishad (< upa *near to, under* + ni-shad *to sit, to lie down*)   **E** *Upanishad*

sorbeo, sorbui, sorptum, sorbēre 빨아들이다,

흡수하다   **E** (ad *'to'* + *-sorption >) adsorption, (adsorption >) adsorb*

> absorbeo, **absorbui**, absorptum, absorbēre (< ab- *off, away from* + sorbēre *to suck*

　in) 흡수하다   **E** *absorb, absorbent, absorptive; absorbance*

　> absorptio, absorptionis, f. 흡수   **E** *absorption, (absorption >) malabsorption*

　> reabsorbeo, **reabsorbui**, reabsorptum, reabsorbēre (< re- *back, again* + absorbēre

　　to absorb) 재흡수하다   **E** *reabsorb*

　　> reabsorptio, reabsorptionis, f. 재흡수   **E** *reabsorption*

> resorbeo, **resorbui**, resorptum, resorbēre (< re- *back, again* + sorbēre *to suck in*)

　제거를 위해 흡수하다   **E** *resorb, resorbent*

　> resorptio, resorptionis, f. (제거를 위한) (재)흡수   **E** *resorption*

< IE. srebh- *to suck, to absorb*

splendeo, splendui, –, splendēre 빛나다, 화려하다   **E** *splendent*

> splendor, splendoris, m. 광휘, 화려   **E** *splendor (splendour)*

> splendidus, splendida, splendidum 눈부신, 화려한   **E** *splendid*

> resplendeo, **resplendui**, –, resplendēre (< re- *back, again; intensive* + splendēre

　to shine) 눈부시게 빛나다, 휘황찬란하다   **E** *resplendent*

< IE. splend- *to shine, to glow*

spondeo, spopondi, sponsum, spondēre 서약하다, 약혼하다, 보증하다, 미리 알리다,

단언하다　　　**E** (sponsus, sponsa (*masculine and feminine past participles*) '*engaged*' >) *spouse*

> sponsor, sponsoris, m. (sponstrix, sponstricis, f.) 보증인, 후견인　　　　**E** *sponsor*

> sponso, −, −, sponsare 약혼하다, 맞아들이다, 받아들이다　　　　**E** *espouse*

> despondeo, **despondi**, desponsum, despondēre (< de- *apart from, down, not; intensive*
　+ spondēre *to pledge*) 약속하다; 낙심하다　　**E** *despond, despondent, despondence*

> respondeo, **respondi**, responsum, respondēre (< re- *back, again* + spondēre *to pledge*)
　(상대방의 약속에 대하여 이쪽에서도) 약속하다, 대응하다, 반응하다,
　대답하다　　　　**E** *respond, response, responsible, irresponsible*

　　[용례] Respondeat superior. (< *Let the superior answer.*) 윗사람이 답하리라
　　　　(문법) respondeat 대답하리라: 능동태 가정법 현재 단수 삼인칭
　　　　　　superior 윗사람이: 형용사의 명사적 용법, 남성 단수 주격
　　　　　　　　< superior, superior, superius

> correspondeo, **correspondi**, corresponsum, correspondēre (< cor- (< cum)
　with, together + respondēre *to answer*) 대응하다, 상응하다,
　부합하다　　　　**E** *correspond, correspondent, correspondence*
< IE. spend- *to make an offering, to perform a rite, hence to engage oneself by a ritual act*
> G. spondē, spondēs, f. *libation, offering*
　> L. spondeus, spondei, m. (헌주시의) 장장격(長長格), 강강격(强强格)　　**E** *spondee*

suadeo, suasi, suasum, suadēre 충고하다, 설득하다,

권유하다　　　　**E** *suasion, suasive*, (ad '*to*' > '*on the pattern of persuasive*' >) *assuasive*

> dissuadeo, **dissuasi**, dissuasum, dissuadēre (< dis- *apart from, down, not* + suadēre
　to advise) (설득·권유하여) 그만두게 하다　　　**E** *dissuade*

> persuadeo, **persuasi**, persuasum, persuadēre (< per- *through, thoroughly* + suadēre
　to advise) 설득하다, 권유하다　　　　**E** *persuade, persuasive*
　> persuasio, persuasionis, f. 설득, 권유　　　　**E** *persuasion*
< IE. swad- *sweet, pleasant*　　　　**E** *sweet*
> L. suavis, suave 입에 당기는, 기분 좋은, 상냥한　　　　**E** *suave*
　> L. *assuavio, *assuaviavi, *assuaviatum, *assuaviare (< ad- *to, toward, at,*
　　according to + suavis *sweet*) 만족시키다, 완화시키다　　　**E** *assuage*
> G. hēdys, hēdeia, hēdy *sweet, pleasant*
　> G. aēdēs, aēdēs, aēdes (< a- *not*) *unpleasant*
　　> L. aedes, aedis, m. 에데스모기, 숲모기　　　**E** *aedes*
　> G. hēdonē, hēdonēs, f. *pleasure*　　**E** *hedonic, hedonism, hedonophobia*
　　> L. anhedonia, anhedoniae, f. (< G. an- *not*) 무쾌감증　　**E** *anhedonia*

taceo, tacui, tacitum, tacēre 침묵하다

> tacitus, tacita, tacitum (*past participle*) 무언의, 묵시적인　　　**E** *tacit*
　> taciturnus, taciturna, taciturnum 무언의, 과묵한　　　**E** *taciturn*
> reticeo, **reticui**, −, reticere (< re- *back, again; intensive* + tacēre *to be silent*)

침묵하다, 비밀로 하다　　　　　　　　　　　　　　　　　　　　　　　**E** *reticent*

　< IE. tak- *to be silent*

taedet, taeduit (taesum est), –, taedēre (비인칭동사) 싫증이 나다

　　> taedium, taedii, n. 싫증　　　　　　　　　　　　　　　　　　　**E** *tedium*

　　　　> taediosus, taediosa, taediosum 싫증이 나는, 싫증을 느끼는　　**E** *tedious*

teneo, tenui, tentum, tenēre 잡다, 지키다, 소유하다, 깨닫다

> **E** (*third personal singular, present indicative, active 'he/she holds'* >) **tenet, tenant, tenable, tennis,** (intertenēre *'to maintain'* > *'to maintain in a certain condition, to treat in a certain way'* > *'to show hospitality'* >) **entertain,** (manu tenēre *'to hold in the hand'* >) **maintain, maintenance,** (locum tenens *'holding the place (of another)'* >) **lieutenant**

　　> tenor, tenoris, m. 진행, 어조(語調)　　　　　　　　　　　　　**E** *tenor*

　　> tenetura, teneturae, f. (tenitura, teniturae, f.) 보유　　　　　　**E** *tenure*

　　> tenementum, tenementi, n. 보유재산, 보유권　　　　　　　　　**E** *tenement*

　　> tenax, (gen.) tenacis 꼭 잡고 있는, 강인한　　　　　　　　　　**E** *tenacious*

　　　　> tenacitas, tenacitatis, f. 강인성　　　　　　　　　　　　　**E** *tenacity*

　　　　> tenaculum, tenaculi, n. 지지구(支持鉤)　　　　　　　　　**E** *tenaculum*

　　　　> pertinax, (gen.) pertinacis (< per- *through, thoroughly* + tenax *holding fast*)

　　　　　　꼭 잡고 있는, 강인한, 집요한　　　　　　　　　　　　　**E** *pertinacious*

　　　　　　> pertinacitas, pertinacitatis, f. 강인, 집요　　　　　　**E** *pertinacity*

　　> abstineo, **abstinui,** abstentum, abstinēre (< abs- (< ab) *off, away from* + tenēre

　　　　to hold) 멀리하다, 끊다　　　　　　　　　　　　　　　**E** *abstain, abstinent*

　　　　> abstinentia, abstinentiae, f. 절제, 중단, 금단(禁斷)　　　　**E** *abstinence*

　　　　> abstentio, abstentionis, f. 억제, 제지　　　　　　　　　　**E** *abstention*

　　> contineo, **continui,** contentum, continēre (< con- (< cum) *with, together; intensive*

　　　　+ tenēre *to hold*) 포함하다, 붙잡아 두다, 억제하다　　**E** *contain, containment*

　　　　> continens, (gen.) continentis (*present participle*) 붙어 있는; 자제력 있는, 절제하는

　　　　　> **E** (terra continens *'continuous land'* >) **continent, continental, subcontinent;** (continens *'restraining oneself'* >) **continent**

　　　　　> continentia, continentiae, f. 내용; 인접; 자제(自制), 금제(禁制)

　　　　　> **E** *countenance* (< *'manner of holding oneself, bearing, behaviour, aspect'*); *continence* (< *'holding together, restraining oneself'*)

　　　　　> incontinens, (gen.) incontinentis (< in- *not* + continens *holding together*)

　　　　　　붙잡아 두지 못하는, 자제력 없는, 절제 없는　　　　　**E** *incontinent*

　　　　　　> incontinentia, incontinentiae, f. 무절제, 실금(失禁), 세기, 찔끔증,

　　　　　　　실조(失調)　　　　　　　　　　　　　　　　　　**E** *incontinence*

　　　　> contentus, contenta, contentum (*past participle*) 포함된, 충족된,

　　　　　만족해하는　　　　　　　　**E** (*adjective*) **content,** (content >) **discontent**

　　　　　> contentum, contenti, n. 내용, 함량　　　　**E** (*noun*) **content**

　　　　> continuus, continua, continuum 붙어 있는, 연속적인　　**E** *continuous, continual*

> continuum, continui, n. 연속, 연속체   **E** *continuum, (pl.) continua*

> continuitas, continuitatis, f. 연속   **E** *continuity*

> continuo, **continuavi,** continuatum, continuare 잇다, 계속하다,

지속하다   **E** *continue, continuant, continuance*

> continuatio, continuationis, f. 계속, 지속   **E** *continuation*

> detineo, **detinui,** detentum, detinēre (< de- *apart from, down, not* + tenēre *to hold*)

억류하다, 점유하다   **E** *detain, (detain >) detainee, detinue*

> detentio, detentionis, f. 억류, 점유   **E** *detention*

> obtineo, **obtinui,** obtentum, obtinēre (< ob- *before, toward(s), over, against, away* +

tenēre *to hold*) 차지하다, 얻다   **E** *obtain*

> pertineo, **pertinui,** pertentum, pertinēre (< per- *through, thoroughly* + tenēre *to hold*)

귀속하다, 관계되다, 적합하다   **E** *pertain, pertinent, impertinent*

> retineo, **retinui,** retentum, retinēre (< re- *back, again* + tenēre *to hold*) 붙잡다, 머물러

있게 하다   **E** *retain, retinue, rein*

> retentio, retentionis, f. 보유; 잔류, 정체, 축적   **E** *retention*

> retinaculum, retinaculi, n. 붙들어 매는 끈, 지대(支帶), 지지구(支持鉤)   **E** *retinaculum*

> sustineo, **sustinui,** sustentum, sustinēre (< sus- (< sub) *under, up from under* +

tenēre *to hold*) 받쳐주다, 견디다, 먹여 살리다   **E** *sustain, sustention, sustenance*

> sustento, **sustentavi,** sustentatum, sustentare (*frequentative*) 지탱하다,

부양하다   **E** *sustentation*

> sustentaculum, sustentaculi, n. 지탱물, 부양물,

버팀   **E** *sustentaculum (sustentacle), sustentacular*

< IE. ten- *to stretch*   **E** *thin*

> L. tendo, **tetendi,** tentum (tensum), tendĕre 뻗치다, 향하다   **E** *tend, tensive, tent*

> L. tendentia, tendentiae, f. 경향, 성향, 소인   **E** *tendency*

> L. tensus, tensa, tensum (*past participle*) 빳빳이 퍼진, 팽팽한, 긴장된   **E** *tense*

> L. tensio, tensionis, f. 빳빳하게 폄, 신장(伸張), 긴장, 장력(張力)

E *tension; hypertension, hypertensive, hypotension, hypotensive, normotension, normotensive, angiotensin*

> L. tensor, tensoris, m. 장근(張筋), 긴장근; (수학) 텐서   **E** *tensor*

> L. tensilis, tensile 펼 수 있는, 장력이 있는   **E** *tensile*

> L. tentorium, tentorii, n. 천막, 야영   **E** *tentorium, tentorial*

[용례] tentorium cerebelli 소뇌천막   **E** *tentorium cerebelli*

(문법) tentorium: 단수 주격

cerebelli 소뇌의: 단수 속격 < cerebellum, cerebelli, n.

> L. tenuis, tenue 가는, 엷은   **E** *tenuous*

> L. pertenuis, pertenue (< per- *through, thoroughly* + tenuis *thin*) 아주

가는, 아주 엷은, 빈약한

> L. tenuitas, tenuitatis, f. 가늚, 엷음, 빈약, 박약, 희박, 미약   **E** *tenuity*

> L. tenuo, **tenuavi,** tenuatum, tenuare 가늘게 하다, 엷게 하다, 약화시키다

> L. attenuo, **attenuavi,** attenuatum, attenuare (< at- (< ad) *to,*

toward, at, according to + tenuare *to make thin*) 약화시키다,
감쇠시키다, 잦아들게 하다   **E** *attenuate, attenuator*

> L. attenuatio, attenuationis, f. 약화, 감쇠, 마멸   **E** *attenuation*

> L. extenuo, **extenuavi**, extenuatum, extenuare (< ex- *out of, away
from* + tenuare *to make thin*) (결점 · 벌 등을) 가볍게 하다,
정상을 참작하다   **E** *extenuate*

> L. tener, tenera, tenerum 부드러운, 연한, 연약한,
민감한   **E** *tender, tenderness, tendril*

> L. *intenero, *inteneravi, *inteneratum, *intenerare (< in- *in, on,
into, toward* + tener *tender*) 부드럽게 하다, 누그러뜨리다   **E** *intenerate*

> L. tento, **tentavi**, tentatum, tentare (tempto, temptavi, temptatum, temptare)
(*frequentative*) 만지다, 시도하다, 시험하다, 유혹하다   **E** *tentative*

> L. tentaculum, tentaculi, n. 촉수, 선모(腺毛)   **E** *tentacle*

> L. temptatio, temptationis, f. 유혹   **E** *temptation*

> L. attento, **attentavi**, attentatum, attentare (attempto, attemptavi,
attemptatum, attemptare) (< at- (< ad) *to, toward, at, according to*
+ tentare (temptare) *to try, to test*) 시도하다   **E** *attempt*

> L. attendo, **attendi**, attentum, attendĕre (< at- (< ad) *to, toward, at, according
to* + tendĕre *to stretch*) 내뻗다, 주의를 기울이다, 집중하다

E *attend, (attend >) tend, attender, (bar + attender >) bartender, attentive;*
attendant, attendance

> L. attentio, attentionis, f. 주의   **E** *attention*

> L. contendo, **contendi**, contentum, contendĕre (< con- (< cum) *with, together*
+ tendĕre *to stretch*) 잡아당기다, 추구하다, 애쓰다, 경쟁하다, 싸우다   **E** *contend*

> L. contentio, contentionis, f. 경쟁, 다툼   **E** *contention*

> L. contentiosus, contentiosa, contentiosum 다투기 좋아하는, 논쟁을
불러일으키는   **E** *contentious*

> L. detendo, **detendi**, detensum, detendĕre (< de- *apart from, down, not* + tendĕre
to stretch) 늦추다, 누그러지게 하다, (천막을) 걷다   **E** *detent, detente*

> L. distendo, **distendi**, distentum (distensum), distendĕre (< dis- *apart from,
down, not* + tendĕre *to stretch*) 넓히다, 팽창시키다   **E** *distend, distensible*

> L. distentio, distentionis, f. (distensio, distensionis, f.) 팽창, 팽만,
확장   **E** *distention (distension)*

> L. extendo, **extendi**, extentum (extensum), extendĕre (< ex- *out of, away from* +
tendĕre *to stretch*) 펴다, 확장하다

E *extend, extent, extensive, extensible, extensile, standard (< 'a flag raised on
a pole as a rallying point, the authorized exemplar of a unit of measurement,
an upright timber'), (standard >) standardize*

> L. extensio, extensionis, f. 폄, 확장   **E** *extension*

> L. extensor, extensoris, m. 폄근, 신근(伸筋), 폄쪽   **E** *extensor*

> L. intendo, **intendi**, intentum (intensum), intendĕre (< in- *in, on, into, toward*
+ tendĕre *to stretch*) 향하게 하다, 의도하다; 집중시키다,

증대시키다   **E** *intend, intensive*

     > L. intensus, intensa, intensum (*past participle*) 센, 강렬한   **E** *intense*

         > L. *intensifico, *intensificavi, *intensificatum, *intensificare (<

             intensus *intense* + –ficare (< facĕre) *to make*) 강하게 하다   **E** *intensify*

            > L. intensitas, intensitatis, f. 세기, 강도(強度)   **E** *intensity*

         > L. intentio, intentionis, f. 의도(意圖),

             기도(企圖)   **E** *intention, intentional, unintentional*

         > L. superintendo, –, –, superintendĕre (< super– *above* + intendĕre

             to turn one's attention) 감시하다   **E** *superintend*

   > L. ostendo, **ostendi**, ostentum (ostensum), ostendĕre (< os– (< obs– < ob)

       before, toward(s), over, against, away + tendĕre *to stretch*) 앞에 내놓다,

       드러내다   **E** *ostensive, ostensible*

     > L. ostento, **ostentavi**, ostentatum, ostentare (*frequentative*) 과시하다,

         겉치레하다   **E** *ostentatious*

         > L. ostentatio, ostentationis, f. 과시, 겉치레   **E** *ostentation*

   > L. portendo, **portendi**; portentum, portendĕre (< por– (< pro) *forth* + tendĕre

       to stretch) 예고하다, 전조로 나타내다   **E** *portend, portent, portentous*

   > L. praetendo, **praetendi**, praetentum (praetensum), praetendĕre (< prae– *before,*

       beyond + tendĕre *to stretch*) 앞으로 뻗치다,

       표면에 내세우다   **E** *pretend, ((past parciple*) praetensus >) *pretense (pretence)*

        > L. praetentio, praetentionis, f. (praetensio, praetensionis, f.) 요구, 자처,

           허세, 겉치레   **E** *pretension, pretentious*

   > L. subtendo, **subtendi**, subtentum (subtensum), subtendĕre (< sub– *under,*

       up from under + tendĕre *to stretch*) 밑에 퍼지다, 밑에 펴다   **E** *subtend*

> G. teinein (*with strong grade of verbal ablaut series* ten–, ton–, ta–) *to stretch,*

   to strain

     > G. anateinein (< an(a)– *up, upward; again, throughout; back, backward;*

         against; according to, similar to) *to stretch out, to stretch forth*

         > (*suggested*) L. antenna, antennae, f. 삼각돛, 촉각(觸角)

            E *antenna,* (pl.) *antennae,* (L. antenna + L. pes, pedis, m. > '*a homeotic gene controlling development of the antennae and legs in* Drosophila melanogaster' >) *antennapedia*

     > G. parateinein (< par(a)– *beside, along side of, beyond*) *to stretch out beside,*

         to protract   **E** *paratenic*

     > G. teinesmos, teinesmou, m. (tēnesmos, tēnesmou, m.) *straining*

        > L. tenesmus, tenesmi, m. 이급후중(裏急後重), 후중(後重), 뒤무직,

           결리(結痢)   **E** *tenesmus*

     > G. tenōn, tenontos, m. (< *stretched sinew*) *sinew, tendon*

        > L. tenon, tenontis, m. 힘줄,

           건(腱)   **E** *tenotomy, tenorrhaphy, tenontoplasty (tenoplasty)*

        > L. tendo, tendinis, m. (*form influeced by* L. tendĕre *to stretch*) 힘줄,

           건(腱)   **E** *tendon; tendinocyte, epitendineum, endotendineum*

[용례] tendo calcaneus (tendo Achillis) (< *calcaneal tendon,*
Achilles tendon) 발꿈치힘줄, 아킬레스힘줄

(문법) tendo 힘줄: 단수 주격

calcaneus 발꿈치의: 형용사, 남성형 단수 주격

< calcaneus, calcanea, calcaneum

Achillis 아킬레스의: 단수 속격

< Achilles, Achillis, m.

< G. Achilleus, Achilleōs, m.

> L. tendineus, tendinea, tendineum 힘줄의, 건(腱)의

> L. tendinosus, tendinosa, tendinosum 힘줄의, 힘줄 모양의 　**E** *tendinous*

　> L. semitendinosus, semitendinosa, semitendinosum (< semi-

half) 반힘줄 모양의 　**E** *semitendinosus (muscle), semitendinous*

> G. tonos, tonou, m. *stretching, rope, chord, tone*

　> L. tonus, toni, m. 긴장(緊張), 장력(張力), (정신·건강·물질의) 정상 상태;

음조(音調), 어조(語調), 색조(色調), 기풍(氣風)

E *tonus, tone, toner, (tone >) tune, tuner, (tune >) attune, tonofilament,*
tonofibril, calcitonin (thyrocalcitonin) (< 'involved in the regulation of
the normal 'tone' of calcium in the body fluids')

　　> L. intono, **intonavi**, intonatum, intonare (< in- *in, on, into, toward*)

음조를 붙이다, 영창을 하다, 억양을 붙이다 　**E** *intone, intonation*

　> G. tonikos, tonikē, tonikon *of or for stretching*

　　> L. tonicus, tonica, tonicum 긴장성의, 장력의, 지속 긴장의, 강직

성의, 몸을 강하게 하는, 기력을 돋우어 주는

E *tonic, (tonic >) tonicity, -tonic, isotonic, hypertonic, hypotonic;*
serotonin (< 'its source from serum and its activity of smooth
muscle constriction'), melatonin (< 'the active pineal gland factor
that can lighten the color of frog melanocytes by causing
aggregation of melanin granules about the nuclei of the cells')

　> G. barytonos, barytonos, barytonon (< barys *heavy, deep* + tonos)

deep-toned 　**E** *barytone (baritone)*

　> G. atonos, atonos, atonon (< a- *not*) *without tone*

　　> G. atonia, atonias, f. *atony*

　　　> L. atonia, atoniae, f. 무긴장증, 이완증 　**E** *atony*

　　> L. atonicus, atonica, atonicum 긴장력이 없는, 이완된, 힘이 없는,

(음성) 강세가 없는 　**E** *atonic, (atonic >) atonicity*

　> L. catatonia, catatoniae, f. (< G. kat(a)- *down, mis-, according to, along,*
thoroughly) 긴장증, 긴장병 　**E** *catatonia*

　> L. dystonia, dystoniae, f. (< G. dys- *bad*) 근육긴장이상 　**E** *dystonia, dystonic*

　> L. myotonia, myotoniae, f. (< G. my(o)- *muscle*) 근육긴장증,

근강직증 　**E** *myotonia, myotonic*

　> G. opisthotonos, opisthotonou, m. (< opisth(o)- (< opisthen) *behind*)

spasm in which the body is drawn back and stiffens

> L. opisthotonus, opisthotoni, m. 활모양강직, 후궁반장(後弓反張),

반궁긴장(反弓緊張)　　　　　　　　E *opisthotonos (opisthotonus)*

> G. peritonaion, peritonaiou, n. (< peri- *around, near, beyond, on account*

of + tonos *stretching*) *stretching-over*

> L. peritonaeum, peritonaei, n. (peritoneum, peritonei, n.)

복막(腹膜)　　　　　　　　　　　E *peritoneum, peritoneocentesis*

[용례] carcinomatosis peritonei 복막 암종증　E *carcinomatosis peritonei*

pseudomyxoma peritonei 복막

거짓점액종　　　　　　　　　　E *pseudomyxoma peritonei*

(문법) carcinomatosis 암종증: 단수 주격

< carcinomatosis, carcinomatosis, f.

pseudomyxoma 거짓점액종: 단수 주격

< pseudomyxoma, pseudomyxomatis, n.

< pseudomucin (*obsolete*) (< *mucin not*

precipitated by acetic acid, like ovarian

cyst mucin) + -ōma (*noun suffix denoting*

tumor)

peritonei 복막의: 단수 속격

> L. peritonaealis, peritonaeale (peritonealis, peritoneale)

복막의　　　　　　　　　　　E *peritoneal, intraperitoneal*

> L. retroperitoneum, retroperitonei, n. (< retro- *backward,*

behind) 배막뒤공간, 복막뒤공간, 복막후강,

후복막강　　　　　　　E *retroperitoneum, retroperitoneal*

> G. tasis, taseōs, f. *stretching*　　　　　　　　E *myotatic*

> G. ektasis, ektaseōs, f. (< ek- *out of, away from* + tasis) *extension,*

dilatation

> L. ectasis, ectasis, f. (ectasia, ectasiae, f. (< + -ia)) 확장,

확장증　　　　　　　　　　E *ectasis (ectasia), ectatic*

> L. atelectasis, atelectasis, f. (< G. atelēs (< a- *not* + telos

completion, end) *incomplete*)

무기폐(無氣肺)　　　　　　E *atelectasis, atelectatic*

> L. bronchiectasis, bronchiectasis, f. (-ectasia, -ectasiae, f.)

(< G. bronchos *windpipe*) 기관지

확장증　　　E *bronchiectasis (bronchiectasia), bronchiectatic*

> L. telangiectasis, telangiectasis, f. (-ectasia, -ectasiae, f.)

(< G. telos *end* + angeion *vessel*) 모세혈관확장, 모세

혈관확장증, 실핏줄확장,

실핏줄확장증　E *telangiectasis (telangiectasia), telangiectatic*

> G. entasis, entaseōs, f. (< *stretching tight* < en- *in* + tasis) *a delicate*

and almost imperceptible swelling of the shaft of a column

> L. entasis, entasis, f. 배흘림　　　　　　　　E *entasis*

> G. tanyein *to stretch*　　　　　　　　　　　　　　　　　　　　 **E** *tanycyte*

> G. (*reduplicated form*) tetanos, tetanē, tetanon *stretched, rigid*

> L. tetanus, tetani, m. 파상풍(破傷風), 강축(强縮),

테타너스　　**E** *tetanus, tetanic,* (tetanus > 'hypocalcemic spasm' >) *tetany*

> G. tainia, tainias, f. *head-band, ribbon, tape*

> L. taenia, taeniae, f. (tenia, teniae, f.) 머리띠, 띠, 붕대; 촌충(寸蟲), 조충(條蟲)

> **E** *taenia (tenia),* (pl.) *taeniae (teniae), -tene, leptotene* (< 'stage of thin ribbons'), *zygotene* (< 'stage of yoked ribbons'), *pachytene* (< 'stage of thick ribbons'), *diplotene* (< 'stage of double ribbons'), *polytene* (< 'a chromosome of many chromatids' < 'many ribbons'), *synteny* (< 'the presence of genes on the same chromosome')

> L. taeniola, taeniolae, f. (< + -ola *diminutive suffix*) 작은 띠　　**E** *taeniola*

> IE. tenk- *to stretch*

> **E** *thing* (< 'matter' < 'affair' < 'assembly' < 'meeting time for an assembly' < 'stretch of time')

> IE. temp- *to stretch* (Vide TEMPUS; *See* E. *tense*)

torqueo, torsi, tortum (torsum), torquēre 비틀다, 비틀어 돌리다, 꼬다,

고문하다　　**E** *torque, torch* (< 'made of twisted tow dipped in pitch, or the like')

> tortus, tortus, m. 비틂, 비틀림, 꼬임, 주름, 고문

> tortuosus, tortuosa, tortuosum 비틀린, 꼬인, 꼬불꼬불한, 고통을 주는　　**E** *tortuous*

> tortuositas, tortuositatis, f. 굽이, 굴절　　**E** *tortuosity*

> torsio, torsionis, f. 비틀림, 꼬임, 고문, 고통, 회선(回旋),

염전(捻轉)　**E** *torsion,* (torsion >) *detorsion* (< 'correction of torsion', 'no normal twisting')

> tortura, torturae, f. 비틀림, 고문, 고통　　**E** *torture*

> tormentum, tormenti, n. 둥근 기둥에 밧줄을 감고 밧줄이 풀리는 힘으로 활이나 창을

쏘는 무기, 고문기, 고통　　**E** *torment*

> (*suggested*) torus, tori, m. 새끼를 칭칭 감아서 뭉친 것; 결절, 융기　　**E** *torus,* (pl.) *tori*

> torulus, toruli, m. (< + -ulus *diminutive suffix*) 작은 결절, 작은 융기　**E** *torulus,* (pl.) *toruli*

> torula, torulae, f. (< + -ula *diminutive suffix*) 크립토콕쿠스(cryptococcus)

효모균의 옛 명칭

> torulopsis, torulopsis, f. (< + G. opsis *appearance*) 토룰롭시스 효모균　**E** *torulopsis*

> torticollis, torticollis, f. (< tortus *crooked, twisted* + collum *neck*) 기운목,

사경(斜頸)　　**E** *torticollis*

> contorqueo, **contorsi**, contortum, contorquēre (< con- (< cum) *with, together; intensive*

+ torquēre *to twist*) 비틀다, 일그러지게 하다, 왜곡하다　　**E** *contort, contortion, contortionist*

> distorqueo, **distorsi**, distortum, distorquēre (< dis- *apart from, down, not; intensive*

+ torquēre *to twist*) 비틀다, 일그러지게 하다, 왜곡하다　　**E** *distort*

> distortio, distortionis, f. 비틀림, 왜곡　　**E** *distortion*

> extorqueo, **extorsi**, extortum, extorquēre (< ex- *out of, away from* + torquēre *to twist*)

밖으로 비틀다, 주리 틀다, 빼앗다　　**E** *extort*

> extortio, extortionis, f. 강탈, 착취　　**E** *extortion*

> extorsio, extorsionis, f. (< *outward torsion*) 외회선(外回旋), 바깥돌림
E *extorsion*

> intorqueo, **intorsi**, intortum, intorquēre (< in- *in, on, into, toward* + torquēre *to twist*)
안으로 비틀다, 뒤틀다
E *intort*

> intorsio, intorsionis, f. (< *inward torsion*) 내회선(外回旋), 안쪽돌림
E *intorsion*

> retorqueo, **retorsi**, retortum, retorquēre (< re- *back, again* + torquēre *to twist*)
뒤틀다, 되밀다, 되받아치다, 보복하다
E *retort, retortion*

< IE. terk^w- *to twist*
E *queer, thwart, (thwart >) athwart*

urgeo, ursi, –, urgēre 세게 떼밀다, 급박해지게 하다, 임박하다
E *urge, urgent, urgency*

< IE. wreg- *to push, to shove, to drive, to track down*
E *wreak, wreck, wrack, wretch*

> G. rhēgnynai (-rrhag- *stem*) *to break, to burst*

> G. rhēxis, rhēxeōs, f. *breaking, bursting*

> L. rhexis, rhexis, f. 파열, 찢김
E *rhexis, rhectic, -rrhexis, karyorrhexis*

> G. rhēgma, rhēgmatos, n. *break, burst, rupture, rent, fracture*
E *rhegma, rhegmatogenous*

> G. -rrhagia, -rrhagias, f. *break, burst*
E *-rrhagia (-rrhage), menorrhagia, metrorrhagia, thelorrhagia, hemorrhage, -rrhagic*

> G. rhagas, rhagados, f. *rent, chink, fissure on the skin*

> L. rhagas, rhagadis, f. 균열(龜裂), 열(裂), 열구(裂溝)
E *rhagas, (pl.) rhagades*

video, vidi, visum, vidēre 보다

E (vidēre licet *'it is permitted to see'* >) **videlicet (viz.)**, **video**, ((*feminine past participle*) *'seen'* >) **visa, view, preview, review, interview, overview**, (ad + visum (*neuter past participle*) > *'view, opinion'* >) **advice, advise**, (clarus + videns (*present participle*) > *'clear seeing'* >) F. **clairvoyant**, F. **voyeur**, F. **deja vu** (< *'already seen'*), F. **jamais vu** (< *'never seen'*), It. **vista** (< *'view'* < *'seen'*)

[용례] vide supra 위에서 보라
E *vide supra*

vide infra 아래에서 보라
E *vide infra*

(문법) vide 보라: 능동태 명령법 현재 단수 이인칭
supra 위에서: 부사
infra 아래에서: 부사

> visus, visus, m. 보는 행위, 시각(視覺), 외양(外樣)
E F. *vis-a-vis* (< *'face-to-face'*), *visage*

> visualis, visuale 시각의, 시력의
E *visual*

> visio, visionis, f. 보는 행위, 시각; 지각, 계시, 전망(展望)
E *vision*

> visibilis, visibile 볼 수 있는, 보이는
E *visible*

> invisibilis, invisibile (< in- *not*) 볼 수 없는, 보이지 않는
E *invisible*

> evidens, (gen.) evidentis (< e- *out of, away from* + videns (*present participle*) *seeing*) 보이는, 분명한, 명백한
E *evident*

> evidentia, evidentiae, f. 분명함, 명백함, 명료, 근거
E *evidence*

> invideo, **invidi**, invisum, invidēre (< in- *in, on, into, toward* + vidēre *to see*) 선망

하다, 질투하다

> invidia, invidiae, f. 선망, 질투　　　　　　　　　　　　　　　　**E** *envy*

> provideo, **providi**, provisum, providēre (< pro- *before, forward, for, instead of* +
vidēre *to see*) 예견하다, 대비하다, 준비하다,

필요한 것을 제공하다　　　　　　**E** *provide, purvey, purview, improvise (< 'unforeseen')*

> providens, (gen.) providentis (*present participle*) 미리 내다보는,

선견이 있는　　　　　　　　　　　　　　　　　　　**E** *provident*

> providentia, providentiae, f. 선견, 섭리　　　　**E** *providence*

> (*contracted*) prudens, (gen.) prudentis 미리 내다보는, 현명한　**E** *prudent*

> prudentia, prudentiae, f. 예견, 현명, 지혜　　**E** *prudence, prudential*

> provisio, provisionis, f. 선견, 예지, 준비, 식량 장만　　　　**E** *provision*

> supervideo, **supervidi**, supervisum, supervidēre (< super- *above* + vidēre *to see*)

감독하다, 조사하다　　　　　　　　　　　　　　　　**E** *supervise, survey*

> viso, **visi**, visum, visēre (*intensive*) 유심히 보다, 검토하다, 방문하다

> visito, **visitavi**, visitatum, visitare (*frequentative*) 방문하다　　**E** *visit, visitation*

> reviso, **revisi**, revisum, revisēre (< re- *back, again* + visēre *to look at*) 재검토

하다, 다시 방문하다, 정정하다, 교정하다　　　　　　**E** *revise, revision*

> vitrum, vitri, n. 유리(琉璃), 초자(硝子)

[용례] in vitro 유리 안에서 > 시험관내　　　　　　　　　　**E** *in vitro*

(문법) in (소재) 안에, 안에서: 전치사, 탈격지배

(방향) 안으로: 전치사, 대격지배

vitro 유리: 단수 탈격

> vitreus, vitrea, vitreum 유리의, 유리로 만든, 유리 같은　　　　**E** *vitreous*

> vitreolus, vitreola, vitreolum (< + -olus *diminutive suffix*)

섬세한 유리의　　**E** *vitriol (< 'the glassy appearance of sulfuric compounds')*

< IE. weid- *to see, to know*

E *guide, guy (< 'to guide'), guise, disguise, -wise, likewise, otherwise, clockwise, counter-clockwise; wise, wisdom, wizard, witness, wit*

> G. eidein (idein *aorist infinitive*) *to see*

> G. eidos, eidous, n. *act of seeing, appearance, shape*　**E** *eidetic, kaleidoscope*

> G. eidyllion, eidylliou, n. (< + -ion *diminutive suffix*) *a short descriptive
poem*

> L. idyllium, idyllii, n. 이야기체의 시, 목가, 전원시　**E** *idyll (idyl), idyllic*

> G. -o-eidēs, -o-eidēs, -o-eides *-shaped, -like, resembling*

> G. geoeidēs, geoeidēs, geoeides (< gē *earth*) *earthy, earth-
like*　　　　　　　　　　　　　　　　　　　　**E** *geoid*

> G. sphairoeidēs, sphairoeidēs, sphairoeides (< sphaira *ball*)
ball-shaped

> L. sphairoides, (gen.) sphairoidis 구형의, 둥근　**E** *spheroid*

> G. thyreoeidēs, thyreoeidēs, thyreoeides (< thyreos *door-stone,
large shield*) *shield-shaped*

> L. thyroideus, thyroidea, thyroideum 방패 모양의　　　　　　E *thyroid*

> L. ‐oides, (gen.) ‐oidis (‐oideus, ‐oidea, ‐oideum) ~ 모양의

> **E** *‐oid, deltoid, lambdoid, sigmoid, hypsiloid, hyoid, asteroid, cricoid, cycloid, ellipsoid, cuboid, rhomboid, discoid, placoid, tactoid, clinoid, condyloid, ethmoid, scaphoid, sphenoid, xiphoid, glenoid, pterygoid, anthropoid, android, gynecoid, arachnoid, coronoid, coracoid, dendroid, phylloid, adenoid, amygdaloid, sesamoid, choroid, mastoid, myeloid, myoid, crystalloid, hyaloid, myxoid, osteoid, chondroid, odontoid, epithelioid, alkaloid, amyloid, colloid, lipoid, opioid, steroid, toxoid, carcinoid, sarcoid, leukemoid, polypoid, cirsoid, pemphigoid, rheumatoid, typhoid, bacteroid (bacterioid), ameboid; humanoid, ovoid, sinusoid, lymphoid, chancroid, viroid, fungoid, fibrinoid, ceroid, corticoid, flavonoid, retinoid, nucleoid; ‐ide, nuclide*

> G. ‐ōdēs, ‐ōdēs, ‐odes (< (*earlier*) *having the smell of, from* od‐ (< ozein) *to smell*) *‐shaped, ‐like, resembling*

> **E** *iodine (I) (< 'violet-colored vapor'), phyllodes, plasmodium, collodion, ‐ode, phyllode, placode (< 'a plaquelike structure of ectoderm in the early embryo, from which a sense organ develops'), nematode, trematode, cestode*

> G. geōdēs, geōdēs, geodes (< gē *earth*) *earthy, earth-like*

> L. geodes, geodis, m. 정동(晶洞)　　　　　E *geode*

> G. eidōlon, eidōlou, n. *image, phantom, idol*

> L. idolum, idoli, n. 우상　　　　　E *idol*

[용례] idola tribus 종족의 우상
idola specus 동굴의 우상
idola fori 광장의 우상
idola theatri 극장의 우상
(문법) idola 우상들: 복수 주격
　　　 tribus 종족의: 단수 속격 < tribus, tribus, f.
　　　 specus 지하 동굴의: 단수 속격 < specus, specus, m.
　　　 fori 시장의, 광장의: 단수 속격 < forum, fori, n.
　　　 theatri 극장의: 단수 속격 < theatrum, theatri, n.

> G. eidōlolatreia, eidōlolatreias, f. (< + latreia *worship*) *the worship of idols*

> L. idololatria, idololatriae, f. (idolatria, idolatriae, f.) 우상 숭배　E *idolatry*

> L. *pareidolia, *pareidoliae, f. (< G. par(a)‐ *beside, along side of, beyond* + eidōlon + ‐ia) 환각　　　　　E *pareidolia*

> G. idea, ideas, f. *look, species, nature, (in Platonic philosophy) a general or ideal form, model; the word being thus analogous in derivation and original sense to* L. species (< specĕre *to see*)

> L. idea, ideae, f. 형상, 본(本), 원형, 이상, 관념, 이념　　　E *idea*

> L. idealis, ideale 이상적, 관념적, 이념적　　　E *ideal, idealize*

> G. histōr, historos, m. *knowledge, judge*

   > G. historia, historias, f. *inquiry, information, knowledge*

      > L. historia, historiae, f. 역사, 진실된 이야기, 옛날이야기   **E** *history, historian*

         > L. storia, storiae, f. historia의 속어   **E** *story*

      > G. historikos, historikē, historikon *of history*

         > L. historicus, historica, historicum 역사의, 역사적인

E *historic* (< 'famous or important in history or potentially so'), **historical** (< 'of or pertaining to history'), **prehistoric** (< 'of or pertaining to the time before written historical records'), (historicus >) **historicity**

   > (*Sanskrit*) veda *knowledge, sacred knowledge, sacred book*

E *Veda*, (rc 'brightness, praise, poem' >) **Rigveda**, (yaus 'sacrifice' >) **Yajurveda**, (saman 'chant' >) **Samaveda**, (atharva 'priest' >) **Atharvaveda**, (ayuh 'life, health' >) **Ayurveda**

voveo, vovi, votum, vovēre (신에게) 서약하다, 맹세하다, 원하다, 청하다

   > votum, voti, n. (신에 대한) 서약, 맹세, 서원, 간청   **E** *vow, votary, votive; vote*

   > devoveo, **devovi**, devotum, devovēre (< de- *apart from, down, not;* intensive + vovēre *to vow*) (신에게) 바치다, 헌신하다

                                        E *devote, devout*

< IE. weg^{w}h- *to preach, to speak solemnly*

●●● 정형 제3변화 A 식

능동태 현재부정법이 –ĕre로, 능동태 직설법 현재 단수 일인칭이 –o로 끝나는 동사.

lego, legi, lectum, legĕre 모으다, 뽑다, 읽다

능동태	부정법	현재				leg-ĕre	모으다, 뽑다, 읽다
	직설법	현재	단수	일인칭		leg-o	나는 ~한다
				이인칭		leg-is	너는 ~한다
				삼인칭		leg-it	그는 ~한다
			복수	일인칭		leg-imus	우리는 ~한다
				이인칭		leg-itis	너희는 ~한다
				삼인칭		leg-unt	그들은 ~한다
		과거	단수	일인칭		leg-ebam	나는 ~하였다
		미래	단수	일인칭		leg-am	나는 ~하겠다
		완료	단수	일인칭		leg-i	나는 ~하였다
	가정법	현재	단수	일인칭		leg-am	나는 ~하리라

	명령법	현재	단수	이인칭	leg-e	너는 ~하라
			복수	이인칭	leg-ite	너희는 ~하라
	분 사	현재			legens, (gen.) legent-is	~하는, ~하고 있는
	목적분사				lect-um	~하러, ~하기 위하여
수동태	부정법	현재			leg-i	모아지다, 읽히다
	분 사	미래			legend-us, legend-a, legend-um	~받아야 할
		과거			lect-us, lect-a, lect-um	~받은, ~받고서

lego, legi, lectum, legĕre 모으다, 뽑다, 읽다

> **E** (lectus (*past participle*) *'chosen'* >) *lectin* (< *'a protein, found primarily in plant seeds, which binds specifically to the branching sugar molecules of glycoproteins and glycolipids on the cell surface')*, (*selected lectin* >) *selectin*

> legio, legionis, f. 군단, 떼   **E** *legion*

> > legionarius, legionaria, legionarium 군단의   **E** *legionary, legionnaire*

> > Legionella, Legionellae, f. (< + -ella *diminutive suffix*) (세균) 레지오넬라속(屬)

> > > **E** *Legionella* (< *'first identified at an American Legion Convention in Philadelphia in 1976')*, *legionellosis*

> legumen, leguminis, n. (< *in allusion to the fact that the fruit may be gathered by hand*) 콩류   **E** *legume, leguminous*

> sacrilegus, sacrilega, sacrilegum (< sacer *holy* + legĕre *to choose*) 성물(聖物)을 훔치는, 신전을 터는, 신성모독의   **E** *sacrilege*

> colligo, **collegi**, collectum, colligĕre (< col- (< cum) *with, together* + legĕre *to choose*) 한데 모으다

> > **E** *collect, collection, collective,* (*collect* >) *collectible (collectable), cull, coil* (< *'gathered up into a number of concentric rings')*

> diligo, **dilegi**, dilectum, diligĕre (< di- (< dis-) *apart from, down, not* + legĕre *to choose*) 고르다, 애착을 가지다

> > diligens, (gen.) diligentis (*present participle*) 꼼꼼히 돌보는, 주의 깊은, 열심인, 근면한   **E** *diligent*

> > > diligentia, diligentiae, f. 근면   **E** *diligence*

> > praediligo, **praedilegi**, praedilectum, praediligĕre (< prae- *before, beyond* + diligĕre *to choose*) 좋아하다, 편애하다   **E** *predilection*

> eligo, **elegi**, electum, eligĕre (< e- *out of, away from* + legĕre *to choose*) 뽑아내다, 선택하다, 선출하다   **E** *elect, election, elective, elite*

> > elegans, (gen.) elegantis (*as if* < *elegare) 뛰어난, 우아한   **E** *elegant*

> > eligibilis, eligibile 적임의, 적격의   **E** *eligible,* (*eligible* >) *eligibility*

> intelligo, **intellexi**, intellectum, intelligĕre (< inter- *between, among* + legĕre *to choose*) 깨닫다   **E** *intelligent, intelligible, intelligibility*

> > intellectus, intellectus, m. 깨달은 것, 지력   **E** *intellect*

> intellectualis, intellectuale 깨달은 것의, 지력의　　　**E** *intellectual, intellectualize*

　　> intelligentia, intelligentiae, f. 깨달음, 지성, 지능　　**E** *intelligence*

> negligo, **neglexi**, neglectum, negligĕre (neglego, **neglexi**, neglectum, neglegĕre)

　(< neg- *not* + legĕre *to choose*)

　소홀히 하다　　　　　　　**E** *negligent, negligence, negligible, negligee, neglect*

> seligo, **selegi**, selectum, seligĕre (< se- *apart, without* + legĕre *to choose*) 가려

　내다, 선택하다　　　　　　**E** *select, selection, selective*

> legenda, legendae, f. (legenda, legendorum, n. **(pl.)**) (< legendum (*neuter gerundive*)

　thing to be read) 읽을거리, 전기, 성인전　　　　**E** *legend*

　　> legendarius, legendaria, legendarium 전설의, 전설적인　　**E** *legendary*

> legibilis, legibile 읽을 수 있는, 판독할 수 있는, 명료한　**E** *legible, legibility, illegible, illegibility*

> lectio, lectionis, f. 수집, 선택, 독서, 낭독, (교과서) 과(課), 수업　**E** *lesson*

> lectura, lecturae, f. 강의　　　　　　　　　　　　**E** *lecture*

> lectrum, lectri, n. 독서대　　　　　　　　　　　　**E** *lectern*

< IE. leg- *to collect; with derivatives meaning 'to speak'*

　> L. lex, legis, f. (< *(possibly) collection of rules*) 법(法), 법칙(法則)

　　> L. legalis, legale 법률상의, 법적인　　　　　**E** *legal, loyal, loyalty*

　　　> L. illegalis, illegale (< *againt the law* < il- (< in-) *not*) 불법의　**E** *illegal*

　　> L. legitimus, legitima, legitimum 합법적인, 정당한

　　　> L. legitimo, **legitimavi**, legitimatum, legitimare 합법화하다, 정당한 것으로

　　　만들다　　　　　　　　**E** *legitimate, (legitimate >) legitimacy*

　　　> L. illegitimus, illegitima, illegitimum (< *not by the law* < il- (< in-) *not*)

　　　비합법적인, 정당하지 못한, 사생(私生)의　　**E** *illegitimate*

　> L. lego, **legavi**, legatum, legare (사명을 주어) 파견하다, (유언으로) 맡기다

　　　> L. legatus, legati, m. 사절, 특사, 보좌관　　**E** *legate*

　　　> L. legatum, legati, n. 유산(遺産), 유증(遺贈)　**E** *legacy*

　　　> L. collega, collegae, f. (< col- (< cum) *with, together* + legare *to depute*)

　　　동료, 동업자　　　　　　**E** *colleague*

　　　　> L. collegium, collegii, n. 단체, 조합, 협회

　　　　　E *collegium, college* (< '*a body of scholars and students within a*

　　　　　university')

　　　> L. allego, **allegavi**, allegatum, allegare (< al- (< ad) *to, toward, at,*

　　　according to + legare *to depute*) 파견하다, (증거로) 제시하다,

　　　(변명으로) 내세우다　　　　　　**E** †*allegate*

　　　　> L. allegatio, allegationis, f. 파견, 제시, 주장　**E** *allegation*

　　　> L. delego, **delegavi**, delegatum, delegare (< de- *apart from, down, not*

　　　+ legare *to depute*) 대표시키다, 위임하다　　**E** *delegate*

　　　> L. relego, **relegavi**, relegatum, relegare (< re- *back, again* + legare *to*

　　　depute) 멀리 보내다, 이관하다　　　　**E** *relegate*

　> L. legislatio, legislationis, f. (< + latio, lationis, f. *bringing, proposing*) 입법,

　법률 제정　　　　　　　　　　　　**E** *legislate*

> L. privilegium, privilegii, n. (< privus, priva, privum *separate, peculiar*) 예외
법규, 특권

E *privilege*

> L. lignum, ligni, n. (< *that which is gathered*) 장작, 목재 　　E *lignin,* (lignum >) *lignify*

> L. ligneus, lignea, ligneum 목재의 　　E *ligneous*

> G. legein *to pick, to gather, to speak;* legesthai (*middle*) *to gather for oneself, to count up, to converse, to discourse*

> G. lexis, lexeōs, f. *speech, word*

> G. lexikos, lexikē, lexikon *of speech, of word*

> L. lexicon, lexici, n. (< G. lexikon biblion *word book*) 사전, 어휘

E *lexicon,* (lexicon >) *lexical, lexeme* (< 'on the pattern of phoneme')

> L. alexia, alexiae, f. (< G. a- *not*) (G. legein (*to speak*) *was confused with* L. legĕre (*to read*)) 읽기언어상실증, 독서불능증, 실독증(失讀症) 　E *alexia*

> L. dyslexia, dyslexiae, f. (< G. dys- *bad*) (G. legein (*to speak*) *was confused with* L. legĕre (*to read*)) 읽기곤란, 읽기장애 　E *dyslexia*

> G. logia, logias, f. *collection* 　　E *pentalogy* (< 'on the pattern of tetralogy')

> G. anthologia, anthologias, f. (< anthos *flower*) *collection of poems*

> L. anthologia, anthologiae, f. 시선집(詩選集), 작품집 　E *anthology*

> G. trilogia, trilogias, f. (< tri- *three* + logia *collection*) *a series of three tragedies (originally connected in subject), performed at Athens at the festival of Dionysus* 　E *trilogy*

> G. tetralogia, tetralogias, f. (< tetr(a)- *four* + logia *collection*) *a series of four dramas, three tragic (the trilogy) and one satyric, exhibited at Athens at the festival of Dionysus; any series of four related compositions; a set of four symptoms jointly characteristic of a disorder, chiefly with reference to Fallot's tetralogy* 　E *tetralogy*

> G. karphologia, karphologias, f. (< karphos, karpheos, n. (karphē, karphēs, f. *twig, straw, bit of wool*) + logia *collection*) *the movements of delirious patients, as if searching for or grasping at imaginary objects, or picking the bed-clothes* 　E *carphology* (floccillation)

> G. logos, logou, m. *word, speech, discourse, reason, account, ratio, proportion*

E *logic, logical, logistic, -logue (-log),* (hoi deka logoi 'the ten words' >) *Decalogue (Decalog), autologous* (< 'on the pattern of homologous')

> G. prologos, prologou, m. (< pro- *before, in front* + logos) *introduction to a play*

> L. prologus, prologi, m. 서언(序言), 서사(序詞) 　E *prologue* (prolog)

> G. epilogos, epilogou, m. (< ep(i)- *upon* + logos) *peroration of a speech*

> L. epilogus, epilogi, m. 맺음말, 결어(結語) 　E *epilogue* (epilog)

> G. monologos, monologos, monologon (< monos *alone* + logos) *speaking alone* 　E *monologue* (monolog)

> G. analogos, analogos, analogon (< an(a)- *up, upward; again, throughout; back, backward; against; according to, similar to* + logos) *according*

to due ratio, proportionate, conformable

> L. analogus, analoga, analogum 유사(類似)한,

상사(相似)한   **E** *analogous, analogue (analog)*

> G. analogia, analogias, f. *equality of ratios, proportion*

> L. analogia, analogiae, f. 유사(類似), 유추(類推), 유비(類比),

비유, 상사(相似)   **E** *analogy*

> G. homologos, homologos, homologon (< homos *of the same* + logos)

agreeing

> L. homologus, homologa, homologum (구조·위치·성질 등이) 일치

하는, 상응하는, 상동(相同)의,

동종(同種)의   **E** *homologous, homologue (homolog)*

> G. homologia, homologias, f. *agreement, assent*

> L. homologia, homologiae, f. 상응, 상동(相同), 동종(同種),

상동성(相同性)   **E** *homology*

> G. heterologos, heterologos, heterologon (< heteros *different* + logos)

disagreeing

> L. heterologus, heterologa, heterologum (구조·위치·성질 등이)

일치하지 않는, 비상동성(非相同性)의,

이종(異種)의   **E** *heterologous, heterologue (heterolog), heterology*

> G. –logia, –logias, f. *speaking, study*   **E** *–logy*

> G. apologia, apologias, f. (< ap(o)– *away from, from* + –logia

speaking) *defence, a speech in defence*

> L. apologia, apologiae, f. 변명   **E** *apology, apologize*

> G. eulogia, eulogias, f. (< eu– *well* + –logia *speaking*) *fair-

speaking, praise, blessing*

> L. eulogia, eulogiae, f. 찬사, 축복   **E** *eulogy, eulogize*

> G. logizesthai *to reckon, to calculate, to compute, to conclude, to infer*

> G. –logismos, –logismou, m. *–logism*   **E** *–logism*

> L. syllogismus, syllogismi, m. (< G. syl– (< syn) *with,

together*) 삼단논법   **E** *syllogism*

> L. paralogismus, paralogismi, m. (< G. par(a)– *beside, along

side of, beyond*) 오류 추리, 배리(背理)   **E** *paralogism*

> G. analegein (< an(a)– *up, upward; again, throughout; back, backward;

against; according to, similar to* + legein) *to pick up, to gather,

to collect*   **E** *analects (analecta)* (< *'things gathered up'*)

> G. eklegein (< ek– *out of, away from* + legein) *to pick out*

     E *eclectic* (< *'selected such doctrines as pleased them in every school'*), *eclecticism*

> G. dialegesthai (< dia– *through, thoroughly, apart* + legesthai) *to converse,

to discourse*

> G. dialektos, dialektou, f. *conversation, speech, dialect*

> L. dialectus, dialecti, f. 사투리, 방언(方言)   **E** *dialect*

> G. dialektikos, dialektikē, dialektikon *of conversation, of discourse*

> L. dialecticus, dialectica, dialecticum 논법의, 변증법의　　E *dialectic*

> G. dialogos, dialogou, m. *conversation, dialogue*

> L. dialogus, dialogi, m. 대화(對話)　　E *dialogue (dialog)*

ago, egi, actum, agĕre 하다, 움직이다, 몰다, 무게를 달다

> E *(verb)* **act, agent, enact, actin, actinin; react, reagent, reaction, reactive, reactant,** *(reagent + -in >* the antibody, IgE, that mediates immediate hypersensitivity reaction' >) **reagin;** *(active in advance, not reactive >)* **proactive; interact, interaction, interactive**

> acta, actorum, n. (pl.) (< actum (*neuter past participle*) *driven, done*) 행적, 법령, 법적 기록, 관보(官報)

> actus, actus, m. 행위　　E *(noun) act*

　> actualis, actuale 현행의, 사실상의, 실제적인　　E *actual*

　　> actualitas, actualitatis, f. 현행, 사실, 실제　　E *actuality*

　> actuarius, actuarii, m. 서기, 속기사　　E *actuary, actuarial*

> actio, actionis, f. 행동, 작용　　E *action, inaction (< 'lack of action')*

> actor, actoris, m. 움직이게 하는 자, 실행자, (법률) 원고, (남자) 배우　　E *actor, actress*

　> actrix, actricis, f. (법률) 여자 원고, 여배우

> activus, activa, activum 활동적인, 활성의, 진행성의, 능동의; (문법) 능동태의　　E *active, activate, inactive, inactivate, retroactive*

　> activitas, activitatis, f. 활동, 활성도　　E *activity, inactivity; hyperactivity*

> agentia, agentiae, f. 작용력, 기관(機關), 기구(機構)　　E *agency*

> agenda, agendorum, n. (pl.) (< agendum (*neuter gerundive*) *thing to be done*) 협의 사항, 의사 일정, 안건　　E *(pl.) agenda*

> agmen, agminis, n. (줄지어 움직이는) 무리, 떼, 대열　　E *agminate*

> agilis, agile 민첩한, 민활한, 기민한　　E *agile*

　> agilitas, agilitatis, f. 민첩, 민활, 기민　　E *agility*

> exagium, exagii, n. (< ex- *out of, away from* + agĕre *to drive, to do*) 계량, 측정, 분석　　E *assay, essay*

> examen, examinis, n. (< ex- *out of, away from* + agĕre *to drive, to do*) 저울의 지침 (指針), 조사, 시험

　> examino, examinavi, examinatum, examinare 저울에 달다, 조사하다, 시험하다　E *examine*

　　> examinatio, examinationis, f. 계량, 조사, 시험　　E *examination*

> agito, agitavi, agitatum, agitare (*frequentative*) 흔들다, 동요시키다, 선동하다, 곰곰이 생각하다　　E *agitate*

　[용례] paralysis agitans (< *shaking palsy, Parkinson disease*) 떨림마비　E *paralysis agitans*
　(문법) paralysis 마비: 단수 주격 < paralysis, paralysis, f.
　　agitans 흔드는: 현재분사, 남·여·중성형 단수 주격
　　　< agitans, (gen.) agitantis

　> cogito, cogitavi, cogitatum, cogitare (< co- (< cum) *with, together* + agitare *to put in motion*) 생각하다　　E *cogitate*

> ambigo, −, −, ambigĕre (< amb(i)- *on both sides, around* + agĕre *to drive, to do*)
   어느 것을 할지 망설이다, 결정을 못 내리다
      > ambiguus, ambigua, ambiguum 망설이는,
         모호한   **E** *ambiguous, (ambiguous >) disambiguate*
            > ambiguitas, ambiguitatis, f. 모호, 애매, 불분명, 다의성(多義性)   **E** *ambiguity*
> exigo, exegi, exactum, exigĕre (< ex- *out of, away from* + agĕre *to drive, to do*)
   내몰다, 받아내다, 요구하다, 끝내다, 정확히 계산하다   **E** *exigent, exigible, exact*
      > exigentia, exigentiae, f. 요구, 필요, 긴요, 긴박   **E** *exigency*
> prodigo, prodegi, prodactum, prodigĕre (< prod- (< pro) *before, forward, for, instead*
   of + agĕre *to drive, to do*) 앞으로 몰다, 아까운 줄 모르고 쓰다, 낭비하다
      > prodigus, prodiga, prodigum 아까운 줄 모르고 쓰는, 낭비하는
         > prodigalis, prodigale 아까운 줄 모르고 쓰는, 낭비하는, 사치한, 방탕한   **E** *prodigal*
> transigo, transegi, transactum, transigĕre (< trans- *over, across, through, beyond*
   + agĕre *to drive, to do*) 지나가게 하다, 관통시키다, 거래를 하다,
   처리하다   **E** *transact, transaction, intransigent*
> cogo, coegi, coactum, cogĕre (< co- (< cum) *with, together* + agĕre *to drive, to do*)
   한 곳으로 몰다, 집결시키다, 응결시키다, 응고시키다   **E** *squat, cogent*
      > coagulum, coaguli, n. 응결물, 응혈   **E** *coagulum, (pl.) coagula*
         > coagulo, coagulavi, coagulatum, coagulare 응결시키다, 응고시키다
            E *coagulate, coagulant, procoagulant, anticoagulant, hypercoagulability,*
            coagulopathy
               > coagulatio, coagulationis, f. 응고   **E** *coagulation*
      > coacto, −, −, coactare 억지로 시키다, 강요하다
         > *coactico, *coacticavi, *coacticatum, *coacticare (*frequentative*) 누르다,
            모으다   **E** *cachet (< 'seal' < 'to compress'), cache (< 'to hide' < 'to store up')*
> fumigo, fumigavi, fumigatum, fumigare (< fumus, fumi, m. *smoke* + agĕre *to drive,*
   to do) 연기 내다, 연기를 쐬다   **E** *fumigate, fumigant*
> fustigo, −, fustigatum, fustigare (< fustis, fustis, m. *stick* + agĕre *to drive, to do*)
   몽둥이로 때리다, 혹평하다   **E** *fustigate*
> laevigo, laevigavi, laevigatum, laevigare (levigo, levigavi, levigatum, levigare) (< laevis,
   laeve (levis, leve) *smooth* + agĕre *to drive, to do*) 매끈하게 하다, 갈고 닦다   **E** *levigate*
> litigo, litigavi, litigatum, litigare (< lis, litis, f. *dispute* + agĕre *to drive, to do*)
   다투다, 소송하다   **E** *litigate*
      > *exlitigo, *exlitigavi, *exlitigatum, *exlitigare (< ex- *out of, away from* + litigare
         to bring suit) (확실한 증거 없이) 주장하다   **E** *allege, alleged, allegedly*
> mitigo, mitigavi, mitigatum, mitigare (< mitis, mite *mild* + agĕre *to drive, to do*)
   완화시키다   **E** *mitigate, mitigable, immitigable*
> navigo, navigavi, navigatum, navigare (< navis, navis, f. *ship* + agĕre *to drive, to do*)
   항해하다   **E** *navigate*
      > navigatio, navigationis, f. 항해   **E** *navigation*
         > circumnavigo, circumnavigavi, circumnavigatum, circumnavigare (< circum-
            around + navigare *to sail*) 배로 일주하다   **E** *circumnavigate*

> purgo, **purgavi,** purgatum, purgare (< purus, pura, purum *pure* + agĕre *to drive, to do*) 깨끗이 하다 `E` *purge, purgative*

> purgatio, purgationis, f. 정화, 배설 `E` *purgation*

> variego, **variegavi,** variegatum, variegare (< varius, varia, varium *various* + agĕre *to drive, to do*) 여러 가지(색깔)로 변화시키다 `E` *variegate*

< IE. ag- *to drive, to draw, to move*

> G. agein *to drive, to lead, to weigh*

`E` (agōn (*present participle*) *'driving'* >) **glucagon** (< *'hyperglycemic substance, driving glucose'*)

> G. agōn, agōnos, m. (< agōn (*present participle*) *driving*) assembly, contest, game `E` *agon, agonal*

[용례] hoi Olympiakoi agōnes 올림픽 경기
(문법) hoi *the*: 정관사, 남성형 복수 주격
Olympiakoi 올림피아의: 형용사, 남성형 복수 주격
< Olympiakos, Olympiakē, Olympiakon *of Olympia*
< Olympia, Olympias, f. *the name of a district of Elis in southern Greece, site of the chief pan-Hellenic sanctuary of the god Zeus and the location for the ancient Olympic Games*
agōnes 경기들: 복수 주격

> G. agōnia, agōnias, f. *struggle, fear, agony*

> L. agonia, agoniae, f. 사투, 고통, 고뇌 `E` *agony*

> G. agōnizesthai *to contend for a prize, to struggle* `E` *agonize*

> G. agōnistēs, agōnistou, m. *prize-fighter, rival*

> L. agonista, agonistae, m. 시합자, 경기자, 작용제, 작용근 `E` *agonist*

> G. prōtagōnistēs, prōtagōnistou, m. (< prōtos *first*) *actor who plays the first part, leader*

> L. protagonista, protagonistae, m. 주역, 주동자 `E` *protagonist*

> G. antagōnizesthai *to struggle against* `E` *antagonize, antagonism*

> G. antagōnistēs, antagōnistou, m. (< ant(i)- *before, against, instead of*) *opponent, rival*

> L. antagonista, antagonistae, m. 대항제, 길항제, 맞버팀제 `E` *antagonist*

> G. agōgos, agōgē, agōgon *leading, drawing* `E` *-agogue, -agogic, -agogy; secretagogue*

> G. paidagōgos, paidagōgou, m. (< G. pais, paidos, m., f. *child* + agōgos) *slave who took children to and from school*

> L. paedagogus, paedagogi, m. (pedagogus, pedagogi, m.) 어린이의 가정교육을 담당하던 교사, 교육자; 현학자 `E` *pedagogue, pedagogic,* (perhaps) *pedant*

> G. paidagōgia, paidagōgias, f. (< paidagōgos + -ia) *office of a*

pedagogue, teaching, training

　　> L. paedagogia, paedagogiae, f. 교육, 교육학　　**E** *pedagogy*

　> G. dēmagōgos, dēmagōgou, m. (< dēmos *people* + agōgos) *a popular*
　　leader, a leader of the mob　　**E** *demagogue, demagogic*

　　> G. dēmagōgia, dēmagōgias, f. (< dēmagōgos + -ia) *leadership*
　　　of the people　　**E** *demagogy*

　> G. mystagōgos, mystagōgou, m. (< mystēs *one initiated* + agōgos) *a*
　　priest who initiates people in sacred mysteries　**E** *mystagogue, mystagogic*

　　> G. mystagōgia, mystagōgias, f. (< mystagōgos + -ia) *initiation*
　　　into the mysteries, mystical doctrine　　**E** *mystagogy*

　> L. sialagogum, sialagogi, n. (< G. sialon *saliva* + agōgos)
　　침분비제　　**E** *sialagogue (sialogogue)*

> G. synagein *to lead together, to assemble*

　> G. synagōgē, synagōgēs, f. (< syn- *with, together*) *assembly, meeting,*
　　synagogue

　　> L. synagoga, synagogae, f. 교회당, (유대교) 회당　　**E** *synagogue*

> G. stratēgos, stratēgou, m. (< stratos, stratou, m. *army* + agein) *general (in*
　Athens, the title of ten officers elected each year to command the army
　and navy)

　> G. stratēgia, stratēgias, f. (*at Athens*) *the office of* stragēgos, *command,*
　　generalship

　　> L. strategia, strategiae, f. 군사령부, 용병술, 작전,
　　　전략(戰略)　　**E** *strategy, strategic*

　> G. stratēgein (stratēgeein) *to be a general, to command*

　　> G. stratēgēma, stratēgēmatos, n. *a piece of generalship,*
　　　stratagem

　　　> L. strategema, strategematis, n. 술책(術策), 책략(策略)　**E** *stratagem*

> G. agra, agras, f. *hunting, capture, game, seizing, seizure*

　> G. podagra, podagras, f. (< pous, podos, m. *foot*) *foot disease, gout, trap for*
　　the feet

　　> L. podagra, podagrae, f. 무지통풍(拇趾痛風)　　**E** *podagra*

　> It. pellagra (< *skin disease; dermatitis due to niacin deficiency*) < L. pellis
　　skin + G. agra) 펠라그라　　**E** *pellagra*

> G. axios, axia, axion *worthy, right and proper*　　**E** *axiology*

　> G. axioun (axioein) *to think worthy, to esteem*

　　> G. axiōma, axiōmatos, n. *valuation, that which commends itself as*
　　　self-evident

　　　> L. axioma, axiomatis, n. 공인된 도리, 자명한 이치, 격언, 금언; (수학)
　　　　공리(公理)　　**E** *axiom, axiomatic*

> (*Celtic*) amb(i)actos (< IE. ambhi- *around* + IE. ag-) *messenger,*
　servant　　**E** *ambassador, embassy*

> IE. agro- *field*　　　　　　　　　　　　　　　　　　　　　**E** *acre*

　　> L. ager, agri, m. (< *place where cattle are driven*) 밭

　　　　> L. agrarius, agraria, agrarium 밭의, 토지의, 농사의　　　**E** *agrarian*

　　　　> L. agricultura, agriculturae, f. (< + colĕre *to cultivate*)

　　　　　　농업　　　　**E** *agriculture,* ('agriculture + inflation' >) *agflation*

　　　　> L. agricola, agricolae, m. (< + colĕre *to cultivate*) 농부

　　　　> L. pereger, (gen) peregris (< per- *through, thoroughly* + ager *field*)

　　　　　　멀리 여행 떠난, 외국에

　　　　　　> L. peregrinus, peregrina, peregrinum 나그네의, 순례자의,

　　　　　　　　외국의　　　　　　　　　　　　　**E** *peregrine, pilgrim*

　　> G. agros, agrou, m. *field*　　　　　　　　　　　　　　**E** *agr(o)-*

　　　　> G. agrios, agria, agrion *living in the fields, wild*

ango, anxi, anctum, angĕre 조이다, 조르다, 괴롭히다

　　> angustus, angusta, angustum 꼭 끼는, 좁은, 옹색한, 곤란한, 간결한

　　　　> angustiae, angustiarum, f. (pl.) 협소, 옹색, 궁색, 곤란, 간결　　**E** *anguish*

　　　　> angusto, **angustavi**, angustatum, angustare 좁게 하다, 제한하다

　　> anxius, anxia, anxium 조바심치는, 걱정하는, 쓰라린　　　　　**E** *anxious*

　　　　> anxietas, anxietatis, f. 조바심, 걱정, 불안　　　　　**E** *anxiety; anxiolytic*

< IE. angh- *tight, painfully constricted, painful*　　　　　　**E** *anger,* D. *Angst*

　　> G. anchein *to throttle, to strangle*　　　　　　　　　　**E** *quinsy*

　　　　> G. anchonē, anchonēs, f. *throttling, strangulation, hanging*

　　　　　　> L. angina, anginae, f. 조임, 구협염(口峽炎), 안지나　**E** *angina, anginal*

　　　　　　　　[용례] angina pectoris 협심증(狹心症), 가슴조임증　**E** *angina pectoris*

　　　　　　　　(문법) angina 조임: 단수 주격

　　　　　　　　　　pectoris 가슴의: 단수 속격 < pectus, pectoris, n.

　　　　　　> L. herpangina, herpanginae, f. (< G. herpēs *shingles*) 포진성

　　　　　　　　(疱疹性) 안지나　　　　　　　　　　　　　　**E** *herpangina*

apo (apio), –, aptum, apĕre 붙들어 매다, 동여매다

　　> aptus, apta, aptum (*past participle*) 동여매인, 갖추어진,

　　　　알맞은　　　　　　　　　　**E** *apt,* (suggested) *artillery* (< 'to set aright')

　　　　> aptitudo, aptitudinis, f. 적합성, 적성, 소질, 기질　　　　**E** *aptitude*

　　　　　　> attitudo, attitudinis, f. 태도, 자세, 마음가짐, 몸가짐　　**E** *attitude*

　　　　> ineptus, inepta, ineptum (< in- *not* + aptus *fit*) 적합지 않은, 적성이 아닌, 서투른　**E** *inept*

　　　　　　> ineptitudo, ineptitudinis, f. 부적합　　　　　　　　**E** *ineptitude*

　　> apto, **aptavi**, aptatum, aptare 맞추다

　　　　E (illa *reaptata (< re- 'again' + aptare 'to fit') > Sp. la reata 'to tie again' >) *lariat*

　　　　> adapto, **adaptavi**, adaptatum, adaptare (< ad- *to, toward, at, according*

　　　　　　to + aptare *to fit*) 적응시키다, 순응시키다　**E** *adapt, adaptor (adapter), adaptive*

> adaptatio, adaptationis, f. 적응, 순응　　　　**E** *adaptation*

> copula, copulae, f. (< coapula < co- (< cum) *with, together* + apĕre *to fasten* + -ula
　　diminutive suffix) 밧줄, 연결, 유대, 성교, 교미;
　　(문법) 계사(繫辭)　　　　**E** *copula, copulin, (noun) couple, couplet*

　　> copulo, copulavi, copulatum, copulare 매다, 결합하다, 교접하다

　　　　E *copulate, copulative, copulatory, (verb) couple, (couple >) coupler, (couple >)*
　　　　uncouple, (uncouple >) uncoupler

< IE. ap- *to fasten, to tie, to reach*

　> L. apiscor, aptus sum, apisci 다다르다, 얻다

　　> L. adipiscor, adeptus sum, adipisci (< ad- *to, toward, at, according to* + apisci
　　　to reach) 다다르다, 얻다　　　　**E** *adept*

　> L. apex, apicis, m. (< *something reached*) 꼭대기, 꼭지, 끝, 정점(頂點), 첨단(尖端)　　**E** *apex*
　　> L. apicalis, apicale 첨단의　　　　**E** *apical*

　> G. haptein *to fasten, to join; (middle) to grasp, to touch; (passive) to catch fire, to
　　be kindled*　　　　**E** *hapten, haptoglobin (< 'able to fasten with free haemoglobin')*

　　> G. hapsis, hapsidos, f. *fastening, felloe, joining; wheel, arch, vault*

　　　> L. apsis, apsidis, f. 아취, 둥근 천장;
　　　　(천문) 장축단(長軸端)　　　　**E** *apsis, (pl.) apsides, apse*

　　　> L. synapsis, synapsis, f. (< G. syn- *with, together* + hapsis *joining*)
　　　　연접, 시냅스; (염색체) 접합; 신경세포접합부

　　　　E *synapsis, (pl.) synapses, synaptonemal (< 'of conjoined threads');*
　　　　synapse, synaptic, presynaptic, postsynaptic, synuclein (< 'normally
　　　　localized to neuronal nucleus and presynaptic terminals')

　　　　> L. asynapsis, asynapsis, f. (< G. a- *not* + synapsis *connexion,*
　　　　　junction) (염색체) 비접합　　　　**E** *asynapsis*

　　　　> G. ephapsis, ephapsidos, f. (< eph- (< epi) *upon* + hapsis *joining*)
　　　　　touch　　　　**E** *ephapse (< 'electrical synapse'), ephaptic*

　　> G. haptikos, haptikē, haptikon *able to grasp, able to touch*　　**E** *haptic, haptics*

　　> G. aphtha, aphthas, f. (< *to catch fire*) *eruption, thrush*

　　　> L. aphtha, aphthae, f. 아프타　　　　**E** *aphtha, aphthous, aphthoid*

battuo, battui, –, battuĕre 때리다, 치다, 싸우다

　E *batter (< in part, frequentative of 'bat'), battery (< 'a number of pieces of artillery used
　together, a number of Leyden jars connected up so as to discharge simultaneously' <
　'metal articles wrought by hammering'), battle, battalion, combat, debate, abate (< 'to beat
　down'), rebate (< 'to beat back, to deduct')*

< IE. bhat- *to strike*　　　　**E** *(probably) bat*

　> (*suggested*) L. fatuus, fatua, fatuum 얼빠진, 어리석은, 실체 없는　　**E** *fatuous*

　　> L. infatuo, infatuavi, infatuatum, infatuare (< in- *in, on, into, toward* + fatuus
　　　foolish) 바보로 만들다, 홀리게 하다　　　　**E** *infatuate*

cado, cecidi, casum, cadĕre 떨어지다, 죽다

> casus, casus, m. 낙하, 추락, 몰락; 우연, 경우, 상황; (문법) (G. ptōsis) 격(格); (의학)

　　증례(症例), 사례(事例)　　　　　　　　　　　　　　　　**E** *chance, case*

　　> casualis, casuale 우연한, 무심결의, 되는 대로의; (문법) 격변화 하는　**E** *casual*

　　　　> casualitas, casualitatis, f. 뜻하지 않은 사고, 재해, 사상자　**E** *casualty*

> caducus, caduca, caducum 떨어지는, 떨어지기 쉬운, 덧없는　　　**E** *caducous*

> cadaver, cadaveris, n. 주검, 시체, 시신　　　　　　　　　　**E** *cadaver*

> accido, accidi, –, accidĕre (< ac- (< ad) *to, toward, at, according to* + cadĕre *to fall*) 일어나다, 닥치다

　　> accidens, accidentis, n. (< *present participle*) 사고, 재해, 우발,

　　　　우연　　　　　　　　　　　　　　　　　　　　**E** *accident, accidental*

> decido, decidi, –, decidĕre (< de- *apart from, down, not* + cadĕre *to fall*) 떨어지다,

　　쓰러지다, 빠지다　　　　　　　　　　**E** *decay;* (de- + cadĕre >) *decadent*

　　> deciduus, decidua, deciduum 탈락하는　　　　　　　　**E** *deciduous*

　　　　[용례] dentes decidui (< *deciduous teeth*) 젖니

　　　　　　(문법) dentes 이[齒]들: 복수 주격 < dens, dentis, m.

　　　　　　　decidui: 형용사, 남성형 복수 주격

　　　　[용례] membrana decidua (< *decidual membrane*) (자궁) 탈락막

　　　　　　(문법) membrana 막: 단수 주격 < membrana, membranae, f.

　　　　　　　decidua: 형용사, 여성형 단수 주격

　　　　> decidua, deciduae, f. (< membrana decidua *deciduous membrane*)

　　　　　　(자궁) 탈락막　　　　　　　　　　　　　**E** *decidua, decidual*

　　　　　　[용례] decidua basalis 바닥쪽탈락막, 기저탈락막　**E** *decidua basalis*

　　　　　　　　decidua capsularis 피막탈락막　　　　**E** *decidua capsularis*

　　　　　　　　decidua parietalis 벽쪽탈락막, 벽측탈락막　**E** *decidua parietalis*

　　　　　　　　(문법) decidua: 명사, 단수 주격

　　　　　　　　　basalis 바닥의: 남·여성형 단수 주격

　　　　　　　　　　< basalis, basale

　　　　　　　　　capsularis 피막의: 남·여성형 단수 주격

　　　　　　　　　　< capsularis, capsulare

　　　　　　　　　parietalis 벽의: 남·여성형 단수 주격

　　　　　　　　　　< parietalis, parietale

　　　　　　> deciduatus, deciduata, deciduatum 탈락막을 가진, 탈락막의　**E** *deciduate*

> incido, incidi, incasum, incidĕre (< in- *in, on, into, toward* + cadĕre *to fall*) 떨어

　　지다, 빠지다, 걸리다, (사건·질병 등이) 발생하다　　**E** *incident, incidental*

　　> incidentia, incidentiae, f. (물리) 입사, 입사각; (사건·질병 등의) 발생　**E** *incidence*

　　> coincido, coincidi, –, coincidĕre (< co- (< cum) *with, together* + incidĕre

　　　　to fall upon) 동시에 발생하다, 합치하다　　**E** *coincide, coincident, coincidental*

> *coincidentia, *coincidentiae, f. 동시 발생, 합치　　　　　　　**E** *coincidence*

> occido, **occidi**, occasum, occidĕre (< oc- (< ob) *before, toward(s), over, against, away* + cadĕre *to fall*) 저물다, 사라지다　　　　　**E** *occident, occidental*

> occasio, occasionis, f. (특수한) 경우(境遇), (*falling together of favorable circumstances* >) 기회(機會), 호기(好機)　　　**E** *occasion, occasional*

> recido, **recidi**, recasum, recidĕre (< re- *back, again* + cadĕre *to fall*) 다시 떨어지다

> recidivus, recidiva, recidivum 재발하는, 재범의, 상습법의　　　**E** *recidivism*

< IE. kad- *to fall*

caedo, cecidi, caesum, caedĕre 베다, 후려치다, 도살하다　　　**E** *chisel, scissor*

> caesura, caesurae, f. 벤 자리, (나무의) 절단부; (운율) 중간 휴지　　**E** *caesura*

> caedimentum, caedimenti, n. (Vide infra)

> caementum, caementi, n. (cementum, cementi, n.) 자른 돌, 건축 석재, 벽돌, 모르타르, 석회, 시멘트　　　　　　　　　　　　**E** *cementum, cement*

> cementiculum, cementiculi, n. (< + -culum *diminutive suffix*) 시멘트 과립　　　　　　　　　　　　　　**E** *cementicle*

> circumcido, **circumcidi**, circumcisum, circumcidĕre (< circum- *around* + caedĕre *to cut, to kill*) 주위를 베다, 할례(割禮)를 베풀다　　**E** *circumcise*

> circumcisio, circumcisionis, f. 환상절제, 할례, 포경(包莖)수술　　**E** *circumcision*

> concido, **concidi**, concisum, concidĕre (< con- (< cum) *with, together; intensive* + caedĕre *to cut, to kill*) 베어 넘기다, 짤막하게 나누다, 간결하게 구분하다　**E** *concise*

> concisio, concisionis, f. 절단, 간결　　　　　　　　　**E** *concision*

> decido, **decidi**, decisum, decidĕre (< de- *apart from, down, not* + caedĕre *to cut, to kill*) 잘라내다, 결정하다　　　　　　　　**E** *decide, decisive*

> decisio, decisionis, f. 절단, 결정　　　**E** *decision, (decision >) indecision*

> excido, **excidi**, excisum, excidĕre (< ex- *out of, away from* + caedĕre *to cut, to kill*) 떼어내다, 절제(切除)하다　　　　　　　　　**E** *excise*

> excisio, excisionis, f. 절제, 적출(摘出)　　　　**E** *excision, excisional*

> incido, **incidi**, jncisum, incidĕre (< in- *in, on, into, toward* + caedĕre *to cut, to kill*) 베다, 칼로 새기다, 베어내다, 절개(切開)하다　　　　**E** *incise, incisive*

> incisio, incisionis, f. 베어냄, 절개　　　　　**E** *incision, incisional*

> incisura, incisurae, f. 베어낸 자리, 패임, 절흔(切痕)　　　**E** *incisure*

[용례] incisura angularis (gastris) (위)모패임, (위)각절흔(角切痕)　**E** *incisura angularis*

(문법) incisura 패임: 단수 주격

angularis 각의, 각이 있는, 모난: 형용사, 남·여성형 단수 주격

< angularis, angulare

gastris 위의: 단수 속격 < gaster, gastris, f. 위, 배

> incisor, incisoris, m. 베어내는 사람, 앞니, 절치(切齒)　　　**E** *incisor*

> praecido, **praecidi**, praecisum, praecidĕre (< prae- *before, beyond* + caedĕre *to cut, to kill*) 앞(뒤)을 베어내다, 절단하다, 요약하다, 명확하게 하다　　**E** *precise*

> praecisio, praecisionis, f. 절단, 요약, 명확 **E** *precision*

> -cida, -cidae, m. ~살해자

> **E** *-cide, suicide, homicide, filicide, uxoricide, pesticide, rodenticide, insecticide, vermicide, larvicide, parasiticide, herbicide, microbicidal, bactericidal, fungicidal; phytocide (< 'agent lethal to plants'), phytoncide (< 'lethal agent from plants')*

< IE. kaəid- *to strike*

carpo, carpsi, carptum, carpĕre 따다, 즐기다, 뜯다,
보풀을 세우다   **E** *carp, carpet (< 'thick woolen cloth')*

[용례] Carpe diem! 날을 따라! > 오늘에 충실하라!
    (문법) carpe 따라!: 능동태 명령법 현재 단수 이인칭
       diem 날을: 단수 대격 < dies, diei, m. 날; f. 날짜

> excerpo, **excerpsi**, excerptum, excerpĕre (< ex- *out of, away from* + carpĕre *to pluck*)
뜯어내다, 골라내다, 발췌하다, 정선하다   **E** *excerpt, scarce (< 'plucked out and therefore rare')*

< IE. kerp- *to gather, to pluck, to harvest*   **E** *harvest*

> G. karpos, karpou, m. *fruit, corn, harvest*   **E** *carpel, carp(o)-, -carp, exocarp*

> G. perikarpion, perikarpiou, n. (< peri- *around, near, beyond, on account of* + karpos + -ion *neuter suffix forming adjective*) *pod, husk, shell*

> L. pericarpium, pericarpii, n. 과피(果皮)   **E** *pericarp*

> L. endocarpium, endocarpii, n. (< G. end(o)- < endon *within*)
내과피(內果皮)   **E** *endocarp*

> L. mesocarpium, mesocarpii, n. (< G. mes(o)- < mesos *middle*)
중과피(中果皮)   **E** *mesocarp*

> L. pilocarpus, pilocarpi, m. (< *felt cap-shaped fruit* < G. pilos *felt, felt cap* + karpos *fruit*) 남미산의 운향과 나무   **E** *pilocarpine*

> L. -carpus, -carpa, -carpum ~ 열매를 맺는   **E** *-carpous*

> (*probably*) L. carpinus, carpini, f. 서어나무(서나무), 개서어나무(개서나무)

cedo, cessi, cessum, cedĕre 가 버리다, ~에게 돌아가다, 되어 버리다, 굴복하다, 양보하다,
인정하다   **E** *cede*

> cesso, **cessavi**, cessatum, cessare (*frequentative*) 그치다, 중지하다   **E** *cease*

> cessatio, cessationis, f. 중지   **E** *cessation*

> incessans, (gen.) incessantis (< in- *not* + cessans (*present participle*) *ceasing*)
(좋지 않은 일이) 그칠 새 없는, 부단한   **E** *incessant*

> necesse (< *no drawing back* < ne- *not* + cess- *past participial stem of* cedĕre)
(형용사, 불변화; 서술적으로만 사용) 필수적, 필연적

> necessarius, necessaria, necessarium 필요한   **E** *necessary*

> necessitas, necessitatis, f. 필요, 필요성   **E** *necessity*

> antecedo, antecessi, antecessum, antecedĕre (< ante- *before* + cedĕre *to go, to yield*)
(시간·관계에서) 앞서다   **E** *antecede, antecedent*

> antecessor, antecessoris, m. 앞서 가는 등불잡이, 선임자,

　　선발대　　　　　　　　　　　　　　　E *ancestor, ancestral, ancestry*

> praecedo, **praecessi**, praecessum, praecedĕre (< prae- *before, beyond* + cedĕre *to go, to yield*) (시간·장소·순서에서) 앞서다, 선행하다　　　　E *precede, precedent*

　　> praecessio, praecessionis, f. 선행; (물리) 섭동(攝動), (천문) 세차(歲差)　E *precession*

> procedo, **processi**, processum, procedĕre (< pro- *before, forward, for, instead of* + cedĕre *to go, to yield*) 나아가다, 잘되다　　E *proceed, proceedings, procedure*

　　> processus, processus, m. 전진, (일련의) 과정, 절차;

　　　　(생물) 돌기(突起)　　　　　　　　　　　E *process, processor*

　　> processio, processionis, f. 전진, 진행, 행진　　　E *procession*

> recedo, **recessi**, recessum, recedĕre (< re- *back, again* + cedĕre *to go, to yield*) 뒤로 무르다, 뒤로 기울다, 후퇴하다, 쇠퇴하다　　　E *recede*

　　> recessus, recessus, m. 들어간 곳, 오목한 곳, 구석진 곳, 휴식; 오목, 함요(陷凹),

　　　　와(窩), 동(洞)　　　　　　　　　　　　E *recessus, recess*

　　> recessio, recessionis, f. 뒤물림, 후퇴　　　　E *recession*

　　> recessivus, recessiva, recessivum 후퇴하는, 역행의, 퇴행성의, 열성(劣性)의　E *recessive*

> retrocedo, **retrocessi**, retrocessum, retrocedĕre (< retro- *backward, behind* + cedĕre *to go, to yield*) 물러가다　　　　　　　　　E *retrocede*

　　> retrocessio, retrocessionis, f. 후퇴, 후진　　　E *retrocession*

> abscedo, **abscessi**, abscessum, abscedĕre (< abs- (< ab) *off, away from* + cedĕre *to go, to yield*) 멀리 떠나가다, 도피하다

　　> abscessus, abscessus, m. (< *from the notion formerly held that humors 'go from' the body into the swelling*) 고름집,

　　　　농양(膿瘍)　　　　E *abscess* (< *a collection of pus in a newly formed cavity*)

> accedo, **accessi**, accessum, accedĕre (< ac- (< ad) *to, toward, at, according to* + cedĕre *to go, to yield*) 접근하다, 응하다, 참가하다, 덧붙이다　　E *accede, accessible*

　　> accessus, accessus, m. 접근 방법, 진입로, 통로, 증대, 부가물　　E *access*

　　> accessio, accessionis, f. 도달, 획득, 증대, 부가　　E *accession, accessional*

　　> accessorius, accessoria, accessorium 부가적인, 부대적인　E *accessory (accessary)*

> concedo, **concessi**, concessum, concedĕre (< con- (< cum) *with, together* + cedĕre *to go, to yield*) 양보하다, 인정하다　　　　　　　　E *concede, concessive*

　　> concessio, concessionis, f. 양보, 인정　　　　E *concession*

> decedo, **decessi**, decessum, decedĕre (< de- *apart from, down, not* + cedĕre *to go, to yield*) 물러서다, 사라지다, 죽다　　E *decease, deceased, decedent, predecessor*

> excedo, **excessi**, excessum, excedĕre (< ex- *out of, away from* + cedĕre *to go, to yield*) (밖으로) 물러가다, 물러나다; (기준을) 넘기다, 뛰어나다　E *exceed, excessive*

　　> excessus, excessus, m. 초과, 과잉　　　　　E *excess*

> intercedo, **intercessi**, intercessum, intercedĕre (< inter- *between, among* + cedĕre *to go, to yield*) 끼어들다, 중재하다　　　　E *intercede, intercession*

> secedo, **secessi**, secessum, secedĕre (< se- *apart, without* + cedĕre *to go, to yield*) 떨어져 나가다, 탈퇴하다　　　　　　　　E *secede, secession*

> succedo, **successi**, successum, succedĕre (< suc- (< sub) *under, up from under*

+ cedĕre *to go, to yield*) 아래로 들어가다, 받아들이다, 뒤따라 일어나다, 잇따르다,

계승하다, (*getting near to something, doing well* >) 성공하다

> successus, successus, m. 성공 **E** *success*

> successio, successionis, f. 연속, 계승; (식물) 천이(遷移); (농업) 윤작(輪作) **E** *succession*

> succedaneus, succedanea, succedaneum 뒤따라 일어나는,

대신한 **E** *succedaneous, succedaneum*

[용례] caput succedaneum 산류(産瘤), 출산머리부종 **E** *caput succedaneum*

(문법) caput 머리: 단수 주격 < caput, capitis, n.

succedaneum: 형용사, 중성형 단수 주격

< IE. ked- *to go, to yield*

cerno, crevi, cretum (certum), cernĕre 체로 치다, 분별하다, 판결하다, 이해하다

> (*suggested*) creta, cretae, f. (< (*probably*) terra creta *sifted earth*) 백악질(白堊質)

점토, 백토(白土), 분필 **E** *crayon*

> cretaceus, cretacea, cretaceum 백악질의 **E** *cretaceous*

> cribrum, cribri, n. 체[篩], 어레미 **E** *cribriform, garble*

> crimen, criminis, n. 범죄, 위반 행위, 고소, 비난 **E** *crime*

> criminalis, criminale 범죄의 **E** *criminal*

> certus, certa, certum (*past participle*) 확실한

> certanus, certana, certanum 확실한 **E** *certain, certainty, ascertain*

> certitudo, certitudinis, f. 확실성 **E** *certitude*

> incertitudo, incertitudinis, f. (< in- *not*) 불확실성 **E** *incertitude*

> certifico, certificavi, certificatum, certificare (< -ficare (< facĕre) *to make*)

증명하다, 보증하다 **E** *certify, certificate*

> certo, certavi, certatum, certare 논쟁하다, 다투다

> concerto, concertavi, concertatum, concertare (< con- (< cum) *with,*

together + certare *to contend*) 논쟁하다, 다투다 **E** (*possibly*) *concert*

> concerno, concrevi, concretum, concernĕre (< con- (< cum) *with, together* + cernĕre

to sift, to separate, to decide) 관계하다 **E** *concern*

> decerno, decrevi, decretum, decernĕre (< de- *apart from, down, not* + cernĕre *to*

sift, to separate, to decide) 판결을 내리다,

공포하다 **E** (decretum (*neuter past participle*) 'thing decided' >) *decree*

> discerno, discrevi, discretum, discernĕre (< dis- *apart from, down, not* + cernĕre

to sift, to separate, to decide) 가리다, 분간하다

E *discern, discernible, discrete* (< 'separate'), *discreet* (< 'careful and circumspect')

> discretio, discretionis, f. 사려 분별, 신중 **E** *discretion*

> discrimen, discriminis, n. 구별, 분별, 식별, 판별

> discrimino, discriminavi, discriminatum, discriminare 구별하다, 분별하다,

식별하다, 판별하다 **E** *discriminate, indiscriminate, discriminant*

> excerno, excrevi, excretum, excernĕre (< ex- *out of, away from* + cernĕre *to sift,*

to separate, to decide) 선별하다, 키질하다, 배설하다 **E** *excrete, excretory*

> excretus, excreta, excretum (*past participle*) 선별한, 키질한,

배설한

> excretio, excretionis, f. 선별, 키질, 배설   **E** *(neuter pl.)* ***excreta***

     E ***excretion***

> excrementum, excrementi, n. 겨, 싸라기, 포도의 찌꺼기, 분비물, 배설물, 똥   **E** ***excrement***

> secerno, **secrevi**, secretum, secernĕre (< se- *apart, without* + cernĕre *to sift, to*

separate, to decide) 분리하다, 분비하다

> secretus, secreta, secretum (*past participle*) 분리한, 호젓한, 혼자뿐인, 비밀의;

분비한   **E** ***secret,*** *(neuter pl.)* ***secreta***

> secretum, secreti, n. 호젓한 곳, 혼자 지냄, 비밀

> secretarius, secretarii, m. 비서, 서기   **E** ***secretary***

> secretio, secretionis, f. 분리, 분비

> **E** ***secretion,*** *(secretion >)* ***secrete,*** *(secrete >)* ***secretory, hypersecretion,***
hyposecretion, secretin *(< 'stimulating pancreatic acinar cells to secrete*
bicarbonate and water')

< IE. krei- *to sieve, to discriminate, to distinguish*

> (*probably*) L. crena, crenae, f. 홈

     E ***crenocyte***

> L. crenatus, crenata, crenatum 홈이 있는, 무딘 톱니 모양의   **E** ***crenate***

> L. crenula, crenulae, f. (< + -ula *diminutive suffix*) 작은 홈

> L. crenulatus, crenulata, crenulatum 작은 홈이 있는,

작은 무딘 톱니 모양의   **E** ***crenulate***

> G. krinein *to separate, to decide, to judge*

> **E** ***-crine*** *(< 'secreting'),* ***endocrine*** *(< 'secreting inwardly, into blood or lymph'),*
paracrine *(< 'of a hormone which affects the cells in the vicinity of the cell*
secreting it'), ***autocrine*** *(< 'of a hormone which affects the same cell secreting*
it'), ***exocrine*** *(< 'secreting outwardly'),* ***merocrine*** *(< 'secreting partly'),* ***apocrine***
(< 'secreting away'), ***holocrine*** *(< 'secreting wholly')*

> G. diakrinein (< di(a)- *through, thoroughly, apart*) *to distinguish*   **E** ***diacritic***

> G. ekkrinein (< ek- *out of, away from*)

to secrete   **E** ***eccrine*** *(< 'merocrine sweat gland')*

> G. krisis, kriseōs, f. *separation, deciding, judgement*

> L. crisis, crisis, f. 위기, 고비, 발증(發症), 발작, 급통증   **E** ***crisis,*** *(pl.)* ***crises, critic***

> G. kritēs, kritou, m. *judge*

> **E** ***hematocrit*** *(< 'a centrifuge used to estimate the volume occupied by the red*
blood cells in a sample of blood; the value obtained, expressed as a
percentage of the volume of the sample')

> G. kritērion, kritēriou, n. (< + -erion *neuter suffix of means*) *means*
for judging, test   **E** ***criterion,*** *(pl.)* ***criteria***

> L. criterium, criterii, n. 기준

> G. kritikos, kritikē, kritikon *of judge, able to judge*

> L. criticus, critica, criticum 판단의, 비평의, 결정적인, 위기의, 위독한;

(물리) 임계(臨界)의   **E** ***critic, critical, criticize, criticism***

> G. hypokrinesthai (< hyp(o)- *under*) (*middle*) *to answer, to play a part on*
the stage, to pretend

> G. hypokrisis, hypokriseōs, f. *the acting of a part on the stage, pretence*

> L. hypocrisis, hypocrisis, f. 흉내, 겉꾸밈, 위선   **E** *hypocrisy*

> G. hypokritēs, hypokritou, m. *an actor on the stage, pretender, dissembler*

> L. hypocrita, hypocritae, m. 흉내 내는 배우, 겉꾸미는 자,

위선자   **E** *hypocrite, hypocritical*

claudo, clausi, clausum, claudĕre 닫다,

막다   **E** *(verb) close, closet, claudin(s); eclosion (< 'emergence from concealment')*

> clausus, clausa, clausum (*past participle*)

닫힌   **E** *(adjective) close (< 'with the intervening space closed up')*

> clausa, clausae, f. 맺는 말,

결론   **E** *clause (< 'closing of a formula, containing a subject and predicate')*

> clausura, clausurae, f. 폐쇄, 봉쇄   **E** *closure*

> claustrum, claustri, n. 폐쇄, 봉쇄, 빗장, 자물쇠, 우리, 담장,

수도원   **E** *claustrum, claustral, cloister, cloistral; claustrophobia*

> concludo, conclusi, conclusum, concludĕre (< con- (< cum) *with, together*

+ claudĕre *to shut*) 종결하다, 결론짓다   **E** *conclude, conclusive*

> conclusio, conclusionis, f. 종결, 결론   **E** *conclusion*

> excludo, exclusi, exclusum, excludĕre (< ex- *out of, away from* + claudĕre

to shut) 제외하다, 배제하다   **E** *exclude, exclusive*

> exclusio, exclusionis, f. 배제   **E** *exclusion*

> includo, inclusi, inclusum, includĕre (< in- *in, on, into, toward* + claudĕre

to shut) 가두다, 포함하다   **E** *include, inclusive, enclose, enclosure*

> inclusio, inclusionis, f. 포함   **E** *inclusion*

> occludo, occlusi, occlusum, occludĕre (< ob- *before, toward(s), over, against,*

away + claudĕre *to shut*) 가두다, 막다   **E** *occlude, occlusive, occlusal, occludin*

> occlusio, occlusionis, f. 폐색(閉塞), 폐쇄(閉鎖); (치의학) 교합(咬合), 맞물림

E *occlusion, malocclusion, disto-occlusion (distoclusion) (< 'malocclusion in which the mandibular arch is in a distal (posterior) position in relation to the maxillary arch')*

> praecludo, praeclusi, praeclusum, praecludĕre (< prae- *before, beyond* +

claudĕre *to shut*) 미리 막다   **E** *preclude, preclusion, preclusive*

> recludo, reclusi, reclusum, recludĕre (< re- *back, again* + claudĕre *to shut*)

(열다), 닫다   **E** *recluse, reclusion, reclusive*

> secludo, seclusi, seclusum, secludĕre (< se- *apart, without* + claudĕre *to*

shut) 떼어 놓다, 가두어 두다   **E** *seclude, seclusion, seclusive*

∞ claudus, clauda, claudum 절뚝거리는

> claudico, claudicavi, claudicatum, claudicare 절뚝거리다, 파행(破行)하다   **E** *claudication*

< IE. klau- (*possibly*) *hook, peg*   **E** *lot, allot*

> L. clavus, clavi, m. 못, (배의) 키, (로마인의 겉옷) 튜니카(tunica)에 맨 주홍색의

세로띠; 티눈   **E** *clove (< 'resemblance of a flower bud to a nail'); clavus, (pl.) clavi; cloy*

> L. clava, clavae, f. 곤봉; 추자(槌子)   **E** *clavate, claviform; clava*

> L. clavis, clavis, f. 열쇠, 빗장

> **E** *clavier, clavichord, clef, autoclave (< 'a self-fastening apparatus'), subclavian (< 'subclavian vessel, nerve, or muscle')*

> L. clavicula, claviculae, f. (< + -cula *diminutive suffix*) 작은 열쇠, 작은 빗장;
(식물의) 덩굴손; 빗장뼈, 쇄골(鎖骨)

> **E** *clavicle (< 'compared to the key of a vault or the ancient bolt'), clavicular, supraclavicular, infraclavicular (subclavicular)*

> L. conclave, clonclavis, n. (< con- (< cum) *with, together* + clavis *key*) 잠글
수 있는 방, 감옥; 비밀회의 　　　　　**E** *conclave*

> L. inclavo, inclavavi, inclavatum, inclavare (< in- *in, on, into, toward* + clavis
key) 가두다 　　　　　**E** *enclave, (enclave >) exclave*

> G. kleiein *to close*

> G. kleisis, kleiseōs, f. *closure* 　　　　　**E** *-cleisis*

> L. vulvocleisis, vulvocleisis, f. (< L. vulva *covering*) 음문폐쇄술 **E** *vulvocleisis*

> G. kleis, kleidos, f. *hook, hook of a clasp, key, bar,*
collar bone 　　　　　**E** *cleid(o)-, sternocleidomastoid*

> G. kleithron, kleithrou, n. *bar, lattice*

> L. clathri, clathrorum, m. (pl.) 창살, 격자(格子) 　　**E** *clathrin*

> L. clathro, -, -, clathrare 창살로 막다

> L. clathratus, clathrata, clathratum (*past participle*) 창살로
막은, 창살 모양의 　　　　　**E** *clathrate*

colo, colui, cultum, colĕre 경작하다, 가꾸다, 연마하다, 돌보다, 숭배하다, 거주하다

> colonus, coloni, m. 농부, 소작인, 정착민

> colonia, coloniae, f. 농경지, 식민지, 정착민 　　**E** *colony, colonial, colonize*

> -colus, -cola, -colum 서식하는

E *-colous, arenicolous (< 'sand-inhabiting'), rupicolous (< 'rock-inhabiting'), saxicolous (< 'stone-inhabiting')*

> *sanguicolus, *sanguicola, *sanguicolum (< sanguis, sanguinis, m. *blood* +
-colus *inhabiting*) 혈액 안에 기생하는 　　　　　**E** *sanguicolous*

> cultus, cultus, m. (경작, 양식), 숭배 　　　　　**E** *cult, cultism*

> cultura, culturae, f. 경작, 양식, 문화, (숭배)

E *culture, (ager 'field' >) agriculture, (hortus 'garden' >) horticulture, (pomum 'fruit' >) pomiculture, (silva (sylva) 'forest' >) silviculture (sylviculture), (vitis 'vine' >) viticulture, (apis 'bee' >) apiculture, (sericum 'silk' > sericiculture >) sericulture, (aqua 'water' >) aquaculture, (mare 'sea' >) mariculture, (piscis 'fish' >) pisciculture, acculturation (< 'the adoption and assimilation of an alien culture')*

> cultivus, cultiva, cultivum 경작할 수 있는

> cultivo, cultivavi, cultivatum, cultivare (< cultiva terra *arable land*)
경작하다 　　　　　**E** *cultivate, (cultivated variety >) cultivar*

> domicilium, domicilii, n. (< domus *house* + colĕre *to cultivate, to dwell*) 거처, 주소 **E** *domicile*

< IE. kʷel-, kʷelə- *to turn, to be around, to dwell*
　　　　　E *wheel*

> L. collum, colli, n. (< *that on which the head turns*) 목

> **E** *collar, collarette,* (*accollare (< ad *'to, toward, at, according to'* + collum *'neck'*) *'to embrace about the neck'* >*accollata (*past participle*) >) *accolade*

> > L. torticollis, torticollis, f. (< tortus *crooked, twisted* + collum *neck*) 기운목, 사경(斜頸) **E** *torticollis*

> L. anculus, anculi, m. (< an- (< am- < amb(i)-) *on both sides, around*) 하인

> > L. ancula, anculae, f. 여자 하인

> > > L. ancilla, ancillae, f. (< + -illa *diminutive suffix*) 작은 여자 하인 **E** *ancillary*

> G. kyklos, kyklou, m. *wheel, cycle, orbit, circle*

> **E** (*noun*) *cycle, cyclic, cycloid, cyclone* (< *'circular wind'*), *cyclotron* (< *'on the pattern of electron'*), *Cyclops, polycyclic, cyclin* (< *'a protein found in cell nuclei, in amounts which fluctuate during the cell cycle, being greatest during DNA replication'*), *cycl(o)-; cycloplegia* (< *'paralysis of the ciliary circle (ciliary muscle) of the eye'*); *bicycle*

> > G. kyklein (kykleein) *to move round and round* **E** (*verb*) *cycle; recycle*

> G. pelein *to be in motion*

> > G. polos, polou, m. *axis of a sphere, pivot, pole, firmament, sundial* **E** (*probably*) (*polidion *'little axis, little pivot'* >) *pulley*

> > > L. polus, poli, m. 극(極) **E** *pole, dipole*

> > > > L. polaris, polare 극(極)의, 극성(極性)의, 분극(分極)의, 극지(極地)의

> > > > **E** *polar, unipolar, bipolar, multipolar,* (*polar* >) *polarity, polarize, polarization, depolarization, repolarization, polariscope (polarimeter); dipolar*

> > > > [용례] Stella Polaris 북극성 **E** *Polaris*

> > > > > (문법) stella 별: 단수 주격 < stella, stellae, f.

> > > > > polaris 극의: 형용사, 남·여성형 단수 주격

> G. palin (< *revolving*) (*adverb*) *back, backwards, again* **E** *palin- (pali-)*

> > L. palingenesis, palingenesis, f. (< + G. genesis *birth*) 재생, 윤회, 반복발생 **E** *palingenesis*

> > > L. *palinopsia, *palinopsiae, f. (< + G. -opsia *seeing*) 반복시(反復視) **E** *palinopsia*

> G. telos, telous, n. (< *completion of a cycle*) *consummation, perfection, end, result* **E** *telomere* (< *'end part'*), *telophase* (< *'end phase'*)

> > G. telikos, telikē, telikon *final*

> > **E** *telic, ammonotelic* (< *'excreting amino nitrogen as ammonia'*), *ureotelic* (< *'excreting amino nitrogen as urea'*), *uricotelic* (< *'excreting amino nitrogen as uric acid'*)

> > G. teleos, telea, teleon (teleios, teleia, teleion) *complete, finished*

> > > L. Teleostei, Teleosteorum, m. (pl.) 경골어류(硬骨魚類)

> > > **E** *teleost* (< *'osseous fish, having the skeleton (usually) completely ossified'*)

> > G. atelēs, atelēs, ateles (< a- *not* + telos) *incomplete, imperfect*

> > > L. atelectasis, atelectasis, f. (< + G. ektasis *extension*) 무기폐(無氣肺) **E** *atelectasis, atelectatic*

> G. telein (teleein) *to complete, to fulfil, to perform (rites), to officiate (in the mysteries), to consecrate*

　　> G. telesma, telesmatos, n. *completion, performance, religious rite, a consecrated object endowed with a magic virtue to avert evil*　　　　**E** *(probably)* **talisman**

> *(probably)* G. telson, telsou, n. *boundary, limit*　　　　**E** *telson*

> L. teleologia, teleologiae, f. (< + G. ‑logia *study*) 목적론(目的論)　　　**E** *teleology*

contemno, contempsi, contemptum, contemnĕre (< con‑ (< cum) *with, together; intensive +* *temnĕre *to slight, to scorn*) 업신여기다　　　**E** *contemn*

　．> contemptus, contemptus, m. 경멸, 모욕　　　　**E** *contempt*

　　> contemptuosus, contemptuosa, contemptuosum 경멸적인, 모욕적인　　**E** *contemptuous*

coquo, coxi, coctum, coquĕre 익히다, 요리하다, 소화(消化)되게 하다

> **E** (*biscoctus panis *'twice baked bread'* >) **biscuit**, (L. terra cocta *'cooked earth'* >) It. **terra cotta**

> coctio, coctionis, f. 삶음, 소화, 숙성(熟成)　　　　**E** *coction*

> coquus, coqui, m. 요리사　　　　**E** *cook*

> coquina, coquinae, f. 부엌, 주방, 요리법　　　　**E** *kitchen, cuisine*

　> *(deformed)* culina, culinae, f. 부엌　　　　**E** *culinary, kiln*

> concoquo, concoxi, concoctum, concoquĕre (< con‑ (< cum) *with, together; intensive + coquĕre to cook*) 푹 삶다, 잘 익히다, 소화시키다　　　**E** *concoct*

　> concoctio, concoctionis, f. 소화　　　　**E** *concoction*

> decoquo, decoxi, decoctum, decoquĕre (< de‑ *apart from, down, not; intensive + coquĕre to cook*) 푹 삶다, 졸이다, 달이다, (재산을) 탕진하다　　　**E** *decoct*

　> decoctio, decoctionis, f. 졸임, 달임, 탕약, 탕진　　　　**E** *decoction*

> praecox, (gen.) praecocis (< prae‑ *before, beyond*) 일찍 익는, 조생종(早生種)의, 조숙(早熟)한　　　　**E** *precocious*, (praecox >) *precocity*

　> praecoquum, praecoqui, n. (< *early ripe*) 살구　　　　**E** *apricot*

< IE. pek^w‑ *to cook, to ripen*

> G. pessein ((*Attic*) peptein) (*base* pep‑) *to make ripe, to cook, to digest*

　> G. peptos, peptē, pepton *cooked*

> **E** *peptone* (< *'digested protein'*), (peptone >) **peptide(s)** (< *'any compound in which two or more amino acids are linked together, typically in a linear sequence, the carboxyl group of each acid usually being joined to the amino group of the next; according to the number of amino-acid residues, peptides are classed as dipeptides, tripeptides, etc., oligopeptides, or polypeptides'*), **neuropeptide(s)** (< *'any peptide with neurohormonal activity'*), **peptidase**, (peptone >) **peptize**

　> G. peptikos, peptikē, peptikon *promoting digestion, able to digest*

　　> L. pepticus, peptica, pepticum 소화성(消化性)의　　　　**E** *peptic*

> G. dyspeptos, dyspeptos, dyspepton (< dys- *bad*) *difficult of digestion*   **E** *dyspeptic*

　　　> G. dyspepsia, dyspepsias, f. *indigestion*

　　　　> L. dyspepsia, dyspepsiae, f. 소화불량   **E** *dyspepsia*

　> G. eupeptos, eupeptos, eupepton (< eu- *well*) *of good digestion*   **E** *eupeptic*

　　　> G. eupepsia, eupepsias, f. *good digestion*

　　　　> L. eupepsia, eupepsiae, f. 소화양호   **E** *eupepsia*

> G. pepsis, pepseōs, f. *digestion*   **E** *pepsin*

> G. pepōn, pepōn, pepon *ripe, gourd or melon eaten when ripe*   **E** *pepo, pumpkin*

curro, cucurri, cursum, currĕre 달리다, 뛰다, (줄 · 선 · 열이)

뻗어 나가다   **E** *current, countercurrent, currency, cursive, corridor, corral, courier*

> cursus, cursus, m. 달림, 진로, 궤도, 역정(歷程), 과정, 경과   **E** *course, coarse* (< *'ordinary'*)

> cursor, cursoris, m. 경주자, 배달부, (주인의 마차 앞에서 뛰는) 길잡이 노예   **E** *cursor*

> currus, currus, m. 수레, 경주마차, 전투마차

　> curriculum, curriculi, n. (원래는 curriculus였음 < + -ulus *diminutive suffix*)

　　작은 수레, 경주, 역정(歷程), 과정   **E** *curriculum,* (pl.) *curricula, extracurricular*

　　[용례] curriculum vitae 이력, 이력서   **E** *curriculum vitae*

　　　(문법) curriculum 역정: 단수 주격

　　　　vitae 삶의: 단수 속격 < vita, vitae, f.

> concurro, concucurri (concurri), concursum, concurrĕre (< con- (< cum) *with, together*
　+ currĕre *to run*) 함께 뛰다, 마주치다, 모여들다, 동시에 일어나다

　경쟁하다   **E** *concur, concurrent, concurrence*

　> concursus, concursus, m. 뛰어 몰려듦, 합류, 군집, 경쟁   **E** *concourse,* F. *concours*

> discurro, discucurri (discurri), discursum, discurrĕre (< dis- *apart from, down, not*
　+ currĕre *to run*) 사방으로 뛰어가다, 퍼지다, 논하다

　> discursus, discursus, m. 사방으로 뛰어다님, 확산, 누구와 이야기함, 추리   **E** *discourse*

> excurro, excucurri (excurri), éxcursum, excurrĕre (< ex- *out of, away from* + currĕre
　to run) 뛰어나가다, 뻗어 나가다, 출격하다, 발휘하다   **E** *excurrent*

　> excursio, excursionis, f. 짧은 여행, 탈선; (천문) 일탈(逸脫)   **E** *excursion*

> incurro, incucurri (incurri), incursum, incurrĕre (< in- *in, on, into, toward* + currĕre
　to run) 뛰어들다, 침략하다, 걸려들다, 초래하다, 발생하다   **E** *incur, incurrent, incursive*

　> incursio, incursionis, f. 뛰어들기, 침략   **E** *incursion*

> intercurro, intercucurri (intercurri), intercursum, intercurrĕre (< inter- *between, among*
　+ currĕre *to run*) 사이를 뛰다, 개입하다, 섞이다   **E** *intercurrent*

　> intercursus, intercursus, m. 개입, 중재, 간섭   **E** *intercourse*

> occurro, occucurri (occurri), occursum, occurrĕre (< oc- (< ob) *before, toward(s),*
　over, against, away + currĕre *to run*) 마주치다   **E** *occur, occurrent, occurrence*

> praecurro, praecucurri (praecurri), praecursum, praecurrĕre (< prae- *before, beyond*
　+ currĕre *to run*) 앞서 달리다, 앞서다

　> praecursor, praecursoris, m. 전구자(前驅者), 선구자, 선봉, 정탐자   **E** *precursor*

> recurro, **recurri**, recursum, recurrĕre (< re- *back, again* + currĕre *to run*) 원래의

자리로 돌아가다, 재발하다　　　　　**E** *recur, recurrent, recurrence, recursive*

　> recursio, recursionis, f. 반복, 재귀, 회귀, 귀납　　　　**E** *recursion*

> succurro, **succurri**, succursum, succurrĕre (< suc- (sub) *under, up from under* +

currĕre *to run*) 밑에 뛰어들다, 무릅쓰다, 돕다　　　　**E** *succor (succour)*

< IE. kers- *to run*

> (*Gaulish*) carros *wagon, cart*

> L. carrus, carri, m. (carrum, carri, n.) (네 바퀴 달린)

화물마차　　　　**E** *car, chariot, (carriole (diminutive) >) carryall*

> L. carrico, **carricavi**, carricatum, carricare 짐을 싣다; 마차로 나르다

E Sp. *cargo, charge (< 'to load a wagon'), discharge (< 'to unload'),*
caricature (< 'overloading, exaggeration'); carry, carrier, carriage,
miscarriage, career (< 'road, racecourse')

> L. carpentum, carpenti, n. 갈리아군의 전차, 이륜마차, 마차

> L. carpentarius, carpentarii, m. 마차 만드는 사람　　　**E** *carpenter*

dico, **dixi**, dictum, dicĕre (< *to show in words*) 말하다, 정하다　**E** It. ((*past participle*) *'said'* >) *ditto*

> dictum, dicti, n. (< dictum (*neuter past participle*) *something said*) 선언, 격언,

금언　　　　**E** *dictum,* (pl.) *dicta*

> verdictum, verdicti, n. (< verus *true* + dictum *something said*) 판정, 평결　**E** *verdict*

> dictio, dictionis, f. 말씨, 말투, 어법, 용어법,

문체　　　　**E** *diction, benediction, malediction, valediction*

> dictionarium, dictionarii, n. 사전(辭典)　　　　**E** *dictionary*

> jurisdictio, jurisdictionis, f. (< jus, juris, n. *law* + dictio *saying*) 재판권,

사법권　　　　**E** *jurisdiction*

> judex, judicis, m. (< jus, juris, n. *law* + dicĕre *to say*) 재판관, 심판자　**E** (*noun*) *judge*

> judico, **judicavi**, judicatum, judicare 재판하다,

판단하다　　　　**E** (*verb*) *judge, judgement (judgment)*

> judicium, judicii, n. 재판, 심리, 판단　　　　**E** *judicious*

> judiciarius, judiciaria, judiciarium 재판의, 사법의　　**E** *judiciary*

> judicialis, judiciale 재판의, 사법의　　　　**E** *judicial*

> praejudicium, praejudicii, n. (< prae- *before, beyond* + judicium *judge-*
ment) 선입견, 예단(豫斷), 편견　　　　**E** *prejudice*

> dicto, **dictavi**, dictatum, dictare (*frequentative*) 반복해서 말하다, 구수(口授)하다,

받아쓰게 하다, 위엄을 부리며 지시하다　　　　**E** *dictate*

> dictator, dictatoris, m. 구수자(口授者), 명령자, 독재자　　**E** *dictator*

> addico, **addixi**, addictum, addicĕre (< ad- *to, toward, at, according to* + dicĕre

to say) 편들어 말하다, 몸과 마음을 바치다, 탐닉하다　　　**E** *addict*

> addictio, addictionis, f. 탐닉, 중독, 마약중독, 마약상습　**E** *addiction*

> condico, **condixi**, condictum, condicĕre (< con- (< cum) *with, together* + dicĕre

to say) 합의 결정하다, 협정하다

> condicio, condicionis, f. (conditio, conditionis, f.) 협정, 협정 조항, 협정 조건, 조건, 제약, 형편　　　　　　　　　　　　　　E *condition, conditional, unconditional*

> contradico, **contradixi**, contradictum, contradicĕre (< contra- *against* + dicĕre *to say*) 반대하다, 반박하다　　　　　　　　　　　　　　E *contradict*

　　> contradictio, contradictionis, f. 반대, 반박, 모순　　　　E *contradiction*

　　> contradictor, contradictoris, m. 반대론자　　　　E *contradictor*

　　　> contradictorius, contradictoria, contradictorium 반대되는; (논리) 모순되는　　　　　　　　　　　　　　E *contradictory*

> edico, edixi, edictum, edicĕre (< e- *out of, away from* + dicĕre *to say*) 공포하다, 포고하다, 칙령을 내리다　　　　　　　　　　　　　　E *edict*

> indico, **indixi**, indictum, indicĕre (< in- *in, on, into, toward* + dicĕre *to say*) 지정하여 통고하다, ~하도록 지시하다, 부과하다　　　　　　　E *indict*

> interdico, **interdixi**, interdictum, interdicĕre (< inter- *between, among* + dicĕre *to say*) 금지하다, 정지하다　　　　　　　　　　　　　　E *interdict*

> praedico, **praedixi**, praedictum, praedicĕre (< prae- *before, beyond* + dicĕre *to say*) 미리 말하다　　　　　　　　　　　　　　E *predict, predictive, predictable*

> dico, **dicavi**, dicatum, dicare 알리다, 헌신하다

　　> abdico, **abdicavi**, abdicatum, abdicare (< ab- *off, away from* + dicare *to make know*) 거부하다, (법정기한 전에) 사임하다　　　　　E *abdicate*

　　> dedico, **dedicavi**, dedicatum, dedicare (< de- *apart from, down, not; intensive* + dicare *to make know*) 신고하다, (종교적으로 신에게) 봉헌하다, 바치다　　　E *dedicate*

　　> indico, **indicavi**, indicatum, indicare (< in- *in, on, into, toward* + dicare *to make know*) 가리키다, 고발하다　　　　E *indicate*

　　　> index, indicis, m., f. 고발자, 집게손가락, 지침, 지표(指標), 지수(指數), 색인(索引)　　　　　　　　　　E *index,* (pl.) *indices*

　　　> indicatio, indicationis, f. 지시, 표시, 징조, 조치　　　E *indication*

　　　> indicator, indicatoris, m. 지시자, 지시기, 지표　　　E *indicator*

　　　> indicativus, indicativa, indicativum 지시하는, 표시하는, 나타내는; (문법) 직설법의　　　　　　　　　　　E *indicative*

　　　> contraindico, **contraindicavi**, contraindicatum, contraindicare (< contra- *against* + indicare *to proclaim*) 금기를 나타내다　　E *contraindicate*

　　　　> contraindicatio, contraindicationis, f. 금기　　E *contraindication*

　　> praedico, **praedicavi**, praedicatum, praedicare (< prae- *before, beyond* + dicare *to make know*) 드러나게 말하다, 설교하다, 단정하다, 서술하다　　　　　　　　　E *preach, predicate, predicative*

　　　> praedicamentum, praedicamenti, n. (< *something predicated*) 범주, 상태, 곤경　　　　　　　　　　E *predicament*

　　> vindico, **vindicavi**, vindicatum, vindicare (< vim dicare *to show authority* < vis, viris, f. *force* + dicare *to make know*) 법적 권리를 요구하다, 주장하다, 복수하다　　　　　　E *vindicate, vindicative, vengeance, avenge, revenge*

　　　> vindicta, vindictae, f. 복수　　　E It. *vendetta, vindictive*

< IE. deik-, deig- *to show, to pronounce solemnly; also in derivatives referring to the directing of words or objects* **E** *teach, token, betoken,* (possibly) *toe*

> L. digitus, digiti, m. (< *pointer, indicator*) 손가락, 발가락 **E** *digit*

　> L. digitalis, digitale 손가락의, 손가락만 한

　　E *digital,* (D. Fingerhut *'thimble'* >) digitalis herba *'digital herb'* >) *digitalis,* (digitalis + toxin >) *digitoxin,* (digitoxin >) *digoxin,* (digoxin > *'obtained by hydrolysis of digoxin'* >) *digoxigenin*

　> L. digitatus, digitata, digitatum 손가락이 있는, 발가락이 있는, 손가락 모양의 **E** *digitate,* (digitate >) *interdigitate*

> G. deiknynai *to show* **E** *deictic*

　> G. deixis, diexēos, f. *display, demonstrable reference* **E** *deixis*

　> G. deigma, deigmatos, n. *sample, pattern*

　　> G. paradeigma, paradeigmatos, n. (< par(a)- *beside, along side of, beyond* + deigma) *example, pattern, model*

　　　> L. paradigma, paradigmatis, n. 보기, 견본, 범례, 모범, 틀; 품사 변화표 **E** *paradigm*

> G. dikein (*to direct an object* >) *to throw*

　> G. diskos, diskou, m. *disc*

　　> L. discus, disci, m. 원반, 디스크, 접시 **E** *discus, disc (disk), discoid, discotheque, diskette, dish, desk*

　> G. diktyon, diktyou, n. *net, fishing net* **E** *dicty(o)-, dictyosome*

> G. dikē, dikēs, f. *justice, right, court case*

　> G. syndikos, syndikou, m. (< syn- *with, together*) *defendant's advocate*

　　> L. syndicus, syndici, m. 변호인, 구역 대표, 이사 **E** *syndic, syndicate*

divido, divisi, divisum, dividĕre (< di- (< dis-) *apart from, down, not; intensive* + < -vidĕre *to separate*) 나누다, 분배하다, 분류하다

E *divide,* (dividendum (*neuter gerundive*) *'which is to be divided'* >) *dividend, divisor, divisible*

> divisio, divisionis, f. 나누기, 분할, (분할된) 부분, 분열 **E** *division*

> *diviso, *divisavi, *divisatum, *divisare (*frequentative*) 생각해내다, 궁리하다, 계획하다, 고안하다, 발명하다 **E** *devise, device*

> dividuus, dividua, dividuum 나뉘는, 갈라놓은

　> individuus, individua, individuum (< in- *not* + dividuus *divisible, separated*) 나눌 수 없는, 개체의, 개인의, 제각기 다른, 개별의

　　> individualis, individuale 개체의, 개인의, 제각기 다른 **E** *individual*

　　> individuo, individuavi, individuatum, individuare 개별화하다, 특징화하다 **E** *individuate*

　　　> individuatio, individuationis, f. 개별화, 특징화 **E** *individuation*

< IE. weidh- *to divide, to separate*

E *widow* (< *'(woman) separated (from her husband by death)'*), (widow >) *widower,* (widow >) *widowhood*

> L. viduus, vidua, viduum 짝 잃은, 혼자된, 과부의

duco, duxi, ductum, ducĕre 이끌다

> dux, ducis, m. 지도자, 공작(公爵)   **E** It. *il Duce, duke*

    > ducissa, ducissae, f. 공작부인(孔雀夫人), 화려하게 차린 여인   **E** *duchess*

> ductus, ductus, m. 인도, 안내, 도관(導管),

    관(管)   **E** *ductus (duct),* (pl.) *ductus, ductal, ductless, douche, aqueduct, oviduct*

    [용례] ductus arteriosus 동맥관   **E** *ductus arteriosus*

        ductus venosus 정맥관   **E** *ductus venosus*

        ductus choledochus (< *common bile duct*) 총담관, 온쓸개관   **E** *ductus choledochus*

        (문법) ductus: 단수 주격

          arteriosus 동맥이 많은, 동맥이 두드러진: 형용사, 남성형 단수 주격

            < arteriosus, arteriosa, arteriosum

          venosus 정맥이 많은, 정맥이 두드러진: 형용사, 남성형 단수 주격

            < venosus, venosa, venosum

          choledochus 담즙을 담는: 형용사, 남성형 단수 주격

              < choledochus, choledocha, choledochum

              < G. cholē, cholēs, f. *bile* + G. dochē, dochēs, f. *receptacle*

    > ductulus, ductuli, m. (< + -ulus *diminutive suffix*)

      소관(小管)   **E** *ductulus,* (pl.) *ductuli, ductule, ductular*

> ductilis, ductile 지도하기 쉬운; (금속 등이) 길게 늘일 수 있는, 두들겨 펼 수 있는   **E** *ductile*

> abduco, abduxi, abductum, abducĕre (< ab- *off, away from* + ducĕre *to lead*)

  끌어내다, 납치하다, 떼어놓다, 벌리다, 외전(外轉)하다

     E *abduct,* ((*present participle*) *'leading away*' >) *abducens,* (abducens >) *abducent*

  > abductio, abductionis, f. 납치, 벌림, 외전(外轉)   **E** *abduction*

  > abductor, abductoris, m. 벌림근, 외전근(外轉筋)   **E** *abductor*

> adduco, adduxi, adductum, adducĕre (< ad- *to, toward, at, according to* + ducĕre

  to lead) 끌어대다, 당기다, 모으다, 내전(內轉)하다   **E** *adduct, adducent, adduce*

  > adductio, adductionis, f. 모음, 내전(內轉)   **E** *adduction*

  > adductor, adductoris, m. 모음근, 내전근(內轉筋)   **E** *adductor*

> circumduco, circumduxi, circumductum, circumducĕre (< circum- *around* + ducĕre

  to lead) 주위로 끌고 돌아다니다, 원회전을 하다   **E** *circumduct*

  > circumductio, circumductionis, f. 원회전   **E** *circumduction*

> conduco, conduxi, conductum, conducĕre (< con- (< cum) *with, together* + ducĕre

  to lead) 이끌다, 인도하다; 도움이 되다

     E (*verb*) *conduct, conductor, conductive, conductivity; conduce, conducive, conducible*

  > conductus, conductus, m. 도관(導管), 통로   **E** (*noun*) *conduct, conduit*

  > conductio, conductionis, f. 전도(傳導)   **E** *conduction*

> deduco, deduxi, deductum, deducĕre (< de- *apart from, down, not* + ducĕre *to*

  lead) 끌어내리다, 빼다, 이끌어 내다, 추론하다   **E** *deduct, deductive, deduce*

  > deductio, deductionis, f. 빼기, 공제, 추론, 연역(演繹)   **E** *deduction*

> educo, **eduxi**, eductum, educĕre (< e- *out of, away from* + ducĕre *to lead*)
끌어내다   E *educe*

> educo, **educavi**, educatum, educare (< *to lead out*) 기르다, 교육하다   E *educate*

> induco, **induxi**, inductum, inducĕre (< in- *in, on, into, toward* + ducĕre *to lead*)
끌어들이다, 초래하다, 하게 하다, 유도하다   E *induce, inducer*

> inductio, inductionis, f. 유도, 귀납(歸納)   E *induction*

> introduco, **introduxi**, introductum, introducĕre (< intro- *inwards* + ducĕre *to lead*)
받아들이다, 도입하다, 안내하다, 소개하다   E *introduce*

> introductio, introductionis, f. 도입, 안내, 소개   E *introduction*

> introductorius, introductoria, introductorium 소개하는, 입문적인   E *introductory*

> produco, **produxi**, productum, producĕre (< pro *forward* + ducĕre *to lead*) 이끌어
내다, 생산하다, 낳다

E *produce, producer, production, productive; reproduce, reproduction, reproductive,*
reproducible

> productum, producti, n. 산물(産物), 생산품, 제품, 성과; (수학) 곱;
(화학) 생성물   E *product, (addition + product >)* **adduct**

> reduco, **reduxi**, reductum, reducĕre (< re- *back, again* + ducĕre *to lead*) 되돌려
놓다, 뒤로 물러나게 하다, 줄어들게 하다   E *reduce, reducer, redux, reductive, reducible*

> reductio, reductionis, f. 환원, (탈구의) 교정,
감소   E *reduction, (reduction 'on the pattern of oxidant' >)* **reductant**

> seduco, **seduxi**, seductum, seducĕre (< se- *apart, without* + ducĕre *to lead*) 따로
떼어내다, 유혹하다, 미혹케 하다   E *seduce, seductive*

> seductio, seductionis, f. 유혹, 미혹   E *seduction*

> subduco, **subduxi**, subductum, subducĕre (< sub- *apart, without* + ducĕre *to lead*)
밑에서 끄집어내다, 들어올리다, 뽑아내다, 떼어버리다, 훔치다   E *subdue*

> subductio, subductionis, f. 제거; (지질) 침입(沈入)   E *subduction*

> transduco, **transduxi**, transductum, transducĕre (< trans- *over, across, through, beyond*
+ ducĕre *to lead*) 변환시키다   E *transduce, transducer, transducin*

> transductio, transductionis, f. 변환   E *transduction*

< IE. deuk- *to lead*

E *tow, tug, taut (< 'drawn'),* **tie, team** *(< 'set of draft animals tied together'),* **teem** *(< 'to*
beget'), (wan + ton > 'badly led' >) **wanton**

edo, edi, esum, edĕre 먹다

> edibilis, edibile 먹을 수 있는   E *edible*

> esca, escae, f. 먹거리, 식품

> esculentus, esculenta, esculentum 식용에 알맞은   E *esculent*

> comedo, **comedi**, comesum, comedĕre (< com- (< cum) *with, together; intensive* +
edĕre *to eat*) 먹어치우다

> comedo, comedonis, m. (< *a comparison of the worm-like shape of the waxy*
material that can be squeezed from a blackhead to a worm believed to

feed on the body) 대식가, 여드름,

면포(面皰)   **E** *comedo,* (pl.) *comedones (comedos), comedocarcinoma*

> *obedo, *obedi, *obesum, *obedĕre (< ob- *before, toward(s), over, against, away*

+ edĕre *to eat*) 게걸스레 먹다

> obesus, obesa, obesum 살찐, 비대한   **E** *obese*

> obesitas, obesitatis, f. 살찜, 비대, 비만   **E** *obesity*

< IE. ed- *to eat; original meaning 'to bite'*   **E** *eat, etch, etching, fret, fretful*

> L. prandium, prandii, n. (< IE. per *first* + IE. ed-) 첫 식사, 점심(원래는 조반·점심

전의 간단한 곁두리였음), 식사   **E** *prandial, preprandial (anteprandial), postprandial*

> G. odynē, odynēs, f. *gnawing care* > *pain, grief* (Vide ODYNĒ: *See* E. *odyn(o)–*)

emo, emi, emptum, emĕre 획득하다, 사다, 구매하다, 매입하다

> emptio, emptionis, f. 구매,

매입   **E** *emption, (emption >) preemption, preemptive, (preemption >) preempt*

> emptor, emptoris, m. 구매자, 매입자

> praemium, praemii, n. (< prae- *before, beyond* + emĕre *to take, to obtain, to buy*)

노획물, 전리품, 벌이, 상   **E** *premium*

> demo, dempsi, demptum (demtum), demĕre (< de- *apart from, down, not* + emĕre

to take, to obtain, to buy) 덜어내다, 떼어내다

> vindemia, vindemiae, f. (< vinum *wine* + demĕre *to remove*) 포도추확, 추수,

수확   **E** *vintage*

> eximo, exemi, exemptum, eximĕre (< ex- *out of, away from* + emĕre *to take,*

to obtain, to buy) 꺼내다, 뽑아내다, 뺏다, 제거하다, 면제하다   **E** *exempt*

> exemptio, exemptionis, f. 제거, 면제   **E** *exemption*

> exemplum, exempli, n. 보기, 예;

모범   **E** *example, (aphetic) sample, exemplify; exemplar, exemplary*

[용례] exempli gratia 예를 위하여 > 예를 들자면   **E** *(exempli gratia >) e.g.*

(문법) exempli: 단수 속격 (원인의 속격, 목적의 속격)

gratia 때문에, 위하여: 단수 탈격, 원인의 속격 또는 목적의

속격을 요구 < gratia, gratiae, f. 호의, 은혜, 감사

> perimo, peremi, peremptum, perìmĕre (< per- *through, thoroughly* + emĕre *to take,*

to obtain, to buy) 제거하다, 전멸하다

> peremptorius, peremptoria, peremptorium 전멸의; 결정적인, 단호한   **E** *peremptory*

> promo, prompsi, promptum, promĕre (< pro- *before, forward, for, instead of* + emĕre

to take, to obtain, to buy) (준비되어 있는 것을 즉각) 꺼내다, 제시하다   **E** *prompt*

> promptus, promptus, m. 준비된 상태, 제시   **E** *(in promptu 'in readiness' >) impromptu*

> promptitudo, promptitudinis, f. 기민, 민첩   **E** *promptitude*

> redimo, redemi, redemptum (redemtum), redimĕre (< red- *back, again* + emĕre *to*

take, to obtain, to buy) 되사다, 몸값을 치르고 구해내다, 대가를 지불하고 사다,

속죄하다   **E** *redeem*

> redemptio, redemptionis, f. 되사기, 변제, 상환, 속죄 　　E *redemption (ransom)*

> sumo, **sumpsi**, sumptum, sumĕre (< sus- (< sub) *under, up from under* + emĕre

to take, to obtain, to buy) 획득하다, 사다, 소비하다

> sumptus, sumptus, m. 가짐, 취함; 비용, 소비; 허비, 낭비

> sumptuarius, sumptuaria, sumptuarium 비용의, 소비의; 비용을 덜 들이는,

절약의 　　E *sumptuary*

> sumptuosus, sumptuosa, sumptuosum 돈이 많이 드는, 호사스런 　　E *sumptuous*

> sumptio, sumptionis, f. 가짐, 받음, 취함, 훔침; (논리) 전제(前提) 　　E *sumption*

> assumo, **assumpsi**, assumptum, assumĕre (< as- (< ad) *to, toward, at, according*

to + sumĕre *to take*) 받아들이다, 취하다, 가정하다 　　E *assume, assumptive*

> assumptio, assumptionis, f. 받아들임, 취함, 인수, 찬탈, 가정 　　E *assumption*

> consumo, **consumpsi**, consumptum, consumĕre (< con- (< cum) *with, together;*

intensive + sumĕre *to take*) 소비하다, 소모하다,

쇠약하게 하다 　　E *consume, consumptive*

> consumptio, consumptionis, f. 소비, 소모, 소모성 질환, 결핵, 쇠약 　　E *consumption*

> praesumo, **praesumpsi**, praesumptum, praesumĕre (< prae- *before, beyond* +

sumĕre *to take*) 먼저 취하다, 짐작하다, 추정(推定)하다, 추론(推論)하다 　　E *presume*

> praesumptivus, praesumptiva, praesumptivum 추정적 　　E *presumptive*

> praesumptio, praesumptionis, f. 추정, 추론; 넘겨짚음, 주제넘음 　　E *presumption*

> praesumpti(u)osus, praesumpti(u)osa, praesumpti(u)osum

주제넘은 　　E *presumptuous*

> resumo, **resumpsi**, resumptum, resumĕre (< re- *back, again* + sumĕre *to*

take) 다시 차지하다, 되찾다, 회복하다,

다시 시작하다 　　E *resume, resumptive,* F. *résumé* (< 'summed up' < 'taken back')

> resumptio, resumptionis, f. 회복, 재개 　　E *resumption*

> subsumo, **subsumpsi**, subsumptum, subsumĕre (< sub- *under, up from under*

+ sumĕre *to take*) 밑으로 가져가다, 포섭하다, 포함하다 　　E *subsume, subsumptive*

> subsumptio, subsumptionis, f. 포섭, 포함 　　E *subsumption*

< IE. em- *to take, to distribute*

fendo, fendi, fensum, fendĕre (*obsolete; exclusively in compounds*) 치다

> defendo, **defendi**, defensum, defendĕre (< de- *apart from, down, not* + fendĕre

to strike) 방어하다

E *defend,* (defensum (*past participle*), defensa (*past participle*) >) *defense*
(defence), defensive, defendant, (defend >) fend, (fend >) fender, (defence
>) fence, (fence >) fencing

> offendo, **offendi**, offensum, offendĕre (< of- (< ob) *before, toward(s), over,*

against + fendĕre *to strike*)

공격하다 　　E *offend,* (offensa (*past participle*) >) *offense (offence), offensive*

< IE. gʷhen- *to strike, to kill* 　　E *bane, gun* (< 'war')

> (*Persian*) zahr *poison*

> (*Persian*) padzahr *counter-poison* (< pad *protecting against* (< IE. pa- *to protect, to feed*) + zahr)

> **E** **bezoar** (< '*a small stony concretion found in the stomachs of ruminants, once used as an antidote for various ailments*'), **phytobezoar, trichobezoar**

fido, fisus sum, fidĕre (반탈형동사) 믿다　　　**E** F. *fiancé,* F. *fiancée, defy, defiant, defiance*

> fides, fidei, f. 믿음, 신앙, 신빙, 신용, 마음, 약속, 보호　　　**E** *faith*

[용례] bona fide 좋은 믿음으로 > 진정한, 성실한　　　**E** *bona fide*

(문법) bona 좋은: 형용사, 여성형 단수 탈격

fide 믿음으로: 단수 탈격

> fidelis, fidele 미더운, 충실한

> fidelitas, fidelitatis, f. 충실, 성실, 정절　　　**E** *fidelity*

> infidelis, infidele (< in- *not*) 믿지 않는, 배신하는, 부정(不貞)한　　　**E** *infidel*

> infidelitas, infidelitatis, f. 믿지 않음, 배신, 부정　　　**E** *infidelity*

> perfidus, perfida, perfidum (< (*deceiving*) *through faith* < per- *through, thoroughly* + fides *faith*) 배신하는　　　**E** *perfidy, perfidious*

> fiducia, fiduciae, f. 믿음, 자신, 저당, 신탁　　　**E** *fiducial, fiduciary*

> confido, confisus sum, confidĕre (< con- (< cum) *with, together; intensive* + fidĕre *to trust*) 믿다, 자신을 갖다　　　**E** *confide, confident*

> confidentia, confidentiae, f. 신뢰, 자신, 당돌함　　　**E** *confidence*

> diffido, diffisus sum, diffidĕre (< dif- (< dis-) *apart from, down, not* + fidĕre *to trust*) 믿지 않다, 자신을 잃다　　　**E** *diffident*

> diffidentia, diffidentiae, f. 불신, 소심, 의구심　　　**E** *diffidence*

< IE. bheidh- *to trust*　　　**E** *abide* (< '*to wait trustingly*'), *abode* (< '*waiting trustingly*')

> L. foedus, foederis, n. 조약, 동맹, 연합

> L. *foederalis, *foederale 동맹의, 연합의, 연방의　　　**E** *federal*

> L. foedero, foederavi, foederatum, foederare 연합하다　**E** *federate, federation, federacy*

> L. confoedero, confoederavi, confoederatum, confoederare (< con- (< cum) *with, together* + foederare *to league together, to establish by league or treaty*) 동맹시키다, 연합시키다　　　**E** *confederate, confederation, confederacy*

figo, fixi, fixum, figĕre 박다, 고정하다, (마음속에) 깊이 간직하다, 주시하다　　**E** *fix* (< '*to fasten*')

> fixo, fixavi, fixatum, fixare 고정하다, (마음속에) 깊이 간직하다, 주시하다　　　**E** *fix* (< '*to preserve with a fixative*'), *fixative*

> fixatio, fixationis, f. 고정, 집착, 주시　　　**E** *fixation*

> crucifigo, crucifixi, crucifixum, crucifigĕre (< crux, crucis, f. *cross* + figĕre *to fix*) 십자가에 못 박다, 십자가형에 처하다　　　**E** *crucify*

> crucifixio, crucifixionis, f. 십자가 처형　　　**E** *crucifixion*

> transfigo, transfixi, transfixum, transfigĕre (< trans- *over, across, through, beyond*

+ figĕre *to fix*) 꿰뚫어 고정시키다   **E** *transfix*

> affigo, **affixi**, affixum, affigĕre (< ad- *to, toward, at, according to* + figĕre *to fix*)
꿰어 박다, 고착시키다, 부착시키다, 첨부하다

  > affixum, affixi, n. 부착물, 첨부물, 첨가물; (문법) 접사(接辭)   **E** *affix*

> infigo, **infixi**, infixum, infigĕre (< in- *in, on, into, toward* + figĕre *to fix*) 박아 넣다

  > infixum, infixi, n. 삽입사(揷入辭)   **E** *infix*

> praefigo, **praefixi**, praefixum, praefigĕre (< prae- *before, beyond* + figĕre *to fix*)
앞에 박다

  > praefixum, praefixi, n. 접두사(接頭辭)   **E** *prefix*

> suffigo, **suffixi**, suffixum, suffigĕre (< suf- (< sub) *under, up from under* + figĕre
to fix) 밑에 붙들어 매다, 매달다

  > suffixum, suffixi, n. 첨가물; 접미사(接尾辭)   **E** *suffix*

< IE. dhig^{w}- *to stick, to fix*   **E** *dig, dike, ditch*

> L. fivĕre *archaic variant of* figĕre

  > L. fivibula, fivibulae, f.

    > L. fibula, fibulae, f. 물림쇠, 걸쇠; 종아리뼈, 비골(腓骨)   **E** *fibula*

      > L. fibularis, fibulare 종아리뼈의, 비골의   **E** *fibular*

      > L. infibulo, infibulavi, infibulatum, infibulare (< in- *in, on, into,
toward*) 물림쇠로 묶다, 단추를 끼우다, 금속 실로 묶다

        > L. infibulatio, infibulationis, f. 봉쇄, 음부봉쇄   **E** *infibulation*

> L. finis, finis, m. 경계, 끝, 목적

E *(noun)* *fine* (< '*payment for ending a lawsuit*'), *(fine > 'fine for debt, compensation, or
ransom' > 'taxation, revenue' >)* **finance, financial,** *(tres fines 'three ends' >)* **trephine**

> L. finalis, finale 경계에 관한, 최종의, 목적의   **E** *final*

> L. finio, finivi (finii), finitum, finire 경계를 정하다, 한정하다, 끝내다

E **finish**, *(adjective, verb)* **fine**, *(fine >)* **refine**, *(refine >)* **refinery**, *(F. 'refined sugar'
>)* **raffinose**

  > L. finitus, finita, finitum *(past participle)* 한정된   **E** *finite*

    > L. infinitus, infinita, infinitum (< in- *not*) 무한한   **E** *infinite*

      > L. infinitas, infinitatis, f. 무한   **E** *infinity*

      > L. *infinitudo, *infinitudinis, f. 무한, 무궁   **E** *infinitude*

    > L. infinitesimus, infinitesima, infinitesimum (< + -esimus, *on the
pattern of* centesimus '*one hundredth*') 무한소(無限小)의   **E** *infinitesimal*

  > L. †finitivus, †finitiva, †finitivum 한정하는

    > L. infinitivus, infinitiva, infinitivum (< in- *not* + †finitivus *defining,
definitive*) (문법) 부정법의, 부정사의   **E** *infinitive*

  > L. definio, definivi (definii), definitum, definire (< de- *apart from, down,
not; intensive*) 경계를 정하다, 정의(定義)하다   **E** *define*

    > L. definitus, definita, definitum *(past participle)* 한정된, 명확한   **E** *definite*

    > L. definitio, definitionis, f. 정의   **E** *definition*

    > L. definitivus, definitiva, definitivum 한정적, 명확한, 결정적,

최종적   **E** *definitive*

> L. affinis, affine (< af- (< ad) *to, toward, at, according to* + finis *limit, end*)

인접한, 관여한, 인척관계에 있는

> **E** *-affin, argentaffin, chromaffin,* (parum *'little'* + affinis *'closely related, akin'* > *'neutral quality and low chemical reactivity'* >) *paraffin*

> L. affinitas, affinitatis, f. 이웃, 인척관계, 밀접한 관련,

친화력   **E** *affinity,* (affinity >) *affinitive*

> L. confinis, confine (< con- (< cum) *with, together* + finis *limit, end*) 경계를

두고 이웃한, 한정된   **E** *confine, confinement*

fingo, finxi, fictum, fingĕre 꾸미다,

제작하다   **E** *feign, feint, faint* (< *'weak'* < *'avoiding one's duty by pretending'*)

> fictitius, fictitia, fictitium (ficticius, ficticia, ficticium) 허구의   **E** *fictitious*

> fictio, fictionis, f. 조형(造形), 허구, 가상, 꾸며낸 이야기   **E** *fiction*

> figmentum, figmenti, n. 조형, 허구, 가상, 꾸며낸 이야기   **E** *figment*

> figura, figurae, f. 모양, 형상, 그림, 도형, 숫자 (< *a numerical symbol; originally*

applied to the ten symbols of the Arabic notation)   **E** *figure, figurine*

> figuro, figuravi, figuratum, figurare 모양을 만들다, 형용하다, 마음에 그리다, 비유

하여 표현하다

> figurativus, figurativa, figurativum 형용적인, 비유적인   **E** *figurative*

> configuro, configuravi, configuratum, configurare (< con- (< cum) *with,*

together + figurare *to figure*) (배치하여) 모양을 이루게 하다   **E** *configure*

> configuratio, configurationis, f. 형상, 윤곽   **E** *configuration*

> diffiguro, diffiguravi, diffiguratum, diffigurare (< dif- (< dis-) *apart from,*

down, not + figurare *to figure*) 모양을 손상하다   **E** *disfigure*

> transfiguro, transfiguravi, transfiguratum, transfigurare (< trans- *over,*

across, through, beyond + figurare *to figure*) 형상을 바꾸다, 변모

시키다   **E** *transfigure*

> transfiguratio, transfigurationis, f. 변모   **E** *transfiguration*

> effingo, effinxi, effictum, effingĕre (< ef- (< ex) *out of, away from* + fingĕre *to form*)

모양을 나타내다, 표상하다

> effigies, effigiei, f. 모습, 초상, 조상, 유사   **E** *effigy*

< IE. dheigh- *to form, to build*

> **E** *dairy* (< *'bread kneader'*), *lady* (< *'loaf (bread) kneader'*), *dough, doughnut (donut), doughy*

> (*Avestan*) pairi-daeza (< pairi *around* (< IE. per *basic meanings of 'forward', 'through'*)

+ daeza *wall, originally made of clay or mud bricks* (< IE. dheigh-)) *enclosure,*

park, garden   **E** *paradise*

flecto, flexi, flexum, flectĕre 굽히다, 꿇다   **E** *flex*

> flexio, flexionis, f. 굽힘, 꿇음   **E** *flexion, dorsiflexion, plantarflexion*

> flexura, flexurae, f. 굽이, 굴곡, 곡, 만곡부　　　　　**E** *flexure, flexural*

> flexor, flexoris, m. 굽힘근, 굴근(屈筋), 굽힘쪽　　　　　**E** *flexor*

> flexilis, flexile 굽어지는, 꺾이는, 유연한　　　　　**E** *flexile*

> flexibilis, flexibile 굽히기 쉬운, 꺾이기 쉬운,

유연한　　**E** *flexible, (flexible time >) flexitime (flextime), (flexible place >) flexiplace*

　　> flexibilitas, flexibilitatis, f. 굽히기 쉬움, 굴곡성, 유연성　　**E** *flexibility*

> circumflecto, circumflexi, circumflexum, circumflectĕre (< circum- *around* + flectĕre

to bend) 휘돌다, 회선(回旋)하다, 만곡(彎曲)하다　　　　**E** *circumflex*

> deflecto, deflexi, deflexum, deflectĕre (< de- *apart from, down, not* + flectĕre *to*

bend) 빗나가게 하다, 편향(偏向)시키다, 빗나가다, 기울다　　**E** *deflect*

　　> deflexio, deflexionis, f. 비낌, 편향, 왜곡; (광선의) 굴절　　**E** *deflexion (deflection)*

> inflecto, inflexi, inflexum, inflectĕre (< in- *in, on, into, toward* + flectĕre *to bend*)

굽히다, 돌리다, 바꾸다　　　　　**E** *inflect*

　　> inflexio, inflexionis, f. 굽힘, 굽음, 만곡, 굴곡, 굴절;

　　　(문법) 어미변화　　　**E** *inflexion (inflection), inflectional*

> reflecto, reflexi, reflexum, reflectĕre (< re- *back, again* + flectĕre *to bend*) 반사

하다, 반영하다, 곰곰이 생각하다　**E** *reflect, (verb) reflex, reflective, (reflect >) reflectance*

　　> reflexus, reflexus, m. 반사, 반사작용, 반사운동　　**E** *(noun) reflex; areflexia*

　　> reflexio, reflexionis, f. 반사, 반영, 숙고　　**E** *reflexion (reflection)*

　　　> *reflexivus, *reflexiva, *reflexivum 반사의; (문법) 재귀용법의　　**E** *reflexive*

fligo, flixi, flictum, fligĕre 치다, 때리다, 부딪치다

> affligo, afflixi, afflictum, affligĕre (< af- (< ad) *to, toward, at, according to* + fligĕre

to strike) 부딪히게 하다, 괴롭히다　　　　**E** *afflict*

> confligo, conflixi, conflictum, confligĕre (< con- (< cum) *with, together* + fligĕre

to strike) 맞부딪히다, 갈등하다　　　　**E** *conflict*

> infligo, inflixi, inflictum, infligĕre (< in- *in, on, into, toward* + fligĕre *to strike*) (상처를)

입히다, (고통을) 가하다　　　　**E** *inflict*

< IE. bhlig- *to strike*

fluo, fluxi, fluxum, fluĕre 흐르다

　　　　　E *fluent, fluency*

> fluxus, fluxus, m. 흐름　　　**E** *flux, (flux >) reflux*

> fluor, fluoris, m. 흘러내림, 유출(流出)

E *fluorite (fluorspar) (< calcium fluoride, CaF$_2$, used as a flux to lower the melting point of raw materials in metallurgy), (fluorite >) fluorine (F), (fluorine >) fluorinate, (fluorine >) fluor(o)-, 5-fluorouracil (5-FU), fluoroapatite, fluoride, (fluoride >) fluoridate*

> *fluoresco, *fluorui, −, *fluorescĕre (< fluorspar (CaF$_2$) + -escĕre

suffix of inceptive (inchoative) verb) 형광(螢光)을 내다

E *fluorescent, fluorescence, (fluorescence >) fluoresce, (fluoresce >) fluorescein, (fluorescence >) fluor(o)-, fluorochrome, fluoroscopy*

> fluidus, fluida, fluidum 흐르는, 유동성의, 액체의　　　**E** *fluid, fluidic, fluidics*

> -fluus, -flua, -fluum 흐르는　**E** *-fluous, lactifluous (< 'on the pattern of mellifluous')*

　　> mellifluus, melliflua, mellifluum (< mel, mellis, n. *honey* + -fluus

　　　　flowing) 꿀이 흐르는　　　　　　　　　　　　　　　**E** *mellifluous*

> fluvius, fluvii, m. 강　　　　　　　　　　　　　　　　　　　**E** *fluvial*

> fluctus, fluctus, m. 물결, 파도

　　> fluctuo, fluctuavi, fluctuatum, fluctuare 물결치다,

　　　　동요하다　　　　　　　　　　　　　　　**E** *fluctuate, fluctuant*

　　　　> fluctuatio, fluctuationis, f. 파동, 동요, 기복, 변동　**E** *fluctuation*

> affluo, affluxi, affluxum, affluĕre (< af- (< ad) *to, toward, at, according*

　　to + fluĕre *to flow*) ~로 흐르다, 흘러들다, 몰려들다,

　　풍요하다　　　　　　　　**E** *affluent, (affluent + influenza >) affluenza*

　　> affluxus, affluxus, m. 유입, 쇄도　　　　　　　　　　**E** *afflux*

　　> affluentia, affluentiae, f. 유입, 쇄도, 풍요　　　　　**E** *affluence*

> confluo, confluxi, confluxum, confluĕre (< con- (< cum) *with, together*

　　+ fluĕre *to flow*) 합류하다, 모여들다　　　　　　　**E** *confluent*

　　> confluxus, confluxus, m. 합류　　　　　**E** *conflux (confluence)*

　　> confluentia, confluentiae, f. 합류　　　**E** *confluence (conflux)*

> effluo, effluxi, effluxum, effluĕre (< ef- (< ex) *out of, away from* + fluĕre

　　to flow) 흘러 나가다　　　　　　　　　　　　　　　**E** *effluent*

　　> effluxus, effluxus, m. 유출　　　　　　　　　　　　**E** *efflux*

> influo, influxi, influxum, influĕre (< in- *in, on, into, toward* + fluĕre *to*

　　flow) 흘러 들어가다, 물밀듯이 들이닥치다, 젖어 들어가다　　**E** *influent*

　　> influxus, influxus, m. 유입　　　　　　　　　　　　**E** *influx*

　　> influentia, influentiae, f. (점성술) (별의) 감응력; 영향　**E** *influence, influential*

　　　　> It. influenza *influence, epidemic*　**E** *influenza, (influenza >) flu (flue)*

　　　　　　> L. influenza, influenzae, f. 인플루엔자

> profluo, profluxi, profluxum, profluĕre (< pro- *before, forward, for, instead*

　　of + fluĕre *to flow*) 흘러 나오다, 거침없이 나오다　　　**E** *profluent*

> refluo, refluxi, —, refluĕre (< re- *back, again* + fluĕre *to flow*) 역류하다　**E** *refluent*

> superfluo, superfluxi, —, superfluĕre (< super- *above* + fluĕre *to flow*)

　　위로 흐르다, 넘치다

　　> superfluus, superflua, superfluum 넘치는　　　　　**E** *superfluous*

< IE. bhleu- *to swell, to well up, to overflow*　　　　　　　　**E** *bloat*

　> G. phlyein (phlyzein) *to boil over*

　　> G. phlyktaina, phlyktainēs, f. *blister, pustule*

　　　> L. phlyctaena, phlyctaenae, f.

　　　　수포(水疱)　　　　　　　　　　**E** *phlyctena, (pl.) phlyctenae, phlyctenar*

　　　　　> L. phlyctaenula, phlyctaenulae, f. (< + -ula *diminutive*

　　　　　　suffix) 소수포(小水疱)　　　　　**E** *phlyctenule, phlyctenular*

　> (*possibly*) G. phloios, phloiou, m. (< *swelling with growth*) *smooth bark*　**E** *phloem*

> (*possibly*) G. phellos, phellou, m, *cork*　　　　　　　　　　　`E phell(o)-`

< IE. bhel- *to blow, to swell; with derivatives referring to various round objects and to the notion of tumescent masculinity* (Vide FOLLIS: *See* E. *folly*)

frigo, frixi, frictum (frixum), frigĕre 굽다, 튀기다, 볶다, 지지다　　`E fry, frizz, trizzle`

< IE. bher- *to cook, to bake*

fundo, fudi, fusum, fundĕre 물을 붓다, 녹여 넣다　　`E fuse, font (fount) (< 'melting, casting')`

> fusio, fusionis, f. 융합, 융해, 고정술, 유합술(癒合術)　　`E fusion`

> futilis, futile 그릇이 새는, 헛수고의, 경박한　　`E futile`

> futilitas, futilitatis, f. 헛수고, 경박　　`E futility`

> confundo, **confudi**, confusum, confundĕre (< con- (< cum) *with, together* + fundĕre *to pour, to melt*) 함께 부어 넣다, 교란시키다, 혼란시키다, 혼동하다　　`E confuse, confound`

> confusio, confusionis, f. 혼란, 혼동　　`E confusion`

> diffundo, **diffudi**, diffusum, diffundĕre (< dif- (< dis-) *apart from, down, not* + fundĕre *to pour, to melt*) 퍼뜨리다, 발산하다, 확산하다　　`E diffuse`

> diffusio, diffusionis, f. 확산　　`E diffusion`

> effundo, **effudi**, effusum, effundĕre (< ef- (< ex) *out of, away from* + fundĕre *to pour, to melt*) 쏟다, 쏟아 놓다　　`E effuse`

> effusio, effusionis, f. 삼출(滲出), 삼출물, 유출　　`E effusion`

> infundo, **infudi**, infusum, infundĕre (< in- *in, on, into, toward* + fundĕre *to pour, to melt*) 부어 넣다　　`E infuse`

> infusio, infusionis, f. 주입, 유입, 즙　　`E infusion`

> infundibulum, infundibuli, n. 깔때기, 누두(漏斗), 누두상(漏斗狀)의 관(管)　　`E infundibulum, infundibular, funnel`

> interfundo, **interfudi**, interfusum, interfundĕre (< inter- *between, among* + fundĕre *to pour, to melt*) 사이에 붓다, 안에 붓다, 스며들게 하다, 섞이게 하다　　`E interfuse`

> perfundo, **perfudi**, perfusum, perfundĕre (< per- *through, thoroughly* + fundĕre *to pour, to melt*) 끼얹다, 흠뻑 적시다, 관류(灌流)하다　　`E perfuse, perfusate`

> perfusio, perfusionis, f. 물 끼얹음, 물 뿌림, 적심, 관류(灌流)　　`E perfusion, reperfusion; hypoperfusion`

> profundo, **profudi**, profusum, profundĕre (< pro- *before, forward, for, instead of* + fundĕre *to pour, to melt*) 쏟아 내다, 낭비하다, 발산하다　　`E profuse`

> profusio, profusionis, f. 흘림, 낭비　　`E profusion`

> refundo, **refudi**, refusum, refundĕre (< re- *back, again* + fundĕre *to pour, to melt*) 다시 부어 넣다, 거꾸로 부어 넣다, 되돌리다　　`E refund`

> *refuso, *refusavi, *refusatum, *refusare (< refusum (*past participle*)) 거절하다　　`E refuse, refusal`

> suffundo, **suffudi**, suffusum, suffundĕre (< suf- (< sub) *under, up from under* + fundĕre *to pour, to melt*) 아래로 붓다, 쏟아 붓다, 뒤덮다　　`E suffuse`

> suffusio, suffusionis, f. 광범피하출혈, 액체조직확산, 충만, 홍조 **E** *suffusion*

> transfundo, **transfudi**, transfusum, transfundĕre (< trans- *over, across, through,*

beyond + fundĕre *to pour, to melt*) 옮겨 붓다, 쏟다 **E** *transfuse*

> transfusio, transfusionis, f. 수혈(輸血) **E** *transfusion*

< IE. gheu- *to pour, to pour a libation*

E *gut, foregut, midgut, hindgut, catgut (< 'the dried and twisted intestines of sheep, also of the horse and ass; used for the strings of musical instruments; also as bands in lathes, clocks, etc.'), gush, geyser (< 'to gush'), gust (< 'a cold blast of wind'), (perhaps) god (< 'one to whom libations are poured'), (L. semideus >) demigod, goodbye (< 'God be with you!'), gossip (< 'idle talk' < 'familiar acquaintance' < 'godparent'), giddy (< 'possessed by a god'), ((perhaps) by god >) bigot, (bigot >) bigotry*

> G. chein (cheein) *to pour*

> G. chymeia, chymeias, f. *pouring, infusion*

> (*possibly*) (*Arabic*) al-kimiya *alchemy*

> L. alchimia, alchimiae, f. 연금술 **E** *alchemy*

> L. alchimista, alchimistae, m. 연금술사 **E** *alchemist*

> L. chimista, chimistae, m. 연금술사, 화학자,

약사 **E** *chemist, chemistry, biochemistry, chem(o)- (chemi-)*

> L. alchimicus, alchimica, alchimicum 연금술의

> L. chimicus, chimica, chimicum *chemic* **E** *chemical*

> G. chymos, chymou, m. *juice (juice in its raw or natural state), flavor*

> L. chymus, chymi, m. 미즙(糜汁), 유미(乳糜)

E *chyme, chymification, chymotrypsin (< 'a proteolytic enzyme secreted in the pancreatic juice, activated by trypsin')*

> G. ekchymoesthai (< ek- *out of, away from* + chymos) *to extravasate*

blood

> G. ekchymōsis, ekchymōseōs, f. (< + -ōsis *condition*) *ecchymosis*

> L. ecchymosis, ecchymosis, f. 출혈반(出血斑),

출혈얼룩 **E** *ecchymosis, (pl.) ecchymoses, ecchymosed*

> G. chylos, chylou, m. *juice (juice produced by decoction or digestion)*

> L. chylus, chyli, m. 암죽, 유미(乳糜) **E** *chyle, chylous, chylomicron, chylemia*

[용례] cisterna chyli 유미조(乳糜槽), 가슴림프관팽대 **E** *cisterna chyli*

(문법) cisterna 물통, 수조(水槽), 조(槽): 단수 주격

< cisterna, cisternae, f.

chyli 유미의: 단수 속격

> L. chyluria, chyluriae, f. (< G. chylos + ouron *urine* + -ia) 암죽뇨,

쌀뜨물오줌, 유미뇨(乳糜尿) **E** *chyluria*

> G. choanē, choanēs, f. *funnel*

> L. choana, choanae, f. 깔때기, 누두(漏斗); 뒤콧구멍,

후비공(後鼻孔) **E** *choana, (pl.) choanae*

> G. enchein (encheein) (< en- *in*) *to pour in*

> G. enchyma, enchymatos, n. (< + -ma *resultative noun suffix*) *infusion*

> G. parenchyma, parenchymatos, n. (< *something poured in beside*
< par(a)- *beside, along side of, beyond* + enchyma) (*the substance
of the liver, lungs, etc. being anciently supposed to be formed
of blood strained through the blood vessels and coagulated
>) the functional tissue of an organ, as distinguished from
its connective and supporting tissue*

> L. parenchyma, parenchymatis, n. 실질(實質)

E *parenchyma (parenchyme), parenchymal, parenchymatous*

> G. mesenchyma, mesenchymatos, n. (< mesos *middle* + enchyma) *a
loosely organized tissue, chiefly mesodermal in origin, especially
the embryonic tissue which develops into connective and skeletal
tissues, including blood, lymph, and muscles*

> L. mesenchyma, mesenchymatis, n. 중간엽(中間葉)

E *mesenchyma (mesenchyme), mesenchymal, (ectodermal
mesenchyme >) ectomesenchyme*

gero, gessi, gestum, gerĕre 지니다, 행하다, 생기다

> -ger, -gera, -gerum 지니는, 생기는　　　　　　　　　　　　　**E** *-gerous*

> dentiger, dentigera, dentigerum (< dens, dentis, m. *tooth* + -ger *bearing*)
이를 지니는, 이가 생기는　　　　　　　　　　　　　　　**E** *dentigerous*

> spiniger, spinigera, spinigerum (< spina, spinae, f. *spine* + -ger *bearing*)
가시를 지니는, 가시가 생기는, 유극성(有棘性)의　　　　　**E** *spinigerous*

> gestus, gesta, gestum (*past participle*) 지닌, 행한, 생긴

E *(gesta (neuter pl.) 'actions, exploits'>) jest (< 'The original sense was 'heroic deeds',
hence 'a narrative of such deeds'; later the term denoted an idle tale, hence a joke')*

> gestus, gestus, m. 몸짓, 손짓

> gesticulus, gesticuli, m. (< + -culus *diminutive suffix*) 몸짓, 손짓

> gesticulor, gesticulatus sum, gesticulari 몸짓하다, 손짓하다　**E** *gesticulate*

> gestura, gesturae, f. 몸짓, 동작　　　　　　　　　　　　　　**E** *gesture*

> gerundium, gerundii, n. 동명사, 동사적 중성명사　　　　　　**E** *gerund*

> gerundivum, gerundivi, n. 수동태 미래분사, 수동태 당위분사, 동사적 형용사　**E** *gerundive*

> gesto, gestavi, gestatum, gestare (< gest- *to bear* + -are) 지니고 있다, 짊어지다,
잉태하다　　　　　　　　　　　　　　　　　　　　　　　　**E** *gestate*

> gestatio, gestationis, f. 운반, 나르기, 임신(姙娠)

E *gestation, gestational, progestational, progestogen(s) (progestin(s)), (progestin +
luteosterone >) progesterone*

> aggero, aggessi, aggestum, aggerĕre (< ag- (< ad) *to, toward, at, according to* +
gerĕre *to bear*) 가져오다, 날라 오다, 날라다 쌓다, 쌓아 올리다

> agger, aggeris, m. 쌓아 올린 것, 더미, 퇴적, 둑

> aggero, aggeravi, aggeratum, aggerare 쌓아 올리다, 크게 만들다

> exaggero, **exaggeravi**, exaggeratum, exaggerare (< ex- *out of,*
away from; intensive + aggerare *to heap up*) 쌓아 올리다, 크게
만들다, 과장하다 　　　　　　　　　　　　　　　　　E *exaggerate*

> congero, **congessi**, congestum, congerĕre (< con- *with, together* + gerĕre *to bear*)
쌓다, 집합시키다 　　　　　　　　　E *congest, congestive, congeries, decongestant*

> congestio, congestionis, f. 밀집, 정체, 울혈(鬱血) 　　　　　E *congestion*

> digero, **digessi**, digestum, digerĕre (< di- (< dis-) *apart from, down, not* + gerĕre
to bear) 분산(分散)시키다, 소화(消化)시키다 　　　　　　E *digest, digestive*

> digestio, digestionis, f. 소화 　　　　　　　　　　　　E *digestion*

> indigestio, indigestionis, f. (< in- *not*) 소화장애, 소화불량 　E *indigestion*

> ingero, **ingessi**, ingestum, ingerĕre (< in- *in, on, into, toward* + gerĕre *to bear*)
안에 지니다, 섭취하다 　　　　　　　　　　　　　　　E *ingest, ingestive*

> ingestio, ingestionis, f. 섭취 　　　　　　　　　　　　E *ingestion*

> regero, **regessi**, regestum, regerĕre (< re- *back, again* + gerĕre *to bear*) 다시 나르다,
쌓다, 모아서 기록하다, 등록하다

> regesta, regestorum, n. (pl.) (< (*past participle*) *things recorded*) 목록

> registrum, registri, n. 등록, 등록부 　　　　E *register, registry, registration*

> suggero, **suggessi**, suggestum, suggerĕre (< sub- *under, up from under* + gerĕre
to bear) 밑으로 가져다주다, 제안하다 　　　　　　　E *suggest, suggestive*

> suggestio, suggestionis, f. 제안, 암시, 시사 　　　　　E *suggestion*

gigno, genui, genitum, gignĕre (타동사) (~을) 낳다, 출산하다 　　E *benign, malign*

> genitus, genita, genitum (*past participle*) 태어난 　　E *gingerly* (< '*well-born*')

> congenitus, congenita, congenitum (< con- (< cum) *with, together* +
genitus *born*) 같은 배에서 태어난; 타고난, 선천적인 　　E *congenital*

> genitalis, genitale 출산의, 생식의,
생식기관의 　　　　　E *genital*, (*neuter* pl.) *genitalia, genito-, genitourinary*

> genitivus, genitiva, genitivum (genetivus, genetiva, genetivum) 낳는, 타고난;
(문법) 속격(屬格)의 (< casus genitivus *genitive case, case of origin* <
mistranslation of G. genikē ptōsis *generic case, case of relation*) 　E *genitive*

> indigenus, indigena, indigenum (< (*Old Latin*) indu *in* + gignĕre *to beget*)
토착의, 토박이의, 고유한 　　　　　　　　　　　E *indigene, indigenous*

> ingenium, ingenii, n. (< in- *in, on, into, toward* + gignĕre *to beget*) 성품,
재능 　　　　　　　　　　　　　　　　　　　　E *engine*

> ingeniosus, ingeniosa, ingeniosum 타고난 재능을 지닌,
정교하게 만들어진 　　　　　　　　　　　　　E *ingenious*

> ingigno, **ingenui**, ingenitum, ingignĕre (< in- *in, on, into, toward* + gignĕre
to beget) 가지고 태어나게 하다, 천부적으로 가지게 하다

> ingenuus, ingenua, ingenuum 토착의, 토박이의, 타고난, 소박한 　E *ingenuous*

> ingenuitas, ingenuitatis, f. 타고난 품성, 소박, 재간 　　　E *ingenuity*

> progigno, **progenui**, progenitum, progignĕre (< pro- *before, forward, for,*

instead of + gignĕre *to beget*) 생기게 하다, 발생시키다

> progenitor, progenitoris, m. 선조　　　　　　　　　　　**E** *progenitor*

> progenies, progeniei, f. 가계, 후예　　　　　　　　　　**E** *progeny*

∽ genuinus, genuina, genuinum 타고난, 혈통이 순수한, 진짜의　　**E** *genuine*

∽ (*archaic*) geno, –, –, genĕre (타동사) (~을) 낳다, 출산하다

> gens, gentis, f. 씨족, 종족, 민족

> gentilis, gentile 씨족의, 같은 씨족에 속한, 동포의; (로마인 편에서) 이민족의,
（그리스도교인의 편에서) 이교도 민족의

> **E** *gentle, genteel, gentry, (gentry >) gentrify, gentrification, jaunty, gentility; gentile*

< IE. genǝ-, gen- *to give birth, to beget; with derivatives referring to aspects and results of procreation and to familial and tribal groups*

> **E** *kin, (of kin >) akin, kindred (< kin + -red 'condition'), kinship (< kin + -ship 'state, condition'), kind, king (< 'head of a kin or son of noble kin'), kingdom, (King Herla 'a mythical figure sometimes identified with Woden' > 'the leader of a legendary troop of demon horsemen' >) harlequin*

> L. nascor, natus sum, nasci (자동사) 태어나다, 출생하다,
생기다　　　　　**E** *(F. (past participle) 'born' >) nee, (F. puine 'born after' >) puny*

[용례] pro re nata (p.r.n.) 생겨난 일을 위하여 > 필요에 따라　　**E** *p.r.n.*
(문법) pro 위하여: 전치사, 탈격지배
re 일: 단수 탈격 < res, rei, f.
nata 생긴: 과거분사, 여성형 단수 탈격
< natus, nata, natum

> L. nascens, (gen.) nascentis (*present participle*) 출생하는, 돋아나는, 발생하는　**E** *nascent*
> L. nascentia, nascentiae, f. 탄생　　　　　　**E** *Renaissance*

> L. natus, natus, m. (식물) 싹틈, (사람) 나이

> L. natus, nati, m. 자식, 아들
> L. natalis, natale 출생의, 출생과
관계되는　　　　**E** *natal, Noel, prenatal (antenatal), postnatal; perinatal*
> L. neonatus, neonati, m. (< G. neos *new* + L. natus *a born*)
신생아　　　　　　　　　　　　**E** *neonate, neonatal*

[용례] icterus neonatorum 신생아황달(新生兒黃疸)　　**E** *icterus neonatorum*
(문법) icterus 황달: 단수 주격
< icterus, icteri, m.
< G. ikteros, ikterou, m. *jaundice*
neonatorum 신생아들의: 복수 속격

> L. nativus, nativa, nativum 태어난 그대로의, 천부(天賦)의,
토박이의　　　　　　　　　**E** *native, naive, (naive >) naivety*
> L. nativitas, nativitatis, f. 출생, 탄생　　　　**E** *nativity*

> L. natura, naturae, f. 태어남, 태어난 그대로의 상태, 천성,
자연　　　　　　　　　　　　**E** *nature, denature, renature*

> L. naturalis, naturale 자연의,

자연적   **E** *natural, naturalize, unnatural, preternatural, supernatural*

> L. natio, nationis, f. 출생, 민족, 국민

E *nation, (nation >) national, (national >) nationality, (national >) international*

> L. connascor, connatus sum, connasci (< con- (< cum) *with, together* + nasci
to be born) (자동사) 타고나다, 동시에 발생하다   **E** *connate*

> L. innascor, innatus sum, innasci (< in- *in, on, into, toward* + nasci *to be born*)
(자동사) 타고나다   **E** *innate*

> L. gnascor, gnatus sum, gnasci (*archaic of* nasci) (자동사) 태어나다, 출생하다

> L. agnascor, agnatus sum, agnasci (< a- (< ad) *to, toward, at, according to*
+ gnasci *to be born*) 덧붙어 나다

> agnatus, agnata, agnatum 덧붙어 난, 부계(父系)의   **E** *agnate*

> L. cognatus, cognata, cognatum (< co- (< cum) *with, together* + gnatus *born*)
조상이 같은, 동족(同族)의, 동계(同系)의   **E** *cognate*

> L. praegnans, (gen.) praegnantis (praegnas, (gen.) praegnatis) (< prae- *before,
beyond* + gnasci *to be born*) 태어나기 전의 >
임신(姙娠)한   **E** *pregnant, (pregnant >) pregnancy*

> L. praegnatus, praegnata, praegnatum (< prae- *before, beyond* + gnasci *to
be born*) 태어나기 전의 > 임신한

> L. impraegno, impraegnavi, impraegnatum, impraegnare (< im- (< in)
in, on, into, toward) 임신시키다, 수정(受精)시키다, 수태(受胎)시키다, 충만
시키다, 스며들게 하다, (사상·감정 등을) 주입하다   **E** *impregnate, impregnation*

> L. genus, generis, n. 혈통, 족속, 종류,

속(屬)   **E** *genus, (pl.) genera, generic, gender, genre, miscegenation*

> L. generalis, generale 종족의, 전체적인, 일반적인   **E** *general, generalize*

> L. generalitas, generalitatis, f. 일반성, 보편성   **E** *generality*

> L. generosus, generosa, generosum 귀족 출신의, 고결한, 관대한   **E** *generous*

> L. generositas, generositatis, f. 귀족 출신, 고결, 관대   **E** *generosity*

> L. genero, generavi, generatum, generare 낳다, 만들어내다   **E** *generate, generative*

> L. generatio, generationis, f. 생식, 세대(世代, *generally considered to
be about thirty years, in which children grow up, become adults,
and have children of their own*), 생성, 발생   **E** *generation*

> L. degenero, degeneravi, degeneratum, degenerare (< de- *apart from,
down, not* + generare *to beget, to produce*) 타락하다, 퇴화하다, 변성
되다, 퇴행하다   **E** *degenerate, degenerative, (degenerate >) degeneracy*

> L. degeneratio, degenerationis, f. 변성, 퇴행   **E** *degeneration*

> L. regenero, regeneravi, regeneratum, regenerare (< re- *back, again*
+ generare *to beget, to produce*) 재생하다   **E** *regenerate, regenerative*

> L. regeneratio, regenerationis, f. 재생   **E** *regeneration*

> L. (*possibly*) naevus, naevi, m. 몸의 반점, 모반(母斑),
오점   **E** *naevus (nevus), (pl.) naevi (nevi); nevoid*

> L. Genius, Genii, m. (로마 신화) (사람·가족·출생·장소·조직의) 수호신; (genius) 재능, 천재, (고장의) 기풍　　E *genius, (pl.) geniuses; genie, (pl.) genii (genies)*

> > L. genialis, geniale (수호신의 보호를 받아) 온화한　　E *genial, (genial >) congenial*

> L. germen, germinis, n. 종자(種子), 싹[芽], 배아(胚芽), 미생물　　E *germ*

> > L. germinalis, germinale 종자(種子)의, 배아(胚芽)의　　E *germinal*

> > L. germino, germinavi, germinatum, germinare 싹트다, 나게 하다, 낳다　　E *germinate*

> > > L. germinatio, germinationis, f. 발아(發芽)　　E *germination*

> > > L. germinativus, germinativa, germinativum 움트는, 발아성(發芽性)의　E *germinative*

∽ L. germanus, germana, germanum 같은 부모에게서 태어난, 밀접한 관계가 있는　　E *german (germane)*

> > G. gen- (*root*) *to give birth, to beget*

E (D. Pangen > D. Gen >) *gene, genotype, genotoxic, oncogene, -genic, polygenic, transgenic;* (D. Gen + D. Chromosom >) *genome, genomic, genomics; eugenics*

> > G. -geneia, -geneias, f. *producing*　　E *-geny, ontogeny, phylogeny*

> > G. -genēs, -genēs, -genes *born, produced, of a specified kind; producing, inducing*

E *-gen, oxygen (O), hydrogen (H), nitrogen (N), halogen(s), carcinogen(s),* (antibody >) *antigen(s), -genic, carcinogenic, antigenic, neurogenic, psychogenic, iatrogenic, -genicity, carcinogenicity, antigenicity; -genous, (* endogen >) *endogenous, (* exogen >) *exogenous; -geneous; anagen, catagen, telogen*

> > > G. autogenēs, autogenēs, autogenes (< autos *self*) *self-produced, independent*　　E *autogenous*

> > > G. homogenēs, homogenēs, homogenes (< homos *of the same*) *of the same kind*

> > > > L. homogeneus, homogenea, homogeneum 같은 종류의, 동종의, 동질의, 균질의, 균일한

E *homogeneous, homogeneity, homogenize, homogenate, inhomogeneous, inhomogeneity*

> > > G. heterogenēs, heterogenēs, heterogenes (< heteros *different*) *of different kind*

> > > > L. heterogeneus, heterogenea, heterogeneum 다른 종류의, 이종의, 이질의, 불균질의, 불균일한　　E *heterogeneous, heterogeneity*

> > L. -genus, -gena, -genum 태어난, 만들어진, 종류의; 만드는, 일으키는

> > G. gennan (gennaein) *to beget*

> > G. gignesthai (ginesthai) *to be born, to become*

> > > G. genesis, geneseōs, f. *birth, origin, creation, generation*

> > > > L. genesis, genesis, f. 탄생, 생성, 발생, 형성; (Genesis) 창세기

E *genesis, -genesis, androgenesis (< 'reproduction from an ovum that contains only paternal chromosomes'), parthenogenesis (< 'reproduction from an ovum without fertilization, as naturally occurs in some plants and animals'), carcinogenesis, oncogenesis*

> > > > > L. pangenesis, pangenesis, f. (< G. pan- *all*) 범생설(凡生說)　　E *pangenesis*

> L. epigenesis, epigenesis, f. (< *the additament of parts budding one out of another* < G. epi– *upon*) 후생설(後生說)

> **E** *epigenesis, (epigenesis > 'altering the activity of genes without changing their structure' >) epigenetic*

> L. pathogenesis, pathogenesis, f. (< G. pathos, pathous, n. *suffering, emotion, feelings, passion*) 발병기전(發病機轉), 발병론(發病論)　　**E** *pathogenesis, (pathogenesis >) pathogen*

> L. agenesis, agenesis, f. (< G. a– *not*) 무발생(無發生)　**E** *agenesis*

> L. dysgenesis, dysgenesis, f. (< G. dys– *bad*) 발생장애(發生障碍)　　　　　　　　　　　　　　**E** *dysgenesis*

> G. genetikos, genetikē, genetikon *genetic*

> L. geneticus, genetica, geneticum 발생의, 기원의; 유전의, 유전자의　　　　　　**E** *genetic, genetics, -genetic*

> G. gonē, gonēs, f. ((*ancient Greek*) gonos) *begetting, birth, origin; offspring, seed*

> **E** *gonorrhoea (gonorrhea) (<'supposed to be a discharge of semen'), (gonorrhoea >) gonococcus*

> G. –gonia, –gonias, f. *begetting*

> **E** *-gony, gametogony (< 'gametogenesis; reproduction by gameto-genesis'), sporogony (<'sporulation, reproduction by sporulation'), merogony (schizogony) (<'reproduction by splitting'), schizogony (merogony)*

> G. theogonia, theogonias, f. (< G. theos *god*) *birth of gods*

> L. theogonia, theogoniae, f. 신들의 계보　　**E** *theogony*

> G. gonimos, gonimos, gonimon *productive, fertile, vigorous*

> L. Metagonimus, Metagonimi, m. (< G. met(a)– *between, along with, across, after*) (흡충) 메타고니무스속(屬)　　**E** Metagonimus, *metagonimiasis*

> L. Paragonimus, Paragonimi, m. (< G. par(a)– *beside, along side of, beyond*) (흡충) 폐흡충속(屬)　　**E** Paragonimus, *paragonimiasis*

> L. gonas, gonadis, f. 생식샘

> **E** *gonad, gonadal, gonadotropin(s), gonadotrope, gonadocorticoid(s)*

> L. gonium, gonii, n. 생식원세포(生殖原細胞)　　**E** *gonium,* (pl.) *gonia*

> L. oogonium, oogonii, n. (< G. ōion *egg*) 난조세포(卵祖細胞), 난원세포(卵原細胞)　　　　**E** *oogonium,* (pl.) *oogonia*

> L. spermatogonium, spermatogonii, n. (< G. sperma, spermatos, n. *seed*) 정조세포(精祖細胞), 정원세포(精原細胞)　　**E** *spermatogonium,* (pl.) *spermatogonia*

> G. genos, genous, n. (genea, geneas, f.) *birth, descent, family, kindred, race; sex, gender*

> **E** *syngeneic (< 'together'), allogeneic (< 'other'), xenogeneic (< 'foreign'); genocide*

> G. genlkos, genikē, genikon *general, generic*

> G. genealogia, genealogias, f. (< + -logia *study*) *tracing of descent*

> L. genealogia, genealogiae, f. 가계, 족보, 계보, 계보학   `E` *genealogy*

†hendo, †hendi, †hensum, †hendĕre 쥐다

> prehendo, **prehendi**, prehensum, prehendĕre (prendo, **prendi**, prensum, prendĕre)

(< prae- *before, beyond* + †hendĕre *to grasp*) 부여잡다, 체포하다, 파악하다

`E` *prehensile, pregnable, impregnable,* (super *'above'* + prehendĕre *'to seize'* >) *'unexpected seizure of a place, unexpected attack on troops'* >) *surprise,* (inter- *'between, among'* + prehendĕre *'to seize'* > *'something undertaken'* >) *enterprise,* (inter- *'between, among'* + prehendĕre *'to seize'* > *'one who undertakes'* >) *entrepreneur*

> prehensio, prehensionis, f. (prensio, prensionis, f.) 잡기, 체포, 파악 `E` *prehension, prison*

> apprehendo, **apprehendi**, apprehensum, apprehendĕre (< ap- (< ad) *to, toward, at, according to* + prehendĕre *to seize*) 붙잡다, 차지하다, 파악하다

`E` *apprehend, apprentice* (< *'of learning'*)

> comprehendo, **comprehendi**, comprehensum, comprehendĕre (< com- (< cum) *with, together* + prehendĕre *to seize*) 붙잡다, 체포하다, 파악하다, 총괄하다, 포괄하다   `E` *comprehend, comprise (comprize), comprehensive, comprehensible*

> reprehendo, **reprehendi**, reprehensum, reprehendĕre (< re- *back, again* + prehendĕre *to seize*) 붙들다, 제지하다, 꾸짖다, 비난하다

`E` *reprehend, reprise* (< *'to take back'*), *reprieve* (< *'to take back'*), *reprehensible*

> (*perhaps*) hedera, hederae, f. (식물) 담쟁이   `E` *hederaceous*

< IE. ghend-, ghed- *to seize, to take*   `E` *get, beget, forget, guess* (< *'to try to get'*)

> L. praeda, praedae, f. 습득물, 노획물, 포획물   `E` *prey*

> L. praedor, praedatus sum, praedari 노획하다, 포획하다, 약탈하다

> L. praedator, praedatoris, m. 노획자, 약탈자, 사냥꾼, 탐욕자   `E` *predator*

> L. depraedor, depraedatus sum, depraedari (< de- *apart from, down, not; intensive*) 약탈하다, 모조리 휩쓸어가다   `E` *depredate*

ico (icio), ici, ictum, icĕre 치다, 찌르다, 쏘다, 강타하다

> ictus, ictus, m. 침, 찌름, 쏨, 일격, 발작(發作)   `E` *ictus, ictal, preictal*

[용례] ictus solis (< *sun stroke*) 일사병(日射病)

ictus epilepticus (< *epileptic seizure*) 뇌전증발작

(문법) ictus 발작: 단수 주격

solis 태양의: 단수 속격 < sol, solis, m.

epilepticus 뇌전증의: 형용사, 남성형 단수 주격

< epilepticus, epileptica, epilepticum

jungo, junxi, junctum, jungĕre (*root* jug-) (마소에게) 멍에를 메우다, 잇다   `E` *join,* (junctus (*past participle*) *'yoked'* >) *joint*

> jugum, jugi, n. 멍에, 포도넌출을 얹어 잡아매는 가로장, 천칭대

> jugulum, juguli, n. (< + -ulum *diminutive suffix*) 쇄골; (쇄골 >) 멱, 목

> jugularis, jugulare 목의   **E** *jugular*

> conjux, conjugis, m., f. (conjunx, conjungis, m., f.) (< con- (< cum) *with,*
together) 배우자, 같은 처지에 있는 동료   **E** *conjugal*

> conjugo, **conjugavi**, conjugatum, conjugare (< con- (< cum) *with, together*)
하나로 묶다, 결합하다, 접합하다;
동사변화를 하다   **E** *conjugate, conjugated, unconjugated, (conjugate >) conjugacy*

> conjugatio, conjugationis, f. 결합, 접합; 동사변화   **E** *conjugation*

> junctio, junctionis, f. 이음, 연결   **E** *junction, junctional*

> junctura, juncturae, f. 이음매, 관절   **E** *juncture*

> adjungo, **adjunxi**, adjunctum, adjungĕre (< ad- *to, toward, at, according to* +
jungĕre *to yoke*) 짝지어 놓다, 인접해 놓다   **E** *adjoin, adjoint, adjunct, adjunction*

> conjungo, **conjunxi**, conjunctum, conjungĕre (< con- (< cum) *with, together* +
jungĕre *to yoke*) 짝지어 멍에 메우다, 연결시키다,
잇다   **E** *conjoin, conjoint, conjunct, conjunction*

> conjunctivus, conjunctiva, conjunctivum 연결시키는, 잇는, 접속어의   **E** *conjunctive*

[용례] tunica conjunctiva (< *conjoining the eyeball with the eyelid*)
결막(結膜), 이음막   **E** *conjunctiva, conjunctival*
(문법) tunica 막: 단수 주격 < tunica, tunicae, f. 층, 막
conjunctiva: 형용사, 여성형 단수 주격

> disjungo, **disjunxi**, disjunctum, disjungĕre (< dis- *apart from, down, not* + jungĕre
to yoke) 떼어 놓다, 분리시키다   **E** *disjoin, disjoint, disjunct, disjunction, nondisjunction*

> injungo, **injunxi**, injunctum, injungĕre (< in- *in, on, into, toward* + jungĕre *to yoke*)
박아넣다, 부과하다, (하도록) 명하다   **E** *enjoin, injunct, injunction*

> subjungo, **subjunxi**, subjunctum, subjungĕre (< sub- *under, up from under* + jungĕre
to yoke) 밑에 매다, 덧붙이다, 추가하다   **E** *subjoin, subjoint, subjunction*

> subjunctivus, subjunctiva, subjunctivum 덧붙이는, 접속(接續)시키는

[용례] modus subjunctivus (< *so named because it was regarded as
specially appropriate to 'subjoined' or subordinate clauses*
< G. hypotaktikē enklisis) 접속법, 가정법   **E** *subjunctive (mood)*
(문법) modus 절도, 양식, 척도, 기준: 단수 주격 < modus, modi, m.
subjunctivus: 형용사, 남성형 단수 주격

< IE. yeug- *to yoke*   **E** *yoke*

> L. juxta (전치사, 대격지배) 바로 곁에

E *juxta-, juxtapose, juxtaposit, juxtaposition, juxtaglomerular, juxtamedullary,
juxtanuclear, jostle*

> L. adjuxto, **adjuxtavi**, adjuxtatum, adjuxtare (< ad- *to, toward, at, according
to* + juxta- *near to*) ~을 ~에 맞추다, 적응하다, 조절하다, 조정하다   **E** *adjust*

> G. zygon, zygou, n. *yoke, crossbar, pair*

E *zyg(o)-, zygotene, zygospore, zygomorphic* (< 'applied to a flower that is symmetrical about a single plane, i.e. divisible into similar lateral halves in only one way, monosymmetrical; opposed to actinomorphous')

> L. zygon, zygi, n. 자이곤 (*the bar or stem connecting the two branches of a zygal fissure*)

E *zygon, zygal*

> G. zygoun (zygoein) *to yoke*

   > G. zygōsis, zygōseōs, f. (< + -ōsis *condition*) *zygosis*

      > L. zygosis, zygosis, f. 접합(接合), 접합자형성(接合子形成)

E *zygosis, (zygosis >) zygosity, homozygosity* (< 'the state of homozygote'), *heterozygosity* (< 'the state of heterozygote')

   > G. zygōma, zygōmatos, n. (< + -ōma *resultative noun suffix*) *zygoma*

      > L. zygoma, zygomatis, n. 광대뼈, 광대활

E *zygoma*

         > L. zygomaticus, zygomatica, zygomaticum 광대뼈의, 광대활의

E *zygomatic*

   > G. zygōtos, zygōtē, zygōton *yoked*

E *zygote* (< 'the cell resulting from union of a male and a female gamete (sperm and ovum)'), *homozygote* (< 'a diploid individual that has a pair of identical alleles'), *heterozygote* (< 'a diploid individual that has a pair of different alleles'), *zygotic, monozygotic* (< 'from one zygote, as identical twins'), *dizygotic* (< 'from two separate zygotes, as fraternal twins')

  > G. zeugnynai *to yoke*

    > G. zeugma, zeugmatos, n. *yoking*

E *zeugma*

    > G. azygos, azygos, azygon (< a- *not*) *unyoked, not paired*

E *azygos (azygous), azygospore*

    > G. syzygos, syzygos, syzygon (< sy- (< syn) *with, together*) *yoked, paired*

       > G. syzygia, syzygias, f. (< -ia *noun suffix*) *yoke, pair, conjunction, copulation*

         > L. syzygia, syzygiae, f. (천문) 합(合), 삭망; (생물) 연접(連接)

E *syzygy*

> (*Sanskrit*) yogah *union*

E *yoga* (< (Hindu) 'union with the Supreme Spirit')

laedo, laesi, laesum, laedĕre 치다, 상하게 하다

  > laesio, laesionis, f. 상해, 병변, 병소(病巢), 병터

E *lesion, intralesional*

  > collido, **collisi**, collisum, collidĕre (< col- (< cum) *with, together* + laedĕre *to strike, to injure*) 충돌하다

E *collide*

    > collisio, collisionis, f. 충돌

E *collision*

 > elido, **elisi**, elisum, elidĕre (< e- *out of, away from* + laedĕre *to strike, to injure*) 처내다, 때려 내쫓다, 깨부수다

E *elide*

    > elisio, elisionis, f. 짜냄; (문법) 모음탈락

E *elision*

linquo, liqui, lictum, linquĕre (남겨 두고) 떠나다, 포기하다, 버리다

> delinquo, **deliqui**, delictum, delinquĕre (< *to leave undone* < de- *apart from, down, not* + linquĕre *to leave*) 불이행하다, 태만히 하다, 잘못하다　　**E** *delinquent*

> relinquo, **reliqui**, relictum, relinquĕre (< re- *back, again; intensive* + linquĕre *to leave*) (남겨 두고) 떠나다, 포기하다, 버리다　　**E** *relinquish, relict, derelict*

　　> reliquiae, reliquiarum, f. (pl.) 남은 것, 유물, 유적　　**E** *relic*

< IE. leik^w- *to leave*　　**E** *loan, lend, eleven* (< 'one left (beyond ten)'), **twelve** (< 'two left (beyond ten)')

> G. leipein *to leave*

　　> G. ekleipein (< ek- *out of, away from* + leipein) *to leave out, to forsake its accustomed place, to fail to appear*

　　　　> G. ekleipsis, ekleipseōs, f. *forsaking, disappearing, loss, eclipse*

　　　　　　> L. eclipsis, eclipsis, f. 생략법;

　　　　　　　　식(蝕: 일식 · 월식)　　**E** *eclipsis, eclipse, ecliptic (ecliptical)*

　　> G. elleipein (< en- *in* + leipein) *to come short, to leave undone*

　　　　> G. elleipsis, elleipseōs, f. *deficiency*

　　　　　　> L. ellipsis, ellipsis, f. 생략법

　　　　　　　　E *ellipsis, ellipse* (< 'the inclination of the cutting plane to the base comes short of the inclination of the side of the cone'), **elliptic** (elliptical), **ellipsoid**

ludo, **lusi**, lusum, ludĕre 놀다, 놀이하다, 유희하다

> ludens, (gen.) ludentis (*present participle*) 노는, 놀이하는　　**E** Homo ludens (< 'playing man')

> lusus, lusus, m. 놀이, 장난, 유희

　　[용례] lusus naturae 자연의 장난, 조화의 장난, 기형
　　　　(문법) lusus: 단수 주격
　　　　　　naturae 자연의: 단수 속격 < natura, naturae, f.

> ludicrum, ludicri, n. 희극　　**E** *ludicrous*

> praeludium, praeludii, n. (< prae- *before, beyond*) 서막, 전주, 서곡　　**E** *prelude*

> interludium, interludii, n. (< inter- *between, among*) 막간극, 간주곡　　**E** *interlude*

> alludo, **allusi**, allusum, alludĕre (< al- (< ad) *to, toward, at, according to* + ludĕre *to play*) 장난치다, 스스럼없이 접근하다, 넌지시 말하다　　**E** *allude*

　　> allusio, allusionis, f. 장난스러운 접근, (간접적) 언급, 암시; (수사) 인유(引喩)　　**E** *allusion*

> colludo, **collusi**, collusum, colludĕre (< col- (< cum) *with, together* + ludĕre *to play*) 함께 놀다, 공모하다, 결탁하다　　**E** *collude*

> deludo, **delusi**, delusum, deludĕre (< de- *apart from, down, not* + ludĕre *to play*) 우롱하다, 기만하다　　**E** *delude, delusive*

　　> delusio, delusionis, f. 우롱, 기만, 망상(妄想)　　**E** *delusion*

> eludo, **elusi**, elusum, eludĕre (< e- *out of, away from* + ludĕre *to play*) 놀기를 마치다; 속이다　　**E** *elude, elusive*

> illudo, **illusi**, illusum, illudĕre (< il- (< in) *in, on, into, toward* + ludĕre *to play*) 가지고 놀다　　**E** *illude, illusive, illusory*

　　> illusio, illusionis, f. 반어(反語), 빈정됨, 속음, 착각　　**E** *illusion, (illusion >) disillusion*

mergo, mersi, mersum, mergĕre 잠기다, 잠그다, 합병하다   `E merge`

> emergo, **emersi**, emersum, emergĕre (< e- *out of, away from* + mergĕre *to plunge*)
수면 위로 나타나다, 나타나다, 불쑥 일어나다   `E emerge`

>> emersio, emersionis, .f. 출현, 재현   `E emersion`

>> emergentia, emergentiae, f. 출현, 발생; (곤충) 우화(羽化); 긴급,
응급   `E emergence; emergency`

> immergo, **immersi**, immersum, immergĕre (< im- (< in) *in, on, into, toward* + mergĕre
to plunge) 물에 잠그다, 액체에 담그다, 몰두시키다   `E immerge (immerse)`

>> immersio, immersionis, .f. 잠금, 담금, 몰두   `E immersion`

> submergo, **submersi**, submersum, submergĕre (< sub- *under, up from under* +
mergĕre *to plunge*) 물 속에 가라앉히다, 은폐하다   `E submerge (submerse)`

mitto, misi, missum, mittĕre 보내다,
던지다   `E (missum (past participle) 'something put on the table'>) mess, messmate`

> missio, missionis, f. 파견, 사명   `E mission`

> missilis, missile 던질 만한, 발사되는   `E missile`

> missaticum, missatici, n. 전갈   `E message, messenger`

> admitto, **admisi**, admissum, admittĕre (< ad- *to, toward, at, according to* + mittĕre
to send) 접근시키다, 들여놓다, 인정하다   `E admit, admission`

> committo, **commisi**, commissum, committĕre (< com- (< cum) *with, together* + mittĕre
to send) 잇다, 겨루게 하다, 저지르다, 내맡기다   `E commit, committee, commission`

>> commissura, commissurae, f. 교련(交聯), 연합(聯合), 맞교차,
경계   `E commissure, commissural, intercommissural`

> demitto, **demisi**, demissum, demittĕre (< de- *apart from, down, not* + mittĕre *to
send*) 내려 보내다   `E demise, demit, demission`

> dimitto, **dimisi**, dimissum, dimittĕre (< di- (< dis-) *apart from, down, not* + mittĕre
to send) 해산시키다, 면직시키다   `E dismiss, dismissal`

> emitto, **emisi**, emissum, emittĕre (< e- *out of, away from* + mittĕre *to send*) 내
보내다, 파견하다, 내쏟다, 방출하다, 방사하다   `E emit`

>> emissio, emissionis, f. 내보냄, 방출, 방사   `E emission`

>> emissarius, emissaria, emissarium 내보내는, 도출(導出)하는   `E emissary`

> intermitto, **intermisi**, intermissum, intermittĕre (< inter- *between, among* + mittĕre
to send) 사이에 집어넣다, 간격을 두다, 잠시 중단하다   `E intermit, intermittent, intermission`

> intromitto, **intromisi**, intromissum, intromittĕre (< intro- *into, within* + mittĕre *to
send*) 들여보내다, 삽입시키다   `E intromit, intromittent, intromission`

> omitto, **omisi**, omissum, omittĕre (< o- (< ob) *before, toward(s), over, against, away;
reversely, inversely* + mittĕre *to send*) 놓아 보내다, 내버리다, 빠뜨리다,
생략하다   `E omit, omission`

> permitto, **permisi**, permissum, permittĕre (< per- *through, thoroughly* + mittĕre
to send) 드나들게 하다, 허락하다   `E permit, permission, permissive`

> praemitto, praemisi, praemissum, praemittĕre (< prae- *before, beyond* + mittĕre *to send*) 먼저 보내다   **E** (praemissa propositio *'proposition set in front'* >) *premise*

> praetermitto, praetermisi, praetermissum, praetermittĕre (< praeter- *past, beyond* + mittĕre *to send*) 지나가게 하다, 소홀히 하다, 간과하다   **E** *pretermit, pretermission*

> promitto, promisi, promissum, promittĕre (< pro- *before, forward, for, instead of* + mittĕre *to send*) 뻗어 나가게 하다, 기대하게 하다, 약속하다   **E** (promissum (*neuter past participle*) *'thing promised'* >) *promise*

     > compromitto, compromisi, compromissum, compromittĕre (< con- (< cum) *with, together* + promittĕre *to promise*) 타협하다, 중재자의 결정에 맡기도록 서로 합의하다, 약속으로 꼼짝 못하게 하다, 위태롭게 하다   **E** *compromise, immunocompromised*

> remitto, remisi, remissum, remittĕre (< re- *back, again* + mittĕre *to send*) 돌려 보내다, 사면하다, 늦추다, 완화하다   **E** *remit, remittent, (remit >) remittance*

     > remissio, remissionis, f. 사면, 완화, 관해(寬解)   **E** *remission*

> submitto, submisi, submissum, submittĕre (< sub- *under, up from under* + mittĕre *to send*) 복종시키다, 대리로 보내다, 제출하다   **E** *submit, submission, submissive*

> supermitto, supermisi, supermissum, supermittĕre (< super- *above* + mittĕre *to send*) 위에 놓다, 추측하다   **E** *surmise*

> transmitto, transmisi, transmissum, transmittĕre (< trans- *over, across, through, beyond* + mittĕre *to send*) 옮기다, 전달하다   **E** *transmit, transmitter, transmissible*

     > transmissio, transmissionis, f. 전달, 투과, 전파, 유전(遺傳)   **E** *transmission*

necto, nexui (nexi), nexum, nectĕre 매다   **E** *fibronectin*

> nexus, nexus, m. 붙들어 맴, 결합; 교통반점(交通斑點)   **E** *nexus, (pl.) nexus, nexin*

> adnecto, adnexui, adnexum, adnectĕre (< ad- *to, toward, at, according to* + nectĕre *to bind, to tie*) 덧붙이다

     > adnexa, adnexorum, n. (pl.) (< adnexum (*neuter past participle*) *binded to*) 부속기(附屬器), 부속기관(附屬器官)   **E** (pl.) *adnexa, adnexal*

> annecto, annexui, annexum, annectĕre (< an- (< ad) *to, toward, at, according to* + nectĕre *to bind, to tie*) 덧붙이다   **E** *annex*

> connecto, connexui, connexum, connectĕre (< con- (< cum) *with, together* + nectĕre *to bind, to tie*) 연결하다, 결합하다

     E *connect, connexion (connection); connexin (< 'gap junction protein'), connexon (< 'assembly of 6 connexins')*

     > connectivus, connectiva, connectivum 연결하는, 결합하는, 연계(連繫)의   **E** *connective*

< IE. ned- *to bind, to tie*   **E** *net, network, nettle (< 'a source of fiber'), (internet + citizen >) netizen*

   > L. nodus, nodi, m. 매듭, 결절(結節), 절(節)   **E** *node, nodal, noose, denouement (< 'unknotting')*

     > L. nodosus, nodosa, nodosum 매듭이 많은   **E** *nodose*

       > L. nodositas, nodositatis, f. 결절상(結節狀)   **E** *nodosity*

     > L. nodulus, noduli, m. (< + -ulus *diminutive suffix*) 소절(小節), 소결절(小結節), 결절(結節)   **E** *nodule, nodular, multinodular, nodulose*

nubo, nupsi, nuptum, nuběre 시집가다

> nubilis, nubile (여성이) 결혼 적령기의, 성적 매력이 있는   **E** *nubile*

> nuptiae, nuptiarum, f. (pl.) 결혼, 결혼식   **E** *nuptial*

> connubium, connubii, n. (< con- (< cum) *with, together*) (로마법상 정당한) 결혼

  < IE. sneubh- *to marry*

    > G. nymphē, nymphēs, f. *bride, maiden, nymph*

      > L. nympha, nymphae, f. 신부, 소녀, 요정; (불완전 변태를 하는 곤충의) 애벌레,
약충(若蟲); 소음순(小陰脣)

        E *nymph, nympholepsy (< 'on the pattern of epilepsy'), nymphomania; nymphotomy, nymphectomy*

      > L. nymphaea, nymphaeae, f. 수련(睡蓮)   **E** *nymphaea*

nuo, nui, –, nuěre 끄덕이다

> nuto, nutavi, nutatum, nutare (*frequentative*) 끄덕거리다, 흔들거리다   **E** *nutation*

> annuo, annui, annutum, annuěre (< an- (< ad) *to, toward, at, according to* + nuěre
to nod) 시인하다, 승낙하다

> innuo, innui, innutum, innuěre (< in- *in, on, into, toward* + nuěre *to nod*) 머리를
끄덕이다, 넌지시 비추다, 암시하다, 의사표시하다   **E** *innuendo*

  < IE. neu- *to nod*

    > L. numen, numinis, n. 머리 끄덕임, 하느님의 뜻, 신성, 신령   **E** *numen, (pl.) numina, numinous*

pello, pepuli, pulsum, pelleře 때리다, 밀치다   **E** *(probably) pelt (< 'to strike')*

> pulsus, pulsus, m. 때림, 충격, 밀침, 추진력, 고동, 맥박   **E** *pulse*

> pulso, pulsavi, pulsatum, pulsare (*frequentative*) 두드리다, 맥동 치다

    E *push, pulsate, (pulsating star >) pulsar (< 'on the pattern of quasar'), pursy (< 'to breathe with difficulty')*

  > pulsatilis, pulsatile 두드리는, 맥동 치는   **E** *pulsatile*

> compello, compuli, compulsum, compelleře (< com- (< cum) *with, together* + pelleře
to drive) 억지로 시키다, 강요하다   **E** *compel, compulsive, compulsory*

  > compulsio, compulsionis, f. 강제, 강박, 충동, 강박 충동   **E** *compulsion*

> dispello, dispuli, dispulsum, dispelleře (< dis- *apart from, down, not* + pelleře *to drive*) 털어 버리다   **E** *dispel*

> expello, expuli, expulsum, expelleře (< ex- *out of, away from* + pelleře *to drive*)
밀어내다, 축출하다   **E** *expel, expellent (expellant), expulsive*

  > expulsio, expulsionis, f. 축출   **E** *expulsion*

> impello, impuli, impulsum, impelleře (< im- (< in) *in, on, into, toward* + pelleře
to drive) 때리다, 움직이게 하다, 추진하다, 충동하다   **E** *impel, impellent, impulsive*

  > impulsus, impulsus, m. 추진, 충동; (물리) 충격, 충격량   **E** *impulse*

  > impulsio, impulsionis, f. 추진, 충동   **E** *impulsion*

> propello, propuli, propulsum, propelleře (< pro- *before, forward, for, instead of* +

pellĕre *to drive*) 앞으로 쫓다, 격동시키다,

추진시키다   **E** *propel, propellent (propellant), propeller, propulsive*

    > propulsio, propulsionis, f. 추진   **E** *propulsion*

   > repello, repuli, repulsum, repellĕre (< re- *back, again* + pellĕre *to drive*) 물리치다,

격퇴하다, 구축(驅逐)하다, 반발하다   **E** *repel, repellent, repulsive, repulse*

     > repulsio, repulsionis, f. 격퇴, 구축, 반발   **E** *repulsion*

   > appello, appellavi, appellatum, appellare (< ad- *to, toward, at, according to* +

pellĕre *to drive*) (*frequentative*) 말을 붙이다, 이름 부르면서 간청하다, 공소하다,

명칭을 붙이다   **E** *appeal, appellant, appellee, (appeal >) peal, (re-appeal >) repeal*

     > appellatio, appellationis, f. 명칭, 호칭   **E** *appellation*

  < IE. pel- *to beat, to drive, to thrust*   **E** *anvil (< 'something beat on'), felt (< 'cloth made by beating')*

    > L. filtrum, filtri, n. 펠트(*felt*, 모전 毛氈), 거르개, 여과지, 여과기, 필터   **E** *(noun) filter*

     > L. filtro, filtravi, filtratum, filtrare 거르다,

여과시키다   **E** *(verb) filter, (filter >) filterable (filtrable), filtrate, ultrafiltrate*

       > L. filtratio, filtrationis, f. 거름, 여과   **E** *filtration*

       > L. infiltro, infiltravi, infiltratum, infiltrare (< in- *in, on, into, toward* +

filtrare *to filtrate*) 침윤(浸潤)하다   **E** *infiltrate, infiltrative*

         > L. infiltratio, infiltrationis, f. 침윤(浸潤)   **E** *infiltration*

    > L. polio, polivi (polii), politum, polire 모직물을 다듬이질하여 끝마무리하다, 다듬다,

연마하다, 세련되게 하다   **E** *polish, polite*

      > L. interpolo, interpolavi, interpolatum, interpolare (< inter- *between, among* +

polire *to polish*) 다시 고치다, 변조하다, 가필하다,

써넣다   **E** *interpolate, (interpolate >) extrapolate*

pendo, pependi, pensum, pendĕre 매달다, 저울로 무게를 달다, 무게가 나가다, 지불하다

(주화가 나오기 전에는 구리 등을 저울로 달아서 치렀음); (*to weigh in mind* >) 깊이

생각하다, 평가하다

   > pensum, pensi, n. (*neuter past participle*) 무게, 분량,

과제   **E** *(noun) poise, equipoise (< 'equal poise'), Sp. peso*

   > pensio, pensionis, f. 저울질, 지불, 연금(年金), 집세   **E** *pension*

   > pondus, pondi, m. 무게, 무게 단위(453.6g)   **E** *(libra pondo (abl.) 'by pound weight' >) pound*

   > pondus, ponderis, n. 무게, 무게 단위(453.6g); 많음, 짐

     > pondero, ponderavi, ponderatum, ponderare 무게를 달다, 숙고하다   **E** *ponder*

       > aequipondero, aequiponderavi, aequiponderatum, aequiponderare (< aequus

equal + ponderare *to weigh*) 균형 잡히게 하다   **E** *equiponderate*

       > praepondero, praeponderavi, praeponderatum, praeponderare (< prae-

before, beyond + ponderare *to weigh*) (무게가) 능가하다, 우세하다,

우위에 있다   **E** *preponderance*

   > penso, pensavi, pensatum, pensare (*frequentative*) 무게를 달다, 숙고하다,

보상하다   **E** *(verb) poise, pensive, F. pensée, pansy*

     > compenso, compensavi, compensatum, compensare (< com- (< cum) *with,*

together + pensare *to weigh*) 보상하다, 보정하다 　　`E` *compensate, compensatory*

　　> compensatio, compensationis, f. 보상,

　　　　보정　　　　　　　　　　`E` *compensation, (compensation >) decompensation*

　　　　> recompenso, **recompensavi**, recompensatum, recompensare (< re-

　　　　　　back, again + compensare *to weigh together*) 보답하다, 변상하다,

　　　　　　배상하다　　　　　　　　　　　　　　`E` *recompense*

> pendeo, **pependi**, −, pendēre 매달리다, 늘어지다,

　　미결 상태로 있다　　　　　　`E` *pend, pendent; pendant, (pendant + pennon >) pennant*

　　> pendulus, pendula, pendulum 매달린, 흔들리는, 확실하지 않는, 미결의　　`E` *pendulous*

　　　　> pendulum, penduli, n. (시계 등의) 추, 진자(振子)　　　　　　`E` *pendulum*

　　> pensilis, pensile 매달린　　　　　　　　　　　　　　　`E` *pensile*

　　> dependeo, **dependi**, −, dependēre (< de- *apart from, down, not* + pendēre

　　　　to hang) 매달려 있다, 속하다

　　　　`E` *depend, dependent, independent, interdependent, dependence, dependency*

　　> impendeo, **impendi**, −, impendēre (< im- (< in) *in, on, into, toward* + pendēre

　　　　to hang) 가까이 있다, 임박하다, 절박하다　　　　　　`E` *impend*

　　> propendeo, **propendi**, −, propendēre (< pro- *before, forward, for, instead of*

　　　　+ pendēre *to hang*) 앞으로 기울다, 마음이 기울다　　　`E` *propensity*

> stipendium, stipendii, n. (< stips, stipis, f. *wages* + pendēre *to weigh, to pay*) 급여　`E` *stipend*

> appendo, **appendi**, appensum, appendēre (< ap- (< ad) *to, toward, at, according to*)

　　+ pendēre *to cause to hang*) 매달다　　　　　　`E` *append, appendage*

　　> appendix, appendicis, f. (< + -ix *noun suffix*) 부속기, 부속물, 부록; 충수(蟲垂),

　　　　막창자꼬리　　　　　　　　　`E` *appendix, (pl.) appendices, appendiceal*

　　　　> mesoappendix, mesoappendicis, f. (< G. mesos *middle*) 충수간막,

　　　　　　막창자꼬리간막　　　　　　　　　　　`E` *mesoappendix*

　　　　> appendicula, appendiculae, f. (< + -cula *diminutive suffix*) 소부속기,

　　　　　　작은 부록　　　　　　　　　　`E` *appendicle, appendicular*

　　> appendicium, appendicii, n. 추가, 부록　　　`E` *penthouse (< 'attached building')*

> compendo, **compependi**, compensum, compendēre (< com- (< cum) *with, together*

　　+ pendēre *to weigh*) 함께 저울에 달다

　　> compendium, compendii, n. 함께 저울에 달기, (노력·시간의) 단축, 요약, 개요,

　　　　첩경　　　　　　　　　　　`E` *compendium*

> dispendo, **dispendi**, dispensum, dispendēre (< dis- *apart from, down, not* + pendēre

　　to weigh) 저울에 달다, 할당하다, 배당하다

　　> dispenso, **dispensavi**, dispensatum, dispensare (*frequentative*) (저울에 달아)

　　　　분배하다, 처방에 따라 약을 조제하다, (재정·가사를) 관리하다, 특별 면제를

　　　　하다　　　　　　　　　　`E` *dispense*

　　　　> dispensatio, dispensationis, f. 분배, 관리, 면제　　`E` *dispensation*

　　　　> dispensator, dispensatoris, m. 분배인, 관리인

　　　　　　> dispensatorius, dispensatoria, dispensatorium 분배의, 관리의

　　　　　　　　> dispensatorium, dispensatorii, n. 조제 지침, 약품 해설서,

약전(藥典)   **E** *dispensatory*

    > dispensarium, dispensarii, n. 조제실, 약국, 진료소   **E** *dispensary*

    > dispensabilis, dispensabile 특별 면제를 할 수 있는,

      없어도 되는   **E** *dispensable, indispensable*

> expendo, **expendi**, expensum, expendĕre (< ex- *out of, away from* + pendĕre *to weigh,*

  to pay) 지출하다   **E** *expend,* (expensa pecunia *'spent money'* >) *expense, expensive, spend*

    > expenditus, expendita, expenditum 지출한   **E** *expenditure*

> perpendo, **perpendi**, perpensum, perpendĕre (< per- *through, thoroughly* + pendĕre

  to weigh, to consider) 무게를 정확히 달다, 심사숙고하다   **E** *perpend*

    > perpendiculum, perpendiculi, n. 연추(鉛錘), 규범

      > perpendicularis, perpendiculare 수직(垂直)의   **E** *perpendicular*

> suspendo, **suspendi**, suspensum, suspendĕre (< sus- (< sub) *under, up from under*

  + pendĕre *to cause to hang*) 매달다, 지지(支持)하다, 미결 상태로 두다,

  정지시키다   **E** *suspend, suspense*

    > suspensio, suspensionis, f. 매달음, 미결, 부유액(浮遊液), 현탁액(懸濁液)   **E** *suspension*

    > suspensorius, suspensoria, suspensorium 매다는   **E** *suspensory*

> vilipendo, −, −, vilipendĕre (< vilis *vile* + pendĕre *to weigh, to consider*) 얕보다,

  헐뜯다   **E** *vilipend*

< IE. (s)pen- *to draw, to stretch, to spin*   **E** *span, spider, spin* (< *'to draw out and to twist'), spindle*

> L. spons, spontis, f. 자유의사, 자기, 자체

    > L. sponte (부사 < 단수 탈격) 자유의사로, 자발적으로, 저절로

      > L. spontaneus, spontanea, spontaneum 자유의사의, 자발적인,

      자연적인   **E** *spontaneous, spontaneity*

> G. span (spaein) *to draw, to tug, to tear, to rend, to drain*

    > G. spasmos, spasmou, m. (spasma, spasmatos, n.) *spasm*

      > L. spasmus, spasmi, m. 경련수축(痙攣收縮), 경축(痙縮),

      연축(攣縮)   **E** *spasm, spasmolytic*

      > G. spasmōdēs, spasmōdēs, spasmōdes (< -ōdēs *like, resembling*)

      spasmodic

        > L. spasmodicus, spasmodica, spasmodicum 연축(攣縮)의   **E** *spasmodic*

    > G. spastikos, spastikē, spastikon *spastic*

      > L. spasticus, spastica, spasticum 경직(硬直)의   **E** *spastic, (spastic >) spasticity*

    > G. spadix, spadikos, m. *palm-branch*

      > L. spadix, spadicis, m. 열매가 달린 채로 꺾인 종려 나뭇가지;

      육수화서(肉穗花序)   **E** *spadix*

    > G. spadōn, spadōnos, m. *eunuch*

      > (*probably*) G. -spadias, -spadiou, m. -*eunuch*

        > G. hypospadias, hypospadiou, m. (< hyp(o)- *under*) *hypospadiac*

        man

          > L. hypospadias, hypospadiae, m. 요도밑열림증,

          요도하열(尿道下裂)   **E** *hypospadias*

> L. epispadias, epispadiae, m. (< ep(i)- *upon*) 요도위열림증,
요도상열(尿道上裂)
E *epispadias*

> G. spadion, spadiou, n. *stadium*

> (*suggested*) G. stadion, stadiou, n. (*influenced by* stadios *standing* <
histanai (sta- *root of* histanai) *to make stand*) *ancient Greek measure
of length, about 185 meters, a track for a foot race or chariot race
(that at Olympia being one stadion long)*

> L. stadium, stadii, n. 거리 단위(약 185m), 경기장
E *stadium*

> G. penia, penias, f. (< *strain, exhaustion*) *poverty, need*

E -*penia*, -*penic*, *leukopenia, neutropenia, lymphopenia, thrombocytopenia, pan-
cytopenia, osteopenia* (< *'bone deficiency'*), *sarcopenia* (< *'flesh deficiency'*),
sideropenia (< *'iron deficiency'*)

> G. penesthai (*root* pon-) *to toil*

> G. ponein (poneein) *to toil*

E (G. hydōr *'water'* > *hydro-* > *'on the pattern of geoponics'* >) *hydroponics*

> G. geōponein (geōponeein) (< geō- < gē *earth*)
to till the soil
E *geoponic, geoponics*

> G. ponos, ponou, m. *toil, hardship, suffering, pain*

> G. aponia, aponias, f. (< *absence of suffering* < a- *not*) *Epicureanism*

> L. aponia, aponiae, f. 에피쿠로스주의; 쾌락주의, 무통
E *aponia*

peto, petivi (petii), petitum, petĕre 날아가다, (어느 방향으로) 가다, 찾아다니다, 청하다

> petitio, petitionis, f. 청원
E *petition*

> appeto, appetivi (appetii), appetitum, appetĕre (< ap- (< ad) *to, toward, at, according
to* + petĕre *to go toward, to seek*) 잡으려고 가까이 가다, 몹시 원하다

> appetitus, appetitus, m. 침입, 욕망, 탐욕, 식욕, 입맛
E *appetite, appetizer*

> competo, competivi (competii), competitum, competĕre (< com- (< cum) *with, together*
+ petĕre *to go toward, to seek*) 같은 곳으로 가다, 함께 얻으려고 힘쓰다, 경쟁하다,
적합하다, 자격이 있다, 능력이 있다 E *compete, competent, immunocompetent, competitive*

> competitio, competitionis, f. 경쟁
E *competition*

> competitor, competitoris, m. 경쟁자
E *competitor*

> competentia, competentiae, f. 적격, 능력, 적임
E *competence, immunocompetence*

> incompetentia, incompetentiae, f. (< in- *not*) 부적격, 무능력,
부적임
E *incompetence, immunoincompetence*

> impeto, impetivi (impetii), impetitum, impetĕre (< im- (< in) *in, on, into, toward* +
petĕre *to go toward, to seek*) 공격하다, 습격하다

> impetus, impetus, m. 공격, 습격, 충격, 충동
E *impetus, impetuous*

> impetigo, impetiginis, f. (< *contagious skin infection*) 고름딱지증,
농가진(膿痂疹)
E *impetigo, impetiginous*

> repeto, repetivi (repetii), repetitum, repetĕre (< re- *back, again* + petĕre *to go toward,
to seek*) 반복하다
E *repeat, repetitive, repetitious, repeatable*

> repetitio, repetitionis, f. 반복   **E** *repetition*

> *petulo, *petulavi, *petulatum, *petulare 주제넘다, 안달하다   **E** *petulant*

> perpetuus, perpetua, perpetuum (< per- *through, thoroughly* + petĕre *to go toward, to seek*) 영속하는, 영구적인

  > perpetuitas, perpetuitatis, f. 영속, 영구   **E** *perpetuity*

  > perpetualis, perpetuale 영속하는, 불후의, 끊임없는   **E** *perpetual*

  > perpetuo, **perpetuavi**, perpetuatum, perpetuare 영속시키다, 영구화하다, 끊지 않고 계속하다   **E** *perpetuate*

> propitius, propitia, propitium (< pro- *before, forward, for, instead of* + petĕre *to go toward, to seek*) 호의적인   **E** *propitious*

  > propitio, **propitiavi**, propitiatum, propitiare 호의를 갖게 하다, 달래다   **E** *propitiate*

> centripetus, centripeta, centripetum (< centrum *center* + petĕre *to go toward, to seek*) 구심(求心)의, 들[入]   **E** *centripetal*

< IE. pet- *to fly, to rush*   **E** *feather*

> L. penna, pennae, f. 깃, 날개, 깃펜   **E** *penna, pen, pennon,* (pendant + pennon >) *pennant*

  > L. pennatus, pennata, pennatum 깃이 있는, 날개가 있는   **E** *pennate*

  > L. pinna, pinnae, f. 깃, 날개, 투구 꼭대기의 장식 깃털, 뾰족탑, 귓바퀴   **E** *pinna*

    > L. pinnatus, pinnata, pinnatum 깃 모양의 (대칭적) 구조를 갖는   **E** *pinnate*

    > L. pinnaculum, pinnaculi, n. (< + -culum *diminutive suffix*) 작은 뾰족탑, 뾰족한 봉우리, (불안한) 절정   **E** *pinnacle, panache*

    > L. Pinnipedia, Pinnipediorum, n. (pl.) (< + pes, pedis, m. *foot*) (동물) (물개 등) 기각목(鰭脚目)   **E** *pinniped*

> G. pteron, pterou, n. *feather, wing, flight, anything like wings*

E *pter(o)-, helicopter* (< 'spiral wing'), *pterin* (< 'first identified in the butterfly wings'), *pteridine*

  > G. pterion, pteriou, n. (< + -ion *diminutive suffix*) *pterion*

    > L. pterion, pterii, n. 관자놀이점   **E** *pterion*

  > G. pteris, pteridos, f. (< *having feathery fronds*) *fern*   **E** *pterid(o)-, pteridophyte, pteridology*

  > L. Pterosaurus, Pterosauri, m. (< G. pteron *wing* + sauros *lizard*) (익룡) 익룡속(翼龍屬)   **E** *pterosaurus (pterosaur)*

  > L. Pterodactylus, Pterodactyli, m. (< G. pteron *wing* + dactylos *finger*) (익룡) 익수룡속(翼手龍屬)   **E** *pterodactyl*

  > L. Lepidoptera, Lepidopterorum, n. (pl.) (< G. lepis, lepidos, f. *scale* + pteron *wing*) (곤충) (나비·나방 등) 인시목(鱗翅目)   **E** *Lepidoptera*

> G. pteryx, pterygos, f. *feather, wing, flight, anything like wings*

E *archaeopteryx* (< 'the oldest known fossil bird'), *apteryx* (< 'a New Zealand bird with merely rudimentary wings and no tail, called by the natives Kiwi'), *pterygoid*

  > G. pterygion, pterygiou, n. (< + -ion *diminutive suffix*) *little wing*

    > L. pterygium, pterygii, n. 군날개, 익상편(翼狀片)   **E** *pterygium,* (pl.) *pterygia*

> G. piptein *to fall, to fail, to be killed, to happen*

> G. ptōsis, ptōseōs, f. (< + -sis *feminine noun suffix*) *fall, ruin, disaster,
corpse;* (*grammar*) *case*

  > L. ptosis, ptosis, f. 처짐, 하수증(下垂症); 눈꺼풀처짐,
안검(眼瞼) 하수증
                                       E *ptosis, ptotic, -ptosis, -ptotic*

> G. ptōma, ptōmatos, n. (< + -ma *resultative noun suffix*) *fall, ruin, disaster;
corpse*
                                               E *ptomaine*

> G. apopiptein (< ap(o)- *away from, from* + piptein) *to fall off*

  > G. apoptōsis, apoptōseōs, f. (< + -sis *feminine noun suffix*) *falling off*

    > L. apoptosis, apoptosis, f. (< *regulated cell death, contrasted with
unregulated necrosis*) 세포자멸사(細胞自滅死), 아포프토시스   **E** *apoptosis*

      > L. necroptosis, necroptosis, f. (< *regulated cell death,
necrosome-dependent, with a necrotic morphotype* <
G. nekros *dead*) 네크로프토시스   **E** *necroptosis*

      > L. pyroptosis, pyroptosis, f. (< *regulated cell death,
pyroptosome (inflammasome)-dependent, with an apoptotic
and necrotic morphotype* < G. pyr *fire*)
피로프토시스   **E** *pyroptosis*

      > L. ferroptosis, ferroptosis, f. (< *regulated cell death, iron-
dependent, with a necrotic morphotype* < L. ferrum *iron*)
페로프토시스   **E** *ferroptosis*

> G. propiptein (< pro- *before, in front* + piptein) *to fall forwards*

  > G. proptōsis, proptōseōs, f. (< + -sis *feminine noun suffix*)
falling forward, prolapse

    > L. proptosis, proptosis, f. 돌출(突出)   **E** *proptosis*

> G. sympiptein (< sym- (< syn) *with, together* + piptein) *to fall together, to
happen*

  > G. symptōma, symptōmatos, n. (< + -ma *resultative noun suffix*) *chance,
accident, misfortune*

    > L. symptoma, symptomatis, n. 증상(症狀)

      E *symptom, symptomatic, asymptomatic, symptomatology, symptomato-
lytic*

> G. peripiptein (< peri- *around, near, beyond, on account of* + piptein) *to
befall, to change suddenly*

  > G. peripeteia, peripeteias, f. *sudden change*

    > L. peripeteia, peripeteiae, f. 급변(急變)   **E** *peripeteia*

> G. potamos, potamou, m. (< *rushing water*) *river*   **E** *potamology*

  > G. hippopotamos, hippopotamou, m. (< hippos *horse*) *river horse*

    > L. hippopotamus, hippopotami, m. 하마(河馬)   **E** *hippopotamus*

  > G. Mesopotamia, Mesopotamias, f. (< mesos *middle*) *the region between the
Tigris and Euphrates rivers*

    > L. Mesopotamia, Mesopotamiae, f. 메소포타미아   **E** *Mesopotamia*

plaudo, plausi, plausum, plaudĕre (plodo, plosi, plosum, plodĕre) 소리 나게 치다,
손뼉 치다, 갈채하다

E ((second personal plural, present imperative, active) Plaudite! 'Applaud' >) *plaudits, plausible,*
implode (< 'on the pattern of explode'), implosion (< 'on the pattern of explosion')

> applaudo, **applausi**, applausum, applaudĕre (applodo, **applosi**, applosum, applodĕre)

(< ap- (< ad) *to, toward, at, according to* + plaudĕre *to clap*)
박수갈채하다　　　　　　　　　　　　　　　　　**E** *applaud, applause, applausive*

> explaudo, **explausi**, explausum, explaudĕre (explodo, **explosi**, explosum, explodĕre)

(< ex- *out of, away from* + plaudĕre *to clap*) (손뼉을 치거나 고함질러서) 내쫓다,
퇴장시키다, 폭발시키다　　　　　　**E** *explode, explosion, explosive, (explosive >) plosive*

pono, posui, positum, ponĕre 놓다, 건설하다, 제출하다, 가정하다

E *pose, (pose >) juxtapose, (past participial stem) posit, (posit >) juxtaposit, (posit >)*
oviposit, (posita (feminine past participle) 'place where one is supposed to be', 'mail
system, with riders and horses placed at intervals along a route' >) post

> positio, positionis, f. 위치, 상태, 지위, 배치, 자세

E *position, (position >) positional, (position >) malposition, (malposition >) malposed,*
(position >) juxtaposition

> positura, positurae, f. 위치, 배치, 자세　　　　　　　**E** *posture, (posture >) postural*

> positivus, positiva, positivum 실제의, 명확한, 긍정적, 적극적, 양(陽)의, 정(正)의; (반응)
양성(陽性)인

E *positive, (positive >) positivity, positivism, positron (< 'on the pattern of electron')*

> appono, apposui, appositum, apponĕre (< ap- (< ad) *to, toward, at, according to*
+ ponĕre *to put, to place*) 곁에 놓다, 나란히 놓다　　　**E** *appose, apposite*

  > appositio, appositionis, f. 병치(竝置), 병렬(竝列), 부가, 첨부;
  (문법) 동격(同格)　　　　　　　　　　　　　　**E** *apposition, appositional*

> compono, **composui**, compositum, componĕre (< com- (< cum) *with, together* +
ponĕre *to put, to place*) 함께 놓다, 갖추게 하다, 진정시키다, 구성하다, 짓다, 합성하다

E *compose, compound, component, composite; (compose >) decompose, decomposite,*
decomposition

  > compositio, compositionis, f. 구성, 합성, 창작, 작품　　　　　**E** *composition*

> contrapono, **cotraposui**, contrapositum, contraponĕre (< contra- *against* + ponĕre
to put, to place) 대치시키다, 대립시키다　　　　　　　**E** *contrapose*

  > cotrapositio, cotrapositionis, f. 대치, 대립; (논리) 대우(對偶)　　**E** *contraposition*

> depono, **deposui**, depositum, deponĕre (< de- *apart from, down, not* + ponĕre *to
put, to place*) 제쳐 놓다, 내려놓다, 내놓다, 보관하다, 기탁하다　**E** (verb) *deposit, deponent*

  > depositum, depositi, n. 보관품, 기탁품, 침착물(沈着物), 침전물
  (沈澱物)　　**E** (noun) *deposit (< 'thing deposited')*, F. *depot (< 'where deposited')*

  > depositio, depositionis, f. 보관, 직위 박탈, 유기(遺棄); 침착(沈着), 침전(沈澱)　**E** *deposition*

  > depositarius, depositarii, m. 보관자, (보관소)　　　　　　　**E** *depositary*

> depositorium, depositorii, n. 보관소, (보관자)   **E** *depository*

> dispono, **disposui**, dispositum, disponĕre (< dis- *apart from, down, not* + ponĕre
   to put, to place) 사이를 고르게 떼어 놓다, 배치하다, 태세를
   갖추게 하다   **E** *dispose, disposal, disposable, (dispose > 'not disposed' >) indisposed*
   > dispositio, dispositionis, f. 배치, 처분, 성향   **E** *disposition*
     > praedispono, **praedisposui**, praedispositum, praedisponĕre (< prae- *before,*
        beyond + disponĕre *to put apart, to arrange*) 미리 배치하다, 태세를 갖추다,
        ~의 소지(素地)를 만들다, 병에 걸리게 쉽게 하다   **E** *predispose*
        >praedispositio, praedispositionis, f. 소인(素因), 소질(素質),
          체질(體質)   **E** *predisposition*

> expono, **exposui**, expositum, exponĕre (< ex- *out of, away from* + ponĕre *to put,*
   to place) 내놓다, 노출시키다, 전시하다, 표명하다,
   설명하다   **E** *expose, expound, exponent, (exponent >) exponential, (expose >) exposure*
   > expositio, expositionis, f. 노출, 유기, 전시, 설명   **E** *exposition (expo)*
   > expositorius, expositoria, expositorium 설명적인, 해설적인   **E** *expository*

> impono, **imposui**, impositum, imponĕre (< im- (< in) *in, on, into, toward* + ponĕre
   to put, to place) 얹다, 짊어지우다, 떠맡기다, 임명하다, 속이다   **E** *impose, impost*
   > impositio, impositionis, f. 부과, 강요   **E** *imposition*
   > impostura, imposturae, f. 기만, 사기   **E** *imposture*
   > impostor, impostoris, m. 기만자, 사기꾼   **E** *impostor (imposter)*
     > superimpono, **superimposui**, superimpositum, superimponĕre (< super- *above*
       + imponĕre *impose*) 얹다, 짊어지우다, 떠맡기다,
       임명하다   **E** *superimpose, (superimpose >) superimposition*

> interpono, **interposui**, interpositum, interponĕre (< inter- *between, among* + ponĕre
   to put, to place) 사이에 놓다, 중재하다
   > interpositio, interpositionis, f. 삽입, 중재, 간섭   **E** *interpose*
                                          E *interposition*

> oppono, **opposui**, oppositum, opponĕre (< op- (< ob) *before, toward(s), over, against,*
   away + ponĕre *to put, to place*) 맞서게 하다   **E** *oppose, opponent, opposite, opposable*
   > oppositio, oppositionis, f. 맞섬, 대립   **E** *opposition*

> praepono, **praeposui**, praepositum, praeponĕre (< prae- *before, beyond* + ponĕre
   to put, to place) 앞에 놓다   **E** *prepose*
   > praepositio, praepositionis, f. 전치사(前置辭)   **E** *preposition*

> propono, **proposui**, propositum, proponĕre (< pro- *before, forward, for, instead of*
   + ponĕre *to put, to place*) 내놓다, 제안하다, 작정하다, 기도(企圖)하다

      E *propose, (propose >) proposal, propone, (propone >) propound, proponent,*
     purpose, (purpose >) purposive, (purpose >) repurpose

   > propositus, propositi, m. 창시자, (유언장의) 본인, 발단자   **E** *propositus, (pl.) propositi*
   > propositio, propositionis, f. 제안, 주제, 명제   **E** *proposition*

> postpono, **postposui**, postpositum, postponĕre (< post- *after* + ponĕre *to put, to place*)
   뒤에 놓다, 미루어 놓다, 제쳐 놓다, 경시하다   **E** *postpose, postpone*
   > postpositio, postpositionis, f. (문법) 후치(後置)   **E** *postposition*

> repono, **reposui**, repositum, reponĕre (< re- *back, again* + ponĕre *to put, to place*)

제자리에 도로 놓다   **E** *repose*

> reposito, repositionis, f. 복위(復位), 보관, 저장   **E** *reposition*

> repositorium, repositorii, n. (요리 접시·과일 그릇 등을 얹어 놓기 위해 식탁에

비치한) 큰 쟁반, 목판; (일반 주택의) 보관 장소, 곡물 저장소; 납골당   **E** *repository*

> suppono, **supposui**, suppositum, suppon ĕre (< sup- (< sub) *under, up from under*

+ pon ĕre *to put, to place*) 밑에 놓다, 예속시키다, 가정하다   **E** *suppose, suppositive*

> suppositio, suppositionis, f. 가정, 상상   **E** *supposition*

> suppositorius, suppositoria, suppositorium 밑에 둔

>suppositorium, suppositorii, n. 받침대, 좌약(坐藥)   **E** *suppository*

> transpono, **transposui**, transpositum, transpon ĕre (< trans- *over, across, through,*

beyond + pon ĕre *to put, to place*) 옮겨 놓다   **E** *transpose, transposable*

> transpositio, transpositionis, f. 옮김,

전위(轉位)   **E** *transposition, (transposition >) transposon*

< IE. apo-, ap- *off, away* (Vide ᴀʙ; *See* E. *ab-*)

premo, pressi, pressum, prem ĕre 누르다, 압박하다   **E** *print, reprint*

> pressura, pressurae, f. 압박, 압착, 압력, 압, 재난, 진통   **E** *pressure, pressurize*

> presso, −, −, pressare (*frequentative*) 꼭 누르다, 짜다,

압착하다   **E** *press, (press >) pressor, vasopressor, vasopressin*

> comprimo, **compressi**, compressum, comprim ĕre (< com- (< cum) *with, together* +

prem ĕre *to press*) 누르다, 압박하다, 압축하다   **E** *compress, decompress*

> compressio, compressionis, f. 압박, 압축   **E** *compression, decompression*

> deprimo, **depressi**, depressum, deprim ĕre (< de- *apart from, down, not* + prem ĕre

to press) 내리누르다, 함몰시키다, 억누르다, 억압하다

     E *depress, (depress + -ant (Latin present participle suffix) >) depressant, antidepressant*

> depressio, depressionis, f. 내리누름, 함몰, 오목, 우울(증)   **E** *depression*

> depressor, depressoris, m. 내리누르는 자, 억압자, 누르개, 내림근   **E** *depressor*

> exprimo, **expressi**, expressum, exprim ĕre (< ex- *out of, away from* + prem ĕre *to*

press) 짜내다, 나타내다, 표현하다, 발현하다

     E *express, (expressed + -on 'a termination of Greek neuter nouns and adjectives' >) exon, (It. caffe espresso 'pressed out coffee' >) espresso*

> expressio, expressionis, f. 표현, 발현   **E** *expression*

> *expressivus, *expressiva, *expressivum 표현의, 표현하는,

의미 있는   **E** *expressive, (expressive >) expressivity*

> imprimo, **impressi**, impressum, imprim ĕre (< im- (< in) *in, on, into, toward* +

prem ĕre *to press*) 눌러 찍다, 새겨 넣다, 인상(印象)을

박아주다   **E** *impress, imprint, (impress >) impressive*

> impressio, impressionis, f. 찍음, 색임, 자국, 인상   **E** *impression*

> opprimo, **oppressi**, oppressum, opprim ĕre (< op- (< ob) *before, toward(s), over,*

against, away + prem ĕre *to press*) 짓누르다, 억누르다   **E** *oppress*

> oppressio, oppressionis, f. 압박   **E** *oppression*

> reprimo, **repressi,** repressum, reprimĕre (< re- *back, again* + premĕre *to press*)

억압하다

> **E** *repress, repressor,* (reprimenda (pl. *neuter gerundive*) *'things to be held in check'* >) *reprimand*

> repressio, repressionis, f. 억압　　　　　　　　　　　　　　　**E** *repression*

> supprimo, **suppressi,** suppressum, supprimĕre (< sup- (< sub) *under, up from under*

+ premĕre *to press*) 억제하다

> **E** *suppress, (suppress >) suppressor, (suppress* + *-ant (Latin present participle*

suffix) >) suppressant

> suppressio, suppressionis, f. 억제　　　　　　　　　　　　　　**E** *suppression*

< IE. per- *to strike; a verbal root belonging to the group of* IE. per *forward, through*

quaero, quaesivi (quaesii), quaesitum, quaerĕre 찾다, 묻다

> **E** ((*second personal singular, present imperative, active*) quaere >) *query, (query >) Q fever*
(< *'to denote the febrile disease until fuller knowledge should allow a better name'), quest*

> quaestio, quaestionis, f. 찾음, 물음, 질문, 문제　　　　**E** *question, questionnaire*

> acquiro, **acquisivi,** acquisitum, acquirĕre (< ac- (< ad) *to, toward, at, according to*

+ quaerĕre *to seek, to ask*) 얻다, 취득하다, 획득하다, 습득하다　　**E** *acquire, acquest*

·> acquisitio, acquisitionis, f. 취득, 획득, 습득　　　　　**E** *acquisition*

> conquiro, **conquisivi,** conquisitum, conquirĕre (< con- (< cum) *with, together; intensive*

+ quaerĕre *to seek, to ask*) 두루 찾다, 찾아내다　　　　**E** *conquer, conquest*

> exquiro, **exquisivi,** exquisitum, exquirĕre (< ex- *out of, away from* + quaerĕre *to seek,*

to ask) 열심히 찾다, 엄선하다　　　　　　　　　　　　**E** *exquisite*

> inquiro, **inquisivi,** inquisitum, inquirĕre (< in- *in, on, into, toward* + quaerĕre *to seek,*

to ask) 물어보다, 조사하다, 탐구하다　　**E** *inquire (enquire), inquiry (enquiry), inquest*

> inquisitivus, inquisitiva, inquisitivum 탐구적인, 캐묻기 좋아하는　　**E** *inquisitive*

> inquisitio, inquisitionis, f. 조사, 탐구, 심문; (역사) 종교재판　　**E** *inquisition*

> inquisitor, inquisitoris, m. 조사자, 탐구자, 심문자; (역사) 종교재판관　　**E** *inquisitor*

> perquiro, **perquisivi,** perquisitum, perquirĕre (< per- *through, thoroughly* + quaerĕre

to seek, to ask) 깊이 조사하다　　　　　　　　**E** *perquisite (< 'thing thought after')*

> requiro, **requisivi,** requisitum, requirĕre (< re- *back, again; intensive* + quaerĕre *to*

seek, to ask) 요구하다, 요청하다　**E** *require, requirement, requisite, prerequisite, request*

> requisitio, requisitionis, f. 요구, 요청　　　　　　　　　　**E** *requisition*

rado, rasi, rasum, radĕre 깎다, 긁다, 문지르다, 지우다　　　**E** *raze, razor*

> rasor, rasoris, m. 현악기 연주자, 면도해 주는 사람, 이발사; (닭·꿩 등) 먹이를 찾아 땅을

파헤치는 동물　　　　　　　　　　　　　　　　　　　　　**E** *rasorial*

> abrado, **abrasi,** abrasum, abradĕre (< ab- *off, away from* + radĕre *to scrape*) (날

있는 도구로) 벗기다, 찰과(擦過)하다　　　　**E** *abrade, (abrade >) abradant, abrasive, abrasor*

> abrasio, abrasionis, f. 찰과상(擦過傷), 개갠 상처, 마멸(磨滅), 마모(磨耗)　　**E** *abrasion*

> corrado, **corrasi**, corrasum, corradĕre (< cor- (< cum) *with, together* + radĕre
   to scrape) 깎아내다   **E** *corrade*
   > *corrasio, *corrasionis, f. (지질) 마식(磨蝕)   **E** *corrasion*
> erado, **erasi**, erasum, eradĕre (< e- *out of, away from* + radĕre *to scrape*)
   지우다   **E** *erase, (erase >) eraser, (erase >) erasure*
   > *erasio, *erasionis, f. 지움, 말소, 삭제, 제거   **E** *erasion*
   > *rasico, *rasicavi, *rasicatum, *rasicare 긁다   **E** *rash, (probably) rascal*
< IE. red- *to scrape, to scratch, to gnaw*   **E** *rat*
   > L. raster, rastri, m. 갈퀴, 쇠스랑, 써레   **E** *raster*
   > L. rodo, **rosi**, rosum, rodĕre 갉아먹다, 잠식(蠶食)하다   **E** *(adjective) rodent*
      > L. Rodentia, Rodentium, n. (pl.) 설치목(齧齒目)   **E** *(noun, adjective) rodent, rodenticide*
      > L. rostrum, rostri, n. 부리, 주둥이, 문(吻), 취(嘴), 뱃부리;
         (pl.) 연단   **E** *rostrum, rostral, rostrad (<+ -ad 'toward')*
         > L. rostellum, rostelli, n. (< + -ellum *diminutive suffix*) 작은 부리,
            작은 주둥이, 액취(額嘴)   **E** *rostellum*
      > L. corrodo, **corrosi**, corrosum, corrodĕre (< cor- (< cum) *with, together* +
         rodĕre *to gnaw*) 쏠다, 부식(腐蝕)하다, 침식(浸蝕)하다   **E** *corrode, corrosive*
         > L. corrosio, corrosionis, f. 부식, 침식   **E** *corrosion*
      > L. erodo, **erosi**, erosum, erodĕre (< e- *out of, away from* + rodĕre *to gnaw*)
         쏠다, 미란(糜爛)하다, 침식(浸蝕)하다   **E** *erode, erosive*
         > L. erosus, erosa, erosum (*past participle*) 울퉁불퉁한   **E** *erose*
         > L. erosio, erosionis, f. 까짐, 짓무름, 미란, 침식   **E** *erosion*

rego, rexi, rectum, regĕre 올바로 이끌다, 다스리다   **E** *regent*
   > regentia, regentiae, f. 지배, 섭정   **E** *regency*
   > rectus, recta, rectum (*past participle*) 곧은, 옳은

      [용례] musculus rectus 곧은근, 직근(直筋)   **E** *rectus (muscle)*
         (문법) musculus 근육, 근: 단수 주격 < musculus, musculi, m.
            rectus: 과거분사, 남성형 단수 주격

      [용례] intestinum rectum 곧창자, 직장(直腸)   **E** *rectum, rectal*
         (문법) intestinum 장(腸): 단수 주격 < intestinum, intestini, n.
            rectum: 과거분사, 중성형 단수 주격

      > rectitudo, rectitudinis, f. 곧음, 옳음   **E** *rectitude*
      > rectilineus, rectilinea, rectilineum (< rectus *straight* + linea *line*) 직선의,
         직선으로 된   **E** *rectilinear (rectilineal)*
      > rectifico, **rectificavi**, rectificatum, rectificare (< rectus *straight* + -ficare
         (< facĕre) *to make*) 바로잡다, 교정하다; (화학) 정류(精溜)하다; (전기) (교류를
         직류로) 정류(整流)하다   **E** *rectify*
   > rector, rectoris, m. 지도자, (남자) 장(長); 키잡이   **E** *rector*
      > rectrix, rectricis, f. 지도자, (여자) 장(長); (pl.) (rectrices) (키잡이 역할을 하는)

새의 꽁지깃　　　　　　　　　　　　　　　　　　　　　**E** *rectrix*

> regula, regulae, f. 곧은 자, 척도, 규칙　　　　　　　**E** *rule, rail (< 'iron rod')*

　　> regularis, regulare 규칙에 맞는, 규칙적, 정규적, 통상의, 보통의　　**E** *regular*

　　　　>irregularis, irregulare (< ir- (< in- *not*) 불규칙적, 비정규적　**E** *irregular*

　　> regulo, −, −, regulare 바로잡다, 조절하다, 규정하다　　**E** *regulate, regulatory*

　　　　>regulatio, regulationis, f. 조절, 규정　　　**E** *regulation; dysregulation*

> regimen, regiminis, n. 지휘, 조타(操舵), 통치, 요법(療法); (문법) 격지배　**E** *regimen, regime*

　　> regimentum, regimenti, n. 통치, 통치권　　　　　　　　**E** *regiment*

> regio, regionis, f. (로마 본토 이외의) 통치지역, 지방(地方), 부위　　**E** *region*

　　> regionalis, regionale 지역의, 지방의, 부위의　　　　　　**E** *regional*

> rex, regis, m. 왕　　　　　　　　　　　　**E** *Rex, regicide, viceroy*

　　> regius, regia, regium 왕의

　　> regalis, regale 왕의, 왕에게 속한　　　　　　**E** *regal, royal, royalty*

　　　　>*regalimen, *regaliminis, n. 왕국, 영역, 범위, 분야　　**E** *realm*

　　> regnum, regni, n. 왕국, 왕권　　**E** *reign,* (inter regna *'between reigns'* >) *interregnum*

　　　　> regno, regnavi, regnatum, regnare 통치하다　　　**E** *regnant*

　　> regina, reginae, f. 여왕　　　　　　　　　　**E** *regina*

> arrigo, **arrexi**, arrectum, arrigĕre (< ar- (< ad) *to, toward, at, according to* + regĕre *to lead straight, to guide, to rule*) 일으켜 세우다

　　> arrector, arrectoris, m. 세움근　　　　　　　　　**E** *arrector*

> corrigo, **correxi**, correctum, corrigĕre (< cor- (< cum) *with, together* + regĕre *to lead straight, to guide, to rule*) 곧게 하다, 바로 잡다, 교정하다, 보정하다

　　E (*verb*) **correct,** ((*neuter gerundive*) *'that which is to be corrected'* >) *corrigendum, corrigible, incorrigible*

　　> correctus, correcta, correctum (*past participle*) 올바른　　**E** (*adjective*) *correct*

　　　　> incorrectus, incorrecta, incorrectum (< in- *not*) 옳지 않은　**E** *incorrect*

　　> correctio, correctionis, f. 교정, 보정　　　　　　　**E** *correction*

> dirigo, **direxi**, directum, dirigĕre (< di- (< dis-) *apart from, down, not* + regĕre *to lead straight, to guide, to rule*) 정렬시키다, 배치하다, 목표를 향해 가게 하다, 지도하다, 지시하다

　　E (*verb*) **direct, directive,** (dirige *'the first word of Latin antiphon* Dirige, Domine, Deus meus, in conspectu tuo viam meam *'Direct, O Lord, my God, my way in thy sight'* (*Psalm*)' >) *dirge*

　　> directus, directa, directum (*past participle*) 똑바른, 직접의, 직접적인　**E** (*adjective*) *direct*

　　　　>indirectus, indirecta, indirectum (< in- *not*) 에두르는, 간접의, 간접적인　**E** *indirect*

　　　　>*directio, *directiavi, *directiatum, *directiare 바로세우다, 배치하다, 정돈하다　**E** *dress*

　　　　　　> *addirectio, *addirectiavi, *addirectiatum, *addirectiare (< ad- *to, toward, at, according to* + *directiare *to straighten, to set up, to arrange*) 바로세우다, 배치하다, 정돈하다　　**E** *address*

　　> directio, directionis, f. 곧게 함, 방향 잡아줌, 방향,

　　　　지도(指導)　**E** *direction, directional, unidirectional, bidirectional, multidirectional*

> erigo, **erexi**, erectum, erigĕre (< e- *out of, away from* + regĕre *to lead straight,*

to guide, to rule) 곧추 세우다, 긴장시키다　**E** *(verb) **erect**, (erect >) **erectile***

　　> erectus, erecta, erectum *(past participle)*

　　　　곧추 선　**E** *(adjective) **erect**, (ad illam erectam 'to the watch tower' >) **alert***

　　> erectio, erectionis, f. 직립, 기립, 건립, 발기　**E** ***erection***

> surgo, **surrexi**, **surrectum**, surgĕre (< sub- *under, up from under* + regĕre *to lead*

straight, to guide, to rule) 일어나다, 솟다, 소생하다　**E** ***surge, source***

　　> insurgo, **insurrexi**, **insurrectum**, insurgĕre (< in- *in, on, into, toward* + surgĕre

　　to rise) 일어나다, 폭동을 일으키다　**E** ***insurge, insurgent***

　　　> insurrectio, insurrectionis, f. 폭동　**E** ***insurrection***

　　> resurgo, **resurrexi**, **resurrectum**, resurgĕre (< re- *back, again* + surgĕre *to rise*)

　　다시 일어나다, 부활하다

　　　　E ***resurge, resurgent, resource***, It. ***Risorgimento***, *(suggested)* ***resort*** (< *to go*
　　　　　frequently)

　　　> resurrectio, resurrectionis, f. 소생, 부활　**E** ***resurrection***

< IE. reg- *to move in a straight line, with derivatives meaning 'to direct in a straight line,*

to lead, to rule'

　　E *right, upright, aright, **rich** (< 'powerful'), **rack** (< 'straight bar'), **rake** (< 'implement with*
　　*straight pieces of wood'), **rank** (< 'haughty, overbearing'), **reckon** (< 'to arrange in order,*
　　*to recount'), **reck, reckless***

> L. ergo (< *(perhaps)* *e rogo (< e- *out of, away from* + *rogus *extension, direction*)

　(접속사) 그러므로　**E** ***ergo***

> L. rogo, **rogavi**, **rogatum**, rogare (손을 쭉 뻗어) 구하다, 부탁하다, 묻다; (로마 역사)

　(민의를 묻기 위해) 법률안을 제출하다　**E** *(probably) **rogue***

　　> L. rogatio, rogationis, f. 요청, 기원, 질문; (민의를 묻기 위한) 법률안의 제출,

　　　제출한 법률안　**E** ***rogation***

　　> L. rogatorius, rogatoria, rogatorium 심문하는, 조사하는; 증인 심문권이 있는　**E** ***rogatory***

　　> L. abrogo, **abrogavi**, **abrogatum**, abrogare (< ab- *off, away from* + rogare

　　　to ask) (권위·평판 등을) 떨어뜨리다, 폐기하다　**E** ***abrogate***

　　> L. arrogo, **arrogavi**, **arrogatum**, arrogare (< ar- (< ad) *to, toward, at,*

　　　according to + rogare *to ask*) (당연한 권리로서) 요구하다, 부당하게 사용

　　　하다　**E** ***arrogate, arrogant***

　　> L. derogo, **derogavi**, **derogatum**, derogare (< de- *apart from, down, not* +

　　　rogare *to ask*) (권위·평판 등을) 떨어뜨리다, (표준·원리 등에서) 일탈하다　**E** ***derogate***

　　　> L. derogatorius, derogatoria, derogatorium (권위·평판 등을) 떨어뜨리는,

　　　　(말 등이) 경멸적인　**E** ***derogatory***

　　> L. interrogo, **interrogavi**, **interrogatum**, interrogare (< inter- *between, among*

　　　+ rogare *to ask*) 질문하다, 캐묻다　**E** ***interrogate, interrogative***

　　> L. praerogo, **praerogavi**, **praerogatum**, praerogare (< prae- *before, beyond*

　　　+ rogare *to ask*) 먼저 청하다, 선불하다, 미리 배정하다　**E** ***prerogative***

　　> L. subrogo, **subrogavi**, **subrogatum**, subrogare (surrogo, **surrogavi**, **surrogatum**,

　　　surrogare) (< sub- (sur-) *under, up from under* + rogare *to ask*) 대신

　　　누구를 뽑다, 대리로 세우다　**E** ***subrogate, surrogate***

> G. oregein *to stretch out, to reach out for*
>> G. orexis, orexeōs, f. *desire, longing*
>>> G. anorexia, anorexias, f. (< G. an- *not*) *anorexia*
>>>> L. anorexia, anorexiae, f. 식욕부진(食慾不振),
입맛 없음

E *anorexia, anorectic*

E *anorexia nervosa*

[용례] anorexia nervosa 신경성 식욕부진
(문법) anorexia 식욕부진: 단수 주격
nervosa 신경성의: 형용사, 여성형 단수 주격
< nervosus, nervosa, nervosum

rumpo, rupi, ruptum, rumpĕre 터뜨리다, 터져 나오게 하다, (약속·신용·침묵을) 깨다, 갈라 놓다, 뚫고 나가다, 길을 열다

E (ruptus (*past participle*) *'broken'* >) **rout**, (rupta (*past participle*) > It. banca rupta *'bank broken'* >) **bankrupt**

[용례] rupta via (< *a road opened up by force*) 신작로(新作路),
새 길 **E** *route, routine (< 'regular way of doing things'),* F. **en route** (< *'on the way'*)
(문법) rupta 열어 놓은: 과거분사, 여성형 단수 주격
< ruptus, rupta, ruptum
via 길: 단수 주격 < via, viae, f.

> ruptura, rupturae, f. 터짐, 파열

E *rupture*

> abrumpo, **abrupi**, abruptum, abrumpĕre (< ab- *off, away from* + rumpĕre *to break*)
(덩어리로부터 갑작스레) 끊어 놓다

E *abrupt*

>> abruptio, abruptionis, f. (덩어리로부터 갑작스런) 분리

E *abruption*

[용례] abruptio placentae 태반조기박리

E *abruptio placentae*

(문법) abruptio 분리: 단수 주격
placentae 태반의: 단수 속격
< placenta, plancentae, f. (납작하고 둥근) 케이크, 태반

> corrumpo, **corrupi**, corruptum, corrumpĕre (< cor- (< cum) *with, together* + rumpĕre *to break*) 변질되게 하다, 부패시키다, 타락시키다

E *corrupt, corruptive, corruptible*

>> corruptio, corruptionis, f. 변질, 부패, 타락

E *corruption*

> disrumpo, **disrupi**, disruptum, disrumpĕre (< dis- *apart from, down, not* + rumpĕre *to break*) 붕괴시키다, 분열시키다

E *disrupt, disruptive, (disrupt >) disrupture*

>> disruptio, disruptionis, f. 붕괴, 분열

E *disruption*

> erumpo, **erupi**, eruptum, erumpĕre (< e- *out of, away from* + rumpĕre *to break*)
분출시키다, 터져 나오다

E *erupt, eruptive*

>> eruptio, eruptionis, f. 분출, 폭발, 발진, 이돋이, 맹출(萌出)

E *eruption*

> interrumpo, **interrupi**, interruptum, interrumpĕre (< inter- *between, among* + rumpĕre *to break*) 중단시키다, 훼방 놓다, 중절시키다, 단속(斷續)시키다

E *interrupt, interruptive*

>> interruptio, interruptionis, f. 중단, 훼방, 중절, 단속(斷續)

E *interruption*

> irrumpo, irrupi, irruptum, irrumpĕre (< ir- (< in) *in, on, into, toward* + rumpĕre
　　to break) 밀려닥치다, 덮치다, 난입하다　　　　　　　　　　　**E** *irrupt, irruptive*
　　　> irruptio, irruptionis, f. 난입, (동물 개체 수의) 급증　　　　　　**E** *irruption*
> rupes, rupis, f. 바위, 암벽　　　　　　　　　　　　　**E** *rupicolous* (< *'rock-inhabiting'*)
　　> rupestris, rupestre 바위의, 암벽의　　　　　　　　　　　**E** *rupestrine*
< IE. reup-, reub- *to snatch*

> **E** *rip, reave, bereave, rob, robe* (< *'clothes taken as booty'*), *rover* (< *'pirate'*), *rub,*
> *rubber, loot*

> L. usurpo, usurpavi, usurpatum, usurpare (< *usu-rupare < usus *use* + IE. reup-,
　　reub- *to snatch*) 불법 사용하다, 강탈하다　　　　　　　　**E** *usurp, usurpation*

sarpo, sarpsi, sarptum, sarpĕre 가지를 쳐내다, 전지(剪枝)하다
　　> sarmentum, sarmenti, n. 곁가지, 삭정이, 나뭇가지
　　　　> sarmentosus, sarmentosa, sarmentosum 넌출이 무성한, 덩굴이 많은　**E** *sarmentose*
< IE. serp- *sickle, hook*
　　> G. harpē, harpēs, f. *sickle; falcon, kite*
　　　　> L. harpe, harpes, f. 초승달 모양의 칼; 매　　　　　　　**E** *harpoon*

scalpo, scalpsi, scalptum, scalpĕre 긁어내다, 깎아내다, 조각하다
　　> scalprum, scalpri, n. (갈대펜 깎는) 주머니 칼, 조각도, 수술 칼
　　　　> scalpellum, scalpelli, n. (< + -ellum *diminutive suffix*) (책장 찢는) 작은 칼,
　　　　　작은 수술 칼　　　　　　　　　　　　　　　　**E** *scalpel*
　　> sculpo, sculpsi, sculptum, sculpĕre 새기다, 조각하다
　　　　> sculptura, sculpturae, f. 조각술, 조각품, 조각　**E** *sculpture, (sculpture >) sculpt*
　　　　> sculptor, sculptoris, m. 조각가　　　　　　　　　　　**E** *sculptor*
< IE. (s)kel- *to cut*

> **E** *shell* (< *'hard outer covering that splits off'*), *scale* (< *'something split off', 'bowl made*
> *from something split off'*), *skoal* (< *'a cup made from a shell'*), (*probably related to 'shell'*
> >) *skull, scalp* (< *'sheath'*), *shelf* (< *'split piece of wood'*), *shelve, shield* (< *'board'*),
> *shelter* (< *'shield'*), *skill* (< *'distinction' < 'to cut apart'*), *school* (< *'division'*), *half, halve*

> L. culter, cultri, m. 작은 칼, 쟁기 날　　　　　　　　**E** *cutlass, coulter (colter)*
　　> L. cultratus, cultrata, cultratum 칼처럼 생긴, 날카로운　　**E** *cultrate*
> L. silex, silicis, m., f. 돌멩이, 차돌, 부싯돌, 규석

> **E** *silica* (< *'silicon dioxide, on the pattern of alumina'*), (*silica >*) *silicify*, (*silica >*)
> *silicosis; silicon (Si)* (< *'on the pattern of carbon, because of chemical resemblances'*),
> *silicone(s)* (< *'semi-organic silicon polymers'*), (*silica, silicon >*) *silic(i)- (silico-)*

> L. siliqua, siliquae, f. 꼬투리, 껍질　　　　　　　　　　　　**E** *siliqua*
> G. skallein *to dig, to hoe*
　　> G. skalēnos, skalēnē, skalēnon *uneven, unequal*
　　　　> L. scalenus, scalena, scalenum 비스듬한, 부등변의; 사각근(斜角筋)의　**E** *scalene*
> IE. skldhra *shoulder blade used as a spade*　　　　　　　　**E** *shoulder*

scando, scandi, scansum, scandĕre 오르다   `E scan, scandent`

> scala, scalae, f. (주로 복수) 사다리, 층계, 계단

> `E scale (<'flight of stairs'), escalator (<'on the pattern of elevator'), (escalator >) escalate, echelon`

[용례] scala media 중간계단   `E scala media`

scala tympani 고실계단   `E scala tympani`

scala vestibuli 전정계단   `E scala vestibuli`

(문법) scala: 단수 주격

media 가운데의: 형용사, 여성형 단수 주격 < medius, media, medium

tympani 고실(鼓室)의: 단수 속격 < tympanum, tympani, n.

vestibuli 전정(前庭)의: 단수 속격 < vestibulum, vestibuli, n.

> scalaris, scalare 사다리의, 층계의, 계단의, 단계적인; (수학) 스칼라의   `E scalar`

> scansorius, scansoria, scansorium 기어오르는, 기어오르기에 알맞은   `E scansorial`

> ascendo, ascendi, ascensum, ascendĕre (< a- (< ad) to, toward, at, according to) + scandĕre to climb) 올라가다   `E ascend, ascendent (ascendant), ascent`

> ascensus, ascensus, m. 오름, 상승

> ascensio, ascensionis, m. 오름, 상승, 승천   `E ascension`

> descendo, descendi, descensum, descendĕre (< de- apart from, down, not + scandĕre to climb) 내려가다   `E descend, decendent (decandant), descent`

> descensus, descensus, m. 내려감, 하강

> descensio, descensionis, m. 내려감, 하강   `E descension`

> condescendo, condescendi, condescensum, condescendĕre (< con- (< cum) with, together; intensive + descendĕre to descend) 자기를 낮추다   `E condescend`

> transcendo, transcendi, transcensum, transcendĕre (< tran- (< trans) over, across, through, beyond + scandĕre to climb) 건너가다, 초월하다   `E transcend, transcendent, transcendentalism`

< IE. skand-, skend- to leap, to climb

> G. skandalon, skandalou, n. trap, snare for an enemy, offense, cause of moral stumbling, scandal

> L. scandalum, scandali, n. 걸려 넘어지게 하는 장애물, 추문   `E scandal, slander`

sero, serui, sertum, serĕre 엮다, 잇달게 하다, 말을 주고받다

> series, seriei, f. 열(列), 계열, 연쇄, 연속   `E series, (pl.) series`

> serialis, seriale 일련의, 연속적   `E serial`

> assero, asserui, assertum, asserĕre (< as- (< ad) to, toward, at, according to + serĕre to join) 뻗대어 말하다, 주장하다   `E assert`

> assertio, assertionis, f. 주장, 단언   `E assertion`

> desero, deserui, desertum, deserĕre (< de- apart from, down, not + serĕre to join) 버리다, 돌보지 않다, 도망치다, 탈주하다

> desertum, deserti, n. (< *neuter past participle*) 황야, 사막　　**E** *(noun) desert*

> desertio, desertionis, f. 유기, 탈주　　**E** *desertion*

> deserto, **desertavi**, desertatum, desertare (< *frequentative*) 버리다, 돌보지

않다, 도망치다, 탈주하다　　**E** *(verb) desert*

> dissero, **disserui**, dissertum, disserĕre (< dis- *apart from, down, not; intensive*

+ serĕre *to join*) 논술하다

> disserto, **dissertavi**, dissertatum, dissertare (*frequentative*) 논술하다　　**E** *dissertate*

> dissertatio, dissertationis, f. 논술, 논문　　**E** *dissertation*

> exsero, **exserui**, exsertum, exserĕre (< ex- *out of, away from* + serĕre *to join*)

뻗치다　　**E** *exsert, exert*

> *exertio, *exertionis, f. 발휘, 노력, 활동　　**E** *exertion, exertional*

> insero, **inserui**, insertum, inserĕre (< in- *in, on, into, toward* + serĕre *to join*)

끼우다, 접하다, 게재하다　　**E** *insert*

> insertio, insertionis, f. 끼워 넣기, 삽입, 닿는 곳, 부착　　**E** *insertion*

< IE. ser- *to line up*

> L. sermo, sermonis, m. (< *stringing together of words*) 말, 이야기, 설교　　**E** *sermon*

> (*perhaps*) L. sera, serae, f. (< *that which aligns*) 빗장, 걸쇠　　**E** *serried*

> L. sors, sortis, f. 추첨널쪽, 추첨, 추첨에 의해 배분된 몫, 신분, 운; (Sors) (로마 신화)

운명의 여신　　**E** *sort, (sort >) sorter, (sort >) assort*

> L. *sortiarius, *sortiarii, m. 마술사　　**E** *sorcerer*

> L. consors, consortis, m., f. (< con- (< cum) *with, together* + sors *lot*) 동료,

배우자　　**E** *consort*

> L. consortium, consortii, n. 공동체, 제휴, 연합　　**E** *consortium*

solvo, solvi, solutum, solvĕre 풀다, 용해시키다

E *solve*, (solvens (*present participle*) 'loosening' >) *solvent*, (solutus (*past participle*)
'loosened' >) *solute*, (solve >) *solvable*, (solvable >) *insolvable*

> solutio, solutionis, f. 해결, 해석, 용해, 용액　　**E** *solution (sol), cytosol (cytoplasmic matrix)*

> solubilis, solubile 풀 수 있는, 용해하는, 용해될 수 있는　　**E** *soluble, solubility, solubilize*

> insolubilis, insolubile (< in- *not*) 풀 수 없는, 불용성의　　**E** *insoluble, insolubility*

> absolvo, **absolvi**, absolutum, absolvĕre (< ab- *off, away from* + solvĕre *to loosen*)

풀어주다, 사면하다, 하던 일을 끝내다　　**E** *absolve*

> absolutus, absoluta, absolutum (*past participle*) 사면된, 완결된, 무조건의,

절대적인　　**E** *absolute*

> absolutio, absolutionis, f. 사면, 사죄, 면죄, 방면　　**E** *absolution*

> dissolvo, **dissolvi**, dissolutum, dissolvĕre (< dis- *apart from, down, not* + solvĕre

to loosen) 용해시키다, 분해시키다, 사라지게 하다　　**E** *dissolve*

> dissolutio, dissolutionis, f. 용해, 분해, 해소, 해체, 파멸　　**E** *dissolution*

> resolvo, **resolvi**, resolutum, resolvĕre (< re- *back, again* + solvĕre *to loosen*) 풀다,

용해시키다, 분해시키다, 끝내다, 해결하다　　**E** *resolve, resolvent*

> resolutus, resoluta, resolutum (*past participle*) 풀린, 해결된, 결심이 굳은   **E** *resolute*

> irresolutus, irresoluta, irresolutum (< ir- (< in- *not*) 풀리지 않은, 해결
되지 않은, 결심이 서지 않은   **E** *irresolute*

> resolutio, resolutionis, f. 해소, 해결, 결의; (물리) 분해능, 해상도   **E** *resolution*

< IE. leu- *to loosen, to divide, to cut*   **E** *lose, lost, loss, loose, loosen, lorn, forlorn, -less*

> L. lues, luis, f. (< *dissolution, putrefaction*) 진창, 재난, 역병, 매독   **E** *lues, luetic*

> G. lyein *to loosen, to release, to dissolve* (Vide LYSIS; *See* E. *lysis*)

spargo, sparsi, sparsum, spargĕre 씨앗을 뿌리다, 흩어지게 하다   **E** *sparge, sparse*

> aspergo, aspersi, aspersum, aspergĕre (< a- (< ad) *to, toward, at, according to*
+ spargĕre *to sprinkle, to strew*) 뿌리다, 퍼뜨리다, 몰래 집어넣다   **E** *asperse*

> aspergillum, aspergilli, n. 물뿌리개

> aspergillus, aspergilli, m. (< *from the resemblance of its fructification
to the brush used for sprinkling holy water*) 누룩곰팡이   **E** *aspergillus*

[용례] Aspergillus flavus 아스페르질루스
플라부스   **E** Aspergillus flavus, (A. flavus + *toxin* >) *aflatoxin*
(문법) aspergillus: 단수 주격
flavus 노란: 형용사, 남성형 단수 주격
< flavus, flava, flavum

> dispergo, dispersi, dispersum, dispergĕre (< di- (< dis-) *apart from, down, not*
+ spargĕre *to sprinkle, to strew*) 사방에 흩어지게 하다, 분산시키다   **E** *disperse*

> dispersio, dispersionis, f. 분산, 산란, 산포도   **E** *dispersion*

> interspergo, interspersi, interspersum, interspergĕre (< inter- *between, among* +
spargĕre *to sprinkle, to strew*) 흩뿌리다   **E** *intersperse*

< (*European root*) (s)preg- *to jerk, to scatter*   **E** *sprinkle, freckle (< 'that which is scattered on the face')*

*stinguo, *stinxi, *stinctum, *stinguĕre 쑤시다, 끄다

> distinguo, distinxi, distinctum, distinguĕre (< di- (< dis-) *apart from, down, not* +
*stinguĕre *to stick, to quench*) 구별하다   **E** *distinguish, distinctive*

> distinctus, distincta, distinctum (*past participle*) 구별된, 뚜렷한, 전혀 다른   **E** *distinct*

> ex(s)tinguo, ex(s)tinxi, ex(s)tinctum, ex(s)tinguĕre (< ex- *out of, away from* + *stinguĕre
to stick, to quench) 불을 끄다, 소멸하다   **E** *extinguish*

> ex(s)tinctus, ex(s)tincta, ex(s)tinctum (*past participle*) (불·빛 등이) 꺼진,
소멸된   **E** *extinct*

> instinguo, instinxi, instinctum, instinguĕre (< in- *in, on, into, toward* + *stinguĕre
to stick, to quench) 충동하다   **E** *instinctive*

> instinctus, instinctus, m. 충동, 본능   **E** *instinct*

< IE. steg-; stegh-; steig- (stei-) *stick, pointed, to stick, to prick*

> L. stimulus, stimuli, m. (가축을 몰거나 노예를 부릴 때 사용한) 끝이 뾰족한 막대,
자극물, 자극   **E** *stimulus,* (pl.) *stimuli*

> > L. stimulo, stimulavi, stimulatum, stimulare 찌르다, 자극하다, 흥분시키다,
격려하다   **E** *stimulate, stimulant,* (stimulate >) *stimulatory*

> > > L. stimulatio, stimulationis, f. 자극, 흥분, 격려   **E** *stimulation*

> > > L. stimulator, stimulatoris, m. 자극을 주는 사람, 자극기, 자극 물질 **E** *stimulator*

> L. stilus, stili, m. (stylus, styli, m. (*spelling and meaning influenced by unrelated*
G. stylos *pillar*)) 뾰족한 것, 철필, 문체, 형(型), 말뚝; (곤충) 침(針); (식물) 암술대,
화주(花柱) **E** *stylus, style, stylish, stylist, stylistic,* (It.) *stiletto,* (It. stiletto >) *stylet*

> L. instigo, instigavi, instigatum, instigare (< in- *in, on, into, toward* + *stigare
to spur on, to prod) 격려하다, 충동하다   **E** *instigate*

> G. stizein *to prick, to tattoo, to brand*

> > G. stiktos, stiktē, stikton *spotted, tattooed*

> > G. stigma, stigmatos, n. *prick, point, blemish, tattoo-mark, brand*

> > > L. stigma, stigmatis, n. 자국, 점, 오점, 낙인(烙印), 징표; (곤충의) 기공
(氣孔); 암술머리

> > > > L. physostigma, physostigmatis, n. (< *the style of the flower
becomes inflated above the stigma* < G. physa, physēs, f.
bellows, bladder, bubble + stigma) (나이지리아 지방에서 나는)
칼라바르 콩(*Calabar bean*)

> G. stachys, stachyos, m. *ear of corn, spike* **E** *stachyose* (< 'sugar from 'ear' of Stachys')

> G. stochos, stochou, m. (< *pointed stake used as a target for archers*) *target, aim,
guess*

> > G. stochazesthai (*middle*) *to aim at a mark, to guess*

> > > G. stochastikos, stochastikē, stochastikon *of guessing*   **E** *stochastic*

> (*suggested*) G. tigris, tigrios, f. (tigris, tigridos, f.) (< *from its sharp, pointed stripes*)
tiger

> > L. tigris, tigris, m., f. (tigris, tigridis, m., f.) 호랑이   **E** *tiger, tigroid*

strepo, strepui, strepitum, strepĕre 소란하다, 소란한 소리가 나다

> strepitus, strepitus, m. 잡음   **E** *strepitus*

strido, –, –, stridĕre (strideo, –, –, stridēre) 소음이 나다, 된소리 나다   E *strident*

> stridor, stridoris, m. 그렁거림, 협착음   E *stridor*

< IE. (s)trei- (*imitative root*) *to hiss, to buzz*

    > G. trismos, trismou, m. *grinding, scream*

        > L. trismus, trismi, m. (< *spasm of the muscles of the neck and lower jaw, causing the jaw to close rigidly*) 입벌림장애   E *trismus*

stringo, strinxi, strictum, stringĕre 조이다   E *strain, stringent, stringency*

> strictus, stricta, strictum (*past participle*) 조인, 좁은, 엄격한   E *strict, strait*

> strictura, stricturae, f. 조임, 협착   E *stricture*

> strigilis, strigilis, f. (고대 로마의) 때 미는 기구, 글겅이   E *strigil*

> astringo, astrinxi, astrictum, astringĕre (< ad- *to, toward, at, according to* + stringĕre *to draw tight*) 비끄러매다, 좁히다, (신맛·떫은 맛 등이) 혀를 죄어들게 하다, 수렴(收斂)시키다 (피부나 점막의 상처에 얇은 막을 만들어 보호하며, 혈관을 수축하고 체액의 분비를 억제하여 상처를 건조시킴으로써 저절로 낫도록 해주다)   E *astringent*

> constringo, constrinxi, constrictum, constringĕre (< con- (< cum) *with, together* + stringĕre *to draw tight*) 조이다, 졸라매다, 오그라들게 하다, 수렴(收斂)시키다, 제약 하다   E *constrain, constringent, constrict, constrictive, constraint*

    > constrictio, constrictionis, f. 조임, 수축(收縮), 협착(狹窄), 수렴(收斂)   E *constriction*

    > constrictor, constrictoris, m. 수축제, 수축근, 협착기   E *constrictor*

> distringo, distrinxi, districtum, distringĕre (< dis- *apart from, down, not* + stringĕre *to draw tight*) 벌리다, 분산시키다, 분주히 지내게 하다, 일에 얽매이게 하다, 정신 못 차리게 하다   E *distrain, district* (< '*territory drawn apart*'), ***distress***, ((*probably*) *distress* >) ***stress***

> praestringo, praestrinxi, praestrictum, praestringĕre (< prae- *before, beyond* + stringĕre *to draw tight*) 졸라매다, 눈부시게 하다, 홀리게 하다

    > praestigium, praestigii, n. (praestigiae, praestigiarum, f. (**pl.**)) 눈속임, 현혹   E *prestige* (< '*dazzling influence*')

> restringo, restrinxi, restrictum, restringĕre 제한하다 (< re- *back, again* + stringĕre *to draw tight*)   E *restrain, restrict, restrictive, restraint*

    > restrictio, restrictionis, f. 제한   E *restriction*

< (*European root*) streig- *to stroke, to rub, to press*   E *strike, stroke, streak*

    > L. stria, striae, f. 도랑, 밭이랑, 좁은 폭의 띠 구조, 선조(線條), 조(條), 줄, 선(線)   E *stria,* (*pl.*) *striae*

      [용례] striae distensae (pl.) 팽창선   E (*pl.*) *striae distensae*

        (문법) striae 선: 복수 주격

          distensae 팽창된: 과거분사, 여성형 복수 주격

            < distensus, distensa, distensum

              < distendo, distendi, distentum (distensum), distendĕre 넓히다, 팽창시키다

> L. striola, striolae, f. (< + -ola *diminutive suffix*) 작은 줄, 작은 선   **E** *striola*

> L. strio, **striavi**, striatum, striare 도랑 치다, 줄 치다   **E** *striatum, striate*

[용례] corpus striatum (< *from the intermixture of the medullary matter,*
which gives the appearance of furrows) 줄무늬체, 선조체

(線條體)   **E** *corpus striatum, palaeostriatum (paleostriatum), neostriatum*

(문법) corpus 몸, 체(體): 단수 주격 < corpus, corporis, n.

striatum 줄 쳐진: 과거분사, 중성형 단수 주격

< striatus, striata, striatum

struo, struxi, structum, struĕre 세우다, 짓다

> structura, structurae, f. 건축, 구조물,

구조   **E** *structure, structural, (structure >) infrastructure, (structure >) ultrastructure*

> struma, strumae, f. (< *swelling, tumor*) 갑상샘종   **E** *struma, strumal*

> industrius, industria, industrium (< *indu-struus < indu- *within* + struĕre *to build*)

부지런한

> industria, industriae, f. 근면, 산업   **E** *industry, (industry >) industrial, industrialize*

> industriosus, industriosa, industriosum 부지런한   **E** *industrious*

> construo, **construxi**, constructum, construĕre (< con- *with, together; intensive* + struĕre

to build) 짓다, 건설하다, 구성하다

E *construct, constructive, reconstructive; construe* (< *to analyze the construction of a*
sentence'), (construe >) misconstrue

> constructio, constructionis, f. 건설, 구성   **E** *construction, reconstruction*

> destruo, **destruxi**, destructum, destruĕre (< de- *apart from, down, not* + struĕre

to build) 파괴하다   **E** *destroy, destructive*

> destructio, destructionis, f. 파괴   **E** *destruction*

> instruo, **instruxi**, instructum, instruĕre (< in- *in, on, into, toward* + struĕre *to build*)

만들다, 배치하다, 교육하다   **E** *instruct, instructive*

> instructio, instructionis, f. 교육, 지시, 명령   **E** *instruction*

> instrumentum, instrumenti, n. 도구, 기구, 기기,

장비   **E** *instrument, instrumental, instrumentation*

> obstruo, **obstruxi**, obstructum, obstruĕre (< ob- *before, toward(s), over, against, away*

+ struĕre *to build*) 막다, 폐쇄하다, 방어하다   **E** *obstruct, obstructive, obstruent*

> obstructio, obstructionis, f. 막음, 막힘, 폐쇄   **E** *obstruction*

> substruo, **substruxi**, substructum, substruĕre (< sub- *under, up from under* + struĕre

to build) 짓다, 건축하다   **E** *substructure*

< IE. sterə-, ster- *to spread* **E** *strain* (< *'offspring'), strew, straw* (< *'that which is scattered'), strawberry*

> L. sterno, **stravi**, stratum, sternĕre 펴다, 평탄케 하다, 깔다, 덮다,

넘어뜨리다   **E** *(strata via 'paved road' >) street*

> L. stratum, strati, n. 요, 이불, 층, 지층, 계층   **E** *stratum, (pl.) strata, stratosphere*

[용례] stratum basale (stratum germinativum) (< *basal layer,*

Malphigian layer) 바닥층, 기저층(基底層),

배아층(杯芽層)　　　　　E *stratum basale (stratum germinativum)*

stratum spinosum (< *spinous layer, prickle cell layer*) 유극(有棘)

세포층　　　　　　　　E *stratum spinosum*

stratum granulosum (< *granular layer*) 과립층(顆粒層)　E *stratum granulosum*

stratum lucidum (< *clear layer*) 담명층(淡明層)　　　E *stratum lucidum*

stratum corneum (< *horny layer, cornified layer, keratinized layer*)

각질층(角質層)　　　　　　E *stratum corneum*

(문법) stratum 층: 단수 주격

basale 기초의, 기본적인, 바닥의: 형용사, 중성형

단수 주격 < basalis, basale

germinativum 움트는, 발아성(發芽性)의: 형용사, 중성형

단수 주격 < germinativus, germinativa, germinativum

spinosum 가시 많은, 가시의, 뾰족한, 까다로운: 형용사, 중성형

단수 주격 < spinosus, spinosa, spinosum

granulosum 작은 알맹이가 많은, 과립의: 형용사, 중성형

단수 주격 < granulosus, granulosa, granulosum

corneum 뿔의, 뿔로 만든, 각질(角質)의: 형용사, 중성형

단수 주격 < corneus, cornea, corneum

> L. stratifico, **stratificavi**, stratificatum, stratificare (< stratum *something spread, something laid down* + -ficare (< facĕre) *to make*) 층으로 배열하다, 층을 이루다, 계층화하다　　　　　E *stratify*

> L. stratus, strati, n. 층운(層雲)　　　E *stratus,* (pl.) *strati*

> L. consterno, **consternavi**, consternatum, consternare (< con- *with, together; intensive* + sternĕre *to lay flat*) 놀라게 하다, 당황하게 하다　E *constrate*

> L. prosterno, **prostravi**, prostratum, prosternĕre (< pro- *before, forward, for, instead of* + sternĕre *to lay flat*) 쓰러뜨리다, 부복시키다, 탈진시키다, 타락시키다　　　　　　　　　　　　　E *prostrate*

> L. prostratio, prostrationis, f. 엎드림, 부복, 쇠약, 허탈　E *prostration*

> L. substerno, **substravi**, substratum, substernĕre (< sub- *under, up from under* + sternĕre *to lay flat*) 밑에 깔다, 굴복시키다

> L. substratum, substrati, n. 기반, 기체(基體), 하층, 기층(基層), 기질(基質)　　　　　E *substratum,* (pl.) *substrata, substrate*

> G. sternon, sternou, n. *breast, breastbone*

> L. sternum, sterni, n. 흉골(胸骨), 복장뼈　　　E *sternum, stern(o)-, sternocleidomastoid; sternoclavicular*

> L. sternalis, sternale 흉골의, 복장뼈의　　　E *sternal*

> G. stratos, stratou, m. *army*　　　E *stratocracy*

> G. stratēgos, stratēgou, m. (< + agein *to lead*) *general (in Athens, the title of ten officers elected each year to command the army and navy)*

> G. stratēgia, stratēgias, f. (*at Athens*) *the office of* stragēgos, *command,*

generalship

> L. strategia, strategiae, f. 군사령부, 용병술, 작전,
전략(戰略)　　　　　　　　　　　　　　　　　　　**E** *strategy, strategic*

> G. stratēgein (stratēgeein) *to be a general, to command*

> G. stratēgēma, stratēgēmatos, n. *a piece of generalship,
stratagem*

> L. strategema, stratematis, n. 술책(術策), 책략(策略)　　**E** *stratagem*

> G. strōma, strōmatos, n. *mattress, bed*

> L. stroma, stromatis, n. 침대요, 버팀질

E *stroma*, (pl.) *stromata, stromal*, (stroma + -lite (< G. lithos) *'stone'* > *'layered
stone'* >) *stromatolite*

sugo, suxi, suctum, sugĕre 빨다, 흡인하다, 흡입하다

> L. suctio, suctionis, f. 빨기, 흡인, 흡입　　　　　　　　**E** *suction*

> L. suctorius, suctoria, suctorium 빠는, 흡인하는, 흡인기관이 있는　　**E** *suctorial*

< IE. seuə- *to take liquid*　　　　　**E** *sup, supper, soup, sip, suck, suckling, soak*

> L. succus, succi, m. (sucus, suci, m.) 즙, 맛, 활력소

> L. succulentus, succulenta, succulentum (suculentus, suculenta, suculentum)

즙이 많은　　　　　　　　　　　　　　　　　　　　**E** *succulent*

> G. hyein *to rain*

> G. hyetos, hyetou, m. *rain*　　　　　　　　　　　　　**E** *hyetometer*

suo, sui, sutum, suĕre 바느질하다, 깁다, 꿰매다, 기우다, 붙이다

> sutura, suturae, f. 봉합, 봉합술　　　　　　　　　　　**E** *suture, sutural*

< IE. syu-, su- *to bind, to sew*　　　　　　　　　　　**E** *sew, seam*

> L. subula, subulae, f. 바늘, 침(針), 송곳

> L. subulatus, subulata, subulatum 송곳 모양의　　　**E** *subulate*

> G. hymēn, hymenos, m. *thin skin, membrane;* (Hymēn) (*Greek mythology*) *the god
of marriage*

> L. hymen, hymenis, m. 처녀막　　　**E** *hymen, (hymen >) hymenal, hymen(o)-*

> L. Hymen, Hymenis, m. (그리스 신화) 결혼의 신　　　**E** *Hymen*

> G. hymenaios, hymenaia, hymenaion *of wedlock*

> L. hymenaeus, hymenaea, hymenaeum 결혼의　　　　**E** *hymeneal*

> (*Sanskrit*) sutram *thread, string,*
(*hence*) *rule*　　　　**E** *sutra*, ((*Sanskrit*) kamah *'love'* + sutram *'rule'* >) *Kamasutra*

tango, tetigi, tactum, tangĕre 만지다, 접촉하다, 접(接)하다; 감동시키다, 취급하다

> tangens, (gen.) tangentis (*present participle*) 접하는　　　**E** *tangent*

> *tangentia, *tangentiae, f. 접함; (수학) 접선(接線)

> tangentialis, tangentiale 접하는, 접선의, 스치는, 탈선하는   E *tangential*

> tactus, tactus, m. 접촉, 촉각; 솜씨   E *tactus, tactual; tact*

> tactilis, tactile 접촉할 수 있는, 촉감의, 촉각의   E *tactile*

> tangibilis, tangibile 만질 수 있는, 접촉할 수 있는   E *tangible*

> intangibilis, intangibile (< in- *not*) 만질 수 없는, 실체가 없는, 막연한   E *intangible*

> taxo, **taxavi**, taxatum, taxare (*frequentative*) 자주 세게 손대다, 만져 보고 감정하다,

값을 매기다, 세금을 매기다,

부과하다   E *tax, (taximeter cab >) taxi, task (< 'imposing a tax on'); taste, tastant*

> taxatio, taxationis, f. 감정(鑑定), 과세   E *taxation*

> intactus, intacta, intactum (< in- *not* + tactus (*past participle*) *touched*) 손을 대지

않은, 손상 없는, 원래대로의, 완전한   E *intact*

> integer, **integra**, integrum (< in- *not* + tag- *stem of* tangĕre *to touch*) 손을 대지

않은, 옹근, 통째로의; (수학) 정수의   E *integer (< 'not fractional'), integrin, entire*

> integritas, integritatis, f. 온전함, 완전, 무결   E *integrity, entirety*

> integralis, integrale 통합된, 일체화된, (전체의 일부로서) 필수의; (수학) 정수의,

적분의   E *integral*

> integro, **integravi**, integratum, integrare 옹글게 하다,

통합하다   E *integrate, integrant, integrase, (integrate >) disintegrate*

> redintegro, **redintegravi**, redintegratum, redintegrare (< red- *back, again*

+ integrare *to make whole*) 전의 완전한 상태로 되돌리다, 원상복구

하다   E *redintegrate*

> attingo, **attigi**, attactum, attingĕre (< ad- *to, toward, at, according to* + tangĕre

to touch) 다다르다, 마주치다, 손에 넣다   E *attain, attainable*

> contingo, **contigi**, contactum, contingĕre (< con- (< cum) *with, together* + tangĕre

to touch) 닿다, 접촉하다; 닥치다, 일어나다   E *contact, (contact >) contactant*

> contigens, (gen.) contigentis (*present participle*) 부수적으로 일어나는, 우연의,

우발적   E *contingent*

> contigentia, contigentiae, f. 부수적 사건, 우연, 우발   E *contingency*

> contiguus, contigua, contiguum 닿는 거리에 있는, 인접한, 연속된   E *contiguous*

> contiguitas, contiguitatis, f. 접촉, 인접, 연속   E *contiguity*

> contagio, contagionis, f. (contagium, contagii, n.) 관련성, 접촉감염,

병폐   E *contagion (contagium)*

> contagiosus, contagiosa, contagiosum 접촉성의, 접촉감염의   E *contagious*

> contamino, **contaminavi**, contaminatum, contaminare (< con- (< cum) *with, together*

+ tag- *stem of* tangĕre *to touch*) 더럽히다   E *contaminate, contaminant*

> contaminatio, contaminatioionis, f. 오염   E *contamination*

< IE. tag- *to touch, to handle*

tego, texi, tectum, tegĕre 덮다, 은폐하다, 보호하다

> tectum, tecti, n. 지붕, 거처, 소굴; 덮개, 개(蓋)   E *tectum*

> tector, tectoris, m. 도장(塗裝), 미장이

> tectorius, tectoria, tectorium 덮는 데 쓰는, 칠하는 데 쓰는   **E** *tectorial*

> tegula, tegulae, f. 지붕, 기와, 타일   **E** *tile, tegular*

> tegmen, tegminis, n. (tegumen, teguminis, n.) 덮개, 보호물, 옷   **E** *tegmen*

> tegmentum, tegmenti, n. (tegumentum, tegumenti, n.) 덮개, 보호물, 옷   **E** *tegmentum, tegument*

> detego, **detexi**, detectum, detegĕre (< de- *apart from, down, not* + tegĕre *to cover*)

     벗기다, 드러나게 하다, 탐지하다, 검출하다   **E** *detect, detective*

     > detectio, detectionis, f. 탐지, 검출   **E** *detection*

> intego, **intexi**, intectum, integĕre (< in- *in, on, into, toward* + tegĕre *to cover*) 덮다,

     보호하다

     > integumentum, integumenti, n. 덮개, 옷, 외피, 피부   **E** *integument, integumentary*

> protego, **protexi**, protectum, protegĕre (< pro- *before, forward, for, instead of* +

     tegĕre *to cover*) 앞을 가리다, 보호하다   **E** *protect, protective; osteoprotegerin*

     > protectio, protectionis, f. 보호   **E** *protection*

< IE. (s)teg- *to cover*   **E** *deck, thatch*

     > L. toga, togae, f. 로마 시민의 겉옷, 로마 시민권   **E** *toga, togavirus* (< 'enveloped virus')

     > G. stegein *to cover, to conceal, to protect*

         > G. stegē, stegēs, f. (stegos, stegou, n.) *covering, roof, shelter*

            > L. Stegodon, Stegodontis, m. (< *ridged teeth* < + G. odous, odontos, m.

                tooth) (대형 화석 코끼리) 스테고돈속(屬)   **E** *stegodon*

            > L. Stegosaurus, Stegosauri, m. (< *roof lizard, armored lizard* < + G.

                sauros, saurou, m. *lizard*) 검룡속(劍龍屬)   **E** *stegosaurus (stegosaur)*

tero, trivi, tritum, terĕre 비비다, 분쇄하다   **E** *trite*

     > tritus, tritus, m. 마찰, 분쇄, 방아질

         > triticum, tritici, n. 밀, 보리, 소맥, 곡식

            > triticeus, triticea, triticeum 밀의, 밀알을 닮은, 곡식의   **E** *triticeous*

                > triticeum, triticei, n. (< cartilago triticea *triticeous cartilage*)

                    밀알 모양 연골   **E** *triticeum*

     > tritura, triturae, f. 마찰, 분쇄, 방아질   **E** *triturate*

     > tribulum, tribuli, n. (알곡을 찧는) 맷돌

         > tribulo, **tribulavi**, tribulatum, tribulare 맷돌로 찧다, 짓누르다

            > tribulatio, tribulationis, f. 고난   **E** *tribulation*

     > teres, (gen.) teretis 가늘고 둥그런 원통 모양의   **E** *terete*

         [용례] musculus teres 원근(圓筋)   **E** *teres (muscle)*

         ligamentum teres 원인대(圓靭帶)   **E** *ligamentum teres*

         (문법) musculus 근육, 근: 단수 주격 < musculus, musculi, m.

            ligamentum 인대: 단수 주격 < ligamentum, ligamenti, n.

            teres: 형용사, 남·여·중성형 단수 주격

     > termes, termitis, f. 나무 먹는 벌레, 흰개미   **E** *termite*

     > attero, **attrivi**, attritum, atterĕre (< ad- *to, toward, at, according to* + terĕre *to rub*)

닳게 하다, 마모시키다

> attritio, attritionis, f. 마모, 마손; (죄로 인한 영혼의 마모에 대한) 뉘우침, 참회(懺悔)

E *attrite*

E *attrition*

> contero, **contrivi**, contritum, conterĕre (< con- (< cum) *with, together; intensive* + terĕre *to rub*) 가루로 만들다, 분쇄하다

E *contrite*

> contritio, contritionis, f. 분쇄; (죄로 인한 영혼의 분쇄에 대한) 아픈 뉘우침, 통회(痛悔)

E *contrition*

> detero, **detrivi**, detritum, deterĕre (< de- *apart from, down, not* + terĕre *to rub*) 닳아지게 하다, 탈곡하다

> detritus, detritus, m. 퇴폐물(頹廢物), 치구(齒垢)

E *detritus*

> detritio, detritionis, f. 마멸

E *detrition*

> detrimentum, detrimenti, n. 손실, 상해

E *detrimental*

> retero, **retrivi**, retritum, reterĕre (< re- *back, again* + terĕre *to rub*) 몹시 닳게 하다, 키질하다

> retrimentum, retrimenti, n. 찌꺼기, 배설물

E *retrimentum*

< IE. terə- *to rub, to turn; with some derivatives referring to twisting, boring, drilling, and piercing; and others referring to the rubbing of cereal grain to remove the husks, and thence to the process of threshing either by the trampling of oxen or by flailing with flails*

E *thrash, thresh, threshold* (< '*sill of a door over which one treads*'), *drill, throw* (< '*to turn, to twist*'), *thread* (< '*twisted yarn*')

> L. tergeo, **tersi**, tersum, tergēre 씻다, 깨끗이 하다

> L. tersus, tersa, tersum (*past participle*) 씻은, 산뜻한

E *terse*

> L. detergeo, **detersi**, detersum, detergēre (< de- *apart from, down, not* + tergēre *to wipe*) 씻어내다, 세척하다

E *deterge, detergent*

> G. tribein *to rub*

E *triboelectricity*

> G. tripsis, tripseōs, f. *rubbing*

E *tripsis, -tripsis, syntripsis* (< '*comminution of a bone*' < '*rubbing together*'); *trypsin* (< '*first obtained by rubbing down the pancreas with glycerin*'), (*trypsin* >) *tryptic, trypsinogen, chymotrypsin* (< '*a proteolytic enzyme secreted in the pancreatic juice, activated by trypsin*'), *tryptophan (Trp, W)* (< '*appeared during pancreatic (tryptic) digestion of proteins*')

> G. thripsis, thripseōs, f. *shattering into pieces*

E *thripsis, -thripsis,* (chromosome + thripsis >) *chromothripsis*

> G. trypan (trypaein) *to bore*

> G. trypanon, trypanou, n. *borer*

> L. trepanum, trepani, n. 관상톱(*crown saw*), 원통톱(*hole saw*)

E *trepan,* (trepan >) *trepanation*

> L. Trypanosoma, Trypanosomatis, n. (< *corkscrew-like motion* < G. trypanon + soma *body*) (원충 原蟲) 트리파노소마속(屬); 트리파노소마, 파동편모충(波動鞭毛蟲)

E *Trypanosoma, trypanosome*

> G. tresis, treseōs, f. *holing*

> L. atresia, atresiae, f. (< G. a- *not*) 폐쇄(閉鎖), 폐쇄증　E *atresia, atretic*

> G. trēma, trēmatos, n. *hole*

　　> L. Trematoda, Trematodorum, n. (pl.) (< + G. -ōdēs *like, resembling*)

　　　(편형동물) 흡충강(吸蟲綱)　E *trematode*

　　> L. Monotremata, Monotrematorum, n. (pl.) (< G. monos *alone*)

　　　(동물) (오리너구리 등) 단공목(單孔目)　E *monotreme*

　　> L. helicotrema, helicotrematis, n. (< G. helix, helikos, f. *winding,*

　　　spire, coil, anything twisted) 달팽이구멍, 와우공(蝸牛孔)　E *helicotrema*

> G. trauma, traumatos, n. *wound, loss*

　> L. trauma, traumatis, n. 외상(外傷), 손상(損傷)

　　E *trauma,* (pl.) *traumata, traumatize, traumatology, barotrauma* (< *'injury caused by pressure changes'*)

　> G. traumatikos, traumatikē, traumatikon *of wound, of loss*

　　> L. traumaticus, traumatica, traumaticum 외상의, 손상의　E *traumatic, atraumatic*

> G. tornos, tornou, m. *lathe, compasses*

　> L. tornus, torni, m. 도공용(陶工用) 녹로(轆轤), 선반(旋盤), 회전, 주위, 일주

　　> L. torno, **tornavi**, tornatum, tornare 손질하다, 돌리다, 모서리를 깎다,

　　　둥글게 하다, 회전하다

　　　E *turn, return, turnover, tour, tournament, tourniquet* (< *'a bandage tightened by twisting a rigid bar put through it'*), *contour, detour, attorney* (< *'one appointed or constituted'*)

> IE. treg- *to gnaw*

　> G. tragos, tragou, m. *he-goat*

　　> G. tragōidia, tragōidias, f. (< (*suggested*) *goatskin dress of the performers,*

　　　representing satyrs; goat-song < tragos + ōidē *song*) *tragedy*

　　　> L. tragoedia, tragoediae, f. 비극(悲劇)　E *tragedy*

　　> G. tragikos, tragikē, tragikon (< *of he-goat, but in sense associated*

　　　with tragedy) *tragic*

　　　> L. tragicus, tragica, tragicum 비극의　E *tragic*

　　> G. tragakantha, tragakanthēs, f. (< + akantha *thorn, thistle*) *goat's-*

　　　thorn, tragacanth-shrub

　　　> L. tragacantha, tragacanthae, f. 트래거캔스 고무나무, 그 수액　E *tragacanth*

　　> L. tragus, tragi, m. 귀구슬,

　　　이주(耳珠)　E *tragus* (< *'hair tuft like a goat's beard'*), *intertragic*

　　　> L. antitragus, antitragi, m. (< G. ant(i)- *before, against, instead*

　　　　of) 맞구슬, 대주(對珠)　E *antitragus*

> (*suggested*) IE. treik- *to rub, to turn*

　> L. tricae, tricarum, f. (pl.) 하찮은 일, 객쩍은 소리; 곤혹, 난관

　　> L. tricor, tricatus sum, tricari 말썽을 일으키다, 트집 잡다,

　　　빈정대다　E (*suggested*) *trick, tricky, treachery, treacherous*

　　　> L. extrico, **extricavi**, extricatum, extricare (< ex- *out of, away*

from + tricari *to raise difficulties, to play tricks*) 벗어나게 하다, 해결하다

> L. extricabilis, extricabile 벗어나게 할 수 있는, 해결할 수 있는 `E` *extricable*

　　> L. inextricabilis, inextricabile (< in- *not*) 벗어나게 할 수 없는, 해결할 수 없는 `E` *inextricable*

　> L. intrico, intricavi, intricatum, intricare (< in- *in, on, into, toward* + tricari *to raise difficulties, to play tricks*) 당황케 하다, 엉키게 하다 `E` *intricate, intricacy, intrigue*

texo, texui, textum, texĕre 짜다, 엮다, 얽다, 집을 짓다, 이야기 속에 엮어 넣다 `E` *tissue*

> textus, textus, m. 엮음, 베, 구조, 문맥 `E` *text, textual*

> textura, texturae, f. 베, 구조, 조직 `E` *texture, textural*

> textilis, textile 짠, 엮은, 얽은, 베의 `E` *textile*

> tela, telae, f. 베, 직물, 거미줄, 날실, 막, 조직 `E` *toilet, (toilet >) toiletry*

　> subtilis, subtile (< sub- *under, up from under* + tela *web, net, warp of a fabric*) (날실 밑을 지나는) 씨실의, (*the finest thread* >) 가는, 섬세한, 정교한, 예민한, 미묘한 `E` *subtle*

　　[용례] Bacillus subtilis (< *fine rod*) 고초균(枯草菌) `E` Bacillus subtilis
　　(문법) Bacillus 바실루스속(屬): 단수 주격
　　　　< bacillus, bacilli, m. 작은 막대기, 막대균, 간균(桿菌), 바실루스; (Bacillus) (세균) 바실루스속(屬)
　　　　< baculus, baculi, m. (baculum, baculi, n.) 지팡이, 막대기
　　　　subtilis 가는: 형용사, 남·여성형 단수 주격

　　>subtilitas, subtilitatis, f. 가냘픔, 섬세함, 정교, 예민, 미묘 `E` *subtlety*

> contexo, contexui, contextum, contexĕre (< con- (< cum) *with, together* + texĕre *to weave*) 짜다, 짜 맞추다, 연결하다, (전후 관계·문맥을) 결부시키다 `E` *context*

> praetexo, praetexui, praetextum, praetexĕre (< prae- *before, beyond* + texĕre *to weave*) 앞자락을 짜다, 첫머리에 엮어 놓다, 앞을 장식하다, 앞을 가리다, 호도(糊塗)하다, 빙자(憑藉)하다 `E` *pretext*

< IE. teks- *to weave; also to fabricate, especially with an ax; also to make wicker or wattle fabric for (mud-covered) house walls*

> G. tektōn, tektonos, m. *carpenter, builder*

　> G. tektonikos, tektonikē, tektonikon *pertaining to building*

　　> L. tectonicus, tectonica, tectonicum 축조의, 구조의; (지질) 지각 구조의 `E` *tectonic, (tectonic >) tectonism*

　> G. architektōn, architektonos, m. (< archē *beginning, principle, power, rule, magistracy* + tektōn) *architect, engineer* `E` *architectonic*

　　> L. architectus, architecti, m. 건축가 `E` *architect*

　　　> L. architectura, architecturae, f. 건축 `E` *architecture*

> G. technē, technēs, f. *craft (of weaving or fabricating),*
>> *art*　　　　　　　　　　　　　　　　　　　　　E *technology, technocracy, technocrat*
>> > G. technikos, technikē, technikon *skillful, artistic*
>> >> > L. technicus, technica, technicum 기술적인,
>> >>> 숙달된　　　　　　　　　　　　　　E *technic, technical,* F. *technique, polytechnic*
>> > G. technasthai *to make by art*
>> >> > G. technētos, technētē, technēton
>> >>> *artificial*　　　　　E *technetium (Tc)* (< *'the first artificially made element'*)
> (*Sanskrit*) tasta (tashta) *cup*
>> > L. testa, testae, f. 질그릇, 질그릇 조각, 기와; 겉껍질,
>>> 거북딱지　　　　　　　　　E *testa, test* (< *'jug, shell'*), *testy* (< *'headstrong'*)
>>> > L. testaceus, testacea, testaceum 겉껍질의, (동물·식물) 적갈색의　E *testaceous*
>>> > L. testudo, testudinis, f. 거북딱지, 거북이, 남생이, 거북 등 모양으로 만든
>>>> 악기, 귀갑(龜甲) 방어　　　　　　　　　　　　　　　　E *testudo*
>>> > L. testum, testi, n. 질그릇 > 골회(骨灰) 도가니
>>>> E *test* (< *'from the use of the cupel in treating or examining the metals'*)

traho, traxi, tractum, trahĕre 잡아당기다, 견인하다

E *train* (< *'that which drags or trails or is trailed, a suite or sequence of persons or things; to treat or manipulate so as to bring to the proper or desired form, specifically in gardening, to manage a plant or branch so as to cause it to grow in some desired form or direction, especially against a wall or upon a trellis or the like'*)

> tractus, tractus, m. 잡아당김, 관(管), 도(道), 로(路), 속(束), 삭(索), 인대(靭帶), 끌림,
> 흔적

　E *tract, trait* (< *'a particular feature of mind or character'* < *'stroke of the pen or pencil in a picture'*), *trace* (< *'path that someone or something takes'*), *tracer, traceable*

> tractio, tractionis, f. 잡아당김, 견인　　　　　　　　　　　　E *traction*
> tractor, tractoris, m. 끄는 것, 견인에 쓰는 것, 트랙터　　　　　E *tractor*
> tragula, tragulae, f. 끝에 가죽 끈이 달린 창, 사립짝, 끌그물[曳網]　E *trail, trailer*
> tracto, tractavi, tractatum, tractare (*frequentative*) 다루다, (사람을) 대하다,
> 논하다　　　　　E *treat,* (treat >) *treatment, treatise, entreat, entreaty*
>> > tractatus, tractatus, m. 다루기, 취급, 검토, 논(論), 조약　　E *treaty*
>> > tractabilis, tractabile 다룰 수 있는　　　　　　　　　　E *tractable*
>> >> >intractabilis, intractabile (< in- *not*) 다루기 어려운, 난치의　E *intractable*
> abstraho, abstraxi, abstractum, abstrahĕre (< abs- (< ab) *off, away from* + trahĕre
> *to draw*) 다른 데로 끌어내다, 다른 데로 빼내다, 추출(抽出)하다,
> 추상(推象)하다　　　　　　　　　　　　　E *abstract, abstractive*
>> > abstractio, abstractionis, f. 추출, 추상　　　　　　　　E *abstraction*
> attraho, attraxi, attractum, attrahĕre (< at- (< ad) *to, toward, at, according to* +
> trahĕre *to draw*) 끌어당기다

E *attract,* *(attract* + *-ant* (*Latin present participle suffix*) >) *attractant, chemoattractant,* *attractive*

> attractio, attractionis, f. 끌어당기기, 유인, 인력, 매력   **E** *attraction*

> contraho, **contraxi**, contractum, contrahĕre (< con- (< cum) *with, together* + trahĕre *to draw*) 서로 잡아당기다, 좁히다, 수축(收縮)시키다, 한데 모으다, (계약을) 체결 하다, 저지르다, 병에 걸리다   **E** *contract, contractile, contractility, subcontract*

> contractio, contractionis, f. 수축(收縮), 축약(縮約)   **E** *contraction*

> contractura, contracturae, f. 구축(拘縮)   **E** *contracture*

> detraho, **detraxi**, detractum, detrahĕre (< de- *apart from, down, not* + trahĕre *to draw*) 떼어내다, 헐뜯다, 훼손시키다   **E** *detract*

> distraho, **distraxi**, distractum, distrahĕre (< dis- *apart from, down, not* + trahĕre *to draw*) 사방으로 잡아당기다, 떼어내다, 마음을 산만하게 하다, 주의를 산만하게 하다   **E** *distract, distraught*

> extraho, **extraxi**, extractum, extrahĕre (< ex- *out of, away from* + trahĕre *to draw*) 밖으로 잡아당기다, 뽑아내다, 적출(摘出)하다, 추출(抽出)하다, 발췌(拔萃)하다

E *(verb)* *extract,* *(extract* + *-ant* (*Latin present participle suffix*) >) *extractant, extractor*

> extractum, extracti, n. 적출물(摘出物), 추출물(抽出物), 발췌물(拔萃物)   **E** *(noun) extract*

> extractio, extractionis, f. 적출, 추출, 발췌   **E** *extraction*

> protraho, **protraxi**, protractum, protrahĕre (< pro- *before, forward, for, instead of* + trahĕre *to draw*) 끌어내다, 밀어내다, 늘이다; 오래 끌다; 드러내 보이다, 묘사하다, 제도(製圖)하다   **E** *protract, protractor, portray, portrait*

> protractio, protractionis, f. 적출(摘出), 돌출(突出), 신장(伸長); 오래 끌기, 연장; 제도(製圖)   **E** *protraction*

> retraho, **retraxi**, retractum, retrahĕre (< re- *back, again* + trahĕre *to draw*) 다시 잡아당기다, 움츠리다, 철회하다, 퇴축(退縮)하다   **E** *retract, retreat, retractor, retractile, retractable*

> retractio, retractionis, f. 뒷당김, 움츠림, 철회, 퇴축   **E** *retraction*

> subtraho, **subtraxi**, subtractum, subtrahĕre (< sub- *under, up from under* + trahĕre *to draw*) 밑에서 잡아당기다, 빼다, 빼앗다   **E** *subtract*

> subtractio, subtractionis, f. 빼기   **E** *subtraction*

< IE. tragh- *to draw, to drag, to move*

> IE. dhragh- (*rhyming variant of* tragh-) *to draw, to drag on the ground*   **E** *draw, withdraw, withdrawal, drag, draggle, dray, draught (draft)*

> IE. dhreg- *to draw, to glide*

E *drink* (< '*to draw into the mouth*'), *drunkard, drench* (< '*to cause to drink*'), *drown*

trudo, trusi, trusum, trudĕre 밀치다, 쫓아내다

> trusio, trusionis, f. 밀치기, 뻐드렁니   **E** *trusion*

> abstrudo, **abstrusi**, abstrusum, abstrudĕre (< abs- (< ab) *off, away from* + trudĕre *to thrust*) 숨기다

> abstrusus, abstrusa, abstrusum (< *past participle*) 숨겨진, 난해한, 심오한　**E** *abstruse*

> detrudo, **detrusi**, detrusum, detrudĕre (< de- *apart from, down, not* + trudĕre
to thrust) 밀어젖히다, 빠뜨리다, 밀어내다　**E** *detrude*

　> detrusio, detrusionis, f. 밀어젖힘, 밀어냄　**E** *detrusion*

　> detrusor, detrusoris, m. 압박기(壓迫器), 배뇨근(排尿筋)　**E** *detrusor*

> extrudo, **extrusi**, extrusum, extrudĕre (< ex- *out of, away from* + trudĕre *to thrust*)
밀어내다, 내밀다, 돌출하다, 분출하다　**E** *extrude*

　> *extrusio, *extrusionis, f. 밀어냄, 내밀기, 돌출, 분출　**E** *extrusion*

> intrudo, **intrusi**, intrusum, intrudĕre (< in- *in, on, into, toward* + trudĕre *to thrust*)
들이밀다, 밀어 넣다, 끼어들다　**E** *intrude*

　> intrusio, intrusionis, f. 들이밀기, 밀어 넣기, 끼어들기　**E** *intrusion*

> obtrudo, **obtrusi**, obtrusum, obtrudĕre (< ob- *before, toward(s), over, against, away*
+ trudĕre *to thrust*) 떼밀다, 강요하다　**E** *obtrude, obtrusive*

　> obtrusio, obtrusionis, f. 강요　**E** *obtrusion*

> protrudo, **protrusi**, protrusum, protrudĕre (< pro- *before, forward, for, instead of*
+ trudĕre *to thrust*) 내밀다, 튀어나오다　**E** *protrude*

　> protrusio, protrusionis, f. 튀어나옴, 돌출　**E** *protrusion*

> retrudo, **retrusi**, retrusum, retrudĕre (< re- *back, again* + trudĕre *to thrust*) 뒤로
밀치다, 밀쳐 넣다　**E** *retrude, retrusive*

　> *retrusio, *retrusionis, f. 후퇴, 후방 전위　**E** *retrusion*

< IE. treud- *to squeeze*　**E** *thrust, threat*

tundo, tutudi, tunsum (tusum), tundĕre 때리다, 바수다, 녹초가 되게 하다, 괴롭히다

　> contundo, **contudi**, contunsum (contusum), contundĕre (< con- (< cum) *with, together;
intensive* + tundĕre *to beat*) 때려 부수다, 멍들게 하다　**E** *contuse*

　　> contusio, contusionis, f. 짓이김, 타박상　**E** *contusion*

　> obtundo, **obtudi**, obtunsum (obtusum), obtundĕre (< ob- *before, toward(s), over,
against, away* + tundĕre *to beat*) 두들기다, (칼날·각을) 무디게 하다, (감각·
기능을) 둔하게 하다　**E** *obtund, obtundent, (obtund >) obtundation*

　　> obtusus, obtusa, obtusum (*past participle*) 얻어맞은, (칼날·각이) 무딘; (식물)
(잎·꽃잎 등의) 끝이 둥그스름한, 둔한　**E** *obtuse*

　> pertundo, **pertudi**, pertunsum (pertusum), pertundĕre (< per- *through, thoroughly*
+ tundĕre *to beat*) 꿰뚫다, 관통하다　**E** *pierce*

　> retundo, **retudi**, retunsum (retusum), retundĕre (< re- *back, again* + tundĕre *to beat*)
눌러 놓다, 둔화시키다, 약화시키다　**E** *retuse*

< IE. (s)teu- *to push, to stick, to knock, to beat; with derivatives referring to projecting
objects, fragments, and certain related expressive notions and qualities*

E *steep, steeple, stoop, step- (< 'bereft' < 'pushed out'), stub (< 'tree stump'), stock (<
'tree trunk'), stoker (< 'one who pokes a furnace'), (stoker >) stoke, stutter (< 'to knock'),
stucco (< 'piece, crust')*

> L. studeo, studui, −, studēre (< *to be pressing forward*) 몰두하다, 노력하다, 공부

하다, 연구하다

> L. studium, studii, n. 몰두, 노력, 공부,

연구, 연구실 　　　　　　　　　　　　E *study*, It. *studio*, F. *etude*, *student*

> L. stupeo, stupui, –, stupēre 경탄하다, 넋을 잃다,

감각을 잃다 　　　　　　　E (stupendus (*gerundive*) *'to be wondered at'* >) *stupendous*

> L. stupor, stuporis, m. 경탄, 놀람, 혼미 　　　　　　　E *stupor*

> L. stuporosus, stuporosa, stuporosum 혼미한 　　　E *stuporous*

> L. stupidus, stupida, stupidum 정신 빠진, 무감각한, 어리석은 　　E *stupid*

> L. stupiditas, stupiditatis, f. 정신 빠짐, 어리석음 　　E *stupidity*

> L. stupefacio, stupefeci, stupefactum, stupefacĕre (< stupēre *to be amazed*

+ facĕre *to make*) 경탄하게 하다, 멍하게 하다, 둔하게 하다 　　E *stupefy*

> L. stuprum, stupri, n. 치욕

> L. stupro, stupravi, stupratum, stuprare (명예를) 더럽히다, 모독하다

> (*suggested*) L. masturbor, masturbatus sum, masturbari (< manus *hand*

+ stuprare *to defile*) 자독(自瀆)행위를 하다, 자위(自慰)행위를 하다,

수음(手淫)행위를 하다 　　　　　　　E *masturbate, masturbation*

> L. tudes, tudis, f. (tudes, tuditis, f.) 쇠망치, 쇠방망이

> L. tudicula, tudiculae, f. (< + –cula *diminutive suffix*) 올리브 열매를 빻는

기계, 제분기

> tudiculo, tudiculavi, –, tudiculare 빻다, 바수다 　　E *toil*

> L. tussis, tussis, f. 기침, 해소(咳嗽) 　　　E *tussive, antitussive*

> L. pertussis, pertussis, f. (< per– *through, thoroughly* + tussis *cough*)

백일해(百日咳) 　　　　　　　　　　　E *pertussis*

> G. stygein *to hate, to fear*

> G. Styx, Stygos, f. (*Greek mythology*) *Styx* (*a river of the lower world or*

Hades, over which the shades of the departed were ferried by Charon, and

by which the gods swore their most solemn oaths)

> L. Styx, Stygis, f. (Styx, Stygos, f.) (그리스 신화) 지하세계의 강, 삼도

(三途)내, 황천(黃泉) 　　　　　　　　　　E *Styx*

> G. typtein *to strike*

> G. typos, typou, m. *blow, mold, die*

> L. typus, typi, m. 형(型), 활자(活字), 표준

E *typ(o)–, typology, type, stereotype* (< *'a duplicate solid plate of an*
original typographical element, used for printing instead of the
original'), *idiotype* (< *'own'*), *isotype* (< *'equal'*), *homotype* (< *'same'*),
homotypic, allotype (< *'other'*), *heterotype* (< *'different'*), *heterotypic,*
antitype (< *'against'*), *atypism; subtype, typify*

> L. atypia, atypiae, f. (< G. a– *not*) 비정형성(非定型性),

이형성(異型性) 　　　　　　　　　　E *atypia*

> G. typikos, typikē, typikon *typical, figurative*

> L. typicus, typica, typicum 표상적(表象的), 전형적(典型的)

> L. typicalis, typicale 표상적, 전형적 　E *typical, (typical >) atypical*

> G. archetypon, archetypou, n. (< archē *beginning*) *the original pattern or model from which copies are made*

> L. archetypum, archetypi, n. 원형(原型), 본, 원본　　**E** *archetype*

> G. prōtotypon, prōtotypou, n. (< prōtos *first*) *the first form, original, primitive, especially in grammatical context*

> L. prototypum, prototypi, n. 원형, 본, 원본　　**E** *prototype*

> G. tympanon, tympanou, n. *kettledrum*

> L. tympanum, tympani, n. 고실(鼓室), 중이(中耳), 고막(鼓膜)　　**E** *tympanum, tympanic, tympan(o)-,* It. *timpani,* F. *timbre*

> G. tympanitēs, tympanitou, m. (tympanias, tympaniou, m.) *gaseous distention*

> L. tympanites, tympanitae, m. (tympanias, tympaniae, m.) 고창(鼓脹), 가스팽만　　**E** *tympanites (tympany), tympanitic*

uro, ussi, ustum, urĕre 태우다

> ustulo, **ustulavi**, ustulatum, ustulare 태우다, 데게 하다, 굽다, 눋다

> ustulatio, ustulationis, f. 태우기, 데치기, 굽기, 눌리기　　**E** *ustulation*

> comburo, **combussi**, combustum, comburĕre (< com- (< cum) *with, together; intensive* + -burĕre (< urĕre) *to singe, to burn*) 태우다

> combustio, combustionis, f. 연소

E *combustion;* ((*Japanese*) moe-kusa *'burning herb'* > mokusa *'mugwort'* > moxa >) *moxibustion*

> combustibilis, combustibile 가연성(可燃性)의　　**E** *combustible*

> urtica, urticae, f. (< *burning itch*) 쐐기풀, 담마(蕁麻), 가려움, 색욕

> urticaria, urticariae, f. 두드러기, 담마진(蕁麻疹)　　**E** *urticaria, urticarial*

< IE. eus- *to burn*

vado, vasi, vasum, vadĕre 가다, 앞으로 나아가다, 전진하다

> invado, **invasi**, invasum, invadĕre (< in- *in, on, into, toward* + vadĕre *to go*) 침입하다, 침범하다, 침습하다　　**E** *invade, invasive*

> invasio, invasionis, f. 침입, 침범, 침습　　**E** *invasion*

> evado, **evasi**, evasum, evadĕre (<e- *out of, away from* + vadĕre *to go*) 빠져 나가다　　**E** *evade, evasive*

> evasio, evasionis, f. 탈주, 도주, 도피, 회피　　**E** *evasion*

> pervado, **pervasi**, pervasum, pervadĕre (< per- *through, thoroughly* + vadĕre *to go*) 뚫고 지나가다, 침투하다, 휩쓸고 지나가다　　**E** *pervade, pervasive*

> pervasio, pervasionis, f. 침투, 침략　　**E** *pervasion*

< IE. wadh- *to go*　　**E** *wade*

veho, vexi, vectum, vehĕre 나르다, 운반하다

> vector, vectoris, m. 운반자, 짐꾼, 운수업자, 매개체, 벡터　　　　　E *vector*

> vehiculum, vehiculi, n. (수레·배 등) 운반기구, 운반체　　　　　E *vehicle*

　　> vehicularis, vehiculare 운반기구의, 운반체의　　　　　E *vehicular*

> vehemens, (gen.) vehementis 사정없이 몰아대는, 격렬한　　　　　E *vehement*

> vexo, **vexavi**, vexatum, vexare 사정없이 몰아대다, 격렬하게 흔들다, 괴롭히다　　　　　E *vex*

　　> vexatio, vexationis, f. 괴롭힘　　　　　E *vexation*

> via, viae, f. 길

> **E** ((abl. sing.) *'by way of, by means of* >) **via, viaduct** (< *'on the pattern of aqueduct'*), **convey, convoy,** (in via *'on the way'* >) **envoy,** (envoy >) **invoice**

> viaticus, viatica, viaticum 여행에 관한

　　> viaticum, viatici, n. 여행에 필요한 것　　　　　E *viaticum, voyage*

> obviam (< ob- *before, toward(s), over, against, away* + via *way*) (부사) 마주치어

　　> obvius, obvia, obvium 마주치는　　　　　E *obvious*

　　　　> obvio, **obviavi**, obviatum, obviare 마주치다, 대항하다, 미연에 방지
　　　　하다　　　　　E *obviate*

> trivium, trivii, n. (< tri- *three* + via *way*) 삼거리, 광장; (역사) 삼학(三學, 중세
대학에서 7교양과목 중 문법·수사(修辭)·변증법의 세 학과)　　　　　E *trivium*, (pl.) *trivia*

　　> trivialis, triviale 보통 있는, 하찮은, 저속한, 야비한; 삼학의　　　　　E *trivial*

> pervius, pervia, pervium (< per- *through, thoroughly* + via *way*) 통행할 수
있는, 통과시키는　　　　　E *pervious*

　　> impervius, impervia, impervium (< im- (< in-) *not* + pervius *pervious*)
　　통행할 수 없는, 통과시키지 않는　　　　　E *impervious*

> praevius, praevia, praevium (previus, previa, previum) (< prae- *before, beyond*
+ via *way*) 앞서 가는, 앞선　　　　　E *previous*

　　[용례] placenta previa 전치(前置)태반　　　　　E *placenta previa*

　　　　(문법) placenta 태반: 단수 주격 < placenta, placentae, f.

　　　　previa 앞서 가는: 형용사, 여성형 단수 주격

> devius, devia, devium (< de- *apart from, down, not; intensive* + via *way*)
길에서 벗어난, 탈선한　　　　　E *devious*

> devio, **deviavi**, –, deviare (< de- *apart from, down, not; intensive* + via *way*)
길에서 벗어나다, 일탈(逸脫)하다, 치우치다, 편향(偏向)하다　　　　　E *deviate, deviant*

　　> deviatio, deviationis, f. 탈선, 일탈, 편향, 편차　　　　　E *deviation*

> conveho, **convexi**, convectum, convehĕre (< con- (< cum) *with, together* + vehĕre
to carry) 함께 실어 나르다, 농산물을 실어다 창고에 쟁이다

　　> convectio, convectionis, f. 운송; 전달, 대류　　　　　E *convection*

　　> convexus, convexa, convexum (< *in forming an arch the extremities of the
　　surface are brought together*) 아취형의,
　　볼록한　　　　　E *convex, convexity, biconvex, biconvexity*

< IE. wegh- *to go, to transport in a wheeled vehicle*

> **E** *way, always, away, wain, wagon, wagon-lit, wag, waggle, wiggle, vogue* (< *'to row, to sail'*), *weigh* (< *'to carry, to balance in a scale'*), *weight*

> G. ochlos, ochlou, m. (< *moving mass*) *throng, crowd, the common people,*
mob　　　　　　　　　　　　　　　　　　　　　　　　　　E *ochlocracy, ochlophobia*

verto, verti, versum, vertĕre (vorto, vorti, vorsum, vortĕre) 돌리다, 돌다,
바꾸다　　　　　　　　　　　E *introvert, introversion, extrovert, extroversion*
　　> versus, versa, versum (*past participle*) *turned*
　　　　> versus, versus, m. 돌아옴, 밭고랑; 시의 행(行), 시　　　E *verse*
　　　　> versus (부사) 향하여, 대하여　　　　　　　　　E *versus (vs., v.)*
　　　　　　> introrsus (< intro- *inwards* + versus *towards*) (부사) 안을 향하여　E *introrse*
　　　　　　> extrorsus (< extro- (< extra) *outwards* + versus *towards*) (부사) 밖을
　　　　　　　　향하여　　　　　　　　　　　　　　　　　　E *extrorse*
　　　　　　> dextrorsus (< dexter *right* + versus *towards*) (부사) 오른쪽을 향하여　E *dextrorse*
　　　　　　> sinistrorsus (< sinister *left* + versus *towards*) (부사) 왼쪽을 향하여　E *sinistrorse*
　　　　> controversus, controversa, controversum (< contro- (< contra) *against* + versus
　　　　　　turned) 대립되는, 논쟁하는　　　　　　　　　　E *controvert*
　　　　　　> controversia, controversiae, f. 논쟁　　　　　E *controversy*
　　　　　　　　> controversialis, controversiale 논쟁의, 논쟁거리의　E *controversial*
　　　　> universus, universa, universum (< unus *one* + versus *turned*) 전체적, 보편적
　　　　　　> universum, universi, n. 전체, 온 누리, 우주　　　E *universe*
　　　　　　> universitas, universitatis, f. 전체, 보편, 공동체, 종합대학교　E *university*
　　　　　　> universalis, universale 전체적, 보편적　　　　E *universal*
　　　　> anniversarius, anniversaria, anniversarium (< annus *year* + versus *turned*)
　　　　　　해마다 돌아오는　　　　　　　　　　　　　　E *anniversary*
　　> versio, versionis, f. 번역, 판(版); (의학) 회전(回轉)　　　E *version*
　　> vertex, verticis, m. 회오리, 꼭대기, 머리끝, 마루점, 두정(頭頂)　E *vertex*
　　　　> verticalis, verticale 꼭대기의, 수직의　　　　　　E *vertical*
　　　　> verticillus, verticilli, m. 작은 회오리, 물렛가락, 방추(紡錘)　E *verticil*
　　　　　　> verticillatus, verticillata, verticillatum 작은 회오리 모양의; (생물) 윤생
　　　　　　　　(輪生)의, 환생(環生)의　　　　　　　　　　E *verticillate*
　　> vortex, vorticis, m. **vertex**; 가마[旋毛]　　　　　　E *vortex*
　　> vertebra, vertebrae, f. (< *the hinge of the body* < + -bra *instrumental suffix*) 관절;
　　　　등마루뼈, 척추(脊椎)뼈, 추골(椎骨)　　　　　　　E *vertebra,* (pl.) *vertebrae*
　　　　> vertebralis, vertebrale 등마루뼈의, 척추뼈의, 추골의　E *vertebral*

　　　　　　[용례] columna vertebralis (< *vertebral column, backbone, spine*
　　　　　　　　(*spinal column*)) 등뼈, 척추(脊椎), 척주(脊柱)
　　　　　　　　(문법) columna (둥근) 기둥, 원주(圓柱), 주(柱): 단수 주격
　　　　　　　　　　< columna, columnae, f.
　　　　　　　　　　vertebralis: 형용사, 남·여성형 단수 주격

　　　　> vertebratus, vertebrata, vertebratum 척추가 있는　　E *vertebrate*
　　　　> invertebratus, invertebrata, invertebratum (< in- *not*) 척추가 없는　E *invertebrate*
　　> vertigo, vertiginis, f. 회전운동, 회전기구, 현기증, 어지러움, 현혹　E *vertigo*

> verso, **versavi**, versatum, versare (*frequentative*) 빙빙 돌리다, (마음을) 쏟다
> versor, versatus sum, versari 늘 한 자리에 있다, 살다, 있다, 종사하다, 연루
되어 있다
> malversor, malversatus sum, malversari (< mal- *badly, bad* + versari
to behave) 배임행위를 하다 **E** *malversation*
> versatilis, versatile 잘 도는, 방향이 자유로운, 융통성 있는, 다용도의,
변덕스러운 **E** *versatile, versatility*
> averto, **averti**, aversum, avertĕre (< a- (< ab) *off, away from* + vertĕre *to turn*)
딴 데로 돌리다, 회피하다 **E** *avert, avertible*
> aversus, aversa, aversum (*past participle*) 반대쪽을 향한, 회피하는, 싫어하는 **E** *averse*
> aversio, aversionis, f. 회피, 기피, 혐오 **E** *aversion*
> adverto, **adverti**, adversum, advertĕre (< ad- *to, toward, at, according to* + vertĕre
to turn) 방향을 돌리다, 주의를 돌리다
E *advert* (< 'to turn the attention to'), ***advertize (advertise)*** (< 'to turn the attention to'),
advertent (< 'turning the attention to'), ***inadvertent*** (< 'not turning the attention to')
> adversus, adversa, adversum (*past participle*) 맞은편에 있는, 거스르는, 역경의 **E** *adverse*
> adversitas, adversitatis, f. 역경, 불우 **E** *adversity*
> adversarius, adversaria, adversarium 맞은편에 있는, 반대의, 거스르는,
적대하는 **E** *adversary, adversarial*
> anteverto, **anteverti**, anteversum, antevertĕre (< ante- *before* + vertĕre *to turn*)
앞지르다; 앞으로 기울다 **E** *antevert*
> anteversio, anteversionis, f. 앞으로 기욺, 전경(前傾) **E** *anteversion*
> converto, **converti**, conversum, convertĕre (< con- (< cum) *with, together; intensive*
+ vertĕre *to turn*) 방향을 전환시키다 **E** *convert, converter (convertor)*
> conversus, conversa, conversum (*past participle*) 거꾸로 된, 반대의,
역(逆)의 **E** *(adjective) converse*
> conversio, conversionis, f. 전환(轉換) **E** *conversion*
> convertibilis, convertibile 전환
할 수 있는 **E** *convertible, (convertible aeroplane >) convertiplane*
> converso, –, –, conversare (*frequentative*) 돌리다, 회전시키다
> conversor, conversatus sum, conversari 교제하다, 대화하다 **E** *(verb) converse*
> conversatio, conversationis, f. 교제, 대화 **E** *conversation*
> diverto, **diversi**, diversum, divertĕre (< di- (< dis-) *apart from, down, not* + vertĕre
to turn) 갈라지다, 이탈하다, 이혼하다 **E** *divert*
> diversus, diversa, diversum (*past participle*) 서로 다른, 다양한 **E** *diverse*
> diversitas, diversitatis, f. 상반, 상이, 다양성 **E** *diversity*
> diversio, diversionis, f. 전환(轉換), 전환술(轉換術) **E** *diversion*
> divertium, divertii, n. (divortium, divortii, n.) 옆길, 분기(分岐), 이혼 **E** *divorce*
> diverticulum, diverticuli, n. 옆길, 곁주머니,
게실(憩室) **E** *diverticulum*, (pl.) *diverticula, diverticular; pseudodiverticulum*
> everto, **eversi**, eversum, evertĕre (< e- *out of, away from* + vertĕre *to turn*) 뒤집어
엎다, 외전(外轉)시키다 **E** *evert, evertor*

> eversio, eversionis, f. 뒤집음, 외전, 외번(外飜)　　　　**E** *eversion*

> inverto, **inversi**, inversum, invertĕre (< in- *in, on, into, toward* + vertĕre *to turn*)
　안과 밖을 뒤집다, 자리바꿈하다, 전도(轉倒)시키다, 도치(倒置)시키다, 전화(轉化)시키다,
　내전(內轉)시키다　　　　**E** *invert, inverter, invertor, invertase*

　　> inversus, inversa, inversum (*past participle*) (위치·순서 등이) 뒤집힌, 역(逆)의　**E** *inverse*

　　> inversio, inversionis, f. 자리바꿈, 전도, 도치, 전화, 내전, 내번(內飜)　**E** *inversion*

> obverto, **obversi**, obversum, obvertĕre (< ob- *before, toward(s), over, against, away*
　+ vertĕre *to turn*) 향해 돌리다; (수동태) 향하다, 향해 있다　　**E** *obvert*

　　> obversus, obversa, obversum (*past participle*) 앞면의, 상대되는; (식물) (잎의)
　　　끝이 넓은　　　　**E** *obverse*

　　> obversio, obversionis, f. (앞면이 보이도록) 뒤집기　　**E** *obversion*

> perverto, **perversi**, perversum, pervertĕre (< per- *through, thoroughly* + vertĕre
　to turn) 거꾸러뜨리다, 붕괴시키다, 타락시키다　　**E** *pervert*

　　> perversus, perversa, perversum (*past participle*) 그릇된　　**E** *perverse*

　　> perversio, perversionis, f. 악용, 변절, 타락, 변태, 도착(倒錯)　**E** *perversion*

　　> perversitas, perversitatis, f. 심술궂음, 고집불통, 사악(邪惡)　**E** *perversity*

> proverto, **proversi**, proversum, provertĕre (< pro- *before, forward, for, instead of*
　+ vertĕre *to turn*) (*obsolete*) 앞으로 향해 가다　　**E** *prose*

> reverto, **reversi**, reversum, revertĕre (< re- *back, again* + vertĕre *to turn*) 되돌아
　가다, 복귀하다　　　　**E** *revert, reversal, reversible, irreversible*

　　> reversus, reversa, reversum (*past participle*) 역전된, 거꾸로 된, 뒷면의

　　　　E *reverse, (reverse transcriptase >) revertase, (reverse transcriptase >) retrovirus*

　　> reversio, reversionis, f. 복귀, 회귀, 전환, 역전　　**E** *reversion*

> retroverto, **retroversi**, retroversum, retrovertĕre (< retro- *backward, behind* + vertĕre
　to turn) 뒤로 (반대로) 돌려놓다　　**E** *retrovert*

　　> retroversus, retroversa, retroversum (*past participle*) 뒤를 향한　**E** *retrorse*

　　> retroversio, retroversionis, f. 뒤로 굽힘, 후경(後傾), 후굴(後屈), 퇴행　**E** *retroversion*

> subverto, **subversi**, subversum, subvertĕre (< sub- *under, up from under* + vertĕre
　to turn) 뒤집어엎다, 파괴하다, 무효화하다　　**E** *subvert*

　　> subversio, subversionis, f. 전복, 파괴　　**E** *subversion*

> transverto, **transversi**, transversum, transvertĕre (< trans- *over, across, through,*
　beyond + vertĕre *to turn*) 바꾸다, 가로지르다

　　> transversus, transversa, transversum (*past participle*) 가로지르는, 횡단하는　**E** *transverse*

　　　　> transverso, **transversavi**, transversatum, transversare 가로지르다,
　　　　횡단하다　　　　**E** *traverse*

　　> transversio, transversionis, f. 전위, 변위　　**E** *transversion*

< IE. wer- *to turn, to bend, to wind*

E *-ward, toward, forward, backward, outward, inward, (inwards >) innards, worth (< 'price given in turn for something'), weird (< 'that which befalls one'), writhe, wreath, awry, wrath (< 'twisted, tormented'), worry, wring, wrong, wrangle, wrench, wrinkle, wry, wryneck, wriggle, wrist, wrest, wrestle, warp (< 'to fling by turning the arm, to throw away'), wrap (< 'to turn, to wind'), ((suggested) wrap >) develop, ((suggested) wrap >) envelop, worm*

> L. vergo, **versi**, −, vergĕre ~로 기울다, 향해 있다, ~까지 펼쳐 있다

> L. convergo, −, −, convergĕre (< con- (< cum) *with, together* + vergĕre *to bend, to turn, to incline*) (한 점으로) 모여들다, 수렴(收斂)하다   **E** *converge, convergent*

> L. *convergentia, *convergentiae, f. 수렴   **E** *convergence*

> L. divergo, −, −, divergĕre (< di- (< dis-) *apart from, down, not* + vergĕre *to bend, to turn, to incline*) (한 점에서) 갈라지다, 분기(分岐)하다, 퍼지다, 발산(發散)하다, 분화(分化)하다   **E** *diverge, divergent*

> L. divergentia, divergentiae, f. 분기, 발산, 분화   **E** *divergence*

> L. verber, verberis, n. 채찍

> L. verbero, **verberavi**, verberatum, verberare 채찍질하다

> L. reverbero, **reverberavi**, reverberatum, reverberare (< re- *back, again* + verberare *to beat*) 튀겨 돌려보내다, 반사시키다   **E** *reverberate, reverberant*

> L. vermis, vermis, m. 벌레   **E** *vermis, vermicide, vermifuge*

> L. vermiculus, vermiculi, m. (< + -culus *diminutive suffix*) 작은 벌레

E *vermicular, vermilion (< 'the cochineal insect from which the color crimson was obtained'),* It. (pl.) *vermicelli*

> L. vermiformis, vermiforme 벌레 모양의   **E** *vermiform*

[용례] appendix vermiformis 충수(蟲垂), 막창자꼬리   **E** *appendix vermiformis*
(문법) appendix 부속기, 부속물: 단수 주격
     < appendix, appendicis, f.
     vermiformis: 형용사, 남·여성형 단수 주격

> L. *vermina, *verminae, f. 구더기, 벌레

> L. verminosus, verminosa, verminosum 구더기가 득실거리는, 벌레 먹은   **E** *verminous*

> L. vermino, −, −, verminare (몸에) 벌레가 생기다   **E** *verminate*

> L. *verminum, *vermini, n. 벌레, 해충, 해로운 작은 동물   **E** *vermin*

> G. rhembein *to turn, to whirl*

> G. rhombos, rhombou, m. *object that can be turned, magic wheel*

> L. rhombus, rhombi, m. 마술용 방추(紡錘), 마름모꼴, 능형(菱形), 사방형(斜方形)   **E** *rhombus, rhombic*

> L. rhomboideus, rhomboidea, rhomboideum (< + G. eidos *shape*) 마름모꼴의, 능형의, 사방형의   **E** *rhomboid*

> G. rhabdos, rhabdou, f. *rod*

E *rhabdomancy, rhabdovirus (< 'rod- or bullet-shaped virus'), rhabd(o)-, rhabdomy(o)-*

> L. Rhabditis, Rhabditis, f. (< *rod-shaped organism*) (선충) 선충속(線蟲屬)   **E** Rhabditis

> L. Caenorhabditis, Caenorhabditis, f. (< G. kainos *new*) 꼬마선충속(屬)   **E** Caenorhabditis

> (*perhaps*) G. rhopalon, rhopalou, n. *club*   **E** *rhopal(o)-*

> G. rhaptein *to sew, to stitch*   **E** *rhapsody*

> G. rhaphē, rhaphēs, f. *seam*

E *rhaphe, -(r)rhaphy, episiorrhaphy, herniorrhaphy, orchiorrhaphy (orchiopexy), tenorrhaphy, dysrhaphism (< 'incomplete closure of a rhaphe; defective fusion, particularly of the neural tube')*

> L. raphe, raphes, f. ((pl.) raphae) 솔기,
봉선(縫線)　　　　　　　**E** *raphe (rhaphe), dysraphism (dysrhaphism)*

> G. rhaphis, rhaphidos, f. *needle*

> IE. wret- (*metathetical variant*) *to turn back*

> L. re-, red- (*before* bowel *and* h) (*back, again*) 다시, 도로　　**E** *re- (red-)*

> L. retro (장소) 뒤로, 뒤에서; (시간) 지나간;
(관계) 거슬러, 되돌려　　**E** *(ad retro 'backward' >) (pl.) arrears, (arrear >) rear*

> L. retro- (*backward, behind*) 뒤로, 지나간　　**E** *retro-*

> L. reciprocus, reciproca, reciprocum (< re- *back, again* + pro- *before, forward, for, instead of*) 왔다갔다하는, 주고받는, 상호의　　**E** *reciprocal, reciprocity*

> L. reciproco, reciprocavi, reciprocatum, reciprocare 왔다갔다하게 하다, 주고받다　　**E** *reciprocate*

---

vinco, vici, victum, vincĕre 이기다　　**E** *vanquish*

[용례] Vincit omnia veritas. (< *Truth conquers all.*) 진리는 모든 것을 제압한다
　[문법] vincit 이긴다: 능동태 직설법 현재 단수 삼인칭
　　omnia 모든 것을: 형용사의 명사적 용법, 중성 복수 대격 < omnis, omne
　　veritas 진리는: 단수 주격 < veritas, veritatis, f.

> victor, victoris, m. 승리자　　**E** *victor*
　> victoria, victoriae, f. 승리　　**E** *victory*
> vincibilis, vincibile 이길 수 있는　　**E** *vincible*
　> invincibilis, invincibile (< in- *not*) 이길 수 없는, 무적의　　**E** *invincible*
> convinco, convici, convictum, convincĕre (< con- (< cum) *with, together; intensive* + vincĕre *to conquer*) 승복시키다, 확신시키다, 유죄를 증명하다, 유죄로 판결하다　　**E** *convince, convict*
> evinco, evici, evictum, evincĕre (< e- *out of, away from* + vincĕre *to conquer*) 완승하다, (꼼짝 못하게) 증명하다, (재판을 통해) 소유권을 되찾다, (법적 수단에 의해) 퇴거시키다　　**E** *evince, evict*

---

vivo, vixi, victum, vivĕre 살다

> vivus, viva, vivum 살아 있는　　**E** *vivisection (< 'on the pattern of dissection')*
　> vivarium, vivarii, n. 동물 사육장, (동물) 우리　　**E** *vivarium*
　> viviparus, vivipara, viviparum (< vivus *alive, living* + -parus (< parĕre *to bring forth, to bear*) *bearing*) (동물) 태생(胎生)의; (식물) 모체 발아의　　**E** *viviparous, (vivipara > vipera > 'ovo-viviparous snake' >) viper*
　> vivifico, vivificavi, vivificatum, vivificare (< vivus *alive, living* + -ficare (< facĕre) *to make*) 생명을 주다, 활기차게 하다　　**E** *vivify*

> vividus, vivida, vividum 살아 있는, 살아 있는 것처럼 보이는   **E** *vivid*

> vivax, (gen.) vivacis 활기 있는, 오래 사는   **E** *vivacious,* It. *vivace*

    > vivacitas, vivacitatis, f. 활기, 생명력, 장수   **E** *vivacity*

> victus, victus, m. 생활 필수품, 양식(養食), 식량(食糧), 생활 양식(樣式)

    > victualis, victuale 식량의   **E** *victual*

> convivo, **convixi**, convictum, convivĕre (< con- (< cum) *with, together* + vivĕre
to live) 함께 살다, 공존하다

    > convivium, convivii, n. 연회, 회식   **E** *convivial*

> revivo, **revixi**, revictum, revivĕre (< re- *back, again* + vivĕre *to live*) 되살아나다,
부흥하다   **E** *revive, revival*

> supervivo, **supervixi**, –, supervivĕre (< super- *above* + vivĕre *to live*) 살아남다,
생존하다   **E** *survive, survival*

< IE. gʷeiə-, gʷei- *to live*   **E** *quick, quicksilver,* (possibly) *quiver*

    > L. vita, vitae, f. 생명, 삶

> **E** F. *vie, viable, viability,* (vita *'life'* + amine > *vitamine 'a mistaken belief about the chemical nature of the compounds'* >) *vitamin(s)*

[용례] aqua vitae (< *aquavit*) 생명의 물, 생명수

(문법) aqua 물: 단수 주격 < aqua, aquae, f.

vitae 생명의: 단수 속격

    > L. vitalis, vitale 생명의, 생명 있는, 활력 있는

> **E** *vital, supravital* (< *'staining living tissue, especially blood, outside the body'*), *devitalize*

    > G. bios, biou, m. *life*

> **E** *bi(o)-, biology, biochemistry,* (bios + -ome >) *biome,* (bios + topos *'place'* >) *biotope (biotop)* (< *'the smallest subdivision of a habitat, characterized by a high degree of uniformity in its environmental conditions and in its plant and animal life'*), *biotron* (< *'cyclotron'* < *'electron'*); *biowarfare, bioclean, biodegradable, biofuel, biochip, biobank, biofeedback;* (*mikrobios >) *microbe, microbial, microbicidal,* (aēr *'air'* >) *aerobe* (< *'perhaps, on the pattern of microbe'*), *aerobic, anaerobe, anaerobic,* (sapros *'putrid'* >) *saprobe, saprobic*

    > G. biotē, biotēs, f. (biotos, biotou, m.) *life*

> **E** *biotin* (< *'the chief component of life, originally described as a necessary growth factor for yeast'*)

    > L. biota, biotae, f. 생물상(相)

> **E** *biota* (< *'fauna and flora considered collectively'*), *microbiota* (< *'microfauna and microflora considered collectively'*)

    > G. bioun (bioein) *to live*

    > G. biōsis, biōseōs, f. (< + -ōsis *condition*) *way of life*   **E** *-biosis*

      > L. parabiosis, parabiosis, f. (< G. par(a)- *beside, along side of, beyond*) 부생(副生)   **E** *parabiosis, parabiotic*

    > G. biōtikos, biōtikē, biōtikon *of life*   **E** *biotic, -biotic*

    > G. symbios, symbios, symbion (< sym- (< syn) *with, together*) *living together*

      > G. symbioun (symbioein) *to live together*

> G. symbiōn, (gen.) symbiountos (*masculine present participle*)
　　living together　　　　　　　　　　　　　　　　　　**E** *symbiont*

> G. symbiōsis, symbiōseōs, f. (< + -ōsis *condition*) *living together*

　　> L. symbiosis, symbiosis, f. 공생　　　　　　　**E** *symbiosis, symbiotic*

　　　　> L. antibiosis, antibiosis, f. (< G. ant(i)- *before,*
　　　　　　against, instead of + symbiosis) 항생(抗生),
　　　　　　항생작용　　　　　　　　　　　　　　　**E** *antibiosis, antibiotic*

> G. amphibios, amphibios, amphibion (< amphi- *on both sides, around*) *living*
　　in both (in water and on land)　　　　　　　　　　　　　　**E** *amphibious*

　　> L. Amphibia, Amphibiorum, n. (pl.) 양서류(兩棲類)　　**E** *amphibian*

> L. -bius, -bia, -bium 사는　　　　　　　　　　　　**E** *-bius (-bia, -bium)*

　　> L. Enterobius, Enterobii, m. (< G. enteron *gut*)
　　　　(선충) 요충속(蟯蟲屬)　　　　　　　　　　**E** Enterobius, *enterobiasis*

> G. zōē, zōēs, f. *life, subsistence, goods*　　　　　　　　　　**E** *hylozoism*

　　> F. azote (< *the gas unable to support life* < G. a- *not* + zōē *life*) *nitrogen*

> **E** *azote,* (azote >) *azo, az(o)-, diaz(o)-, azide,* (tetra- + azote + oleum >)
> *tetrazolium*

　　> L. azotaemia, azotaemiae, f. (< + G. haima, haimatos, n. *blood* + -ia)
　　　　질소혈증(窒素血症)　　　　　　　　　　　　**E** *azotaemia (azotemia)*

　　> L. azotobacter, azotobacteris, m. (< *nitrogen-fixing bacterium*
　　　　< + G. -bacter *bacterium*) 아조토박터　　　　　**E** *azotobacter*

> G. zōion, zōiou, n. (zōon, zōou, n.) *living being, animal*

　　> L. zoon, zoi, n. (동물의) 개체

> **E** *zoon,* (pl.) *zoa, zoology,* (zoological garden >) *zoo, zoopery* (< 'the performing
> of experiments on animals, especially the lower animals'), *zo(o)-, -zoon,* (pl.)
> *-zoa,* (zōion + -itēs 'adjective suffix' >) *-zoite, sporozoite* (< 'a protozoon
> resulted from sporogony'), *merozoite (schizozoite)* (< 'a protozoon resulted
> from merogony or schizogony'), *hypnozoite* (< 'a protozoon that sleeps'),
> *trophozoite* (< 'a protozoon that feeds'), *tachyzoite* (< 'a quickly multiplying
> trophozoite of Toxoplasma gondii'), *bradyzoite* (< 'a slowly multiplying
> trophozoite of Toxoplasma gondii')

　　> L. zoonosis, zoonosis, f. (< + G. nosos *disease*) 인수공통감염증(人獸共通
　　　　感染症), 인수전염병　　　　　　　**E** *zoonosis,* (pl.) *zoonoses, zoonotic*

　　> L. spermatozoon, spermatozoi, n. (< G. sperma, spermatos, n. *seed*)
　　　　정자(精子)　　　　　　　　　　　**E** *spermatozoon,* (pl.) *spermatozoa*

　　> L. Protozoa, Protozoorum, n. (pl.) (< G. prōtos *first*) 원생동물문(門);
　　　　원충류(原蟲類)

> **E** Protozoa, (Protozoa >) *protozoal;* (sing.) *protozoon,* (protozoon >) *protozoan*

　　> L. Metazoa, Metazoorum, n. (pl.) (< G. met(a)- *between, along with,*
　　　　across, after) 후생동물문(門)

> **E** Metazoa, (Metazoa >) *metazoal;* (sing.) *metazoon,* (metazoon >) *metazoan*

　　> L. Sporozoa, Sporozoorum, n. (pl.) (< G. spora *spore*) 포자충강(胞子蟲

綱)

E Sporozoa; (sing.) *sporozoon, (sporozoon >) sporozoan*

> G. zōidion, zōidiou, n. (< zōion *animal* + -idion *diminutive suffix*) *small animal, sculptured animal figure*

> G. zōidiakos, zōidiakē, zōidiakon *zodiac*

E zodiac

> G. hygiēs, hygiēs, hygies (< IE. aiw-, ayu- *vital force* + IE. g^{w}eiə-, g^{w}ei-) *healthy*

(Vide JUVENIS; *See* E. *juvenile*)

volvo, volvi, volutum, volvĕre 말다[捲], 싸다, 감다

E vault

> voluta, volutae, f. (< *feminine past participle*) 소용돌이 모양 장식, 권패류(卷貝類)

E volute

> volumen, voluminis, n. 둘둘 만 것, 두루마리 책; 부피, 용적;
소용돌이, 인간사의 부침

E volume, voluminal, volumetric

> voluminosus, voluminosa, voluminosum 권수가 많은; 부피가 큰

E voluminous

> volubilis, volubile 빙빙 도는, 소용돌이치는, 감기는; 혀가 잘 돌아가는, 유창한, 달변의

E voluble

> volubilitas, volubilitatis, f. (식물의) 감기는 습성; 달변, 다변

E volubility

> volvox, volvocis, m. (< *a fresh-water organism having a spherical form and provided with cilia which enable them to roll over in the water*) 볼복스

E volvox

> volvulus, volvuli, m. 창자꼬임증, 장축염전증(腸軸捻轉症)

E volvulus

> convolvo, **convolvi**, convolutum, convolvĕre (< con- (< cum) *with, together* + volvĕre *to roll*) 휘말다, 감싸다, 휘감다, 돌리다, 회전시키다

E convolve, convolute

> convolutio, convolutionis, f. 나선(螺旋), 선회(旋回), 회(回), 뇌회(腦廻), 이랑

E convolution, convolutional (convolutionary)

> devolvo, **devolvi**, devolutum, devolvĕre (< de- *apart from, down, not* + volvĕre *to roll*) 굴러 떨어지게 하다, 넘겨주다, 굴러 떨어지다, 넘어가다

E devolve

> devolutio, devolutionis, f. 추이, 이전, 이양, 양도; (생물) 퇴화

E devolution

> evolvo, **evolvi**, evolutum, evolvĕre (< e- *out of, away from* + volvĕre *to roll*) 굴려 내다, 굴려 가져가다, (만 것·접은 것을) 펼치다, 전개시키다, 발전시키다

E evolve

> evolutio, evolutionis, f. 펼침, 전개; (생물) 진화

E evolution, evolutional (evolutionary)

> involvo, **involvi**, involutum, involvĕre (< in- *in, on, into, toward* + volvĕre *to roll*) 말아 넣다, 휘말리게 하다, 포함시키다, (펼친 것을) 접어 넣다,
(펼치기 전으로) 되돌아가다

E involve, involvement, involute

> involutio, involutionis, f. 말아 넣음, 퇴화, 퇴축

E involution, involutional

> involucrum, involucri, n. 보자기, 싸개, 덮개, 봉투; 피막, (식물의) 총포(總苞), 골구(骨柩)

E involucrum, involucrin (< 'envelope protein of keratinocytes')

> revolvo, **revolvi**, revolutum, revolvĕre (< re- *back, again* + volvĕre *to roll*) 다시 뒤로 돌리다, 회전시키다, 소용돌이치게 하다, 변혁시키다

E revolve, revolver

> revolutio, revolutionis, f. 회전, 변혁, 혁명

E revolution, revolutionary

< IE. wel- *to turn, to roll; with derivatives referring to curved, enclosing objects*

E waltz, welter, walk, vagrant, well (< 'rolling or bubbling water, spring'), **wallow** (< 'to roll in mud'), **wallet**

> L. vola, volae, f. 요면(凹面), 손바닥, 발바닥

E volar

> L. valgus, valga, valgum 가쪽 들린, 밖으로 구부러진, 외번(外飜)의　　　　　　**E** *valgus*

> L. valva, valvae, f. (< *leaf of a door* < *that which turns*) 두 짝으로 된 접는 문의

　　한 짝, 쌍문의 한 짝, 판(瓣), 판막(瓣膜)　　　　　　　　　　　　**E** *valve*

　　> L. valvula, valvulae, f. (< + -ula *diminutive suffix*) 작은 문짝,

　　　　작은 판막　　　　　　　　　　　　　　　　**E** *valvula, valvular*

> L. volva, volvae, f. (vulva, vulvae, f.) 봉지, 덮개; 음문(陰門)　**E** *volva, vulva, vulval (vulvar)*

> L. valles, vallis, f. (< *that which is surrounded by hills*) 골짜기　　**E** *valley, vale, vail*

　　> L. vallecula, valleculae, f. (< + -cula *diminutive suffix*) 작은 계곡　**E** *vallecula*

> (*possibly*) L. lorum, lori, n. 가죽 끈, 고삐

　　> L. lorica, loricae, f. 갑옷, 흉갑(胸甲); (동물) 갑각(甲殼)　　**E** *lorica, loricrin*

> G. eilein *to turn, to roll, to squeeze*

　　> G. eileos, eilea, eileon (ileos, ilea, ileon) *colic*

　　　　> L. ileus, ilei, m. 장폐색증(腸閉塞症)　　　　　　　**E** *ileus, ileac*

　　> G. eilēma, eilēmatos, n. *coil,*

　　　　covering　　　**E** *neurolemma (neurilemma)* (< '*by association of* G. lemma *husk*')

> G. e(i)lyein *to roll round, to wrap up*

　　> G. elytron, elytrou, n. *covering, sheath*

　　　　> L. elytrum, elytri, n. (갑충류의) 시초(翅鞘), 겉날개; (해부)

　　　　　　질(膣)　　　　　**E** *elytrum (elytron),* (pl.) *elytra, elytrorrhagia*

> G. helissein *to turn round, to twist*

　　> G. helix, helikos, f. *winding, spire, coil, anything twisted*

　　　　> L. helix, helicis, f. 나선(螺旋), 나선 구조, 기둥머리의 소용돌이 장식; (식물)

　　　　　　담쟁이; 귓바퀴, 귓바퀴, 이륜(耳輪)

　　　　　　E *helix,* (pl.) *helices, helic(o)-, helicoid, helicase, helicopter* (< '*spiral*
　　　　　　wing'), *helicab*

　　　　　　> L. *helicalis, *helicale 나선의, 나선 모양의　　　　**E** *helical*

　　　　　　> L. helicinus, helicina, helicinum 나선 모양의

　　　　　　　　E *helicine* (< '*applied to certain small arteries of the penis and*
　　　　　　　　clitoris and to the helix of the ear')

　　　　> L. anthelix, anthelicis, f. (antihelix, antihelicis, f.) (< G. anth- (*before*

　　　　　　aspirate), ant(i)- (< anti) *before, against, instead of*) 맞둘레, 대륜

　　　　　　(對輪), 대이륜(對耳輪)　　　　　　　　　**E** *anthelix (antihelix)*

> G. helmins, helminthos, m. *parasitic*

　　worm　　　　　**E** *helminth, helminthology, anthelminthic (anthelmintic)*

　　> G. helminthian (helminthiaein) *to suffer from worms*

　　　　> L. helminthiasis, helminthiasis, f. (< + G. -sis *feminine noun suffix*)

　　　　　　연충증(蠕蟲症), 기생충증　　　　　　　　　　**E** *helminthiasis*

　　> L. Nemathelminthes, Nemathelminthium, m. (pl.) (< G. nēma, nēmatos, n. *thread*

　　　　(기생충) 선형동물문(線形動物門)　　　　　　　　**E** *nemathelminth*

　　> L. Platyhelminthes, Platyhelminthium, m. (pl.) (< G. platys *flat*) (기생충)

　　　　편형동물문(扁形動物門)　　　　　　　　　　　**E** *platyhelminth*

> (*possibly*) G. Helenē, Helenēs, f. ((*oldest form*) Welena) *Helen*   **E** *Helen*

       > G. (*possibly commemorating Helen of Troy*) helenion, heleniou, n. *elecampane*

          > L. helenium, helenii, n. 목향(木香, Inula helenium)

          > L. inula, inulae, f. 목향(木香, Inula helenium)   **E** *inulin,* (Inula campania >) *elecampane*

vomo, vomui, vomitum, voměre 토(吐)하다

E *vomit*

    > vomitus, vomitus, m. 구토(嘔吐), 구토물(嘔吐物)   **E** *vomitus*

< IE. weme- *to vomit*

    > G. emein (emeein) *to vomit*

      > G. emetos, emetou, m. *vomiting*   **E** *emetic, antiemetic, emetine*

      > G. emesis, emeseōs, f. *the act of vomiting*

        > L. emesis, emesis, f. 구토(嘔吐)   **E** *emesis*

          > L. hyperemesis, hyperemesis, f. (< G. hyper- *over*) 입덧,
          과다구토   **E** *hyperemesis*

            [용례] emesis gravidarum 임신구토   **E** *emesis gravidarum*

              hyperemesis gravidarum 임신과다구토   **E** *hyperemesis gravidarum*

              (문법) emesis, hyperemesis: 단수 주격

                gravidarum 임신부들의: 형용사의 명사적 용법,

                  여성 복수 속격 < gravidus, gravida, gravidum

                  가득한, 임신한

          > L. haematemesis, haematemesis, f. (< G. haima, haimatos, n.
          blood) 토혈(吐血), 혈액구토   **E** *haematemesis (hematemesis)*

frango, fregi, fractum, frangěre 분지르다, 깨트리다

    > fractus, fracta, fractum (*past participle*) 깨진, 조각난,
    파괴된   **E** *fractal, defray* (< 'pay for breakage')

    > fractio, fractionis, f. 깨트림, 쪼갬, 분획; 분수   **E** *fraction, fractional, fractionate*

    > fractura, fracturae, f. 부러진 자리, 깨진 금, 골절, 조각   **E** *fracture*

    > fragmentum, fragmenti, n. 부서진 조각, 파편, 단편,
    잔해   **E** *fragment, fragmental, fragmentary, fragmentation*

    > fragilis, fragile (섬세하게 만들어져) 깨지기 쉬운   **E** *fragile, frail*

      > fragilitas, fragilitatis, f. 깨지기 쉬움, 여림, 취약성   **E** *fragility, frailty*

    > frangibilis, frangibile (사용 도중에) 깨지기 쉬운   **E** *frangible*

      > infrangibilis, infrangibile (< in- *not* + frangibilis *breakable*) 파괴할 수 없는,
      침범해서는 안 되는   **E** *infrangible*

    > diffringo, **diffregi**, diffractum, diffringěre (< dif- (< dis-) *apart from, down, not* +
    frangěre *to break*) 분산시키다, 회절(廻折)시키다   **E** *diffract*

      > diffractio, diffractionis, f. 회절   **E** *diffraction*

    > refringo, **refregi**, refractum, refringěre (< re- *back, again* + frangěre *to break*)
    짓부수다, 굴절(屈折)하다, 반사하다, 제지하다

E *refract, refringent, birefringent, refractive, refrain* (< *'the refrain breaking the sequence'*)

　　　> refractio, refractionis, f. 굴절　　　　　　　　　　　　　　　　**E** *refraction*

　　　　> refractarius, refractaria, refractarium 완강한　　　**E** (⁺*refractary* >) *refractory*

　　> infringo, **infregi**, **infractum**, infringĕre (< in- *in, on, into, toward* + frangĕre *to break*)

　　　　파괴하다, 침해하다, 위반하다　　　　　　　　　　　　　　　　**E** *infract, infringe*

　　　　> infractio, infractionis, f. 침해, 위반　　　　　　　　　　　　**E** *infraction*

　　> perfringo, **perfregi**, **perfractum**, perfringĕre (< per- *through, thoroughly* + frangĕre

　　　to break) 깨트리다

< IE. bhreg- *to break* **E** *break, breakthrough, breach, brake* (< *'flax brake'*), *brick, briquette (briquet)*

　　> (*probably*) L. fragor, fragoris, m. 깨짐, 깨지는 소리, 요란한 소리, (군중의) 찬성하는

　　　소리

　　　> L. suffragor, suffragatus sum, suffragari (< *out-break of shouts, as of approval*

　　　　of a crowd < suf- (< sub) *under, up from under* + fragor *a noise of breaking*)

　　　　찬성투표하다, 지지하다, 돕다

　　　　> L. suffragium, suffragii, n. 투표에 쓰던 사금파리, 찬성투표, 지지　　**E** *suffrage*

　　　　> L. refragor, refragatus sum, refragari (< re- *back, again*) 반대투표를 하다

　　　　　> L. irrefragabilis, irrefragabile (< ir- (< in-) *not* + refragari *to*

　　　　　oppose) 논박할 수 없는　　　　　　　　　　　　　**E** *irrefragable*

∽ IE. bheg- *to break*

E *bang* (< *'hammering'*), *bank* (< *'feature where the contour of the ground is broken'*), *bench*, (It. banca *'moneychanger's table'* >) *bank*, (It. banca rotta *'bank broken'* >) *bankrupt, banquet*

plango, **planxi**, **planctum**, plangĕre 치다, 가슴이나 무릎을 치며 울다, 통곡하다　　**E** *plangent*

　　> planctus, planctus, m. 가슴을 치며 통곡함　　　　　　　　　　　　　**E** *plaint*

　　> planctivus, planctiva, planctivum 가슴을 치며 통곡하는　　　　　　　**E** *plaintiff*

　　> complango, **complanxi**, complanctum, complangĕre (< com- (< cum) *with, together;*

　　　intensive + plangĕre *to lament*) 몹시 슬퍼하다, 비탄에 잠기다　**E** *complain, complaint*

< IE. plak- *to strike*　　　　　　　　　　　　　　　　　　　　　　　　　**E** *fling*

　　> L. plaga, plagae, f. 타격, 재앙, 역병　　　　　　　　　　　　　　　**E** *plague*

　　> G. plēssein (plēk- *root of* plēssein) *to beat, to strike*

　　　　> G. plēxis, plēxeōs, f. *stroke,*

　　　　percussion　　**E** *-plexy, plexor* (< *'small hammer'* < *'on the pattern of flexor'*)

　　　> G. plēgē, plēgēs, f. *blow, stroke, wound*　　**E** *-plegia* (< *'paralysis or stroke'*), *-plegic*

　　　　> G. hemiplēgia, hemiplēgias, f. (< hemi- *half*) *hemiplegia*

　　　　　> L. hemiplegia, hemiplegiae, f. 반마비(半癩痹), 편마비　　**E** *hemiplegia*

　　　　> L. diplegia, diplegiae, f. (< G. di- *two*) 양측마비　　　　　**E** *diplegia*

　　　　> L. cycloplegia, cycloplegiae, f. (< G. cycl(o)- *circle; ciliary circle*

　　　　　(*ciliary muscle*) *of the eye*) 모양근(毛樣筋)마비, 조절마비　　**E** *cycloplegia*

　　　> G. plēktron, plēktrou, n. *plectrum; spear-point, oar, paddle*

　　　　> L. plectrum, plectri, n. (현악기를 탈 때 사용하던 상아로 만든) 채;

칠현금; 서정시　　　　　　　　　　　　　　　　　　**E** *plectrum*

> G. paraplēssein (< par(a)- *beside, along side of, beyond*) *to strike at the side*

> G. paraplēgia, paraplēgias, f. *paraplegia*

> L. paraplegia, paraplegiae, f. 하반신마비　　　　　**E** *paraplegia*

> G. apoplēssein (< ap(o)- *away from, from*) *to disable by a stroke*　**E** *apoplectic*

> G. apoplēxia, apoplēxias, f. *apoplexy*

> L. apoplexia, apoplexiae, f. 뇌출혈, 중풍(中風), 졸중(卒中)　**E** *apoplexy*

> G. kataplēssein (< kat(a)- *down, mis-, according to, along, thoroughly*) *to strike down with terror or the like*

> G. kataplēxis, kataplēxeōs, f. *stupefaction*

> L. *cataplexis, *cataplexis, f. 허탈발작　　　　**E** *cataplexy*

> G. plazein *to drive away, to turn aside*

> G. planktos, planktē, plankton *wandering, roaming, mad*　**E** *plankton*

pando, pandi, pansum (passum), pandĕre 펴다, 벌리다

> passus, passus, m. (< *a stretching out of the leg in walking*) 걸음

> **E** *(verb)* **pass** *(< 'to pass'), (pass > passed >)* **past, passage, passable, impassable, passenger, passport,** *(pass + time >)* **pastime; compass** *(< 'a pair of compasses, measure, circle'),* **encompass;** F. **en passant** *(< 'in passing'),* F. **passé** *(< 'passed'),* F. **impasse** *(< 'no passing');* **pace, pacemaker,** *(noun) (pace > 'narrow path' >)* **pass, bypass**

> passim (부사) 여기저기　　　　　　　　　　　**E** *passim*

> expando, **expandi,** expansum (expassum), expandĕre (< ex- *out of, away from* + pandĕre *to spread out*) 펼치다, 벌려 놓다, 팽창시키다　**E** *expand, spawn*

> expansum, expansi, n. (< *neuter past participle*) 넓게 펼쳐짐, 광활한 장소, 광활한 공간　　　　　　　　　　　　　**E** *expanse*

> expansio, expansionis, f. 팽창　　　　　　　　**E** *expansion*

< IE. petə- *to spread*　　**E** *fathom (< 'length of two arms stretched out'), fathomable, unfathomable*

> L. pateo, **patui,** -, patēre 열리다, 열려 있다

> L. patens, (gen.) patentis (*present participle*) 열려 있는　**E** *patent, (patent >) patency*

> L. patulus, patula, patulum 열린, 개방된　　　**E** *patulous*

> G. petannynai *to spread out, to unfold*

> G. petalon, petalou, n. *leaf, tablet*

> L. petalum, petali, n. 꽃잎, 화판(花瓣)　　　　　**E** *petal*

> G. petasos, petasou, m. *broad-brimmed hat*

> L. petasus, petasi, m. 창이 넓은 여행용 모자　　**E** *petasos (petasus)*

> G. patanē, patanēs, f. (< *thing spread out*) *platter*

> L. patina, patinae, f. (patera, paterae, f.) 운두 얕은 접시, 제물 담는 접시　**E** *paten, pan*

> L. patella, patellae, f. (< + -ella *diminutive suffix*) 작은 접시; 종지뼈, 무릎뼈, 슬개골(膝蓋骨)　　　　**E** *pail, patella, (patella >) patellar*

pango, pepigi (panxi, pegi), pactum (panctum), pangĕre 박다, 든든하게 고정시키다,
(나무 등을) 심다, 협정을 맺다

> compingo, compegi, compactum, compingĕre (< com- (< cum) *with, together* + pangĕre *to fasten*) 꽉 짜이게 하다　　　**E** *compact*

> impingo, impegi, impactum, impingĕre (< im- (< in) *in, on, into, toward* + pangĕre *to fasten*) 박아 넣다, 부딪히다, 영향을 미치다　　　**E** *impinge, impact*

< IE. pag-, pak- *to fasten*　　　**E** *fang (< 'to seize')*

> L. pala, palae, f. 삽, 가래, 부삽　　　**E** *palette*

> L. palus, pali, m. 말뚝, (*fixed in the ground* >) (경계선의)
푯말　　　**E** *pale, pole,* (*palisatus* >) *palisade*

> L. trepalium, trepalii, n. (< tres *three* + palus *stake*) (세 개의 말뚝처럼 생긴)
고문 도구　　　**E** *travail (< 'to trouble', 'to put to torture'), (travail >) travel*

> L. impalo, impalavi, impalatum, impalare (< im- (< in) *in, on, into, toward* + palus *stake*) (말뚝으로) 둘러싸다, (둘러싸서) 합하다, 꿰뚫다, (꿰뚫어) 고정
시키다　　　**E** *impale*

> L. pagus, pagi, m. (말뚝으로 경계를 표시한, 성으로 둘러싸이지 않은) 촌락, 촌사람

> L. paganus, pagana, paganum 시골의, 이교도의, 신앙이 없는 사람의　　　**E** *pagan*

> L. pagensis, pagensis, m. 시골 사람, 농부　　　**E** *peasant*

> L. pagina, paginae, f. (< *trellis to which a row of vines is fixed, hence (by metaphor) column of writing, page*)
페이지　　　**E** *page, paginate, pageant (< 'scene displayed on a stage')*

> L. pax, pacis, f. (< *a binding together by treaty or agreement*) 평화　　　**E** *peace, appease*

> L. paco, pacavi, pacatum, pacare 평화롭게 하다,
조정하다　　　**E** *pay (< 'to appease a creditor')*

> L. pacificus, pacifica, pacificum (< pax *peace* + -ficus (< facĕre) *making*)
평화로운, 태평한　　　**E** *pacific*

> L. pacifico, pacificavi, pacificatum, pacificare 평화롭게 하다　　　**E** *pacify*

> L. paciscor, pactus sum, pacisci 계약하다, 합의하다

> L. pactum, pacti, n. (< *neuter past participle*) 계약, 합의　　　**E** *pact*

> L. compaciscor, compactus sum, compacisci (< con- (< cum) *with, together*)
계약을 맺다　　　**E** *compact*

> L. propago, propagavi, propagatum, propagare (< *to fix before* < pro- *before* + pangĕre *to fasten, to fix*) 휘묻이하다, 자손을 증식시키다,
전파하다　　　**E** *propagate, ((feminine gerundive) 'faith' to be spread' >) propaganda*

> L. propagatio, propagationis, f. 증식, 전파　　　**E** *propagation*

> G. pēgnynai *to fasten, to coagulate*

> G. pēxis, pēxeōs, f. *fastening*

E *pexis, -pexis (-pexy), cryopexy (< 'fastening by cold'), orchiopexy (orchiorrhaphy) (< 'fastening in the scrotum of an undescended testis'), hemopexin (< 'a protein binding free heme in plasma')*

> G. pēktos, pēktē, pēkton *congealed*

> **E** *pectin* (< '*polysaccharides present in ripe fruits and used to gel various food, drugs, and cosmetics*'), (amylon '*starch*' + pēktos > '*a water-insoluble congealing glycan of starch*' >) **amylopectin**

> G. pagos, pagou, m. *that which is fastened, mass, hill*

> **E** (Areios pagos '*the hill of Ares, the hill at Athens where the highest judicial court of the city held its sittings*' >) **Areopagus**

> L. -pagus, -pagi, m. 결합체　　　　　**E** *-pagus*

> L. thoracopagus, thoracopagi, m. (< *Siamese twins joined at the thorax* < G. thōrax *chest*) 가슴 붙은 쌍둥이　　　**E** *thoracopagus*

pingo, pinxi, pictum, pingĕre 그리다, 묘사하다

> **E** *paint*, ((probably) picta (*feminine past participle*) '*the painted mark on a vessel showing the level that indicates the standard measure*' >) **pint**, Sp. **pinto**, Sp. **pinta**; *pictogram*

> pictor, pictoris, m. 화가　　　　　　**E** *pictorial, picturesque*
> pictura, picturae, f. 그림, 얼굴 화장　　　　**E** *picture*
> pigmentum, pigmenti, n. 그림물감, 화장품, 향료, 약재, 문채(文彩)

> **E** *pigment, pimiento (pimento)*, (pigment >) **pigmentation**, (pigmentation >) **de-pigmentation**

> pigmentarius, pigmentaria, pigmentarium 색소의　　**E** *pigmentary*
> pigmentosus, pigmentosa, pigmentosum 색소가 많은, 색깔이 많은, 색소성의　**E** *pigmentous*
> depingo, depinxi, depictum, depingĕre (< de- *apart from, down, not; intensive* + pingĕre *to paint*) 그리다, 묘사하다, 서술하다　　**E** *depict*

< IE. peig-, peik- *to cut, to mark by incision*　　**E** *file* (< '*cutting instrument*')
> G. pikros, pikra, pikron *sharp, bitter*　　**E** *picric acid*
> G. poikilos, poikilē, poikilon *colored, pied, variegated*

> **E** *poikil(o)-, poikiloderma* (< '*skin of mottled pigmentation*'), *poikilotherm* (< '*organism with variegated temperature*'), *poikilocyte* (< '*red blood cell with irregular shape*')

pungo, pupugi, punctum, pungĕre 찌르다, 꿰뚫다, 점을 찍다

> **E** *pungent, poignant*, (suggested) *pivot* (< '*tooth of a fax comb*'), (pivot >) **pivotal**

> punctus, punctus, m. 찌름, 찔린 자국, 점(點)

> punctuo, punctuavi, punctuatum, punctuare 점을 찍다, 구두점을 찍다　**E** *punctuate*
> punctuatio, punctuationis, f. 구두점 찍기, 구두법, 구두점　**E** *punctuation*
> punctualis, punctuale 점의, 시점을 지키는, 시간을 지키는, 규칙적인　**E** *punctual*
> punctum, puncti, n. 찌름, 찔린 자국, 점, 시점(時點), 요점(要點)

> **E** *punctum*, (pl.) *puncta, point*, (acupuncture point >) **acupoint**, *appoint* (< '*to come to a point about a matter*'), **appointment**, *disappoint* (< '*to undo the appointment of*'), **disappointment, pointillism**, (suggested) *pun* (< '*fine point*')

> punctatus, punctata, punctatum 점이 있는　　**E** *punctate*, (punctate >) **punctation**
> punctio, punctionis, f. 찌름　　　　**E** *punch* (< '*to prick*'), **pounce**

> punctura, puncturae, f. 찌름, 천자(穿刺), 찔린

자국　　　**E** *puncture, venipuncture,* (acu (abl.) *'with a needle'* + *puncture* >) *acupuncture*

> compungo, **compunxi**, compunctum, compungĕre (< com- (< cum) *with, together;*

intensive + pungĕre *to prick*) 날카롭게 찌르다

> compunctio, compunctionis, f. (바늘·송곳으로) 찌름, 회한,

가책　　　　**E** *compunction, (compunction* >) *compunctious*

> expungo, **expunxi**, expunctum, expungĕre (< *to mark for deletion by means of points*

< ex- *out of, away from* + pungĕre *to prick*) 삭제하다, 말소하다　**E** *expunge, expunction*

< IE. peuk-, peug- *to prick*

> L. pugnus, pugni, m. 주먹, 주먹질

> L. pugil, pugilis, m. 권투경기자

> L. pugilisticus, pugilistica, pugilisticum 권투경기자의　　**E** *pugilistic*

> L. pugno, **pugnavi**, pugnatum, pugnare 싸우다,

논쟁하다　　　　**E** *impugn, oppugn, repugn, repugnant*

> L. pugnax, (gen.) pugnacis 호전적인, 전투적인　　**E** *pugnacious*

> G. pygmē, pygmēs, f. *fist, boxing; the length measured*

from elbow to knuckles　　**E** *pygmy* (< *'not taller than a cubit'*), *pygmaean (pygmean)*

strepo, **strepui**, strepitum, strepĕre 소란하다, 소리 지르다, 불평 터뜨리다

> obstrepo, **obstrepui**, obstrepitum, obstrepĕre (< ob- *before, toward(s), over, against,*

away + strepĕre *to make a noise*) 요란하게 하다, 요란하게 해 중단시키다　**E** *obstreperous*

< (*Imitative European root*) strep- *to make a noise*

−esco, −evi, −etum, −escĕre *suffix of inceptive (inchoative) verb*

E *luminescence, luminescent, luminesce, phosphorescence, phosphorescent, phosphoresce, fluorescence, fluorescent, fluoresce, iridescence, iridescent, iridesce, opalescence, opalescent, opalesce*

cresco, **crevi**, cretum, crescĕre (< IE. ker- *to grow* + -escĕre *suffix of inceptive (inchoative)*

verb) 자라다

E *crescent, (crescent* >) *crescentic,* It. *crescendo,* F. *croissant, crew* (< *'an organized band'* < *'a band of soldiers serving as reinforcements'*)

> procerus, procera, procerum (< pro- *before, forward, for, instead of* + *stem of*

crescĕre *to grow*) 높은, 긴, 가느다란　　　　**E** *procerus (muscle)*

> accresco, **accrevi**, accretum, accrescĕre (< ac- (< ad) *to, toward, at, according to*

+ crescĕre *to grow*) (부착에 의해) 자라다, 더해가다　　**E** *accrete, accrue, accrual*

> accretio, accretionis, f. (부착에 의한) 증대　　　　**E** *accretion*

> incresco, **increvi**, incretum, increscĕre (< in- *in, on, into, toward* + crescĕre *to grow*)

(점점) 자라나다　　**E** *increase, increscent, incretin(s)* (< *'insulinotropic gut hormones'*)

> incrementum, incrementi, n. 증가, 증가량, 증가분　　**E** *increment*

> percresco, **percrevi,** percretum, percrescĕre (< per- *through, thoroughly* + crescĕre *to grow*) 많이 자라다

    [용례] placenta accreta 유착(癒着)태반   **E** *placenta accreta*
            placenta increta 함입(陷入)태반, 감입(嵌入)태반   **E** *placenta increta*
            placenta percreta 천공(穿孔)태반, 전감입(全嵌入)태반   **E** *placenta percreta*
            (문법) placenta 태반: 단수 주격 < placenta, placentae, f.
               accreta 자란: 과거분사, 여성형 단수 주격
                 < accretus, accreta, accretum
               increta 더 자란: 과거분사, 여성형 단수 주격
                 < incretus, increta, incretum
               percreta 많이 자란: 과거분사, 여성형 단수 주격
                 < percretus, percreta, percretum

> concresco, **concrevi,** concretum, concrescĕre (< con- (< cum) *with, together* + crescĕre *to grow*) 장성하다, 견고해지다   **E** *concrete, concretion, concrescence*

> decresco, **decrevi,** decretum, decrescĕre (< de- *apart from, down, not* + crescĕre *to grow*) (점점) 줄어들다   **E** *decrease, decrescent,* It. *decrescendo*

    [용례] Valetudo decrescit, accrescit labor. 건강은 줄어들고 병고는 더해 간다
            (Titus Maccius Plautus, 254?-184 B.C.E.)
            (문법) valetudo 건강은: 단수 주격 < valetudo, valetudinis, f.
               decrescit 줄어든다: 능동태 직설법 현재 단수 삼인칭
               accrescit 늘어난다: 능동태 직설법 현재 단수 삼인칭
               labor 병고는: 단수 주격
                 < labor, laboris, m. 일, 노동, 병고, 진통(陣痛), 분만통(分娩痛),
                   산통(産痛), 분만

    > decrementum, decrementi, n. 감소, 감소량, 감소분   **E** *decrement*

> excresco, **excrevi,** excretum, excrescĕre (< ex- *out of, away from* + crescĕre *to grow*) 커지다, (병적으로) 군더더기 살이 생기다   **E** *excrescent*

    > excrescentia, excrescentiae, f. 돌출, 돋이, 병적 증식물, 췌생(贅生), 식육(息肉),
         사마귀   **E** *excrescence*

> recresco, **recrevi,** recretum, recrescĕre (< re- *back, again* + crescĕre *to grow*)
     다시 자라다   **E** (recretus (*masculine past participle*) >) *recruit,* (recruit >) *rookie*

< IE. ker- *to grow*

    > L. creo, **creavi,** creatum, creare 창조하다,
         낳다   **E** *create, creative,* (creative >) *creativity, creole*
        > L. creatio, creationis, f. 창조   **E** *creation*
        > L. creatura, creaturae, f. 창조물, 산물   **E** *creature*
        > L. creator, creatoris, m. 창조자   **E** *creator*
        > L. procreo, **procreavi,** procreatum, procreare (< pro- *before, forward, for,*
             instead of + creare *to create*) 낳다, 생산하다, 나게 하다, 만들어 내다   **E** *procreate*
        > L. recreo, **recreavi,** recreatum, recreare (< re- *back, again* + creare *to*

create) 다시 창조하다, 고쳐 만들다, 소생시키다,

회복시키다　　　　　　　　　**E** *re-create, re-creation, recreate, recreation*

> L. ceres, cereris, f. 곡물; (Ceres) (로마 신화) 곡물의 여신, 농업의

여신　**E** *Ceres, cerium (Ce) (< 'named after the asteroid Ceres discovered shortly before')*

　> L. cerealis, cereale 곡물의　　　　　　　　　　　　**E** *cereal*

　> L. cerevisia, cerevisiae, f. (cervisia, cervisiae, f.) 맥주

> L. sincerus, sincera, sincerum (< *of one growth* < IE. sem- *one* + IE. ker- *to grow*)

자연 그대로의, 순수한, 성실한　　　　　　　　　　　　**E** *sincere*

> G. koros, korou, m. (kouros, kourou, m.) *boy, son*

　G. korē, korēs, f. (kourē, kourēs, f.) *girl, daughter, doll, pupil of eyeball*　**E** *hypocorism*

　　> L. isocoria, isocoriae, f. (< G. isos *equal* + korē *pupil* + -ia *noun suffix*)

양안동공동등　　　　　　　　　　　　　　**E** *isocoria*

　　　> L. anisocoria, anisocoriae, f. (< G. an- *not*) 동공부등　**E** *anisocoria*

　　> L. *leukocoria, *leukocoriae, f. (*leukokoria, *leukokoriae, f.) (< G. leukos

white + korē *pupil* + -ia *noun suffix*) 백색동공　　**E** *leukocoria (leukokoria)*

alesco, -, -, alescĕre (< alĕre *to nourish* + -escĕre *suffix of inceptive (inchoative) verb*)

(동·식물이) 자라다

　> adolesco, adolevi, adultum, adolescĕre (< ac- (< ad) *to, toward, at, according*

to + alescĕre *to grow up*) 자라다　　　　　　　　　**E** *adolesce*

　　> adolescens, adolescentis, m., f. (< *present participle*) 젊은이, 젊은 여자,

청소년　　　　　　　　　　　　　　　**E** *adolescent*

　　> adolescentia, adolescentiae, f. (< *present participle*) 청춘, 청소년기　**E** *adolescence*

　　> adultus, adulta, adultum (*past participle*) 성장한　　　　**E** *adult*

　> coalesco, coalui, coalitum, coalescĕre (< co- (< cum) *with, together* + alescĕre

to grow up) 엉겨 붙어 자라다, 아물어 붙다,

유합(癒合)하다　　　　　　　　　　**E** *coalesce, coalescent, coalescence*

　　> coalitio, coalitionis, f. 연합, 제휴　　　　　　　　**E** *coalition*

< alo, alui, altum (alitum), alĕre 기르다, 자라게 하다

　> alimonia, alimoniae, f. 양육, 생계비, 부양비　　　　　　**E** *alimony*

　> alimentum, alimenti, n. 식량, 영양물, 생활 필수품　　　　**E** *aliment*

　　> alimentarius, alimentaria, alimentarium 양식이 되는, 영양의, 음식물의　**E** *alimentary*

　　> alimento, alimentavi, alimentatum, alimentare 영양을 주다, 영양이 되다

　　　> alimentatio, alimentationis, f. 영양, 영양법　　　　**E** *alimentation*

　> almus, alma, almum 자양분을 주는, 생명을 길러주는

[용례] alma mater 모교　　　　　　　　　　　　**E** *alma mater*

(문법) alma: 형용사, 여성형 단수 주격

mater 모교: 단수 주격 < mater, matris, f. 어머니; (어머니의

역할을 하는) 모교(母校)

　> alumnus, alumni, m., alumna, alumnae, f. 양육되는 어린 것, 생도

E (pl.) *alumni, warfarin* (< 'Wisconsin Alumni Research Foundation, on the pattern of coumarin')

> aboleo, **abolevi**, abolitum, abolēre (< ab- *off, away from* + alĕre *to nourish*)

　폐지하다, 지워 버리다 　　　　　　　　　　　　　　　　　　　　　　**E** *abolish*

　　> L. abolitio, abolitionis, f. 폐지 　　　　　　　　　　　　　　**E** *abolition*

< IE. al- *to grow, to nourish* 　　　　　　　　　　　　　　　**E** *old, elder, eldest*

　> L. altus, alta, altum (< *grown tall*) 높은

E It. *alto, haughty*, (*inaltiare (< in- *'in, on, into, toward; intensive'* + altus *'high'*) *'to elevate'* >) *enhance*

　　> L. altitudo, altitudinis, f. 높이, 고도, 표고 　　　　　　　　**E** *altitude*

　　> L. exalto, **exaltavi**, exaltatum, exaltare (< ex- *out of, away from* + altus *high*)

　　　높이다 　　　　　　　　　　　　　　　　　　　　　**E** *exalt, exaltation*

　> L. proles, prolis, f. (< pro- *before, forward, for, instead of* + al- *to grow, to nourish*)

　　자손, 후손

　　> L. proletarius, proletarii, m. 최하층 시민(평상시에는 병역 의무가 없고 인구

　　　증가에만 기여하는 계급), 천민, 빈민 　　　　　　**E** *proletarian*, F. *proletariat*

　　> L. prolificus, prolifica, prolificum (< proles *offspring* + -ficus (< facĕre) *making*)

　　　다산(多産)의 　　　　　　　　　　　　　　　　　　　　**E** *prolific*

　　> L. prolifer, prolifera, proliferum (< proles *offspring* + -fer (< ferre *to carry, to bear*) *carrying, bearing*) 번식하는, 증식하는

E *proliferous*, (proliferous >) *proliferation*, (proliferation >) *proliferate*, (proliferate >) *proliferative*

convalesco, convalui, –, convalescĕre (< con- (< cum) *with, together; intensive* + valēre *to be strong* + -escĕre *suffix of inceptive (inchoative) verb*) 병이 나아가다 　**E** *convalescent*

　> convalescentia, convalescentiae, f. 회복, 회복기 　　　　　**E** *convalescence*

< valeo, **valui**, valitum, valēre 건강하게 잘 있다, 힘이 있다, 가치가 있다

E (valens (*present participle*) >) *valiant*, (valita (*feminine past participle*) >) *value*, (value >) *valuable*, (valuable >) *invaluable* (< *'priceless'*), (value >) *valueless* (< *'worthless'*), (value >) *evaluate, avail, available*, (contra valēre *'to be of worth against'* >) *countervail; univalent, bivalent, trivalent, quadrivalent, quinquevalent, sexivalent, multivalent; monovalent, divalent, trivalent, tetravalent, pentavalent, hexavalent, polyvalent; ambivalent* (< *'on the pattern of equivalent'*), *ambivalence* (< *'on the pattern of equivalence'*)

[용례] Si vales, valeo. 네가 잘 있다면 나도 잘 있다

　　　(문법) si 만일 ~면, ~거든: 종속접속사

　　　　　vales 너는 잘 있다: 능동태 직설법 현재 단수 이인칭

　　　　　valeo 나는 잘 있다: 능동태 직설법 현재 단수 일인칭

　> valetudo, valetudinis, f. 건강 　　　　　　　　　　　　**E** *valetudinarian*

　> valor, valoris, m. 용기, (전쟁터 등에서의) 용맹, 가치 　　　　**E** *valor (valour)*

　> validus, valida, validum 건장한, 유효한, 타당한 　　　　　　　**E** *valid*

> validitas, validitatis, f. 건장, 유효, 타당성   **E** *validity*

> valido, −, −, validare 굳세게 하다, 인증하다   **E** *validate*

> invalidus, invalida, invalidum (< in- *not* + validus *strong*) 병약한, 허약한,

효력이 없는, 타당치 않는   **E** *invalid*

> invalido, −, −, invalidare 무효로 하다   **E** *invalidate*

> valide (valde) (부사) 매우

> valentia, valentiae, f. 건장, 힘, 능력; 가(價), 원자가,

결합가   **E** *valence (valency), covalence (covalency), (covalence >) covalent*

> aequivaleo, −, −, aequivalēre (< aequus *equal* + valēre *to be worth*) 힘이

같다, 가치가 같다   **E** *equivalent*

> aequivalentia, aequivalentiae, f. (힘·가치·의의 등이) 같음, 동등,

등가(等價)   **E** *equivalence*

> praevaleo, praevalui, −, praevalēre (< prae- *before, beyond* + valēre *to be*

worth) 매우 건장하다, 더 힘 있다, 우세하다   **E** *prevail, prevalent*

> praevalentia, praevalentiae, f. 우세, 우월, 유병율(有病率)   **E** *prevalence*

< IE. wal- *to be strong*   **E** *wield, wieldy, unwieldy*

gnosco, gnovi, gnotum, gnoscĕre (< IE. gno- *to know* + -escĕre *suffix of inceptive*

(inchoative) verb) (*obsolete*) 알다

> ignotus, ignota, ignotum (< i- (< in-) *not* + gnotus *known*) 알려지지 않은, 모르는

[용례] ignotum per ignotius 모르는 것을 더욱 모르는 것을 통하여 (설명함)

(문법) ignotum 모르는 것을: 형용사의 명사적 용법, 중성 단수 대격

per 통하여: 전치사, 대격지배

ignotius 더 모르는 것을: 형용사의 명사적 용법, 중성 단수 대격

< ignotior, ignotior, ignotius (비교급) 더 모르는

> cognosco, cognovi, cognitum, cognoscĕre (< co- (< cum) *with, together; intensive*

+ gnoscĕre *to know*) 인식하다,

인지하다   **E** (cognitus (*past participle*) 'known' >) *quaint, acquaint, acquaintance*

> cognoscens, (gen.) cognoscentis (*present participle*) 인식하고 있는

> *cognoscentia, *cognoscentiae, f. 인식,

인지   **E** *cognizance, (cognizance >) cognize*

> cognitio, cognitionis, f. 인식, 인식력, 인식작용, 인식의 소산, 지식   **E** *cognition*

> cognitivus, cognitiva, cognitivum 인식의, 인지되는   **E** *cognitive*

> cognoscitor, cognoscitoris, m. 감정가, 감식가   **E** *connoisseur*

> recognosco, recognovi, recognitum, recognoscĕre (< re- *back, again* +

cognoscĕre *to know*) 재인식하다, 인정하다, 승인하다,

검증하다   **E** *recognize, recognizance, reconnaissance*

> recognitio, recognitionis, f. 인식, 인정, 승인, 검증   **E** *recognition*

> nosco, novi, notum, noscĕre 알다, 알게 되다, 배우다, 깨닫다

> notus, nota, notum (*past participle*) 잘 알려진, 악명 높은

> notio, notionis, f. 앎, 인식, 개념   **E** *notion*

> notitia, notitiae, f. 알려져 있음, 알림   **E** *notice*

> notorius, notoria, notorium 잘 알려진, 악명 높은   **E** *notorious*

     > notorietas, notorietatis, f. 악명   **E** *notoriety*

> notifico, **notificavi**, notificatum, notificare (< notus *known* + -ficare

     (< facĕre) *to make*) 알리다   **E** *notify*

     > notificatio, notificationis, f. 통지, 공시, 신고   **E** *notification*

< IE. gno- *to know*

> **E** *know, knowledge, acknowledge, can, (can >) canny, (canny >) uncanny, cunning, uncouth, (uncouth >) couth, ken, kenning, keen*

> L. gnarus, gnara, gnarum 알고 있는, 알려진

     > L. ignoro, **ignoravi**, ignoratum, ignorare (< i- (< in-) *not* + gnarus *knowing*

     + -are) 모르다   **E** *ignore, ignorant*

     > L. narro, **narravi**, narratum, narrare 이야기하다,

       서술하다   **E** *narrative, narration, narrator*

> L. gnobilis, gnobile 알려진, 귀족의, 고귀한

     > L. ignobilis, ignobile (< i- (< in-) *not* + gnobilis *noble*) 알려지지 않은, 무명의,

     천한   **E** *ignoble*

     > L. nobilis, nobile 알려진, 귀족의, 고귀한   **E** *noble,* F. *noblesse oblige*

> L. nota, notae, f. 표, 기호, 음부(音符), 인장, 평점, 주(註)   **E** *(noun) note*

     > L. noto, **notavi**, notatum, notare 표시를 하다, 주를 달다,

     주의하다   **E** *(verb) note, notate, notable*

       [용례] nota bene (n.b.) 잘 주의하라   **E** *nota bene (n.b.)*

       (문법) nota 주의하라: 능동태 명령법 현재 단수 이인칭

         bene 잘: 부사

       > L. notatio, notationis, f. 표기, 표기법; (수학) 기수법(記數法);

       (음악) 기보법(記譜法)   **E** *notation*

       > L. annoto, **annotavi**, annotatum, annotare (< an- (< ad) *to, toward,*

       at, according to + notare *to note*) 주석(註釋)을 달다,

       주해(註解)하다   **E** *annotate, annotation*

       > L. connoto, **connotavi**, connotatum, connotare (< con- (< cum) *with,*

       together + notare *to note*) (말이 원래의 의미 외에 부수적 의미를)

       내포(內包)하다   **E** *connote, connotation*

       > L. denoto, **denotavi**, denotatum, denotare (< de- *apart from, down,*

       not; intensive + notare *to note*) 명시하다, 외연(外延)을

       나타내다   **E** *denote, denotation*

     > L. notarius, notarii, m. 서기, 비서, 공증인   **E** *(notary public >) notary*

> G. gignōskein (ginōskein) (gnō- *root of* gignōskein) *to know, to think, to judge*

   (Vide GNOSIS; *See* E. *gnosis*)

••• 정형 제 3 변화 B 식

> 능동태 현재부정법이 –ĕre로, 능동태 직설법 현재 단수 일인칭이 –io로 끝나는 동사.

capio, cepi, captum, capĕre 잡다, 붙잡다, 획득하다

능동태	부정법	현재			cap-ĕre	붙잡다
	직설법	현재	단수	일인칭	cap-io	나는 ~한다
				이인칭	cap-is	너는 ~한다
				삼인칭	cap-it	그는 ~한다
			복수	일인칭	cap-imus	우리는 ~한다
				이인칭	cap-itis	너희는 ~한다
				삼인칭	cap-iunt	그들은 ~한다
		과거	단수	일인칭	cap-iebam	나는 ~하였다
		미래	단수	일인칭	cap-iam	나는 ~하겠다
		완료	단수	일인칭	cep-i	나는 ~하였다
	가정법	현재	단수	일인칭	cap-iam	나는 ~하리라
	명령법	현재	단수	이인칭	cap-e	너는 ~하라
			복수	이인칭	cap-ite	너희는 ~하라
	분 사	현재			capiens, (gen.) capient-is	~하는, ~하고 있는
	목적분사				capt-um	~하러, ~하기 위하여
수동태	부정법	현재			cap-i	붙잡히다
	분 사	미래			capiend-us, capiend-a, capiend-um	~받아야 할
		과거			capt-us, capt-a, capt-um	~받은, ~받고서

capio, cepi, captum, capĕre 잡다, 붙잡다, 획득하다   **E** *cop, copper*

> [용례] capias (< *Thou mayest take.*) 구인장   **E** *capias*
> (문법) capias (집행관 귀하는 이 구인장에 적힌 사람을) 붙잡아야 할 것이다:
> 능동태 가정법 현재 단수 이인칭

> captio, captionis, f. 포착, 계교, 궤변   **E** *caption*
>> captiosus, captiosa, captiosum 트집 잡는, 계교의, 궤변의   **E** *captious*
> captura, capturae, f. 포획, 노획물   **E** *capture*
> captivus, captiva, captivum 사로잡힌, 포로가 된, 감금당한   **E** *captive*
>> captivitas, captivitatis, f. 사로잡힘, 포로, 감금   **E** *captivity*
>> captivo, captivavi, captivatum, captivare 사로잡다, 포로로 잡다, 감금하다   **E** *captivate*

> capax, (gen.) capacis 수용할 수 있는, 널따란, 차지할 수 있는   **E** *capacious*

   > capabilis, capabile 수용할 만한, 포용할 만한, 능력 있는   **E** *capable,* (capable >) *capability*

    > incapabilis, incapabile (< in- *not*) 수용할 수 없는, 포용할 수 없는,

        능력 없는   **E** *incapable,* (incapable >) *incapability*

  > capacitas, capacitatis, f. 수용력, 용량, 능력

    E *capacity,* (capacity reactance >) *capacitance,* (capacity >) *capacitate,* (capacitate >) *capacitation,* (capacitation >) *decapacitation,* (decapacitation >) *decapacitate*

> capsa, capsae, f. 상자

    E *case, encase, caisson, cash* (< 'cash box'), *lowercase* (< 'small-letter type kept in the lower case'), *uppercase* (< 'capital-letter type kept in the upper case"), *capsid* (< 'protein shell that protects the nucleic acid of a virus'), *capsomere* (< 'morphological unit of the viral capsid'), (diminutive of F. cassee >) *cassette,* (suggested) *casket*

  > capsula, capsulae, f. (< + -ula *diminutive suffix*) 작은 상자, 캡슐, 피낭(被囊),

    피막(皮膜)   **E** *capsule,* (capsula >) *encapsulate, encapsulation*

    > capsularis, capsulare 꼬투리 모양 삭과(蒴果)의, 캡슐의, 피낭(被囊)의,

      피막(被膜)의   **E** *capsular*

   > (*perhaps*) Capsicum, Capsici, n. (< *podlike fruit*)

    고추속(屬)   **E** *capsicum,* (alteration of capsicine >) *capsaicin*

> capulum, capuli, n. 널, 관(棺), 손잡이, 칼자루, 고삐   **E** *cable*

> capto, **captavi**, captatum, captare (*frequentative*) 사냥하다, 걸려들게 하다, 꾀다, 힘쓰다

    E *catch, chase, cater,* (pro- 'before, forward, for, instead of' + captare 'to chase' >) *purchase,* (mercurium captans 'catching mercury' >) *mercapt(o)-*

> -ceps, (gen.) -cipis 잡는

  > forceps, forcipis, m., f. (< formus, forma, formum *hot* + -ceps *taking*) 부집게,

    집게, 족집게, 집게발, 겸자(鉗子), 학익진(鶴翼陣)   **E** *forceps,* (forceps >) *forcipate*

  > manceps, mancipis, m. (< manus, manus, f. *hand* + -ceps *taking*) 소유자,

    매입자

    > mancipium, mancipii, n. (법적 절차를 밟은) 취득, 소유권, 노예

     > emancipo, **emancipavi**, emancipatum, emancipare (< ex- *out of, away*

       from) (법적 소유권을) 해제하다, 해방하다   **E** *emancipate*

  > municeps, municipis, m., f. (< munus, muneris, n. *duty* + -ceps *taking*) 자유

    시민

    > municipium, municipii, n. 자유도시, 자치도시, 지자체

     > municipalis, municipale 자유도시의, 자치도시의, 지자체의   **E** *municipal*

  > particeps, (gen.) participis (< pars, partis, f. *part* + -ceps *taking*) 한몫 끼는,

    참가하는

    > participium, participii, n. 참여; (문법) 분사(分詞)   **E** *participle*

     > participialis, participiale (문법) 분사의   **E** *participial*

    > participo, **participavi**, participatum, participare 한몫 끼다,

      참가하다   **E** *participate, participant*

  > princeps, (gen.) principis (< *taking first place* < primus *first* + -ceps *taking*)

으뜸의 　　　　　　　　　　　　　　　　　　　　　　　　　　　E *prince*

> principalis, principale 주요한 　　　　　　　　　　　　　E *principal*

> principium, principii, n. 개시(開始), 원리 　　　　　　　E *principle*

> accipio, **accepi**, acceptum, accipĕre (< ad- *to, toward, at, according to* + capĕre
to take) 받아들이다, 용납하다 　　　　　　　　　　　E *accept, acceptance*

> concipio, **concepi**, conceptum, concipĕre (< con- (< cum) *with, together; intensive*
+ capĕre *to take*) 붙잡다, 받아들이다, 마음에 품다, 개념을 가지다, 임신하다

　E *conceive, conceit* (< '*on the pattern of deceit*'), *conceptive,* (contra- '*against*' +
conceptive 'conceiving' >) *contraceptive*

> conceptum, concepti, n. 개념, 태아 　　　　　　　　　　E *concept*

> conceptus, conceptus, m. 수용, 개념, 수태물, 태아 　　　E *conceptus*

> conceptualis, conceptuale 개념상의 　　　　　　　E *conceptual*

> conceptio, conceptionis, f. 개념, 수태,

임신 　E *conception,* (contra- '*against*' + *conception 'conceiving*' >) *contraception*

> decipio, **decepi**, deceptum, decipĕre (< de- *apart from, down, not* + capĕre *to take*)
속이다 　　　　　　　　　　　　　　　　　E *deceive, deceit, deceptive*

> deceptio, deceptionis, f. 기만 　　　　　　　　　　　　E *deception*

> excipio, **excepi**, exceptum, excipĕre (< ex- *out of, away from* + capĕre *to take*)
빼내다, 제외하다 　　　　　　　　　　　　　　　　　　E *except*

> exceptio, exceptionis, f. 제외, 예외 　　　　　E *exception, exceptional*

> incipio, **incepi**, inceptum, incipĕre (< in- *in, on, into, toward* + capĕre *to take*)
시작하다 　　　　　　　　　　　　　　　　　　　E *incept, incipient*

> inceptio, inceptionis, f. 시작, 개시, 발단 　　　　　　E *inception*

> inceptivus, inceptiva, inceptivum 개시의, 발단의; (문법) 동작의 개시를 뜻하는,
기동동사(起動動詞)의 　　　　　　　　　　　　　　　E *inceptive*

> intercipio, **intercepi**, interceptum, intercipĕre (< inter- *between, among* + capĕre
to take) 가운데서 가로채다, 횡령하다 　　　　　　　E *intercept*

> percipio, **percepi**, perceptum, percipĕre (< per- *through, thoroughly* + capĕre *to take*)
꽉 잡다, 온전히 받아들이다, 감지하다,
지각하다 　E *perceive, percept, perceptive, perceptual* (< '*on the pattern of conceptual*')

> perceptio, perceptionis, f. 지각(知覺) 　　　　　　　E *perception*

> perceptibilis, perceptibile 지각할 수 있는 　　　　　E *perceptible*

> appercipio, **appercepi**, apperceptum, appercipĕre (< ap- (< ad) *to, toward,
at, according to* + percipĕre *to perceive*) 통각(統覺)하다 　E *apperceive*

> appèrceptio, apperceptionis, f. 통각(統覺) 　　　　E *apperception*

> praecipio, **praecepi**, praeceptum, praecipĕre (< prae- *before, beyond* + capĕre *to
take*) 먼저 잡다, 미리 알다, 미리 일러주다, 가르치다, 지도하다 　E *precept*

> preceptor, preceptoris, m. 미리 일러주는 사람, 스승, 지도자 　E *preceptor*

> recipio, **recepi**, receptum, recipĕre (< re- *back, again* + capĕre *to take*)
받다 　　　　　E *receive,* (recepta (*feminine past participle*) '*received*' >) *receipt*

[용례] Recipe! 받으십시오! 　　　　　　　　　　　　　E *recipe*

(문법) recipe 당신께서는 받으십시오: 능동태 명령법 현재 단수 이인칭

> receptio, receptionis, f. 받아들이기, 접수, 수용(受容)　　　　E *reception*

> receptor, receptoris, m. 받아들이는 사람, 수용체(受容體), 수용기(受容器)　　E *receptor*

> receptivus, receptiva, receptivum 수용력 있는, 감수성 있는　　E *receptive, receptivity*

> recepto, **receptavi**, receptatum, receptare (*frequentative*) 도로 잡다, 자주 받아
　　들이다

　　　> receptaculum, receptaculi, n. 그릇, 용기(容器), 저장소　　E *receptacle*

> recupero, **recuperavi**, recuperatum, recuperare 도로 찾다,
　　회복하다　　　　E *recuperate, recover, recovery*

> suscipio, **suscepi**, susceptum, suscipĕre (< sus- (< sub) *under, up from under* +
　　capĕre *to take*) 받아들이다, 환영하다

　　> susceptivus, susceptiva, susceptivum 받아들이는, 용납되는,
　　　감수성 있는　　　　E *susceptive, susceptivity*

　　> susceptibilis, susceptibile 받아들일 만한, 용납될 만한,
　　　감수성 있는　　　　E *susceptible, susceptibility*

　　> intussuscipio, **intussuscepi**, intussusceptum, intussuscipĕre (< intus *within*
　　　+ suscipĕre *to take up*) 겹치게 하다, 중첩(重疊)시키다, 감입(嵌入)시키다

　　　　E *intussuscept*, (*present participle*) *intussuscipiens*, (*neuter past participle*)
　　　　intussusceptum

　　　> intussusceptio, intussusceptionis, f. 창자겹침증, 장겹침증, 장중첩,
　　　　중첩　　　　E *intussusception*

> anticipo, **anticipavi**, anticipatum, anticipare (< anti- *before* + -cipare (< capĕre)
　　to take) 미리 차지하다, 앞지르다, 예견하다, 예기하다　　E *anticipate, anticipant, anticipatory*

　　> anticipatio, anticipationis, f. 앞지르기, 선취, 선행(先行), 예견, 예기　　E *anticipation*

> occupo, **occupavi**, occupatum, occupare (< oc- (< ob) *toward(s), to, on, over, against*
　　+ -cupare (< capĕre) *to take*) 차지하다, 점령하다, (마음을) 사로잡다, 종사하게
　　하다　　　　E *occupy, occupant, occupier*

　　> occupatio, occupationis, f. 점령, 종사, 직업　　E *occupation, occupational*

< IE. kap- *to grasp*

　　E *have, behave, misbehave, behavior (behaviour), behavioral, heavy* (< '*containing something*'),
　　haven (< '*place that holds ships*'), *hawk, heave* (< '*to lift*'), *upheave, behoove;* (*probably*)
　　gaff (< '*hook*'), *gaffe* (< '*hook*')

cupio, **cupivi (cupii)**, cupitum, cupĕre 몹시 원하다, 탐하다

　　> cupido, cupidinis, f. 욕망

　　　> Cupido, Cupidinis, m. (로마 신화) 사랑의 신, 큐피드　　E *Cupid*

　　> cupidus, cupida, cupidum 욕망하는, 욕정적인

　　　> cupiditas, cupiditatis, f. 탐욕　　E *cupidity, covet*

　　> concupisco, **concupivi (concupii)**, concupitum, concupiscĕre (< con- (< cum) *with,*

together; intensive + cupĕre *to long for, to desire* + -escĕre *suffix of inceptive (inchoative) verb*) 탐욕하다　　　　　　　**E** *concupiscent, concupiscence*

< IE. kwep- *to smoke, to cook, to move violently, to be agitated emotionally*

    > L. vapor, vaporis, m. 김, 수증기　　　　　　　**E** *vapor*

      > L. vapidus, vapida, vapidum 김빠진, 맥없는　　　　**E** *vapid*

      > L. evaporo, **evaporavi**, evaporatum, evaporare (< e- *out of, away from* + vapor *steam*) 증발시키다　　　　　　　**E** *evaporate*

    > G. kapnos, kapnou, m. *smoke, steam, vapor*

      > L. hypercapnia, hypercapniae, f. (< *excess of carbon dioxide in the blood* < G. hyper- *over*) 고탄산혈증　　　　　　　**E** *hypercapnia*

facio, feci, factum, facĕre 만들다

> **E** (Fac simile! *'Make a similar thing!'* >) *facsimile,* *(facsimile* >) *fax,* (Fac totum! *'Do all!'* >) *factotum, -facient,* (sorbĕre *'to absorb'* >) *sorbefacient, -faction, feasible, infeasible;* (manu facĕre *'to make by hand'* >) *manufacture,* (contra-facĕre *'to make in opposition'* >) *counterfeit,* (foris facĕre *'to do outside'* > *'to transgress'* >) *forfeit,* (superficĕre *'to do in excess'* >) *surfeit;* (disfacĕre *'to undo'* >) *defeat, defeasance, defeasible*

> factum, facti, n. 사실, 실제 행동, 결과, 규정　　**E** *factum,* (pl.) *facta, fact, feat, factual* (< *'on the pattern of actual'*)

> factio, factionis, f. 행위, 집단, 도당　　　　**E** *faction, fashion*

> factura, facturae, f. 제조, 제작, 제품, 작품　　**E** *facture, feature*

> factor, factoris, m. 제조인, 행위자, 요인(要因), 소인(素因), 인자(因子); (수학) 인수(因數); (물리) 계수(係數)　　**E** *factor,* (*factor* >) *cofactor, factorial, multifactorial*

  > factoria, factoriae, f. 제조소, 공장　　　　**E** *factory*

> factitius, factitia, factitium (facticius, facticia, facticium) 인위적인　**E** *factitious, fetish, fetishism*

> facilis, facile 쉬운, ~하기 쉬운, 다루기 쉬운　　**E** *facile*

  > facilitas, facilitatis, f. 쉬움, 용이　　　　**E** *facility, facilitate*

  > facultas, facultatis, f. 능력, 기능　　　**E** *faculty,* (*faculty* >) *facultative*

  > difficilis, difficile (< dif- (< dis-) *apart from, down, not* + facilis *easy*) 어려운, 다루기 힘든　　　　　　**E** *difficile*

    > difficultas, difficultatis, f. 어려움, 곤경　　**E** *difficulty,* (*difficulty* >) *difficult*

> (*probably*) facies, faciei, f. 얼굴, 면(面)

> **E** *facies, face,* (*face* >) *interface,* (F. face *'face'* > (*diminutive*) facette *'little face'* >) *facet, demifacet* (< *'half facet'*), F. *en face* (< *'facing forwards'* < *'in face'*), (de- + facies > *'to mar the face'* >) *deface, defacement,* (ex- + facies > *'to rub out from the surface'* >) *efface, effacement*

[용례] facies hippocratica 히포크라테스 안모(顏貌), 빈사(瀕死) 안모　　**E** *facies hippocratica*

  (문법) facies: 단수 주격

    hippocratica 히포크라테스의: 형용사, 여성형 단수 주격

      < Hippocraticus, Hippocratica, Hippocraticum

> facialis, faciale 얼굴의, 면(面)의 **E** *facial*

> superficies, superficiei, f. (< super- *above* + -ficies (< facies) *face*) 겉, 허울,
   표면; (법률) 지상권 **E** *superficies, surface, (surface active agent >) surfactant*
   > superficialis, superficiale 표면의, 표재의, 얕은 **E** *superficial*

> -facio, -feci, -factum, -facĕre 만들다

> benefacio, **benefeci**, benefactum, benefacĕre (< bene *well*) 좋은 일을 하다 **E** *benefaction*
   > benefactum, benefacti, n. 선행, 은혜, 업적 **E** *benefit*
> malefacio, **malefeci**, malefactum, malefacĕre (< male *badly*)
   나쁜 일을 하다 **E** *malefaction*

> -ficio, -feci, -fectum, -ficĕre 만들다

> afficio, **affeci**, affectum, afficĕre (< af- (< ad) *to, toward, at, according to*)
   어떤 상태에 이르게 하다, 영향을 주다, 느끼게 하다,
   병 걸리게 하다 **E** *affect (< 'to influence'), affective, affair*
   > affectio, affectionis, f. 상태, 작용, 영향, 감정, 정동(情動), 애정,
      질병 **E** *affection, (affection >) affectionate*
   > affecto, **affectavi**, affectatum, affectare (*frequentative*) (목적 달성을
      위한) 방법을 마련하다, 열망하다, 추구하다 **E** *affect (< 'to aim at')*
      > affectatio, affectationis, f. 열망, 추구 **E** *affectation*
> conficio, **confeci**, confectum, conficĕre (< con- (< cum) *with, together*) 섞어
   만들다, 제조하다, 조제하다 **E** *confect, (disconficĕre 'to undo' >) discomfit*
   > confectum, confecti, n. 제조물, 조제물 **E** *confetti, comfit*
   > confectio, confectionis, f. 제조, 조제 **E** *confection, confectionery*
> deficio, **defeci**, defectum, deficĕre (< de- *apart from, down, not*) 떨어져
   나가다, 모자라다, 결핍되다
   E *(verb) defect, (third personal singular, present indicative, active 'it is lacking' >) deficit, deficient, defective*
   > defectus, defectus, m. 결함, 결손, 결여 **E** *(noun) defect*
   > deficientia, deficientiae, f. 결핍(증) **E** *deficiency*
> efficio, **effeci**, effectum, efficĕre (< ef- (< ex) *out of, away from*) 이루다,
   성과를 거두다, 효과를 거두다 **E** *(verb) effect*
   > effectus, effectus, m. (이루어 낸) 결과, 효과, 작용 **E** *(noun) effect*
      > effectualis, effectuale (결정적 결과를 만들어 내는 데) 효력 있는 **E** *effectual*
   > efficiens, (gen.) efficientis (*present participle*) (경제적으로 결과를 만들어
      내어서) 능률적인,
      효율적인 **E** *efficient, (efficient >) inefficient, (efficient >) coefficient*
      > efficientia, efficientiae, f. 능률,
         효율 **E** *efficiency, (efficiency >) inefficiency*
   > effectivus, effectiva, effectivum (예기한 결과를 만들어 내는 데)
      효과적인 **E** *effective, (effective >) ineffective, (effective >) effectiveness*
   > efficax, (gen.) efficacis (바라는 결과를 만들어 내는 데) 효능적인 **E** *efficacious*
      > efficacia, efficaciae, f. 효능 **E** *efficacy*

> inficio, infeci, infectum, inficĕre (< in- *in, on, into, toward*) 물들이다, 얼룩
지게 하다, 감염(感染)시키다

> **E** *infect, infective, (infective >) infectivity, (infect >) disinfect, disinfectant, disinfection*

> infectio, infectionis, f. 감염

> **E** *infection, (infection >) infectious, infectiousness, superinfection, (trans-, transfer + infection >) transfection*

> perficio, **perfeci**, perfectum, perficĕre (< per- *through, thoroughly*) 완성하다,
완전하게 하다

> perfectus, perfecta, perfectum (*past participle*) 완성된, 완료된,
완전한   **E** *perfect, pluperfect*

> imperfectus, imperfecta, imperfectum (< im- (< in-) *not*) 미완
성의, 불완전한   **E** *imperfect*

[용례] fungi imperfecti (pl.) 불완전곰팡이   **E** (pl.) *fungi imperfecti*
(문법) fungi 곰팡이들: 복수 주격 < fungus, fungi, m.
imperfecti: 형용사, 남성형 복수 주격

> perfectio, perfectionis, f. 완성, 완전, 완벽   **E** *perfection*

> praeficio, **praefeci**, praefectum, praeficĕre (< prae- *before, beyond*) 지휘하게
하다, 감독하게 하다

> praefectus, praefecti, m. 지휘관, 감독관, (고대 로마) 지방장관   **E** *prefect*

> praefectura, praefecturae, f. 지휘관의 직책, 감독직, (고대 로마)
지방 자치도시, 주(州)   **E** *prefecture*

> proficio, **profeci**, profectum, proficĕre (< pro- *before, forward, for, instead of*)
앞으로 나아가다, 성과를 거두다, 값이 오르다, 이롭다, 유리하다

> proficiens, (gen.) proficientis (*present participle*) 숙달한,
능숙한   **E** *proficient, proficiency*

> profectus, profecti, m. 향상, 성과, 이익   **E** *profit*

> reficio, **refeci**, refectum, reficĕre (< re- *back, again*) 복구하다, 기운을 회복
시키다, 쉬게 하다   **E** *refect, refectory*

> sufficio, **suffeci**, suffectum, sufficĕre (< suf- (< sub) *under, up from under*)
밑에 두다, 제공하다, 견디다, 넉넉하다   **E** *suffice*

> sufficiens, (gen.) sufficientis (*present participle*) 넉넉한, 충족한   **E** *sufficient*

> sufficientia, sufficientiae, f. 충족   **E** *sufficiency*

> insufficiens, (gen.) insufficientis (< in- *not*) 넉넉지 못한,
부족한   **E** *insufficient*

> insufficientia, insufficientiae, f. 부족   **E** *insufficiency*

> -ficus, -fica, -ficum ~ 만드는, ~ 하는   **E** *-fic*

> beneficus, benefica, beneficum (< bene *well* + -ficus *making*)
선행을 행하는   **E** *benefic*

> beneficium, beneficii, n. 선행, 은혜, 성직록(聖職祿)   **E** *benefice*

> beneficiarius, beneficiaria, beneficiarium 은혜의, 은혜를 받는,

성직록을 받는, 수익자의　　　　　　　　　　`E beneficiary`

> prolificus, prolifica, prolificum (< proles *offspring* + -ficus *making*)

다산(多産)의　　　　　　　　　　　　　　　`E prolific`

> specificus, specifica, specificum (< species *appearance, kind* + -ficus *making*)

특유한, 특이한　　　　　　　　　`E specific, (specific >) specificity`

> specifico, **specificavi**, specificatum, specificare 종류를 구분하다, 명시

하다, 한정짓다, 규명하다　　　　　　　　　`E specify`

> specificatio, specificationis, f. 명시, 내역,

세목　　　　　　　`E specification, (specification >) specs`

> vulnificus, vulnifica, vulnificum (< vulnus *wound* + -ficus *making*) 상처

입히는, 살해하는　　　　　　　　　　`E (obsolete) vulnific`

> falsificus, falsifica, falsificum (< falsus *false* + -ficus *making*) 속이는,

위조의　　　　　　　　　　　　`E (obsolete) falsific`

> falsifico, **falsificavi**, falsificatum, falsificare 속이다, 위조하다　`E falsify`

> falsificatio, falsificationis, f. 위조, 조작, 꾸며냄　`E falsification`

> -fico, -ficavi, -ficatum, -ficare 만들다

`E -fy, -fication, classify, glorify, identify, modify, ossify, ramify, signify; acidify, gratify, intensify, justify, notify, purify, rectify, simplify, verify`

< IE. dhe- *to put, to set*

`E do, (do on >) don, (do off >) doff, (at do > 'to do' >) ado, deed (< 'thing laid down or done'), indeed, doom (< 'judgement' < 'what is laid down'), deem, -dom`

> L. multifarius, multifaria, multifarium (< multus *many*) 여러 군데의, 여러 종류의　`E multifarious`

> L. condo, **condidi**, conditum, condĕre (< con- (< cum) *with, together*) 세우다,

간직하다, 감추다　　　　　　　　　`E recondite, incondite`

> L. abscondo, **abscondidi**, absconditum, abscondĕre (< abs- (< ab) *off, away*

from + condĕre *to put together*) 감추다, 숨다　`E abscond`

> L. condio, **condivi (condii)**, conditum, condire (< con- (< cum) *with, together*)

절이다, 양념하다　　　　　　　　　　`E condiment`

> L. abdomen, abdominis, n. (< *part placed away, concealed part*) 배[腹], 복부(腹部)　`E abdomen`

> L. abdominalis, abdominale 배[腹]의, 복부의　`E abdominal`

> G. thēkē, thēkēs, f. *repository, receptacle, box, chest, tomb, coffin, sheath*　`E discotheque`

> L. theca, thecae, f. 막(膜), 초(鞘), 난포막(卵胞膜), 건초(腱鞘), 경막(硬膜),

수막(髓膜)　　　　　　　　　　　　`E theca, intrathecal`

[용례] theca interna 속난포막, 내난포막　　　　`E theca interna`

theca externa 바깥난포막, 외난포막　　　`E theca externa`

(문법) theca 난포막: 단수 주격

interna 안의: 형용사, 여성형 단수 주격

< internus, interna, internum

externa 바깥의: 형용사, 여성형 단수 주격

< externus, externa, externum

> G. apothēkē, apothēkēs, f. (< ap(o)- *away from, from* + thēkē) *storehouse, granary, receptacle, magazine*

>> L. apotheca, apothecae, f. 저장실, 창고, 포도주 창고　　　　　**E** *boutique (< 'shop')*

>>> L. apothecarius, apothecarii, m. 창고지기　　　　　**E** *apothecary*

> G. bibliothēkē, bibliothēkēs, f. (< biblion *book* + thēkē *repository*) *book-case, library*

>> L. bibliotheca, bibliothecae, f. 책장, 서재, 서고, 도서실　　　**E** *bibliotheca*

> G. tithenai (the- *root of* tithenai) *to put, to place* (Vide THESIS; *See* E. *thesis*)

> (*suggested*) IE. dhemo- *house*

>> L. famulus, famuli, n. 노예, 하인

>>> L. familia, familiae, f. 한 집안 권속으로서의 노예 무리, 식솔, 가족, 가정, 가문, 집단; (생물) 과(科); (언어) 어족(語族)　　　**E** *family, (family >) familial, superfamily*

>>>> L. familiaris, familiare 한 집안 노예 무리에 속하는, 집안의, 잘 아는, 친숙한　　　**E** *familiar*

>>>>> L. familiaritas, familiaritatis, f. 가까운 사이, 친숙　**E** *familiarity*

fodio, fodi, fossum, fodĕre 파다, 채굴하다

> fossa, fossae, f. 구덩이, 오목, 우묵, 와(窩)　　　　　　　　　　　**E** *fossa*

[용례] fossa ovalis 난원와(卵圓窩)　　　　　　　　　　　**E** *fossa ovalis*

(문법) fossa 오목, 와(窩): 단수 주격

　　ovalis 난원형의: 형용사, 남·여성형 단수 주격 < ovalis, ovale

> fossula, fossulae, f. (< + -ula *diminutive suffix*) 작은 오목, 소와(小窩)　　　　　　　　　　　**E** *fossula, (pl.) fossulae*

> fossor, fossoris, m. 땅 파는 사람, 농부, 광부

>> fossorius, fossoria, fossorium 땅 파는, 땅 파는 데 쓰는, 땅 파기에 알맞은　**E** *fossorial*

> fossilis, fossile 땅에서 파낸, 땅에서 캐낸, 화석의　　　　**E** *fossil*

< IE. bhedh- *to dig*　　　　　**E** *bed (< 'garden plot, sleeping place')*

> (*perhaps*) G. bothros, bothrou, m. *hole, pit, a hole or pit into which drink offerings to the nether gods were poured by the ancient Greeks*　**E** *bothr(o)-*

>> G. bothrion, bothriou, n. (< + -ion *diminutive suffix*) *small pit*

>>> L. bothrium, bothrii, n. 작은 홈　**E** *bothrium, (pl.) bothria, bothri(o)-, -bothrium*

>>>> L. Diphyllobothrium, Diphyllobothrii, n. (< G. di- *two* + phyllon *leaf* + bothrium) 열두조충속(裂頭條蟲屬)

E *diphyllobothrium (< 'two bilateral grooves (bothria) of their scolex')*

fugio, fugi, fugitum, fugĕre 도망하다, 피하다

[용례] Tempus fugit. 세월은 유수 같다

(문법) tempus 시간은: 단수 주격 < tempus, temporis, n.

fugit 도망한다: 능동태 직설법 현재 단수 삼인칭

> fugitivus, fugitiva, fugitivum 도망하는, 달아나는, 덧없는 　　　　　**E** *fugitive*

> refugio, **refugi**, refugitum, refugĕre (< re- *back, again* + fugĕre *to flee*) 퇴각하다,
　도망하다, 피하다
　　> refugium, refugii, n. 피신, 피신처 　　**E** *refugium,* (pl.) *refugia, refuge, refugee*

> subterfugio, subterfugi, –, subterfugĕre (< subter- *below* + fugĕre *to flee*) 몰래 도
　망하다, 몰래 피하다, 빠져나가다
　　> subterfugium, subterfugii, n. 구실, 핑계, 발뺌, 속이기 　　**E** *subterfuge*

> -fugus, -fuga, -fugum 도망하는, 피하는
　　> centrifugus, centrifuga, centrifugum (< centrum *center* + -fugus *fleeing*)
　　　원심(遠心)의, 날 [出] 　　**E** *centrifuge, centrifugal*

> fuga, fugae, f. 도망, 둔주(遁走), 둔주곡(遁走曲) 　　**E** *fugue,* It. *fuga*
　　> fugo, **fugavi**, fugatum, fugare 도망가게 하다, 물리치다, 쫓다
　　　> febrifuga, febrifugae, f. (febrifugia, febrifugiae, f.) (< febris *fever* +
　　　　fugare *to put to flight*) 해열제;
　　　　쑥국화 (Tanacetum parthenium) 　　**E** *febrifuge, febrifugal; feverfew*
　　　> -fugus, -fuga, -fugum 도망가게 하는, 물리치는, 쫓는 　　**E** *vermifuge, vermifugal*

> fugax, (gen.) fugacis 쉽게 달아나는, 잠시 지나가 버리는, 덧없는,
　조락성(凋落性)의 　　**E** *fugacious,* (fugacious >) *fugacity*

< IE. bheug- *to flee*
　> G. pheugein *to flee*
　　> G. phygē, phygēs, f. *flight* 　　**E** *apophyge*

jacio, jeci, jactum, jacĕre 던지다, 발사하다

[용례] Jacta est alea. (< *The die is cast.*) 주사위는 던져졌다 (Gaius Julius Caesar,
　　100-44 B.C.E.)
　　(문법) jacta est 던져졌다: 수동태 직설법 완료 단수 삼인칭, 여성형 단수 주격
　　　　< jactus, jacta, jactum
　　　alea 주사위는: 단수 주격 < alea, aleae, f.

> jaculum, jaculi, n. (던지는) 창
　　> ejaculor, ejaculatus sum, ejaculari (< e- *out of, away from* + jaculum *dart* +
　　　-ari *suffix for deponent verb*) 앞으로 쏘아 보내다, 갑작스레 부르짖다,
　　　내뿜다, 사출(射出)하다, 사정(射精)하다 　　**E** *ejaculate*
　　　> *ejaculatio, *ejaculationis, f. 절규, 사출, 사정 　　**E** *ejaculation*
　　　> ejaculator, ejaculatoris, m. 절규하는 사람, 사출기
　　　　> ejaculatorius, ejaculatoria, ejaculatorium 절규하는, 사정의 　　**E** *ejaculatory*
> jacto, **jactavi**, jactatum, jactare (*frequentative*) 내던지다, 팽개치다,
　떠들어대다 　　**E** *jet, jut, jettison*
　　> jactito, **jactitavi**, jactitatum, jactitare (*frequentative*) 내던지다, 내팽개치다,
　　　사칭(詐稱)하다

> jactitatio, jactitationis, f. 몸부림, 뒤척임, 전전반측(轉轉反側), 사칭   **E** *jactitation*

> abjicio, **abjeci**, abjectum, abjicěre (< ab- *off, away from* + -jicěre (< jacěre) *to throw*) 멀리 던지다, 내리 던지다, 내동댕이치다, 비굴하게 만들다   **E** *abject, abjective*

> abjectio, abjectionis, f. 영락, 비굴, 천함   **E** *abjection*

> adjicio, **adjeci**, adjectum, adjicěre (< ad- *to, toward, at, according to* + -jicěre (< jacěre) *to throw*) ~로 던지다, ~에 덧붙이다

> adjectivus, adjectiva, adjectivum (< nomen adjectivum *adjective name* < G. onoma epitheton *attributive name*) 부수적, 형용사의   **E** *adjective*

> conjicio, **conjeci**, conjectum, conjicěre (< con- (< cum) *with, together* + -jicěre (< jacěre) *to throw*) 한 곳에 집중적으로 던지다, 처넣다, (생각 속에 함께 처넣다) 짐작하다

> conjectura, conjecturae, f. 짐작, 추측   **E** *conjecture, conjectural, conjecturable*

> dejicio, **dejeci**, dejectum, dejicěre (< de- *apart from, down, not* + -jicěre (< jacěre) *to throw*) 내려 던지다, 떨어뜨리다, 배설하다, 낙담시키다   **E** *deject*

> dejecta, dejectorum, n. (pl.) 배설물   **E** *(pl.) dejecta*

> ejicio, **ejeci**, ejectum, ejicěre (< e- *out of, away from* + -jicěre (< jacěre) *to throw*) 밖으로 내던지다, 쫓아내다, 분출시키다, 박출시키다   **E** *eject, ejector*

> ejectio, ejectionis, f. 쫓아냄, 분출, 박출   **E** *ejection*

> injicio, **injeci**, injectum, injicěre (< in- *in, on, into, toward* + -jicěre (< jacěre) *to throw*) 안으로 던지다, 주입하다   **E** *inject, injector*

> injectio, injectionis, f. 주입, 주사   **E** *injection*

> interjicio, **interjeci**, interjectum, interjicěre (< inter- *between, among* + -jicěre (< jacěre) *to throw*) 사이에 끼워 넣다   **E** *interject*

> interjectio, interjectionis, f. 끼워 넣기, 끼워 넣는 말, 탄성; (문법) 감탄사   **E** *interjection*

> objicio, **objeci**, objectum, objicěre (< ob- *before, toward(s), over, against, away* + -jicěre (< jacěre) *to throw*) 앞에 내던지다, 보이게 하다, 맞세우다, (방어하기 위해) 반대하다

> objectum, objecti, n. (< *thing presented to the mind*) 대상, 객관; (문법) 목적어   **E** *(noun) object*, F. *objet*

> objectivus, objectiva, objectivum 대상의, 객관적인, 목적에 관한; (문법) 목적어의   **E** *objective*

> objectio, objectionis, f. 앞에 내던짐, 맞세움, 반대, 이의(異議)   **E** *objection*

> objecto, **objectavi**, objectatum, objectare (*frequentative*) 앞에 내던지다, 논박하다, 반대하다   **E** *(verb)* (objicěre *and* objectare >) *object*

> obex, obicis, m., f. 빗장, 방책, 장애   **E** *obex*

> projicio, **projeci**, projectum, projicěre (< pro- *before, forward, for, instead of* + -jicěre (< jacěre) *to throw*) 앞으로 내던지다, 두드러지게 하다   **E** *(verb) project, projective*

> projectum, projecti, n. (< *neuter past participle*) 돌출부, 기획, 계획   **E** *(noun) project*

> projectio, projectionis, f. 돌출, 사출, 발사, 투사, 투영, 계획   **E** *projection*

> projector, projectoris, m. 투사기, 투영 장치, 계획자   **E** *projector*

> projectilis, projectile 돌출된, 사출하는, 발사되는, 추진하는   **E** *projectile*

> rejicio, **rejeci**, rejectum, rejicĕre (< re- *back, again* + -jicĕre (< jacĕre) *to throw*)
되던지다, 물리치다, 거절하다, 거부하다 **E** *reject*

> rejectio, rejectionis, f. 거절, 거부 **E** *rejection*

> subjicio, **subjeci**, subjectum, subjicĕre (< sub- *under, up from under* + -jicĕre
(< jacĕre) *to throw*) 밑에 던져두다, 종속시키다, (어떤) 의미를 가지게 하다, 생각
나게 하다 **E** *(verb, adjective) subject*

> subjectum, subjecti, n. (< *neuter past participle*) 주제; (문법) 주어 **E** *(noun) subject*

> subjectivus, subjectiva, subjectivum 주관적인; (문법) 주어의 **E** *subjective*

> subjectio, subjectionis, f. 종속 **E** *subjection*

> subex, subicis, m. 발판

> subiculum, subiculi, n. (< + -ulum *diminutive suffix*) 작은 발판, 지지체,
지각(支脚) **E** *subiculum*

> trajicio, **trajeci**, trajectum, trajicĕre (< tra- (< trans) *over, across, through, beyond*
+ -jicĕre (< jacĕre) *to throw*) 저쪽으로 던지다, 옮기다, 건너다 **E** *traject*

> trajectorius, trajectoria, trajectorium 궤도의 **E** *trajectory*

< IE. ye- *to throw, to impel*

> L. jaceo, **jacui**, jacetum, jacĕre 넘어져 있다, 누워 있다

> L. adjaceo, **adjacui**, adjacetum, adjacēre (< ad- *to, toward, at, according to*
+ jacēre *to lie*) 옆에 위치하다, 인접하다

E *adjacent, ease* (< *'lying nearby, hence easy to reach'*), *disease* (< *'no ease'*),
malaise (< *'bad ease'*), *easy*, ((It.) ad agio *'at ease'* >) *adagio*

> L. subjaceo, **subjacui**, subjacetum, subjacēre (< sub- *under, up from under*
+ jacēre *to lie*) 아래에 있다 **E** *subjacent*

> G. hienai (he- *stem of* hienai) *to throw, to send, to let go, to set in motion*

> G. aphienai (< aph- (< apo) *away from, from*) *to let go away*

> G. aphesis, apheseōs, f. *letting go away*

E *aphesis* (< *'gradual and unintentional loss of a short unaccented vowel
at the beginning of a word'*), *aphetic*

> G. enienai (< en- *in*) *to send in*

> G. enema, enematos, n. (< -ma *resultative noun suffix*) *a liquid or
gaseous substance (either medicinal or alimentary) introduced
mechanically into the rectum*

> L. enema, enematis, n. 관장제(灌腸劑), 관장(灌腸) **E** *enema*

> G. kathienai (< kath- (< kata) *down, mis-, according to, along, thoroughly*)
to send down

> G. kathetēr, kathetēros, m. *anything let down into, catheter*

> L. catheter, catheteris, m. 카테터, 도관(導管), 이끌관 **E** *catheter, catheterize*

> G. parienai (< par(a)- *beside, along side of, beyond*) *to let fall at the side,
to relax, to forgive, to remit*

> G. paresis, pareseōs, f. *forgiveness, remission, slackening, partial
paralysis*

> L. paresis, paresis, f. 불완전마비, 부전마비(不全痲痺)　　**E** *paresis, paretic*

　　> L. hemiparesis, hemiparesis, f. (< G. hemi- *half*) 반불

　　　완전마비, 반부전마비　　**E** *hemiparesis*

　　> L. paraparesis, paraparesis, f. (< G. par(a)- *beside, along*

　　　side of, beyond) 하반신 불완전마비　　**E** *paraparesis*

quatio, quassi, quassum, quatĕre 흔들다, 진동시키다

> quasso, quassavi, quassatum, quassare (*frequentative*) 뒤흔들다, 부스러뜨리다　　**E** *squash*

> concutio, concussi, concussum, concutĕre (< con- (< cum) *with, together* + -cutĕre

　　(< quatĕre) *to shake*) 충격을 주다　　**E** *concuss*

　　> concussio, concussionis, f. 진탕(震盪), 뇌진탕　　**E** *concussion*

> discutio, discussi, discussum, discutĕre (< dis- *apart from, down, not* + -cutĕre

　　(< quatĕre) *to shake*) 깨트리다, (안개·구름을) 흩어지게 하다, 떨쳐 버리다, 검토

　　하다, 토론하다　　**E** *discuss, discussant*

　　> discussio, discussionis, f. 검토, 토론　　**E** *discussion*

> excutio, excussi, excussum, excutĕre (< ex- *out of, away from* + -cutĕre (< quatĕre)

　　to shake) 털어내다, 흔들어 떨어뜨리다, (병·악습을) 떨어지게 하다　**E** (*reexcutĕre >) *rescue*

> percutio, percussi, percussum, percutĕre (< per- *through, thoroughly* + -cutĕre

　　(< quatĕre) *to shake*) 세게 흔들어 대다, 치다, 쳐서 울리다　　**E** *percuss*

　　> percussio, percussionis, f. 충격, 충격에 의한 진동, 타진(打診)　　**E** *percussion*

> succutio, succussi, succussum, succutĕre (< suc- (< sub) *under, up from under* +

　　-cutĕre (< quatĕre) *to shake*) 뒤엎다, 출렁이게 하다, 환자를 흔들어 출렁이는

　　액체 소리를 듣다　　**E** *succuss*

　　> succussio, succussionis, f. 진탕(震盪)　　**E** *succussion*

< IE. kwet- *to shake*

> G. passein *to sprinkle upon, to interweave, to embroider*

　　> G. pastos, pastē, paston *sprinkled, salted*

　　　> G. pasta, pastōn, n. (*neuter pl.*) (< *salted food*) *barley porridge*

　　　　> L. pasta, pastae, f. 가루 반죽, 풀[糊], 연고

　　　　E It. *pasta, paste, pastry, pastel* (< '*the plant's leaves were made*

　　　　into a paste in producing the dye')

　　　　> L. pasticium, pasticii, n. 가루 반죽 과자　　**E** *patisserie, pastiche*

rabio, -, -, rabĕre 미쳐 있다, 실성하다, 격분하다

> rabies, rabiei, f. 광기, 실성, 격분, 광견병, 미친개병, 공수병(恐水病)　　**E** *rabies, rage*

> rabidus, rabida, rabidum 미친, 미친 듯한, 과격한, 열광적인, 광견병의　　**E** *rabid*

< IE. rebh- *violent, impetuous*

rapio, rapui, raptum, rapĕre 날쌔게 잡다, 잡아채다, 빼앗다, 약탈하다,

　　납치하다　　**E** *rape, ravish, rapt, ravage*

> rapina, rapinae, f. 약탈, 약탈품   **E** *raven, ravenous*

> raptor, raptoris, m. 약탈자, 납치자, 강간자, 육식조(肉食鳥), 맹금(猛禽)   **E** *raptor*

    > velociraptor, velociraptoris, m. (< velox, (gen.) velocis *swift*) 벨로시랩터   **E** *velociraptor*

> raptura, rapturae, f. (사람을 다른 곳, 특히 천국으로) 보내기, 황홀경   **E** *rapture*

> rapax, (gen.) rapacis 강탈하는   **E** *rapacious*

> rapidus, rapida, rapidum 날쌘, 맹렬한   **E** *rapid*

> surripio, surripui, surreptum, surripĕre (< sur- (< sub) *under, up from under* +

    -ripĕre (< rapĕre) *to seize*) 훔치다

    > surreptitius, surreptitia, surreptitium 남의 눈을 피해서 하는, 은밀한, 부정한   **E** *surreptitious*

< IE. rep- *to snatch*

sapio, sapivi (sapii, sapui), -, sapĕre 맛있다, 맛을 알다, 알다,

지혜롭다   **E** *sage, sapient,* (sapiens (*present participle*) 'sapient' >) F. *savant*

> sapor, saporis, m. 맛, 멋   **E** *sapor (sapour), saporific, savor (savour), savory (savoury)*

> sapidus, sapida, sapidum 맛있는   **E** *sapid*

    > insipidus, insipida, insipidum (< in- *not* + -sipidus (< sapidus) *sapid*) 맛없는   **E** *insipid*

> sapientia, sapientiae, f. 지혜   **E** *sapiential*

< IE. sep-, sap- *to taste, to perceive*   **E** *sap*

specio (spicio), spexi, spectum, specĕre 바라보다

> species, speciei, f. 외형, 형상, 종류, 종(種), 향신료

E *species (sp.),* (pl.) *species (spp.),* (species >) *speciation, spice* (< 'assorted goods, wares')

> subspecies, subspeciei, f. (< sub- *under, up from under*) 아종(亞種)   **E** *subspecies (ssp.)*

> speciosus, speciosa, speciosum 외관이 좋은, 허울 좋은   **E** *specious*

> specialis, speciale 특별한, 특유한

E *special* (< 'different from usual'), *specialist, specialize, especial* (< 'better or greater than usual')

    > specialitas, specialitatis, f. 특성, 전문성   **E** *speciality (specialty)*

> specificus, specifica, specificum (< species *appearance, kind* + -ficus (<

facĕre) *making*) 특유한, 특이한   **E** *specific,* (specific >) *specificity*

    > specifico, specificavi, specificatum, specificare 종류를 구분하다, 명시

      하다, 한정 짓다, 규명하다   **E** *specify*

      > specificatio, specificationis, f. 명시, 내역,

      세목   **E** *specification,* (specification >) *specs*

> specimen, speciminis, n. 특징, 검증, 견본, 표본, 검사물, 검체   **E** *specimen*

> specula, speculae, f. 망대, 초소, 감시, 관찰

    > speculor, speculatus sum, speculari 살피다, 숙고하다, 추측하다   **E** *speculate, speculative*

      > speculatio, speculationis, f. 숙고, 추측   **E** *speculation*

> speculum, speculi, n. 거울, 영상, 반영, 경(鏡), 검경(檢鏡)   **E** *speculum, specular*

> spectrum, spectri, n. 환영(幻影), 유령, 스펙트럼, 분광상, 전역(全域), 범위

> > **E** *spectre (specter), (spectre > 'isolated from 'ghosts' of red blood cells' >) spectrin, spectrum, (pl.) spectra, spectrometer, spectrophotometer, spectroscope*

> > spectralis, spectrale 유령의, 스펙트럼의   **E** *spectral*

> specto, spectavi, spectatum, spectare (*frequentative*) 응시하다, 구경하다

> > **E** *spectate, spectator, (spectator + -itis 'noun suffix denoting inflammation' >) spectatoritis*

> > spectaculum, spectaculi, n. (spectaclum, spectacli, n.) 광경, 장관,
> > 구경거리   **E** *spectacle, spectacular*

> > ex(s)pecto, ex(s)pectavi, ex(s)pectatum, ex(s)pectare (< ex- *out of, away*
> > *from* + spectare *to look*) 기대하다, 예상하다   **E** *expect, expectant*

> > > ex(s)pectatio, ex(s)pectationis, f. 기대, 예측   **E** *expectation*

> > > ex(s)pectantia, ex(s)pectantiae, f. 기대, 예측   **E** *expectancy*

> -spex, -spicis, m. 점쟁이

> > auspex, auspicis, m., f. (< avispex, avispicis, m., f. *inspector of birds*) 새
> > 점쟁이, 가호자   **E** *auspex*

> > > auspicium, auspicii, n. 새 점, 조짐, (일의 상서로운) 시작,
> > > 가호   **E** *auspice, auspicious*

> > haruśpex, haruspicis, m. (< *inspector of entrails* < (*of Etruscan origin*) haru-
> > *entrails* (< IE. gherǝ- *gut, entrail*) + -spex, -spicis, m. *inspector*) (희생
> > 동물의 내장을 보고 점치는) 장복(臟卜) 점쟁이   **E** *haruspex*

> frontispicium, frontispicii, n. (< frons, frontis, f. *front* + specĕre *to look*) 앞면,
> 정면   **E** *frontispiece*

> aspicio, aspexi, aspectum, aspicĕre (< ad- *to, toward, at, according to* + -spicĕre
> (< specĕre) *to look*) 똑바로 쳐다보다, (어느 쪽을) 향해 있다   **E** *aspect*

> circumspicio, circumspexi, circumspectum, circumspicĕre (< circum- *around* +
> -spicĕre (< specĕre) *to look*) 사방을 살펴보다,
> 신중히 생각하다   **E** *circumspect, circumspection, circumspective*

> conspicio, conspexi, conspectum, conspicĕre (< con- (< cum) *with, together;*
> *intensive* + -spicĕre (< specĕre) *to look*) 주목하다, 괄목하다

> > conspectus, conspectus, m. (일목요연한) 개관   **E** *conspectus*

> > conspicuus, conspicua, conspicuum 주목할 만한, 두드러진   **E** *conspicuous*

> despicio, despexi, despectum, despicĕre (< de- *apart from, down, not* + -spicĕre
> (< specĕre) *to look*) 내려다보다, 업신여기다   **E** *despise, despite, spite, spiteful*

> despicor, despicatus sum, despicare (< de- *apart from, down, not* + specĕre *to look*)
> 멸시하다, 경멸하다, 천대하다   **E** *despicable*

> inspicio, inspexi, inspectum, inspicĕre (< in- *in, on, into, toward* + -spicĕre (<
> specĕre) *to look*) 들여다보다, 살펴보다

> > inspecto, inspectavi, inspectatum, inspectare (*frequentative*) 자세히 들여다보다,
> > 시찰하다   **E** *inspect, inspective*

> > > inspectio, inspectionis, f. 검사, 조사, 시찰   **E** *inspection*

> introspicio, introspexi, introspectum, introspicĕre (< intro *inward(s)* + -spicĕre

(< specĕre) *to look*) 안을 들여다보다

> introspecto, **introspectavi**, introspectatum, introspectare (*frequentative*) 자기

성찰을 하다, 내성(內省)하다, 내관(內觀)하다 　　　　**E** *introspect, introspective*

> perspicio, **perspexi**, perspectum, perspicĕre (< per- *through, thoroughly* + -spicĕre

(< specĕre) *to look*) 꿰뚫어 보다, 전체를 파악하다, 통찰(洞察)하다 　**E** *perspective*

> perspicuus, perspicua, perspicuum 명료한 　　　　　**E** *perspicuous*

> perspicax, (gen.) perspicacis 통찰력이 있는 　　　**E** *perspicacious*

> prospicio, **prospexi**, prospectum, prospicĕre (< pro- *before, forward, for, instead of*

+ -spicĕre (< specĕre) *to look*) 내다보다, 예견하다 　**E** *prospect, prospective*

> respicio, **respexi**, respectum, respicĕre (< re- *back, again* + -spicĕre (< specĕre)

to look) 돌아보다, 돌이켜 보다, 돌보다

> respecto, **respectavi**, respectatum, respectare (*frequentative*) 지켜보다,

소중히 여기다 　　　　**E** *respect, respectful, respectively, respite*

> retrospicio, **retrospexi**, retrospectum, retrospicĕre (< retro- *backward, behind* +

-spicĕre (< specĕre) *to look*) 뒤돌아보다, 회고하다, 소급하다 　**E** *retrospect, retrospective*

> suspicio, **suspexi**, suspectum, suspicĕre (< sus- (< sub) *under, up from under* +

-spicĕre (< specĕre) *to look*) 올려보다, 의심하다 　　**E** *suspect*

> suspectio, suspectionis, f. 경탄, 의혹, 낌새 　　　**E** *suspicion*

> suspiciosus, suspiciosa, suspiciosum 의심스러운 　**E** *suspicious*

> transpicio, **transpexi**, transpectum, transpicĕre (< tran- (< trans) *over, across,*

through, beyond + -spicĕre (< specĕre) *to look*) 건너다보다, 꿰뚫어 보다 　**E** *transpicuous*

< IE. spek- *to observe* 　　　　　　　　**E** *spy, espionage*

> G. skopein (skopeein) *to observe*

> G. skopos, skopou, m. *watcher, spy, mark, object* 　　　**E** *scope*

> G. episkopos, episkopou, m. (< ep(i)- *upon*) *overlooker, overseer*

> L. episcopus, episcopi, m. 감독, 주교 　　　**E** *bishop*

> L. episcopalis, episcopale 주교의 　　　**E** *episcopal*

> G. skopē, skopēs, f. (skopia, skopias, f.) *observation* 　**E** *-scopy, microscopy*

> G. -skopion, -skopiou, n. *instrument for observing*

E *scope, -scopic, periscope, otoscope, rhinoscope, laryngoscope, retinoscope, endoscope, microscope, microscopic, macroscopic (< 'on the pattern of microscopic')*

> G. skeptesthai (*middle*) *to examine, to consider*

> G. skeptikos, skeptikē, skeptikon *reflective, inquiring*

> L. scepticus, sceptica, scepticum 회의적인, 회의론의

E *sceptic (skeptic), sceptical (skeptical), scepticism (skepticism)*

> G. skepsis, skepseōs, f. *examining, observation, consideration*

> L. scepsis, scepsis, f. 명상, 회의 　　**E** *omphaloscepsis (omphaloskepsis)*

••• 정형 제 4 변화

> 능동태 현재부정법이 –ire로, 능동태 직설법 현재 단수 일인칭이 –io로 끝나는 동사.

audio, audivi (audii), auditum, audire 듣다

능동태	부정법	현재			aud-ire	듣다
	직설법	현재	단수	일인칭	aud-io	나는 ~한다
				이인칭	aud-is	너는 ~한다
				삼인칭	aud-it	그는 ~한다
			복수	일인칭	aud-imus	우리는 ~한다
				이인칭	aud-itis	너희는 ~한다
				삼인칭	aud-iunt	그들은 ~한다
		과거	단수	일인칭	aud-iebam	나는 ~하였다
		미래	단수	일인칭	aud-iam	나는 ~하겠다
		완료	단수	일인칭	audiv-i	나는 ~하였다
	가정법	현재	단수	일인칭	aud-iam	나는 ~하리라
	명령법	현재	단수	이인칭	aud-i	너는 ~하라
			복수	이인칭	aud-ite	너희는 ~하라
	분 사	현재			audiens, (gen.) audient-is	~하는, ~하고 있는
	목적분사				audit-um	~하러, ~하기 위하여
수동태	부정법	현재			aud-iri	들리다
	분 사	미래			audiend-us, audiend-a, audiend-um	~받아야 할
		과거			audit-us, audit-a, audit-um	~받은, ~받고서

audio, audivi (audii), auditum, audire 듣다

> **E** *audient, audile* (< 'on the pattern of tactile'), ***audi(o)-***, *(audi(o)- >)* ***audio, audio-visual, audiometer, audiogram***

> auditus, auditus, m. 청각, 들음, 듣고 앎, 들은 내용; 회계 감사,

　　감사(監査)　　**E** *audit* (< 'audit of an account, originally being presented orally')

> auditio, auditionis, f. 들음, 청취; 시청(試聽), 심사　　　　　　　　**E** *audition*

> audientia, audientiae, f. 경청, 알현, 청중　　　　　　　　　　　**E** *audience*

> auditor, auditoris, m. 청취자　　　　　　　　　　　　　　　　**E** *auditor*

> auditorius, auditoria, auditorium 청취의, 청각의　　　　　　**E** *auditory*

> auditorium, auditorii, n. 청중, 강당　　　　　　**E** *auditorium*

어원론을 위한 라틴어 • 601

> audibilis, audibile 들리는, 들을 수 있는   **E** *audible*

> oboedio, oboedivi (oboedii), oboeditum, oboedire (obedio, obedivi (obedii),

     obeditum, obedire) (< ob- *before, toward(s), over, against, away* + audire

     to hear) 경청하다, 복종하다   **E** *obey, obedient, disobey, disobedient*

     > oboedientia, oboedientiae, f. (obedientia, obedientiae, f.) 경청,

         복종   **E** *obedience, disobedience*

<IE. au-dh-, awis-dh- (< au- *to perceive* + dhe- *to put, to set*) *to put perception*

< IE. au-, awis- *to perceive*

> G. aisthanesthai (*middle*) *to perceive, to sense, to feel*   **E** *aesthetic (esthetic)*

   > G. aisthēsis, aisthēseōs, f. *perception, sensation, feeling*   **E** *-aesthesia (-esthesia)*

     > G. anaisthēsia, anaisthēsias, f. (< an- *without* + aisthēsis *feeling*)

       anesthesia

       > L. anaesthesia, anaesthesiae, f. (anesthesia, anesthesiae, f.)

         마취(痲醉), 무감각,

         지각소실   **E** *anaesthesia (anesthesia), anesthetic, anesthesiology*

     > G. dysaisthēsia, dysaisthēsias, f. (< dys- *bad* + aisthēsis *feeling*)

       dysesthesia

       > L. dysaesthesia, dysaesthesiae, f. (dysesthesia, dysesthesiae, f.)

         감각장애, 감각이상   **E** *dysaesthesia (dysesthesia), dysesthetic*

     > L. hyperaesthesia, hyperaesthesiae, f. (hyperesthesia, hyperesthesiae, f.)

       (< G. hyper- *over*) 감각과민   **E** *hyperaesthesia (hyperesthesia), hyperesthetic*

     > L. hypaesthesia, hypaesthesiae, f. (hypesthesia, hypesthesiae, f.)

       (< G. hyp(o)- *under*)

       감각저하   **E** *hypaesthesia (hypesthesia, hypoesthesia), hypesthetic*

     > L. paraesthesia, paraesthesiae, f. (paresthesia, paresthesiae, f.)

       (< G. par(a)- *beside, along side of, beyond*) 감각이상,

       이상감각   **E** *paraesthesia (paresthesia), paresthetic*

     > L. kinaesthesia, kinaesthesiae, f. (kinesthesia, kinesthesiae, f.)

       (< G. kinein (kineein) *to set in motion, to move*)

       운동감각   **E** *kinaesthesia (kinesthesia), kinesthetic*

     > L. thermaesthesia, thermaesthesiae, f. (thermesthesia, thermesthesiae, f.)

       (< G. thermē *warmth, heat*)

       온도감각   **E** *thermaesthesia (thermesthesia), thermesthetic*

     > L. synaesthesia, synaesthesiae, f. (synesthesia, synesthesiae, f.)

       (< G. syn- *with, together*) 동반감각, 공감;

       (심리) 공감각(共感覺)   **E** *synaesthesia (synesthesia), synesthetic*

dormio, dormivi (dormii), dormitum, dormire 잠자다

     > dormans, (gen.) dormantis (*present participle*) 잠자는   **E** *dormant, (dormant >) dormancy*

     > dormitorius, dormitoria, dormitorium 잠에 관한, 침실의

       > dormitorium, dormitorii, n. 침실   **E** *dormitory*

> dormito, **dormitavi**, dormitatum, dormitare (*frequentative*) 졸다

[용례] Dormitat Homerus. (> *Even Homer sometimes nods.*) 호머도 실수한다
(Quintus Horatius Flaccus, 65-8 B.C.E.)
(문법) dormitat 졸다: 능동태 직설법 현재 단수 삼인칭
Homerus 호머가: 단수 주격 < Homerus, Homeri, m. 호머
< G. Homēros, Homērou, m. *Homer*

< IE. drem- *to sleep*

farcio, farsi, fartum (farctum), farcire 처넣다, 틀어막다　　　　　**E** *farce, forcemeat*
> infarcio, **infarsi**, infarsum (infartum, infarctum), infarcire 빈틈없이 채워 넣다,
다져 넣다　　　　　　　　　　　　　　　　　　　　　**E** (*verb*) *infarct*
> infarctus, infarctus, m. 경색(梗塞)　　　　　　　　　**E** (*noun*) *infarct*
> infarctio, infarctionis, f. 경색증(梗塞症)　　　　　　　　**E** *infarction*
< IE. bhrek^w- *to cram together*
> L. frequens, (gen.) frequentis 가득 들어찬, 많이 모이는, 자주 모이는, 잦은,
빈번한　　　　　　　　　　　　　　　　　　　**E** (*adjective*) *frequent*
> L. frequentia, frequentiae, f. 군집, 빈도; 주파수, 진동수　　　**E** *frequency*
> L. frequento, **frequentavi**, frequentatum, frequentare 자주 드나들다,
반복하다　　　　　　　　　　　　　　**E** (*verb*) *frequent, frequentative*
> G. phrassein *to block up, to fence in, to enclose*
> G. phragma, phragmatos, n. *fence, hedge*　　　　　　**E** *phragmoplast*
> G. diaphragma, diaphragmatos, n. (< di(a)- *through, thoroughly, apart*)
partition wall, diaphragm
> L. diaphragma, diaphragmatis, n. 칸막이, 격막(隔膜);
가로막, 횡격막　　　　　　　**E** *diaphragm, diaphragmatic*

garrio, garrivi (garrii), garritum, garrire 지껄이다, (새들이) 지저귀다,
(개구리가) 개골개골하다　　　　　　　　　　　　　　　　**E** *garrulous*
< IE. gar- *to call, to cry; expressive root*
E *care* (< *'grief'*), *chary* (< *'sorrowful, anxious'*), ((*Gaelic*) sluagh-ghairm *'army-cry'* >) *slogan*

glutio, glutivi (glutii), glutitum, glutire (gluttio, gluttivi (gluttii), gluttitum, gluttire)
꿀꺽 삼키다, 게걸스레 먹다　　　　　　　　　　　　　　　　**E** *glut*
> glutto, gluttonis, m. 대식가, 탐식가　　　　　　　　**E** *glutton, gluttony*
> deglutio, **deglutivi (deglutii)**, deglutitum, deglutire (< de- *apart from, down, not;*
intensive + glutire *to swallow*) 삼키다, 참다
> deglutitio, deglutitionis, f. 삼키기, 연하(嚥下)　　　　**E** *deglutition*
< IE. g^{w}elə- *to swallow*　　　　　　　　　　　　　**E** *keel* (< *'beak of a ship'*)
> L. gula, gulae, f. 목구멍, 탐식, 식도락　　　　　　　　**E** *gullet, gully*

∽ IE. gʷerə- *to swallow*

> L. gurges, gurgitis, m. 목구멍, 끝없이 깊은 곳, 심연, 소용돌이,

방탕아　　　**E** *gorge, (suggested) gorgeous (< 'adorning the neck'), engorge, disgorge*

> L. gurgito, gurgitavi, gurgitatum, gurgitare 목까지 채우다, 잔뜩 먹이다　　**E** *gurgitate*

> L. ingurgito, ingurgitavi, ingurgitatum, ingurgitare (< in- *in, on, into,*
toward + gurgitare *to engulf*) 폭식하다　　**E** *ingurgitate*

> L. regurgito, regurgitavi, regurgitatum, regurgitare (< re- *back, again*
+ gurgitare *to engulf*) 역류하다　　**E** *regurgitate, regurgitant*

> L. regurgitatio, regurgitationis, f. 역류　　**E** *regurgitation*

> L. voro, voravi, voratum, vorare 탐식하다　　**E** *-vore, devour*

> L. vorax, (gen.) voracis 탐식하는, 탐욕의　　**E** *voracious*

> L. -vorus, -vora, -vorum

먹는　　**E** *-vorous, frugivorous, graminivorous, piscivorous, formicivorous*

> L. carnivorus, carnivora, carnivorum (< caro, carnis, f. *flesh* + -vorus
devouring) 육식의　　**E** *carnivorous*

> L. herbivorus, herbivora, herbivorum (< herba, herbae, f. *grass* + -vorus
devouring) 초식의　　**E** *herbivorous*

> L. omnivorus, omnivora, omnivorum (< omnis, omne *all* + -vorus *de-
vouring*) 잡식의　　**E** *omnivorous*

> L. *sanguivorus, *sanguivora, *sanguivorum (< sanguis, sanguinis, m.
blood + -vorus *devouring*) 흡혈성의　　**E** *sanguivorous*

> G. brōsis, brōseōs, f. *eating*

> G. abrōsia, abrōsias, f. (< a- *not*) *fasting*　　**E** *abrosia*

> G. brōma, brōmatos, n. *food*　　**E** *bromatology*

> L. Theobroma, Theobromatis, n. (< G. theos *god* + brōma *food*)

카카오나무속(屬)　　**E** *(Theobroma cacao >) theobromine*

> G. bronchos, bronchou, m. (< *throat*) *windpipe*

> L. bronchus, bronchi, m. 기관지　　**E** *bronchus, (pl.) bronchi, bronchial, bronchogenic*

> L. bronchiolus, bronchioli, m. (< + -olus *diminutive suffix*)

세기관지　　**E** *bronchiolus, (pl.) bronchioli, bronchiole, bronchiolar*

> G. branchion, branchiou, n. *fin;* (pl. branchia) *gills*

> L. branchiae, branchiarum, f. (pl.) 아가미,

새(鰓)　　**E** *branchia, (pl.) branchiae, branchial, branchi(o)-*

micturio, micturivi, micturitum, micturire (*desiderative*) 소변보고 싶다, 오줌 마렵다

> micturitio, micturitionis, f. 배뇨(排尿)　　**E** *micturition, (micturition >) micturate*

< mejo, mixi, mictum, mejĕre (mingo, minxi, mictum (minctum), mingĕre) 오줌 누다

< IE. meigh- *to urinate*　　**E** *mist, mistletoe (< 'propagated through the droppings of the mistle thrush')*

nutrio, nutrivi (nutrii), nutritum, nutrire (젖으로) 기르다, 영양분을 주어 키우다, 양육하다,

보살피다　　　　　　　　　　　　　　　　　　　　　　　**E** *nourish, nutrient, nutritive*

> nutritio, nutritionis, f. 영양, 영양 섭취　　　　　　**E** *nutrition, nutritional, nutritionist, malnutrition*

> nutritura, nutriturae, f. 영양 상태, 양육, 양성　　　　**E** *nutriture, nurture, (nurture >) nurturant*

> nutrimentum, nutrimenti, n. 영양분, 자양물　　　　　　**E** *nutriment, nutrimental*

> nutrix, nutricis, f. 젖어미, 유모, 보살피는 여자

　　> nutricius, nutricia, nutricium (nutritius, nutritia, nutritium) 먹이는, 기르는,

　　　　양육하는　　　　　　　　　　　　　　　　　　**E** *nutritious*

　　　　> nutricia, nutriciae, f. 양육 맡은 여자　　　　**E** *nurse, nursing, nursery*

< IE. (s)na, (s)nau- *to swim, to flow, to let flow, to suckle*

> L. no, navi, −, nare 헤엄치다, 부유하다

　　> L. nato, **natavi**, natatum, natare (*frequentative*) 헤엄치다, 표류하다　　**E** *natant*

　　　　> L. natatio, natationis, f. 헤엄, 수영, 유영　　　　　　　　**E** *natation*

　　　　> L. natatorius, natatoria, natatorium 헤엄치는 데 쓰이는,

　　　　　　헤엄치는 데 적합한　　　　　　　　　　　　　**E** *natatorium, natatorial*

　　　　> L. supernato, **supernatavi**, supernatatum, supernatare (< super- *above*

　　　　　　+ natare *to swim*) 위를 헤엄치다, 표면에 뜨다　　　**E** *supernatant*

> G. nein (neein) *to swim*

　　> G. neustos, neustē, neuston *swimming*

　　　　E *neuston (< 'the minute organisms inhabiting the surface layer of water or moving on the surface film')*

> G. nēchein *to swim*

　　> G. nēktos, nēktē, nēkton *swimming*

　　　　E *nekton (< 'aquatic animals that are able to swim and move independently of water movements')*

> G. nēsos, nēsou, f. *island, peninsula*

　　　　E *Indonesia, Melanesia (< 'the region of islands inhabited by dark-skinned peoples'), Micronesia, Polynesia*

　　> G. nēsidion, nēsidiou, n. (< nēsos + -idion *diminutive suffix*)

　　　　little island　　　　　　**E** *nesidioblast (< 'pancreatic islet-forming cell')*

> G. nan (naein) *to flow, to flow over*

　　> G. Naias, Naiados, f. *water nymph*

　　　　> L. Naias, Naiadis, f. 물의 요정　　　　　　　　**E** *naiad*

perio, perui, pertum, perire (*obsolete*) 덮다

> aperio, aperui, apertum, aperire (< a- (< ab) *off, away from* + perire (*obsolete*) *to cover*) 열다, 개통시키다, 드러내다,

밝히다　　　　　　　**E** *aperient, (aperitivus 'of opening' >) aperitif, overt, pert*

[용례] spina bifida aperta 개방이분척추, 드러난 척추갈림증　　**E** *spina bifida aperta*

(문법) spina 척추: 단수 주격 < spina, spinae, f. 가시, 등마루

bifida 두 갈래의: 형용사, 여성형 단수 주격

< bifidus, bifida, bifidum

aperta 드러난: 과거분사, 여성형 단수 주격

< apertus, aperta, apertum

> apertura, aperturae, f. 입구, 구멍　　　　　　　　　**E** *aperture, overture*

> operio, operui, opertum, operire (< op- (< ob) *toward(s), to, on, over, against* +
perire (*obsolete*) *to cover*) 덮다, 가리다

> operculum, operculi, n. 덮개, 뚜껑,
마개　　　　　　　　　　　　　　　**E** *operculum, (pl.) opercula, opercular, operculate*

> cooperio, cooperui, coopertum, cooperire (< co- (< cum) *with, together* +
operire *to hide*) 뒤덮다, 가리다, 파묻히게 하다

E *cover, covert, coverage, uncover, curfew (< 'to cover fireplace'), kerchief (<
'a cloth used to cover the head, formerly a woman's head-dress'), (kerchief
>) handkerchief*

> *coopertura, *cooperturae, f. 덮개, 보호물, 숨는 곳, 외관　　　**E** *coverture*

> discooperio, discooperui, discoopertum, discooperire (< dis- *apart from,
down, not* + cooperire *to cover*) 벗기다, 발견하다, 깨닫다　**E** *discover, discovery*

< IE. wer- *to cover*　　　　　　**E** *warn, warrant, warranty, warrantee, guaranty, garage, garment*

salio, salui (salivi, salii), saltum, salire 뜀뛰다, 도약하다, 튀다, 솟구치다, (동물의 수컷이)
흘레하다

E *sally, salient, saute (< 'fried in a pan with a little butter over a high heat, while being
tossed from time to time'), (supra 'above' + saltus 'leap' >) somersault, (con- (< cum)
'with, together' + salire 'to leap' >) consilience*

> salto, saltavi, saltatum, saltare (*frequentative*) 춤추다, 도약하다

> saltatio, saltationis, f. 춤, 도약　　　　　　　　　　　**E** *saltation*

> saltator, saltatoris, m. 춤추는 사람, 도약하는 사람

> saltatorius, saltatoria, saltatorium 춤추는, 도약하는　**E** *saltatory, saltatorial*

> assilio, assilui, assultum, assilire (< as- (< ad) *to, toward, at, according to* + salire
to leap) 덤벼들다, 공격하다　　　　　　　　　　　　　　　**E** *assail*

> assulto, assultavi, assultatum, assultare (*frequentative*) 힘껏 덤벼들다, 강습
하다, 폭행하다　　　　　　　　　　　　　　　　　　　**E** *assault*

> exsilio, exsilui, exsultum, exsilire (< ex- *out of, away from* + salire *to leap*) 뛰어
오르다, 솟구치다

> exsulto, exsultavi, exsultatum, exsultare (exulto, exultavi, exultatum, exultare)
(*frequentative*) 뛰어 오르다, 기뻐 날뛰다　　　　　　　　**E** *exult*

> insilio, insilui, insultum, insilire (< in- *in, on, into, toward* + salire *to leap*) 올라
타다, 달려들다　　　　　　　　　　　　　　　　　　　**E** *insult*

> resilio, resilui (resilii), resultum, resilire (< re- *again, back* + salire *to leap*) 되튀다,
움츠러들다　　　　　　　　　　　　　　　　　**E** *resile, resilient, resilin*

> *resilientia, *resilientiae, f. 탄력성, 탄성, 복원력　　　**E** *resilience (resiliency)*

> resulto, resultavi, resultatum, resultare (*frequentative*) (< re- *again, back* +

resilire *to rebound*) 되튀다, 움츠러들다 **E** *result, resultant, resultative*

< IE. sel- *to jump*

> (*probably*) L. salmo, salmonis, m. (< *leaping fish*) 연어 **E** *salmon*

sentio, sensi, sensum, sentire (< *to go mentally*) 느끼다, 생각하다, 깨닫다

E *sentient, sensor, scent* (< 'with unexplained addition of -c-'), *resent,* (*suggested*) *sentinel,* (*suggested*) *sentry*

> sensus, sensus, m. 감각, 감각기관, 감정, 생각, 의미 **E** *sense, sensuous*

[용례] sensu stricto 좁은 의미로, 협의(狹義)로 **E** *sensu stricto*

sensu lato 넓은 의미로, 광의(廣義)로 **E** *sensu lato*

(문법) sensu 뜻으로: 단수 탈격

stricto 좁은: 과거분사, 여성형 단수 탈격

< strictus, stricta, strictum 조인, 좁은, 엄격한

< stringo, strinxi, strictum, stringĕre 조이다

lato 넓은: 형용사, 여성형 단수 탈격 < latus, lata, latum

> sensualis, sensuale 감각적인, 관능적인, 육욕의 **E** *sensual, sensualism*

> sensualitas, sensualitatis, f. 관능성, 육욕성 **E** *sensuality*

> sensatus, sensata, sensatum 지각 있는, 사려 분별이 있는

> sensatio, sensationis, f. 감각, (감각을 통한) 지각 **E** *sensation, sensational*

> sensorium, sensorii, n. 감각, 감각중추 **E** *sensorium, sensorial, sensory*

> sensitivus, sensitiva, sensitivum 감각이 예민한,

민감한 **E** *sensitive,* (*sensitive* >) *sensitize, desensitize; hypersensitive*

> sensitivitas, sensitivitatis, f. 민감성, 민감도 **E** *sensitivity; hypersensitivity*

> insensitivus, insensitiva, insensitivum (< in- *not*) 둔감한 **E** *insensitive*

> insensitivitas, insensitivitatis, f. 둔감 **E** *insensitivity*

> sensibilis, sensibile 감각으로 파악할 수 있는, 감각 능력을 갖춘 **E** *sensible*

> sensibilitas, sensibilitatis, f. 감각 **E** *sensibility*

> insensibilis, insensibile (< in- *not*) 감각으로 파악할 수 없는,

감각 능력이 없는 **E** *insensible*

> insensibilitas, insensibilitatis, f. 무감각 **E** *insensibility*

> sentimentum, sentimenti, n. 감각, 감정, 정서, 감상(感想), 감상(感傷) **E** *sentiment, sentimental*

> sententia, sententiae, f. 의견, 의도, 의미; (문법) 문장, (철학) 명제, (법률) 판결 **E** *sentence*

> sententialis, sententiale (문법) 문장의, (법률) 판결의 **E** *sentential*

> sententiosus, sententiosa, sententiosum 금언의, 함축성 있는, 점잔 부리는 **E** *sententious*

> assentio, **assensi**, assensum, assentire (< ad- *to, toward, at, according to* + sentire

to feel) 찬성하다

> assentor, assentatus sum, assentari 찬성하다 **E** *assent*

> consentio, **consensi**, consensum, consentire (< con- (< cum) *with, together* + sentire

to feel) 의견을 같이하다, 동의하다 **E** *consent*

> consensus, consensus, m. (의견 등의) 일치, 합의, 다수의 의견 **E** *consensus, consensual*

> dissentio, **dissensi**, dissensum, dissentire (< dis- *apart from, down, not* + sentire
to feel) 의견을 달리하다, 반대하다, 불화하다   **E** *dissent, dissension*

> praesentio, **praesensi**, praesensum, praesentire (< prae- *before, beyond* + sentire
to feel) 예감하다   **E** *presentiment*

< IE. sent- *to head for, to go*   **E** *send*

venio, veni, ventum, venire 오다   **E** *(feminine past participle > verbal noun 'coming' >) venue*

> advenio, **adveni**, adventum, advenire (< ad- *to, toward, at, according to* + venire
to come) 도착하다, 도래하다, (뜻하지 않게) 생기다   **E** *avenue*

   > adventus, adventus, m. 도착, 도래   **E** *advent*

   > adventura, adventurae, f. 돌발적인 일, 이상한 사건,
모험   **E** *adventure, (adventure >) venture*

   > adventitius, adventitia, adventitium (밖에서부터) 다가오는, 외래의, 우발적인   **E** *adventitious*

     > adventitia, adventitiae, f. 외막(外膜), 바깥막   **E** *adventitia, adventitial*

> circumvenio, **circumveni**, circumventum, circumvenire (< circum- *around* + venire
to come) 에워싸다, 걸려들게 그물을 치다, 속이다   **E** *circumvent*

   > circumventio, circumventionis, f. 포위, 유혹, 기만   **E** *circumvention*

> convenio, **conveni**, conventum, convenire (< con- (< cum) *with, together* + venire
to come) 같이 오다, 만나다, 모이다; 뜻이 맞다, 협정을 맺다, 계약하다; 들어맞다,
적합하다   **E** *convene, convent; covenant; convenient*

   > conventio, conventionis, f. 모임, 집회; 협정, 계약, 관습   **E** *convention, conventional*

   > convenientia, convenientiae, f. 적합, 편의, 편리   **E** *convenience*

> evenio, **eveni**, eventum, evenire (< e- *out of, away from* + venire *to come*) 나오다,
(결과로서) 나타나다, (어떤 결과를) 가져오다, 일어나다

   > eventus, eventus, m. (어떤 일의 결과로 생겨나는) 사건   **E** *event, eventful, uneventful*

     > eventualis, eventuale 결과로서 일어나는, 최종적인   **E** *eventual*

> intervenio, **interveni**, interventum, intervenire (< inter- *between, among* + venire
to come) 끼어들다, 개입하다, 중재하다   **E** *intervene*

   > interventio, interventionis, f. 개입, 중재   **E** *intervention, interventional*

> invenio, **inveni**, inventum, invenire (< in- *in, on, into, toward* + venire *to come*)
찾아내다, 밝혀내다, 발견하다, 발명하다; (수동) ~이 있다, ~하다   **E** *invent*

   > inventio, inventionis, f. 발견, 발명   **E** *invention*

   > inventarium, inventarii, n. (inventorium, inventorii, n.) (< *a list of what are
found*) 물품 목록, 목록에 있는 물품, 목록   **E** *inventory*

> praevenio, **praeveni**, praeventum, praevenire (< prae- *before, beyond* + venire *to
come*) 먼저 오다, 앞지르다, 선수를 치다   **E** *prevent, prevenient, preventive*

   > praeventio, praeventionis, f. 먼저 옴, 앞지름, 선수를 침, 예방   **E** *prevention*

> provenio, **proveni**, proventum, provenire (< pro- *before, forward, for, instead of* +
venire *to come*) 나오다, 발생하다   **E** *provenience (provenance)*

> revenio, **reveni**, reventum, revenire (< re- *back, again* + venire *to come*)

돌아오다   **E** *revenant* (< *'coming back'*), ***revenue*** (< *'returned to the government'*)

> subvenio, **subveni**, subventum, subvenire (< sub- *under, up from under* + venire *to come*) 도우러 오다, 고치다, (일이) 일어나다,

(생각이) 떠오르다   **E** *souvenir* (< *'to come into the mind'*)

> supervenio, **superveni**, superventum, supervenire (< super- *above* + venire *to come*)

잇따라 일어나다   **E** *supervene, supervenient*

> superventio, superventionis, f. 속발, 병발   **E** *supervention*

< IE. gʷa-, gʷem- *to go, to come*   **E** *come, become, welcome*

> G. bainein (ba- *stem*) *to go, to walk, to step*

> G. basis, baseōs, f. *stepping, tread, base*   **E** *dysbasia* (< *'bad stepping'*)

> L. basis, basis, f. 바닥, 기저, 바탕, 기초, 기본

E *basis, base,* (base >) *basic, basically, basement, platybasia* (< *'flat base'*), ***basophil*** (< *'a cell or element staining readily with basic dyes'*)

> L. basalis, basale 바닥의, 기저의, 기초의, 기본적인   **E** *basal*

> L. basilaris, basilare 바닥의   **E** *basilar (basilary), basilad* (< + -ad *'toward'*)

> G. basidion, basidiou, n. (< + -idion *diminutive suffix*) *little pedestal (supporting the spores)*

> L. basidium, basidii, n. 담자(擔子), 담자기(擔子器)

E *basidium,* (pl.) *basidia, basidi(o)-, basidiospore,* (pl.) *basidiomycetes*

> G. -batos, -batos, -baton *going*

> G. akrobatos, akrobatos, akrobaton (< akros *point, highest*) *walking on tiptoe, climbing aloft*

> G. akrobatēs, akrobatou, m. *tightrope walker, acrobat*   **E** *acrobat*

> G. -batēs, -batou, m. *one that goes or treads, one that is based*

> G. diabētēs, diabētou, m. (< di(a)- *through, thoroughly, apart* + bainein *to go*) *passer through, siphon*

> L. diabetes, diabetae, m. 수도관, 파이프;

당뇨병   **E** *diabetes, diabetic, diabetogenic*

탈형동사의 변화

탈형동사는 꼴이 수동태이나 뜻은 능동태인 동사이다. 그러나 탈형동사라고 해서 모든 꼴이 다 수동태의 꼴은 아니다. 현재분사와 수동형 미래분사는 정형 동사처럼 능동태의 꼴을 갖는다.

라틴어사전은 직설법 현재 단수 일인칭, 직설법 완료 단수 일인칭 남성형, 그리고 현재부정법을 차례대로 제시한다.

●●● 탈형 제1변화

현재부정법이 –ari로, 직설법 현재 단수 일인칭이 –or로 끝나는 동사.

imitor, imitatus sum, imitari 모방하다, 본받다

부정법	현재				imit-ari	모방하다
직설법	현재	단수	일인칭		imit-or	나는 ~한다
			이인칭		imit-aris	너는 ~한다
			삼인칭		imit-atur	그는 ~한다
		복수	일인칭		imit-amur	우리는 ~한다
			이인칭		imit-amini	너희는 ~한다
			삼인칭		imit-antur	그들은 ~한다
	과거	단수	일인칭		imit-abar	나는 ~하였다
	미래	단수	일인칭		imit-abor	나는 ~하겠다
	완료	단수	일인칭		imitat-us, -a, -um sum	나는 ~하였다
가정법	현재	단수	일인칭		imit-er	나는 ~하리라
명령법	현재	단수	이인칭		imit-are	너는 ~하라
		복수	이인칭		imit-amini	너희는 ~하라
분 사	현재				imitans, (gen.) imitant-is	~하는, ~하고 있는
	과거				imitat-us, imitat-a, imitat-um	~한
수동형	미래분사				imitand-us, imitand-a, imitand-um	~받아야 할

imitor, imitatus sum, imitari 모방하다, 본받다

    < IE. aim- *to copy* (Vide IMAGO; *See* E. *image*)

E *imitate, imitable, inimitable*

conor, conatus sum, conari 하려 하다, 애쓰다, 노력하다

    < IE. ken- *to set oneself in motion, to arise, to make an effort*

        > G. diakonos, diakonou, m. (< di(a)- *through, thoroughly, apart*) *servant, attendant;*

          deacon

E *conatus, conative, conation*

E *deacon*

cunctor, cunctatus sum, cunctari 주저하다, 지체하다, 지연시키다

    < IE. konk- *to hang*

E *cunctator*

E *hang, hanker, hinge*

for, fatus sum, fari 말하다, 이야기하다, 읊다, 예언하다

      > infans, infantis, m., f. (< in- *not* + fans (*present participle*) *speaking*) 영아(嬰兒),

유아(乳兒), 젖먹이

> **E** *infant, infanticide, infantry (< 'foot-soldiery' < 'young servant or attendant serving on foot'), infantryman*

> infantia, infantiae, f. 말하지 못함, 표현 능력 없음, 어릴 때, 햇것, 영아기, 유아기　**E** *infancy*

> infantilis, infantile 영아의, 유아의, 아기 같은, 천진난만한, 유치한　**E** *infantile, infantilism*

> fatum, fati, n. (< fatum (*neuter past participle*) *that which has been spoken*) 천명, 예언, 운명, 불길　**E** *fate*

　> fatalis, fatale 운명에 관한, 운명을 결정하는, 숙명적인, 생명에 관계되는, 치명적인, 파멸적인　**E** *fatal*

　　> fatalitas, fatalitatis, f. 운명적임, 치명적임, (생명에 관계되는) 재난, (재난에 의한) 죽음　**E** *fatality*

　　> Fata, Fatae, f. (< fata, fatorum, n. pl.) (로마 신화) 운명의 세 여신(*the three Fates*: Nona, Decima, Morta)의 하나　**E** *fay, fairy*

> fabula, fabulae, f. 떠도는 이야기, 동화, 우화(寓話)　**E** *fable, ((possibly) fable >) fib*

　> fabulosus, fabulosa, fabulosum 동화 같은, 우화에 나오는, 믿기지 않는　**E** *fabulous*

　> fabulor, fabulatus sum, fabulari 이야기하다, 꾸며낸 이야기를 하다

　　> confabulor, confabulatus sum, confabulari (< con- (< cum) *with, together* + fabulari *to converse, to chat*) 서로 이야기하다, 대화하다　**E** *confabulate*

　　　> confabulatio, confabulationis, f. 이야기; 작화증(作話症), 말짓기증　**E** *confabulation, confabulatory*

> fateor, fassus sum, fateri 고백하다, 공언하다

　> confiteor, confessus sum, confiteri (< con- (< cum) *with, together; intensive* + fateri *to acknowledge, to avow*) 고백하다　**E** *confess*

　> profiteor, professus sum, profiteri (< pro- *before* + fateri *to acknowledge, to avow*) 공언하다, 신봉하다, (자기가 ~임을) 밝히다, (직업적으로) 가르치다　**E** *profess, professor*

　　> professio, professionis, f. 공언, 전문직, 직업　**E** *profession*

　　　> professionalis, professionale 전문직의, 직업적인　**E** *professional*

> affor, affatus sum, affari (< af- (< ad) *to, toward, at, according to* + fari *to speak*) 정답게 말을 걸다

　> affabilis, affabile 더불어 말할 만한, 붙임성 있는　**E** *affable*

> effor, effatus sum, effari (< ef- (< ex) *out of, away from* + fari *to speak*) 말로 표현하다, 격식을 갖추어 말하다

　> effabilis, effabile 말로 표현할 수 있는　**E** *effable, ineffable*

> praefor, praefatus sum, praefari (< prae- *before, beyond* + fari *to speak*) (무엇을) 하기에 앞서 말하다, 서두에서 말하다

　> praefatio, praefationis, f. 서언, 서문　**E** *preface, prefatory*

< IE. bha- *to speak*

> **E** *ban (< 'to proclaim'), banal (< 'common to all' < 'compulsory' < 'to proclaim to arms'), banish (< 'to proclaim as an outlaw'), bandit (< 'to have been summoned'), abandon (< 'to someone else's proclamation'), contraband (< 'against the proclamation'), boon (< 'prayer, request')*

> L. fas, n. (< *divine law* < *divinely spoken*) (불변화) 신의 계율, 천명, 적법

　> L. nefas, n. (< ne- *not*) (불변화) 법도에 어긋남

　　> L. nefarius, nefaria, nefarium 흉악한, 끔찍한　　　　**E** *nefarious*

> L. fama, famae, f. 소문, 명성　　　　**E** *fame*

　> L. famosus, famosa, famosum 유명한　　　　**E** *famous*

　> L. infamis, infame (< in- *not* + fama *fame*) 평판 나쁜

　　> L. infamosus, infamosa, infamosum 평판 나쁜　　　　**E** *infamous*

　　> L. infamia, infamiae, f. 오명, 악명, 비행　　　　**E** *infamy*

　> L. diffamo, **diffamavi**, diffamatum, diffamare (< dif- (< dis-) *apart from, down, not* + fama *fame*) 명예를 훼손하다, 나쁜 소문을 퍼뜨리다　　**E** *defame, defamatory*

> G. phanai *to speak*

　> G. phasis, phaseōs, f. *information, assertion, denunciation*

　　> G. -phasia, -phasias, f. *speaking*　　　　**E** *-phasia*

　　　> G. aphasia, aphasias, f. (< a- *not*) *speechlessness*

　　　　> L. aphasia, aphasiae, f. 언어상실증, 실어증　　　　**E** *aphasia*

　　　> L. dysphasia, dysphasiae, f. (< G. dys- *bad*) 언어장애　　**E** *dysphasia*

　　　> L. paraphasia, paraphasiae, f. (< G. par(a)- *beside, along side of, beyond*) 착어증, 말이상증　　　　**E** *paraphasia*

　> G. phēmē, phēmēs, f. *voice, speech, saying*

　　> G. blasphēmos, blasphēmos, blasphēmon (< (*perhaps*) blas- < IE. mel- *false, bad, wrong*) *evil-speaking, blasphemous*

　　　> G. blasphēmein (blasphēmeein) *to speak profanely*

　　　　> L. blasphemo, **blasphemavi**, blasphematum, blasphemare 욕설하다, 저주하다　　　　**E** *blaspheme, blame*

　　> G. euphēmos, euphēmos, euphēmon (< eu- *well*) *speaking words of good omen*

　　　> G. euphēmizein *to speak fair*　　　　**E** *euphemize*

　　　　> G. euphēmismos, euphēmismou, m. *substitution of a word or expression of comparatively favorable implication or less unpleasant associations, instead of the harsher or more offensive one*

　　　　　　　　E *euphemism, dysphemism* (< *on the pattern of euphemism*)

　> G. prophētēs, prophētou, m. (< pro- *before, in front* + phanai) *prophet*

　　> L. propheta, prophetae, m. (prophetes, prophetae, m.) 예언자　　**E** *prophet*

　　> G. prophēteia, prophēteias, f. *action or faculty of prophesying*

　　　> L. prophetia, prophetiae, f. 예언　　**E** (*noun*) **prophecy**, (*verb*) **prophesy**

　> G. apophanai (< ap(o)- *away from, from*) *to speak off, to deny*

　　> G. apophasis, apophaseōs, f. *denial*

　　　> L. apophasis, apophasis, f. 형식적 부정, 언급을 피한다고 하면서 슬쩍 암시하는 말　　　　**E** *apophasis*

> G. phōnē, phōnēs, f. *voice, vocal sound*

> **E** *phon(o)-, phonic, phonology,* (phōnē >) *phonation, (phonation >) phonate, -phone, telephone (phone),*

> G. -phōnos, -phōnos, -phōnon *sounding*

> G. antiphōnos, antiphōnos, antiphōnon (< ant(i)- *before, against, instead of; in return*) *sounding in response*

> **E** (ta antiphōna *'things sounding in response' > 'musical accords' >*) *antiphon, anthem*

> G. symphōnos, symphōnos, symphōnon (< sym- (< syn) *with, together*) *harmonious*

> G. symphōnia, symphōnias, f. *agreement or concord of sound, concert of vocal or instrumental music*

> L. symphonia, symphoniae, f. 화음, 교향악　　　**E** *symphony*

> G. -phōnia, -phōnias, f. *sounding*

> G. euphōnia, euphōnias, f. (< eu- *well*) *euphony*

> L. euphonia, euphoniae, f. 듣기 좋은 음조, 듣기 좋음, 음편(音便)　　　**E** *euphony, euphonic*

> G. kakophōnia, kakophōnias, f. (< kakos *bad*) *cacophony*

> L. cacophonia, cacophoniae, f. 불협화음　　　**E** *cacophony*

> G. aphōnia, aphōnias, f. (< a- *not*) *aphony*

> L. aphonia, aphoniae, f. 소리못냄증, 발성불능증　　　**E** *aphonia (aphony)*

> L. dysphonia, dysphoniae, f. (< G. dys- *bad*) 발성장애　　　**E** *dysphonia*

> L. paraphonia, paraphoniae, f. (< G. par(a)- *beside, along side of, beyond*) 발성이상, 이성증(異聲症)　　　**E** *paraphonia*

> G. phōnein (phōneein) *to produce a sound, to speak*

> G. phōnēma, phōnēmatos, n. *sound, speech*

> L. phonema, phonematis, n. 음소(音素), 말　　　**E** *phoneme, phonemics,* (G. allos *'other'* + *phoneme >*) *allophone*

> G. phōnētikos, phōnētikē, phōnētikon *relating to speech*

> L. phoneticus, phonetica, phoneticum 음성의　　　**E** *phonetic, phonetics*

solor, solatus sum, solari 위로하다, 위안시키다

> solacium, solacii, n. 위로, 위안　　　**E** *solace*

> consolor, consolatus sum, consolari (< con- (< cum) *with, together; intensive* + solari *to soothe*) 위로하다, 위안시키다　　　**E** *console*

> consolatio, consolationis, f. 위로, 위안　　　**E** *consolation*

> consolator, consolatoris, m. 위로자

> consolatorius, consolatoria, consolatorium 위로가 되는　　　**E** *consolatory*

< IE. sel-, selə- *of good mood, to favor* **E** *silly (< 'foolish' < 'unworldly' < 'innocent' < 'blessed' < 'happy')*

> G. hilaros, hilara, hilaron *cheerful, merry*

> L. hilarus, hilara, hilarum (hilaris, hilare) 즐거운, 쾌활한   **E** *hilarious*

  > L. hilaritas, hilaritatis, f. 즐거움, 쾌활   **E** *hilarity*

  > L. exhilaro, **exhilaravi**, exhilaratum, exhilarare (< ex- *out of, away from*

    + hilarus *cheerful*) 즐겁게 하다, 쾌활하게 하다   **E** *exhilarate*

●●● 탈형 제 2 변화

현재부정법이 –eri로, 직설법 현재 단수 일인칭이 –eor로 끝나는 동사.

tueor, tuitus (tutus) sum, tueri 지켜보다, 주시하다, 보살피다

부정법	현재			tu-eri	지켜보다, 보살피다
직설법	현재	단수	일인칭	tu-eor	나는 ~한다
			이인칭	tu-eris	너는 ~한다
			삼인칭	tu-etur	그는 ~한다
		복수	일인칭	tu-emur	우리는 ~한다
			이인칭	tu-emini	너희는 ~한다
			삼인칭	tu-entur	그들은 ~한다
	과거	단수	일인칭	tu-ebar	나는 ~하였다
	미래	단수	일인칭	tu-ebor	나는 ~하겠다
	완료	단수	일인칭	tuit-us (tut-us), -a, -um sum	나는 ~하였다
가정법	현재	단수	일인칭	tu-ear	나는 ~하리라
명령법	현재	단수	이인칭	tu-ēre	너는 ~하라
		복수	이인칭	tu-emini	너희는 ~하라
분 사	현재			tuens, (gen.) tuent-is	~하는, ~하고 있는
	과거			tuit-us, tuit-a, tuit-um (tut-us, -a, -um)	~한
수동형	미래분사			tuend-us, tuend-a, tuend-um	~받아야 할

tueor, tuitus (tutus) sum, tueri 지켜보다, 주시하다, 보살피다

> tuitio, tuitionis, f. 후견, 교육   **E** *tuition*

> tutor, tutoris, m. 후견인, 개별 지도교사, 교사   **E** *tutor*

> tutela, tutelae, f. 후견, 교육   **E** *tutelar (tutelary), tutelage*

> intueor, intuitus sum, intueri (< in- *in, on, into, toward*) 들여다보다, 곰곰이 생각

  해 보다

  > intuitio, intuitionis, f. 직관(直觀), 직관적 통찰, 직관적 지식   **E** *intuition, intuitional*

  > intuitivus, intuitiva, intuitivum 직관의, 직관에 의한   **E** *intuitive, counterintuitive*

< IE. teuə- *to pay attention to, to pay*

medeor, -, mederi 치료하다

> medicus, medica, medicum 치료의, 의술의

[용례] digitus medicus 약손가락, 무명지 (Gaius Plinius Caecilius Secundus,
61-c.113)
(문법) digitus 손가락: 단수 주격 < digitus, digiti, m. 손가락, 발가락
medicus 치료의, 의술의: 형용사, 남성형 단수 주격

> medicus, medici, m. 의사   **E** *medic, paramedics*
> medicinus, medicina, medicinum 의사의, 의학의
> medicina, medicinae, f. 의학, 약   **E** *medicine*
> medicinalis, medicinale 의학의, 약의   **E** *medicinal*
> medicalis, medicale 치료의, 의술의   **E** *medical, paramedical*
> medicor, medicatus sum, medicari (medico, **medicavi**, medicatum, medicare)
치료하다   **E** *medicate*
> medicatio, medicationis, f. 치료, 약물처치, 투약   **E** *medication, premedication*
> medicamentum, medicamenti, n. 치료제, 약물, 약   **E** *medicament*
> remedium, remedii, n. (< re- *back, again*) 치료제, 치료법, 치료   **E** *remedy*
> remedialis, remediale 치료의   **E** *remedial*
> remedio, **remediavi**, remediatum, remediare 치료하다   **E** *remediation*

< IE. med- *to take appropriate measures*

E *mete* (< '*to measure*'), *must* (< '*to have occasion, to be permitted or obliged*'), *empty*
(< '*unoccupied*')

> L. meditor, meditatus sum, meditari 깊이 생각하다   **E** *meditate*
> L. meditatio, meditationis, f. 심사숙고, 명상   **E** *meditation*
> L. modus, modi, m. 양식(樣式), 방식, 척도, 기준, 절도(節度);
(문법) (동사의) 법(法)   **E** *modus, mode,* (*mode* >) *mood*
> L. modalis, modale 양식의, 방식의   **E** *modal*
> L. modalitas, modalitatis, f. 양식, 방식   **E** *modality*
> L. modulus, moduli, m. (< + -ulus *diminutive suffix*) 척도,
규범   **E** *modulus, module, modular, model, modeling, remodeling, mold (mould)*
> L. modulor, modulatus sum, modulari 조정하다

E *modulate, calmodulin* (< '*calcium-binding protein that modulates a variety
of cellular responses to calcium*')

> L. modo (부사) (제한) 다만, (시간) 방금
> L. modernus, moderna, modernum 요즈음의, 현대의, 신식의   **E** *modern*
> L. modius, modii, m. (곡식이나 액체를 재는) 말 (약 7리터)
> L. modiolus, modioli, m. (< + -ulus *diminutive suffix*) 되, 잔, (물레방아
식의, 급수기에 고정된) 두레박; (수레의) 바퀴통, 굴대, 축(軸), 달팽이축,
와우축(蝸牛軸)   **E** *modiolus*

> L. modestus, modesta, modestum 적절한, 온당한, 겸손한   **E** *modest*

> L. modestia, modestiae, f. 적절, 온당, 겸손   **E** *modesty*

> L. immodestus, immodesta, immodestum (< im- (< in-) *not*) 적절치

못한, 천박한, 뻔뻔스러운   **E** *immodest*

> L. moderor, moderatus sum, moderari 절도를 지키다, 조정하다

> L. moderatus, moderata, moderatum (*past participle*) 절도 있는,

중등도의   **E** *moderate,* It. *moderato*

> L. immoderatus, immoderata, immoderatum (< im- (< in-) *not*)

절도 없는, 지나친, 터무니없는   **E** *immoderate*

> L. moderator, moderatoris, m. 조정자, 중재자, 조절기, 사회자   **E** *moderator*

> L. modifico, **modificavi**, modificatum, modificare (< modus *measure, due*

measure + -ficare (< facĕre) *to make*) 수정하다, 변경하다, 변화시키다,

수식(修飾)하다   **E** *modify*

> L. modificatio, modificationis, f. 수정, 변경, 변화, 수식   **E** *modification*

> L. commodus, commoda, commodum (< com- (< cum) *with, together* + modus

measure, due measure) 알맞은, 편리한, 유익한

> L. commoditas, commoditatis, f. 편리, 유익; 일용품, 상품, 산물   **E** *commodity*

> L. accommodo, **accommodavi**, accommodatum, accommodare (< ac-

(< ad) *to, toward, at, according to* + commodare *to suit*) 알맞게

만들다, 조절하다, 적응시키다   **E** *accommodate, accommodative*

> L. accommodatio, accommodationis, f. 조절, 적응, 숙소   **E** *accommodation*

> G. medein *to rule*

> G. medousa, medousas, f. (< *feminine present participle of* medein) *(female)*

ruler; (Medousa) (*Greek mythology*) *the name of the only mortal gorgon,*

killed by Perseus

> L. Medusa, Medusae, f. (그리스 신화) 메두사   **E** *Medusa*

reor, ratus sum, reri ~라고 생각하다

> ratus, rata, ratum (*past participle*) 생각한, 산정(算定)된, 일정한, 고정된, 인정된

[용례] pro rata (parte) 산정된 몫에 따라, 그에 비례하여   **E** *rate*

(문법) pro 위하여, 따라: 전치사, 탈격지배

rata 산정된: 과거분사, 여성형 단수 탈격

parte 부분: 명사, 단수 탈격 < pars, partis, f. 부분, 부(部)

> ratifico, **ratificavi**, ratificatum, ratificare (< ratus *fixed, valid* + -ficare (<

facĕre) *to make*) 승인하다, 인가하다, 비준하다, 재가하다   **E** *ratify*

> ratio, rationis, f. 고려, 계산, 방법, 근거;

비(比), 비율(比率)   **E** *ratio, reason, ration* (< '*provisions fixed by ratios*')

> rationalis, rationale 계산의, 이성적, 합리적;

(수학) 유리수(有理數)의   **E** *(neuter sing.) rationale, rational, rationalize*

> irrationalis, irrationale (< ir- < in- *not*) 비이성적, 불합리적; (수학)

무리수(無理數)의   **E** *irrational*

> ratiocinor, ratiocinatus sum, ratiocinari 계산하다, 추론하다, 추리하다   **E** *ratiocinate*

< IE. re(i)- *to reason, to count*

> **E** *read (< 'to explain'), dread (< 'to fear < 'to advise against'), riddle (< 'to reason'), -red (< 'condition'), (hate + -red 'condition' >) hatred, (kin + -red 'condition' >) kindred, (hund '100' + -red 'count' >) hundred, rhyme (< 'number, series')*

> L. ritus, ritus, f. 종교의식, 전례(典禮), 관례   **E** *rite*

    > L. ritualis, rituale 의식의, 전례의   **E** *ritual*

> G. arithmos, arithmou, m. *number, amount*   **E** *arithmetic*

    > L. logarithmus, logarithmi, m. (< G. logos, logou, m. *word, speech, discourse, reason, account, ratio, proportion* + arithmos) 대수(對數)   **E** *logarithm (log)*

vereor, veritus sum, vereri 존경하다, 경외하다

> verecundus, verecunda, verecundum 어려워하는, 부끄러워하는

> revereor, reveritus sum, revereri (< re- *back, again; intensive*) 존경하다, 경외하다

> **E** *revere, (reverens, (gen.) reverentis (present participle) 'revering' >) reverent, (reverendus (masculine gerundive) 'person to be revered' >) reverend (Rev.)*

> reverentia, reverentiae, f. 존경, 경외   **E** *reverence*

< IE. wer- *to perceive, to watch out for*

> **E** *wary, aware, ward (< 'watching'), warden, wardrobe (< 'robe keeper'), steward (< 'house keeper'), lord (< 'loaf keeper'), award (< 'to give after careful watching'), guard (< 'to watch'), guardian, regard (< 'to watch'), regardless, disregard, reward (< 'to regard'), ware (< 'what is kept safe')*

> G. ouros, ourou, m. *watcher, warder*

    > G. Arktouros, Arktourou, m. (< *from its situation at the tail of the Bear* < arktos, arktou, m., f. *bear* + ouros) *the Bear guardian*

       > L. Arcturus, Arcturi, m. (천문) 목동자리, 대각성(大角星)   **E** *Arcturus*

    > G. pylōros, pylōrou, m., f. (pylouros, pylourou, m.) (< G. pylē, pylēs, f. *gate* + ouros) *gatekeeper, porter*

       > L. pylorus, pylori, m. 날문(-門), 유문(幽門)   **E** *pylorus*

         > L. pyloricus, pylorica, pyloricum 날문의, 유문의   **E** *pyloric*

> G. horan (horaein) *to see*

    > G. horama, horamatos, n. (< -ma *resultative noun suffix*) *that which is seen, sight, view*   **E** *panorama, (panorama >) pan, panoramic, diorama*

••• 탈형 제 3 변화 A 식

현재부정법이 -i로, 직설법 현재 단수 일인칭이 -or로 끝나는 동사.

loquor, locutus sum, loqui 말하다

부정법	현재			loqu-i	말하다
직설법	현재	단수	일인칭	loqu-or	나는 ~한다
			이인칭	loqu-eris	너는 ~한다
			삼인칭	loqu-itur	그는 ~한다
		복수	일인칭	loqu-imur	우리는 ~한다
			이인칭	loqu-imini	너희는 ~한다
			삼인칭	loqu-untur	그들은 ~한다
	과거	단수	일인칭	loqu-ebar	나는 ~하였다
	미래	단수	일인칭	loqu-ar	나는 ~하겠다
	완료	단수	일인칭	locut-us, -a, -um sum	나는 ~하였다
가정법	현재	단수	일인칭	loqu-ar	나는 ~하리라
명령법	현재	단수	이인칭	loqu-ĕre	너는 ~하라
		복수	이인칭	loqu-imini	너희는 ~하라
분 사	현재			loquens, (gen.) loquent-is	~하는, ~하고 있는
	과거			locut-us, locut-a, locut-um	~한
수동형	미래분사			loquend-us, loquend-a, loquend-um	~받아야 할

loquor, locutus sum, loqui 말하다

> locutio, locutionis, f. 말씨, 말투, 화법, 관용어법   **E** *locution*

   > circumlocutio, circumlocutionis, f. (< circum- *around* + locutio *speaking*

      < G. periphrasis) 에둘러 말하기, 완곡어법   **E** *circumlocution*

> loquax, (gen.) loquacis 수다스러운, 지저귀는, 우짖는   **E** *loquacious*

   > loquacitas, loquacitatis, f. 수다, 다변   **E** *loquacity*

> colloquium, colloquii, n. (< col- (< cum) *with, together* + loqui *to speak*)

   대화   **E** *colloquy, colloquium, colloquial*

> soliloquium, soliloquii, n. (< solus *alone* + loqui *to speak*) 혼잣말, 독백   **E** *soliloquy*

> ventriloquium, ventriloquii, n. (< venter, ventris, m. *belly* + loqui *to speak*)

   복화술   **E** *ventriloquy (ventriloquism)*

> eloquor, elocutus sum, eloqui (< e- *out of, away from* + loqui *to speak*) 터놓고

   이야기하다, 웅변적으로 말하다   **E** *eloquent*

   > elocutio, elocutionis, f. 연설 태도, 연설법   **E** *elocution*

     > eloquentia, eloquentiae, f. 웅변, 능변, 웅변법   **E** *eloquence*

> interloquor, interlocutus sum, interloqui (< inter- *between, among* + loqui *to speak*)

   말을 가로채다, 대화하다   **E** *interlocutor*

     > interlocutio, interlocutionis, f. 대화   **E** *interlocution*

< IE. tolk^w- *to speak*

fungor, functus sum, fungi 이행(履行)하다; 완수하다, 기능을 다하다, 생애를 마치다

> functio, functionis, f. 이행, 기능, 작용, 직분;

(수학) 함수　**E** *function, (function >) malfunction; hyperfunction, hypofunction, dysfunction*

[용례] functio laesa 기능상실　**E** *functio laesa*

(문법) functio 기능: 단수 주격

laesa 다친: 과거분사, 여성형 단수 주격

< laesus, laesa, laesum

< laedo, laesi, laesum, laedĕre 치다, 상하게 하다

> functionalis, functionale 기능상의, 기능적; (수학) 함수의　**E** *functional*

> fungibilis, fungibile (< **fungi** *vice to serve in place of*) 바꿀 수 있는, 대체할 수 있는　**E** *fungible*

> defungor, defunctus sum, defungi (< **de-** *apart from, down, not; intensive* + fungi *to perform*) 이행하다; 완수하다, 기능을 다하다, 생애를 마치다　**E** *defunct*

> perfungor, perfunctus sum, perfungi (< **per-** *through, thoroughly* + fungi *to perform*) 완수하다

> perfunctorius, perfunctoria, perfunctorium (< *(deceiving) through performance*) 형식적으로 하는, 되는 대로의　**E** *perfunctory*

< IE. bheug- *to enjoy*

irascor, iratus sum, irasci 분노하다　**E** *irate, irascible*

< ira, irae, f. 분노　**E** *ire*

< IE. eis- *in words denoting passion*　**E** *iron (< 'holy metal')*

> G. hieros, hiera, hieron *vigorous, strong, holy, sacred*　**E** *hier(o)-, hierarchy, hierocracy (< 'on the pattern of democracy'), hieroglyph*

> G. oistros, oistrou, m. *gadfly, sting, pain, madness*

> L. oestrus, oestri, m. 등에, 쇠파리, 광증, 격렬한 욕망, 심한 충동, 시인의 영감, 동물의 발정, 발정기

E *oestrus (estrus), oestrous (estrous), oestrogen(s) (estrogen(s)) (< 'maintaining the estrous cycle'), estrane (< 'the 18-carbon tetracyclic hydrocarbon nucleus; used for steroid hormone nomenclature'), (estrane + di- + -ol >) estradiol, (estrane + tri- + -ol >) estriol*

> L. pro-oestrus, pro-oestri, m. (< G. pro- *before, in front*) 발정전기　**E** *pro-oestrus (proestrus)*

> L. metoestrus, metoestri, m. (< G. met(a)- *between, along with, across, after*) 발정후기　**E** *metoestrus (metestrus)*

> L. dioestrus, dioestri, m. (< G. di(a)- *through, thoroughly, apart*) 발정사이기　**E** *dioestrus (diestrus)*

labor, lapsus sum, labi 미끄러지다, (강물이) 흐르다, (시간이) 지나가다, 해이해지다, 나빠지다

> lapsus, lapsus, m. 미끄러짐, 흘러 내려감, 무너짐, 실수, 타락, 범죄　**E** *lapse*

[용례] lapsus linguae 실언(失言)

    (문법) lapsus 실수: 단수 주격

        linguae 혀의, 언어의: 단수 속격 < lingua, linguae, f.

> labilis, labile 미끄러지기 쉬운, 곧 변화하는, 불안정한, 유연한   **E** *labile, (labile >) lability*

> lapso, **lapsavi**, lapsatum, lapsare (*frequentative*) 계속 미끄러지다, 비틀거리다   **E** *lapse*

> collabor, collapsus sum, collabi (< col- (< cum) *with, together* + labi *to slip, to totter*) 무너지다, 허탈상태에 빠지다   **E** *collapse*

> elabor, elapsus sum, elabi (< e- *out of, away from* + labi *to slip, to totter*) 미끄러져 나가다   **E** *elapse*

> prolabor, prolapsus sum, prolabi (< pro- *before, forward; for; instead of* + labi *to slip, to totter*) 미끄러져 나오다   **E** *(verb) prolapse*

    > prolapsus, prolapsus, m. 탈출   **E** *prolapsus, (noun) prolapse*

        [용례] prolapsus uteri 자궁탈출   **E** *prolapsus uteri*

          (문법) prolapsus: 단수 주격

             uteri 자궁의: 단수 속격 < uterus, uteri, m.

> relabor, relapsus sum, relabi (< re- *back, again* + labi *to slip, to totter*) (예전의 상태로) 되돌아가다, (병이) 도지다   **E** *relapse*

> (*probably*) labor, laboris, m. 일, 노동, 병고, 진통(陣痛), 분만통(分娩痛), 산통(産痛), 분만   **E** *labor (labour)*

    > laboriosus, laboriosa, laboriosum 수고스러운, 힘든, 고된   **E** *laborious*

    > laboro, **laboravi**, laboratum, laborare 일하다, 수고하다

        > laboratorium, laboratorii, n. 실험실   **E** *laboratory*

        > collaboro, –, –, collaborare (< col- (< cum) *with, together* + laborare *to work*) 함께 일하다, 합작하다   **E** *collaborate*

        > elaboro, **elaboravi**, elaboratum, elaborare (< e- *out of, away from* + laborare *to work*) 정성스레 만들다   **E** *elaborate*

< IE. leb-, lab-, lob- *to hang down*

E *lap (< 'fold or hanging part of a garment'), (lap (diminutive) >) lapel, label (< 'rag, shred')*

> G. lobos, lobou, m. (< *a roundish projecting part*) *vegetable pod, lobe of the ear, more or less-well defined portion of an organ*

    > L. lobus, lobi, m. (콩) 깍지, (누에) 고치, (호두·계란·조개 등) 껍질, 귓불, 엽(葉), 대엽(大葉)   **E** *lobe*

        > L. lobaris, lobare 엽(葉)의, 대엽(大葉)의   **E** *lobar, interlobar*

        > L. lobatus, lobata, lobatum 엽상(葉狀)의, 열편(裂片) 모양의   **E** *lobate, bilobate, trilobate, (lobate >) lobation*

        > L. lobulus, lobuli, n. (< + -ulus *diminutive suffix*) 소엽(小葉)   **E** *lobule, lobular, interlobular, multilobular, lobulate, (lobulate >) lobulation*

    > D. Trilobit, Trilobiten, m. (< G. tri- (< treis) *three* + lobos *lobe* + -itēs *adjective suffix*) 삼엽충(三葉蟲)   **E** *trilobite*

> IE. (s)lemb- *to hang down*　　　　**E** *limp* (< *'to walk lamely'*), *lump; lumpectomy*

　　> L. limbus, limbi, m. 가장자리, 변연(邊緣),

　　　　연(緣)　　**E** *limb* (< *'border'*), *limbic*, (abl. sing. *'on the border of Hell'* >) *limbo*

sequor, secutus sum, sequi (sec- *root of* sequi *to follow*) 뒤따르다, 잇따르다, 추구(追求)

하다, 누구에게 (유산·상속으로) 돌아가다, 누구의 차지가 되다　　**E** *sequent, sue, suit, suite*

> sequentia, sequentiae, f. 후속, 연속, 결과, 순서, 연쇄　　**E** *sequence, sequential*

> sequela, sequelae, f. 후속, 결과, 귀결, (군대를) 따라다니는 사람,

　　후유증　　**E** *sequela*, (pl.) *sequelae, sequel*, (pre- *'before, beyond'* + *sequel* >) *prequel*

> secta, sectae, f. (행동) 원칙, 방침, 분파, 당파, 학파, 종파　　**E** *sect, sectarian*

> secus, seca, secum (< sec- + -us, -a, -um *adjective suffix*) 직후에, 가까이, 곁에

　　> intrinsecus, intrinseca, intrinsecum (< intra- *inside* + secus *following*) 내부로

　　　　부터의, 내적인, 내재(內在)하는, 내인(內因)의, 본질적인　　**E** *intrinsic*

　　> extrinsecus, extrinseca, extrinsecum (< extra- *outside* + secus *following*)

　　　　외부로부터의, 외적인, 비본질적인　　**E** *extrinsic*

> secundus, secunda, secundum (< sec- + -undus, -unda, -undum *adjective suffix*)

　　뒤따르는, 순조로운, 둘째의

　　　　E *secund, second* (< *'following'*), (secunda pars minuta *'second minute part'* >) *second*

　　　　> secondarius, secondaria, secondarium 2차적인, 부차적인, 속발한, 제2기의　　**E** *secondary*

> sequester, sequestra, sequestrum 뒤쫓는 > 알선하는, 중재하는, 중개하는, 계쟁물

　　(係爭物) 공탁의

　　> sequestrum, sequestri, n. (분리해서 제3자에게 맡겨 놓는) 계쟁물(係爭物); 분리

　　　　뼛조각, 부골(腐骨), 죽은 뼈　　**E** *sequestrum*

　　> sequestro, **sequestravi**, sequestratum, sequestrare 계쟁물을 공탁하다, 계쟁

　　　　물을 격리하다, 격리하다, 분리하다　　**E** *sequestrate (sequester), sequestrant*

　　　　> sequestratio, sequestrationis, f. 격리, 분리　　**E** *sequestration*

> consequor, consecutus sum, consequi (< con- (< cum) *with, together* + sequi *to*

　　follow) 뒤따르다, 논리적(필연적) 귀결로 ~되다, 도달하다, 성취하다　　**E** *consequent, consecutive*

　　> consecutio, consecutionis, f. 뒤따름, 수반, 논리적 일관성; (문법) 일치　　**E** *consecution*

　　> consequentia, consequentiae, f. 귀추, 귀결, 결과,

　　　　예후　　**E** *consequence, consequential*, (*consequential* >) *inconsequential*

> ex(s)equor, ex(s)ecutus sum, ex(s)equi (< ex- *out of, away from* + sequi *to follow*)

　　끝까지 따라가다, 장례식에 따라가다, 완수하다, 응징하다, 집행하다,

　　실행하다　　**E** *execute, executive*

　　> ex(s)ecutio, ex(s)ecutionis, f. 집행, 실행　　**E** *execution*, (*execution* >) *executioner*

> insequor, insecutus sum, insequi (< in- *in, on, into, toward* + sequi *to follow*)

　　잇따르다, 잇달아 일어나다　　**E** *ensue*

> obsequor, obsecutus sum, obsequi (< ob- *before, toward(s), over, against, away* +

　　sequi *to follow*) 순종하다, 아부하다　　**E** *obsequious*

> persequor, persecutus sum, persequi (< per- *through, thoroughly* + sequi *to follow*)

　　끈덕지게 뒤쫓다, 박해하다　　**E** *persecute, persecutive, persecutory*

> persecutio, persecutionis, f. 추적, 박해   **E** *persecution*

> prosequor, prosecutus sum, prosequi (< pro- *before, forward, for, instead of* +

sequi *to follow*) 따라가다(오다), 추적하다, 기소하다   **E** *prosecute, pursue, pursuant, pursuit*

> prosecutor, prosecutoris, m. 동반자, 수행원, 추적자, 검사(檢事)   **E** *prosecutor*

> subsequor, subsecutus sum, subsequi (< sub- *under, up from under* + sequi *to*

follow) 바로 뒤따르다   **E** *subsequent, subsequently*

< IE. sek^w- *to follow*

> L. signum, signi, n. (< *standard that one follows; (also suggested) incised mark*

< IE. sek- *to cut* (Vide SECARE: *See* E. *secant*)) 군기, 표, 신호,

징후(徵候)   **E** *sign, cosign* (< '*to sign jointly*'), *signet* (< '*small seal*')

> L. sigillum, sigilli, n. (< + -illum *diminutive suffix*) 작은 초상, 작은 조상(彫像),

인장, 봉인   **E** *sigil, seal*

> L. signalis, signale 표의, 신호의   **E** *signal*

> L. insignis, insigne (< in- *in, on, into, toward* + signum *sign*) (몸에) 특징

있는 표를 타고 난, 뚜렷한, 뛰어난

> L. insigne, insignis, n. 표지, 기장, 훈장   **E** *insigne, (*pl.*) insignia, ensign*

> L. signo, **signavi**, signatum, signare 표를 하다, 서명하다

> L. signatura, signaturae, f. 서명   **E** *signature*

> L. signatorius, signatoria, signatorium 서명하는, 서명한   **E** *signatory*

> L. assigno, **assignavi**, assignatum, assignare (< ad- *to, toward, at,*

according to + signare *to sign*) 봉인하다, (법적으로) 지정하다, 배정

하다, 분배하다, 맡기다   **E** *assign*

> L. consigno, **consignavi**, consignatum, consignare (< con- (< cum)

with, together; intensive + signare *to sign*) 서명날인하다, 위임하다,

넘겨주다   **E** *consign*

> L. designo, **designavi**, designatum, designare (< de- *apart from, down,*

not + signare *to sign*) 명시하다, 지정하다, 지명하다, 표시하다, 도면을

그리다   **E** *designate, design*

> L. resigno, **resignavi**, resignatum, resignare (< re- *back, again* + signare

to sign) 사임하다   **E** *resign*

> L. significo, **significavi**, significatum, significare (< signum *sign* + -ficare

(< facĕre) *to make*) 드러내다, 뜻하다   **E** *signify, significant, insignificant*

> L. significatio, significationis, f. 신호, 표시   **E** *signification*

> L. significantia, significantiae, f. 의미, 함축성, 중요성   **E** *significance*

> L. socius, socii, m. 동료   **E** *socio-; socioeconomic*

> L. societas, societatis, f. 공동체, 집단, 사회, 모임, 사교   **E** *society, (*society >*) societal*

> L. socialis, sociale 집단의, 사회의, 사회적, 사교적   **E** *social, antisocial*

> L. socio, **sociavi**, sociatum, sociare 함께 하다

> L. sociabilis, sociabile 사교적인, 붙임성 있는   **E** *sociable*

> L. associo, **associavi**, associatum, associare (< as- (< ad) *to, toward,*

at, according to + sociare *to ally*) 연합하다,

연관시키다   **E** *associate, associative*

> L. associatio, associationis, f. 연합, 협회, 연관, 연상(聯想)

> **E** *association, soccer* (< 'the game of football as played under Association rules')

> L. dissocio, **dissociavi**, dissociatum, dissociare (< *dis-* *apart from, down, not* + sociare *to ally*) (관계를) 단절하다, 분리하다, 해리(解離)하다　　　**E** *dissociate, dissociative*

> L. dissociatio, dissociationis, f. 분리, 해리, 분열　　**E** *dissociation*

utor, usus sum, uti 이용하다

> usus, usus, m. 사용, 행사(行使), 실천　　**E** *use, usage, useful, useless, misuse, peruse* (< 'to use up')

> usura, usurae, f. 사용, 이자, 고리(高利)　　**E** *usury*

> usurpo, **usurpavi**, usurpatum, usurpare (< *usu-rupare* < usus *use* + IE. reup-, reub- *to snatch*) 불법 사용하다, 강탈하다　　**E** *usurp*

> usualis, usuale 흔히 사용하는, 일반적인　　**E** *usual, unusual*

> utilis, utile 유용한　　**E** *utilize*

> utilitas, utilitatis, f. 유용성　　**E** *utility, (utility >) utilitarian*

> utensilis, utensile 유용하고 필요한　　**E** *utensil*

> abutor, abusus sum, abuti (< *ab-* *off, away from* + uti *to use*) 마구 쓰다, 남용하다, 범하다　　**E** *(verb) abuse, abusive, abusage*

> abusus, abusus, m. 남용, 학대　　**E** *(noun) abuse*

●●● 탈형 제 3 변화 B 식

현재부정법이 -i로, 직설법 현재 단수 일인칭이 -ior로 끝나는 동사.

patior, passus sum, pati 당하다, 견디다, 참다, 고통받다, 내버려 두다

부정법	현재			pat-i	참다, 고통받다
직설법	현재	단수	일인칭	pat-ior	나는 ~한다
			이인칭	pat-eris	너는 ~한다
			삼인칭	pat-itur	그는 ~한다
		복수	일인칭	pat-imur	우리는 ~한다
			이인칭	pat-imini	너희는 ~한다
			삼인칭	pat-iuntur	그들은 ~한다
	과거	단수	일인칭	pat-iebar	나는 ~하였다
	미래	단수	일인칭	pat-iar	나는 ~하겠다
	완료	단수	일인칭	pass-us, -a, -um sum	나는 ~하였다

가정법	현재	단수	일인칭	pat-iar	나는 ~하리라
명령법	현재	단수	이인칭	pat-ĕre	너는 ~하라
		복수	이인칭	pat-imini	너희는 ~하라
분 사	현재			patiens, (gen.) patient-is ~하는, ~하고 있는	
	과거			pass-us, pass-a, pass-um ~한	
수동형	미래분사			patiend-us, patiend-a, patiend-um ~받아야 할	

patior, passus sum, pati 당하다, 견디다, 참다, 고통받다, 내버려 두다

> patiens, (gen.) patientis (*present participle*) 참는, 고통받는, 병 앓는,
꿋꿋한   **E** *patient, inpatient, outpatient*
>> patientia, patientiae, f. 인내   **E** *patience*
>> impatiens, (gen.) impatientis (< im- (< in-) *not* + patiens *patient*)
참지 못하는   **E** *impatient*
>>> Impatiens, Impatientis, f. (< *the ripe seed-pods readily burst open when touched*) 봉선화속(屬)   **E** *impatiens*
>>> impatientia, impatientiae, f. 참지 못함, 성급함, 조바심, 안달   **E** *impatience*
> passio, passionis, f. 수난, 격정   **E** *passion, passionate*
> passivus, passiva, passivum 당하는, 수동적인, 피동의, 소극적인; (문법) 수동태의   **E** *passive*
> compatior, compassus sum, compati (< com- (< cum) *with, together* + pati *to suffer*)
함께 당하다, 함께 견디다, 동정하다, 양립하다, 적합하다
>> compassio, compassionis, f. 동정, 연민   **E** *compassion, compassionate*
>> compatibilis, compatibile 양립하는, 적합한,
거부반응을 일으키지 않는   **E** *compatible, compatibility*
>>> incompatibilis, incompatibile (< in- *not*) 부적합한 **E** *incompatible, incompatibility*
< IE. pe(i)- *to hurt*   **E** *fiend, archfiend*
> L. paene (pene) (부사) 거의, 하마터면

> **E** *paen(e)- (pen(e)-), peninsula, penumbra, penultimate, penult, antepenultimate, antepenult*

>> (*suggested*) L. paeniteo, paenitui, –, paenitēre 뉘우치다   **E** *penitent, repent*
>>> L. paenitentia, paenitentiae, f. 뉘우침, 회개   **E** *penitence, penance*

gradior, gressus sum, gradi 걷다, 나아가다   **E** *gradient*
> gressus, gressus, m. 걸음, 보행, (선박의) 진로
> gressorius, gressoria, gressorium 보행성의, 보행에 알맞은   **E** *gressorial*
> gradus, gradus, m. 걸음, 계단, 층, 등급, 단계, 도(度), 정도,
학위   **E** *grade, upgrade, grading, centigrade*
>> gradatio, gradationis, f. 점진적 단계, 점진적 이행; (수사) 점층법(漸層法); (언어)
모음 전환(*ablaut*)   **E** *gradation*
>> gradualis, graduale 점진적인   **E** *gradual*

> graduo, **graduavi**, graduatum, graduare 진급시키다, 졸업시키다, 등급을 매기다,
눈금을 매기다 　　　　　　　　　　　　　　　　　　E *graduate*

> *degradus, *degradus, m. (< de- *apart from, down, not; intensive* + gradus
step, grade) 등급, 단계, (각도 · 온도 등의) 도(度); (법률) 촌수;
(문법) (형용사 · 부사의 비교의) 급(級) 　　　　　　　　E *degree*

> degrado, **degradavi**, degradatum, degradare (< de- *apart from, down, not*)
강등시키다; 퇴화시키다, 붕괴시키다, 분해시키다, 분해하다 　E *degrade, degradable*

> degradatio, degradationis, f. 퇴행, 붕괴, 분해 　　　E *degradation*

> -gradus, -grada, -gradum 걷는

> plantigradus, plantigrada, plantigradum (< planta *sole* + -gradus *walking*)
발바닥으로 걷는, 척행(蹠行)의 　　　　　　　　　　　E *plantigrade*

> digitigradus, digitigrada, digitigradum (< digitus *finger, toe* + -gradus *walking*)
발가락으로 걷는, 지행(趾行)의 　　　　　　　　　　　E *digitigrade*

> tardigradus, tardigrada, tardigradum (< tardus *slow* + -gradus *walking*)
느리게 걷는, 완보류(緩步類)의 　　　　　　　　　　　E *tardigrade*

> aggredior, aggressus sum, aggredi (< ag- (< ad) *to, toward, at, according to* +
gradi *to step*) 다가가다, 습격하다, 공격하다 　　　　E *aggress, aggressive*

> congredior, congressus sum, congredi (< con- (< cum) *with, together* + gradi *to step*)
만나다, 회담하다, 접전하다 　　　　　　　　　　　　E *congress*

> degredior, degressus sum, degredi (< de- *apart from, down, not* + gradi *to step*)
내려오다, 떠나가다, 물러가다 　　　　　　　　　　　E *degression*

> digredior, digressus sum, digredi (< di- (< dis-) *apart from, down, not* + gradi
to step) 옆길로 새다, 이탈하다, 탈선하다 　　　　　E *digress*

> egredior, egressus sum, egredi (< e- *out of, away from* + gradi *to step*) 밖으로
나가다 　　　　　　　　　　　　　　　　　　　　　E *egress*

> ingredior, ingressus sum, ingredi (< in- *in, on, into, toward* + gradi *to step*) 들어
가다, 시작하다 　　　　　　　　　　　　　　　　　E *ingress, ingredient*

> introgredior, introgressus sum, introgredi (< intro- *within, into* + gradi *to step*)
안으로 들어가다 　　　　　　　　　　　　　　　　　E *introgression*

> progredior, progressus sum, progredi (< pro- *before, forward, for, instead of* + gradi
to step) 나아가다, 전진하다, 진행하다, 진보하다 　E *prograde, progress, progressive*

> progressio, progressionis, f. 전진, 진행, 진보 　　　E *progression*

> regredior, regressus sum, regredi (< re- *back, again* + gradi *to step*) 물러나다,
후퇴하다, 퇴보하다, 퇴행하다 　　　　　　　　　　　E *regress, regressive*

> regressio, regressionis, f. 퇴행, 역행, 회귀(回歸) 　E *regression*

> retrogradior, retrogressus sum, retrogradi (< retro- *backward, behind* + gradi *to
step*) 뒤로 물러가다, 퇴보하다, 퇴화하다

E *retrograde, retrogress, retrogression* (< '*on the pattern of progression*'), *retrogressive;*
(*retrograde* >) *anterograde* (*antegrade*)

> transgredior, transgressus sum, transgredi (< trans- *over, across, through, beyond*
+ gradi *to step*) 건너가다, 어기다, 범하다 　　　　E *transgress*

< IE. ghredh- *to walk, to go*

morior, mortuus sum, mori 죽다

> mortuus, mortua, mortuum (< *past participle*) 죽은

E *mortgage* (< *'dead pledge: the debt becomes dead when the pledge was redeemed'*)

> mortuarius, mortuaria, mortuarium 죽은 사람에 관한　　　　　　E *mortuary*

> mors, mortis, f. 죽음, 주검; (Mors) (로마 신화) 죽음의 신　　　　E *Mors*

> mortalis, mortale 죽어 없어질, 치명적, 덧없는　　　　　　　E *mortal*

> mortalitas, mortalitatis, f. 죽을 운명, 사멸성, 덧없음, 사망률　E *mortality*

> immortalis, immortale (< im- (< in-) *not*) 죽지 않는, 불사의,

불멸의　　　　　　　　　E *immortal, immortality, immortalize*

> mortifico, mortificavi, mortificatum, mortificare (< +-ficare (< facĕre) *to make*)

죽이다, 정욕을 죽이다, 극기하다　　　　　　　　　E *mortify*

> moribundus, moribunda, moribundum 죽어 가는, 빈사 상태의, 치명적인　E *moribund*

< IE. mer- *to rub away, to harm*　　　　　E *nightmare* (< *'night goblin'*), *murder*

> L. morbus, morbi, m. 병(病)

> L. morbidus, morbida, morbidum 병의, 병든, 병에 잘 걸리는　　E *morbid*

> L. morbiditas, morbiditatis, f. 병적 상태, 이환(罹患), 이환율　E *morbidity, comorbidity*

> L. morbilli, morbillorum, m. (pl.) (< +-illus *diminutive suffix*) 홍역(紅疫)　E *morbilliform*

> L. mordeo, momordi, morsum, mordĕre 물다, 물어뜯다, 괴롭히다, 파고들다

E *mordent,* (mordens (*present participle*) *'biting'* + -ant (*Latin present participle suffix*)
>) *mordant, morsel* (< *'little bite'*)

> L. remordeo, remomordi, remorsum, remordēre (< re- *back, again; intensive*
+ mordēre *to bite*) 물어뜯다, (맛 등을) 얼얼하게 하다, 괴롭히다, 가책을
느끼게 하다　　　　　　　　　　E *remorse*

> L. mortarium, mortarii, n. (< *ground down*) 모르타르, 회반죽; 절구, 회반죽통; 박격포　E *mortar*

> G. marainein (maran- *aorist stem*) *to waste away, to wither*

> G. marasmos, marasmou, m. *marasmus*

> L. marasmus, marasmi, m. 소모증　　　　E *marasmus, marasmic*

> G. marantikos, marantikē, marantikon *wasting away, withering*　E *marantic*

> G. amarantos, amarantos, amaranton (< a- *not*) *everlasting*

> L. amarantus, amaranti, m. 영원히 시들지 않는 꽃, 비름속(屬)의

식물　　　　E *amaranth* (< *'altered on the pattern of -anthus (-flower)'*)

> G. marmaros, marmarou, m. (< *what is breakable, boulder*) *stone, rock, marble* (<
meaning affected by association with marmairein *to sparkle, to glisten, to gleam*)

> L. marmor, marmoris, n. 대리석　　　　　　E *marble*

> G. ambrotos, ambrotos, ambroton (< a- *not* + -mbrotos, brotos *mortal*) *immortal*

> G. ambrosia, ambrosias, f. *ambrosia (food of the gods and immortals)*　E *ambrosia*

> (*Sanskrit*) amrtam (< a- *not* + mrta- *dead*) *immortality*　E *amrita*

> IE. merk- *to decay*

> L. marceo, marcui, –, marcēre 시들다, 이울다, 쇠약해지다

> L. marcesco, **marcui**, –, marcescĕre (< marcēre *to decay, to wither* + -escĕre *suffix of inceptive (inchoative) verb*) 시들다, 이울다, 쇠약 해지다   **E** *marcescent*

> IE. smerd– *pain*

> **E** *smart* (< *'neat in a brisk, sharp style'* < *'keen, brisk'* < *'causing sharp pain'*), (D. Schmerz *'pain'* > D. Mittelschmerz *'mid pain'* >) *mittelschmerz*

●●● 탈형 제 4 변화

현재부정법이 –iri로, 직설법 현재 단수 일인칭이 –ior로 끝나는 동사.

orior, ortus sum, oriri 돋다, 나다, 출현하다

부정법	현재			or-iri	돋다, 나다, 출현하다
직설법	현재	단수	일인칭	or-ior	나는 ~한다
			이인칭	or-iris	너는 ~한다
			삼인칭	or-itur	그는 ~한다
		복수	일인칭	or-imur	우리는 ~한다
			이인칭	or-imini	너희는 ~한다
			삼인칭	or-iuntur	그들은 ~한다
	과거	단수	일인칭	or-iebar	나는 ~하였다
	미래	단수	일인칭	or-iar	나는 ~하겠다
	완료	단수	일인칭	ort-us, -a, -um sum	나는 ~하였다
가정법	현재	단수	일인칭	or-iar	나는 ~하리라
명령법	현재	단수	이인칭	or-ire	너는 ~하라
		복수	이인칭	or-imini	너희는 ~하라
분 사	현재			oriens, (gen.) orient-is	~하는, ~하고 있는
	과거			ort-us, ort-a, ort-um	~한
수동형	미래분사			oriend-us, oriend-a, oriend-um	~받아야 할

orior, ortus sum, oriri 돋다, 나다, 출현하다

> oriens, orientis, m. (< *present participle*) 동쪽, 동양

> **E** *orient*, (orient >) *orientation*, (orientation >) *orientate; disorient (disorientate)*, *disorientation; orienteering*

> orientalis, orientale 동쪽의, 동양의   **E** *oriental*

> origo, originis, f. 기원   **E** *origin*, (origin >) *originate*

[용례] ab origine 기원부터　　　　　　　　　　　　　　　　　　　**E** *ab origine*

　　(문법) ab 부터: 전치사, 탈격지배

　　　origine 기원: 단수 탈격

> aborigines, aboriginum, m. (pl.) (< ab origine *from the beginning*) 원주민,

　토착민, 토착 동식물　**E** *(pl.) aborigines, (sing.) (aborigines >) aborigine, aboriginal*

> originalis, originale 근본의, 원시의, 원본의　　　　　　　　　　**E** *original*

> aborior, abortus sum, aboriri (< ab- *off, away from* + oriri *to arise*) 물거품이 되다,

　좌절하다, 유산(流産)하다　　　　　　　　　　　　　　　　　　　**E** *abort*

　　> abortus, abortus, m. 유산, 낙태; 유산아(流産兒), 낙태아(落胎兒)　**E** *abortus*

　　> abortio, abortionis, f. 좌절, 돈좌(頓挫), 발육정지, 유산, 낙태　　**E** *abortion*

　　> abortivus, abortiva, abortivum 물거품이 된, 불발한, 유산의　　　**E** *abortive*

< IE. er- *to move, to set in motion*

　E *rise, arise, raise, roam, rear (< 'to raise'), (perhaps)* **earnest** *(< 'zealous, serious'), (probably)* **are** *(< 'to be, to exist')*

> L. irrito, irritavi, irritatum, irritare (< ir- (< in) *in, on, into, toward*) 건들다, 안달

　하게 하다　　　　　　　　　　　　　　　　　　　　　　　　　**E** *irritate, irritant*

　　> L. irritatio, irritationis, f. 자극, 과민상태　　　　　　　　　　　**E** *irritation*

　　> L. irritabilis, irritabile 자극에 반응하는, 자극에 과민한, 흥분하기 쉬운　**E** *irritable*

　　　> L. irritabilitas, irritabilitatis, f. 자극반응성, 자극과민성, 흥분성　**E** *irritability*

> G. ornysthai *to urge on, to make rise*

　　> G. hormē, hormēs, f. *impulse, onrush*

　　　> G. horman (hormaein) *to stimulate, to excite*

　　　E *(hormōn, (gen.) hormontos (masculine present participle) >)* **hormone, hormonal,** *(pherein 'to carry' + hormone >)* **pheromone**

　　　> G. hormēsis, hormēseōs, f. *rapid motion, eagerness*

　　　E *hormesis (< 'generally-favorable biological responses to low exposures to toxins and other stressors')*

　　> G. oresthai *to raise oneself*

　　　> G. oros, orous, n. *mountain, mountain range*　　　　　　**E** *oro-*

experior, expertus sum, experiri (< ex- *out of, away from* + periri *to try*) 경험해 보다,

　시험해 보다　　　　　　　　　　　　　　　　　　　　　　　**E** *expert, expertise*

　　> experientia, experientiae, f. 경험　　　　　　　　　　　**E** *experience*

　　> experimentum, experimenti, n. 실험　　　　　　**E** *experiment, experimental*

　< periri (*obsolete*) 경험해 보다, 시험해 보다

　　　> periculum, periculi, n. 시도, 위험　　　　　　　　　　　**E** *peril*

　　　　> periculosus, periculosa, periculosum 위험한　　　　**E** *perilous*

< IE. per- *to try, to risk (< to lead over, to press forward); a verbal root belonging to the*

　group of IE. per *forward, through*　　　　　　　　　　　　　**E** *fear*

　> G. peiran (peiraein) *to try, to attempt*

　　E *zoopery (< 'the performing of experiments on animals, especially the lower animals')*

> G. peira, peiras, f. *trial, attempt*

> G. empeiria, empeirias, f. (< em- (< en) *in* + peira) *experience*

> G. empeirikos, empeirikos, empeirikon *empiric*

> L. empiricus, empirica, empiricum

경험적　　　　　　　　　　　　　　　　**E** *empiric, empirical, empiricism*

> G. peiratēs, peiratou, m. *pirate*

> L. pirata, piratae, m. 해적　　　　　　　　　　　**E** *pirate*

> G. peirateia, peirateias, f. *piracy*

> L. piratia, piratiae, f. 해적질　　　　　　　　　**E** *piracy*

metior, mensus sum, metiri 재다, 측량하다, 측정하다, 판단하다

> immensus, immensa, immensum (< im- (< in-) *not* + mensus (*past participle*)

measured) 잴 수 없는, 끝없는　　　　　　　　　　　**E** *immense*

> immensitas, immensitatis, f. 광대, 무한　　　　**E** *immensity*

> mensura, mensurae, f. 측량, 측정, 척도; (수학) 약수;

(시) 운율　　　　　　　　**E** *(noun) measure, (measure >) measurement*

> mensuralis, mensurale 측량의, 측정의　　　　　**E** *mensural*

> mensuro, **mensuravi**, mensuratum, mensurare 측량하다, 측정하다　　**E** *(verb) measure*

> mensurabilis, mensurabile 측정할 수 있는, 무시 못 할　　**E** *measurable*

> immensurabilis, immensurabile (< im- (< in-) *not*) 측정할 수 없는,

무한한　　　　　　　　　　　　　**E** *immeasurable*

> commensuratus, commensurata, commensuratum (< con- (< cum) *with,*

together) 같은 정도의, 같은 단위를 갖는　　　　　**E** *commensurate*

> dimetior, dimensus sum, dimetiri (< di- (< dis-) *apart from, down, not* + metiri

to measure) 재다, 측량하다

> dimensio, dimensionis, f. 측량, 길이·폭·높이,

차원(次元)　　　　　　　　　**E** *dimension, dimensional, dimensionless*

< IE. me- *to measure*

E *meal (< 'appointed time, time for eating'), piecemeal (< 'quantity taken at one time')*

> G. metron, metrou, n.

measure　　　**E** *metre (meter), metric, metronome, -meter, -metry, -metric, isometric*

> G. diametros, diametrou, f. (< diametros grammē *line measuring across*

< di(a)- *through, thoroughly, apart* + metron) *diagonal of a parallelogram,*

diameter of a circle

> L. diametros, diametri, f. (diametrus, diametri, f.) 지름, 직경, 거리　**E** *diameter*

> G. perimetros, perimetrou, f. (< perimetros grammē *line measuring around*

< peri- *around, near, beyond, on account of* + metron) *circumference*

> L. perimetros, perimetri, f. 둘레, 주위, 주변　**E** *perimeter, (perimeter>) perimetry*

> G. geōmetria, geōmetrias, f. (< gē *earth*) *geometry*

> L. geometria, geometriae, f. 기하학(幾何學)　　　　**E** *geometry*

> G. symmetria, symmetrias, f. (< sym- (< syn) *with, together*) *symmetry*

> L. symmetria, symmetriae, f. 대칭, 균형, 조화　E *symmetry, symmetric, asymmetric*

> L. parametrum, parametri, n. (< *number figuring as a variable in an expression or an equation* < G. par(a)- *beside, along side of, beyond*) 파라미터, 매개변수, 지표; (통계) 모수(母數), 모집단특성치　E *parameter, parametric, nonparametric*

> IE. men-, menen-, menot-, mens- *moon, month (an ancient and universal unit of time measured by the moon)*

E *moon, month,* (G. hēmera Selēnēs *'day of* Selēne*',* L. dies Lunae·*'day of the moon'* >) *Monday*

> L. mensis, mensis, m. (시간의) 달, 월경　E (pl.) *menses*

　　> L. mensalis, mensale 매달의　E *mensal*

　　> L. menstruus, menstrua, menstruum 매달의

　　　　> L. menstrua, menstruorum, n. (pl.) 월경

　　　　　　> L. menstrualis, menstruale 월경의　E *menstrual*

　　　　　　> L. menstruo, menstruavi, menstruatum, menstruare 월경하다　E *menstruate*

　　　　　　　　> L. menstruatio, menstruationis, f. 월경하다　E *menstruation*

　　> L. trimestris, trimestre (trimenstris, trimenstre) (< tri- (< tres) *three* + mensis *month*) 3개월의　E *trimester, trimestral*

　　> L. semestris, semestre (semenstris, semenstre) (< se- (< sex) *six* + mensis *month*) 6개월의　E *semester, semestral*

> G. mēnē, mēnēs, f. *moon*

　　> G. mēniskos, mēniskou, m. (< + -iskos *diminutive suffix*) *crescent*

　　　　> L. meniscus, menisci, m. 초승달, 반달; 반달연골　E *meniscus,* (pl.) *menisci*

> G. mēn, mēnos, m. *month*

　　> L. menarche, menarchae, f. (< G. mēn + archē *beginning*) 초경(初經), 첫월경　E *menarche, menarcheal (menarchial)*

　　> L. menopausis, menopausis, f. (< G. mēn + pausis *cessation*) 폐경(閉經), 폐경기(閉經期)

　　E *menopause, menopausal, premenopausal, perimenopausal, postmenopausal*

　　> L. amenorrhoea, amenorrhoeae, f. (< G. a- *not* + mēn + rhoia, rhoias, f. *flow, flux*) 무월경(無月經)　E *amenorrhoea (amenorrhea), amenorrheal*

　　　　> (*probably*) L. menorrhoea, menorrhoeae, f. 월경, 월경과다

　　　　E *menorrhoea (menorrhea), hypermenorrhea, oligomenorrhea,* (*menorrhea* + *-algia* >) *menorrhalgia* (*dysmenorrhea*)

　　　　　　> L. dysmenorrhoea, dysmenorrhoeae, f. (< G. dys- *bad*) 월경통　E *dysmenorrhoea (dysmenorrhea)* (*menorrhalgia*)

　　> L. menorrhagia, menorrhagiae, f. (< + -rrhagia < -rrhag- *stem of* rhēgnynai *to break, to burst*) 월경과다　E *menorrhagia*

　　> L. catamenia, catameniae, f. (< G. kat(a)- *down, mis-, according to, along, thoroughly*) 월경　E *catamenia*

　　> L. paramenia, parameniae, f. (< G. par(a)- *beside, along side of, beyond*) 월경곤란, 월경불순　E (*rare*) *paramenia*

불규칙 동사의 변화

영어의 *be* 동사에 해당하는 esse 동사, 영어의 조동사 역할을 하는 동사, 이와 비슷한 변화를 하는 동사 등은 불규칙 변화를 한다. 수는 몇 안 되지만 자주 사용하는 동사들이다.

sum, fui, –, esse ~이다, 있다

능동태	부정법	현재				esse	~이다, 있다
	직설법	현재	단수	일인칭		sum	나는 ~이다, 있다
				이인칭		es	너는 ~이다, 있다
				삼인칭		est	그는 ~이다, 있다
			복수	일인칭		sumus	우리는 ~이다, 있다
				이인칭		estis	너희는 ~이다, 있다
				삼인칭		sunt	그들은 ~이다, 있다
		과거	단수	일인칭		er-am	나는 ~이었다, 있었다
		미래	단수	일인칭		er-o	나는 ~이겠다, 있겠다
		완료	단수	일인칭		fu-i	나는 ~이었다, 있었다
	가정법	현재	단수	일인칭		sim	나는 ~이리라, 있으리라
	명령법	현재	단수	이인칭		es	너는 ~이어라, 있어라
			복수	이인칭		es-te	너희는 ~이어라, 있어라
	분 사	현재				없음	
		미래				#futur-us, futur-a, futur-um ~일, 있을	
	목적분사					없음	
수동태						없음	

#futur-us < (*suppletive*) futurus, futura, futurum *that is to be*
  < IE. bheuə- *to be, to exist, to grow* (Vide PHYSIS; *See* E. *physis*)

sum, fui, –, esse ~이다, 있다   **E** *esse*

[용례] Ars (est) longa, vita (est) brevis. 의술은 길고, 인생은 짧다
(문법) ars 의술은: 단수 주격 < ars, artis, f. 기술, 솜씨, 전문직, 예술
   est ~이다: 직설법 현재 단수 삼인칭 (뜻이 분명한 경우, esse 동사를
     생략할 수 있음)
   longa 긴: 형용사, 여성형 단수 주격 < longus, longa, longum
   vita 인생은: 단수 주격 < vita, vitae, f. 생명, 삶

brevis 짧은: 형용사, 남·여성형 단수 주격 < brevis, breve

> ens, entis, f. (< *on the pattern of present participle*) 존재

> entitas, entitatis, f. 존재성, 실체, 본질   **E** *entity*

> futurum, futuri, n. (< futurus, futura, futurum *that is to be*) 미래   **E** *future*

> essentia, essentiae, f. 본질, 요소   **E** *essence*

> essentialis, essentiale 본질의, 필수적인   **E** *essential*

> quintessentia, quintessentiae, f. (< quinta essentia < G. pemptē ousia *the fifth essence*) 제5원(元) (물·불·흙·공기 4원 외의 원), (물질의) 가장 순수한 본질   **E** *quintessence*

> absum, **abfui** (afui), −, abesse (< ab− *off, away from* + esse *to be*) 떨어져 있다, 있지 않다, 결석하다

> absens, (gen.) absentis (*present participle*) 떨어져 있는, 있지 않는, 결석한   **E** *absent*

> absentia, absentiae, f. 결석, 결여   **E** *absence*

> intersum, **interfui**, −, interesse (< inter− *between, among* + esse *to be*) 사이에 있다, 관계 있다   **E** *interest*

> praesum, **praefui**, −, praeesse (< prae− *before, beyond* + esse *to be*) 앞에 있다, 감독하다, 보호하다

> praesens, (gen.) praesentis (*present participle*) 앞에 있는, 출석한, 현재의   **E** *present*

> praesentia, praesentiae, f. 면전, 출석, 현존   **E** *presence*

> praesento, **praesentavi**, praesentatum, praesentare (누구) 앞에 보이다, 제시하다, 바치다, 선물하다   **E** *present (< 'to make present')*

> praesentatio, praesentationis, f. 제시, 제출, 발표, 증정; 태아위치, 태위(胎位)   **E** *presentation, (presentation >) malpresentation*

> repraesento, **repraesentavi**, repraesentatum, repraesentare (< re− *back, again*) 눈앞에 있게 하다, 드러내다, 표현하다, 대표하다   **E** *represent, representative*

> prosum (prodes, prodest), **profui**, −, prodesse (< prod− (< pro) *before, forward, for, instead of* + esse *to be*) 쓸모가 있다, 이롭다   **E** *proud, pride, improve, improvement*

< IE. es− *to be*

E *am, is, yes* (< *'so it be'* < IE. i− *'pronominal stem'* + IE. es− *'to be'), **sooth** (< 'real, true'* < *'that which is'), **soothsayer, soothe** (< *'to say yes to'), **sin** (< *'it is true, the sin is real'*)

> G. einai *to be*

> G. ōn, (gen.) ontos (*masculine present participle*) *being*

E *-ont,* (symbioun *'to live together'* > *'living together'* >) **symbiont,** (hals *'salt'* > *'living in a saline habitat'* >) **halobiont,** (schizein *'to split'* > *'splitting'* >) **schizont,** (gamete > *'producing gametes'* >) **gamont** (< *'on the pattern of schizont'),* (merozoite > *'producing merozoites'* >) **meront** (< *'on the pattern of schizont'),* (spora *'spore'* > *'producing sporoblasts'* >) **sporont** (< *'on the pattern of schizont')*

> G. ousa, (gen.) ousēs (*feminine present participle*) *being*

> G. ousia, ousias, f. *being, essence, substance*

> G. on, (gen.) ontos (*neuter present participle*) *being*   **E** *ont(o)-, ontogeny*

> L. ontologia, ontologiae, f. (< G. ont− + −logia *study*) 존재론   **E** *ontology*

> (*suggested*) G. etymos, etymos, etymon *real, actual, true*

    > G. etymon, etymou, n. *the 'true' literal sense of a word according to its*

        origin, its 'true' or original form

        > L. etymon, etymi, n. 낱말의 원형, 어원(語源), 말밑   **E** *etymon,* (pl.) *etyma*

        > G. etymologia, etymologias, f. (< + -logia *study*) *etymology*

            > L. etymologia, etymologiae, f. 어원론, 어원학   **E** *etymology*

            > G. etymologikos, etymologikē, etymologikon *etymologic*

                > L. etymologicus, etymologica, etymologicum 어원론의,

        어원학의   **E** *etymologic (etymological)*

> (*Sanskrit*) sat-, sant- *existing, true, virtuous*

    E **suttee** (< (*Hindi*) satti *'good, pure'*), (*Sanskrit*) **bodhisattva** (< *'one enlightened with essence'*), (*Hindi*) **Satyagraha** (< *'truth grasping'*)

> (*Sanskrit*) -asti *being*

    > (*Sanskrit*) svasti (< (*Sanskrit*) su- *good* (< IE. (e)su- *good*) + -asti *being*)

        well-being, good luck, benediction

        > (*Sanskrit*) svastika (< + -ka *diminutive suffix*) *fylfot*   **E** *swastika (swastica)*

> IE. (e)su- (< *being true, being good*) *good*

    > G. eus, eus, eu *good, brave*

        > G. eu (*adverb*) *well*

        > G. eu- *well*   **E** *eu-*

    > (*Sanskrit*) su- *good* (Vide supra)

---

possum, potui, -, posse 할 수 있다, 가능성 있다

능동태	부정법	현재				posse	할 수 있다, 가능성 있다
	직설법	현재	단수	일인칭		pos-sum	나는 ~ 있다
				이인칭		pot-es	너는 ~ 있다
				삼인칭		pot-est	그는 ~ 있다
			복수	일인칭		pos-sumus	우리는 ~ 있다
				이인칭		pot-estis	너희는 ~ 있다
				삼인칭		pos-sunt	그들은 ~ 있다
		과거	단수	일인칭		pot-eram	나는 ~ 있었다
		미래	단수	일인칭		pot-ero	나는 ~ 있겠다
		완료	단수	일인칭		potu-i	나는 ~ 있었다
	가정법	현재	단수	일인칭		pos-sim	나는 ~ 있으리라
	명령법	현재	단수	이인칭		없음	
			복수	이인칭		없음	
	분 사	현재				potens, (gen.) potent-is	~ 있는

	목적분사			없음	
수동태				없음	

possum, potui, -, posse (< potis (pote) *able, possible* + esse *to be*) 할 수 있다, 가능성 있다, 힘이 있다, 능력이 있다　　　　　　　　　　　　　　　**E** *posse, power*

> potens, (gen.) potentis 힘 있는, 능력 있는　　　　　　　　　**E** *potent*

　　> potentia, potentiae, f. 힘, 능력, 잠재력, 효능, 역가

　　　　E *potency (potence),* (D. Potenz *'power'* + H• *'former chemical symbol for hydrogen ion'* > *'potency of hydrogen ion (H⁺)'* >) *pH*

　　　　> potentialis, potentiale 힘 있는, 가능한, 가능성을 가진, 잠재력의　**E** *potential*

　　　　　　> potentialitas, potentialitatis, f. 가능성, 잠재력　**E** *potentiality*

　　> impotens, (gen.) impotentis (< im- (< in-) *not* + potens *able, powerful*) 무능한, 무력한, 발기부전의　　　　　　　　　　　　**E** *impotent*

　　　　> impotentia, impotentiae, f. 무능, 무력, 발기부전　**E** *impotence (impotency)*

　　> omnipotens, (gen.) omnipotentis (< omnis *all* + potens *able, powerful*) 전능한　　　　　　　　　　　　　**E** *omnipotent, omnipotence*

　　> *totipotens, (gen.) *totipotentis (< totus *total* + potens *able, powerful*) 만능의, 전능한　　　　　　　　　　　　**E** *totipotent*

　　> pluripotens, (gen.) pluripotentis (< plus, pluris *more* + potens *able, powerful*) 다능한　　　　　　　　　　　**E** *pluripotent*

　　> multipotens, (gen.) multipotentis (< multus *many* + potens *able, powerful*) 다능한, 매우 유능한, 권력이 대단한　　　**E** *multipotent*

< potis (pote) (불변화) 할 수 있는, 능력이 있는

　　> possideo, **possedi**, possessum, possidēre (< potis (pote) *able, possible* + sedēre *to sit*) 차지하다, 소유하다　**E** *possess, possession, possessive*

　　> possibilis, possibile (< pos- (< potis) *able, possible* + -ibilis (< habilis < habēre *to have*) *able*) 있을 수 있는, 일어날 수 있는, 가능한　**E** *possible*

　　　　> possibilitas, possibilitatis, f. 실현성, 가능성　**E** *possibility*

< IE. poti- *powerful, lord*

　　> G. despotēs, despotou, m. (< *house-master* < IE. dem- *house, household* (Vide DOMINUS: *See* E. *domino*) + IE. poti-) *lord, master, owner*　　**E** *despot*

eo, ivi (ii), itum, ire 가다

능동태	부정법	현재				ire	가다
	직설법	현재	단수	일인칭		e-o	나는 간다
				이인칭		i-s	너는 간다
				삼인칭		i-t	그는 간다

		복수	일인칭	i-mus	우리는 간다
			이인칭	i-tis	너희는 간다
			삼인칭	e-unt	그들은 간다
	과거	단수	일인칭	i-bam	나는 갔다
	미래	단수	일인칭	i-bo	나는 가겠다
	완료	단수	일인칭	i-i	나는 갔다
가정법	현재	단수	일인칭	e-am	나는 가리라
명령법	현재	단수	이인칭	i	너는 가라
		복수	이인칭	i-te	너희는 가라
분 사	현재			iens, (gen.) eunt-is	가는, 가고 있는
목적분사				it-um	가려, 가기 위하여
수동태				관용적 비인칭 수동태 외에는 없음	

eo, ivi (ii), itum, ire 가다

> itio, itionis, f. (어디로) 감
>> sedition, seditionis, f. (< sed- (< se-) *apart, without* + itio *going*) 치안 방해,
>> 선동   **E** *sedition*
> iter, itineris, n. 길 떠남, 여행, 여정
>> itinerarius, itineraria, itinerarium 여행의, 여정의   **E** *itinerary*
>> itineror, itineratus sum, itinerari 여행하다, 순회하다   **E** *itinerate, itinerant*
> adeo, adivi (adii), aditum, adire (< ad- *to, toward, at, according to* + ire *to go*)
> ~로 가다, 찾아가다
>> aditus, aditus, m. 접근, 입구   **E** *aditus (adit)*
> ambio, ambivi (ambii), ambitum, ambire (< amb(i)- *on both sides, around* + ire
> *to go*) 돌아다니다, 둘러싸다, 휘감다, 휘감기다, 찾아다니며 (표를) 부탁하다, 얻으
> 려고 애쓰다   **E** *ambient*
>   **E** *ambit*
>> ambitus, ambitus, m. 둘레, 범위, 영역
>> ambitio, ambitionis, f. (로마 역사) 표를 얻기 위한 입후보자의 일주 작전, 공명심,
>> 야망   **E** *ambition*
>>> ambitiosus, ambitiosa, ambitiosum 야망이 있는   **E** *ambitious*
> circumeo, circumivi (circumii), circumitum, circumire (circueo, circuivi (circuii),
> circuitum, circuire) (< circum- *around* + ire *to go*) 돌아다니다
>> circumitus, circumitus, m. (circuitus, circuitus, m.) 순회, 주위, 우회,
>> 회로   **E** *circuit, circuity, (circuit >) circuitry*
>>> circuitosus, circuitosa, circuitosum 우회로의, 에두르는,
>>> 직접적이 아닌   **E** *circuitous*
> coeo, coivi (coii), coitum, coire (< co- (< cum) *with, together* + ire *to go*) 함께 가다,

성교하다, 교미하다

> coitus, coitus, m. 결합, 연합, 성교, 교미, 교배　　　　　　　**E** *coitus, coital, postcoital*

> comes, comitis, m., f. 길동무, 동반자, 수행원, 조신(朝臣),

　　백작(伯爵)　　　**E** *count, countess,* (comes stabuli *'count of the stable'* >) *constable*

　　> comitatus, comitatus, m. 동반, 수행, 백작령(伯爵領)　　　　　**E** *county*

　　> comitor, comitatus sum, comitari 동반하다, 따르다

　　　　　[용례] Tardis mentibus virtus non facile comitatur.

　　　　　　　　더딘 정신에는 덕이 쉽게 따르지 않는다 (Marcus Tullius Cicero,

　　　　　　　　106-43 B.C.E.)

　　　　　　　(문법) tardis 더딘: 형용사, 여성형 복수 여격

　　　　　　　　　　< tardus, tarda, tardum

　　　　　　　　　mentibus 정신들에게: 복수 여격 < mens, mentis, f.

　　　　　　　　　virtus 덕이: 단수 주격 < virtus, virtutis, f.

　　　　　　　　　non 아니: 부사

　　　　　　　　　facile 쉽게: 부사 < facilis, facile 쉬운

　　　　　　　　　comitatur 따른다: 직설법 현재 단수 삼인칭

　　> comitans, (**gen.**) comitantis (*present participle*) 동반하는, 따르는

　　　　　[용례] vena comitans, (pl.) venae comitantes 동반정맥,

　　　　　　　　반행(伴行)정맥　　　　**E** *vena comitans,* (pl.) *venae comitantes*

　　　　　　　(문법) vena 정맥: 단수 주격

　　　　　　　　　　< vena, venae, f. 맥, 혈관, 정맥

　　　　　　　　　comitans 동반하는: 남·여·중성형, 단수 주격

　　　　　　　　　venae 정맥들: 복수 주격

　　　　　　　　　comitantes 동반하는: 남·여성형, 복수 주격

　　> concomitor, concomitatus sum, concomitari (< con- (< cum)

　　　with, together + comitari *to accompany*) 동반하다, 따르다　**E** *concomitant*

　　> vicecomes, vicecomitis, m. (< vice- *in place of*) 자작(子爵)　**E** *viscount, viscountess*

> exeo, exivi (exii), exitum, exire (< ex- *out of, away from* + ire *to go*) 나가다, 출동

　하다, (결과로서) 나오다, 발간되다, 끝나가다

　　E *(verb) (third personal singular, present indicative, active 'he/she goes out'* >) *exit*

　　> exitus, exitus, m. 출구, 말로(末路), 결과　　　　　　　**E** *(noun) exit, issue*

> ineo, inivi (inii), initum, inire (< in- *in, on, into, toward* + ire *to go*) 들어가다,

　시작하다

　> initium, initii, n. 시작

　　　　[용례] ab initio 처음부터　　　　　　　　　　　　　　**E** *ab initio*

　　　　　　(문법) ab 부터: 전치사, 탈격지배

　　　　　　　initio 시작: 단수 탈격

　　> initialis, initiale 시작의, 처음의, 초기의　　　　　　　**E** *initial, initialize*

　　> initio, **initiavi**, initiatum, initiare 시작하다　　　　　**E** *initiate, initiative*

　　　> initiatio, initiationis, f. 시작, 개시　　　　　　　　　**E** *initiation*

> *cominitio, *cominitiavi, *cominitiatum, *cominitiare (< com- (<
cum) *with, together;* *intensive* + initiare *to begin*) 시작하다　**E** *commence*

> introeo, introivi (introii), introitum, introire (< intro *inward* + ire *to go*) 들어가다
> introitus, introitus, m. 들어감, 입장, 시작, 입구, 구(口)　**E** *introitus*

> obeo, obivi (obii), obitum, obire (< ob- *before, toward(s), over, against, away* + ire
to go) 향해서 가다, 맞닥뜨리다, 완수하다,
죽다　**E** *(third personal singular, perfect indicative, active 'he/she died' >)* **obiit (ob.)**
> obitus, obitus, m. 도착, 만남, 완수, 죽음
> obituarius, obituaria, obituarium 죽음의, 죽음을 기록하는　**E** *obituary*

> pereo, perivi (perii), peritum, perire (< per- *through, thoroughly* + ire *to go*) 사라
지다, 죽다, 망하다　**E** *perish, perishable*

> praetereo, praeterivi (praeterii), praeteritum, praeterire (< praeter- *past, beyond* +
ire *to go*) 지나가다, (시간) 지나다, 지나치다, 빠뜨리다, 간과하다　**E** *preterit(e)*
> praeteritio, praeteritionis, f. 간과, 누락　**E** *preterition*

> subeo, subivi (subii), subitum, subire (< sub- *under, up from under* + ire *to go*)
아래로 들어가다, 감당하다, 접근하다, 몰래 들어가다, 침입하다, (일이) 일어나다
> subitus, subita, subitum (*past participle*) 돌발한, 새로운, 서두르는　**E** *sudden,* It. *subito*

> transeo, transivi (transii), transitum, transire (< trans- *over, across, through, beyond*
+ ire *to go*) 지나가다, 통과하다, 이행(移行)하다　**E** *transit, transient, trance*
> transitio, transitionis, f. 통과, 이행, 천이(遷移)　**E** *transition, transitional*
> transitivus, transitiva, transitivum 이행하는; (문법) 타동사의　**E** *transitive*
> transitivus, transitiva, transitivum (< in- *not*) (문법) 자동사의　**E** *intransitive*

< IE. ei- *to go*
> L. janus, jani, m. 덮개 있는 통로, 현관, 입구
> L. Janus, Jani, m. (로마 신화) 야누스 신(문과 도로의 수호신)　**E** *Janus*
> L. Januarius, Januaria, Januarium 야누스 신의,
1월의　**E** *(Januarius mensis 'month of Janus' >)* *January*
> L. janua, januae, f. (집의) 바깥문
> L. janitor, janitoris, m. 문지기　**E** *janitor*

> G. iēnai *to go*
> G. ion, (gen.) iontos (*neuter present participle*) *going*

E *ion (< 'thing going'), ionic, ionize, ionized, nonionized, counterion,* (D. Zwitter
(< 'hybrid' < zwei 'two') + ion >) *zwitterion, ionophore (< 'an agent which is
able to carry ions across a lipid membrane'), iontophoresis (< 'carrying ions
into tissue by electric current')*

> G. aniēnai (< an(a)- *up, upward; again, throughout; back, backward; against;
according to, similar to* + iēnai) *to go up*
> G. anion, (gen.) aniontos (*neuter present participle*)
going up　**E** *anion (< 'thing going up' < 'thing going to the anode'), anionic*
> G. katiēnai (< kat(a)- *down, mis-, according to, along, thoroughly* + iēnai)
to go down
> G. kation, (gen.) kationtos (*neuter present participle*) *going*

down **E** *cation* (< 'thing going down' < 'thing going to the cathode'), *cationic*
> (*Sanskrit*) yanam *way;* (*Buddhism*) *mode of knowledge, vehicle* **E** *Hinayana, Mahayana*

fero, tuli, latum, ferre 옮기다, 가져가다, 가져오다, 지니다, 견디다

능동태	부정법	현재				ferre	가져가다, 견디다
	직설법	현재	단수	일인칭		fer-o	나는 ~한다
				이인칭		fer-s	너는 ~한다
				삼인칭		fer-t	그는 ~한다
			복수	일인칭		fer-imus	우리는 ~한다
				이인칭		fer-tis	너희는 ~한다
				삼인칭		fer-unt	그들은 ~한다
		과거	단수	일인칭		fer-ebam	나는 ~하였다
		미래	단수	일인칭		fer-am	나는 ~하겠다
		완료	단수	일인칭		tul-i	나는 ~하였다
	가정법	현재	단수	일인칭		ferr-em	나는 ~하리라
	명령법	현재	단수	이인칭		fer	너는 ~하라
			복수	이인칭		fer-te	너희는 ~하라
	분 사	현재				ferens, (gen.) ferent-is	~하는, ~하고 있는
	목적분사					lat-um	~하러, ~하기 위하여
수동태	분 사	미래				ferend-us, ferend-a, ferend-um	~받아야 할
		과거				#lat-us, lat-a, lat-um	~받은, ~받고서

#lat-us < (*suppletive*) latus, lata, latum *carried, borne*
< IE. telə- *to lift, to support, to weigh* (Vide TOLERARE: *See* E. *tolerate*)

fero, tuli, latum, ferre 옮기다, 가져가다, 가져오다, 지니다, 견디다
> -fer (-ferus), -fera, -ferum 옮기는, 가져가는, 가져오는, 지니는

E *-ferous, calciferous, cruciferous, culmiferous, lactiferous, laniferous, melliferous, odoriferous, proliferous, seminiferous, somniferous, sudoriferous, uriniferous;* (*calciferous* >) *calciferol(s), cholecalciferol, ergocalciferol*

> fertilis, fertile 산출하는, 비옥한, 임신이 가능한,
가임의 **E** *fertile,* (*fertile* >) *fertilize,* (*fertilize* >) *fertilization, fertilizer, unfertilized*
> fertilitas, fertilitatis, f. 생식력, 출산력 **E** *fertility*
> infertilis, infertile (< in- *not* + fertile *productive*) 불모의, 불임의 **E** *infertile*
> infertilitas, infertilitatis, f. 불임증 **E** *infertility*
> latio, lationis, f. 이동, 전달, 선포

> legislatio, legislationis, f. (< legis (< lex, legis, f. *law*) *of law* + latio *bringing*)

입법, 법률 제정　　　　　　　　　　　　　E *legislation, (legislation >) legislate*

> affero, attuli, allatum, afferre (< af- (< ad) *to, toward, at, according to* + ferre *to carry*) 가져오다, 들다[시]　　　　　　　　　　　E *afferent*

> aufero, abstuli, ablatum, auferre (< au- (< ab) *off, away from* + ferre *to carry*)

가져가다, 빼앗아가다, 제거하다　　　　　　　E *ablate*

　> ablatio, ablationis, f. 제거, 절제　　　　　E *ablation*

　> ablativus, ablativa, ablativum (문법) 탈격(奪格)의　　　E *ablative (abl.)*

> circumfero, cirumtuli, circumlatum, circumferre (< circum- *around* + ferre *to carry*)

돌리다

　　> circumferentia, circumferentiae, f. (둥근 면적의) 둘레　E *circumference, circumferential*

> confero, contuli, conlatum (collatum), conferre (< con- (< cum) *with, together* + ferre *to carry*) 한 곳으로 옮기다, 한데 모으다, 참조하다, 비교하다,

수여하다　　　　　　　　　　　　　　　E *confer, conference, collate*

[용례] confer 참조하라, 비교하라　　　　　E *confer (cf.)*

　　　(문법) confer: conferre의 능동태 명령법 현재 단수 이인칭

> defero, detuli, delatum, deferre (< de- *apart from, down, not* + ferre *to carry*)

나르다; 넘겨주다, 고발하다, (남의 의견·판단에) 따르다,

경의를 표하다　　　　　　　　　　　　E *defer, deferent, delation, deference*

[용례] vas deferens (ductus deferens) 정관(精管),

수정관(輸精管)　　　　　　　　　E *vas deferens (ductus deferens)*

　　　(문법) vas 관(管): 단수 주격 < vas, vasis, n.

　　　　　ductus 관(管): 단수 주격 < ductus, ductus, m.

　　　　　deferens 넘겨주는: 현재분사, 남·여·중성형 단수 주격

　　　　　　< deferens, (gen.) deferentis

> differo, distuli, dilatum, differre (< di- (< dis-) *apart from, down, not* + ferre *to carry*) (타동사) 여기저기 나르다, (*to put off action or procedure to some later time >*) 미루다; (자동사) (*to tend apart or diversely in nature or character >*)

다르다　　　　　　　　　　　　　　E *defer, deferral; differ*

　> differens, (gen.) differentis (*present participle*) 다른, 차이가 있는　E *different*

　　> differentia, differentiae, f. 다름, 차이　　　E *difference*

　　　> differentialis, differentiale 차별적인, 미분(微分)의 (< *the infinites-imal difference between consecutive values of a continuously varying quantity*)　　　　　　　E *differential*

　　　> differentio, differentiavi, differentiatum, differentiare 차별하다, 차이가 나다, 분화(分化)하다, 미분하다

　　　E *differentiate, differentiable, differentiation, dedifferentiate, un-differentiated*

　　> indifferens, (gen.) indifferentis (< in- *not*) 차별을 두지 않는, 아무래도 괜찮은, 무관심한, 냉담한　　　　　　E *indifferent*

> indifferentia, indifferentiae, f. 무차별, 무관심, 냉담　　　　　**E** *indifference*

　> dilatorius, dilatoria, dilatorium 미루는, 지연시키는　　　　　**E** *dilatory*

> effero, **extuli**, elatum, efferre (< ef- (< ex) *out of, away from* + ferre *to carry*)
밖으로 내가다, 쳐들다, 치켜
세우다　　**E** *efferent, elate; efferocytosis* (< *'removal of apoptotic cells by phagocytosis'*)

> infero, **intuli**, illatum, inferre (< in- *in, on, into, toward* + ferre *to carry*) 안으로
끌어들이다, 추론하다　　　　　**E** *infer, inference, illation, illative*

> offero, **obtuli**, oblatum, offerre (< of- (< ob) *before, toward(s), over, against, away*
+ ferre *to carry*) 앞에 갖다 놓다, 제공하다,
바치다　　**E** *offer, oblate,* (pro- *'before'* + offerre *'to offer'* >) *proffer*

> praefero, **praetuli**, praelatum, praeferre (< prae- *before, beyond* + ferre *to carry*)
앞에 지니다, 더 낮게 여기다, 선호하다　　　**E** *prefer, preference, preferential, preferable*

> refero, **re(t)tuli**, relatum, referre (< re- *back, again* + ferre *to carry*) 되돌리다, 가리
키다, 연관시키다, 조회하다,
참고하다　　　**E** *refer, reference,* (refer >) *referral,* (refer >) *referee, relate*

> referendum, referendi, n. (< (*neuter gerundive*) *something to be referred;*
(*gerund*) *referring*) 국민투표, 국민결의권, (외교관이 본국 정부에 보내는)
훈령 청원서　　　　　**E** *referendum*

> relativus, relativa, relativum 관계가 있는, 상관된, 상대적,
비교적　　　　　**E** *relative, relatively, relativity*

> relatio, relationis, f. 연관,
관계　　**E** *relation, relationship,* (relation >) *correlation,* (correlation >) *correlate*

> suffero, **sustuli**, sublatum, sufferre (< suf- (< sub) *under, up from under* + ferre
to carry) 밑에 넣다, 받치다, 가져가다, 견디다, 인내하다　　　**E** *suffer, sublate*

> superfero, **supertuli**, superlatum, superferre (< super- *above* + ferre *to carry*) 위로
가져가다, 최상으로 올리다　　　　　**E** *superlative*

> transfero, **transtuli**, translatum (tralatum), transferre (< trans- *over, across, through,*
beyond + ferre *to carry*) 옮기다, 이전(移轉)하다, 전달하다, 번역하다　**E** *transfer, translate*

> *transferentia, *transferentiae, f. 옮기기, 이전, 양도　　　**E** *transference*

> translatio, translationis, f. 전환, 번역, 해석　　　　　**E** *translation*

< IE. bher- *to carry, also to bear children*

E *bear* (< *'to carry'*), *forbear* (< *'to bear up against'*), *bier,* (*probably*) *bear* > *'adequate sea*
room' >) *berth, barrow, wheelbarrow, bring, burden, born, inborn, newborn, air-borne,*
water-borne, birth, birthmark

> L. fors, fortis f. (< *a bringing, that which is brought*) 우연, (우연한) 기회, 운수,
행운

> L. fortuna, fortunae, f. 운, 행운, (pl.) 재산, 부; (Fortuna) (로마 신화)
행운의 여신　　　　　**E** *fortune, Fortuna*

> L. fortuno, **fortunavi**, fortunatum, fortunare 운 좋게 만들다　　**E** *fortunate*

> L. fortuitus, fortuita, fortuitum 우연한　　　　**E** *fortuitous*

> L. fur, furis, m. 도둑　　　　　**E** *ferret*

> L. furtum, furti, n. 도둑질

> L. furtivus, furtiva, furtivum 도둑질의, 남몰래 하는, 은밀한　　　**E** *furtive*

　　> L. furunculus, furunculi, m. (< *modeled on* latrunculus *robber, diminutive of*
　　　latro, latronis, m. *bandit*) 바늘도둑, 소매치기; (*knob on a vine that 'steals'*
　　　the sap >) 절(癤), 종기(腫氣)　　　**E** *furuncle*

> G. pherein (phorein (phoreein)) ((*future infinitive*) oisein) *to carry, to bear, to rob*

E (pherein *'to carry'* + hormone >) **pheromone,** (tokos *'offspring'* + pherein *'to bear'* +
-ol >) **tocopherol**

　　> G. phernē, phernēs, f. *dowry*

　　　　> G. parapherna, paraphernas, f. (< par(a)- *beside, along side of, beyond*
　　　　　+ phernē *dowry*) *property apart from a dowry*

　　　　　　> L. paraphernalia, paraphernalium, n. (pl.) 아내의 지참금 외 사물
　　　　　　　(私物), 개인 소유물　　　**E** *paraphernalia*

　　> G. pheretron, pheretrou, n. *bier*

　　　　> L. pheretrum, pheretri, n. 들것　　　**E** *feretory*

　　> G. phora, phoras, f. *carrying, bearing*

　　　　> G. anaphora, anaphoras, f. (< an(a)- *up, upward; again, throughout;*
　　　　　back, backward; against; according to, similar to + phora *carrying*)
　　　　　ascent; repetition

　　　　　　> L. anaphora, anaphorae, f. 천체의 떠오름; (수사) 반복;
　　　　　　　(문법) 대용어, 전방대용어　　　**E** *anaphora, anaphor*

　　　　> G. kataphora, kataphoras, f. (< kat(a)- *down, mis-; according to, along,*
　　　　　thoroughly + phora *carrying*) *bringing down*

　　　　　　> L. cataphora, cataphorae, f. (문법) 후방대용어　　　**E** *cataphora (cataphor)*

　　　　> G. metaphora, metaphoras, f. (< met(a)- *between, along with, across,*
　　　　　after + phora *carrying*) *carrying over*

　　　　　　> L. metaphora, metaphorae, f. 은유　　　**E** *metaphor, metaphorically*

　　　　> G. epiphora, epiphoras, f. (< ep(i)- *upon* + phora *carrying*) *carrying*
　　　　　upon

　　　　　　> L. epiphora, epiphorae, f. 넘쳐흐름, 눈물흘림　　　**E** *epiphora*

　　> G. phorēsis, phorēseōs, f. *carrying*

E -phoresis, electrophoresis, electrophoretic, electrophoretogram (electropherogram)
(< *'written result of electrophoresis'*), (electrophoresis >) **electrophorese,**
iontophoresis (< *'carrying ions into tissue by electric current'*)

　　> G. phoreus, phoreōs, m. *carrier, bearer*

　　　　> G. amphiphoreus, amphiphoreōs, m. (< amphi- *on both sides, around*
　　　　　+ phoreus *bearer*) *two-handled pitcher*

　　　　　　> G. amphoreus, amphoreōs, m. *two-handled pitcher*

　　　　　　　> L. amphora, amphorae, f. 손잡이 둘 달린 항아리　　　**E** *amphora*

　　　　　　　　> L. ampulla, ampullae, f. (손잡이가 둘이고 목이 잘록한)
　　　　　　　　　단지; 팽대부　　　**E** *ampulla, ampule (ampoule)*

　　　　　　　　　> L. ampullaris, ampullare 단지의;

팽대부의　　　　　　　　　　　　　**E** *ampullar (ampullary)*

> G. -phoros, -phoros, -phoron *carrying,*

　　　bearing　　　　　　　　　　**E** *-phore,* (tēle *'afar, far off'* >) *telpher (telfer)*

　　> G. Christophoros, Christophoros, Christophoron (< Christos, Christou, m.

　　　　Christ + -phoros) *Christ-bearing*

　　　　> G. Christophoros, Christophorou, m. *Chirst-bearer*

　　　　　　> L. Christophorus, Christophori, m. 크리스토퍼　**E** *Christopher*

　　> G. phōsphoros, phōsphoros, phōsphoron (< phōs, phōtos, n. *light* +

　　　　-phoros) *light-bearing*

　　　　> G. Phōsphoros, Phōsophorou, m. (< phōsphoros astēr)

　　　　　the morning star

　　　　　　> L. Phosphorus, Phosphori, m. 샛별; (phosphorus) 인(燐)

> **E** *Phosphor, phosphorescence; phosphorus (P), phosphorous, phosphoric, (phosphoric* >*) phosphoryl, (phosphoryl* >*) phosphorylation, (phosphorylation* >*) phosphorylase, (phosphoric acid* >*) phosphate, (phosphate* >*) phosphatase, pyrophosphate (< originally produced by heating phosphates'), phosphite, phosphide, phosph(o)- (< 'substances containing phosphorus or phosphates, or involved in the metabolism of phosphates'), phospholipid(s) (< 'any lipid containing a phosphate group')*

　　> G. ōiphoros, ōiphoros, ōiphoron (< ōion, ōiou, n. *egg* + -phoros)

　　　egg-bearing

　　　　> G. ōiphoron, ōiphorou, n. *ovary*

　　　　　> L. oophoron, oophori, n.

　　　　　　난소(卵巢)　　　　　**E** *oophor(o)-, oophoritis, oophorectomy*

　　> L. oophorus, oophora, oophorum 난소의, 난포의

　　　　[용례] cumulus oophorus 난포세포더미, 난구(卵丘)　**E** *cumulus oophorus*

　　　　(문법) cumulus 더미, 퇴적, 구(丘): 단수 주격

　　　　　　< cumulus, cumuli, m.

　　　　　　oophorus: 형용사, 남성형 단수 주격

> L. -phorus, -phora, -phorum 나르는, 지니는

> **E** *-phorous, -phore, chromophore (< 'color radical'), chromatophore (< 'pigment-bearing cell, pigment-bearing plastid'), melanophore (< 'a dermal chromatophore containing melanin, especially such a cell in fishes, amphibians, and reptiles'), luminophore (< 'light radical'), ionophore (< 'an agent which is able to carry ions across a lipid membrane'), -phorin, glycophorin(s) (< 'sugar-bearing protein(s)')*

> G. -phoria, -phorias, f. *bearing*

　　> G. euphoria, euphorias, f. (< eu- *well* + -phoria) *euphoria*

　　　> L. euphoria, euphoriae, f. 다행감, 쾌감, 이상 행복감,

　　　　　이상 황홀감　　**E** *euphoria, euphoric, euphorigenic; euphoriant*

　　> G. dysphoria, dysphorias, f. (< dys- *bad* + -phoria) *dysphoria*

> L. dysphoria, dysphoriae, f. 불행감, 불쾌감　**E** *dysphoria, dysphoric*

> L. orthophoria, orthophoriae, f. (< G. orthos *upright, straight,*
correct) 정위(正位), 정상눈위치　**E** *orthophoria*

> L. heterophoria, heterophoriae, f. (< G. heteros *different*)
사위(斜位)　**E** *heterophoria*

> L. cyclophoria, cyclophoriae, f. (< G. kyklos *circle*)
회선사위(廻旋斜位)　**E** *cyclophoria*

> L. exophoria, exophoriae, f. (< G. exō- *outside, outwards*)
외사위(外斜位)　**E** *exophoria*

> L. esophoria, esophoriae, f. (< G. esō- *within, inwards*)
내사위(內斜位)　**E** *esophoria*

> L. hyperphoria, hyperphoriae, f. (< G. hyper- *over*)
상사위(上斜位)　**E** *hyperphoria*

> L. hypophoria, hypophoriae, f. (< G. hypo- *under*)
하사위(下斜位)　**E** *hypophoria*

> L. phoria, phoriae, f. (< L. -phoria < (*perhaps*) heterophoria)
사위(斜位)　**E** *phoria*

> G. peripherein (< peri- *around, near, beyond, on account of* + pherein) *to*
carry round, to carry about

> G. periphereia, periphereias, f. *circumference, rounded surface, curve,*
arc of a circle　**E** *pi (π)*

> L. peripheria, peripheriae, f. 둘레, 주위, 원주(圓周), 주변,
말초(末稍)　**E** *periphery, (peripherial >) peripheral*

> G. diaphorein (diaphoreein) (< di(a)- *through, thoroughly, apart* + phorein
(phoreein)) *to carry off, to throw off by perspiration*

> G. diaphorēsis, diaphorēseōs, f. *sweat, perspiration, especially, that*
produced by artificial means

> L. diaphoresis, diaphoresis, f. 발한, 발한작용　**E** *diaphoresis*

volo, volui, -, velle 원하다

능동태	부정법	현재			velle	원하다
	직설법	현재	단수	일인칭	vol-o	나는 ~한다
				이인칭	vi-s	너는 ~한다
				삼인칭	vul-t	그는 ~한다
			복수	일인칭	vol-umus	우리는 ~한다
				이인칭	vul-tis	너희는 ~한다
				삼인칭	vol-unt	그들은 ~한다
		과거	단수	일인칭	vol-ebam	나는 ~하였다

	미래	단수	일인칭	vol-am	나는 ~하겠다
가정법	완료	단수	일인칭	vol-ui	나는 ~하였다
	현재	단수	일인칭	vel-im	나는 ~하리라
명령법				없음	
분 사	현재			volens, (gen.) volent-is	~하는, ~하고 있는
목적분사				없음	
수동태				없음	

volo, volui, –, velle 원하다   **E** *benevolent, malevolent*

> vel (< 이것이나 저것 마음대로 취하라: velle의 고형(古形) 명령법) (접속사) 또는, 혹

> voluntas, voluntatis, f. 뜻, 의사, 의도

   > voluntarius, voluntaria, voluntarium 본의에 의한, 수의(隨意)의,

     임의(任意)의   **E** *voluntary, volunteer*

      > involuntarius, involuntaria, involuntarium (< in- *not*) 본의 아닌,

        불수의(不隨意)의   **E** *involuntary*

> volitio, volitionis, f. 의지, 결단, 의지력, 결단력   **E** *volition*

> velleitas, velleitatis, f. (행동으로 나타나지 않는) 불완전 의욕, (노력이 따르지 않는)

   약한 의욕   **E** *velleity*

< IE. wel- *to wish, will*

   E *will, well* (< *'according to one's wish'*), *wealth, gallop* (< *'well run'*), *gallant* (< *'to take it easy'*)

> L. voluptas, voluptatis, f. 쾌락

   > L. voluptuosus, voluptuosa, voluptuosum 쾌락의, 매혹적인   **E** *voluptuous*

   > L. voluptuarius, voluptuaria, voluptuarium 쾌락을 즐기는   **E** *voluptuary*

불비동사의 변화

불비(不備)동사는 법, 시제, 인칭 등이 결여되어 있는 동사이다. 결여동사라고도 한다. 불비동사는 완료어간을 중심으로 변화하며, 완료는 현재의 뜻을 가지고 과거부정법은 현재부정법의 뜻을 갖는다. 모자라는 시칭이나 형은 같은 뜻을 갖는 다른 낱말로 대신한다.

–, memini, –, meminisse (과거부정법 meminisse; 뜻은 현재) 기억하고 있다

   > Minerva, Minervae, f. (*earlier* Menerva) (로마 신화) 지혜의 여신 (그리스 신화의

     Athēnē 여신에 해당함)   **E** *Minerva*

> comminiscor, commentus sum, comminisci (< com- (< cum) *with, together; intensive*
+ meminisse *to keep in mind*) 고안하다, 발명하다, 날조하다
> commentum, commenti, n. (< *past participle*) 창안, 상상   **E** *(noun) comment*
> commentarius, commentaria, commentarium 주석(註釋)의, 기록의   **E** *commentary*
> commentor, commentatus sum, commentari (*frequentative*) 궁리하다   **E** *(verb) comment*
> commentator, commentatoris, m. 주석가(註釋家)   **E** *commentator*
> reminiscor, –, reminisci (< re- *back, again* + meminisse *to keep in mind*) 다시
생각나다, 회상하다   **E** *reminiscent*
> reminiscentia, reminiscentiae, f. 회상   **E** *reminiscence*
< IE. men- *to think; with derivatives referring to various qualities and states of mind and*
thought   **E** *mind, remind,* (D. Minnesinger *'love-singer'* >) *minnesinger*
> L. mens, mentis, f. 정신
> L. mentalis, metale 정신의   **E** *mental*
> L. mentalitas, mentalitatis, f. 정신상태   **E** *mentality*
> L. amens, (gen.) amentis (< a- (< ab) *off, away from*) 정신 나간, 미친   **E** *ament*
> L. amentia, amentiae, f. 아멘티아   **E** *amentia*
> L. demens, (gen.) dementis (< de- *apart from, down, not*) 정신 나간, 미친   **E** *dement*
> L. dementia, dementiae, f. 치매(癡呆)   **E** *dementia*
> L. mentio, mentionis, f. 언급   **E** *mention*
> L. moneo, **monui**, monitum, monēre 생각나게 하다, 권고하다, 경고하다
> L. monitio, monitionis, f. 경고   **E** *monition*
> L. monitor, monitoris, m. 경고자, 경고 장치   **E** *monitor*
> L. monumentum, monumenti, n. 기념물   **E** *monument*
> L. monstrum, monstri, n. (길흉의) 전조, 괴상한 일(것), 괴물   **E** *monster*
> L. monstrosus, monstrosa, monstrosum 괴상한, 괴물 같은   **E** *monstrous, monstrosity*
> L. monstro, **monstravi**, monstratum, monstrare 보여 주다, 가리키다, 증명하다   **E** *muster*
> L. demonstro, demonstravi, demonstratum, demonstrare (< de- *apart
from, down, not; intensive* + monstrare *to show*) 명시하다, 똑똑히
가리키다, 증명하다   **E** *demonstrate*
> L. remonstro, **remonstravi**, remonstratum, remonstrare (< re- *back, again;
intensive* + monstrare *to show*) 충고하다, 항의하다   **E** *remonstrate*
> L. admoneo, **admonui**, admonitum, admonēre (< ad- *to, toward, at, according
to* + monēre *to warn*) 권고하다   **E** *admonish, admonition*
> L. praemoneo, **praemonui**, praemonitum, praemonēre (< prae- *before, beyond*
+ monēre *to warn*) 예고하다   **E** *premonish, premonition*
> L. summoneo, **summonui**, summonitum, summonēre (< sum- (< sub) *under,
up from under* + monēre *to warn*) 비밀히 알려 주다, 귀엣말로 하다   **E** *summon*
> G. mnasthai *to remember*
> G. mnēmē, mnēmēs, f. *memory*

E *mnemonics (mnemotechnics),* (mnēmē + -on *'a termination of Greek neuter
nouns and adjectives'* >) *mnemon* (< *'a unit of memory, the minimum
physical change in the nervous system that encodes one memory')*

> G. mnēmosynē, mnēmosynēs, f. *memory;* (Mnēmosynē) (*Greek mythology*)
  the Goddess of memory, mother of the Muses   `E  Mnemosyne`

> G. mnēmōn, mnēmōn, mnēmon *mindful, remembering, unforgetting*

  > G. mnēmonikos, mnēmonikē, mnēmonikon *relating to memory*

    > L. mnemonicus, mnemonica, mnemonicum 기억의, 기억술의,
      기억을 돕는   `E  mnemonic`

> G. mimnēskein *to remind;* (*passive*) *to remember, to recall*

  > G. amnēstos, amnēstos. amnēston *not remembered*

    > G. amnēstia, amnēstias, f. *oblivion*

      > L. amnestia, amnestiae, f. 사면   `E  amnesty, amnestic`

      > G. amnēsia, amnēsias, f. *forgetfulness*

        > L. amnesia, amnesiae, f. 기억상실,
          건망증   `E  amnesia, amnesic, amnesiac`

          > L. paramnesia, paramnesiae, f. (< G. par(a)- *beside,*
            along side of, beyond + amnesia *loss of memory*)
            기억착오   `E  paramnesia`

> G. anamimnēskein (< an(a)- *up, upward; again, throughout; back, backward;*
  against; according to, similar to) *to remind*

  > G. anamnēsis, anamnēseōs, f. *remembrance*

    > L. anamnesis, anamnesis, f. 회상, 기왕력(旣往歷), 병력(病歷) `E  anamnesis`

> G. mainesthai *to be mad, to rave*

  > G. mania, manias, f. *madness, frenzy, enthusiasm*

    > L. mania, maniae, f. 들뜸, 열광증, 조병(躁病)   `E  mania, -mania`

    > G. manikos, manikē, manikon *mad*

      > L. manicus, manica, manicum 조병(躁病)의   `E  manic, manic-depressive`

    > G. maniakos, maniakē, maniakon *mad, of mad man*

      > L. maniacus, maniaca, maniacum 미친, 미치광이의   `E  maniac, maniacal`

> G. -matos *thinking, willing, acting*

  > G. automatos, automatos (automatē), automaton (< autos *self*) *self-thinking,*
    voluntary, self-acting

    `E` (*neuter* sing.) **automaton,** (*neuter* pl.) **automata, automatic,** (*automatic* >) **automaticity,**
    (*automatic* >) **automation,** (*automation* >) **automate,** (*automatic* >) **automatism**

> G. mantis, manteōs, m., f. *soothsayer, seer, prophet*   `E  mantic`
  > G. manteia, manteias, f. *prophecy, divination*   `E  -mancy`
  > L. mantis, mantis, f. (< *praying mantis*) 사마귀   `E  mantis`

> G. Mentōr, Mentōros, m. (< *adviser, monitor*) *Mentor* (*the name of a character in*
  the Odyssey, in whose likeness Athena appears to Telemachus and acts as his
  guide and adviser)   `E  Mentor, mentor`

> G. Mousa, Mousas, f. *Muse* (*each of nine goddesses, the daughters of Zeus and*
  Mnemosyne, who preside over the arts and sciences)

> G. mousikos, mousikē, mousikon *relating to the Muse or Muses (applied generally to artistic culture, poetry, etc., but also specifically to music)*

E (mousikē technē *'art of the Muses'* >) **music, musical, musician, musicotherapy**

> G. mouseios, mouseia, mouseion *of or belonging to the Muses*

> G. museion, museiou, n. *a place holy to the Muses*

> L. museum, musei, n. 뮤즈의 신전; 박물관, (학문 연구의) 학원 **E** *museum*

> L. Musa, Musae, f. 뮤즈 **E** *Muse*

> L. musaicus, musaica, musaicum 뮤즈의

E (musaicum opus *'work dedicated to the Muses'* >) **mosaic, mosaicism**

> (*probably*) G. martys, martyros, m., f. (martyr, martyros, m., f.) *witness, martyr* **E** *martyr, martyrdom*

> (*Sanskrit*) mantrah *counsel, prayer, hymn* **E** *mandarin*

> (*Avestan*) mazda *wise*

E *Mazda* (< *'the Wise One; the name of the good principle of the Zoroastrian religion'*)

> IE. mendh- *to learn*

> G. manthanein (math- *aorist stem*) *to learn*

> G. mathē, mathēs, f. *learning*

> G. polymathēs, polymathēs, polymathes (< polys *much*) *having learnt much* **E** *polymath*

> G. mathēma, mathēmatos, n. (< ma- *resultative noun suffix*) *what is learned, the act of learning, learning, knowledge*

> G. mathēmatikos, mathēmatikē, mathēmatikon (< -ikos *adjective suffix*) *inclined to learn, mathematical* **E** *mathematical, mathematics*

−, odi, (osus sum), odisse 미워하다, 귀찮게 굴다

> odium, odii, n. 미움, 싫음, 불쾌

E *odium,* (est mihi in odio *'it is to me hateful'* >) **annoy, annoyance,** (annoy ± -some >) **noisome**

> odiosus, odiosa, odiosum 밉살스러운, 싫은, 불쾌한 **E** *odious*

< IE. od- *to hate*

aio (ajo), ais, ait, aiunt (ajunt) 말하다

> adagium, adagii, n. (adagio, adagionis, f.) (< ad- *to, toward, at, according to* + aio *I say*) 옛말, 속담, 격언 **E** *adage*

> prodigium, prodigii, n. (< prod- (< pro) *before, forward, for, instead of* + aio *I say*) 놀라운 일, 불가사의 **E** *prodigy*

> prodigiosus, prodigiosa, prodigiosum 놀라운, 불가사의한 **E** *prodigious*

< IE. ag- *to speak*

동사를 만드는 방법

반복동사

동작의 반복을 나타내는 반복동사(反復動詞, *frequentative, iterative*)는 동사의 과거분사 어간에 -are를 붙여 정형 제1변화 동사로 만든다.

domito, domitavi, domitatum, domitare 길들이다, 억누르다   **E** *daunt*
> indomitabilis, indomitabile (< in- *not*) 굴복하지 않는, 불굴의   **E** *indomitable*
< domo, **domui**, domitum, domare 길들이다, 억누르다
< IE. demə- *to constrain, to force, especially to break in (horses)*   **E** *tame* (< *'domesticated'*)
> G. daman (damaein) *to tame*
> G. adamas, adamantos, m. (< *the unconquerable* < a- *not* + daman) *the hardest metal, steel, diamond*
> L. adamas, adamantis, m. 강철, 금강석; 냉혈한(冷血漢)

> **E** *adamant,* *(adamantane 'a molecular structure composed of three six-sided rings of carbon atoms arranged in the manner of the crystal lattice of diamond' > adamantanamine >)* ***amantadine***

> L. diamas, diamantis, m. (< *on the pattern of* G. di(a)- *through, thoroughly, apart*) 금강석   **E** *diamond*
> G. adamantinos, adamantinē, adamantinon *of steel, steely*
> L. adamantinus, adamantina, adamantinum 강철 같은, 견고한 **E** *adamantine*

nictito, nictitavi, nictitatum, nictitare 눈을 깜박거리다   **E** *nictitate*
< nicto, **nictavi**, nictatum, nictare 눈을 깜박거리다   **E** *nictate*
< IE. kneig^wh- *to lean on*
> L. conniveo, connivi (connixi), –, connivēre (coniveo, conivi (conixi), –, conivēre) 눈을 감다, 눈감아 주다, 묵인하다   **E** *connive*

vegeto, vegetavi, vegetatum, vegetare 활기 있게 하다, 성장하다, 식물처럼 성장하다, 증식하다; 식물처럼 단조롭게 살다   **E** *vegetate*
> vegetatio, vegetationis, f. 식물의 생장, 식물, 증식; 무위도식   **E** *vegetation*
> vegetativus, vegetativa, vegetativum 식물이 생장하는; 식물성의, 아무것도 하지 않고 지내는   **E** *vegetative*
> vegetabilis, vegetabile 활기 있게 해주는, 식물성의, 식물의   **E** *vegetable,* *(vegetable >)* ***vegetarian, vegeburger***
< vegeo, –, –, vegēre 박차를 가하다, 자극하다

< IE. weg- *to be strong, to be lively*

> **E** **wake, awake, waken, watch, wicked, witch, wait, waft,** ((*probably*) D. Beiwacht *'by-watch'* >) **bivouac**

> L. vigor, vigoris, m. 활력   **E** *vigor (vigour)*

>> L. vigorosus, vigorosa, vigorosum 활력 있는   **E** *vigorous*

>> L. vigoro, **vigoravi**, vigoratum, vigorare 기운 나게 하다

>>> L. invigoro, **invigoravi**, invigoratum, invigorare (< in- *in, on, into, toward* + vigorare *to make strong*) 기운 나게 하다   **E** *invigorate, invigorant*

> L. vigil, (gen.) vigilis 잠 안 자고 지키는

>> L. vigilia, vigiliae, f. 철야, 전야, 불침   **E** *vigil*

>> L. vigilo, **vigilavi**, vigilatum, vigilare 잠 안 자고 지키다, 잠 안 자고 하다   **E** *vigilant*, (*supervigilare *'to watch over'* >) *surveillance*

> L. velox, (gen.) velocis 재빠른

>> L. velocitas, velocitatis, f. 신속, 속도   **E** *velocity*

canto, cantavi, cantatum, cantare (*frequentative*) 노래 부르다, 연주하다, 찬송하다

> **E** (It. cantata aria *'sung air'* >) **cantata**, It. **cantabile** (< *'suited for singing'* < *'singable'*), (*verb*) **chant, cant**

> incanto, **incantavi**, incantatum, incantare (< in- *in, on, into, toward* + cantare *to sing*) 노래하다, 주문을 외다, 마술을 걸다, 호리다   **E** *enchant*

> recanto, **recantavi**, recantatum, recantare (< re- *back, again* + cantare *to sing*) 다시 노래하다, 메아리치다; 취소하다, 철회하다   **E** *recant*

>> incantatio, incantationis, f. 주문, 마술   **E** *incantation*

< cano, **cecini**, cantum (cantatum), canĕre 노래하다, 지저귀다, 연주하다

> canor, canoris, m. 노래

>> canorus, canora, canorum 음악적인   **E** *canorous*

> cantus, cantus, m. 노래   **E** (*noun*) *chant*

>> accentus, accentus, m. (< *song added to* (*speech*) < ac- (< ad) *to, toward, at, according to* + cantus *song*) 강세   **E** *accent*

>>> accentuo, **accentuavi**, accentuatum, accentuare 강세를 주어 발음하다, 강조하다, 강화하다   **E** *accentuate*

> cantor, cantoris, m. 가수   **E** *cantor*

>> cantrix, cantricis, f. 여가수

> cantio, cantionis, f. 노래 부르기, 노래   **E** It. *canzone*

> oscen, oscinis, m. (< os- (< ob) *before, toward(s), over, against, away* + canĕre *to sing*) 울음소리로 길흉을 알리는 새 (특히 까마귀)   **E** *oscine*

> incino, –, –, incinĕre (< in- *in, on, into, toward* + canĕre *to sing*) 노래하다, (악기를) 불다

>> incentivus, incentiva, incentivum 선창하는, 선동하는, 격려하는   **E** *incentive*

< IE. kan- *to sing*   **E** *hen*

> L. carmen, carminis, n. 노래, 시가, 기도문, 주문   **E** *charm*

consulto, consultavi, consultatum, consultare 숙고하다, 염려하다,

　　　상담하다　　　　　　　　　　　　　　　　　　　**E** *consult, consultant, (consultant >) consultancy*

　　　< consulo, consului, consultum, consulĕre (< con- (< cum) *with, together*) 숙고하다,

　　　　　염려하다, 문의하다, 의논하다

　　　　　> consul, consulis, m. 집정관, 지방총독, 영사　　　　　　　　　　　**E** *consul*

　　< IE. sel- *to take, to seize*　　　　　　　　　　　　　　　　　　　　　　　**E** *sell*

　　　　> L. consilium, consilii, n. (< con- (< cum) *with, together*) 협의, 조언, 협의회,

　　　　　자문기관　　　　　　　　　　　　　　　　**E** *counsel, counselor (counsellor)*

명사 유래 동사

　　　동사로부터 명사, 형용사, 부사를 만드는 것이 일반적이나, 역으로 명사나 형
용사, 부사로부터 동사를 만들기도 한다. 명사로부터 만드는 경우가 많아 명사
유래 동사(*denominative*)라고 한다. 이 경우, 명사나 형용사의 어간이나 부사에다
-are를 붙여 정형 제1변화 동사로 만드는 것이 보통이다.

••• 정형 제1변화

deliro, deliravi, deliratum, delirare (< de- *apart from, down, not* + lira *furrow*) (곧은)

　　　밭이랑에서 벗어나다; 온전한 정신이 아니다

　　　　> delirium, delirii, n. 섬망(譫妄), 정신착란　　　　**E** *delirium, (delirium >) delirious*

　　　　　　[용례] delirium tremens 떨림섬망, 진전섬망(振顫譫妄)　　　**E** *delirium tremens*

　　　　　　(문법) delirium: 단수 주격

　　　　　　　　　tremens 떨고 있는, 떠는: 현재분사, 남·여·중성형 단수 주격

　　　　　　　　　　　< tremens, (gen.) trementis

　　　　　　　　　　　< tremo, tremui, -, tremĕre 떨다

　　　< lira, lirae, f. 이랑(두둑과 고랑, *a ridge and a furrow*, (옛) 사래), 두둑, 고랑

　　< IE. leis- *track, furrow*

　　　　E *last* (< *'to continue'* < *'to follow a track'*), *learn* (< *'to follow a course of study'*), *lore* (<
　　　　'learning'), *folklore*

serro, serravi, serratum, serrare 톱으로 켜다, 자르다　　　　**E** *(verb) serrate, serration*

　　　< serra, serrae, f. 톱

　　　　　> serratus, serrata, serratum (가장자리나 잎이) 톱니 꼴의　　　**E** *(adjective) serrate*

　　　　　> serrula, serrulae, f. (< + -ula *diminutive suffix*) 작은 톱

　　　　　　> serrulatus, serrulata, serrulatum 가는 톱니 꼴의　　　　**E** *serrulate*

stipo, stipavi, stipatum, stipare 삼[麻] 부스러기로 틀어막다, 쑤셔 넣다, 밀집시키다

> constipo, constipavi, constipatum, constipare (< con- (< cum) *with, together*
+ stipare *to press, to stuff, to cram*) 쑤셔 넣다, 밀집시키다　　　**E** *constipate*

> constipatio, constipationis, f. 밀집시킴, 변비(便祕)　　　**E** *constipation*

> obstipo, −, −, obstipare (< ob- *before, toward(s), over, against, away* +
stipare *to press, to stuff, to cram*) 다져 넣다, 꾹꾹 눌러 밀어 넣다

> obstipatio, obstipationis, f. 운집, 군중, 된변비(便祕)　　　**E** *obstipation*

< stipa, stipae, f. 배의 틈새를 막는 데 쓰는 삼[麻] 부스러기, 지푸라기

< IE. steip- *to stick, to compress*　　　**E** *stipple* (< *'to stick'), stiff*

> L. stipes, stipitis, m. (stipis, stipis, f.) 나무줄기, 막대기　　　**E** *stipes, stipe*

> L. stipula, stipulae, f. (stupula, stupulae, f.) (< +-ula *diminutive suffix*) 작은
줄기, 짚　　　**E** *stubble, stipule, etiolate* (< *'to grow into haulm'*)

> L. stipella, stipellae, f. (< +-ella *diminutive suffix*) 작은 턱잎　　　**E** *stipel*

> L. stipulatus, stipulata, stipulatum 턱잎이 있는,
탁엽(托葉)이 있는　　　**E** *(adjective) stipulate*

> (*suggested*) L. stipulor, stipulatus sum, stipulari 약속의 표시로 짚대를
꺾다, (구두로) 약속하다, 계약하다　　　**E** *(verb) stipulate*

bajulo, −, −, bajulare (짐을) 져 나르다　　　**E** *bail, bailout*

< bajulus, bajuli, m. 짐 져 나르는 사람

nuntio, nuntiavi, nuntiatum, nuntiare (nuncio, nunciavi, nunciatum, nunciare)
통지하다

> annuntio, annuntiavi, annuntiatum, annuntiare (annuncio, annunciavi, annunciatum,
annunciare) (< an- (< ad) *to, toward, at, according to* + nuntiare *to report*)
통지하다, 고지(告知)하다　　　**E** *announce, (announce >) announcement*

> annuntiatio, annuntiationis, f. (annunciatio, annunciationis, f.) 통지,
고지　　　**E** *annunciation*

> denuntio, denuntiavi, denuntiatum, denuntiare (denuncio, denunciavi, denunciatum,
denunciare) (< de- *apart from, down, not* + nuntiare *to report*) 고발하다,
(공공연히) 비난하다, 규탄하다　　　**E** *denounce (denunciate)*

> denuntiatio, denuntiationis, f. (denunciatio, denunciationis, f.) 고발,
(공공연한) 비난, 규탄　　　**E** *denunciation*

> enuntio, enuntiavi, enuntiatum, enuntiare (enuncio, enunciavi, enunciatum,
enunciare) (< e- *out of, away from* + nuntiare *to report*) 분명히 발음하다,
진술하다, 선언하다　　　**E** *enounce (enunciate)*

> enuntiatio, enuntiationis, f. (enunciatio, enunciationis, f.) 발음, 진술,
선언　　　**E** *enunciation*

> pronuntio, pronuntiavi, pronuntiatum, pronuntiare (pronuncio, pronunciavi,
pronunciatum, pronunciare) (< pro- *before, forward, for, instead of* + nuntiare

to report) 공포하다, 낭독하다, 발음하다   **E** *pronounce*

    > pronuntiatio, pronuntiationis, f. (pronunciatio, pronunciationis, f.) 공포

        (公布), 낭독, 발음   ·   **E** *pronunciation*

    > renuntio, **renuntiavi**, renuntiatum, renuntiare (renuncio, **renunciavi**, renunciatum,

        renunciare) (< re- *back, again* + nuntiare *to report*) 부인하다   **E** *renounce*

        > renuntiatio, renuntiationis, f. (renunciatio, renunciationis, f.) 부인 **E** *renunciation*

  < nuntius, nuntii, m. (nuncius, nuncii, m.) 전령, 소식

    > internuntius, internuntii, m. (internuncius, internuncii, m.) (< inter- *between,*

        among) 사절(使節), 중개자   **E** *internuncial, (internuncial neuron >) interneuron*

< IE. neu- *to shout*

minio, miniavi, miniatum, miniare 진사(辰砂)로 붉게 물들이다, 주홍색으로 칠하다

        E *(verb) miniate*

    > miniatus, miniata, miniatum (*past participle*) 진사로 붉게 물들인, 주홍색으로

    ·· 칠한   **E** *(adjective) miniate*

    > miniatura, miniaturae, f. (양피지 등에 붉은 도료로 세밀하게 그린) 작은 그림,

    삽화   **E** *miniature, (miniature >) mini-, mini*

  < minium, minii, n. 진사(辰砂, *cinnabar*), 연단(鉛丹, *red lead*)

< (*perhaps*) *Of Iberian origin*

stagno, stagnavi, stagnatum, stagnare 물이 고이다, 침수되다, 잠기게 하다 **E** *stagnate, stagnant*

    > stagnatio, stagnationis, f. 정체, 침체   **E** *stagnation, stagflation*

  < stagnum, stagni, n. (stagnus, stagni, m.) (물이 흐르지 않고 고여 있는) 늪, 못

< IE. stag- *to seep, to drip*

    > G. stazein *to ooze, to drip, to distill*   **E** *stactometer*

      > G. staxis, staxeōs, f. *dripping*

        > L. staxis, staxis, f. 출혈   **E** *staxis*

      > G. epistazein (< ep(i)- *upon* + stazein) *to bleed at the nose*

        > G. epistaxis, epistaxeōs, f. *nasal bleeding*

          > L. epistaxis, epistaxis, f. 코피, 비(鼻)출혈   **E** *epistaxis*

  > (*suggested, via Celtic*) L. stagnum, stagni, n. (< *being easily fusible*) 주석(朱錫)

    > L. stannum, stanni, n. 주석   **E** *stannum (Sn), stannous (Sn^{++}), stannic (Sn^{++++})*

tanno, tannavi, tannatum, tannare 무두질하다, (무두질한 가죽처럼) 옅은 갈색이 나게 하다,

    햇볕에 태우다   **E** *(verb) tan*

  < tannum, tanni, n. 참나무, (무두질을 하기 위한 참나무 등의 으깬)

    나무껍질   **E** *(noun) tan (< 'the bark of young oak'), tannin(s) (tannic acid(s)), tawny*

< (*probably*) *Of Celtic origin*

formido, formidavi, formidatum, formidare 몹시 무서워하다

> formidabilis, formidabile 무서운, 무시무시한 **E** *formidable*

   < formido, formidinis, f. 공포

< IE. mormo- *to feel horror*

   > G. mormō, mormous, f. (mormōn, mormonos, f.) *a hideous she-monster (used by nurses to frighten children), bugbear, spectre*

grego, gregavi, gregatum, gregare 떼 짓게 하다, 불러 모으다, 모이다

   > aggrego, **aggregavi**, aggregatum, aggregare (< ad- *to, toward, at, according to* + gregare *to herd*) 집합시키다, 응집하다 **E** *aggregate*

     > *aggregatio, *aggregationis, f. 집합, 응집 **E** *aggregation*

   > congrego, **congregavi**, congregatum, congregare (< con- (< cum) *with, together* + gregare *to herd*) 모으다, 모이다 **E** *congregate*

     > congregatio, congregationis, f. 모임, 집합 **E** *congregation*

   > segrego, **segregavi**, segregatum, segregare (< se- *apart, without* + gregare *to herd*) 갈라놓다, 분리시키다 **E** *segregate*

     > segregatio, segregationis, f. 분리, 격리 **E** *segregation*

  < grex, gregis, m. 떼, 무리, 군중

   > gregarius, gregaria, gregarium 떼의, 무리 짓는 **E** *gregarious*

   > egregius, egregia, egregium (< e- *out of, away from* + grex *flock*) 뛰어난 **E** *egregious*

< IE. ger- *to gather* **E** *cram*

   > G. agora, agoras, f. ((*Aeolic*) agyris, agyrios, f.) *meeting, assembly, market, market-place, speech* **E** *agora, agoraphobia*

    > G. agoreuein *to speak in assembly*

     > G. allēgorein (allēgoreein) (< allos *other*) *to speak metaphorically*

      > G. allēgoria, allēgorias, f. *allegory*

       > L. allegoria, allegoriae, f. 비유, 풍유, 우화 **E** *allegory*

     > G. katēgorein (katēgoreein) (< kat(a)- *down, mis-, according to, along, thoroughly*) *to speak against, to accuse, to allege, to predicate*

      > G. katēgoria, katēgorias, f. *accusation; assertion, predication, category*

       > L. categoria, categoriae, f. 비난; 부류, 범주 **E** *category, (category >) categorize*

     > G. parēgorein (parēgoreein) (< par(a)- *beside, along side of, beyond*) *to exhort, to encourage*

      > G. parēgoria, parēgorias, f. *exhortation, consolation*

       > L. paregoria, paregoriae, f. 진정, 완화, 진통 **E** *paregoric*

    > G. panēgyris, panēgyreōs, f. (< pan- *all* + agyris) *public assembly, public festival* **E** *panegyric* (< 'of public eulogy')

glutino, glutinavi, glutinatum, glutinare 풀로 붙이다, 접착시키다, 아물다

> agglutino, **agglutinavi**, agglutinatum, agglutinare (< ag- (< ad) *to, toward, at, according to* + glutinare *to glue*) 교착(膠着)하다, 응집(凝集)하다

E *agglutinate, agglutination, agglutinin; hemagglutinate (< 'to agglutinate red blood cells'), hemagglutination, hemagglutinin*

> agglutinativus, agglutinativa, agglutinativum 교착하는, 응집하는; (언어) 교착성의
E *agglutinative*

> conglutino, **conglutinavi**, conglutinatum, conglutinare (< con- (< cum) *with, together* + glutinare *to glue*) 접착시키다
E *conglutinate*

< gluten, glutinis, n. (glus, glutis, f.) 풀[糊], 갖풀, 아교(阿膠)

E *glue, gluten, (gluten >) glutenin, (gluten > 'amino acid obtained by hydrolysis of gluten' >) glutamic acid (Glu, E), glutamate, (glutamic acid >) glutamine (Gln, Q), (gluten > (probably) 'on the pattern of tartaric acid' >) glutaric acid, glutarate, (glutaric acid + aldehyde >) glutaraldehyde*

> glutinosus, glutinosa, glutinosum 아교질의, 점착성의, 끈적끈적한
E *glutinous*

< IE. glei- *clay*
E *clay*

> G. glia, glias, f. *glue*
E *gliadin (< 'with intrusive -d-')*

> L. neuroglia, neurogliae, f. (< G. neuron *nerve*) 신경아교(神經阿膠), 신경교 (神經膠); 신경아교세포, 신경교세포
E *neuroglia, neuroglial*

> L. glia, gliae, f. (< *short for* neuroglia) 신경아교, 신경교; 신경아교세포, 신경교세포
E *glia, glial*

[용례] glia limitans 경계신경아교
E *glia limitans*
(문법) glia 신경아교: 단수 주격
limitans 경계를 긋는: 현재분사, 남·여·중성형
단수 주격
< limitans, (gen.) limitantis
< limito, limitavi, limitatum, limitare 경계를 긋다, 제한하다, 한정하다

> L. macroglia, macrogliae, f. (< G. makros *long, large*) 큰아교세포, 대교세포(大膠細胞)
E *macroglia*

> L. microglia, microgliae, f. (< G. mikros *small*) 미세아교세포, 소교세포(小膠細胞)
E *microglia*

> L. oligodendroglia, oligodendrogliae, f. (< G. oligos *few, little* + dendron *tree*) 희소돌기아교세포, 핍지교(乏枝膠)
E *oligodendroglia (oligodendrocyte)*

> L. gliosis, gliosis, f. (< + G. -ōsis *condition*) 신경아교증, 교증
E *gliosis*

ulcero, ulceravi, ulceratum, ulcerare 궤양(潰瘍)을 일으키다
E *ulcerate, ulcerative*

> ulceratio, ulcerationis, f. 궤양형성, 궤양화
E *ulceration*

< ulcus, ulceris, n. 상처, 궤양
E *ulcer, ulcerogenic*

< IE. elk-es- *wound*

> G. helkos, helkou, n. *wound, ulcer, evil*
E *-helcosis*

laxo, laxavi, laxatum, laxare 느슨하게 하다, 해이(解弛)해지게 하다, 완화(緩化)시키다,

넓히다   **E** *lease, leash* (< '*to let run on a slack lead*'), *unleash, laxative, lush*

> laxatio, laxationis, f. 느슨함, 완화, 배변   **E** *laxation*

> relaxo, relaxavi, relaxatum, relaxare (< re- *back, again* + laxare *to loosen*)

풀어주다, 해이(解弛)해지게 하다, 완화시키다,

이완(弛緩)하다   **E** *relax, relaxant, release, relish* (< '*something remaining*'

> relaxatio, relaxationis, f. 풀림, 해이, 완화, 이완   **E** *relaxation*

< laxus, laxa, laxum 느슨한, 해이해진   **E** *lax*

> laxitas, laxitatis, f. 느슨함, 해이됨   **E** *laxity*

< IE. (s)leg- *to be slack, to be languid*   **E** *slack*

> L. langueo, langui, −, languēre 나른해지다, 시들다, 쇠약해지다, 앓다   **E** *languish*

> L. languor, languor, m. 나른함, 무기력, 쇠약   **E** *languor*

> L. languidus, languida, languidum 나른한, 무기력한, 쇠약   **E** *languid*

> G. lagneia, lagneias, f. *lust*

> L. algolagnia, algolagniae, f. (< G. algos *pain* + lagneia) 고통음락증(淫樂症)

(마조히즘과 사디즘을 포함)   **E** *algolagnia*

> G. lagōs, lagō, m. (lagōos, lagōou, m.) (< *with drooping ears* < IE. (s)leg- + IE.

ous-) *hare*

    E *lagophthalmos (lagophthalmus)* (< '*being unable to close the eyes, as the hare was supposed to*')

∽ (*possibly*) IE. sleb- *to be weak, to sleep*   **E** *sleep*

luxo, luxavi, luxatum, luxare 제자리에서 물러나게 하다, 관절을 삐게 하다, 탈구(脫臼)시키다   **E** *luxate*

> luxatio, luxationis, f. 어긋남, 이탈, 전위, 탈구   **E** *luxation* (*dislocation*)

> subluxatio, subluxationis, f. (< sub- *under, up from under*) 부분이탈,

부분탈구   **E** *subluxation*

< luxus, luxa, luxum 제자리에서 물러난, 탈구(脫臼)된

< IE. leug- *to bend*

    E (*probably*) *lock* (< '*fastening made by bending two branches until they meet*'), *interlock*

> (*probably*) L. luxus, luxus, m. 외도, 방탕

> L. luxuria, luxuriae, f. 방탕, 무절제, 사치, (말·글의) 현란함, 과잉, 풍성, 무성함   **E** *luxury*

> L. luxuriosus, luxuriosa, luxuriosum 방탕한, 사치스러운, 풍성한,

(문체가) 화려한   **E** *luxurious*

> L. luxurio, luxuriavi, luxuriatum, luxuriare 방탕하다, 무절제하다, 사치에

흐르다, (말·글이) 자유분방하다, 무성하다   **E** *luxuriate, luxuriant*

> L. luctor, luctatus sum, luctari 맞붙잡고 겨루다, 싸우다

> L. eluctor, eluctatus sum, eluctari (< e- (< ex) *out of, away from* + luctari

to struggle) 어려움을 싸워 이기다, 힘들여 빠져 나오다

> L. eluctabilis, eluctabile 빠져 나올 수 있는

> L. ineluctabilis, ineluctabile 빠져 나올 수 없는, 불가피한   **E** *ineluctable*

> L. reluctor, reluctatus sum, reluctari (< re- *back, again; intensive* + luctari *to struggle*) 대항하여 싸우다, 저항하다, 마음 내키지 않다　<u>**E** *reluctant, (reluctant >) reluctance*</u>

> G. loxos, loxē, loxon *slanting, oblique*

lubrico, lubricavi, lubricatum, lubricare 미끄럽게 하다, 원활히 움직이게 하다　<u>**E** *lubricate, lubricant*</u>
　　< lubricus, lubrica, lubricum 미끄러운, 원활하게 움직이는　<u>**E** *lubricious*</u>
　< IE. sleubh- *to slide, to slip*

> <u>**E** *sleeve* (< *'into which the arm slips'*), *sloven* (< *'to put on clothes carelessly'*), *slovenly*, *slop* (< *'dung'*), (slop >) *sloppy*</u>

manifesto, manifestavi, manifestatum, manifestare 드러내다, 표명하다
　　　> manifestatio, manifestationis, f. 드러냄, 표명, 선언, 표현, 표시, 소견(所見)　<u>**E** *manifestation*</u>
　　< manifestus, manifesta, manifestum (< manus *hand*) 현장에서 붙잡힌, 드러난, 명백한　<u>**E** *manifest*, It. *manifesto*</u>
　< (*probably*) IE. dhers- *to be bold, to attack*　<u>**E** *dare*</u>
　　> L. infestus, infesta, infestum (< in- *in, on, into, toward*) 덤벼드는, 괴롭히는, 휩쓰는
　　　> L. infesto, infestavi, infestatum, infestare 휩쓸다, 설치다　<u>**E** *infest, (infest >) disinfest*</u>
　　　　> L. infestatio, infestationis, f. 휩쓺, 들끓음, 횡행, 유린　<u>**E** *infestation, disinfestation*</u>

mutilo, mutilavi, mutilatum, mutilare 지체(肢體)를 절단하다, 불구로 만들다, 훼손하다, (말·글 등의 중요 부분을) 빼먹다　<u>**E** *mutilate*</u>
　　　> mutilatio, mutilationis, f. 절단, 불구, 훼손　<u>**E** *mutilation*</u>
　　< mutilus, mutila, mutilum 지체(肢體)를 잘린, 중요 부분을 잘린, 뿔을 잘린, 불구의

penetro, penetravi, penetratum, penetrare (< penitus *inward* + intrare (< intra- *inside*) *to go into*) 깊숙이 들어가다, 진입하다, 침투하다, 관통하다, 투과하다

> <u>**E** *penetrate*, (penetrans (*present participle*) >) *penetrant*, (penetrans (*present participle*) >) *penetrance*</u>

　　　> penetratio, penetrationis, f. 진입, 침투, 관통, 투과, 간파　<u>**E** *penetration*</u>
　　< penitus, penita, penitum 내부의
　　< penus, peni, m., f. 비축 식량, Vesta 신전의 안채
　< IE. pen- *to feed, food*

●●● 정형 제 2 변화

luceo, luxi, -, lucēre 빛나다, 드러나다, 명백하다　<u>**E** *lucent, translucent, radiolucent*</u>
　　　< lux, lucis, f. 빛
　　< IE. leuk- *light, brightness* (Vide LUX; *See* E. *lux*)

●●● 정형 제3변화

*luminesco, *luminui, *–, *luminescĕre (< + -escĕre *suffix of inceptive (inchoative) verb*)

　　　　냉광(冷光)을 내다　　　　　　　　　　　　　　　E *luminescence, luminescent, luminesce*

　　　< lumen, luminis, n. 빛, 촛불, (창, 틈, 구멍 >) 내강(內腔)

　< IE. leuk- *light, brightness* (Vide LUX: *See* E. *lux*)

●●● 정형 제4변화

ignio, ignivi, ignitum, ignire 불붙이다　　　　　　　　　　　　　E *ignite*

　　　　> ignitio, ignitionis, f. 점화, 발화　　　　　　　　　　E *ignition*

　　　< ignis, ignis, m. 불

　　　　> igneus, ignea, igneum 불의, 불 같은; (지질) 화성(火成)광물의　　E *igneous*

　< IE. egni- (ogni-) *fire*

servio, servivi (servii), servitum, servire 섬기다, 봉사하다

　　　　E *serve, server, servant, sergeant, dessert* (< *'last course'* < *'removal of what has been served'*)

　　　　> deservio, –, –, deservire (< de- *apart from, down, not; intensive* + servire
　　　　　　to serve) 충실히 섬기다, 열심히 돌보다; 보답받을 만한 일을 하다, 보답받을
　　　　　　만하다　　　　　　　　　　　　　　　　　　　　E *deserve, desert*

　　　　> subservio, –, –, subservire (< sub- *under, up from under* + servire *to serve*)
　　　　　　종노릇하다, 복종하다; 도와주다　　　　　　　　　E *subserve, subservient*

　　　< servus, servi, m. 종, 노예　　　E *serf, servomotor, (servomotor >) servo-*

　　　　> servilis, servile 노예의, 비천한　　　　　　　　　　　　E *servile*

　　　　> servitium, servitii, n. 노예의 신분, 예속, 노역, 섬김, 봉사　　E *service*

　　　　> servitudo, servitudinis, f. 노예의 신분, 예속　　　　　　　E *servitude*

　　　　> conservus, conservi, m. (< con- (< cum) *with, together* + servus *slave*) 동료
　　　　　　노예　　　　　　　　　　　　　　　　　　　E *(probably) concierge*

　< *(probably) Of Etruscan origin*

●●● 탈형 제1변화

lamentor, lamentatus sum, lamentari 슬퍼하다, 한탄하다, 비탄하다,

　　　　통곡하다　　　　　　　　　　　　　　　　　　　E *lament, lamentable*

　　　　> lamentatio, lamentationis, f. 애도, 비탄　　　　　　　　E *lamentation*

　　　< lamenta, lamentorum, n. (pl.) 슬픔, 한탄, 비탄, 통곡

< IE. la- (*echoic root*) *crying sound*

●●● 탈형 제4변화

partior, partitus sum, partiri 나누다   **E** (*verb*) *part*

    < pars, partis, f. 부분, 부(部)   **E** (*noun*) *part*

    < IE. perə- *to grant, to allot (reciprocally, to get in turn)* (Vide PAR: *See* E. *par*)

전치사

전치사는 명사나 대명사 앞에 위치하여 형용사구나 부사구를 이룬다. 전치사 뒤에 오는 명사나 대명사는 대격 또는 탈격이어야 하며, 이를 전치사의 격지배 라고 한다.

전치사 중에는 두 가지의 격을 지배하는 전치사가 있다. 뒤에 오는 명사나 대 명사의 격에 따라 뜻도 달라진다.

전치사는 관용구를 이룰 뿐 아니라 여러 합성어를 만들기도 한다. 이때 같은 전치사라도 뜻이 다른 합성어를 만드는 것은, 합성어의 의미가 확장되었기 때문 이기도 하지만, 전치사가 뒤에 오는 명사나 대명사의 격에 따라 다른 뜻을 갖기 때문이다.

대격지배 전치사

ad (대격지배) (장소·시간) ~에, ~으로, ~까지, ~에게로, 부근에; (관계) 관해서; (수반) 따라;

    (목적) 위하여

    [용례] ad litteram 문자를 따라, 문자 그대로   **E** *ad litteram*

        (문법) ad 따라: 전치사, 대격지배

            litteram 글자: 단수 대격 < littera, litterae, f.

    > ad-, ac- (*before* c, k, q), af- (*before* f), ag- (*before* g), al- (*before* l),

      an- (*before* n), ap- (*before* p), ar- (*before* r), as- (*before* s), at- (*before* t),

      a- (*before* sc, scr, sp, st) *to, toward, at, according to*

        E *ad- (ac-, af-, ag-, al-, an-, ap-, ar-, as-, at-, a-), add, accent, acquire, affair, aggressive, ally, announce, appear, arrive, associate, attract, ascend, ascribe, aspect, astringent*

> -ad *toward*

E *-ad, caudad, cephalad, coronad, rostrad, dorsad, ventrad, laterad, mesiad, basilad, dextrad, sinistrad*

< IE. ad- *to, near, at*

E *at, (at one > 'to make or to become united or reconciled' >)* **atone**, *(at one > 'to do' >)* **ado**

ante (대격지배) (장소) 앞에; (시간) 먼저; (관계) 우선하여

[용례] ante meridiem (a.m.) 오전에 (정오 전에)   **E** *ante meridiem (a.m.), antemeridian*
(문법) meridiem 정오, 남쪽: 단수 대격 < meridies, meridiei, m.

[용례] ante cibum (a.c.) 식전(食前)에   **E** *ante cibum (a.c.)*
(문법) cibum 음식, 먹이: 단수 대격 < cibus, cibi, m.

[용례] ante mortem 사전(死前)에   **E** *antemortem*
(문법) mortem 죽음: 단수 대격 < mors, mortis, f. 죽음, 주검

> ante-, anti- *before*

E *ante- (anti-), antebrachial (antibrachial), anticipate, (ab ante 'away before' >)* **advance**, *(ab ante 'away before' >)* **advantage**, *(advantage >)* **vantage, vanguard, avant-garde**

> (비교급) anterior, anterior, anterius ((gen.) anterioris) 앞의, 이전의   **E** *anterior*
> *anteanus, *anteana, *anteanum 옛날의, 고대의 (서로마제국 멸망 이전의)   **E** *ancient*
> antiquus, antiqua, antiquum (< + IE. okʷ- *to see*; Vide OCULUS: *See* E. *oculus*)

(품위 · 가치가) 뛰어난; 오래된   **E** *antique*

> antiquo, antiquavi, antiquatum, antiquare 낡은 것이 되게 하다   **E** *antiquate*

< IE. ant- *front, forehead*   **E** *along, until, end, un- (< 'to undo' < 'against' < 'in front of, before')*

> G. anti (전치사, 속격지배) ~에 대하여, ~ 대신에

> G. ant(i)-, anth- (*before* aspirate) *before, against, instead of*

E *ant(i)- (anth-), antibiotic, antimicrobial, antarctic, anthelix (antihelix), anthelminthic (anthelmintic); antacid, antibody, (antibody >)* **antigen**, **autoantigen** *(< 'self antigen')*, **autoantibody, isoantigen** *(< 'an antigen in one individual which is capable of eliciting immune reaction in other, genetically different, individuals of the same species, called also alloantigen')*, **isoantibody** *(< 'called also alloantibody')*, **alloantigen** *(isoantigen)*, **alloantibody** *(isoantibody)*

> G. enantios, enantia, enantion (< en- *in*) *opposite, facing, hostile*

E *(enantios + meros part > 'an opposite isomer' >)* **enantiomer, enantiomorphic**

> (*probably*) IE. ant-bhi- *from both sides*

> IE. ambhi, mbhi *around* (Vide AMBI-; *See* E. *amb(i)-*)

post (대격지배) 뒤에, 후에

[용례] post meridiem (p.m.) 오후에 (정오 후에)   **E** *post meridiem (p.m.), postmeridian*
(문법) meridiem 정오, 남쪽: 단수 대격 < meridies, meridiei, m.

[용례] post cibum (p.c.) 식후(食後)에   **E** *post cibum (p.c.)*

(문법) cibum 음식, 먹이: 단수 대격 < cibus, cibi, m.

[용례] post mortem 사후(死後)에　　　　　　　　　　　　　　**E** *postmortem*

(문법) mortem 죽음: 단수 대격 < mors, mortis, f. 죽음, 주검

> post- *after*　　　　　　　　　　　　　　　　　　　　　**E** *post-*

< (*probably*) IE. apo-, ap- *off, away* (Vide ᴀʙ: *See* E. *ab-*)

circa (대격지배) 주위에, 무렵에, 경에

> circa- *about*　　　　　　　　　　　　　　　　　　　　**E** *circa-*

< IE. (s)ker- *to turn, to bend* (Vide ᴄᴜʀᴠᴜs: *See* E. *curve*)

circum (대격지배) 둘러싸고, 두루

> circum- *around*　　　　　　　　　　　　　　　　　　**E** *circum-*

< IE. (s)ker- *to turn, to bend* (Vide ᴄᴜʀᴠᴜs: *See* E. *curve*)

cis, citra (대격지배) (장소) 이쪽에; (시간) 이내에

> cis- *on this side*　　　　　　　　**E** *cis-, cislunar, (cis-trans >) cistron, cis*

< IE. ko- *stem of demonstrative pronoun meaning 'this'*　**E** *he, his, him, her, it, here, hence, hither*

> IE. ke- (*deictic particle*) *this, here*

> L. ceterus, cetera, ceterum (< IE. ke- + IE. etero- *a second time, again*

(< IE. i- *pronominal stem*)) 그밖의, 나머지의

[용례] et cetera (etc.) (< *and others*) 등등(等等)　　**E** *et cetera (etc.)*

(문법) et 그리고: 접속사

cetera 나머지들: 형용사의 명사적 용법, 중성 복수 주격

> L. -ce (*deictic particle*) *this, here*

> L. *nunce (< IE. nu- *now* (*related to* IE. newo- *new*))

> L. nunc (부사) 지금

> L. hic, haec, hoc (< IE. gho- *base of demonstrative pronouns and deictic pronouns* + IE. ke-) 이 사람, 이 남자; 이 여자; 이것; 이

trans (대격지배) 저쪽으로, 건너, 너머, 저편

> trans-, tran- (*before* s), tra- (*before* consonant, *occasionally*) *over, across, through, beyond*

> **E** *trans- (tran-, tra-), translunar, (cis-trans >) cistron, trans, transfer, translate, transcribe, tradition, transverse, traverse; traffic*

< IE. terə- *to cross over, to pass through, to overcome*

> **E** *thrill (< 'to pierce'), nostril (< 'nose hole' < 'boring through the nose'), through, thorough*

> L. truncus, trunci, m. (< *deprived of branches and limbs, mutilated*) 그루터기, 몸집,
　　동체(胴體), 간(幹), 체간(體幹), 구간(軀幹)　　　　　　　　　**E** *trunk, (trunk >) truncal*
　　　> L. trunco, truncavi, truncatum, truncare 끊다, .
　　　　절단하다　　　　　　**E** *truncate, trench, entrench, trenchant (< 'cutting')*
> G. nektar, nektaros, n. (< *overcoming death* < IE. nek- *death* + IE. terə- *to overcome*)
　　the drink of the gods, wine or other sweet drink
　　　> L. nectar, nectaris, n. 신들의 음료, 감로주, 달콤한 음료　　　**E** *nectar, nectarine*
> (*Sanskrit*) avatara (< ava *down* + t'r-, tar- *to pass over*) *descent*　　**E** *avatar*

ultra (대격지배) 저쪽으로, 한도를 넘어, 저 너머

　　　> ultra- *on the other side of, beyond*　　　　　　　　　　**E** *ultra-*
　< IE. al- *beyond* (Vide ILLE: *See* E. *alarm*)

contra (대격지배) 맞은편에, 반대하여

　　　> contra- *against*　　　　　　　　　　　　　　　　　　　**E** *contra-*
　< IE. kom *beside, near, by, with* (Vide CUM: *See* E. *con-*)

extra (대격지배) 바깥에, 이외에

　　　　　> extra- *outside*　　　　　　　　　　　　　　　　　**E** *extra-*
　　　　　> extro- (*when opposed to* intro-) *outwards*　　　　**E** *extro-*
　　　< exter (exterus), extera, exterum 바깥의
　　< ex, e (전치사, 탈격지배) 에서, 부터
　< IE. eghs *out* (Vide EX: *See* E. *ex-*)

intra (대격지배) 안에서

　　　　> intra- *inside*　　　　　　　　　　　　　　　　　　**E** *intra-*
　　　< inter (전치사, 대격지배) 가운데에서, 사이에서
　< IE. en *in* (Vide IN: *See* E. *in-*)

inter (대격지배) 사이에, 동안에

　　[용례] inter alia 다른 것들 사이에 > 그 중에서도, 무엇보다도　　**E** *inter alia*
　　　　　inter alios 다른 사람들 사이에 > 그들 중에서도, 누구보다도　**E** *inter alios*
　　　　(문법) alia 다른 것들: 인칭 대명사, 중성 복수 대격
　　　　　　< alius, alia, aliud 다른 사람, 다른 남자; 다른 여자; 다른 것
　　　　　alios 다른 사람들: 인칭 대명사, 남성 복수 대격

　　　> inter- *between, among*　　　　　　　　　　　　　　　**E** *inter-*
　< IE. en *in* (Vide IN: *See* E. *in-*)

infra (대격지배) 아래에

> infra– *below, beneath*　　　　　　　　　　　　　　　　　　**E** *infra-, infrasellar*

< inferus, infera, inferum 아래쪽의, 하부(下部)의

> (비교급) inferior, inferior, inferius ((gen.) inferioris) 더 아래의, 뒤떨어지는,

열등한　　　　　　　　　　　　　　　　　　　　　　　**E** *inferior*

> *inferioritas, *inferioritatis, f. 열등　　　　　　　　**E** *inferiority*

(최상급) infimus, infima, infimum 맨 아래의

imus, ima, imum 맨 아래의　　　　　　　　　　　　　　　**E** *ima*

> infernus, inferna, infernum 아래에 있는, 하계(下界)의, 지옥의　**E** *inferno*

> infernalis, infernale 지옥의, 악마 같은　　　　　　**E** *infernal*

< IE. ndher– *under*　　　　　　　　　　　　　　　　　　　　**E** *under, under-*

supra (대격지배) 위에 (super와 같은 뜻이지만 위치를 강조함)

> supra– *above* (super-와 같은 뜻이지만 위치를 강조함)　　　**E** *supra-*

< superus, supera, superum 위쪽의, 상부(上部)의

< IE. uper *over* (Vide SUPER; *See* E. *super-*)

juxta (대격지배) 바로 곁에

> juxta– *near to*　　　　　　　　　　　　　　　　　　　　**E** *juxta-*

< IE. yeug– *to yoke* (Vide JUNGĔRE; *See* E. *join*)

ob (대격지배) 앞에, 때문에

> ob– (os–), oc– (*before* c), of– (*before* f), o– (*before* m), op– (*before* p) *before,*
toward(s), over, against, away

E *ob- (os-, oc-, of-, o-, op-), obese, ostensible, occipital, offer, omit, opportunistic*

< IE. epi, opi *near, at, against*

> G. epi (전치사, 속격·여격·대격지배) *upon*

> G. ep(i)–, eph– (*before* aspirate) *upon*

E *ep(i)- (eph-), epilogue (epilog), eponym (< '(the one) upon a name'), ephemeral*

> G. piezein (piezeein) (< *to sit upon* < IE. epi + IE. sed– *to sit*)
to press tight　　　　　　　　　　　　　　　　　　**E** *piez(o)-, isopiestic*

> G. opisthen (전치사, 속격지배; 부사) *behind*

> G. opisth(o)– *behind*　　　**E** *opisth(o)-, opisthotonos (opisthotonus), Opisthorchis*

> G. *ops *extra on the side, with*

> G. opson, opsou, n. *anything eaten with bread, condiment, cooked food*

> G. opsōnein *to buy food*　　　**E** *monopsony (< 'on the pattern of monopoly')*

> G. opsōnion, opsōniou, n. *food, provisions*

> L. opsonium, opsonii, n. (obsonium, obsonii, n.) 반찬,
요리

per (대격지배) 통하여, 동안

[용례] per capita 머리들을 통하여 > 머릿수로, 일인당 **E** *per capita*

(문법) capita 머리들을: 복수 대격 < caput, capitis, n.

> per-, pel- *through, thoroughly*

E *per- (pel-), perfect, permanent, paramount, pellucid; perfidy, perfunctory, perjure*

< IE. per *base of prepositions and preverbs with the basic meanings of 'forward', 'through', and wide range of extended senses such as 'in front of', 'before', 'early', 'first', 'chief', 'toward', 'near', 'at', 'around', 'against'*

E *fore, fore-, forehead, forearm, foreskin, before* (< *bi- 'at, by' < IE. ambhi 'around'), *for, forth, (forth > 'to further, to promote' >)* **afford, far, further, former, foremost, first, from, fro, frame** (< 'to prepare (timber) for use (in building)'), **furnish** (< 'to further'), **furniture, veneer** (< 'to furnish'), **perform** (< 'to furnish through'), (perform >) **performance, for-, forbid, forget, forlorn**

> L. prae (전치사, 탈격지배) 앞에, 앞으로; ~보다; 때문에

> L. prae- *before, beyond* **E** *pre-, predict, prevail*

> L. praeter (< + -ter *comparative suffix*) (전치사, 대격지배) 지나서, 외에

> L. praeter- *past,*

beyond **E** *preter-,* (praeter naturam 'beyond nature' >) *preternatural*

> L. pro (전치사, 탈격지배) 앞에, 앞으로; 위하여; 대신에 **E** *pro*

> L. pro-, prod- *before, forward; for; instead of*

E *pro- (prod-), provide,* (pro- + captare 'to chase' >) **purchase,** (prod- + aio 'I say' >) **prodigy,** (prod- + agère 'to drive, to do' > 'driving forth or away' >) **prodigal, pronucleus** (< 'the precursor of a nucleus'); **procure; pronoun, provirus**

> L. pronus, prona, pronum 앞으로 수그린, 엎드린, 엎친, 복와위(腹臥位)의, (~하기) 쉬운 **E** *prone*

> L. prono, pronavi, pronatum, pronare 앞으로 수그리다, 엎드리다, 바닥이 밑으로 가게 하다, 복와위를 취하다 **E** *pronate*

> L. pronatio, pronationis, f. 엎침, 회내(廻內) **E** *pronation*

> L. pronator, pronatoris, m. 엎침근, 회내근(廻內筋) **E** *pronator*

> L. reciprocus, reciproca, reciprocum (< re- *back, again* + pro-) 왔다 갔다 하는, 주고받는, 상호 간의 **E** *reciprocal, reciprocity, reciprocate*

> L. probus, proba, probum (< *growing straightforward, growing well* < pro- + *-bhw- < IE. bheuə-, bheu- to be, to exist, to grow* (Vide PHYSIS; See E. *physis*)) 올곧은, (질적으로) 좋은, 정직한

> L. probo, probavi, probatum, probare 시험하다, 입증하다, 증명하다

E (probandus (*masculine gerundive*) *'one who must be proved'* >) *proband*, *probate* (< *'something proved'*), *prove*, (*prove* >) *proof*, (*prove* >) *disprove*, (*proof* >) *disproof*

> L. proba, probae, f. 시험, 입증, 증명　　　　　　　　　　**E** *probe*

> L. probabilis, probabile 있음직한, 개연성(蓋然性)

있는　　　　　　　　　　**E** *probable, probabilism, probabilistic*

> L. probabilitas, probabilitatis, f. 있음직함, 개연성, 확률　**E** *probability*

> L. approbo, **approbavi**, approbatum, approbare (< ad- *to,
toward, at, according to* + probare *to try, to test*) 승인

하다　　　　　　　　**E** *approve, (approve* >) *approval*

> L. prosum (prodes, prodest), **profui**, –, prodesse (< prod- + esse *to be*)

이롭다　　　　　　　　**E** *proud, pride, improve*

> L. prope (전치사, 대격지배) (장소·시간) 가까이

(부사) 가까이　　　　**E** *reproach* (< *'to rebuke'* < *'to bring back close'*)

> L. (부 사, 비교급) propius 더 가까이

> L. propio, **propiavi**, propiatum, propiare 접근하다

> L. appropio, **appropiavi**, appropiatum, appropiare
(< ap- (< ad) *to, toward, at, according to*
+ propiare *to come nearer*)

접근하다　　　　**E** *approach, rapprochement*

(부 사, 최상급) proxime 가장 가까이

> L. (형용사, 비교급) propior, propior, propius ((gen.) propioris) 더 가까운

(형용사, 최상급) proximus, proxima, proximum 가장 가까운

> L. proximalis, proximale 기점(基點)에 가장 가까운,

몸쪽의, 근위(近位)의　　　　**E** *proximal*

> L. proximitas, proximitatis, f. 근접, 인접

E *proximity, proxemics* (< *'on the pattern of phonemics'*)

> L. proximo, **proximavi**, proximatum, proximare 인접하다,

접근하다　　　　　　**E** *proximate*

> L. approximo, **approximavi**, approximatum, approximare (< ap- (< ad) *to, toward, at, according to* + proximare *to come nearest*)

인접하다, 접근하다　**E** *approximate, approximant*

> (*Old Latin*) pri, pris 이전의

> L. pristinus, pristina, pristinum 지난날의, 소박한　　　**E** *pristine*

> L. (비교급) prior, prior, prius ((gen.) prioris) 먼저의　　**E** *prior*

> L. prioritas, prioritatis, f. 우선, 우선권　　　**E** *priority*

(최상급) primus, prima, primum 첫째의　　**E** *prime, prim, primer*

> L. primarius, primaria, primarium 제1의 **E** *primary, premier, premiere*

> L. primitivus, primitiva, primitivum 최초의, 원시의　　**E** *primitive*

> L. primalis, primale 최초의, 원시의, 가장 중요한, 근본적인　**E** *primal*

> L. primas, (gen.) primatis 으뜸가는　　　　**E** *primate*

> L. primatia, primatiae, f. 으뜸   E *primacy*

> L. privus, priva, privum (< *standing in front, isolated from others*) 각각의, 개인의

   > L. privo, privavi, privatum, privare (공인(公人)의 자격을 박탈해 사인(私人)이
     되게 하다 >) 빼앗다, 박탈하다

     > L. privatus, privata, privatum (*past participle*) (국가에 대한 의무와 권
       리를) 박탈당한, (공공으로부터) 격리된, 사사로운,
       개인적인   E *private, (private >) privacy, privy*

     > L. deprivo, deprivavi, deprivatum, deprivare (< de- *apart from, down,*
       not; intensive + privare *to take away*) 박탈하다, 제한하다, 상실시키다   E *deprive*

       > L. deprivatio, deprivationis, f. 박탈, 제한, 상실   E *deprivation*

   > L. proprius, propria, proprium (< pro privo *for the individual* < pro *for* +
     privus *individual*) 자기 자신에게 속한, 고유한

     E *proper, (proprius 'proper' + receptor > 'a sensory receptor which responds to*
     stimuli arising within the body' >) proprioceptor, (proprioceptor >) proprio-
     ception, (proprioceptor >) proprioceptive

     > L. proprietas, proprietatis, f. 개성, 고유성, 특색, 소유권, 재산권, 소유물,
       재산; (말의) 적절한 표현, 독특한 표현   E *propriety, property*

       > L. proprietarius, proprietaria, proprietarium 소유자의, 소유권의   E *proprietary*

     > L. approprio, appropriavi, appropriatum, appropriare (< ap- (< ad)
       to, toward, at, according to + proprius *own, proper*) 자기 것으로
       만들다   E *appropriate, inappropriate*

   > L. privilegium, privilegii, n. (< privus *separate, peculiar* + lex *law*) 예외 법규,
     특권   E *privilege*

> L. prandium, prandii, n. (< *first eating* < IE. per *first* + IE. ed- *to eat*) (간단한
   조반, 점심 전의 곁두리, 점심 >) 식사   E *prandial, postprandial*

> G. pro (전치사, 속격지배) *before, in front; (for); (instead of)*

   > G. pro- *before, in front*   E *pro-, prologue (prolog)*

   > G. pros (전치사, 속격·여격·대격지배) *towards, near, beside(s)*

     > G. pros- *towards, near, beside(s)*   E *pros-, prosthesis, prosthodontics*

   > G. proteros, protera, proteron (비교급) *former*

     E *proter(o)-, Proterozoic, hysteron proteron (< 'the latter (put as) the former')*

   > G. prōtos, prōtē, prōton *first*

     E *(neuter sing. 'the first thing' > 'the fundamental building block of atomic*
     nuclei' >) proton, prot(o)-, prototype, protophyton, protozoon, protoplasm,
     protamine(s)

     > L. protium, protii, n. (< *the first of the three naturally occurring hydrogen*
       isotopes (protium, deuterium, and tritium)) 프로튬   E *protium (^{1}H)*

   > G. prōteios, prōteia, prōteion *primary, prime*

     E *protein(s) (< 'a primary substance'), apoprotein(s) (< 'the protein moiety of*
     a conjugated protein or protein complex' < 'away' protein), (protein >)
     proteinous (proteinaceous), (proteinous infectious particle > (rearranged) >)
     prion, proteolyis, (protein + -ase 'enzyme' >) protease(s) (proteinase(s)),
     (protease + -some 'body' >) proteasome, (protein + -mer 'part' > 'the
     structural unit of a multimeric protein' >) protomer

> G. prōtistos, prōtistē, prōtiston (*superlative of* prōtos) *the very first, first of all*

> L. Protista, Protistorum, n. (pl.) 원생생물계(原生生物界) **E** *protist*

> G. proira, proiras, f. *prow*

> L. prora, prorae, f. 이물, 뱃머리 **E** *prow*

> G. peri (전치사, 속격·대격지배) *around, near, beyond, on account of*

> G. peri- *around, near, beyond, on account of* **E** *peri-*

> G. perix (전치사, 속격·대격지배; 부사) *round about*

> G. perissos, perissē, perisson *superfluous, redundant, odd, (of numbers) uneven* **E** *perissodactyl*

> G. para (전치사, 속격·여격·대격지배) *beside, along side of, beyond*

> G. par(a)- *beside, along side of, beyond*

E *par(a)-; paralanguage (< 'the non-phonemic component of speech'), Paralympics (< 'games held in parallel with the olympics' < 'games for paraplegics'), Paralympian*

> G. presbys (< *going before* < *pres- (< IE. per) + IE. gʷa- *to go, to come*) *old, elder*

> G. presbys, presbyeōs, m. *old man, elder, someone revered* **E** *presbyopia, presbyacusis (presbycusis, presbyacusia)*

> G. presbyteros, presbytera, presbyteron (비교급) *elder* **E** *presbyterian, priest*

> (*Avestan*) pairi-daeza (< *enclosure* < pairi *around* (< IE. per *around*) + daeza *wall, originally made of clay or mud bricks* (< IE. dheigh-)) **E** *paradise*

> IE. per- *to lead, to pass-over* (Vide PORTARE: *See* E. *portable*)

> IE. per- *to try, to risk* (< *to lead over, to press forward*) (Vide EXPERIRI: *See* E. *expert*)

> IE. per- *to strike* (Vide PREMĔRE: *See* E. *print*)

> IE. per- *to traffic in, to sell* (Vide PRETIUM: *See* E. *price*)

탈격지배 전치사

ab (*before* vowel, h), a (탈격지배) ~부터, ~로부터

[용례] ab initio (< *from the beginning*) 시작부터 **E** *ab initio*
(문법) initio 시작: 단수 탈격 < initium, initii, n.

[용례] a capite ad calcem (< *from head to heal*) 머리부터 발꿈치까지, 모조리
(문법) capite 머리: 단수 탈격 < caput, capitis, n.
ad 한테, 까지: 전치사, 대격지배
calcem: 단수 대격 < calx, calcis, f., m. 발꿈치

[용례] a priori (< *from what is before*) 선천적, 선험적 **E** *a priori*
a posteriori (< *from what is after*) 후천적, 귀납적 **E** *a posteriori*

(문법) priori: 형용사의 명사적 용법, 중성 단수 탈격

    < prior, prior, prius ((gen.) prioris) 먼저의

    posteriori: 형용사의 명사적 용법, 중성 단수 탈격

       < posterior, posterior, posterius ((gen.) posterioris) 더 뒤의

> ab-, abs- (*before* c, q, t), a- (*before* m, p, v), as-, au- *off,*
   away from   **E** *ab- (abs-, a-), abort, abscess, abstain, amentia, aperture, avulsion*

< IE. apo-, ap- *off, away*   **E** *off, of, ebb, aft (< 'behind'), after, awkward (< 'turned backward'), ablaut*

> G. apo (전치사, 속격지배) *away from, from*

   > G. ap(o)-, aph- (*before* aspirate) *away from,*
      from   **E** *ap(o)- (aph-), apology, aphaeresis (apheresis, pheresis)*

> L. (*probably*) post (전치사, 대격지배) 뒤에, 후에

   > L. post- *after*   **E** *post-*

   > L. posterus, postera, posterum 뒤의

      > L. (비교급) posterior, posterior, posterius ((gen.) posteroris) 더 뒤의 **E** *posterior*

      > L. (최상급) postremus, postrema, postremum 맨 뒤의

         postumus, postuma, postumum 맨 뒤의   **E** *posthumous*

      > L. posteritas, posteritatis, f. 미래, 후세, 후예   **E** *posterity*

      > L. posterula, posterulae, f. (< + -ula *diminutive suffix*) 뒷길, 뒷문

         > L. posterna, posternae, f. (< *perhaps on the pattern of*
           internus, externus) 뒷길, 뒷문   **E** *postern*

      > L. praeposterus, praepostera, praeposterum (< prae- *before, beyond*
        + posterus *coming after*) 앞뒤가 뒤바뀐, 도착된, 불합리한   **E** *preposterous*

> L. (*probably*) *posinĕre (< + sinĕre *to leave, to let; of obscure origin*)

   > L. pono, **posui**, positum, ponĕre 놓다, 건설하다, 제출하다, 가정하다 (Vide PONĔRE:
   See E. *posit*)

cum (탈격지배) ~와 함께   **E** *cum*

   > con-, col- (*before* l), com- (*before* m, b, p), cor- (*before* r), co- (*before* vowel, h, gn,
   other consonants) *with, together; intensive*

      E *con- (col-, com-, cor-, co-), conventional, collateral, commensal, combine, complement,
      correlate, coagulate, cohabit, cognate, cosine*

< IE. kom *beside, near, by, with*   **E** *enough*

   > L. contra (전치사, 대격지배) 맞은편에, 반대하여   **E** *contra (con)*

      > L. contra- *against*

        E *contra-, (contrarotulus 'copy of a roll to check accounts' >) control, ((Late
        Latin) contrata terra 'that which lies opposite or fronting the view' >) country,
        counter, counter-, counterion, encounter,* F. *contre,* F. *contrecoup*

      > L. contrarius, contraria, contrarium 맞은편의, 반대편의, 거스르는;
        (논리) 반대되는   **E** *contrary*

   > G. koinos, koinē, koinon *common, public*   **E** *Koine*

de (탈격지배) ~에서, ~로부터; ~한테서; ~에 대하여

[용례] de facto (< *from the fact*) 사실상　　　　　　　　　　　　　　**E** *de facto*
　　　(문법) de ~로부터: 전치사, 탈격지배
　　　　　facto 사실로: 단수 탈격 < factum, facti, n.

[용례] de novo (< *from that which is new*) 처음부터, 새로이　　　　　**E** *de novo*
　　　(문법) de ~로부터: 전치사, 탈격지배
　　　　　novo 새로움으로: 형용사의 명사적 용법, 중성 단수 탈격
　　　　　　　< novus, nova, novum

[용례] De Humani Corporis Fabrica (< *On Fabric of Human Body*) 인체의 구조물에 대하여
　　　　(Andreas Vesalius, 1514-1564)
　　　(문법) de ~에 대하여: 전치사, 탈격지배
　　　　　humani 인간의: 형용사, 중성형 단수 속격 < humanus, humana, humanum
　　　　　corporis 몸의: 단수 속격 < corpus, corporis, n. 몸
　　　　　fabrica 구조물: 단수 탈격
　　　　　　< fabrica, fabricae, f. < faber, fabri, m. 목수

[용례] Exercitatio Anatomica de Motu Cordis et Sanguinis in Animalibus (< *Anatomic
　　　　Exercitation on Motion of Heart and of Blood in Animals*) 동물에서 심장과
　　　　혈액의 운동에 대한 해부 실습 (William Harvey, 1578-1657)
　　　(문법) exercitatio 실습: 단수 주격
　　　　　　< exercitatio, exercitationis, f. 연습, 실습, 실천
　　　　　anatomica 해부의: 형용사, 여성형 단수 주격
　　　　　　　　< anatomicus, anatomica, anatomicum
　　　　　　　< G. anatomikos, anatomikē, anatomikon *anatomic*
　　　　　de ~에 대한: 전치사, 탈격지배
　　　　　motu 움직임, 운동: 단수 탈격
　　　　　　< motus, motus, m. < moveo, movi, motum, movēre 움직이다
　　　　　cordis 심장의: 단수 속격 < cor, cordis, n.
　　　　　et 와, 과: 접속사
　　　　　sanguinis 피의: 단수 속격 < sanguis, sanguinis, m.
　　　　　in ~에: 전치사, 탈격지배
　　　　　animalibus 동물들에서: 복수 탈격 < animal, animalis, n.

　　> de- (*influenced by* dis-) *apart from, down, not; intensive*

　　　　E *de-, defect; debug, defog, deplane, detrain,* F. *debride* (< *'to remove the bridle
　　　　　from'),* F. *debridement,* F. *des-*
　　　> (원급) *deter 못한
　　　　　> (비교급) deterior, deterior, deterius ((gen.) deterioris) 더 못한
　　　　　　　　> deterioro, **deterioravi,** deterioratum, deteriorare
　　　　　　　　　　악화시키다　　　　　　　　　　　　　　　　**E** *deteriorate*
　　　　　> (최상급) deterrimus, deterrima, deterrimum 가장 못한
　　< IE. de- *demonstrative stem, base of prepositions and adverbs*　　**E** *to, too*

ex, e (탈격지배) ~에서, ~부터

> ex- (*before* bowel, c, h, p, q, s, t), e- (*before* b, d, g, j, l, m, n, r, v), ef- (*before* f)
out of, away from; intensive `E ex- (e-, ef-), exacerbate, edit, effect`

> exter (exterus), extera, exterum 바깥의

> extra (전치사, 대격지배) 바깥에, 이외에; (부사) 바깥에, 밖으로

> extra- *outside* `E extra-`

> extro- (*when opposed to* intro-) *outwards* `E extro-, extrovert`

> extraneus, extranea, extraneum 바깥의, 외부의, 외래의,
상관없는 `E extraneous, strange, stranger`

> extraneo, exteraneavi, –, extraneare 외부 사람으로 다루다, 멀리
하다, 상속에서 제외하다 `E estrange`

> externus, externa, externum 바깥의, 외부의, 외래의 `E external`

> (비교급) exterior, exterior, exterius ((gen.) exterioris) 바깥의 `E exterior`

(최상급) extremus, extrema, extremum (extimus, extima, extimum) 가장 먼,
마지막의, 극단의 `E extreme`

> extremitas, extremitatis, f. 끝, 말단, 극단; 팔다리, 사지(四肢) `E extremity`

< IE. eghs *out*

> G. ex, ek (*before* consonant) (전치사, 속격지배) *out of, away from*

> G. ex-, ek- *out of, away from*

`E ex- (ec-) (ec- 'often before c, s of Greek origin'), exodontics, ectopy, eccentric, ecstasy, (ecstrophy >) exstrophy`

> G. exō (전치사, 속격지배; 부사) *outside, outwards*

> G. exō- *outside, outwards* `E exo-, exotic, exotoxin, exocytosis, exotropia`

> (비교급) exōteros, exōtera, exōteron *outer* `E exoteric`

> G. ektos (부사) *outside, without*

> G. ekt(o)- *outside* `E ect(o)-, ectoderm, ectoplasm`

prae (탈격지배) 앞에, 앞으로; ~보다; 때문에

> prae- *before, beyond*
< IE. per *basic meanings of 'forward', 'through'* (Vide PER: *See* E. per-)

pro (탈격지배) 앞에, 앞으로; 위하여, 따라; 대신에

> pro-, prod- *before, forward; for; instead of*
< IE. per *basic meanings of 'forward', 'through'* (Vide PER: *See* E. per-)

sine (탈격지배) 없이, 없는 `E (sine cura 'without care' >) sinecure`

> F. sans (전치사) *without* `E sans`
< IE. sanə-, sen- *apart, separated* `E asunder, sunder, sundry`

대격과 탈격지배 전치사

in (대격지배) ~로, 안으로; (탈격지배) ~에, 안에, 위에

[용례] Mens sana in corpore sano. (< *A sound mind in a sound body.*) 건강한 육체에
　　　건강한 정신이 깃든다 (Decimus Junius Juvenalis, c.60−c.140)
　　　(문법) mens 정신은: 단수 주격 < mens, mentis, f.
　　　　　　sana 건강한: 형용사, 여성형 단수 주격 < sanus, sana, sanum
　　　　　　in ~에: 전치사, 탈격지배
　　　　　　corpore 몸: 단수 탈격 < corpus, corporis, n.
　　　　　　sano 건강한: 형용사, 중성형 단수 탈격 < sanus, sana, sanum

[용례] in vitro 시험관내 < vitro 단수 탈격 < vitrum, vitri, n. 유리(琉璃), 초자(硝子)
　　　in vivo 생체내 < vivo 단수 탈격 < vivum, vivi, n. 생체, 생살, 원금(原金)
　　　in utero 자궁내 < utero 단수 탈격 < uterus, uteri, m. 자궁 < 배[腹]
　　　in situ 제자리, 정위치 < situ 단수 탈격 < situs, situs, m. 위치, 장소
　　　in vacuo 진공내 < vacuo 단수 탈격 < vacuum, vacui, n. 진공, 공허
　　　in silico 컴퓨터 시뮬레이션으로 < E. *silicon*

> in-, il- (*before* l), im- (*before* m, b, p), ir- (*before* r) *in, on, into, toward*

> **E** *in- (il-, im-, ir-), include, illuminate, imminent, imbibe, imprint, irradiate; enclose, encourage, embrace*

< IE. en *in*　　　　　　　　　　**E** *in, (in >* (comparative) *>) inner, inn, into,* (possibly) *and*
　> G. en (전치사, 여격지배)

　　> G. en-, el- (*before* l), em- (*before* m, b, p, ph) *in*

　　　　> **E** *en- (el-, em-), encephalon, parenthesis, ellipsoid, emmetropia, embalm, empiric, emphasis*

　> L. endo (*Archaic Latin*) *within*

　　> L. indu- *within*　　　　　　　　　　　　　　　　　　　**E** *indu-*

　　　　> L. industrius, industria, industrium (< *indu-struus < indu- *within* +
　　　　　struĕre *to build*) 부지런한　　　　**E** *industry, industrial, industrialize*

　　　> L. indigeo, indigui, −, indigēre (< indu- *within* + egēre *to be in need*)
　　　　(누구한테 무엇이) 없다, 필요로 하다, 아쉽다　　　　　**E** *indigent*

> G. endon (전치사, 속격지배; 부사) *within, at home, at heart*

　　> G. end(o)- *within*　　**E** *end(o)-, endotoxin, endocytosis, endoderm* (entoderm)*, endoplasm*

　G. entos (전치사, 속격지배; 부사) *within, inside*

　　> G. ent(o)- *within, inside*　　　　　　　　**E** *ent(o)-, entoderm* (endoderm)

　　　> G. enteron, enterou, n. *gut*

　　　　> L. enteron, enteri, n. 창자, 장(腸)

　　　　　　E *enter(o)-, enteral,* (G. par(a)- *'beside, along side of, beyond'* +
　　　　　　enteron >) *parenteral*

　　　　> L. archenteron, archenteri, n. (< G. archē *beginning*) 원시
　　　　　창자, 원장(原腸)　　　　　　　　　　　　　　　**E** *archenteron*

> L. exentero, **exenteravi**, exenteratum, exenterare (< ex-
　　out of, away from) 창자를 끄집어내다,
　　내용물을 끄집어내다　　　　　　　　　　　　**E** *exenterate*
　　> L. *exenteratio, *exenterationis, f. 내용제거술, 모두
　　　제거술　　　　　　　　　　　　　　　　**E** *exenteration*
> G. enterikos, enterikē, enterikon *of gut*
　　> L. entericus, enterica, entericum 창자의, 장(腸)의　　**E** *enteric*
　　　> L. myentericus, myenterica, myentericum
　　　　(< G. my(o)- < mys, myos, m. *mouse,*
　　　　muscle) 장근(腸筋)의　　　　　　　　**E** *myenteric*
> G. mesenterios, mesenterios, mesenterion (< mesos *middle* +
　　enteron + -ios *adjective suffix*) *of mesentery*
　　> G. mesenterion, mesenteriou, n. *mesentery*
　　　> L. mesenterium, mesenterii, n. 장간막(腸間膜), 창자
　　　간막　　　　　　　　　　　　**E** *mesentery, mesenteric*
> G. dysenteria, dysenterias, f. (< G. dys- *bad* + enteron *gut* + -ia
　　noun suffix) *dysentery*
　　> L. dysenteria, dysenteriae, f. 이질(痢疾)　**E** *dysentery, dysenteric*
> L. Enterococcus, Enterococci, m. (< + G. kokkos *grain, berry*)
　　(세균) 엔테로코쿠스속(屬), 장알균속(屬)　　　**E** *Enterococcus*
> L. Enterobacter, Enterobacteris, m. (< + -bacter, -bacteris, m.
　　< G. baktērion *bacterium*) (세균) 엔테로박터속(屬)　**E** Enterobacter
　　　　　　　　　　　　　　　　　　　　　　　E *episode*
G. eis (대격지배) *into, toward(s), for, for the purpose of*
G. eisō (esō) (부사) *within, inwards*
　> G. esō- *within, inwards*　　　　　　　**E** *eso-, esotropia*
　> G. (비교급) esōteros, esōtera, esōteron *inner*　　**E** *esoteric*
> L. intus (부사) 안에서, 안으로　　　　　　**E** *intussusception*
　> L. intestinus, intestina, intestinum 안의, 안에 있는
　　> L. intestinum, intestini, n. 내장, 장, 창자　　**E** *intestine*
　　　> L. intestinalis, intestinale, n. 내장의, 장의, 창자의　**E** *intestinal*
> L. deintus (< de- *apart from, down, not; intensive* + intus *within*) (부사) 안에,
　　속에; 안으로부터　　　**E** *denizen (< 'one within' < 'on the pattern of citizen')*
> L. inter (전치사, 대격지배) 가운데에서, 사이에서
　> L. inter- *between, among*　　　　　　　**E** *inter-*
　> L. intra (전치사) 안에서
　　> L. intra- *inside*

　　　E *intra-; intragenic, (intragenic + -on 'a termination of Greek neuter*
　　　nouns and adjectives' >) intron

　　> L. intro, intravi, intratum, intrare 들어가다, 들어오다

　　　E (intrare >) ***enter***, (intrata (*feminine past participle*) >) ***entry***, (entrans,
　　　entrantis (*present participle*) >) ***entrant, entrance***

> L. penetro, **penetravi**, penetratum, penetrare (< penitus
inward + intrare (< intra- *inside*) *to go into*) 깊숙이 들어
가다, 진입하다, 침투하다, 관통하다, 투과하다　　**E** *penetrate*

> L. intro (부사) 안으로

> L. intro- *inwards*　　**E** *intro-, introvert*

> L. internus, interna, internum 안의　　**E** *intern, internment*

> L. internalis, internale 안의, 내면적인　　**E** *internal, internalize*

> L. interaneus, interanea, interaneum 내부의, 내장의

> L. interanea, interaneorum, n. **(pl.)** 내장, 오장육부　　**E** *entrails*

> L. interim (부사) 그 사이에, 잠정적으로, 이따금　　**E** *interim*

> L. (비교급) interior, interior, interius (**(gen.)** interioris) 안의　　**E** *interior*

(최상급) intimus, intima, intimum 맨 안쪽의, 친밀한　　**E** *intima*

> L. intimo, **intimavi**, intimatum, intimare 깊숙이 들어가게
하다, 알리다　　**E** *intimate, (intimate >) intimacy*

> L. intimatio, intimationis, f. 알림　　**E** *intimation*

super (대격지배) 위로; (탈격지배) 위에

> super- *above*

E *super-, superficial, surface, sirloin,* (*superanus >) *sovereign,* (sovereign >)
sovereignty

< superus, supera, superum 위쪽의, 상부(上部)의

> (비교급) superior, superior, superius (**(gen.)** superioris) 더 위의, 더 먼저의, 더
나은　　**E** *superior*

> superioritas, superioritatis, f. 우월　　**E** *superiority*

(최상급) supremus, suprema, supremum 맨 위의　　**E** *supreme, (supreme >) supremacy*

summus, summa, summum 맨 위의　　**E** (summum > *'the topmost'* >) *summit*

> summa, summae, f. 가장 높은 곳, 정상, 가장 중요한 부분, 요점,
합계 (< (*probably*) *from the Roman practice of writing the
sum of a column of figures at the top rather than the
bottom*)　　**E** *summa,* (pl.) *summae,* (noun) *sum*

> summarius, summaria, summarium 요점의, 개요의
포괄적인　　**E** *summary, summarize*

> summo, −, −, summare 요약하다,
합계를 내다　　**E** (verb) *sum, summate*

> summatio, summationis, f. 요약, 합계, 가산　　**E** *summation*

> consummo, **consummavi**, consummatum, consummare (<
con- (< cum) *with, together* + summa *sum*) 완성하다,
정점에 이르게 하다　　**E** *consummate*

> consummatio, consummationis, f. 완성, 극치　　**E** *consummation*

> supra (전치사, 대격지배) 위에 (super와 같은 뜻이지만 위치를 강조함)

> supra- *above* (super-와 같은 뜻이지만 위치를

강조함)   **E** *supra‑, suprasellar,* It. *soprano, somersault*

> supernus, superna, supernum 위에 있는, 천상의   **E** *supernal*

> superbus, superba, superbum (< *being above* < + L. **-bhw‑ being*

     < IE. bheuə‑, bheu‑ *to be, to exist, to grow*) 뛰어난, 오만한   **E** *superb*

< IE. uper *over*   **E** *over, over‑*

    > G. hyper (전치사, 속격·대격지배) *on behalf of, over*

      > G. hyper‑ *over*   **E** *hyper‑*

sub (대격지배) 아래로; (탈격지배) 아래

    [용례] sub rosa 장미 아래에서 > 비밀히   **E** *sub rosa*

     (문법) sub 아래에서: 전치사, 탈격지배

       rosa 장미: 단수 탈격 < rosa, rosae, f.

    [용례] Nihil sub sole novum. 태양 아래 새로운 것은 없다

     (문법) nihil 무(無): (단수 주격) < nihil, n. (불변화)

       sub 아래에서: 전치사, 탈격지배

       sole 태양: 단수 탈격 < sol, solis, n.

       novum 새로운: 형용사, 중성형 단수 주격

   > sub‑, suc‑ (*before* c), suf‑ (*before* f), sug‑ (*before* g), sum‑ (*before* m),

   sup‑ (*before* p), sur‑ (*before* r), sus‑ (*often before* c, p, t) *under, up from under;*

     (동작을 뜻하는 동사와 합하여) 아래, 조금, 밑에서 위로

    E *sub‑ (suc‑, suf‑, sug‑, sum‑, sup‑, sur‑, sus‑), subsequent, succumb, sufficient,*
    suggest, summon, suppress, surrogate, susceptible, suspend, sustain

    > subter (< sub *under* + ‑ter *comparative suffix*) (전치사, 탈격지배) 아래

      > subter‑ *below*   **E** *subter‑*

      > sursum (< sub *up from under* + versum *turning*) 밑에서 위로   **E** *sursum‑*

< IE. upo *up from under, over, under*

    E *up, (up >) upper (comparative), up‑, above, open* (< '*put or set up*'), *often (oft), eaves*
    (< '*that which is above or in front*'), *eavesdrop*

   > L. supinus, supina, supinum 위로 향한, 누운, 앙와위(仰臥位)의   **E** *(adjective) supine*

     > L. supinum, supini, n. (< supinum verbum) 목적분사, 동사적 명사   **E** *(noun) supine*

     > L. supino, **supinavi**, supinatum, supinare 자빠트리다, 뒤집다, 땅을 갈다, 위로

       쳐들다, 앙와위를 취하다   **E** *supinate*

       > L. supinatio, supinationis, f. 뒤침, 회외(廻外)   **E** *supination*

       > L. supinator, supinatoris, m. 뒤침근, 회외근(廻外筋)   **E** *supinator*

       > L. resupino, **resupinavi**, resupinatum, resupinare (< re‑ *back, again;*

         intensive + supinare *to supinate*) 뒤집다   **E** *resupinate*

   > L. vassus, vassi, m. (< (*Celtic*) < + IE. sta‑ *to stand*) 하인

     > L. vassallus, vassalli, m. 하인, 가신   **E** *vassal, valet*

   > G. hypo (전치사, 속격·대격지배) *under*

     > G. hyp(o)‑ *under*   **E** *hyp(o)‑*

> G. hypsos, hypsous, n. *height, top*　　　　　　　　　　E *hyps(o)-, hypsarrhythmia*

　　> G. hypsi (*adverb*) *aloft*　　　　　　　　　　　　E *hypsi-*

> (*Sanskrit*) upa *near to, under*

　　> (*Sanskrit*) upanishad (< upa *near to, under* + ni-shad *to sit down, to lie*
　　　　down)　　　　　　　　　　　　　　　　　　E *Upanishad*

> (*Sanskrit*) upala *precious stone*　　　　　　　E (*probably*) *opal, opalescence*

부사, 접속사, 감탄사

부사

etiam (< et *and* + jam *already*) ~도 또한, (단순 의문에 대한 긍정적 대답) 그렇다

　< IE. eti *above, beyond* (Vide ET: *See* E. *eddy*)

non (< ne *not* + oinos *one* (< IE. oi-no- *one*)) 아니, (대답으로서) 아니다

　　　　> non- *not*

　　　　E *non-, nonsense, nonfiction, nongovernmental, nonproliferation, nonsmoker, nonstop, nonprotein*

　　< ne 아니

　　　　> ne- *not*　　　　　　　　　　　　　　　　　　　　E *ne-*
　　　　> neg- *not*　　　　　　　　　　　　　　　　　　　　E *neg-*
　　　　　> nego, negavi, negatum, negare (< + agĕre *to drive, to do;* ajo *I say*)
　　　　　　부정(否定)하다　　　　　　　　　　　　　　　E *negate*
　　　　　　> negatio, negationis, f. 부정　　　　　　E *negation*
　　　　　　> negativus, negativa, negativum 부정적, 소극적, 음(陰)의, 부(負)의;
　　　　　　　(반응) 음성(陰性)인　　E *negative,* (*negative* >) *negativity, negativism*
　　　　　　> denego, denegavi, denegatum, denegare (< de- *apart from, down,*
　　　　　　　not; intensive + negare *to deny*) 완강히 부정하다　E *deny,* (*deny* >) *denial*
　　　　　　> renego, renegavi, renegatum, renegare (< re- *back, again;*
　　　　　　　intensive + negare *to deny*) 부인하다, 약속을 어기다　E *renege, renegade*
　　　　> nullus, nulla, nullum (< ne *not* + ullus, ulla, ullum *any*) 아무 ~도 아니, 하나도
　　　　　없는, 무효의　　　　　　　　　　　　　　　　　　　E *null*
　　　　　> nullifico, nullificavi, nullificatum, nullificare (< nullum *none* + -ficare
　　　　　　(< facĕre) *to make*) 무효로 하다　　　　　　　　E *nullify*
　　　　　> annullo, annulavi, annulatum, annulare (< an- (< ad) *to, toward, at,*
　　　　　　according to + nullum *none*) 무효로 하다　　　　E *annul*
　　　　> neuter, neutra, neutrum (< ne *not* + uter, utra, utrum *either of two*) 둘 다

아닌, 중성의

> **E** *neuter (n.)*; *neutron* (< 'on the pattern of electron'), *neutrophil* (< 'a cell or element staining readily with neutral dyes')

> neutralis, neutrale 어느 편도 아닌,

중립의　　**E** *neutral*, *(neutral >) neutralize*, *(neutralize >) neutralization*

> neutralitas, neutralitatis, f. 중립, 중성　　**E** *neutrality*

> nihilum, nihili, n. (< ne *not* + hilum *a thing, trifle*) 무(無)

> nihil, n. (불변화) 아무것도 ~ 아니, 무(無)　　**E** *nihil, nihilism*

> nil, n. (불변화) 무(無)　　**E** *nil*

[용례] Ex nihilo, nihil fit. 무(無)로부터는 아무것도 만들어지지 않는다

(문법) ex ~로부터: 전치사, 탈격지배

nihilo 무: 단수 탈격 < nihilum, nihili, n.

nihil 무: (단수 주격) < nihil, n. (불변화)

fit 만들어진다: 변칙동사 fio, factus sum, fieri(만들어

지다)의 능동태 직설법 현재 단수 삼인칭

< facio, feci, factum, facĕre 만들다

> annihilo; **annihilavi**, annihilatum, annihilare (< an- (< ad) *to, toward, at, according to*) 무(無)로 돌아가게 하다, 절멸시키다　**E** *annihilate*

< IE. ne *not*

> **E** *no* (< 'not ever'), *never* (< 'not ever'), *nay* (< 'not ever'), *none* (< 'not one'), *neither* (< 'no whether'), *nor* (< 'neither'), *nothing* (< 'no thing'), *nought (naught)* (< 'no thing'), *(nought >) not; un-*

> L. in-, il- (*before* l), im- (*before* m, b, p), ir- (*before* r) *not*　　**E** *in- (il-, im-, ir-)*

> G. ne- *not*　　**E** *ne-*

G. a-, an- (*before* bowel) *not*　　**E** *a- (an-)*

> (*Sanskrit*) a-, an- *not*

> (*Sanskrit*) ahimsa (< a- + himsa (< IE. ghei- *to propel, to prick*) *injury*) *non-injury*

sic 이렇게　　**E** *sic* (< 'thus, so')

< IE. so- *this, that* (Vide HO: See E. *the*)

ut (부사) ~처럼, ~와 같이; (접속사) ~하기 위하여

> **E** (Ut queant laxis resonare fibris ··· 'So that (your servants) may sing at the top of (their) voices ···' > gamma ut 'the name of the lowest note in the medieval scale' > 'the whole range of notes used in medieval music' >) *gamut*

[용례] ut dictum (< *as directed*) 말한 바와 같이, (처방전) 지시에 따라서　　**E** *ut dictum*

(문법) ut ~처럼, ~와 같이: 부사

dictum 말해진 것: 과거분사, 중성형 단수 주격

< dico, dixi, dictum, dicĕre 말하다

등위접속사

et (< *furthermore*) ~와, ~과, 그리고
   < IE. eti *above, beyond*

sed 그러나

vel (이것이나 저것 마음대로 취하라: velle의 고형(古形) 명령법 >) 또는, 혹
     < volo, volui, —, velle 원하다
   < IE. wel- *to wish, will* (Vide VELLE; See E. *voluntary*)

ergo (< (*perhaps*) *e rogo *from the direction of* (< e- *out of, away from* + *rogus *extension, direction*) 그러므로
   < IE. reg- *to move in a straight line* (Vide REGÉRE; See E. *regent*)

종속접속사

quam (접속사) 만큼, ~보다, (부사) 얼마나
   < IE. kʷo-, kʷi- *stem of interrogative and relative pronouns* (Vide IE. kʷo-, kʷi-; See E. *who*)

si 만일 ~면, ~거든

quasi (< *as if as it were, just as* < quam *as, than, how* + si *if, whether*) ~기나 한 듯이, ~처럼

[용례] Quasi mures, semper edimus alienum cibum. 쥐들처럼 늘 남의 음식만
       우리는 먹고 있다 (Titus Maccius Plautus, 254?–184 B.C.E.)
    (문법) quasi ~처럼: 종속접속사
       mures 쥐들: 복수 주격 < mus, muris, m.
       semper 늘, 언제나: 부사
       edimus 우리는 먹는다, 우리는 먹고 있다: 능동태 직설법 현재 복수 일인칭
         < edo, edi, esum, edĕre
       alienum 남의, 낯선: 형용사, 남성형 단수 대격 < alienus, aliena, alienum
       cibum 음식을: 단수 대격 < cibus, cibi, m.

감탄사

ecce (주격 또는 대격과 함께 쓰는 감탄사) 보라; 자, 여기 있다

    [용례] Ecce homo! 보라, (이) 사람이로다!

           Ecce me! 나, 여기 있다!, 내 꼴을 좀 보라!

          (문법) ecce 보라: 감탄사

                homo 사람: 단수 주격 < homo, hominis, m.

                me 나를: 일인칭 인칭대명사, 단수 대격

제 **3** 부

어원론을
위한
그리스어

Etymological Greek

Ἡ Ετυμολογικη
Ἑλληνικη Γλωσσα

제 1 장 역사

발칸 반도 남쪽에 위치한 헬라스(Hellas) 지방의 헬렌족 언어를 그곳 사람들은 헬라어(Hellēnikē)라고 한다. 전설상의 조상인 헬렌의 이름에서 비롯하였다. 바깥 사람들이 헬라스의 라틴어 명칭인 그래치아(Graecia)를 따라 그리스어(*Greek*)라고 부르는 언어이다.

그리스어 문자는 기원전 14~13세기에 미케네 그리스어(*Mycenaean Greek*)에서 사용한 선형문자(線形文字) B(*Linear B*)와 그에 앞서 미노아 그리스어(*Minoan Greek*)에서 사용한 선형문자 A(*Linear A*)로 거슬러 올라간다. 그러나 선형문자는 음절문자로서 표음문자인 그리스어 알파벳과는 전혀 다르다.

그리스어 알파벳의 기원은 페니키아인들의 표음문자로서 알파와 베타라는 문자 이름 자체가 그리스어가 아닌 페니키아어이다. 페니키아 문자는 이집트 상형문자의 영향을 받았다.

페니키아 문자는 자음만으로 이루어져 있었으나 그리스인들은 자기들에게 필요치 않은 문자를 모음으로 전용하고 그래도 아쉬운 문자는 새로 만들어 최초로 자음과 모음을 갖춘 알파벳을 이루었고, 그 알파벳으로 기록을 남겼다. 그때의 그리스어가 고대(古代) 그리스어(*Archaic Greek*)이다. 호머(Homēros)의 언어이기도 하다.

고대 그리스어는 더욱 가다듬어지면서 고전 그리스어(*Classical Greek*)로 발전한다. 고전 그리스어에는 아티카 방언, 도리아 방언을 포함한 서북 방언, 아이올로스 방언, 이오니아 방언 등이 있었으나 그 중 아테네가 위치한 아티카 방언이 표준이 되었다. 아티카 방언은 플라톤(Platōn)의 언어이자 데모스테네스(Dēmosthenes)의 언어이다. 히포크라테스 학파의 언어는 주로 이오니아 방언이다.

마케도니아의 알렉산드로스 3세에 의해 건설된 헬레니즘 세계에서 공용으로 사용된 그리스어를 헬레니즘기 그리스어(*Hellenistic Greek*), 또는 '공통의'라는 뜻의 그리스어 낱말 κοινη를 가져와, 그냥 Koinē(공용어)라고 한다. 고전 그리스어의 아티카 방언이 모태가 되었다. 70인역 구약성경과 신약성경의 언어이자 초기 기독교의 언어이기도 하므로 성서 그리스어(*Biblical Greek*)라고도 한다.

고전 그리스어는 문어(文語)로서 중세의 비잔틴 그리스어(*Byzantine Greek*)를 거쳐 현대 문어(*Καθαρευουσα* 'Katharevousa', 순수어라는 뜻이다)로 이어져 왔다. 이에 비해 구어(口語)로서 그리스어는 중세의 구어(이 또한 Koinē라고 한다)를 거쳐 현대 구어(*Δημοτικη* 'Dimotiki', 민중어라는 뜻이다)로 이어져 왔다. 이로 인해 최근까지만 해도 그리스어에는 문어와 구어라는, 한 뿌리이지만 다른, 두 언어가 있었다. 1976년 그리스는 구어인 민중어를, 문어의 내용을 가미해, 단일 공용어로 선포하였다. 신그리스어(*Νεα Ελληνικα* 'Nea Ellinika', *New Greek*)이다. (신그리스어의 자역(字譯)은 고전 그리스어의 자역과 조금 다르다. 이 책에서 신그리스어의 자역은 이 문단과 아래 시대구분 표에서만 나오며 인용부호('')로 구분하였다.)

9c ~ 6c BCE	5c ~ 4c BCE	4c BCE ~ 4c CE	5c ~ 15c (Medieval G.)	15c ~ 1976 yr (Modern G.)	1976 yr ~ Present
Archaic Greek	Classical Greek	Hellenistic Greek (Koinē)	Byzantine Greek (Written)	'Katharevousa' (Written)	'Nea Ellinika' (Written, spoken)
			Koinē (Spoken)	'Dimotiki' (Spoken)	

학술어로서 그리스어는 고전 그리스어를 뜻한다. 그러나 학술어로서 그리스어가 고전 그리스어라고 해서 그 시대의 어휘만 사용한다는 말은 아니다. 현대에 만들어진 학술용어도 그 기원이 그리스어이면 고전 그리스어의 틀에 담아 사용한다. 학술 그리스어는 고전 그리스어의 틀을 빌린 학술어인 것이다. 〈어원론을 위한 그리스어〉는 당연히 학술 그리스어를 따랐다.

제 2 장 알파벳과 발음

그리스어 문자는 24가지이다. 모음 문자는 α, ε, η, ι, o, υ, ω의 7개이다. 나머지는 자음 문자인데 시그마의 소문자에는 두 가지가 있어 18개가 된다. (시그마 소문자가 낱말의 맨 끝에 올 때는 ς를 쓰고, 그렇지 않는 경우에는 o를 쓴다.) 낱말이나 문장을 적을 때에는 주로 소문자를 쓴다.

글자이름	글자이름 (자역)	대문자	소문자	로마자 소문자
$\alpha\lambda\varphi\alpha$	alpha	A	α	a
$\beta\eta\tau\alpha$	bēta	B	β	b
$\gamma\alpha\mu\mu\alpha$	gamma	Γ	γ	g, n
$\delta\eta\lambda\tau\alpha$	dēlta	Δ	δ	d
$\varepsilon\psi\iota\lambda o\nu$	epsilon	E	ε	e
$\zeta\eta\tau\alpha$	zēta	Z	ζ	z
$\eta\tau\alpha$	ēta	H	η	ē
$\theta\eta\tau\alpha$	thēta	Θ	θ	th
$\iota\omega\tau\alpha$	iōta	I	ι	i
$\kappa\alpha\pi\pi\alpha$	kappa	K	κ	k
$\lambda\alpha\mu\beta\delta\alpha$	lambda	Λ	λ	l
$\mu\upsilon$	my (mu)	M	μ	m
$\nu\upsilon$	ny (nu)	N	ν	n
$\xi\iota$	xi	Ξ	ξ	x
$o\mu\iota\kappa\rho o\nu$	omikron	O	o	o
$\pi\iota$	pi	Π	π	p
$\rho\omega$	rhō	P	ρ	r, rh
$\sigma\iota\gamma\mu\alpha$	sigma	Σ	σ, ς	s
$\tau\alpha\upsilon$	tau	T	τ	t
$\upsilon\psi\iota\lambda o\nu$	ypsilon	Υ	υ	y, u
$\varphi\iota$	phi	Φ	φ	ph
$\chi\iota$	chi (khi)	X	χ	ch, kh
$\psi\iota$	psi	Ψ	ψ	ps
$\omega\mu\varepsilon\gamma\alpha$	ōmega	Ω	ω	ō

그리스어 문자의 소리값은 원칙적으로 해당하는 로마자의 소리값과 같으며 다음을 주의하면 된다.

모음 중에서 ε과 o은 단음이고, η와 ω는 장음이다, 이중모음 αι, αυ, ει, ευ, οι 등의 경우 앞모음을 길게, 뒷모음을 짧게 발음한다. 그러나 ου의 발음은 [ㅜ-]이다. (헬레니즘기 그리스어에서는 이중모음 ευ의 발음이 [ㅠ-]로 바뀐다.)

자음 중에서 ξ(로마자 x)는 [ㅋㅅ], ψ(로마자 ps)는 [ㅍㅅ], χ(로마자 ch 또는 kh)는 톡 튀는 [ㅋ]의 소리값을 갖는다. θ(로마자 th)는 초기에는 톡 튀는 [ㅌ] 소리값을 가졌으나 후에는 국제음성문자 [θ]의 소리값을 가졌으며, φ(로마자 ph)는 초기에는 톡 튀는 [ㅍ] 소리값을 가졌으나 후에는 국제음성문자 [f]의 소리값을 가졌다. 이오타 하기법에 의한 ι의 발음과 [ㅎ] 음이 들어가는 발음은 자역 편에서 설명한다.

제3장 자역

원의 지름에 대한 둘레($\pi\varepsilon\rho\iota\varphi\varepsilon\rho\varepsilon\iota\alpha$)의 비, 즉 원주율을 $\pi\varepsilon\rho\iota\varphi\varepsilon\rho\varepsilon\iota\alpha$의 머리 글자 π 로 표시하듯, 그리스어 문자는 과학에서 기호로 자주 쓰인다. 그러나 과학 기호 외의 그리스어 문자를 읽고 쓴다는 것이 대중적이지 않기 때문에, 어원론을 포함한 대부분의 분야에서는 그리스어 낱말이나 문장을 로마자로 옮겨 놓는다. 자역(字譯, *transliteration*)이라고 한다. 둘레라는 낱말 $\pi\varepsilon\rho\iota\varphi\varepsilon\rho\varepsilon\iota\alpha$를 periphereia로 옮겨 적고, '너 자신을 알라'라는 문장 $\Gamma N\Omega\Theta I\ \Sigma E A\Upsilon T O N$을 GNŌTHI SEAUTON으로 옮겨 적는 것이다.

알파벳 표를 보면 자역이 어렵지는 않으나 그렇다고 간단하지만은 않음을 알 수 있다. 하나의 그리스어 문자가 두 가지 로마자로 옮겨지기도 하고, 두 가지 그리스어 문자가 하나의 로마자로 옮겨지기도 한다. 또, 발음 따라 달리 옮겨지기도 한다. 그러나 자역에는 나름대로 규칙이 있다.

학술용어를 이해하기 위해서는 그리스어 문자로 된 낱말이나 문장을 읽고 해석하기보다도 자역된 낱말을 보고서 어간이 무엇이며, 그 어간으로부터 파생어나 합성어가 어떻게 만들어졌는지를 찾아낼 줄 알면 된다. 〈*Oxford English Dictionary*〉와 그 외 한두 가지를 제외하면, 어원론에서는 자역된 낱말을 가지고서 어원을 밝힌다. 따라서 그리스어 문자와 자역의 규칙을 몰라도 좋다. 그래도 알아둔다면 〈*Oxford English Dictionary*〉를 읽을 수 있으며, 까탈스러운 철자를 이해할 수 있고, 어원론의 묘미를 즐길 수 있다.

모음의 자역

그리스어 낱말을 적을 때에는 모음 위에다 강세를 표시하는 것이 원칙이다. 강세에는 강한 강세(´), 중간 강세(ˆ), 약한 강세(`)의 세 가지가 있다. 그러나 자역할 때에는 특별한 경우를 제외하고는 강세 표시를 하지 않는다.

| $\beta\iota o\varsigma$ | > | bios | 생명 |
| $\beta\iota o\varsigma$ | > | bios | 활 |

ε(e)과 ο(o)은 단모음이고, η(ē)와 ω(ō)는 장모음으로서 서로 다르다. 자역할 때에도 장단의 차이를 표시하는 것이 원칙이다.

장모음 α, η, ω에 ι가 결합하면 장모음을 좀 더 길게 발음한다. 이 때에는 ι를 장모음 밑에다 조그맣게 붙여 쓴다. 이오타 하기법(ι 下記法, iota subscript)이라고 한다. 하기(下記)한 ι는 i로 자역하기도 하나 ι를 발음하라는 의미가 아니므로 생략하기도 한다. ι를 발음해야 하는 경우에는 ι 위에 분음부호(¨)를 붙인다.

$\nu\varepsilon\upsilon\rho o\nu$	>	neuron	신경, 힘줄, 근육
$\delta\eta\mu o\varsigma$	>	dēmos	민중
$\varphi o\nu$	>	ōion (ōon)	알
$\dot{\eta}\rho\omega\ddot{\iota}\kappa o\varsigma$	>	hērōïkos	영웅의

υ은 y로 옮긴다. 그러나 이중모음 속의 υ은 u로 옮긴다(αυ = au, ευ = eu, ου = ou 또는 u). 이중모음이 아닌 υ을 u로 옮겨놓은 어원론도 있다.

| $\alpha\nu\alpha\lambda\upsilon\sigma\iota\varsigma$ | > | analysis | 분석 |
| $\alpha\upsilon\tau o\varsigma$ | > | autos | 자기(自己) |

낱말의 처음에 모음이 올 때에는 모음 위에 숨표(breathing mark)를 붙인다. 이중모음이 올 때에는 두 번째 모음 위에 숨표를 붙인다. 숨표에는 약한 숨표(smooth breathing)와 강한 숨표(rough breathing)가 있다. 약한 숨표는 발음에 영향을 주지 않으며, 보통의 숨표 기호(')로 표시한다. 강한 숨표는 [ㅎ]음을 내게 하는 기호(')로서 약한 숨표 기호의 좌우가 바뀐 것이다. 약한 숨표가 붙은 모음을 자역할 때에는 숨표를 무시하고 자역한다. 강한 숨표가 붙은 모음을 자역할 때에는 h를 덧붙인다. 이 경우, 발음 따라 자역하는 것이므로, 음역(音譯)이라고 할 수 있으나 넓은 의미로는 음역도 자역에 포함시킨다. 자역한 낱말에는, 약한 숨표든 강한 숨표든, 숨표 기호를 붙이지 않는다.

ἄνθος	>	anthos	꽃
αὐτος	>	autos	자기(自己)
ἵππος	>	hippos	말[馬]

모음 υ으로 시작하는 낱말은 첫 부분이 강하게 발음되므로 강한 숨표가 붙으며 hy 또는 hu로 자역한다.

ὕδωρ	>	hydōr	물
ὕπερ	>	hyper	위에

자음의 자역

자음의 자역에서 주의할 점은 다음과 같다.

연구개음 γ는 같은 연구개음인 γ, κ, ξ, χ 앞에서는 비음인 n으로 발음된다. 비음 감마(*nasal gamma*)라고 한다. 이런 경우 γ는 g가 아니라 n으로 음역하는 것이 일반적이다. 음역하지 않은, 일차 자역만을 옮겨놓은 어원론도 있다.

αγγειον	>	aggeion	>	angeion	혈관
αγκων	>	agkōn	>	ankōn	팔꿈치
φαρυγξ	>	pharygx	>	pharynx	인두
βρογχος	>	brogchos	>	bronchos	송풍관

자음 ρ로 시작하는 낱말은, ρ에 강한 숨표가 붙으므로, rh로 자역한다.

ῥοδον	>	rhodon	장미
ῥευμα	>	rheuma	흐름
ῥαχις	>	rhachis	척추

χ는 ch로 옮긴다. 사전에 따라서는 kh로 옮기기도 한다.

$\psi\upsilon\chi\eta$	>	psychē	숨, 정신, 혼, 생명
$\chi\alpha\rho\iota\sigma\mu\alpha$	>	charisma	특별한 은혜, 특별한 능력
$X\rho\iota\sigma\tau\sigma\varsigma$	>	Christos	그리스도

지금부터는 그리스어 낱말을 로마자로 자역해 기술한다. 필요한 몇몇 경우에는 그리스어 문자를 썼으나 그런 경우에도 괄호 안에 자역한 로마자를 덧붙였다.

제 4 장 품사

그리스어 품사에는 명사, 대명사, 정관사, 형용사, 1부터 4까지 수사, 동사 등 변화 품사와 부사, 전치사, 접속사, 1부터 4까지를 제외한 수사, 감탄사 등 불변화 품사가 있다.

명사

그리스어 명사도 성(남성·여성·중성), 수(단수·복수), 격(주격·속격·여격·대격·호격)에 따라 어미변화를 한다. 라틴어에서와 달리 그리스어 명사변화에는 탈격이 없으며 속격과 여격이 탈격의 역할을 분담한다. 그리스어 명사변화에는 크게 세 가지가 있다.

명사변화

●●● 제1변화

단수 주격 어미가 -a 또는 -ē으로 끝나는 여성 명사와 단수 주격 어미가 -ēs 또는 -as로 끝나는 남성 명사. 단수 주격의 어간과 단수 속격의 어간이 같다. 변화할 때 α가 많이 들어가므로 알파변화라고도 한다. (라틴어 명사의 제1변화(cellul-a, cellul-ae, f. 세포)에 해당한다.)

●●● 제1변화 제1식

단수 주격 어미가 -a, 어간의 끝이 -e, -i, -r인 여성 명사의 변화. 단수 속격 어미는 -as 이다.

hōra, hōras, f. *year, season, period, time, hour*

	단 수	복 수	
주격	hōr-a	hōr-ai	~이, ~가, ~은, ~는, ~께서
속격	hōr-as	hōr-ōn	~의
여격	hōr-ai	hōr-ais	~게, ~에게, ~께, ~한테
대격	hōr-an	hōr-as	~을, ~를
호격	hōr-a	hōr-ai	~여, ~이여

hōra, hōras, f. *year, season, period, time, hour;* ((pl.) Horai) (*Greek mythology*) *goddesses of orderly life*
> L. hora, horae, f. 시간; ((pl.) Horae) (그리스 신화) 계절과 질서의 여신들   **E** *hour,* (pl.) *Horae*
>> L. horarius, horaria, horarium 시간의, 시간을 나타내는   **E** *horary*
> hōroskopos, hōroskopou, m. (< hōra *time, hour* + skopos *watcher) observer of the hour of nativity, caster of nativities, nativity*
>> L. horoscopus, horoscopi, m. 점성가, 출생 시간을 가리키는 별의 위치, 12궁도   **E** *horoscope*
< IE. yer- *year, season*   **E** *year*

agyia, agyias, f. *road, path, street*   **E** *agyiophobia*

aitia, aitias, f. *cause, responsibility*
> aitiologia, aitiologias, f. (< + -logia *study) giving a cause*
>> L. aetiologia, aetiologiae, f. 원인(原因), 원인론, 병인(病因), 병인론   **E** *aetiology (etiology)*
< IE. ai- *to give, to allot*
> G. aisa, aisēs, f. *lot, fate, share, dispensation*
>> G. diaita, diaitēs, f. (< *daily allowance* < di(a)- *through, thoroughly, apart* + aisa) *way of life; regimen, food*
>>> L. diaeta, diaetae, f. 일정; 규정식, 섭생, 식이요법   **E** *diet*
>>>> L. diaetarius, diaetaria, diaetarium 규정식의, 섭생의   **E** *dietary*
>>> G. diaitētikos, diaitētikē, diaitētikon *of diet*
>>>> L. diaeteticus, diaetetica, diaeteticum 규정식의, 식이요법의   **E** *dietetic, dietetics*

elegeia, elegeias, f. (< + -ia *noun suffix*) *elegy*

> L. elegia, elegiae, f. 애가(哀歌), 비가(悲歌), 만가(輓歌)　　　　　**E** *elegy*

> elegeiakos, elegeiakē, elegeiakon (< + -akos *adjective suffix*) *of or for an elegy*

> L. elegiacus, elegiaca, elegiacum 애가의, 비가의, 만가의, 애조를 띤　**E** *elegiac*

< elegos, elegou, m. *mournful poem, lament*

< (*perhaps*) *Of Asiatic origin*

eschara, escharas, f. *hearth, fireplace; scab caused by burning*

> L. eschara, escharae, f. 괴사딱지, 가피(痂皮)　　　　**E** *eschar, (eschar >) scar*

> escharōtikos, escharōtikē, escharōtikon *forming an eschar, caustic*

> L. escharoticus, escharotica, escharoticum 괴사딱지의, 부식성의　**E** *escharotic*

hēmera, hēmeras, f. *day*　　　　**E** *(*dekaēmeron (*dechēmeron) >) Decameron*

> ephēmeros, ephēmeros, ephēmeron (< eph- (< epi) *upon* + -ēmera (< hēmera)

lasting one day, for one day, short-lived, during the day　**E** *ephemeral*

> L. ephemera, ephemerae, f. 하루살이, 덧없는 것　**E** *ephemera*

< IE. amer- *day*

lalia, lalias, f. *talking, chat, speech*　　　　**E** *-lalia*

> L. coprolalia, coprolaliae, f. (< G. kopros *dung*) 욕설증　**E** *coprolalia*

> L. echolalia, echolaliae, f. (< G. ēchō *echo*) 메아리증, 반향언어증　**E** *echolalia*

> L. palilalia, palilaliae, f. (< G. palin *back, backwards, again*) 말되풀이증,

동어반복증　**E** *palilalia*

> L. rhinolalia, rhinolaliae, f. (< G. rhis, rhinos, f. *nose*) 콧소리증, 비성증　**E** *rhinolalia*

< lalein (laleein) *to talk, to prattle*

< IE. al- *echoic root*

Magnēsia, Magnēsias, f. *Magnesia, the southeastern area of Thessaly in Central Greece, homeland of Jason and Peleus and his son Achilles; An ancient city of Asia Minor*

> Magnētēs, Magnētēs, Magnētes *Magnesian*

[용례] ὁ μαγνητης λιθος (ho Magnētēs lithos) *the Magnesian stone (magnetic)*
(문법) ho *the*: 정관사, 남성형 단수 주격
Magnētēs *Magnesian*: 형용사, 남·여성형 단수 주격
lithos *stone*: 단수 주격 < lithos, lithou, m.

> L. magnes, magnetis, m. 마그네시아의 돌;

자석(磁石)　　　　**E** *magnet, electromagnet, magnetism*

> L. magneticus, magnetica, magneticum

자석의　　**E** *magnetic, electromagnetic, diamagnetic, paramagnetic*

> magnēsia, magnēsias, f. *Magnesian white/black ores (not magnetic)*

> L. magnesia, magnesiae, f. 마그네시아 광석

[용례] magnesia alba *white magnesia*
(문법) magnesia 마그네시아 광석: 단수 주격
alba 흰: 형용사, 여성형 단수 주격 < albus, alba, album

> L. magnesium, magnesii, n. 마그네슘　　　　　E *magnesium (Mg)*

[용례] magnesia nigra *black magnesia*
(문법) magnesia 마그네시아 광석: 단수 주격
nigra 검은: 형용사, 여성형 단수 주격 < niger, nigra, nigrum

> It. manganese 망간　　　　　E *manganese (Mn)*

Odysseia, Odysseias, f. *Odyssey*　　　E *Odyssey*

< Odysseus, Odysseōs, m. *Odysseus, a king of Ithaca*　　E *Odysseus*
> L. Ulixes, Ulixis, m. (Ulysses, Uliyssis, m.) 율리시즈 (이타카섬의 왕)　　E *Ulysses*

therapeia, therapeias, f. *service, attendance, care, medical treatment*

> L. therapia, therapiae, f. 치료(治療), 요법(療法)

E *therapy, (therapy > 'one who practises in therapy, now especially psychotherapy' >) therapist, -therapy, actinotherapy, aromatherapy, bibliotherapy, bromatotherapy (bromatherapy), chemotherapy, chrysotherapy (aurotherapy), cryotherapy, hydrotherapy, hypnotherapy, kinesitherapy, logotherapy, metallotherapy, musicotherapy, pharmacotherapy, phototherapy, physiotherapy, psychotherapy, pyretotherapy (pyretherapy), thermotherapy, trophotherapy; aurotherapy (chrysotherapy), immunotherapy, radiotherapy; sclerotherapy, brachytherapy*

< therapeuein *to serve, to attend, to take care, to heal*
> therapeutēs, therapeutou, m. *servant, attendant, care-taker, healer*
> therapeutikos, therapeutikē, therapeutikon *therapeutic*
> L. therapeuticus, therapeutica, therapeuticum 치료의, 치료법의

E *therapeutic, therapeutics, therapeutist* (< 'one skilled in therapeutics, a physician')

tiara, tiaras, f. *tiara, turban*

> L. tiara, tiarae, f. Persia와 Media인들의 터번, 관모(冠帽), 교황의 삼층관, 보관(寶冠)　　E *tiara*

●●● **제 1 변화 제 2 식**

단수 주격 어미가 -a, 어간의 끝이 -e, -i, -r가 아닌 여성 명사의 변화. 단수 속격 어미는 -ēs이다.

doxa, doxēs, f. *opinion, glory*

	단 수	복 수	
주격	dox-a	dox-ai	~이, ~가, ~은, ~는, ~께서
속격	dox-ēs	dox-ōn	~의
여격	dox-ēi	dox-ais	~게, ~에게, ~께, ~한테
대격	dox-an	dox-as	~을, ~를
호격	dox-a	dox-ai	~여, ~이여

doxa, doxēs, f. *opinion, glory*　　　　　　　　　　　E *orthodox, heterodox, paradox*
> < dokein *to appear, to seem, to think, to believe* (< *to cause to accept or be accepted*)
> < IE. dek- *to take, to accept* (Vide DOCĒRE: *See* E. *docent*)

Athēna, Athēnēs, f. (*Attic*) (Athēnē, Athēnēs, f. (*Ionic*)) (*Greek mythology*) *goddess of*
　wisdom (로마 신화의 Minerva 여신에 해당함)
> > L. Athena, Athenae, f. (Athene, Athenes, f.) (그리스 신화) 아테나 여신　E *Athena (Athene)*
> > Athēnai, Athēnōn, f. (pl.) *Athens*
> > > L. Athenae, Athenarum, f. (pl.) 아테나이(아테네) (현 그리스의 수도
> > > Aθηνα)　　　　　　　　　　　E *Athens, Athenian*

chalaza, chalazēs, f. *hailstone, hard lump, small knot*
> > L. chalaza, chalazae, f. (동물) 알끈, (식물) 합점(合點)　E *chalaza,* (pl.) *chalazae*
> > chalazion, chalaziou, n. (< + -ion *diminutive suffix*) *chronic sty*
> > > L. chalazion, chalazii, n. 콩다래끼, 산립종(霰粒腫)　E *chalazion*
> < IE. ghelə d- *hail*

dipsa, dipsēs, f. *thirst*
> > L. dipsomania, dipsomaniae, f. (< G. dipsa + mania *madness*)
> > 음주광　　　　　　　　E *dipsomania, dipsomaniac* (< *'on the pattern of maniac'*)
> > L. polydipsia, polydipsiae, f. (< G. polys *much* + -dipsa + -ia) 다갈증(多渴症)　E *polydipsia*

kolla, kollēs, f. *glue*

E F. *collage* (< *'gluing'*), *collagen* (< *'yielding gelatin on boiling'*), (kolla *'glue'* + -oid *'-like'*
　>) *colloid, colloidal*
> > kollōdēs, kollōdēs, kollōdes (< + eidos *shape*) *glue-like*　　　　　E *collodion*
> > prōtokollon, prōtokollou, n. (< prōtos *first*) *the first leaf of a volume, a fly-leaf*
> > *glued to the case and containing an account of the manuscript*
> > > L. protocollum, protocolli, n. (칙서 등의) 첫머리 정식문(定式文), 외교문서, (외교

상의) 의정서(議定書), 공문서의 서식, (공식적 의례의) 의례준칙　　　**E** *protocol*

thalassa, thalassēs, f. *sea, sea-water, inner sea, the Mediterranean*　　　**E** *thalass(o)-*

> L. thalassaemia, thalassaemiae, f. (< *limited almost wholly to Italians, Greeks and Syrians, i.e., to the people originating about the Mediterranean Sea* < G. thalassa *inner sea, the Mediterranean* + haima *blood* + -ia) 지중해빈혈증, 탈라세미아　　　**E** *thalassaemia (thalassemia)*

●●● 제 1 변화 제 3 식

단수 주격 어미가 -ē인 여성 명사의 변화. 단수 속격 어미는 -ēs 이다.

graphē, graphēs, f. *drawing, writing*

	단 수	복 수	
주격	graph-ē	graph-ai	~이, ~가, ~은, ~는, ~께서
속격	graph-ēs	graph-ōn	~의
여격	graph-ēi	graph-ais	~게, ~에게, ~께, ~한테
대격	graph-ēn	graph-as	~을, ~를
호격	graph-ē	graph-ai	~여, ~이여

graphē, graphēs, f. *drawing, writing*

　　< graphein *to scratch, to draw, to write*

　< IE. gerbh- *to scratch* (Vide GRAPHEIN; *See* E. *graph*)

Aphroditē, Aphroditēs, f. (< (*suggested*) aphros, aphrou, m. *foam*) (*Greek mythology*) *Aphrodite*

> L. Aphrodita, Aphroditae, f. (그리스 신화) 아프로디테 여신　　　**E** *Aphrodite*

> aphrodisios, aphrodisia, aphrodision *belonging to Aphrodite, indulging in love*

　　> aphrodisiakos, aphrodisiakē, aphrodisiakon *aphrodisiac*　　　**E** *aphrodisiac*

> (*suggested, via Etruscan*) L. Aprilis, Aprile 아프로디테 여신의, 4월의　　　**E** (Aprilis mensis *'month of Aphrodite'* >) *April*

athērē, athērēs, f. *groats, gruel*

> athērōma, athērōmatos, n. (< + -ōma *noun suffix denoting tumor*) *atheroma*

> L. atheroma, atheromatis, n. 죽종(粥腫), 아테로마

> E *atheroma* (< *'tumor containing matter resembling gruel'*), **atheromatous**, *(atheroma* >*) atherogenesis, atherogenic*

> L. atherosclerosis, atherosclerosis, f. (< + G. sklērōsis *hardness*) 죽상(粥狀)경화증, 죽(粥)경화증

> E *atherosclerosis, atherosclerotic*

Krētē, Krētēs, f. *Crete*

> L. Creta, Cretae, f. (Crete, Cretes, f.) 크레타 섬

> E *Crete, Cretan*

> synkrētismos, synkrētismou, m. (< syn- *with, together* + Krētes *Cretans*) *federation of Cretan cities*

> L. syncretismus, syncretismi, m. (여러 학설, 분파 등의) 통합; 어형 융합

> E *syncretism* (< *"Cretan federation' was presented by Plutarch; etymologically, however, G.* synkrasis *'mixing together' is preferred.'*)

eunē, eunēs, f. *bed, marriage bed, bedroom*

> eunouchos, eunouchou, m. (< eunē + och- (< echein) *to hold*) *eunuch, chamberlain*

> L. eunuchus, eunuchi, m. 고자(鼓子), 내시, 환관

> E *eunuch, eunuchoid*

> pareunazesthai (< par(a)- *beside, along side of, beyond* + eunē) *to lie beside, to lie with*

> pareunos, pareunos, pareunon *lying beside, lying with a bedfellow*

> L. pareunia, pareuniae, f. 성교

> L. dyspareunia, dyspareuniae, f. (< G. dys- *bad*) 성교통증

> E *dyspareunia*

gē, gēs, f. ((*poetic form*) gaia, gaias, f.) *earth, land, soil, ground, field, home;* (Gē, Gaia) (*Greek mythology*) *the goddess of the earth (daughter of Chaos, mother and wife of Uranus, mother of the Titans and the Cyclops)*

> E *Ge (Gaia, Gaea), Pangaea (Pangea), geo-*

> geoidēs, geoidēs, geoides (< gē *earth* + eidos *shape*) *earthy, earth-like*

> E *geoid*

> geōdēs, geōdēs, geōdes (< gē *earth* + eidos *shape*) *earthy, earth-like*

> L. geodes, geodis, m. 정동(晶洞)

> E *geode*

> epigeios, epigeios, epigeion (< ep(i)- *upon* + gē *earth*) *on the earth, earthly*

> E *epigeal*

> hypogeios, hypogeios, hypogeion (< hyp(o)- *under* + gē *earth*) *underground*

> L. hypogeus, hypogea, hypogeum 지하의, 지하성의

> E *hypogeal*

> geōmetria, geōmetrias, f. (< gē *earth* + metron *measure*) *geometry*

> L. geometria, geometriae, f. 기하학(幾何學)

> E *geometry*

> geōgraphia, geōgraphias, f. (< gē *earth* + -graphia *drawing, writing*) *geography*

> L. geographia, geographiae, f. 지리, 지리학, 지지(地誌)

> E *geography*

> L. geologia, geologiae, f. (< G. gē *earth* + -logia *study*) 지질학

> E *geology*

glēnē, glēnēs, f. *eyeball, pupil of the eye; used by Galen to denote a shallow joint-socket*

> E *glenoid*

> L. Euglena, Euglenae, f. (< *a reddish stigma erroneously known as eyespot* < G. eu- *well* + glēnē *pupil of the eye*) 유글레나속(屬), 연두벌레속,

미안충(美顔蟲)속

    < IE. gel- *bright*

> **E** Euglena, *euglenoid*
> **E** *clean, cleanse*

hēbē, hēbēs, f. *youth, prime of youth, vigor, young men, manhood; (Hēbē) (Greek mythology) the goddess of youth and spring, the daughter of Zeus and Hera, the cup-bearer of Olympus*

    > L. Hebe, Hebes, f. (그리스 신화) 청춘의 여신

> **E** *Hebe*

    > hēbētikos, hēbētikē, hēbētikon *youthful, of puberty, happening at puberty*

> **E** *hebetic*

    > L. hebephrenia, hebephreniae, f. (< *a form of insanity incident to the age of puberty* < + G. phrēn, phrenos, f. *mind*) 파과증(破瓜症), 사춘기치매

> **E** *hebephrenia, hebephrenic, hebephreniac*

    < IE. yeg^w-a- *power, youthful strength*

hylē, hylēs, f. *wood, forest; stuff, matter*

> **E** *hylozoism, -yl, (organic acid(s) + -yl >) acyl, (alcohol(s) + -yl > 'hydrocarbon radical(s)' >) alkyl, (aromatic hydrocarbon radical(s) + -yl >) aryl, (ether + -yl >) ethyl, (ethyl + -ēnos 'adjective suffix' >) ethylene, (methy 'wine' + -yl + -ēnos 'adjective suffix' > F. esprit-de-bois 'wood spirit' >) methylene, (methylene >) methyl; (alkyl + L. -anus 'adjective suffix' > 'saturated hydrocarbon(s)' >) alkane, (alkyl + G. -ēnos 'adjective suffix' > 'unsaturated hydrocarbon(s) containing one or more carbon-carbon double bonds' >) alkene, (alkyl + -yne (< 'alteration of -ine' < L. -inus 'adjective suffix') > 'unsaturated hydrocarbon(s) containing one or more carbon-carbon triple bonds' >) alkyne*

kēlē, kēlēs, f. *hernia; swelling, tumor*

> **E** *-cele, encephalocele (< 'brain hernia'), myelocele (< 'spinal cord hernia'), meningocele (< 'meningeal hernia'), enterocele (< 'intestinal hernia'), omphalocele (< 'umbilical hernia'); mucocele (< 'mucus-filled cavity'), hematocele (< 'blood-filled cavity'), chylocele (< 'chyle-filled cavity')*

    > L. cystocele, cystoceles, f. (< G. kystis *bladder*) 주머니혹, 낭류(囊瘤); 방광(낭)류

> **E** *cystocele (< 'vesical hernia')*

    > L. hydrocele, hydroceles, f. (< G. hydōr *water*) 물혹, 수종(水腫), 수류(水瘤); 음낭수종

> **E** *hydrocele (< 'fluid-filled cavity')*

    > L. varicocele, varicoceles, f. (< L. varix *varix*) 정맥류(靜脈瘤)

> **E** *varicocele (< 'varicose swelling')*

    < IE. kaula *hernia, swelling, tumor*

narkē, narkēs, f. *numbness, stupor*

> **E** *narc(o)-, narcolepsy (< 'on the pattern of epilepsy')*

    > (*suggested*) narkissos, narkissou, m. *narcissus, daffodil; (Narkissos) (Greek mythology) the name of a beautiful youth who fell in love with his own reflection in a fountain*

        > L. narcissus, narcissi, m. 수선화;

(Narcissus) (그리스 신화) 나르키서스　　　　　**E** *narcissus, narcissism*

　　> narkoun (narkoein) *to make numb*

　　　　> narkōtikos, narkōtikē, narkōtikon *of making numb*

　　　　　　> L. narcoticus, narcotica, narcoticum 마취성의, 마약의　**E** *narcotic, narcotism*

　　　　> narkōsis, narkōseōs, f. (< + ‑ōsis *condition*) *stupor, drowsiness*

　　　　　　> L. narcosis, narcosis, f. 마취, 혼미(昏迷), 혼수(昏睡)　**E** *narcosis*

　< IE. nerk‑ *to twist, to entwine*

< IE. (s)ner‑ *to twist, to entwine*　　　　　　　　　　　**E** *snare, narrow*

nikē, nikēs, f. *conquest, victory;* (Nikē) (*Greek mythology*) *the goddess of victory*　　**E** *Nike*

　< (*probably*) IE. neik‑ *to attack*

phialē, phialēs, f. *cup, bowl, vessel, urn*

　　> L. phiala, phialae, f. 대접　　　**E** *phiale (vial)* (< *'a small cylindrical glass bottle'*)

posthē, posthēs, f. *foreskin*　　　**E** *balanoposthitis, posthetomy* (*circumcision*)

selēnē, selēnēs, f. *moon, moonshine;* (Selēnē) (*Greek mythology*) *the goddess of the moon,*
　　who fell in love with Endymion

　　E *Selene, selenography, selenium (Se)* (< *'the resemblance of the properties to those of*
　　tellurium (< L. tellus *'earth'*)*'*)

　< (*probably*) IE. swel‑ *to shine, to burn*　　**E** *sultry, swelter, swale* (< *'cool' < 'lukewarm' < 'hot'*)

smilē, smilēs, f. *woodcarving knife*

　　> smileusis, smileuseōs, f. *carving*

　　　　E *keratomileusis, LASIK* (*laser-assisted in situ keratomileusis*), *LASEK* (*laser epithelial*
　　　　keratomileusis)

　　> L. smilodon, smilodonis, m. (< *saber-toothed tiger*) (고생물) 스밀로돈,
　　　　검치호(劍齒虎)　　　　　　　　　　　　　　　　**E** *smilodon*

　< IE. smi‑ *to cut, to work with a sharp instrument*　　**E** *smith, smithy, smithery*

　　> (*perhaps*) G. smilax, smilakos, f. (< *the use of oak in carving*) *a kind of oak, yew,*
　　　　bindweed

　　　　> L. smilax, smilacis, f. 청미래덩굴속(屬)의 식물　　　　　**E** *smilax*

strangalē, strangalēs, f. *halter*

　　> strangalan (strangalaein) *to halter*

　　　　> L. strangulo, strangulavi, stangulatum, strangulare 목 조르다, 교살하다, 교수형에
　　　　　　처하다　　　　　　　　　　　　　　　　**E** *strangle, strangulate*

　　　　　　> L. strangulatio, strangulationis, f. 목조름, 교액(絞扼), 꼬임, 질식　**E** *strangulation*

< IE. strenk- *tight, narrow*

> (*suggested*) G. strongylos, strongylē, strongylon *rounded, round*

> L. Strongylus, Strongyli, m. (선충) 원충속(圓蟲屬)

E *strong, strength, string*

E Strongylus

> L. Strongyloides, Strongyloidis, m. (< + G. -eidēs *like, resembling*

< eidos *shape*) (선충) 스트론질로이디즈속(屬), 분선충속(糞線蟲屬),

간충속(杆蟲屬)

E Strongyloides

●●● 제1변화 제4식

단수 주격 어미가 -ēs로 끝나는 남성 명사. 단수 속격 어미는 -ou이며, 단수 여격과 대격 어미는 제1변화 제3식과 같고, 호격 어미는 제1변화 제1식과 같다.

poiētēs, poiētou, m. *maker, creator, poet*

	단 수	복 수	
주격	poiēt-ēs	poiēt-ai	~이, ~가, ~은, ~는, ~께서
속격	poiēt-ou	poiēt-ōn	~의
여격	poiēt-ēi	poiēt-ais	~게, ~에게, ~께, ~한테
대격	poiēt-ēn	poiēt-as	~을, ~를
호격	poiēt-a	poiēt-ai	~여, ~이여

poiētēs, poiētou, m. *maker, creator, poet*

> L. poëta, poëtae, m. 시인

E *poet*

< poiein (poieein) *to make, to create*

> poiēsis, poiēseōs, f. *making, creating, poetry*

E *-poiesis, angiopoiesis*

> L. poesis, poesis, f. 시작(詩作), 작시법(作詩法), 시

E *poesy*

> L. haematopoiesis, haematopoiesis, f. (haemopoiesis, haemopoiesis, f.)

(< G. haima, haimatos, n. *blood*)

조혈(造血)

E *haematopoiesis (hematopoiesis, hemopoiesis)*

> L. erythropoiesis, erythropoiesis, f. (< G. erythros *red*) 적혈구

생성

E *erythropoiesis*

> poiēma, poiēmatos, n. (< + -ma *resultative noun suffix*) *work, book, poem*

> L. poëma, poëmatis, n. 시

E *poem*

> poiētikos, poiētikē, poiētikon *capable of making, productive, poetic*

E *-poietic, (-poietic >) -poietin, erythropoietic, hematopoietic (hemopoietic), erythropoietin (hematopoietin, hemopoietin), angiopoietic, angiopoietin*

> L. poeticus, poetica, poeticum 시인의, 시의

E *poetic, poetics*

> -poiia, -poiias, f. *making*

> mythopoiia, mythopoiias, f. (< G. mythos *word, speech, story, legend*)

myth making

> L. mythopoeia, mythopoeiae, f. 신화 만들기　　**E** *mythopoeia, mythopoeic*

> onomatopoiia, onomatopoiias, f. (< G. onoma, onomatos, n. *name*)

word making

> L. onomatopoeia, onomatopoeiae, f. 의성어 만들기,

의성어　　**E** *onomatopoeia, onomatopoeic*

> pharmakopoiia, pharmakopoiias, f. (< pharmakon *drug, poison*)

drug making

> L. pharmacopoeia, pharmacopoeiae, f.

약전(藥典)　　**E** *pharmacopoeia (pharmacopeia), pharmacopeic*

< IE. kʷei– *to pile up, to build, to make*

athlētēs, athlētou, m. *prize-fighter, athlete*

> L. athleta, athletae, m. 투기자(鬪技者), 경기자　　**E** *athlete*

< athlein (athleein) *to contest for a prize*

< athlon, athlou, n. (athlos, athlou, m.) *contest, prize*　　**E** *decathlon, biathlon, triathlon*

> pentathlon, pentathlou, n. (< pente *five*) *athletic contest consisting of five*

disciplines (running, jumping, discus throwing, javelin throwing, and wrestling)

E *pentathlon (< 'competition consisting of fencing, shooting, swimming, riding, and cross-country running')*

Hermēs, Hermou, m. (*Greek mythology*) *Hermes*

> L. Hermes, Hermae, m. (그리스 신화) 헤르메스　　**E** *Hermes, hermetic*

margaritēs, margaritou, m. *pearl*

> L. margarita, margaritae, f. 진주

E *Margaret, margarine (< 'on account of its having the appearance of mother-of-pearl')*

< margaron, margarou, n. *pearl*

< *Of Oriental origin, 'bud'*

Prokroustēs, Prokroustou, m. (< *one that stretches*) (*Greek mythology*) *Procrustes (a*

fabulous robber of Attica who is said to have stretched or mutilated his

victims to conform them to the length of his bed)

> L. Procrustes, Procrustae, m. 프로크루스테스　　**E** *Procrustes, procrustean*

< prokrouein (< pro– *before, in front*) *to beat, to hammer out, to stretch out*

< krouein *to strike, to beat*

< IE. kreuə– *to push, to strike*　　**E** *rue, ruth, ruthless*

●●● 제 1 변화 제 5 식

단수 주격 어미가 -as 로 끝나는 남성 명사. 단수 속격 어미는 -ou 이며, 단수 여격, 대격, 호격 어미는 제1변화 제1식과 같다.

neanias, neaniou, m. *young man, youth*

	단 수	복 수	
주격	neani-as	neani-ai	~이, ~가, ~은, ~는, ~께서
속격	neani-ou	neani-ōn	~의
여격	neani-ai	neani-ais	~게, ~에게, ~께, ~한테
대격	neani-an	neani-as	~을, ~를
호격	neani-a	neani-ai	~여, ~이여

neanias, neaniou, m. *young man, youth*
  < IE. newo- *new (related to* IE. nu- *now)* (Vide NOVUS: *See* E. *nova)*

●●● 제 2 변화

단수 주격 어미가 -os 로 끝나는 남성 또는 여성 명사와 -on 으로 끝나는 중성 명사. 단수 속격 어미는 -ou 이다. 단수 주격의 어간과 단수 속격의 어간이 같다. 변화할 때 o 이 많이 들어가므로 오미크론변화라고도 한다.

●●● 제 2 변화 제 1 식

단수 주격 어미가 -os 로 끝나는 남성 또는 여성 명사. 주로 남성 명사이다. (라틴어 명사의 제2변화 제1식(nucle-us, nucle-i, m. 핵)에 해당한다.)

logos, logou, m. *word, speech, discourse, reason, account, ratio, proportion*

	단 수	복 수	
주격	log-os	log-oi	~이, ~가, ~은, ~는, ~께서
속격	log-ou	log-ōn	~의
여격	log-ōi	log-ois	~게, ~에게, ~께, ~한테
대격	log-on	log-ous	~을, ~를
호격	log-e	log-oi	~여, ~이여

logos, logou, m. *word, speech, discourse, reason, account, ratio, proportion*

　< IE. leg- *to collect; with derivatives meaning 'to speak'* (Vide LEGÈRE: *See* E. *lecture*)

alabastros, alabastrou, m. *alabaster, alabaster vase for holding perfumes*

　　> L. alabaster, alabastri, m. 설화석고, 설화석고로 만든 향합　　　　　　　E *alabaster*

　< (*possibly*) (*Egyptian*) a-la-baste *vessel of the goddess Bast in the city of Bubastis*

Asklēpios, Asklēpiou, m. (*Greek mythology*) *Asclepius, son of Apollo, the god of medicine*
　　and healing, father of Panacea and Hygeia

　　> L. Asclepius, Asclepii, m. (Aesculapius, Aesculapii, m.) (그리스 신화)
　　　　아스클레피우스　　　　　　　　　　　　　　　　E *Asclepius (Aesculapius)*

Delphoi, Delphōn, m. (pl.) (*place name*) *a town of ancient Greece on the slope of Mount*
　　Parnassus, the seat of Apollo's oracles

　　> L. Delphi, Delphorum, m. (pl.) 그리스 파르나수스산 기슭의 작은 마을, 신탁으로 유명한
　　　　아폴로 신전이 있음　　　　　　　　　　　　E *Delphi, Delphic (Delphian)*

dēmos, dēmou, m. (< *division of the people*) *the commons, the people,*
　　country　　　E *dem(o)-, demagogue* (< '*a leader of the mob*'), *demography* (< '*writing of people*')
　　> dēmios, dēmia, dēmion *belonging to the common people, public*
　　　　> epidēmios, epidēmios, epidēmion (< ep(i)- *upon*) *spread among the people*
　　　　　　> epidēmia, epidēmias, f. *prevalence of an epidemic*
　　　　　　　> L. epidemia, epidemiae, f. 유행병,
　　　　　　　　전염병　　　　　E *epidemic,* (*epidemic* >) *epidemicity, epidemiology*
　　> endēmos, endēmos, endēmon (< en- *in*) *native, at home*
　　　　> L. endemus, endema, endemum 토착성의, 풍토성의,
　　　　　　풍토병의　　　　　　　　　E *endemic,* (*endemic* >) *endemicity*
　　> pandēmos, pandēmos, pandēmon (< pan- *all*) *of all the people*
　　　　> L. pandemus, pandema, pandemum 범유행의, 세계적
　　　　　　유행의　　　　　　　　　E *pandemic,* (*pandemic* >) *pandemicity*
　　> dēmokratia, dēmokratias, f. (< dēmos *the people* + kratos *rule*) *popular government*
　　　　> L. democratia, democratiae, f. 민주정체(民主政體)　　　　E *democracy*
　　> apodēmein (< ap(o)- *away from, from*) *to go abroad, to be abroad, emigrate*
　　　　> apodēmos, apodēmos, apodēmon *abroad*
　　　　　> L. Apodemus, Apodemi, m. (< *field mice of the Old World*) 들쥐속(屬) E *Apodemus*
　< IE. da- *to divide*

　　E *time, tide,* (*tide* >) *tidal,* (*tide* >) *tidy,* D. *Zeitgeist, tap* (< '*a tapering cylindrical plug, for*
　　closing and opening a hole bored in a vessel'), *tampon* (< '*plug*'), (*tampon* >) *tamponade*

　　> G. daiesthai *to divide*

> G. geōdaisia, geōdaisias, f. (< gē *earth*) *land surveying, measuring of land*
>> L. geodaesia, geodaesiae, f. 측지학(測地學)　　　　　**E** *geodesy*

> G. daimōn, daimōnos, m., f. (< *divider of destinies*) *divine being, guardian spirit,*
one's genius; evil spirit
>> L. daemon, daemonis, m. (그리스 신화) 수호신;
악령　　　　　**E** *daemon (demon, daimon), demonic, demoniac*
>> G. eudaimōn, eudaimōn, eudaimon (< eu- *well*) *blessed with a good genius,*
fortunate, happy　　　　　**E** *eudaemonics (eudemonics)*
> IE. dail- *to divide*

E *deal, ordeal* (< 'a positioning out, judgement' < IE. ud- 'up, out' + IE. dail- 'to divide')

dinos, dinou, m. *rotation, whirling, whirlpool*　　　　　**E** *din(o)-*

> L. Dinoflagellata, Dinoflagellatorum, n. (pl.) (< dinos *whirling* + flagellum *small*
whip) (*protist*) 와편모충문(渦鞭毛蟲門)　　　　　**E** *dinoflagellate*

< IE. deye- *to swing, to whirl*

gamos, gamou, m. *marriage*

E *-gamy, isogamy* (< 'the union of two isogametes in reproduction'), *heterogamy* (< 'the
union of two heterogametes in reproduction')

> monogamos, monogamos, monogamon (< monos *alone*) *marrying once, married once*
> monogamia, monogamias, f. *the practice of marrying once*
>> L. monogamia, monogamiae, f. 단혼제, 일부일처제　　　　　**E** *monogamy*
> polygamos, polygamos, polygamon (< polys *many*) *marrying often, married often*
> polygamia, polygamias, f. *the practice of marrying often*
>> L. polygamia, polygamiae, f. 복혼제, 일부다처제　　　　　**E** *polygamy*
> L. phanerogamus, phanerogama, phanerogamum (< *of visible reproduction*
< G. phaneros *visible*) 현화(顯花)식물의　　　　　**E** *phanerogam*
> L. cryptogamus, cryptogama, cryptogamum (< *of inapparent reproduction*
< G. kryptos *hidden*) 은화(隱花)식물의　　　　　**E** *cryptogam*
> gamein (gameein) *to marry*
> gametēs, gametou, m. *husband*; gametē, gametēs, f. *wife*
>> L. gameta, gametae, f. (< *a haploid reproductive cell, ovum or sperm*)
배우자(配偶子), 생식자(生殖子), 생식세포

E *gamete, isogamete* (< 'a gamete of the same size and structure as the
one with which it unites'), *heterogamete* (< 'a gamete of different size
and structure than the one with which it unites'), *microgamete,
macrogamete, gametogenesis* (< 'development into gametes'), *gametocyte*
(< 'a cell capable of gametogenesis, an oocyte or spermatocyte; gamont'),
gametogony (< 'gametogenesis; reproduction by gametogenesis'),
(gamete >) *gamont* (< 'producing gametes' < 'on the pattern of schizont')

< IE. gemə- *to marry*

Hermaphroditos, Hermaphroditou, m. (< Hermēs + Aphroditē) (*Greek mythology*) *son of Hermes and Aphrodite, who grew together with the nymph Salmacis, while bathing in her fountain, and thus combined male and female characters*

> L. Hermaphroditus, Hermaphroditi, m. (그리스 신화) 헤르마프로디투스

> E Hermaphroditus, hermaphrodite (< *'an individual who has both male and female gonadal tissue'*), hermaphroditism, pseudohermaphrodite (< *'an individual who has gonadal tissue of one sex but has some characteristics of the opposite sex'*).

hymnos, hymnou, m. *song, hymn; melody*   E *hymn*

< IE. sam- *to sing*

kentauros, kentaurou, m. (*Greek mythology*) *a fabulous creature, with the head, trunk, and arms of a man, joined to the body and legs of a horse*

> L. centaurus, centauri, m. (그리스 신화) 반인반마(半人半馬), 켄타우로스; (Centaurus) (천문) 인마좌(人馬座)   E *centaur*

kirsos, kirsou, m. *varix*   E *cirs(o)-, cirsectomy*

> kirsoeidēs, kirsoeidēs, kirsoeides (kirsōdēs, kirsōdēs, kirsōdes) (< + eidos *shape*) *varix-like*   E *cirsoid*

> kirsion, kirsiou, n. (< + -ion *diminutive suffix*) *a kind of thistle, said to heal varix*

> L. cirsium, cirsii, n. 엉겅퀴   E *cirsium*

kolossos, kolossou, m. *gigantic statue*

> L. colossus, colossi, m. 거상(巨像)   E *colossus, colossal*

> L. colosseus, colossea, colosseum 거상의, 거대한

> L. Colosseum, Colossei, m. 콜로세움(로마의 원형 경기장)   E *Colosseum*

< *Of Aegean origin*

kōmos, kōmou, m. *merry-making, festival procession, revel*

> kōmikos, kōmikē, kōmikon *of comedy, comic*

> L. comicus, comica, comicum 희극의, 우스꽝스러운   E *comic*

> kōmōidia, kōmōidias, f. (< kōmos *merry-making* + aoidos *singer*) *comedy*

> L. comoedia, comoediae, f. 희극   E *comedy*

kophinos, kophinou, m. *basket*

> L. cophinus, cophini, m. 바구니, 채롱   E *coffer, coffin*

kopos, kopou, m. *striking, beating, wailing, weariness, trouble, pain*

> osteocopos, osteocopou, m. (< osteon *bone*) *a pain in a bone*

> L. osteocopus, osteocopi, m. 뼈통증, 골통(骨痛)

`E` *osteocope*

> L. *ophthalmocopia, *ophthalmocopiae, f. (< G. ophthalmos *eye*) 눈피로 `E` *ophthalmocopia*

labyrinthos, labyrinthou, m. *maze, labyrinth*

> labyrinthus, labyrinthi, m. 미로

`E` *labyrinth, (labyrinth >) labyrinthine*

< *Of non-Hellenic origin*

laos, laou, m. (leōs, leō, m.) *people, crowd, host, army*

> laikos, laikē, laikon *of the people*

> L. laicus, laica, laicum 속인의,

평신도의 `E` *lay, layman, laywoman, layperson, (lay >) laity*

> leitourgia, leitourgias, f. (< leito- (< leōs) + -urgia (< ergon *work*) *working*) *public
service, expenditure for the state, public service to the gods*

> L. liturgia, liturgiae, f. (고대 그리스에서 부유층 시민에게 부과한) 공공 봉사;

전례(典禮) `E` *liturgy*

lithos, lithou, m. *stone*

`E` *lithium (Li) (< 'mineral origin'), Paleolithic, Neolithic, lith(o)-, -lith, megalith, monolith,
otolith (statolith) (otoconium, statoconium), -lite*

> L. lithiasis, lithiasis, f. (< G. lithos + -iasis *suffering from*)

결석증(結石症) `E` *lithiasis, lithiasic, -lithiasis*

> L. cholelithiasis, cholelithiasis, f. (< G. cholē *bile*) 담석증(膽石症) `E` *cholelithiasis*

> L. nephrolithiasis, nephrolithiasis, f. (< G. nephros *kidney*)

신석증(腎石症) `E` *nephrolithiasis*

> L. sialolithiasis, sialolithiasis, f. (< G. sialon *saliva*) 타석증(唾石症) `E` *sialolithiasis*

> lithotomia, lithotomias, f. (< + temnein *to cut*) *incision of a duct or organ, especially
of the urinary bladder, for removal of stone*

> L. lithotomia, lithotomiae, f. 돌제거술, 결석제거술 `E` *lithotomy*

> L. lithonthrypticus, lithonthryptica, lithonthrypticum (< G. pharmaka tōn en nephrois
lithōn thryptika *drugs comminutive of stones in the kidneys* < + G. thryptein
to crush small, to comminute) 돌을 깨는, 쇄석(碎石)의

`E` *lithotriptic, (lithotriptic >) lithotriptor, (lithotriptor >) lithotrity, lithotripsy (< 'affected
by G. tripsis rubbing')*

> L. *litholapaxis, *litholapaxis, f. (< *an operation for crushing stone in the bladder
and evacuating it* < + G. lapaxis *evacuation* < lapassein *to empty, to evacuate*)
추석술(抽石術), 쇄석술, 돌깸술 `E` *litholapaxy*

mimos, mimou, m. *imitator, actor*

`E` *mime*

> pantomimos, pantomimou, m. (< *all-imitator* < pant(o)- *all*) *a theatrical performer*
who played by gestures and actions without words

> L. pantomimus, pantomimi, m. 무언극 배우   **E** *pantomime*

> mimikos, mimikē, mimikon *of mime*

> L. mimicus, mimica, mimicum 흉내 내는, 모조의   **E** *mimic, mimicry*

> mimeisthai (*middle*) *to imitate*

> mimēsis, mimēseōs, f. *imitation, copy*

> L. mimesis, mimesis, f. 모방, 모사(模寫), 모의(模擬); (생물) 의태(擬態)   **E** *mimesis*

> mimēma, mimēmatos, n. *that which is*
imitated   **E** **meme** (*< 'a cultural analogue of a gene') < 'on the pattern of gene'*)

> mimētikos, mimētikē, mimētikon
imitative   **E** *mimetic, sympathomimetic, parasympathomimetic*

> L. mimus, mimi, m. 풍자극 배우, 풍자극

> L. mimosus, mimosa, mimosum 흉내 내는

> L. mimosa, mimosae, f. (< *mimicking the sensitivity of an animal* <
herba mimosa *mimicking herb*) 미모사, 함수초(含羞草)   **E** *mimosa*

[용례] Mimosa pudica 미모사, 함수초(含羞草)   **E** Mimosa pudica
(문법) mimosa 미모사: 단수 주격
pudica 부끄러워하는: 형용사, 여성형 단수 주격
< pudicus, pudica, pudicum 부끄러워하는, 정숙한,
순결한

mythos, mythou, m. *word, speech, story, legend*   **E** *myth, mythical, mythology, mythopoeic*

noos, noou, m. (nous, nou, m.) *mind*

> G. paranoia, paranoias, f. (< par(a)- *beside, along side of, beyond*) *madness*

> L. paranoia, paranoiae, f. 집착증, 편집증   **E** *paranoia, paranoiac, paranoid*

nostos, nostou, m. *return home, travel, journey*

> L. nostalgia, nostalgiae, f. (< G. nostos *return home* + algos *pain* + -ia *noun suffix*)
향수(鄕愁)   **E** *nostalgia*

< IE. nes- *to return safely*
home   **E** *harness* (*< 'army provisions' < IE. koro- 'war, war-band, host, army' + IE. nes-*)

onkos, onkou, m. *burden, swelling, mass, tumor*

E *onc(o)-, oncology, oncogenesis, oncogene, oncovirus, oncocyte, oncotic (< 'osmotic*
pressure exerted by a colloid, especially plasma protein')

< IE. nek-, enk- *to bring*

ōkeanos, ōkeanou, m. *ocean;* (Ōkeanos) (*Greek mythology*) *the great stream or river supposed to encompass the disc of the earth, and personified as a deity, the son of Uranus and Gaia, husband of Tethys, and father of the river gods and nymphs (hence, the great outer sea, as opposed to the Mediterranean)*

> L. Oceanus, Oceani, m. 대양; (그리스 신화) 대양의 신　 E *ocean, Oceanus, (ocean >) Oceania*

　　> L. Oceanicus, Oceanica, Oceanicum 대양의; 대양의 신의　　　 E *oceanic*

　　> Ōkeanis, Ōkeanidos, f. *any of three thousand ocean nymphs, daughters of Oceanus and Tethys*

　　　　 E *Oceanid,* (pl.) *Oceanides*

Olympos, Olympou, m. *Olympus*

> L. Olympus, Olympi, m. 올림푸스　　　　　　　　　　　 E *Olympus*

> Olympikos, Olympikē, Olympikon *of Olympus*　　　　　 E *Olympic*

> Olympia, Olympias, f. *Olympia, the town in Ancient Greece where the Olympic Games were held.*

　　　　　　　　 E *Olympia*

　　> Olympias, Olympiados, f. *ancient Olympic Games; four-year period between the games*　　　　 E *Olympiad*

< (*probably*) *Of Pre-Greek origin*

ouranos, ouranou, m. *heavens, sky;* (Ouranos) (*Greek mythology*) *personification of heaven or the sky*

> L. Uranus, Urani, m. (그리스 신화) 하늘의 신;

　　천왕성　　 E *uranium (U)* (< '*from the name of the planet, discovered eight years earlier*')

phakelos, phakelou, m. *bundle*　　　　　　　　　　　 E *fagot (faggot)*

satyros, satyrou, m. (*Greek mythology*) *one of lustful and drunken woodland gods, represented as a man with horse's ears and tail, a companion of Dionysus*　 E *satyr, satyric*

sitos, sitou, m. (sition, sitiou, n.) *wheat, grain,*

　　bread, food　　　 E *sitology (sitiology), sitosterol* (< '*a sterol present in grains*')

　　> parasitos, parasitou, m. (< par(a)- *beside, along side of, beyond* + sitos) *a person who eats at the table of another, a person who lives at another's expense and repays him or her with flattery, a person who dines with a superior officer, a priest who is permitted meals at the public expense*

　　　　> L. parasitus, parasiti, m. 식객, (남의 식탁에 참석해서 이야기 등으로 흥을 돋우는 것을 업으로 삼던) 반식자(伴食者); 기생생물, 기생충

　　　　　　 E *parasite, endoparasite, ectoparasite, parasitic, parasitize, parasiticide, parasitology*

　　　　> L. parasitismus, parasitismi, m. 기식, 기생, 기생충감염　 E *parasitism, hyperparasitism*

skotos, skotou, m. (skotos, skoteos, n.) *darkness, blindness*

> **E** *scot(o)-, scotopia, scotopsin* (< *'rod opsin for dim light vision'*), *scotochromogen, scotophilia, scotophobia*

> skoptoun (skoptoein) *to darken, to make dim-sighted*

> skotōma, skotōmatos, n. (< + -ōma *resultative noun suffix*)

dizziness accompanied by dimness of sight

> L. scotoma, scotomatis, n. 현기증; (망막의)

암점(暗點)　　　　　　　　　**E** *scotoma,* (pl.) *scotomata, scotomatous*

< IE. skot- *dark, shadow*　　**E** *shade, shed* (< *'possibly a variant of shade'*), *shadow*

stichos, stichou, m. *row, line, line of verse*　　**E** (akros *'topmost'* + stichos *'line of verse'* >) *acrostic*

< IE. steigh- *to stride, to step, to rise*　　**E** *stair, stile, turnstile, stirrup, sty (stye)* (< *'riser'*)

> G. stoicheion, stoicheiou, n. *element, first principle*

> **E** *stoicheiometry (stoichiometry)* (< *'quantitative measuring of the elements in chemical reaction'*)

Tantalos, Tantalou, m. (*Greek mythology*) *a king of Phrygia, son of Zeus and the nymph Pluto, father of Pelops and Niobe, condemned, for revealing the secrets of the gods, to stand in Tartarus up to his chin in water, which constantly receded as he stooped to drink, and with branches of fruit hanging above him which ever fled his grasp*

> L. Tantalus, Tantali, m. (그리스 신화)

탄탈루스　　　**E** *Tantalus, tantalize, tantalum (Ta)* (< *'frustrating insolubility in acids'*)

taphos, taphou, m. (taphē, taphēs, f.) *tomb, burial*　　　　　　　**E** *taphonomy*

> -taphios, -taphios, -taphion *of tomb, of burial*

> epitaphion, epitaphiou, n. (< ep(i)- *upon*) *speech on the occasion of a burial, writing upon a tomb*

> L. epitaphium, epitaphii, n. 비명(碑銘), 비문, 비석　　　**E** *epitaph*

> kenotaphion, kenotaphiou, n. (< kenos *empty*) *empty tomb*

> L. cenotaphium, cenotaphii, n. 빈 무덤; (전몰용사) 기념비　　**E** *cenotaph*

< IE. dhembh- *to bury*

Tartaros, Tartarou, m. (*Greek mythology*) *the infernal regions*

> L. Tartarus, Tartari, m. 지옥　　**E** (suggested) (*'once symbol of heresy'* >) *tortoise, turtle*

thrēnos, thrēnou, m. *funeral lament*　　　　　　　　　　　　　**E** *threnetic*

> thrēnōidia, thrēnōidias, f. (< thrēnos + ōidē *song*) *song of lamentation, dirge*　　**E** *threnody*

< IE. dher- (*probably imitative*) *to drone, to murmur, to buzz*　　**E** *drone* (< *'male honeybee'*)

thriambos, thriambou, m. *hymn to Dionysus, hymn, procession, triumph*

> (*via Etruscan*) L. triumphus, triumphi, m. 로마로의 개선식, 개선, 승리,

환호성　　　　　　　　　　　　　　　　　　　　　 **E** *triumph, (triumph >) trump*

> L. triumphalis, triumphale 개선의　　　　　　　　 **E** *triumphal*

tokos, tokou, m. *birth, offspring*

E (tokos '*birth*' >) **tocology**, (tokos '*offspring*' + pherein '*to bear*' + -*ol* >) **tocopherol**, **tocolysis** (< '*inhibition of uterine contractions*')

> eutokia, eutokias, f. (< eu- *well*) *normal childbirth*

> L. eutocia, eutociae, f. 순산(順産), 정상분만　　　　 **E** *eutocia*

> dystokia, dystokias, f. (< dys- *bad*) *difficult childbirth, painful childbirth*

> L. dystocia, dystociae, f. 난산(難産)　　　　　　　 **E** *dystocia*

> oxytokia, oxytokias, f. (< oxys *sharp, quick, sour*) *quick delivery*　 **E** *oxytocic, oxytocin*

< IE. tek- *to beget, to give birth to*

thylakos, thylakou, m. *bag, pouch*　　　　　　　　　　　　　　 **E** *thylakoid*

zēlos, zēlou, m. *zeal, eagerness, jealousy*

> L. zelus, zeli, m. 열성, 열망, 질투　　　　　　　　　 **E** *zeal*

> L. zelosus, zelosa, zelosum 열성적인, 열망하는, 질투하는　 **E** *zealous, jealous, jealousy*

> zēloun (zēloein) *to be jealous*

> zēlōtēs, zēlōtou, m. *zealot, admirer, rival*

> L. zelotes, zelotae, m. 열성인 사람　　　　　　 **E** *zealot*

< IE. ya- *to seek, to request, to desire*

ebenos, ebenou, f. *ebony tree, ebony*

> ebenus, ebeni, f. (hebenus, hebeni, f.) 흑단(黑檀)나무, 그 목재　　 **E** *ebony*

< *Of Semitic or Egyptian origin*

hodos, hodou, f. *way*

E *electrode* (< '*a conductor through which electricity enters or leaves an object, substance, or region*' < '*on the pattern of anode and cathode*'), *diode* (< '*of two ways*')

> hodometron, hodometrou, n. (hodometros, hodometrou, f.) (< + metron *measure*)

instrument for measuring distances by land or sea　　 **E** *hodometer (odometer)*

> hodaios, hodaia, hodaion *pertaining to a way, on the road, by the road*

> L. stomodaeum, stomodaei, n. (stomodeum, stomodei, n.) (< G. stoma *mouth*

+ hodaios) 입오목　　　　　　　　　　　　　　 **E** *stomodeum*

> L. proctodaeum, proctodaei, n. (proctodeum, proctodei, n.) (< G. prōktos

anus, anus and rectum + hodaios) 항문오목　　　 **E** *proctodeum*

> eisodos, eisodou, f. (< eis *into, toward(s), for, for the purpose of* + hodos) *entrance,*

vestibule, admission

> epeisodion, epeisodiou, n. (*neuter of* epeisodios *coming in besides* < ep(i)– *upon* + eisodos) *dialogue scene in tragedy*　　　　　　　　**E** *episode*

> exodos, exodou, f. (< ex– *out of, away from* + hodos) *way out, going out*

　> L. exodus, exodi, f. 이스라엘 백성의 이집트 출국; (Exodus) 출애굽기　　**E** *exodus*

> methodos, methodou, f. (< meth– (< meta) *between, along with, across, after* + hodos) *pursuit of knowledge, mode of investigation*

　> L. methodus, methodi, f. (일정한 원칙에 의해 세워진) 방법, 방식, 체계　　　　　　　　　　　　　　　　**E** *method, methodical, methodology*

> periodos, periodou, f. (< peri– *around, near, beyond, on account of* + hodos) *way round, cycle, period, periodic return*

　> L. periodus, periodi, f. 주기(週期), 시기, 시대, (발달 과정의) 기(期), 구분, 단락, 완결문　　　　　　　　　　　　　　　　　　　　　　**E** *period*

　> periodikos, periodikos, periodikon *of or relating to the recurring motion of a celestial object, recurrent, intermittent (of fevers), characterized by the use of rhetorical periods*

　　> L. periodicus, periodica, periodicum 주기적인, 정기적으로 출현하는, 간헐적인, 주기적 발열 질환의　　**E** *periodic, antiperiodic, (periodic >) periodicity, periodical*

> synodos, synodou, f. (< syn– *with, together* + hodos) *assembly, meeting*

　> L. synodus, synodi, f. 회합, 종교회의　　　　　　　　　　　　**E** *synod*

> anodos, anodou, f. (< an(a)– *up, upward; again, throughout; back, backward; against; according to, similar to* + hodos) *way up*　　**E** *anode (< 'the way up (out of the electrolyte) for electrons')*

> kathodos, kathodou, f. (< kath– (< kata) *down, mis–; according to, along, thoroughly* + hodos) *way down*　　**E** *cathode (< 'the way down (into the electrolyte) for electrons')*

< IE. sed– *to go*

nosos, nosou, f. *disease*

E *nos(o)–, nosogeography, nosomania, nosophobia, nosencephaly (< 'defective cranium and brain')*

> nosokomos, nosokomou, m. (< + –komos < kamnein *to work*) *one that tends the sick*

　> nosokomeion, nosokomeiou, n. *hospital*

　　> L. nosocomium, nosocomii, n. 병원　　　　　　　　　　**E** *nosocomial*

> L. nosologia, nosologiae, f. (< + G. –logia *study*) 질병분류학, 질병분류표　**E** *nosology*

> L. zoonosis, zoonosis, f. (< G. zōon *animal* + nosos) 인수공통감염증(人獸共通感染症), 인수전염병　　　　　　　　　　　　　　**E** *zoonosis, (pl.) zoonoses, zoonotic*

parthenos, parthenou, f. *maiden, virgin, young woman; (Parthenos) (Greek mythology) the goddess Parthenos, one of the names of Athena*

E *parthenogenesis* (< 'reproduction from an ovum without fertilization, as naturally occurs in some plants and animals')

> parthenōn, parthenōnos, m. *maiden's apartments;* (Parthenōn) *temple of Athena in Athenian Acropolis*

E *Parthenon*

●●● 제2변화 제2식

단수 주격 어미가 –on으로 끝나는 중성 명사. 단수 및 복수에서 주격, 대격, 호격이 똑같다. (라틴어 명사의 제2변화 제3식(ov-um, ov-i, n. 알)에 해당한다.)

dōron, dōrou, n. *gift*

	단 수	복 수	
주격	dōr-on	dōr-a	~이, ~가, ~은, ~는, ~께서
속격	dōr-ou	dōr-ōn	~의
여격	dōr-ōi	dōr-ois	~게, ~에게, ~께, ~한테
대격	dōr-on	dōr-a	~을, ~를
호격	dōr-on	dōr-a	~여, ~이여

dōron, dōrou, n. *gift*

< IE. do- *to give* (Vide DARE: *See* E. *date*)

Ēlysion, Ēlysiou, n. (< Ēlysion pedion *Elysian field*) (*Greek mythology*) *abode of the blessed after death, where heroes and the virtuous dwell*
> L. Elysium, Elysii, n. (그리스 신화) 엘리시움; 극락정토

E *Elysium, Elysian*

epision, episiou, n. (episeion, episeiou, n.) *pubic region* **E** *episi(o)-, episiotomy, episiorrhaphy*

hoplon, hoplou, n. ((*usually* pl.) hopla) *tool, implement; ship's tackle; arms, harness, armor, weapon; camp*
> hoplitēs, hoplitou, m. *heavy-armed (foot-) soldier, hoplite* **E** *hoplite*
> panoplia, panoplias, f. (< pan- *all* + hopla) *suit of armor, full armor, panoply* **E** *panoply*

pharmakon, pharmakou, n. *drug, poison* **E** *pharmac(o)-, pharmacology*
> pharmakeuein *to administer a drug or medicine*
> pharmakeia, pharmakeias, f. *use of drugs, especially of purgatives; poisoning or witchcraft; (figurative) remedy*

> L. pharmacia, pharmaciae, f. 제약술, 조제술, 약국　　**E** *pharmacy, pharmacist*

> pharmakeutēs, pharmakeutou, m. *druggist, poisoner*

> pharmakeutikos, pharmakeutikē, pharmakeutikon *of druggist, of poisoner*

> L. pharmaceuticus, pharmaceutica, pharmaceuticum 제약의,

조제의　　**E** *pharmaceutics, pharmaceutical*

> pharmakopoiia, pharmakopoiias, f. (< + -poiia *making*) *drug making*

> L. pharmacopoeia, pharmacopoeiae, f.

약전(藥典)　　**E** *pharmacopoeia (pharmacopeia), pharmacopeic*

< (*perhaps*) *Of* non-IE. *origin*

toxon, toxou, n. *bow;* (pl. toxa) *bow and arrows*　　**E** *toxophily*

> toxikos, toxikē, toxikon *of or for the bow and arrows, belonging to archery*

[용례] το τοξικον φαρμακον (to toxikon pharmakon)

(< *the poison for smearing arrows*) 화살독

(문법) to *the*: 정관사, 중성형 단수 주격

toxikon *of arrows*: 형용사, 중성형 단수 주격

pharmakon *drug, poison*: 단수 주격

< pharmakon, pharmakou, n.

> L. toxicum, toxici, n. 화살에 바르는 독, 독

E *toxic, (toxic >) toxicity, toxic(o)-, toxicology, tox(o)- (toxi-), toxin, antitoxin, toxoid, toxaemia (toxemia), -toxic, -toxicity, cytotoxic, genotoxic; detoxify*

> L. toxicosis, toxicosis, f. (< + G. -ōsis *condition*)

중독증　　**E** *toxicosis, -toxicosis*

> L. toxico, toxicavi, –, toxicare 독을 넣다, 독을 먹이다,

중독(中毒)시키다　　**E** *toxicant, toxication*

> L. intoxico, intoxicavi, intoxicatum, intoxicare (< in- *in,*
on, into, toward + toxicare *to poison*) 중독시키다　　**E** *intoxicate*

> L. intoxicatio, intoxicationis, f. 중독　　**E** *intoxication*

> L. Toxoplasma, Toxoplasmatis, n. (< *bow-shaped tachyzoite* < G. toxon *bow* +
plasma, plasmatos, n. *something formed*) (포자충 胞子蟲) 톡소플라스마
속(屬)　　**E** *Toxoplasma*

> L. Toxocara, Toxocarae, f. (< *arrow-shaped head* < G. toxon *arrow* + kara,
karatos, n. *head*) (선충 線蟲) 톡소카라속(屬)　　**E** *Toxocara*

< (*Iranian*) *taksa- (< *those which fly*) *bow, arrow*

> L. taxus, taxi, f. 주목(朱木), 주목 나무로 만든 말뚝창

E *paclitaxel (Taxol®)* (< '*originally isolated from the bark of the Pacific yew*, Taxus
brevifolia, *which interferes with microtubule function and inhibits cell division*')

< IE. tekʷ- *to run, to flee*

●●● 제3변화

단수 주격 어미는 변화 방식에 따라 다르며 단수 속격 어미가 -os (-eōs, -ous) 인 남성, 여성, 중성 명사. 복수 여격의 (n) 은 'movable (n)' 이다. 원칙적으로 단수 주격의 어간과 단수 속격의 어간이 다르다. 어간이 자음으로 끝나는 명사가 많고 그 끝자음에 따라 변화 방식이 달라지므로 자음변화라고도 한다. (라틴어 명사의 제3·4·5변화에 해당한다.)

●●● 제3변화 제1식 a

단수 속격 어간이 치음 자음(d, t, th), 연구개음 자음(g, k, ch), 순음 자음(b, p, ph)으로 끝나는 남성 또는 여성 명사. (라틴어 명사의 제3변화 제1식 a(homo, hominis, m. 사람)에 해당한다.)

geron, gerontos, m. *oldness, old man*

	단 수	복 수	
주격	geron	geront-es	~이, ~가, ~은, ~는, ~께서
속격	geront-os	geront-ōn	~의
여격	geront-i	gerou-si(n)	~게, ~에게, ~께, ~한테
대격	geront-a	geront-as	~을, ~를
호격	geron	geront-es	~여, ~이여

geron, gerontos, m. *oldness, old man*   **E** *gerontology* (< 'the study on the processes of aging')
  < IE. gerǝ- *to grow old*
      > G. gēras, gēraos, n. *old age*

E *geriatrics* (< 'treatment of the ailments that accompany growing older'), *gereology* (< 'the study of the social, economic, and political consequences of old men'), *gerodontics, geromorphism* (< 'premature senility')

      > L. progeria, progeriae, f. (< G. pro- *before, in front* + gēras + -ia) (유전성)
        조로증   **E** *progeria*
      > G. graios, graia, graion *old*
          > G. Graiai, Graiōn, f. (pl.) (< *old women*) (*Greek mythology*) *the three old*
            sisters who have only one eye and one teeth to share among them and
            act as guards for the Gorgons
              > L. Graeae, Graearum, f. (pl.) (그리스신화) 그라이아이   **E** (pl.) *Graeae*

drakon, drakontos, m. (< *monster with the evil eyes*) *dragon, serpent*
        > L. draco, draconis, m. 용, 큰 구렁이, 보물의 수호자, 보병부대의 군기; (Draco)

(천문) 용좌 E *dragon, dragoon*

> L. Dracunculus, Dracunculi, m. (< L. dracun- (< dracon-) *dragon* +
-culus *diminutive suffix*) (선충) 드라쿤쿨루스속(屬); (식물) 쑥의 한
속(屬) E Dracunculus, *dracunculiasis (dracontiasis)*, *rankle*

[용례] Dracunculus medinensis (< *little dragon from Medina*) 메디나
충(*Medina worm*), 기니충(*Guinea worm*) E Dracunculus medinensis
(문법) Dracunculus 드라쿤쿨루스속(屬): 단수 주격
medinensis 메디나 지방의: 형용사, 남·여성형 단수 주격
< Medinensis, Medinense (< + -ensis)
< Medina (< *The Enlightened City*) 메디나 (사우디
아라비아의 도시)

> drakaina, drakainēs, f. *she-dragon*
> L. Dracaena, Dracaenae, f. (< *a reddish resin known as Dragon's blood*)
열대산 용혈수과(龍血樹科) 식물의 한 속(屬) E *dracaena*
> drakontion, drakontiou, n. (< + -ion *diminutive suffix*) *Medina worm, Guinea
worm* E *dracontiasis (dracunculiasis)*

< G. derkesthai *to look, to see, to look at*
< IE. derk- *to see*

gigas, gigantos, m. *giant* E *giant, gigantic, gigantism (giantism); gigabyte*

abbas, abbatos, m. *spiritual father, abbot*

> L. abbas, abbatis, m. 대수도원장 E *abbot*
> L. abbatissa, abbatissae, f. 여자 대수도원장 E *abbess*
> L. abbatia, abbatiae, f. 대수도원, 자치수도원 E *abbey*
< (*Aramaic*) 'abbā *father*

erōs, erōtos, m. *love, desire;* (*Eros*) (*Greek mythology*) *the god
of love* E *Eros, erotism, erotogenous, erotomania*
> erōtikos, erōtikē, erōtikon *of love, prone to love, amorous* E *erotic,* (*neuter* pl.) *erotica*

pemphix, pemphigos, m. *bubble*

> L. pemphigus, pemphigi, m. 천포창(天疱瘡), 물집증 E *pemphigus, pemphigoid*
< IE. bamb-, bhambh- (*echoic root*) *to swell*
> G. pomphos, pomphou, m. *bubble, pustule, blister*
> L. pompholyx, pompholygis, f. 한포(汗疱) E *pompholyx*

abax, abakos, m. *drawing board, calculating table, board*

> L. abacus, abaci, m. 그림판, 셈판, 선반, 주판   **E** *abacus*

< (*possibly*) (*Hebrew*) ' abhaq *dust; dust or sand used as a drawing or writing surface*

perdix, perdikos, m., f. (< *a sharp whirring sound when suddenly flushed*) *partridge*   **E** *partridge*

< IE. perd- *to fart*   **E** *fart*

phoinix, phoinikos, m., f. (m.) (*Egyptian mythology*) *phoenix;* (f.) *date-palm*

> L. phoenix, phoenicis, m., f. (m.) (이집트 신화) 불사조; (f.) 대추야자   **E** *phoenix*

bombyx, bombykos, m. *silkworm; silk, silk garment*

> L. bombyx, bombycis, m. (f.) 누에; 명주실, 명주옷   **E** (Bombyx mori *'silkworm'* >) *bombykol*

< *Of Anatolian origin*

kēryx, kērykos, m. (*Attic*) *herald, town crier;* (*at Athens*) *the crier who made proclamations in the public assemblies*

> kērykeion, kērykeiou, n. (< + -ion *diminutive suffix*) *herald's staff;* (*Greek mythology*) *wand of Hermes,* (*Roman mythology*) *wand of Mercury*

> L. caduceus, caducei, m. (caduceum, caducei, n.) 평화의 기장(旗章); (그리스·로마 신화) Hermes 신과 Mercurius 신의 지팡이   **E** *caduceus*

< IE. kar- *to praise loudly, to extol*

Artemis, Artemidos, f. (*Greek mythology*) *the goddess of the hunt, wild animals, and wilderness; the sister of Apollo*   **E** *Artemis*

> L. artemisia, artemisiae, f. (< *sacred to Artemis*) 쑥

> **E** *artemisia,* (*artemisia* + *quinine* > *'antimalarial drug from* Artemisia annua*'* >) *artemisinin*

Ilias, Iliados, f. *epic of Ilion, Iliad*   **E** *Iliad*

< Ilion, Iliou, n. (Ilios, Iliou, f.) *Troy*

< Ilos, Ilou, m. *the eldest son of* Trōs, *the grandfather of* Priamos

Pallas, Pallados, f. (*Greek mythology*) *the goddess Pallas, one of the names of Athena*

> L. Pallas, Palladis, f. (그리스 신화) (아테나 여신의 다른 이름)

팔라스 여신   **E** *Palladium* (< *'name of an asteroid'*), (*Palladium* >) *palladium (Pd)*

> Palladion, Palladiou, n. (< + -ion *diminutive suffix*) *statue of the goddess Pallas, specifically a Trojan statue*

> L. Palladium, Palladii, n. 트로이에 있던 팔라스 여신의 동상

gynē, gynaikos, f. *woman*

> **E** *gynaec(o)- (gynec(o)-), gynecology, gynecoid, gyn(o)-, gynandromorphism, -gyny, androgyny, monogyny, polygyny*

< IE. gwen- *woman*   **E** *queen*

●●● 제 3 변화 제 1 식 b

단수 속격 어간이 자음으로 끝나는 중성 명사. (라틴어 명사의 제 3 변화 제 1 식 b (caput, capitis, n. 머리)에 해당한다.)

onoma, onomatos, n. *name*

	단 수	복 수	
주격	onoma	onomat-a	~이, ~가, ~은, ~는, ~께서
속격	onomat-os	onomat-ōn	~의
여격	onomat-i	onoma-si(n)	~게, ~에게, ~께, ~한테
대격	onoma	onomat-a	~을, ~를
호격	onoma	onomat-a	~여, ~이여

onoma, onomatos, n. ((Aeolic) onyma, onymatos, n.) *name*

  < IE. no-men- *name* (Vide NOMEN; *See* E. *nominal*)

sēma, sēmatos, n. *sign, signal*   **E** *sematic, semaphore*

  > sēmainein *to give a sign, to explain by a sign, to signify*

      > sēmantikos, sēmantikē, sēmantikon *significant*   **E** *semantic, semantics, semanteme*

      > sēmasia, sēmasias, f. *significance, meaning*   **E** *semasiology*

  > sēmeion, sēmeiou, n. *sign, signal*   **E** *semeiology (semiology)*

      > sēmeioun (sēmeioein) *to interpret as a sign*

          > sēmeiōtikos, sēmeiōtikē, sēmeiōtikon *of interpreting signs, significant* **E** *semiotic*

  < IE. dheiə- *to see, to look*

      > (*Sanskrit*) dhyana (< *observing mentally*) *meditation*

          > (*Chinese*) chan 선(禪)

              > (*Japanese*) zen 선   **E** *zen*

teras, teratos, n. *wonder, monster*   **E** *terat(o)-, teratology, teratogen, tera-, terabyte*

  > L. teratoma, teratomatis, n. (< + G. -ōma *noun suffix denoting tumor*)

      기형종(畸形腫)   **E** *teratoma, teratomatous*

< IE. kʷer- *to make, to cast spell upon*

> (*Sanskrit*) kr *to make, to do*

> (*Sanskrit*) krta *made*

> **E** ((IE. sem- >) sam *'together'* + krta > *'made together'* > *'perfected'* >) *Sanskrit,* ((IE. per >) pra *'before'* + krta > *'before being made'* > *'unrefined'* >) *Prakrit*

> (*Sanskrit*) karma *act, deed*　　　　　　　　　**E** *karma*

thenar, thenaros, n. *flat of the hand (palm), flat of the foot (sole)*

> L. thenar, thenaris, n. 엄지두덩, 무지구(拇指球)　　　**E** *thenar*

> hypothenar, hypothenaros, n. (< hyp(o)- *under*) *the eminence on the inner side of the palm, over the metacarpal bone of the little finger*

> L. hypothenar, hypothenaris, n. 새끼두덩, 소지구(小指球)　　　**E** *hypothenar*

< IE. dhen- *level place*

●●● 제 3 변화 제 2 식

> 단수 속격 어간이 유음 자음(l, r)이나 비음 자음(m, n)으로 끝나는 남성 또는 여성 명사.

anēr, andros, m. *man, male*

	단 수	복 수	
주격	anēr	andr-es	～이, ～가, ～은, ～는, ～께서
속격	andr-os	andr-ōn	～의
여격	andr-i	andr-a-si(n)	～게, ～에게, ～께, ～한테
대격	andr-a	andr-as	～을, ～를
호격	anēr	andr-es	～여, ～이여

anēr, andros, m. *man, male*

> **E** *androgen(s), android, androgenesis* (< *'reproduction from an ovum that contains only paternal chromosomes'*), *gynandromorphism, Alexander* (< *'defender of men'*), *Andromeda* (< *'ruling over men'*)

< IE. ner- *man; basic sense 'vigorous, vital, strong'*

> L. Nero, Neronis, m. (< *magistrate, strong man*) 네로　　**E** *Nero* (< *'magistrate, strong man'*)

> (*suggested*) G. anthrōpos, anthrōpou, m. (< *human-faced* < andr- (< anēr) + ōps, ōpos, f. *eye, face*) *human being (as opposed to gods and beasts)*

> **E** *anthrop(o)-, anthropoid, anthropology, anthropometry, anthropophagy, anthropophobia*

Hellēn, Hellēnos, m. *son of Deucalion and Pyrrha, legendary king of Thessaly, ancestor of all the Hellenes or Greeks*
> Hellēnikos, Hellēnikē, Hellēnikon *Hellenic*   **E** *Hellenic*
> Hellēnizein *to speak Greek, to make Greek*   **E** *Hellenize (hellenize)*
>> Hellēnismos, Hellēnismou, m. *Hellenism*   **E** *Hellenism*

Pan, Panos, m. *(Greek mythology) (probably originally in the sense 'the feeder', i.e., herds-man >) the god of flocks and herds*
> L. Pan, Panis, m. 숲과 들과 목동의 신(神), 목신(牧神)   **E** *Pan*
> Panikos, Panikē, Panikon *of or relating to the god Pan; (panikos) panic (< Pan was thought to frequent mountains, caves, and lonely places, and sounds heard or fears experienced in such places came to be attributed to him)*
>> L. Panicus, Panica, Panicum 목신(牧神)의; (panicus) 당황한   **E** *panic*

Titan, Titanos, m. *(Greek mythology) Titan (any of the older gods who preceded the Olympians and were the children of Uranus and Gaia. Lead by Cronus, they overthrew Uranus; Cronus' son, Zeus, then rebelled against his father and eventually defeated the Titans)*
> L. Titan, Titanos, m. (Titan, Titanis, m.) (그리스 신화)
>> 타이탄
    E *Titan, titanomachy, titanium (Ti) (< 'on the pattern of uranium'), (Titan protein >) titin*
> Titanikos, Titanikē, Titanikon *of Titan*   **E** *Titanic*

Lakōn, Lakōnos, m. *Laconia (Sparta being the capital)*
> Lakōnikos, Lakōnikē, Lakōnikon *of Laconia, of Sparta*   **E** *laconic (< 'the Spartans being known for their terse speech')*

Tritōn, Tritōnos, m. *(Greek mythology) proper name of a sea-deity, son of Poseidon and Amphitrite, or otherwise of Nereus; also, one of a race of inferior sea-deities, or imaginary sea-monsters, of semi-human form*
> L. Triton, Tritonos, m. (Triton, Tritonis, m.) (그리스 · 로마 신화) 반인반어(半人半魚)의 해신 (Neptunus와 Salacia의 아들); (triton) 소라고둥, 도롱뇽   **E** *Triton, triton*

Typhōn, Typhōnos, m. *(Greek mythology) the name of a giant (in the depths), a tempestuous wind*   **E** *Typhon*
< IE. dheub-, dheubh- *deep, hollow*   **E** *deep, depth, dimple, dip, dope (< 'to dip'), (dope >) doping, dive*
> G. Pythōn, Pythōnos, m. *(Greek mythology) the name of a mythological serpent (in the depths) slain near Delphi by Apollo*   **E** *Python*

aktis, aktinos, f. *ray, light*

E *actinic, actinium (Ac)* (< *'glows in the dark with a pale blue light, due to its intense radioactivity'*)

> L. actinomyces, actinomycetis, m. (< *ray-fungus* < + G. mykēs, mykētos, m. *mushroom*) 방선균(放線菌), 바큇살균   **E** *actinomyces*

chelidōn, chelidonos, f. *swallow*

> L. celidonia, celidoniae, f. (< *the flowers appearing at the time of the arrival of the swallows and withering at their departure*) 애기똥풀(*greater celandine*), 미나리아재비의 일종(*lesser celandine*)   **E** *celandine*

> L. Chelidonium, Chelidonii, n. 애기똥풀속(屬)   **E** *Chelidonium*

< IE. ghel- *to call*   **E** *yell, yelp,* (IE. nek^{w}t- *'night'* + -n- + IE. ghel- *'night-singer'* >) *nightingale*

eikōn, eikonos, f. *likeness, image, picture, phantom*

> L. icon, iconis, f. 초상, 유사 기호   **E** *icon, iconolatry* (< *'on the pattern of idolatry'*), *iconoclasm*

> eikonographia, eikonographias, f. (< + -graphia *drawing, writing*) *the description or illustration of any subject by means of drawings or figures*

> L. iconographia, iconographiae, f. 도상(圖像)   **E** *iconography*

> L. iseikonia, iseikoniae, f. (< G. is(o)- *equal* + eikon- *image* + -ia) 양안등상시(兩眼等像視)   **E** *iseikonia (isoeiconia, isoiconia)*

> L. aniseikonia, aniseikoniae, f. (< G. an- *not*) 양안부등상시(兩眼不等像視)   **E** *aniseikonia (anisoeiconia, anisoiconia)*

< IE. weik- *to be like*

phrēn, phrenos, f. *mind, soul, sense, understanding, reason; (where the mind was thought to lie >) heart, breast, midriff*

> phrenitis, phrenitidos, f. *inflammation of the brain, madness*

> phrenitikos, phrenitikē, phrenitikon *suffering from inflammation of the brain, mad*

> L. phreniticus, phrenitica, phreniticum (phreneticus, phrenetica, phreneticum) 섬망(譫妄)의, 정신착란의, 미친, 열광적인   **E** *phrenetic (frenetic), frantic*

> L. phrenesia, phrenesiae, f. 섬망, 정신착란, 광란, 열광   **E** *frenzy*

> L. phrenicus, phrenica, phrenicum 정신의; 횡경막의   **E** *phrenic*

> L. schizophrenia, schizophreniae, f. (< G. schizein *to split*) 정신분열증   **E** *schizophrenia, schizophrenic*

> L. hebephrenia, hebephreniae, f. (< *a form of insanity incident to the age of puberty* < G. hēbē *youth*) 파과증(破瓜症), 사춘기치매   **E** *hebephrenia, hebephrenic*

> L. paraphrenia, paraphreniae, f. (< G. par(a)- *beside, along side of, beyond*) 망상분열증   **E** *paraphrenia, paraphrenic*

< IE. g^{w}hren- *to think*

> G. phrazein *to point out, to indicate, to declare, to tell*

> G. phrasis, phraseōs, f. *speech, way of speaking, style, diction, idiom,*
phrase   **E** *phraseology*

> L. phrasis, phrasis, f. 말투, 어법, 숙어, 구(句)   **E** *phrase, (phrase >) phrasal*

> G. metaphrazein (< met(a)- *between, along with, across, after*)

to translate   **E** *metaphrase*

> G. paraphrazein (< par(a)- *beside, along side of, beyond*)

to tell in other words   **E** *paraphrase*

> G. periphrazein (< peri- *around, near, beyond, on account of*)

to tell in a roundabout way   **E** *periphrase*

Seirēn, Seirēnos, f. (*Greek mythology*) *Siren (one of several fabulous monsters, part woman, part bird, who were supposed to lure sailors to destruction by their enchanting singing*)

> L. Siren, Sirenis, f. (그리스 신화) 사이렌; (siren) 요부, 인어

> L. sirenomelia, sirenomeliae, f. (< siren *mermaid* + melos *limb*)

인어다리증   **E** *sirenomelia*

●●● 제 3 변화 제 3 식

단수 속격의 본디 어간이 치음 자음(s)으로 끝나는 명사 또는 이와 같은 명사. 주로 중성 명사이다.

genos, genous, n. (genes- *original stem*) *race, family, kind, sex, gender*

	단 수	복 수	
주격	gen-os	gen-ē	~이, ~가, ~은, ~는, ~께서
속격	gen-ous	gen-ōn	~의
여격	gen-ei	gen-e-si(n)	~게, ~에게, ~께, ~한테
대격	gen-os	gen-ē	~을, ~를
호격	gen-os	gen-ē	~여, ~이여

genos, genous, n. (genes- *original stem*) *race, family, kind, sex, gender*

< IE. genə-, gen- *to give birth, to beget* (Vide GIGNĔRE; *See* E. *genital*)

melos, melous, n. *limb; hence a musical member or phrase, hence music, song, melody*

E *-melia, -melus;* (melos *'song'* + drama >) *melodrama* (< *'originally, a stage play, usually romantic and sensational in plot, and interspersed with songs, in which the action is accompanied by orchestral music appropriate to the various situations'*)

> melōidia, melōidias, f. (< melos *song* + ōidē *song*) *singing, chanting, choral song, music*

> L. melodia, melodiae, f. 선율   **E** *melody*

> L. phocomelia, phocomeliae, f. (< G. phōkē *seal*) 바다표범발증, 해표상지증(海豹狀肢症)   **E** *phocomelia*

> L. phocomelus, phocomeli, m. (< G. phōkē *seal*) 바다표범발체, 해표상지체(海豹狀肢體)   **E** *phocomelus*

> L. sirenomelia, sirenomeliae, f. (< L. siren *mermaid* < G. Seirēn *Siren*) 인어다리증(症)   **E** *sirenomelia, sirenomelus*

> L. notomelia, notomeliae, f. (< G. nōton *back*) 등팔다리증(症)   **E** *notomelia, notomelus*

> L. symmelia, symmeliae, f. (< G. sym- (< syn) *with, together*) 양지유착증(症)   **E** *symmelia, symmelus*

< IE. mel- *limb*

misos, misous, n. *hatred, enmity, hateful thing, hateful person*

> misein (miseein) *to hate*   **E** *mis(o)-, misogamy, misogyny*

pathos, pathous, n. *suffering, emotion, feelings, passion*   **E** *pathos, amphipathic* (< *'having two different properties'*)

> pathētikos, pathētikē, pathētikon *capable of feeling or emotion, impassioned, emotional*

> L. patheticus, pathetica, patheticum 감상적인, 정서적인, 비창한   **E** *pathetic*

> L. sympatheticus, sympathetica, sympatheticum (< G. sym- (< syn) *with, together*) 공감하는, 교감하는; 교감신경계의 (< *sympathize with the host for fight or flight reaction*)

E *sympathetic, sympathomimetic, sympatholytic; (sympathetic >) parasympathetic* (< *'some running alongside sympathetic nerves'*), *parasympathomimetic, parasympatholytic*

> -patheia, -patheias, f. (*suffix, combining form*) *forming nouns denoting kinds of feeling or ways of being affected; forming nouns denoting diseases and disorders of a specified kind or affecting a specified part, faculty, etc.; forming nouns with the sense 'method of cure, curative treatment'*

E (D. Einfühlung *'feeling-into'* >) *empathy, telepathy; -pathy, -path, -pathic;* (homoios *'like'* >) *homoeopathy (homeopathy)* (< *'Likes are cured by likes.'*), (allos *'other'* >) *allopathy* (< *'Likes are cured by unlikes.'*)

> apatheia, apatheias, f. (< a- *not*) *apathy*

> L. apathia, apathiae, f. 무감동, 무관심, 감정둔마(感情鈍痲), 무욕(無慾), 냉담   **E** *apathy, (apathy > 'on the pattern of pathetic' >) apathetic*

> sympatheia, sympatheias, f. (< sym- (< syn) *with, together*) *sympathy*

> L. sympathia, sympathiae, f. 공감, 동정   **E** *sympathy, sympathize*

> idiopatheia, idiopatheias, f. (< idios *own, private, peculiar*) *idiopathy*

> L. idiopathia, idiopathiae, f. 특발증, 자발증(自發症), 원인불명증   **E** *idiopathy, idiopathic*

> L. pathologia, pathologiae, f. 병리학, 병리   **E** *pathology, pathologic, pathological*

< IE. kʷent(h)- *to suffer*

    > G. penthos, penthous, n. *grief, sorrow; misfortune*

        > G. nepenthēs, nepenthēs, nepenthes (< ne- *not* + penthos) *removing sorrow*

            > L. nepenthes, nepenthis, f. 슬픔을 없애주는 약; (Nepenthes) (식충 식물)

              네펜시스속(屬)   **E** *Nepenthes, nepenthean*

stēthos, stēthous, n. *breast; heart, feelings; understanding*   **E** *stethoscope*

akos, akeos, n. *remedy, healing*   **E** *autacoid*

    > panakēs, panakēs, panakes (< pan- *all*) *all-healing*

        > panakeia, panakeias, f. *plant reputed to have universal healing powers,*
            universal remedy; (Panakeia) (*Greek mythology*) *goddess of healing, the*
            daughter of Asclepius

            > L. panacea, panaceae, f. 만병통치의 약초; (Panacea) (그리스 신화)
                파나케이아(치료의 여신, 아스클레피우스의 딸)   **E** *panacea, Panacea*

        > panax, panakos, m. *plants reputed to have universal healing powers*

            > L. panax, panacis, m. 만병통치의 영약   **E** *panax*

  < IE. yek- *to heal*

••• 제3변화 제4식

> 단수 속격의 본디 어간이 모음(i, y, eu 등)으로 끝나는 남성 또는 여성 명사. (라틴어 명사
> 의 제3변화 제2식 c(auris, auris, f. 귀)에 해당한다.)

polis, poleōs, f. (poli- *original stem*) *city, state*

	단 수	복 수	
주격	poli-s	pol-eis	~이, ~가, ~은, ~는, ~께서
속격	pol-eōs	pol-eōn	~의
여격	pol-ei	pol-e-si(n)	~게, ~에게, ~께, ~한테
대격	poli-n	pol-eis	~을, ~를
호격	poli	pol-eis	~여, ~이여

polis, poleōs, f. (poli- *original stem*) *city, state*   **E** *-polis, cosmopolis, necropolis*

    > politēs, politou, m. *citizen*

        > politeia, politeias, f. *citizenship, government, administration, constitution, polity*

> L. politia, politiae, f. 국가, 공화국, 정부; 정책   **E** *polity, policy, police*

> politikos, politikē, politikon *of or relating to citizens, belonging to the state or its administration, politic, public*

> L. politicus, politica, politicum 정치의, 정치적   **E** *political*

> akropolis, akropoleōs, f. (< akros *extreme, topmost, terminal*) *the elevated part of the town, or the citadel, in a Grecian city;* (Akropolis) *that of Athens*   **E** *acropolis*

> mētropolis, mētropoleōs, f. (< mētēr, mētros, f. *mother*) *mother-city of a colony, capital city*

> L. metropolis, metropolis, f. 모도(母都), 수도(首都)   **E** *metropolis*

> mētropolitēs, mētropolitou, m. *a citizen of a metropolis*

> L. metropolita, metropolitae, m. 수도에 사는 사람   **E** *metropolitan*

> propolis, propoleōs, f. (< pro- *before, in front*) *suburb, bee glue (apparently on account of the material being used by bees to maintain the structure of their hives)*

> L. propolis, propolis, f. 봉랍(蜂蠟)   **E** *propolis*

< IE. pelǝ- *citadel, fortified high place*

> (*Sanskrit*) pur, puram *city*

> (*Sanskrit*) simhapuram (< simhah *lion* + puram) *lion city*   **E** *Singapore*

Promētheus, Promētheōs, m. (< *theft of fire*) (*Greek mythology*) *Prometheus (The name of Prometheus was later interpreted by the Greeks as meaning 'forethought', leading to the creation of the name Epimetheus, 'afterthought', for this brother)*

> L. Prometheus, Prometheos, m. (Prometheus, Promethei, m.) (그리스 신화) 프로메테우스   **E** *Prometheus*

> Epimētheus, Epimētheōs, m. (*Greek mythology*) *Epimetheus*

> L. Epimetheus, Epimethei, m. (그리스 신화) 에피메테우스   **E** *Epimetheus*

< (*possibly*) IE. math- *gnawing vermin, various insect names; to steal*   **E** *maggot, moth*

Prōteus, Prōteōs, m. (*Greek mythology*) *Proteus, a sea-god, the son of Oceanus and Tethys, fabled to assume various shapes*

> L. Proteus, Proteos, m. (Proteus, Protei, m.) (그리스 신화) 프로테우스   **E** *Proteus, protean*

> L. Proteus, Protei, m. (< *forming cocci and rods of variable length*) (세균) 프로테우스속(屬)   **E** Proteus

ēchō, ēchous, f. *echo;* (Ēchō) (*Greek mythology*) *an Oread*

> L. echo, echus, f. 메아리, 반향(反響); (Echo) (그리스 신화) 산의 요정

E *echo,* (*echo* >) *echoic, echo-, echogenic, echocardiography* (< *'recording heart with reflected ultrasound'*)

< IE. (s)wagh- *to resound*   **E** *sough*

> G. ēchē, ēchēs, f. *sound*

> G. ēchein (ēcheein) *to sound, to cause to sound*

　　> G. katēchein (katēcheein) (< kat(a)- *down, mis-, according to, along,*
　　　　thoroughly) *to resound, to teach, to inform*

　　　　> G. katēchizein *to catechize*　　　　　　　　　　**E** *catechism*

halōs, halō, f. (halōs, halōos, f.) *threshing floor, disk of the sun, moon, or a shield*

　> L. halos, halo, f. 달무리, 햇무리, 운영(暈影), 테　　　**E** *halo, (halo >) halation*

● ● ● 불변화 명사

> 수와 격에 따른 어미변화를 하지 않는 명사이다.

iōta, n. *iota (I, ι), the smallest letter, jot*

　> L. iota, n. (불변화) 그리스어의 아홉째 가장 작은 글자 (I, i)　　**E** *jot*

methy, n. *wine*

> **E** (methy *'wine'* + hylē *'wood'* + -ēnos *'adjective suffix'* >) **methylene** (< F. esprit-de-bois
> *'wood spirit'*), (methylene >) **methyl**, (methyl + L. -anus *'adjective suffix'* >) **methane**

　> methyskein *to make drunk;* (*passive*) *to get drunk*

　　> amethystos, amethystos, amethyston *not drunken*

　　　> amethystos, amethystou, f. *amethyst*

　　　　> L. amethystus, amethysti, f. (amethystos, amethysti, f.) 자수정 **E** *amethyst*

< IE. medhu- *honey, also mead*　　　　　　　　　　　　　**E** *mead*

지소사

그리스어에서는 명사 어간에 다음의 지소 접미사를 붙여 지소사(指小辭,
diminutive)를 만든다. 지소사는 지소 접미사에 따라 남성 (-iskos) 또는 중성
(-ion, -idion) 명사가 되며, 제 2 변화 제 1 식 (-iskos) 또는 제 2 변화 제 2 식
(-ion, -idion)의 변화를 따른다.

- -iskos, -iskou, m.
- -ion, -iou, n.
- -idion, -idiou, n.

–iskos, –iskou, m.   E -isk

asteriskos, asteriskou, m. *little star*
> L. asteriscus, asterisci, m. 별표   E asterisk
< astēr, asteros, m. *star*
< IE. ster– *star* (Vide STELLA: *See* E. *stellar*)

mēniskos, mēniskou, m. *crescent*
> L. meniscus, menisci, m. 초승달, 반달; 반달연골   E meniscus, (pl.) menisci
< mēnē, mēnēs, f. *moon*
< IE. me– *to measure* (Vide METIRI: *See* E. *measure*)

obeliskos, obeliskou, m. *small spit, leg of a compass, obelisk*
> L. obeliscus, obelisci, m. 방첨탑(方尖塔), 오벨리스크   E obelisk
< obelos, obelou, m. *spit, nail, needle, pointed pillar*
> L. obelus, obeli, m. (인쇄) 단검표, 의구표(疑句標)   E obelus, (pl.) obeli
> obolos, obolou, m. (*a type of coin as, in early times, nails were used as
money >*) *ancient Greek coin (1/6 drachma), ancient Greek weight
(11 and 1/4 grains)*
> L. obolus, oboli, m. (고대 그리스) 화폐 단위, 돈, 중량 단위,
소량   E obolus, (pl.) oboli, obol

–ion, –iou, n.   E -ium

biblion, bibliou, n. *the inner bark of the papyrus, paper, scroll, roll, book;* (pl. ta biblia)
the books, the canonical books, the Scriptures   E biblio-
> L. biblia, bibliae, f. 책   E Bible
> L. biblicus, biblica, biblicum 책의   E Biblical
> bibliographia, bibliographias, f. (< biblion *book* + -graphia *drawing, writing*)
book-writing
> L. bibliographia, bibliographiae, f. 서지학(書誌學), 도서목록   E bibliography
> bibliothēkē, bibliothēkēs, f. (< biblion *book* + thēkē *repository*) *book-case,
library*
> L. bibliotheca, bibliothecae, f. 책장, 서재, 서고, 도서실   E bibliotheca
< biblos, biblou, f. (byblos, byblou, f.) *the inner bark of the papyrus, paper, scroll,
roll, book*
< (*suggested*) Byblos *Phoenician port from which Egyptian papyrus was exported to Greece*

kollyrion, kollyriou, n. *poultice, eye-salve*
> L. collyrium, collyrii, n. 안약(眼藥), 점안제(點眼劑), 세안제(洗眼劑)   E collyrium
< kollyra, kollyras, f. *roll of coarse bread*

marsypion, marsypiou, n. *little bag*

> L. marsupium, marsupii, n. 돈지갑, 돈주머니   **E** *marsupium*

> L. marsupialis, marsupiale 주머니의, 주머니 모양의, 주머니가 있는;

유대동물(有袋動物)의   **E** *marsupial, marsupialze*

< marsypos, marsypou, m. *pouch*

< (*perhaps*) (*Avestan*) marshu *belly*

–idion, –idiou, n.   **E** *–idium*

---

balantidion, balantidiou, n. *little bag*

> L. Balantidium, Balantidii, n. (섬모충) 발란티듐속(屬)   **E** Balantidium

< balantion, balantiou, n. *bag, pouch, purse*

klōstridion, klōstridiou, n. (< *small spindle-shaped because of the presence of an endospore*) *clostridium*

> L. Clostridium, Clostridii, n. (세균) 클로스트리듐속(屬)   **E** Clostridium, *clostridial*

> L. Clostridioides, Clostridioidis, n. (< *clostridium-like micro-organism* < + G. eidos *shape*) (세균)

클로스트리디오이데스속(屬)   **E** Clostridioides

< klōstēr, klōstēros, m. *spindle*

< klōthein *to spin*

> klōthō, klōthous, f. *spinner;* (Klōthō) (*Greek mythology*) *the youngest of the three Fates, who spins the thread of life*

> L. Clotho, Clothus, f. (그리스 신화) 운명을 맡은 세 여신 중 가장 어린

여신(사람의 출생을 맡음)   **E** *Clotho*

< IE. klo– *to spin*

명사를 만드는 방법

●●● 형용사와 분사의 차용

형용사와 분사의 명사적 용법을 말한다.

---

antidoton, antidotou, n. (< *neuter* sing., *adjective*) *remedy*

> L. antidotum, antidoti, n. 해독제   **E** *antidote*

< antidotos, antidotos, antidoton *given against, given as a remedy*

< antididonai (< ant(i)– *before, against, instead of*) *to give in return*

< didonai (do- *root of* didonai) *to give*

< IE. do- *to give* (Vide DARE: *See* E. *date*)

horizōn, horizontos, m. (< horizōn (kyklos) (*masculine present participle*)) *the bounding circle, horizon*

> L. horizon, horizontis, m. 시계(視界), 지평선, 수평선   **E** *horizon*

> L. horizontalis, horizontale 지평선의, 수평선의, 수평면의,

수평의   **E** *horizontal*

< horizein *to bound, to limit, to define*

> aoristos, aoristos, aoriston (< a- *not*) *undefined, indefinite*

E *aorist* (< '*a simple past occurrence, with none of the limitations as to completion, continuance, etc.*')

> aphorizein (< aph- (< apo) *away from, from*) *to divide by a boundary line, to select, to divide*

> aphorismos, aphorismou, m. *limitation, definition, short pithy sentence*

> L. aphorismus, aphorismi, m. 금언, 격언, 경구, 잠언   **E** *aphorism*

< horos, horou, m. *boundary, limit,*

definition   **E** (horos '*boundary*' + optēr '*viewer*' > '*boundary viewer*' >) *horopter*

● ● ●   명사 접미사의 이용

접미사를 붙여 명사를 만든다.

-tēs, -tou, m.	**E** *-tes*
-tēr, -tēros, m. 동사의 어근에 붙여 행위자나 상태를 가리키는 명사를 만든다.	**E** *-ter*
-tōr, -tōros, m.	**E** *-tor*

diabētēs, diabētou, m. (< di(a)- *through, thoroughly, apart* + bainein *to go*) *passer through, siphon*

> L. diabetes, diabetae, m. 수도관, 파이프; 당뇨병   **E** *diabetes*

< bainein *to go*

< IE. g^{w}a-, g^{w}em- *to go, to come* (Vide VENIRE: *See* E. *venue*)

kautēr, kautēros, m. *branding iron*

> L. cauter, cauteris, m. 낙형(烙刑)하는 인두, 낙인(烙印)

> kautērion, kaukēriou, n. (< + -ion *diminutive suffix*) *small branding iron*

> L. cauterium, cauterii, n. 달군 인두, 낙인, 지짐기, 지짐술, 소작기(燒灼器),

소작술, 부식구(腐蝕具)   **E** *cautery, cauterize*

< kaiein *to burn*

> kaustos, kaustē, kauston *burnt, burnable*

> kaustikos, kaustikē, kaustikon *burning, corrosive, destructive to living tissue*

> L. causticus, caustica, causticum 소작성의, 부식성의, 가성(苛性)의, 신랄한　　**E** *caustic*

> holokaustos, holokaustos, holokauston (< holos *whole*) *burnt in whole, of burnt-offering*

> L. holocaustum, holocausti, n. 번제(燔祭, 희생동물을 통째로 태워 바치던 제사)　　**E** *holocaust*

> kausis, kauseōs, f. *burning*　**E** (byssos *'flax'* + kausis > *'moxibustion'* >) *byssocausis*

> kauma, kaumatos, n. *heat*　**E** (suggested) *calm* (< *'rest during the heat of the day'*)

> kausos, kausou, m. *heat, fever*

> L. causos, causi, m. 심한 열, 고열

> L. causalgia, causalgiae, f. (< + G. algos *pain*) 작열통(灼熱痛)　　**E** *causalgia, causalgic*

> kalon, kalou, n. *wood*

> kalopodion, kalopodiou, n. (< + pous, podos, m. *foot*) *shoemaker's last*

> (Arabic) qalib *mould for casting metal*

E (probably) *caliber (calibre), calibrate,* (caliber >) *calipers (callipers)*

> enkaiein (< en *in* + kaiein) *to burn in*

> enkauston, enkaustou, n. (< *thing burnt in*) *the purple ink used by the Greek kings and Roman emperors for their signatures*

> L. encaustum, encausti, n. 잉크　　**E** *ink*

< IE. kau- *to burn*

praktōr, praktōros, m. *doer*　　　　　**E** *chiropractor*

< prattein (*Attic*) (prassein (*non-Attic*)) *to pass through, to achieve, to do*

(Vide PRATTEIN: *See* E. *practical*)

-istēs, -istou, m.　동사의 어근이나 명사의 어간에 붙여 행위자나 상태를 가리키는 명사를 만든다.　　**E** *-ist*

baptistēs, baptistou, m. *dyer, baptizer*

> L. baptista, baptistae, m. 세례자　　**E** *baptist*

< baptizein *to dip, to dye, to wash, to baptize*

> L. baptizo, **baptizavi,** baptizatum, baptizare 물에 담그다, 씻다, 세례 주다　**E** *baptize*

> baptismos, baptismou, m. (baptisma, baptismatos, n.) *baptism*

> L. baptismus, baptismi, m. (baptisma, baptismatis, n.) 세례　　**E** *baptism*

< baptein *to dip, to dye*

< IE. gʷabh- *to dip, to sink*

buddhistēs, buddhistou, m. *buddhist*

> L. buddhista, buddhistae, m. 불교신자

< (*Sanskrit*) budh *to know*

> (*Sanskrit*) buddha (*past participle*) *enlightened,*
awakened　　　　　　　　　　　　　　E *Buddha, buddhism, buddhist*

< IE. bheudh- *to be aware, to make aware*　　E *bid, forbid,* D. *verboten, bode, forebode, ombudsman*

-sis, -seōs, f.　　동사의 어근에 붙여 행위, 상태, 과정을 가리키는 명사를　　E *-sis, -asis (-iasis)*
만든다.

---

gnōsis, gnōseōs, f. (< + -sis *feminine noun suffix*) *knowledge, wisdom, judicial sentence,*
inquiry

> L. gnosis, gnosis, f. 앎, (신비적) 직관　　　　　　　　　　E *gnosis*

< gignōskein (ginōskein) (gnō- *root of* gignōskein) *to know, to think, to judge*

< IE. gno- *to know* (Vide GNOSIS; *See* E. *gnosis*)

psōriasis, psōriaseōs, f. (< + -sis *feminine noun suffix*) *suffering from itch, psoriasis*

> L. psoriasis, psoriasis, f. 마른비늘증, 건선(乾癬)　　E *psoriasis, psoriatic*

< psōrian (psōriaein) *to suffer from itch*

< psōra, psōras, f. *itch, mange*

-ōsis, -ōseōs, f.　　동사의 어근이나 명사 또는 형용사의 어간에 붙여 상태, 특히　　E *-osis*
비정상 상태를 가리키는 명사를 만든다.

---

necrōsis, necrōseōs, f. *making dead, deadness*

> L. necrosis, necrosis, f. 괴사(壞死)　　　　　　　　E *necrosis*

< nekroun (nekroein) *to kill, to make dead*

< nekros, nekra, nekron *dead*

< IE. nek- *death* (Vide NOCĒRE; *See* E. *noxious*)

thrombōsis, thrombōseōs, f. *thrombosis*

> L. thrombosis, thrombosis, f. 혈전증(血栓症)　　　　　E *thrombosis*

< thrombos, thrombou, m. *lump, piece, curd of milk, blood clot*

< IE. dherebh- *to coagulate* (Vide *TROPHICUS; *See* E. *trophic*)

-ia, -ias, f.
-sia, -sias, f.　　동사의 어근에 붙여 행위, 과정, 상태를 가리키는 명사를 만든다.　　**E** *-ia*
　　　　　　　　　　　　　　　　　　　　　　　　　　　　　　　　　　　　　E *-sia*

mania, manias, f. *madness, frenzy, enthusiasm*

> L. mania, maniae, f. 들뜸병, 조병(躁病), 열광증

> **E** *mania, -mania, choreomania, cleptomania (kleptomania), dipsomania, erotomania, onomatomania, potomania, pyromania; Beatlemania*

< mainesthai *to be mad, to rave*

< IE. men- *to think* (Vide MEMINISSE: *See* E. *comment*)

asphyxia, asphyxias, f. (< *stoppage of the pulse (a misnomer)* < G. a- *not* + sphyg- + -sia) *asphyxia*

> L. asphyxia, asphyxiae, f. 질식(窒息)

> **E** *asphyxia, (asphyxia >) asphyxial, (asphyxia >) asphyxiate, asphyxiation, asphyxiant*

< sphyzein (sphyg- *root of* sphyzein) *to throb*

> sphygmos, sphygmou, m. *pulse*

> L. sphygmus, sphygmi, m. 맥박

> **E** *sphygmus, sphygmic, sphygm(o)-,* (G. manos *'scanty'* >) *'measuring pulse and pressure'* >) *sphygmomanometer,* (G. bolē *'throw, shot'* >) *'measuring pulse and flow'* >) *sphygmobolometer,* (G. dynamis *'power'* >) *'measuring pulse and power'* >) *sphygmodynamometer, sphygmoscope*

-ia, -ias, f.　　명사 또는 형용사의 어간에 붙여 성격이나 상태를 가리키는 명사를 만든다.　　**E** *-ia*

-phobia, -phobias, f. *-phobia*

> L. -phobia, -phobiae, f. ~공포증

> **E** *phobia, -phobic, -phobe,* (G. akari *'mite'* >) *acarophobia,* (G. akros *'topmost'* >) *acrophobia,* (G. agora *'market-place'* >) *agoraphobia,* (G. agyia *'street'* >) *agyiophobia,* (G. algos *'pain'* >) *algophobia,* (G. anthrōpos *'human being'* >) *anthropophobia,* (G. arachnē *'spider'* >) *arachnophobia,* (G. belonē *'needle'* >) *belonephobia,* (G. hēdonē *'pleasure'* >) *hedonophobia,* (G. hydōr *'water'* >) *hydrophobia,* (G. lyssa *'rabies'* >) *lyssophobia,* (G. mysos *'uncleanness'* >) *mysophobia,* (G. nosos *'disease'* >) *nosophobia,* (G. ochlos *'crowd'* >) *ochlophobia,* (G. phōs *'light'* >) *photophobia,* (G. skotos *'darkness'* >) *scotophobia,* (G. triskaideka *'thirteen'* >) *triskaidekaphobia,* (G. xenos *'strange'* >) *xenophobia;* (L. cancer *'cancer'* >) *cancer phobia (cancerphobia, cancerophobia),* (L. claustrum *'closed place'* >) *claustrophobia,* (E. Russia >) *Russophobia*

> L. phobia, phobiae, f. 공포증   E *phobia, phobic*

    < phobos, phobou, m. *flight, fear*

   < phebesthai *to flee, to fear*

  < IE. bheg^w– *to flee*

sikchasia, sikchasias, f. *loathing for food, nausea*

    > L. sicchasia, sicchasiae, f. 욕지기, 구역(嘔逆)   E *sicchasia*

   < sikchos, sikchē, sikchon *squeamish*

–(s)ma, –(s)matos, n.
–(s)mos, –(s)mou, m.
–ismos, –ismou, m.

동사의 어근에 붙여 행위의 결과를 가리키는 명사를 만든다.

E *-ma (-m, -sm)*
E *-m (-sm)*
E *-ism*

---

drama, dramatos, n. *action, deed, play*

    > L. drama, dramatis, n. 연극   E *drama*

    > dramatikos, dramatikē, dramatikon *dramatic*   E *dramatic*

   < dran (draein) *to perform*

    > drastikos, drastikē, drastikon (< *applied to the effect of medicine*) *active,*
      efficacious   E *drastic*

  < IE. derə– *to work*

ēthmos, ēthmou, m. *sieve, strainer*

    > ēthmoeidēs, ēthmoeidēs, ēthmoeides (< + eidos *shape*) *sieve-like,*
      cribriform   E *ethmoid, ethmoidal*

   < ēthein *to sift*

  < IE. se– *to sift*

orgasmos, orgasmou, m. *violent excitement*

    > L. orgasmus, orgasmi, m. 극치감(極致感)   E *orgasm, orgasmic*

   < organ (orgaein) *to swell with moisture, to swell and ripen, to be excited or eager*

  < IE. wrog– *to burgeon, to swell with strength*

priapismos, priapismou, m. *priapism*

    > L. priapismus, priapismi, m. 음란, 호색, 지속발기   E *priapism*

   < priapizein *to act the part of Priapus*

  < Priapos, Priapou, m. (*Greek mythology*) *son of Dionysus and Aphrodite, personifying*
    the male procreative power

> L. Priapus, Priapi, m. (로마 신화) 프리아푸스 (Bacchus와 Venus의 아들, 남성
생식력의 신); (priapus) 남경(男莖), 호색한

-ōma, -ōmatos, n.   명사 또는 형용사의 어간에 붙여 병적 결과인 종창(腫脹)을
가리키는 명사를 만든다.

E *-oma*

---

karkinōma, karkinōmatos, n. (< (*suggested*) *the swollen veins surrounding the part*
affected bear a resemblance to the limbs of a crab (*Galen of Pergamon*) *carcinoma*
> L. carcinoma, carcinomatis, n. 암(癌),
암종(癌腫)

E *carcinoma,* (pl.) *carcinomata (carcinomas)*

< G. karkinos, karkinou, m. *crab*
< IE. kar-, ker- *hard* (Vide CANCER; *See* E. *cancer*)

trachōma, trachōmatos, n. *roughness, rough tumor*
> L. trachoma, trachomatis, n. 트라코마

E *trachoma*

< trachys, tracheia, trachy *rough*
< IE. dher- *to make muddy, darkness* (Vide TRACHYS; *See* E. *trachoma*)

대명사

그리스어에는 아홉 가지 대명사가 있다. 그중 학술용어의 이해에 필요한 대명
사는 삼인칭 인칭대명사이다.

인칭대명사

● ● ● 제 3 인칭

autos (m.), autē (f.), auto (n.) *self, personal, by oneself, together with*

E *aut(o)-, autosome* (<'*the non-aberrant chromosomes previously called ordinary*
chromosomes, unlike allosomes (sex chromosomes)')

> authentēs, authentou, m. (< autos *self* + -hentēs (< IE. senə- *to accomplish, to*
achieve)) *one who does things himself, author*
> authentikos, authentikē, authentikon *of first-hand authority, original*

> L. authenticus, authentica, authenticum 진품의, 믿을 만한   **E** *authentic*

> L. autismus, autismi, m. (< *self-absorbed and out of contact with reality*)

자폐증(自閉症)   **E** *autism,* *(autism >)* *autistic*

정관사

그리스어사전은 정관사의 단수 주격 ὁ (ho), ἡ (hē), το (to)를 써서 명사의 성을 표시한다. 학술용어에서는 그리스어 낱말을 대부분 라틴어화한 후 사용하며 라틴어화할 때 성이 바뀔 수 있으므로 그리스어 명사의 성을 알아둘 필요는 없으며, 정관사도 꼭 알아야 하는 것은 아니다. 부정관사는 없다.

	단 수			복 수		
	남성	여성	중성	남성	여성	중성
주격	ho	hē	to	hoi	hai	ta
속격	tou	tēs	tou	tōn	tōn	tōn
여격	tōi	tēi	tōi	tois	tais	tois
대격	ton	tēn	to	tous	tas	ta
호격	(−)	(−)	(−)	(−)	(−)	(−)

ho (m.), hē (f.) *the*

< IE. so– *this, that*   **E** *the, she*

> L. sic (부사) 이렇게   **E** *sic*

to (n.) *the*

[용례] το αυτο (to auto) *the same (thing)*

> **E** (to auto *'the same'* > (*contracted*) >) ***taut(o)–,*** (tauto– *'the same'* + meros *'part'* > *'one of the structural isomers that readily interconvert'* >) ***tautomer, tautomerism***

(문법) to *the* : 정관사, 중성형 단수 주격

auto *itself* : 인칭대명사, 삼인칭, 중성 단수 주격; 정관사가 삼인칭 인칭대명사

(autos (m.), autē (f.), auto (n.))를 수식하면 '바로 그 자신'을 뜻함

> tautologia, tautologias, f. (< tauto– *the same* + –logia *speaking*) *tautology*

> L. tautologia, tautologiae, f. 동어(同語) 반복, 반복   **E** *tautology*

[용례] $\tau\alpha\ \mu\epsilon\tau\epsilon\omega\rho\alpha$ (ta meteōra) *the heavenly (things)*

   (문법) ta *the*: 정관사, 중성형 복수 주격

     meteōra *heavenly*: 형용사의 명사적 용법, 중성 복수 주격

      < meteōros, meteōros, meteōron (< met(a)- *between, along with, across,*

        after + eōra *suspension*) (Vide ARTERIA: *See* E. *artery*)

< IE. to- *demonstrative pronoun; other cases*

   E *this, that, these, those, they, their, them, than, then, thence, there, thither, thus, both*

> L. tam (지시부사) 이처럼

  > L. tantus, tanta, tantum (지시형용사) 이와 같은, 이렇게 많은,

    이렇게 큰   **E** *tantamount* (< '*amount to as much*')

  > L. tandem (< tam *so* + -dem (*demonstrative suffix*))

    (부사) 마침내   **E** *tandem* (< '*at length*' < '*at length of time*' < '*finally*')

> L. talis, tale (지시형용사) 이러한

형용사

    형용사는 명사나 대명사를 한정적 또는 서술적으로 수식하며, 한정적으로 수식할 경우에는 명사나 대명사의 바로 앞 또는 바로 뒤에 위치한다.

    형용사는 성, 수, 격에 따라 어미를 바꾼다. 수식하는 명사나 대명사에다 성, 수, 격을 맞추어야 하기 때문이다. 형용사의 어미변화는 명사의 어미변화를 따른다. 형용사변화에는, 따르는 명사변화에 따라, 1·2변화, 2변화, 3변화, 1·3변화의 네 가지가 있다.

형용사변화

●●● 제 1·2 변화

남성형과 중성형의 변화는 제2변화 남성 명사와 중성 명사의 변화를 따르고, 여성형의 변화는 제1변화 여성 명사의 변화를 따른다. 형용사의 어간이 -e, -i, -r로 끝나면 여성형 단수 주격 어미는 -a, 단수 속격 어미는 -as가 되고 그렇지 않으면 여성형 단수 주격 어미는 -ē, 단수 속격 어미는 -ēs가 된다. 그리스어사전은 남성형, 여성형, 중성형을 순서대로 표기한다. (라틴어 형용사의 제1·2변화 제1식(bon-us, bon-a, bon-um)에 해당한다.)

katharos, kathara, katharon *clean, pure*

	단 수			복 수		
	남성	여성	중성	남성	여성	중성
주격	kathar-os	kathar-a	kathar-on	kathar-oi	kathar-ai	kathar-a
속격	kathar-ou	kathar-as	kathar-ou	kathar-ōn	kathar-ōn	kathar-ōn
여격	kathar-ōi	kathar-ai	kathar-ōi	kathar-ois	kathar-ais	kathar-ois
대격	kathar-on	kathar-an	kathar-on	kathar-ous	kathar-as	kathar-a
호격	kathar-e	kathar-a	kathar-on	kathar-oi	kathar-ai	kathar-a

dynamikos, dynamikē, dynamikon *powerful*

	단 수			복 수		
	남성	여성	중성	남성	여성	중성
주격	dynamik-os	dynamik-ē	dynamik-on	dynamik-oi	dynamik-ai	dynamik-a
속격	dynamik-ou	dynamik-ēs	dynamik-ou	dynamik-ōn	dynamik-ōn	dynamik-ōn
여격	dynamik-ōi	dynamik-ēi	dynamik-ōi	dynamik-ois	dynamik-ais	dynamik-ois
대격	dynamik-on	dynamik-ēn	dynamik-on	dynamik-ous	dynamik-as	dynamik-a
호격	dynamik-e	dynamik-ē	dynamik-on	dynamik-oi	dynamik-ai	dynamik-a

katharos, kathara, katharon *clean, pure*

> kathairein *to cleanse, to purge*

> katharsis, katharseōs, f. *cleansing, purging*

> L. catharsis, catharsis, f. 정화(淨化), 카타르시스; (하제에 의한) 배변(排便), 설사(泄瀉)

E *catharsis*

> kathartikos, kathartikē, kathartikon *fit for cleansing, purgative*

> L. catharticus, cathartica, catharticum 정화작용이 있는, 변을 잘 통하게 하는

E *cathartic*

amauros, amaura, amauron *dark, dim, blind*

> amauroun (amauroein) *to darken, to weaken*

> amaurōsis, amaurōseōs, f. (< + -ōsis *condition*) *dimming*

> L. amaurosis, amaurosis, f. 흑암시(黑暗視), 흑내장(黑內障)

E *amaurosis*

> *amaurōtikos, *amaurōtikē, *amaurōtikon *amaurotic*

> L. amauroticus, amaurotica, amauroticum 흑암시의, 흑내장의   **E** *amaurotic*

krauros, kraura, krauron *brittle, dry*

> L. kraurosis, kraurosis, f. (< + G. ‐ōsis *condition*) 위축증   **E** *kraurosis*

mōros, mōra, mōron *foolish, stupid, tasteless*   **E** (*neuter* sing.) *moron*, (*moron* >) *moronic*

> L. oxymoron, oxymori, n. (< G. oxys *sharp* + moron) 모순어법   **E** *oxymoron*

skiros, skira, skiron *hard*

> skirrhos, skirrhou, m. *hardened tumor*

> L. scirrhus, scirrhi, m. 경성암(硬性癌)

> L. scirrhosus, scirrhosa, scirrhosum 경성암의   **E** *scirrhous*

myrios, myria, myrion *countless*

> myrioi, myriai, myria (pl.) (*numeral*) *ten thousand*

> myrias, myriados, f. *the number ten thousand, myriad*   **E** *myriad*

< IE. meuə‐ *abundant, reproductively powerful*

> L. muto, mutonis, m. 음경(陰莖)

sardanios, sardania, sardanion *scornful, sarcastic*

> L. sardonius, sardonia, sardonium (< *spelling altered in association with* herba Sardonia *'Sardinian plant' which was said to produce facial convulsions resembling horrible laughter, usually followed by death*) 비웃는, 냉소적인   **E** *sardonic*

< IE. sward‐ *to laugh*

skaios, skaia, skiaon *left, western, awkward, clumsy, silly, unlucky*

E *normoskeocytosis* (< '*a condition of the blood leukocytes in which the number is normal, but many immature forms, deviated to the left, are present'*)

dynamikos, dynamikē, dynamikon *powerful*

> L. dynamicus, dynamica, dynamicum 힘 있는, 동적인, 동력의, 역학의   **E** *dynamic, dynamics*

< dynamis, dynameōs, f. *power*

> L. dynamis, dynamis, f. 힘, 동력   **E** *dynam(o)‐, dynamism, dynamite, dyne*, (*dyne* >) *dynein*

< dynasthai *to be able*

> dynastēs, dynastou, m. *ruler*

> L. dynastes, dynastae, f. 왕자(王者), 지배자   **E** *dynast*

> dynasteia, dynasteias, f. *rule, lordship*

> L. dynastia, dynastiae, f. 왕조, 왕가　　　　　　**E** *dynasty*

gorgos, gorgē, gorgon *terrible, wild, fierce*

> Gorgō, Gorgonos, f. (*Greek mythology*) *one of three sisters, Stheno, Euryale, and Medusa, with snakes for hair, whose look turned the beholder into stone; Medusa was slain by Perseus, and her head fixed on Athene's shield*

> L. Gorgo, Gorgonis, f. (Gorgon, Gorgonis, f.) (그리스 신화) 고르곤　　**E** *Gorgon*

kakos, kakē, kakon *bad, evil*　　　　　　　**E** *cac(o)-, cacography, cacophony*

> kakē, kakēs, f. (kakia, kakias, f.) *badness, evil*　　**E** (spondylos '*vertebra*' + kakē > '*tuberculosis of the vertebra*' >) *spondylocace*

> kachexia, kachexias, f. (< + hexis, hexeōs, f. *condition, state, behavior, habit*) *cachexia*

> L. cachexia, cachexiae, f. 불건전한 정신 상태, 도덕의 타락, 악액질(惡液質)　　　　　　**E** *cachexia, cachectic*

> kakōdēs, kakōdēs, kakōdes (< + -ōdēs (< ozein *to smell*) *smelling*) *stinking*　　　　　　**E** *cacodyl* (< '*disgusting garlic odor*')

< IE. kakka-, kaka- *to defecate; root imitative of glottal closure during defecation*　　**E** *cucking stool*

kalos, kalē, kalon *beautiful, lovely, good*　　　　　**E** *kaleidoscope*

> (*superlative*) kallistos, kallistē, kalliston *of the most beautiful*

> Kallistō, Kallistous, f. (*Greek mythology*) *a nymph of Artemis, beloved of Zeus and hated by Hera; Hera changed her into a bear, and Zeus then placed her in the sky as the constellation Ursa Major*

> L. Callisto, Callistus, f. (그리스 신화) 칼리스토　　**E** *Callisto*

> L. calomelas, calomelae, f. (< (*perhaps*) *obtained from a black mixture* < G. kalos *beuatiful* + melas *black*) 염화 제1수은, 감홍(甘汞)　　**E** *calomel*

< IE. kal- *beautiful*

> G. kallos, kallous, n. *beauty, ornament, excellence*

E (kallikreas '*pancreas*' > '*found in the human pancreas*' >) *kallikrein, prekallikrein, calligraphy*

> G. Kalliopē, Kalliopēs, f. (< *beautiful-voiced* < kallos *beauty* + ops *voice*) (*Greek mythology*) *the ninth of the Muses, presiding over eloquence and heroic poetry*

> L. Calliope, Calliopes, f. (그리스 신화) 칼리오페(웅변과 서사시의 뮤즈)　**E** *Calliope*

> G. kallipygos, kallipygos, kallipygon (< kallos *beauty* + pygē *buttock*) *of well-shaped buttocks; of the name of a famous statue of Aphrodite's*　**E** *callipygian*

kenos, kenē, kenon *empty*

> kenotaphion, kenotaphiou, n. (< taphos *tomb*) *empty tomb*

> L. cenotaphium, cenotaphii, n. 빈 무덤, (전몰용사) 기념비　　**E** *cenotaph*

< IE. ken– *empty*

lordos, lordē, lordon *bent backward*

> lordōsis, lordōseōs, f. (< + -ōsis *condition*) *lordosis*

> L. lordosis, lordosis, f. 척추전만증, 척추앞굽음증   **E** *lordosis*

< IE. lerd– *to make crooked*

orphanos, orphanē, orhanon *orphaned, destitute, bereft*

> L. orphanus, orphani, m., f. 고아

> **E** *orphan, (respiratory enteric orphan virus 'virus not associated with any known disease; even though identified later with various diseases, the original name is still used' >) reovirus*

< IE. orbh– *to change allegiance, to pass from one status to another*

> (*Czech*) robota *compulsory labor, drudgery*   **E** *robot*

pyknos, pyknē, pyknon *dense, thick*   **E** *picn(o)- (pikn(o)-), pyknocyte*

> pyknoun (pyknoein) *to make dense, to make solid*

> pyknōsis, pyknōseōs, f. (< + -ōsis *condition*) *condensation*

> L. pycnosis, pycnosis, f. (pyknosis, pyknosis, f.) (세포핵 · 염색체)

농축   **E** *pycnosis (pyknosis), pyknotic*

> L. karyopyknosis, karyopyknosis, f. (< G. kary(o)– *nucleus*)

(세포) 핵농축   **E** *karyopyknosis*

< IE. puk– *to compress*

monos, monē, monon *alone, only, left alone*

> **E** *mon(o)-, monocyte (< 'uninucleated leukocyte'); mononucleosis (< 'atypical lymphocytosis in infectious mononucleosis')*

> monas, monados, f. *unit*

> L. monas, monadis, f. 단일, 단일성, 개체; (철학) 단자(單子); (생물) 단세포생물   **E** *monad*

> L. Pseudomonas, Pseudomonadis, f. (< G. pseudēs *false* + monas) (세균)

슈도모나스속(屬)   **E** *Pseudomonas, pseudomonad*

> L. Trichomonas, Trichomonadis, f. (< G. thrix, trichos, f. *hair, wool, bristle* + monas) (편모충 鞭毛蟲) 트리코모나스속(屬)   **E** *Trichomonas, trichomoniasis*

> monachos, monachē, monachon *solitary*

> L. monachus, monachi, m. 수도자   **E** *monk*

> monazein *to live alone*

> monastērion, monastēriou, n. *monk's cell, monastery*

> L. monasterium, monasterii, n. 수도원   **E** *monastery, minster*

< IE. men– *small, isolated*

> G. manos, manē, manon *thin, scanty, slack, rare, sparse*   **E** *manometer (< 'an instrument to measure scantiness of the air')*

oligos, oligē, oligon *few, little*　　　　　　　　　　　　　　　　**E** *olig(o)-*
　　< IE. leig- *poor*

isos, isē, ison *equal*

> **E** *is(o)- (< 'equal'), isobar, isotonic, isometric, isotropic (< 'of an object or substance having a physical property which has the same value when measured in different directions'), isotope (< 'an element occupying the same place in the periodic table'), isomer (< 'different chemical compounds that have the same molecular formula'), topoisomer, isoenzyme (isozyme)*

> anisos, anisos, anison (< an- *not) unequal*

> **E** *anis(o)- (< 'unequal'), anisometric, anisotropic (< 'of an object or substance having a physical property which has a different value when measured in different directions')*

homos, homē, homon *of the same, common*

> **E** *hom(o)- (< 'of the same'), homonym, homogeneous, homogeneity, homogenize, homogenate, homologue (homolog), homologous, homology; homosexual (homo)*

> homoios, homoia, homoion *like, similar, resembling,*
　　　of the same　　**E** *homoe(o)- (home(o)-, homoi(o)-), homoeothermic (homeothermic)*
　　> homoiōsis, homoiōseōs, f. (< + -ōsis *condition) likeness*

　　　> L. homoeosis, homoeosis, f. (< *the formation of a body part having the characteristics normally found in a related part at a different body site*) 호메오시스

　　　　> **E** *homoeosis (homeosis), homeotic,* (homeotic genes + box >) *homeobox (< 'a shared nucleotide sequence of developmental control genes for bodily segmentation of Drosophila melanogaster. The sequence is short and, when written on paper, can be enclosed by a box.'), homeodomain (< 'protein domain encoded by homeobox')*

　　　> L. homoeostasis, homoeostasis, f. (< + G. stasis *standing, standstill*)
　　　　항상성(恒常性)　　　　　**E** *homoeostasis (homeostasis), homeostatic*

> homalos, homalē, homalon *even*

　> anōmalos, anōmalos, anōmalon (< an- *not) uneven, unequal*

　　> L. anomalus, anomala, anomalum 이례적, 변칙적, 이상(異常)한,
　　　기형(畸形)의　　　　　　　　　　　　　　　　　　**E** *anomalous*

　　> anōmalia, anōmalias, f. *unevenness, unequality*

　　　> L. anomalia, anomaliae, f. 이례, 변칙, 이상, 기형　　**E** *anomaly*

　> homilos, homilou, m. (homos + ilē *crowd) crowd, throng*

　　> homilia, homilias, f. *living together, assembly, instruction*　　**E** *homily*

< IE. sem- *one; also adverbially 'as one', together with* (Vide IE. sem-; *See* E. *same*)

allos, allē, allo *other (of the same kind)*

E *all(o)-* (< *'other'*), (allos *'other'* + -ergeia *'reactivity'* > *'altered reactivity'* >) *allergy, allergen*

> allēl(o)- (*stem of reciprocal pronoun*) *one another, each other*

E *allel(o)-* (< *'another'*), *allelomorph (allele)* (< *'any alternative form of a gene that can occupy a particular chromosomal locus; in diploid organisms there are two alleles, one on each chromosome of a homologous pair'*), (allele >) *allelic*

> parallēlos, parallēlos, parallēlon (< par(a)- *beside, along side of, beyond* + allēl(o)-) *side by side*

> L. parallelus, parallela, parallelum 평행의, 상사(相似)의, 대응하는　　　　**E** *parallel, antiparallel*

> allassein *to alter, to change*

> parallassein (< par(a)- *beside, along side of, beyond*) *to alter, to vary, to change, to exchange*

> parallaxis, parallaxeōs, f. *alteration, change, exchange*

> L. parallaxis, parallaxis, f. 변이(變異), 변위(變位), 시차(視差)　　　**E** *parallaxis (parallax), odontoparallaxis (odontoloxia)*

> hypallassein (< hyp(o)- *under*) *to exchange*

> hypallagē, hypallagēs, f. *exchange*

> L. hypallage, hypallages, f. 환치(換置)　　　**E** *hypallage*

< IE. al- *beyond* (Vide ILLE: *See* E. *alarm*)

heteros, hetera, heteron (*earlier* hateros) *another, different* (*of different kinds*)

E *heter(o)-* (< *'different'*), *heteronym, heterogeneous, heterogeneity, heterologue (heterolog), heterologous, heterology; heterosexual (hetero)*

< IE. sem- *one; also adverbially 'as one', together with* (Vide IE. sem-; *See* E. *same*)

xenos, xenē, xenon *foreign, strange*

E *xen(o)-* (< *'foreign'*), *xenon (Xe)* (< *'the hitherto unknown inert gas'*), *xenobiotic* (< *'designating a substance foreign to the body'*), *xenophilia, xenophobia*

< IE. ghos-ti- *guest, host, stranger; properly 'someone with whom one has reciprocal duties of hospitality'* (Vide HOSPES: *See* E. *host*)

●●● 제 2 변화

남성형, 여성형, 중성형의 변화가 각각 제 2 변화 남성, 여성, 중성 명사의 변화를 따른다. 제 2 변화 남성 명사와 여성 명사의 변화가 똑같기 때문에 형용사도 남성형과 여성형의 변화가 똑같다. 앞에 다른 낱말이 붙은 파생 형용사나 합성 형용사가 주로 제 2 변화를 한다. 그리스어 사전은 남·여성형 하나와 중성형 하나를 표기한다.

atomos, atomos, atomon *uncut, indivisible*

	단 수			복 수		
	남성	여성	중성	남성	여성	중성
주격	atom-os	atom-os	atom-on	atom-oi	atom-oi	atom-a
속격	atom-ou	atom-ou	atom-ou	atom-ōn	atom-ōn	atom-ōn
여격	atom-ōi	atom-ōi	atom-ōi	atom-ois	atom-ois	atom-ois
대격	atom-on	atom-on	atom-on	atom-ous	atom-ous	atom-a
호격	atom-e	atom-e	atom-on	atom-oi	atom-oi	atom-a

atomos, atomos, atomon (< a- *not*) *uncut, indivisible*

> **E** *atom,* *(atom >)* *atomic*

      < tomos, tomē, tomon *cut*

    < temnein *to cut*

  < IE. tem-, temə- *to cut* (Vide TEMPLUM: *See* E. *temple*)

anekdotos, anekdotos, anekdoton (< an- *not*) *unsurrendered, unmarried,*
       unpublished

> **E** (anekdota (*neuter pl.*) >) *anecdote*

      < ekdotos, ekdotos, ekdoton *surrendered, married, published*

     < ekdidonai (< ek- *out of, away from*) *to surrender, to marry, to publish*

    < didonai (do- *root of* didonai) *to give*

  < IE. do- *to give* (Vide DARE: *See* E. *date*)

barbaros, barbaros, barbaron *not Greek, foreign, uncivilized, cruel*

    > barbarikos, barbarikē, barbarikon *not Greek, foreign, uncivilized, cruel*

> **E** *barbaric*

    > L. barbarus, barbara, barbarum 외국의, 야만의, 미개한, 거친,
       잔인한

> **E** *barbarous, barbarian* (< '*not Christian*'), (*suggested*) *brave*

      > L. barbara, barbarae, f. 외국 여자, 야만인 여자

> **E** *Barbara,* (*suggested*) (Sancta Barbara '*Saint Barbara*' >) *barbituric acid,*
barbiturate, barbital

  < IE. barbar- (*echoic root*) *used to unintelligible speech of foreigners*

> **E** *babble*

●●● 제 3 변화

남성형, 여성형, 중성형 모두 제3변화 명사변화를 따른다. 남성 명사처럼 변하는 형용사와 여성 명사처럼 변하는 형용사 두 가지가 있다. 어느 쪽이나 남성형과 여성형의 어미변화가 똑같기 때문에 그리스어사전은 남·여성형 하나와 중성형 하나를 표기한다.

hygiēs, hygiēs, hygies *healthy*

	단 수			복 수		
	남성	여성	중성	남성	여성	중성
주격	hygi-ēs	hygi-ēs	hygi-es	hygi-eis	hygi-eis	hygi-ē
속격	hygi-ous	hygi-ous	hygi-ous	hygi-ōn	hygi-ōn	hygi-ōn
여격	hygi-ei	hygi-ei	hygi-ei	hygi-e-si(n)	hygi-e-si(n)	hygi-e-si(n)
대격	hygi-ē	hygi-ē	hygi-es	hygi-eis	hygi-eis	hygi-ē
호격	hygi-ēs	hygi-ēs	hygi-es	hygi-eis	hygi-eis	hygi-ē

piōn, piōn, pion *fat, plump, fertile, rich*

	단 수			복 수		
	남성	여성	중성	남성	여성	중성
주격	piōn	piōn	pion	pion-es	pion-es	pion-a
속격	pion-os	pion-os	pion-os	pion-ōn	pion-ōn	pion-ōn
여격	pion-i	pion-i	pion-i	pio-si(n)	pio-si(n)	pio-si(n)
대격	pion-a	pion-a	pion	pion-as	pion-as	pion-a
호격	piōn	piōn	pion	pion-es	pion-es	pion-a

hygiēs, hygiēs, hygies *healthy*   **E** *hygiene*

> < IE. aiw-, ayu- *vital force, life, long life, eternity; also endowed with the acme of vital force, young* (Vide JUVENIS; *See* E. *juvenile*)
>
> + IE. gʷeiə-, gʷei- *to live* (Vide VIVĔRE; *See* E. *vivarium*)

piōn, piōn, pion *fat, plump; fertile; rich*   **E** (pro- *'before, in front'* + piōn >) *propionic acid*

> < IE. peiə- *to be fat, to swell* (Vide PINUS; *See* E. *pine*)

arrhēn, arrhēn, arrhen (arsēn, arsēn, arsen) *male, manly, vigorous, strong*   **E** *arrhen(o)-*

●●● 제 1·3 변화

남성형과 중성형의 변화는 제3변화 남성 명사와 중성 명사의 변화를 따르고, 여성형의 변화는 제1변화 여성 명사의 변화를 따른다. 그리스어사전은 남성형, 여성형, 중성형을 순서대로 표기한다.

pas, pasa, pan *all*

	단 수			복 수		
	남성	여성	중성	남성	여성	중성
주격	pas	pas-a	pan	pant-es	pas-ai	pant-a
속격	pant-os	pas-ēs	pant-os	pant-ōn	pas-ōn	pant-ōn
여격	pant-i	pas-ēi	pant-i	pa-si(n)	pas-ais	pa-si(n)
대격	pant-a	pas-an	pan	pant-as	pas-as	pant-a
호격	(−)	(−)	(−)	(−)	(−)	(−)

pas, pasa, pan *all*

> E *pan- (pant(o)-), panorama, pantomime,* (dia pasōn chordōn *'through all notes'* >) *diapason*
> pantothen (*adverb*)
　　　from all sides　　E *pantothenic acid* (< *'an acid of very widespread occurrence'*)
< IE. pant- *all; root found only in Tocharian and Greek*

bathys, batheia, bathy *deep, high, wide, vehement*

> bathos, bathous, m. *depth*　　E *bathy- (bath(o)-), bathymeter (bathometer)*
< IE. gʷadh- *to sink*
> G. benthos, benthous, n.
　　depth　　E *benthos* (< *'the flora and fauna at or near the bottom of the sea'*)

bradys, bradeia, brady *slow*

> E *brady-, bradycardia, bradypnoea (bradypnea), bradykinin* (< *'slow kinin'* < *'slow contraction produced in isolated guinea pig ileum'*)

tachys, tacheia, tachy *swift*

> E *tachy-, tachycardia, tachypnoea (tachypnea),* (tachy- + -on *'a termination of Greek neuter nouns and adjectives'* >) *tachyon* (< *'a hypothetical particle that travels at superluminal speed'*)
> (*superlative*) tachistos, tachistē, tachiston *swiftest*　　E *tachistoscope*
> tachos, tachous, n. *speed*　　E *tachometer*

eurys, eureia, eury *wide, broad*　　E *eury-*
> eurynein *to widen*
　　> aneurynein (< an(a)- *up, upward; again, throughout; back, backward; against; according to, similar to* + eurynein) *to widen out*
　　　> aneurysma, aneurysmatos, n. (aneurysmos, aneurysmou, m.) *dilatation*

> L. aneurysma, aneurysmatis, n. (aneurysmus, aneurysmi, m.)

자루, 류(瘤), 동맥류(動脈瘤)　　E *aneurysm, aneurysmal, pseudoaneurysm*

> Eurydikē, Eurydikēs, f. (< *wide justice* < + dikē, dikēs, f. *justice*) (*Greek mythology*)

　　Eurydice, the wife of Orpheus

> L. Eurydice, Eurydicis, f. (그리스 신화) 유리디케 (오르페우스의 아내)　　E *Eurydice*

< IE. werə- *wide, broad*

ithys, itheia, ithy (euthys, eutheia, euthy) *straight, direct, plain, honest*　　E *ithyphallic*

< IE. sidh- *to go directly toward*

> G. athroos, athoē, athroon *gathered, crowded, in one body, all at once*

뜻의 비교

---

makros, makra, makron *long, large*　　E (*neuter sing.*) *macron, macr(o)-*

　　[용례] ἡ τεχνη (εστι) μακρα. (hē technē (esti) makra.) *Art is long.*
　　(문법) hē *the*: 정관사, 여성형 단수 주격
　　　　technē *craft*: 단수 주격 < technē, technēs, f.
　　　　esti *is*: einai 동사, 능동태 직설법 현재 단수 삼인칭
　　　　makra *long*: 형용사, 여성형 단수 주격

< IE. mak- *long, thin*

> L. macer, macra, macrum 야윈, 메마른　　E *meager*

> L. maceo, -, -, macēre 야위다, 메마르다

> L. macies, maciei, f. 야윔, 수척, 쇠약

> L. emacio, -, emaciatum, emaciare (< e- *out of, away from*)

　　야위게 하다, 쇠약하게 하다　　E *emaciate*

> G. mēkos, mēkous, n. *length*

> G. paramēkēs, paramēkēs, paramēkes (< par(a)- *beside, beyond, against* +

mēkos *length*) *oblong*

> L. paramecium, paramecii, n. 짚신벌레　　E *paramecium*

mikros, mikra, mikron *small, little, short*

E (*neuter sing.*) *micron, omicron* (< *'little O'*), *chylomicron* (< *'an extremely small particle of lipoprotein visible in the chyle and blood after the ingestion of fat'*), *micr(o)-*

< IE. smik- *small*

> L. mica, micae, f. 작은 조각, 부스러기, 돌비늘, 운모　　E *mica, (mica >) micaceous*

> L. micella, micellae, f. (< + -ella *diminutive suffix*) 미포(微胞), 미셀　　E *micelle*

brachys, bracheia, brachy *short, not far off, little, shallow*　　　　　　　　`E brachy-`

[용례] *ὁ βιος (εστι) βραχυς.* (ho bios (esti) brachys.) *Life is short.*
　　　(문법) ho *the*: 정관사, 남성형 단수 주격
　　　　　　bios *life*: 단수 주격 < bios, biou, m.
　　　　　　esti *is*: einai 동사, 능동태 직설법 현재 단수 삼인칭
　　　　　　brachys *short*: 형용사, 남성형 단수 주격

< IE. mregh-u- *short* (Vide BREVIS: *See* E. *brief*)

trachys, tracheia, trachy *rough*

[용례] *ἡ τραχεια αρτηρια* (hē tracheia artēria) *the rough windpipe*
　　　(문법) hē *the*: 정관사, 여성형 단수 주격
　　　　　　tracheia *rough*: 형용사, 여성형 단수 주격
　　　　　　artēria *windpipe*: 단수 주격 < artēria, artērias, f. 기관(氣管); 동맥

　　　　> L. trachea, tracheae, f. 기관(氣管)　　　`E trachea, tracheal`
　　　　> trachōma, trachōmatos, n. (< + -ōma *noun suffix denoting tumor*) *roughness,*
　　　　　　rough tumor
　　　　　　> L. trachoma, trachomatis, n. 트라코마　　　`E trachoma`
< IE. dher- *to make muddy, darkness*　　　　　　　`E dark, dreg, dross`
　　　> G. tarassein ((*Attic*) tarattein) *to disturb*
　　　　　> G. ataraxia, ataraxias, f. (< a- *not*) *impassiveness*
　　　　　　　> L. ataraxia, ataraxiae, f. 평온, 불안해소, 냉정　　`E ataraxia (ataraxy)`

lissos, lissē, lisson *smooth*　　　　　　`E liss(o)-, lissive, lissencephaly (agyria)`

leios, leia, leion *smooth, polished, bald*　　　　`E leio- (lio-), leiomy(o)-`
< IE. (s)lei- *slimy* (Vide LAEVIS: *See* E. *levigate*)

pachys, pacheia, pachy *thick, fat, rich, dull*　　`E pachy-, pachytene (<'stage of thick ribbons')`
　　　　> L. pachymeninx, pachymeningis, f. (< *the dura* < G. mēninx, mēningos, f.
　　　　　membrane of the brain) 경수막(硬髓膜)　　　`E pachymeninx`
< IE. bhengh- *thick, fat*

leptos, leptē, lepton *cleaned of the husks, thin, slender,*
　　　delicate　　　　　　`E lept(o)-, leptotene (< 'stage of thin ribbons')`
　　　　> L. leptomeninx, leptomeningis, f. (< *the pia-arachnoid* < G. mēninx,
　　　　　mēningos, f. *membrane of the brain*) 연질뇌척수막(軟質腦脊髓膜),
　　　　　연수막(軟髓膜)　　　　　`E leptomeninx, (pl.) leptomeninges`
　　　< lepein *to peel off*

< IE. leup-, lep- *to peel off, to break off, to scale* (Vide LIBER: *See* E. *library*)

ōchros, ōchra, ōchron *pale yellow*

> G. ōchra, ōchras, f. (< *natural earthy materials or clays which are rich in iron oxides
and vary in color from light yellow to deep orange-red or brown*) ochre

> L. ochra, ochrae, f. 황토(黃土)　　　　　　　　　　**E** *ochre (ocher), ochreous (ocherous)*

> L. ochraceus, ochracea, ochraceum 황토의,
담황갈색의　　　　　　　　　**E** *(toxin from Aspergillus ochraceus >) ochratoxin*

> L. ochronosis, ochronosis, f. (< *brown pigmentation of the collagen,
usually secondary to alkaptonuria* < + G. nosos *disease* + -ōsis
condition) 갈색증　　　　　　　　　　　　　　　**E** *ochronosis*

xanthos, xanthē, xanthon *yellow, red-yellow*

E *xanth(o)-, xanthochromic, xanthine* (< *'forming a lemon-yellow compound with nitric
acid'*), *xanthophyll (xanthophyl)* (< *'the yellow colouring-matter of leaves in autumn, a
constituent or derivative of chlorophyll'*)

> L. xanthoma, xanthomatis, n. (< + G. -ōma *noun suffix denoting tumor*)
황색종(黃色腫)　　　　　　　　　　　　**E** *xanthoma, xanthomatous*

> L. xanthelasma, xanthelasmatis, n. (< + G. elasma, elasmatos, n. *metal beaten out,
metal plate*) 황색판종(黃色板腫)　　　　　**E** *xanthelasma* (< *'planar xanthoma'*)

kirrhos, kirrha, kirrhon *orange-yellow, tawny*

> L. cirrhosis, cirrhosis, f. (< *the color of the liver in alcoholic cirrhosis* < + G. -ōsis
condition) 경화(硬化), 경화증(硬化症)　　　　　　　**E** *cirrhosis, cirrhotic*

glaukos, glaukē, glaukon (*originally*) *gleaming, clear, bright; bluish, bluish-green, bluish-
grey, grey-green*　　　　　　　　　　　　　　　　　　　**E** *glaucous*

> glaukōma, glaukōmatos, n. (< *first used in the sense of cataract, the distinction
between cataract and glaucoma not being established until about 1705* <
grey-green haze in the pupil) *cataract, glaucoma*

> L. glaucoma, glaucomatis, n. 녹내장(綠內障)　　　　　　　**E** *glaucoma*

kyanos, kyanē, kyanon (kyaneos, kyanea, kyaneon) *dark-blue*

E *cyan, cyan(o)-, cyanobacteria* (< *'prokaryotic micro-organisms that contain chlorophyll and
phycocyanin, and produce free oxygen in photosynthesis'*), *anthocyanin(s)* (< *'blue, violet,
or red flavonoid pigments in flowers'*); *cyanide(s)*

> L. cyaneus, cyanea, cyaneum 짙푸른
> kyanōsis, kyanōseōs, f. (< + -ōsis *condition*) *dark-blue color*

> L. cyanosis, cyanosis, f. 청색증(靑色症)　　　　**E** *cyanosis, cyanotic, acyanotic*

phaios, phaia, phaion *dusky, gray*

> **E** *phae(o)- (phe(o)-), phaeochromocyte (pheochromocyte) (< 'staining dusky (brown) with chromic salts')*

melas, melaina, melan *dark, dusky, gloomy, black*

> **E** *melan(o)-, melanocyte, melanin(s),* (eu- *'well'* >) *eumelanin,* (phaios *'dusky, gray'* >) *pheomelanin,* (neuron *'nerve'* >) *neuromelanin, melanosome, calomel (< 'mercurous chloride' < 'beautiful black, originally obtained from a black mixture')*

> melaina, melainēs, f. (< melaina nosos *black disease*) *disease characterized by bloody vomit (in the Hippocratic Corpus)*
>> L. melaena, melaenae, f. (melena, melenae, f.) 흑색변, 흑혈변, 혈변　**E** *melaena (melena)*
> melancholē, melancholēs, f. (< melan(o)- *black* + cholē *bile*) *black bile*
>> melancholia, melancholias, f. *condition of having black bile*
>>> L. melancholia, melancholiae, f. 검은 담즙, 우울, 우울증　　**E** *melancholy*
> melainein *to blacken*
>> melasma, melasmatos, n. (< + -sma *extended form of* -ma *resultative noun suffix*) *black spot, chloasma*
>>> L. melasma, melasmatis, n. 기미　　　　**E** *melasma (chloasma)*

< IE. mel- *of a darkish color*

비교급과 최상급

형용사에는 원급·비교급·최상급이 있으며, 어미만 규칙적으로 바뀌는 규칙 형용사와 어간까지 바뀌는 불규칙 형용사 두 가지가 있다.

●●● 규칙 형용사

원급의 형용사 어간에 비교급은 -teros, -tera, -teron을, 최상급은 -tatos, -tatē, -taton을 붙이는 방식과; 비교급은 -ōn, -ōn, -on을, 최상급은 -istos, -istē, -iston을 붙이는 방식이 있다.

원 급　　ne-os, ne-a, ne-on *new, early, young*

비교급　　neō-teros, neō-tera, neō-teron *newer, earlier, younger*

최상급   neō-tatos, neō-tatē, neō-taton *newest, earliest, youngest*

  < IE. newo- *new (related to* IE. nu- *now)* (Vide NOVUS: *See* E. *nova)*

원 급   (없음)

비교급   hysteros, hystera, hysteron *latter,*

       later   **E** *hysteron proteron* (< *'the latter (put as) the former')*

      > hysterein (hystereein) *to be behind, to come late*

          > hysterēsis, hysterēseōs, f. *coming late, coming short, deficiency*

            > L. hysteresis, hysteresis, f. 이력(履歷) 현상   **E** *hysteresis*

    < IE. ud- *up, out*

        E *out, outer, outage, utmost, utter, but, about,* (IE. ud- + IE. dhe- *'to set, to put'* > *'out-set'* >) *odd, (odd* >) *odds,* (IE. ud- + IE. dail- *'to divide'* > *'positioning out, judgement'* >) *ordeal, (suggested) evil* (< *'exceeding due measure, overstepping proper limits')*

최상급   (없음)

원 급   tachy-s, tachei-a, tachy *swift*

비교급   tachy-ōn, tachy-ōn, tachy-on *swifter*

최상급   tach-istos, tach-istē, tach-iston *swiftest*

●●● 불규칙 형용사

원급 형용사의 바뀐 어간에 비교급은 -ōn, -ōn, -on을, 최상급은 -istos, -istē, -iston을 붙인다.

원 급   megas, megalē, mega *large, great, big*

비교급   meiz-ōn, meiz-ōn, meiz-on *larger, greater, bigger*

최상급   meg-istos, meg-istē, meg-iston *largest, greatest, biggest*

    < IE. meg- *great* (Vide MAGNUS: *See* E. *magnum)*

원 급   poly-s, poll-ē, poly *many, much, frequent*

비교급   plei-ōn, plei-ōn, plei-on (ple-ōn, ple-ōn, ple-on) *more*

최상급   ple-istos, ple-istē, ple-iston *most*

    < IE. pelə- *to fill; with derivatives referring to abundance and multitude*

       (Vide PLĒRE: *See* E. *complete)*

형용사를 만드는 방법

••• 형용사 접미사의 이용

접미사를 붙여 형용사를 만든다.

-tikos, -tikē, -tikon 동사의 어근에 붙여 가능성, 자격, 속성을 가리키는 형용사를 만든다. **E** *-tic*

sēptikos, sēptikē, sēptikon *putrefactive*

> L. septicus, septica, septicum 감염된, 패혈증의 **E** *septic, aseptic, antiseptic*

> L. septicaemia, septicaemiae, f. (< + G. haima *blood* + -ia *noun suffix*)

패혈증(敗血症) **E** *septicaemia (septicemia), septicemic*

< sēpein *to make rotten; to rot, to decay*

> sēpsis, sēpseōs, f. (< + -sis *feminine noun suffix*) *sepsis*

> L. sepsis, sepsis, f. 부패증, 패혈증 **E** *sepsis*

> L. asepsis, asepsis, f. (< G. a- *not*) 무균, 방부 **E** *asepsis*

> (*perhaps*) sēpia, sēpias, f. (< *the inky fluid which the cuttlefish secretes*)

cuttlefish

> L. sepia, sepiae, f. 오징어, (오징어 먹의) 암갈색 **E** *sepia*

∽ sapros, sapra, sapron *rotten, decayed, putrid, worthless*

E (-phagos *'eating'* >) *saprophagous*, (phyte *'plant'* >) *saprophyte*, (bios *'life'* >) *saprobe*

-akos, -akē, -akon 명사의 어간에 붙여 가능성, 자격, 관계를 가리키는 형용사를 **E** *-ac*
-ikos, -ikē, -ikon 만든다. **E** *-ic*

kardiakos, kardiakē, kardiakon *of heart* **E** *cardiac*

< kardia, kardias, f. *heart, mind, soul*

< IE. kerd- *heart* (Vide COR; *See* E. *courage*)

basilikos, basilikē, basilikon *royal*

> L. basilicus, basilica, basilicum 왕의, 귀한, 호화로운,

중요한 **E** *basilic*, (G. basilikē stoa *'royal portico'* >) *basilica*

[용례] vena basilica (< *basilic vein* < *vein of great importance, the right and left basilic veins were formerly thought to be in direct communication with the liver and spleen respectively*) 자쪽피부

정맥, 척측피정맥(尺側皮靜脈)　　　　　　　　　　　　　　　**E** *basilic vein*

(문법) vena 정맥: 단수 주격 < vena, venae, f. 맥, 혈관, 정맥

basilica 중요한: 형용사, 여성형 단수 주격

< basileus, basileōs, m. *king*

> basiliskos, basiliskou, m. (< + –iskos *diminutive suffix*) *kinglet*

> **E** *basilisk* (<'a fabulous reptile, also called a cockatrice, alleged to be hatched by a serpent from a cock's egg; ancient authors stated that its hissing drove away all other serpents, and that its breath, and even its look, was fatal; so called, says Pliny, from a spot, resembling a crown, on its head: mediaeval authors furnished it with 'a certain combe or coronet')*

–os, –a (–ē), –on　　　　명사의 어간에 붙여 명사를 형용사로 만든다.　　　　**E** *-on, -um*

---

perikardios, perikardia, perikardion (< peri– *around, near, beyond, on account of*)

> *pericardial*

> L. pericardium, pericardii, n. 심장막, 심외막　　　　**E** *pericardium*

< kardia, kardias, f. *heart, mind, soul*

< IE. kerd– *heart* (Vide COR: *See* E. *courage*)

–ēnos, –ēnē, –ēnon　　　명사의 어간에 붙여 장소, 기원, 소속을 가리키는 형용사를 만든다.　　　　**E** *-ene*

Pergamēnos, Pergamēnē, Pergamēnon *of Pergamon*

> L. Pergamenus, Pergamena, Pergamenum 페르가몬의

> L. pergamena, pergamenae, f. (< Pergamena charta *chart of Pergamum where parchment was supposedly first made*) 양피지　　　　**E** *parchment*

< Pergamon, Pergamou, n. *Pergamon, the city and capital of an ancient kingdom in Asia Minor (now Bergama in Turkey)*

> L. Pergamum, Pergami, n. 페르가몬(소아시아의 도시, 페르가몬 왕국의 수도, 유명한 도서관이 있었음)

–itēs, –itēs, –ites　　　명사의 어간에 붙여 소속이나 성격을 가리키는 형용사를 만든다.　　　　**E** *-ite, -itis*

---

dendritēs, dendritēs, dendrites *of a tree*　　　　**E** *dendrite, (dendrite >) dendritic*

< dendron, dendrou, n. *tree*

< IE. deru–, dreu– *to be firm, solid, steadfast; hence specialized senses 'tree', 'wood', and*

derivatives referring to objects made of wood (Vide DURUS: *See* E. *endure*)

arthritēs, arthritēs, arthrites *of joint*

> [용례] *ἡ ἀρθρίτης νοσος* (hē arthritēs nosos) *the joint disease*
> (문법) hē *the*: 정관사, 여성형 단수 주격
>   arthritēs *of joint*: 형용사, 남·여성형 단수 주격
>   nosos *disease*: 단수 주격 < nosos, nosou, f.

    < arthron, arthrou, n. *joint, limb, article*
  < IE. ar– *to fit together* (Vide ARS: *See* E. *art*)

–oeidēs, –oeidēs, –oeides –odēs, –odēs, –odes	명사의 어간에 붙여 생김새를 뜻하는 형용사를 만든다.	**E** *-oid* **E** *-ode*

deltoeidēs, deltoeidēs, deltoeides (< + eidos *shape*) *Δ-shaped, delta-shaped*

    > L. deltoideus, deltoidea, deltoideum *Δ* 모양의, 델타 모양의   **E** *deltoid*
  < delta *delta*

hyoeidēs, hyoeidēs, hyoeides (< + eidos *shape*) *υ* (*lower case*)*-shaped, hy-shaped*

    > L. hyoideus, hyoidea, hyoideum *υ* 모양의; (os hyoideum 목뿔뼈, 설골(舌骨) >)
    목뿔뼈의, 설골의   **E** *hyoid*
        > L. geniohyoideus, geniohyoidea, geniohyoideum (< G. geneion *chin,*
        lower jaw, beard) 턱끝목뿔뼈의   **E** *geniohyoid*
        > L. mylohyoideus, mylohyoidea, mylohyoideum (< G. mylē (mylos) *molar*)
        턱목뿔뼈의   **E** *mylohyoid*
        > L. omohyoideus, omohyoidea, omohyoideum (< G. ōmos *shoulder*) 어깨
        목뿔뼈의   **E** *omohyoid*
        > L. thyrohyoideus, thyrohyoidea, thyrohyoideum (< G. thyreos *door-*
        stone, large shield) 방패목뿔뼈의   **E** *thyrohyoid*
    < hy psilon (< hy + psilos, psilē, psilon *bare, naked, simple, plain*) upsilon, plain hy

hypsiloeidēs, hypsiloeidēs, hypsiloeides (< + eidos *shape*) *Υ* (*upper case*)*- shaped,* *ypsilon- shaped*

        E *hypsiloid*
    < hy psilon (< hy + psilos, psilē, psilon *bare, naked, simple, plain*) upsilon, plain hy

geōdēs, geōdēs, geōdes (< + eidos *shape*) *earthy, earth-like*

    > L. geodes, geodis, m. 정동(晶洞)   **E** *geode*

< gē, gēs, f. *earth*

수사

기수와 서수가 있다. 합성어의 조어 성분이 되므로 기본 수사는 알아둘 필요가
있다. 그리스어 수사의 어원과 그리스어 수사에서 비롯된 영어 낱말은 라틴어
수사편에 함께 실려 있다.

●●● 기수

1부터 4까지는 성과 격에 따라 어미변화를 하며, 5부터 100까지는 어미변화를 하지 않는
다. 200부터는 성에 따른 어미변화를 한다. 명사로 사용된다.

heis (m.)	mia (f.)	hen (n.)	*one*
dyo (m.)	dyo (f.)	dyo (n.)	*two*
treis (m.)	treis (f.)	tria (n.)	*three*
tessares (m.)	tessares (f.)	tessara (n.)	*four*
pente			*five*
hex			*six*
hepta			*seven*
oktō			*eight*
ennea			*nine*
deka			*ten*
hendeka			*eleven*
dōdeka			*twelve*
eikosi			*twenty*
hekaton			*hundred*
chilioi (m.)	chiliai (f.)	chilia (n.)	*thousand*
myrioi (m.)	myriai (f.)	myria (n.)	*ten thousand*

••• 서수

모든 서수는 성, 수, 격에 따라 형용사 제1·2변화의 어미변화를 한다. 형용사로 사용된다.

prōtos (m.)	prōtē (f.)	prōton (n.)	*first*
deuteros (m.)	deutera (f.)	deuteron (n.)	*second*
tritos (m.)	tritē (f.)	triton (n.)	*third*
tetartos (m.)	tetartē (f.)	tetarton (n.)	*fourth*
pemptos (m.)	pemptē (f.)	pempton (n.)	*fifth*
hektos (m.)	hektē (f.)	hekton (n.)	*sixth*
hebdomos (m.)	hebdomē (f.)	hebdomon (n.)	*seventh*
ogdoos (m.)	ogdoē (f.)	ogdoon (n.)	*eighth*
enatos (m.)	enatē (f.)	enaton (n.)	*ninth*
dekatos (m.)	dekatē (f.)	dekaton (n.)	*tenth*

••• 파생 수사

수 자체 또는 그만큼의 묶음을 가리키는 명사는 다음과 같다.

monas, monados, f.	*unit*	E *monad*
dyas, dyados, f.	*the number two, pair, dyad*	E *dyad*
trias, triados, f.	*the number three, triad*	E *triad*
tetras, tetrados, f.	*the number four, tetrad*	E *tetrad*
pentas, pentados, f.	*the number five, pentad*	E *pentad*
hexas, hexados, f.	*the number six, hexad*	E *hexad*
heptas, heptados, f.	*the number seven, heptad*	E *heptad*
hebdomas, hebdomados, f.	*the number seven, hebdomad*	E *hebdomad*
oktas, oktados, f.	*the number eight, octad*	E *octad*
enneas, enneados, f.	*the number nine, ennead*	E *ennead*
dekas, dekados, f.	*the number ten, decad*	E *decad, decade*
myrias, myriados, f.	*the number ten thousand, myriad*	E *myriad*

동사

   그리스어의 동사는 형과 태(정형 능동태·정형 중간태·정형 수동태·탈형 능동태), 법(직설법·가정법·명령법·희구법·부정법), 시제(현재·미완료·미래·부정과거·현재완료·과거완료), 수(단수·복수), 인칭(일인칭·이인칭·삼인칭), 분사(현재분사·미래분사·과거분사·완료분사)에 따라 어미를 달리하는 변화 품사로서 어미변화가 복잡하다. 그러나 어원을 이해하기 위해서는 어간과 뜻 정도만 알면 되며, 그러기 위해서는 사전이 제시하는 동사를 보고서 어간과 어미를 구분할 수 있을 정도면 된다. 구분에 필요한 것은 다음 네 가지, 형과 태에 따른 종류이다.

- 정형 능동태 (*active*)

- 정형 중간태 (*middle*)

- 정형 수동태 (*passive*)

- 탈형 능동태 (혼동태, *deponent*)

동사의 형과 태

   그리스어 동사의 태에서 정형 능동태는 꼴과 뜻이 모두 능동태인 태로서 라틴어 정형동사의 능동태와 같다. 정형 중간태는 주어의 행위 결과가 다시 주어에게 미치는, 그리스어에만 있는 독특한 태이다. '자신을 위해 무엇을 하다'를 뜻하고자 할 때 쓴다. 정형 수동태는 객어의 행위 결과가 주어에게 미치는 태이며, 라틴어 정형동사의 수동태와 같다. 탈형 능동태는, 어미의 꼴은 정형 중간태이거나 정형 수동태인데 뜻은 능동태인 태이며, 라틴어의 탈형동사(이태동사)에 해당한다. 행위의 대상을 갖는 타동사는 능동태, 중간태, 수동태의 태를 모두 가질 수 있으나 자동사는 그렇지 못한다. 탈형 능동태 동사는 능동태 이외의 태를 갖지 않는다.

그리스어 동사의 형과 태의 예

정형 능동태	ly-ō	나는 풀어준다	직설법 현재 단수 일인칭
중간태	ly-omai	나는 푼다	직설법 현재 단수 일인칭
수동태	ly-omai	나는 풀리운다	직설법 현재 단수 일인칭
정형 능동태	didō-mi	나는 준다	직설법 현재 단수 일인칭
중간태	did-omai	나는 내게 준다	직설법 현재 단수 일인칭
수동태	did-omai	나는 받는다	직설법 현재 단수 일인칭
탈형 능동태	erch-omai	나는 간다/온다	직설법 현재 단수 일인칭

직설법 현재 단수 일인칭에 의한 동사 구분

정형 능동태의 직설법 현재 단수 일인칭은 −ō 아니면 −mi로 끝난다. 이에 따라 정형 동사를 ō 동사와 mi 동사의 두 가지로 구분한다. ō 동사는 가장 일반적인 동사이며 규칙적인 어미변화를 한다. mi 동사는 ō 동사의 고대형으로 수는 적으나 자주 사용되는 동사이며, 사뭇 불규칙한 어미변화를 한다. (ō 동사의 −ō는 고대형 −omi가 변한 것이다.) 정형 중간태, 정형 수동태, 탈형 능동태의 직설법 현재 단수 일인칭의 어미는 모두 −omai로 끝난다. 따라서 직설법 현재 단수 일인칭 어미를 보면 동사가 (1) 정형 능동태의 ō 동사인지, (2) 정형 능동태의 mi 동사인지, (3) 정형 중간태, 정형 수동태, 또는 탈형 능동태의 동사인지를 알 수 있다. 그리스어사전은 동사의 직설법 현재 단수 일인칭을 표제어로 제시함으로써 현재어간과 뜻을 밝힌다.

그리스어사전의 동사 표기 예

ly-ō	나는 풀어준다	직설법 현재 단수 일인칭, 정형 능동태, ō 동사
lou-ō	나는 씻어준다	직설법 현재 단수 일인칭, 정형 능동태, ō 동사
didō-mi	나는 준다	직설법 현재 단수 일인칭, 정형 능동태, mi 동사
ei-mi	나는 ~이다/있다	직설법 현재 단수 일인칭, 정형 능동태, mi 동사
erch-omai	나는 간다/온다	직설법 현재 단수 일인칭, 탈형 능동태

gign-omai　　　나는 태어난다　　　직설법 현재 단수 일인칭, 탈형 능동태

현재부정법에 의한 동사 구분

그리스어 동사의 부정법(부정사, *infinitive*)이란 수와 인칭이 정해지지 않은 동사 형태이며, 형과 태(정형 능동태·정형 중간태·정형 수동태·탈형 능동태), ō 동사와 mi 동사, 시제(현재·미래·부정과거·현재완료)에 따라 어미를 달리한다. 라틴어 동사의 부정법에 해당한다. 현재부정법의 어미는 (1) 정형 능동태 ō 동사의 경우에는 -ein이고, (2) 정형 능동태 mi 동사의 경우에는 -nai이며, (3) 정형 중간태, 정형 수동태, 탈형 능동태 동사의 경우에는 -esthai이다. 어원론에서는, 그리스어사전에서처럼 동사의 직설법 현재 단수 일인칭을 제시함으로써 현재어간과 뜻을 밝히기도 하나, 현재부정법을 제시함으로써 현재어간과 뜻을 밝히는 것이 일반적이다.

어원론의 그리스어 동사 표기 예

ly-ein	풀기는, 풀기를	현재부정법, 정형 능동태, ō 동사
lou-ein	씻기는, 씻기를	현재부정법, 정형 능동태, ō 동사
dido-nai	주기는, 주기를	현재부정법, 정형 능동태, mi 동사
ei-nai	~이기/있기는, ~이기/있기를	현재부정법, 정형 능동태, mi 동사
erch-esthai	가기/오기는, 가기/오기를	현재부정법, 탈형 능동태
gign-esthai	태어나기는, 태어나기를	현재부정법, 탈형 능동태

정형 중간태, 정형 수동태, 탈형 능동태의 구분과 표시

그리스어사전은, 낱말이 만들어지는 과정을 밝히기 위해, 정형 능동태와 함께 정형 중간태나 정형 수동태를 덩달아 보여줄 때가 있다. 또는, 정형 중간태나 정형 수동태로 만들어지는 과정에서 뜻이 바뀌기 때문에 정형 중간태나 정형 수동태가 표제어로 제시될 때가 있다. 이 때에도 그리스어사전은 직설법 현재 단수 일인칭의 꼴을 보여주고, 어원론은 현재부정법을 보여준다.

형과 태에 따른 그리스어 동사의 구분 예

종류	직설법 현재 단수 일인칭	현재부정법	뜻
정형 능동태	skell–ō	skell–ein	*to dry up*
수동태	skell–omai	skell–esthai	*to be dried up*
정형 능동태	phain–ō	phain–ein	*to bring to light, to cause to appear, to show*
수동태	phain–omai	phain–esthai	*to be brought to light, to appear*
정형 능동태	arch–ō	arch–ein	*to lead, to rule*
중간태	arch–omai	arch–esthai	*to begin, to try*
수동태	arch–omai	arch–esthai	*to be ruled*

직설법 현재 단수 일인칭이나 현재부정법 등 현재 시제에서는 정형 중간태, 정형 수동태, 탈형 능동태의 어미가 같다. 그러나 동사의 뜻이 중간, 수동, 능동인지를 보고, 주어진 태 외에 다른 태가 더 있는지를 보면, 동사의 종류를 구분할 수 있다. 그리스어사전이나 어원론은, 얼른 구분되지 않거나 구분을 확실하게 해야 할 필요가 있을 때에는, 그 태를 밝혀 놓는다. *middle*(중간태), *passive*(수동태), *deponent*(탈형 능동태) 등으로 표시해 놓는 것이다.

그리스어 동사에서 태의 표시 예

태	표시	직설법 현재 단수 일인칭	현재부정법	뜻
정형 능동태	표시 않음	arch–ō	arch–ein	*to lead, to rule*
중간태	*middle*	arch–omai	arch–esthai	*to begin, to try*
수동태	*passive*	arch–omai	arch–esthai	*to be ruled*
탈형 능동태	*deponent*	erch–omai	erch–esthai	*to go, to come*

단축동사

모음 ε, α, ο으로 끝나는 어간에 모음으로 시작하는 어미가 붙을 때에는 두 모음이 하나의 장모음이나 하나의 이중모음으로 단축된다. 단축동사(*contracted verb*)라고 한다. 모음 단축은 직설법 현재 단수 일인칭과 현재부정법의 경우에도 일어나므로, 모음이 어떻게 단축되는지를 알고 있어야 동사의 본디 꼴을 찾을 수 있다. 어원론에 따라서는 일부러 단축시키지 않은 꼴을 싣기도 한다.

단축동사의 정형 능동태 현재부정법 어미에는 -ein (< -e- + -ein), -an (< -a- + -ein), -oun (< -o- + -ein)이 있으며 정형 중간태와 정형 수동태의 현재부정법 어미는 각각 -eisthai, -asthai와 -ousthai이다.

그리스어 단축동사의 현재부정법 예

정형 능동태 (단축형)	정형 능동태 (원형)	정형 중간태	정형 수동태	뜻
phil–ein	phile–ein	phil–eisthai	phil–eisthai	*to love*
sp–an	spa–ein	sp–asthai	sp–asthai	*to draw*
zyg–oun	zygo–ein	zyg–ousthai	zyg–ousthai	*to yoke*

형과 태에 따른 동사의 어미

이상을 다음과 같이 정리할 수 있다. 그리스어사전이나 어원론이 표시하는 동사 어미에는 (1) -ō/-ein (-ein, -an, -oun), (2) -mi/-nai, (3) -omai/-esthai (-eisthai, -asthai, -ousthai)의 세 가지가 있는 것이다.

그리스어사전과 어원론에서 표시하는 동사 어미의 종류

형	태	ō, mi 동사	직설법 현재 단수 일인칭 (그리스어사전)	현재부정법 (어원론)		
정형	능동태	ō 동사	–ō	–ein		
				–ein	<	–e–ein
				–an	<	–a–ein
				–oun	<	–o–ein
		mi 동사	–mi	–nai		
	중간태, 수동태	ō, mi 동사	–omai	–esthai		
				–eisthai	<	–e–esthai
				–asthai	<	–a–esthai
				–ousthai	<	–o–esthai
탈형	능동태	(해당 안 됨)	–omai	–esthai		
				–eisthai	<	–e–esthai
				–asthai	<	–a–esthai
				–ousthai	<	–o–esthai

분사

분사에는 현재분사, 미래분사, 과거분사, 완료분사의 네 가지가 있다. 동사처럼 태와 시제를 가지고 형용사처럼 성, 수, 격을 가진다. 어원론에서 필요한 분사는 능동태 현재분사이며, 그 변화꼴 중에서는 남성형과 중성형의 단수 주격 및 속격이 필요하다.

einai *to be*

    > ōn, (gen.) ontos (*masculine present participle*) *being*   **E** *-ont*

    > on, (gen.) ontos (*neuter present participle*) *being*   **E** *ont(o)-, ontogeny*

        > L. ontologia, ontologiae, f. (< G. ont(o)– + –logia *study*)

            존재론   **E** *ontology*

    < IE. es– *to be* (Vide ESSE: *See* E. *esse*)

schizein *to split, to cleave, to separate*

> schizōn, (gen.) schizontos (*masculine present participle*)

splitting

E *schizont*

< IE. skei- *to cut, to split*

< IE. sek- *to cut* (Vide SECARE: *See* E. *secant*)

bioun (bioein) *to live*

> symbioun (symbioein) (< sym- (< syn) *with, together*)

to live together

> symbiōn, (gen.) symbiountos (*masculine present participle*)

living together

E *symbiont*

< bios, biou, m. *life*

< IE. gʷeiə-, gʷei- *to live* (Vide VIVĔRE: *See* E. *vivarium*)

능동태 현재분사는, 규칙동사의 경우, 현재어간에다 영어 *be* 동사에 해당하는 einai 동사의 현재분사를 그대로 갖다 붙여 만든다. 어미변화는 형용사 제 1·3 변화를 따른다. 불규칙동사의 경우에는 사전에 의존할 수밖에 없다.

einai *to live*

능동태	부정법	현재			ei-nai	이다, 있다	
	직설법	현재	단수	일인칭	ei-mi	나는 ~이다, 있다	
	분 사	현재	단수	주 격	ōn (m.)	ousa (f.) ~인, ~있는	on (n.)
				속 격	ontos	ousēs	ontos

lyein *to loosen*

능동태	부정법	현재			ly-ein	풀어주다	
	직설법	현재	단수	일인칭	ly-ō	나는 ~한다	
	분 사	현재	단수	주 격	ly-ōn (m.)	ly-ousa (f.) ~하는, ~하고 있는	ly-on (n.)
				속 격	ly-ontos	ly-ousēs	ly-ontos

동사의 본디 어간

　직설법 현재 단수 일인칭이나 현재부정법에서 어미를 떼어내고 남은 부분이 현재어간이다. 그러나 동사 중에는 불규칙 동사가 있어 현재어간으로는 본디 어간을 알 수 없는 동사가 있다. 수는 적지만 자주 사용하는 동사일수록 그러하다. 그런 동사의 본디 어간을 알려면 부정과거(不定過去, *aorist*)의 어간을 보아야 한다. 본디 어간이 현재 시제에서는 바뀌었으나 부정과거 시제에서는 바뀌지 않고 쓰여 왔기 때문이다.

　그리스어사전은 불규칙동사의 부정과거형을 제시해주나 영어사전은 제시해주지 않는다. 대신 영어사전은 별도로 본디 어간을 제시해 준다. 다음 예는 '배우다'라는 동사 manthanein의 부정과거어간이 math-이며 파생어나 합성어가 math-를 축으로 만들어짐을 보여준다.

manthanein (math- *aorist stem*) *to learn*　　　　　　　　　　　E *polymath*
　　　> mathēma, mathēmatos, n. (< -ma *resultative noun suffix*) *what is*
　　　　　learned, the act of learning, learning, knowledge
　　　　　　> mathēmatikos, mathēmatikē, mathēmatikon (< -ikos *adjective*
　　　　　　　suffix) *inclined to learn, mathematical*　　E *mathematical, mathematics*
　　< IE. mendh- *to learn* (Vide MEMINISSE; *See* E. *comment*)

　드물지만 현재어간이 아닌 부정과거 어간에 현재부정법의 어미를 붙인 부정과거 부정법(*aorist infinitive*)을 제시하는 경우가 있다.

부정과거부정법의 제시 예

직설법 현재 단수 일인칭	부정과거 부정법	뜻
bleph-ō	id-ein	*to see*
hor-ō	id-ein	*to see*
esthi-ō	phag-ein	*to eat*

동사변화

••• 정형 ō 동사

능동태 현재부정법이 –ein (–ein, –an, –oun)으로, 능동태 직설법 현재 단수 일인칭이 –ō 로 끝나는 동사. 능동태 직설법 현재 복수 삼인칭의 (n)은 'movable (n)'이다.

lyein *to loosen, to release, to dissolve*

능동태	부정법	현재			ly-ein	풀어주다
	직설법	현재	단수	일인칭	ly-ō	나는 ~한다
				이인칭	ly-eis	너는 ~한다
				삼인칭	ly-ei	그는 ~한다
			복수	일인칭	ly-omen	우리는 ~한다
				이인칭	ly-ete	너희는 ~한다
				삼인칭	ly-ousi(n)	그들은 ~한다
	분 사	현재	단수	주 격	ly-ōn (m.)	ly-ousa (f.) ly-on (n.)
						~하는, ~하고 있는
				속 격	ly-ontos	ly-ousēs ly-ontos
중간태	부정법	현재			ly-esthai	(주어가 주어에게) 풀어주다
수동태	부정법	현재			ly-esthai	풀리우다

lyein *to loosen, to release, to dissolve*

< IE. leu– *to loosen, to divide, to cut* (Vide LYSIS; *See* E. *lysis*)

aeidein ((*Attic*) aidein) *to sing, to praise*

> aoidē, aoidēs, f. ((*Attic*) ōidē, ōidēs, f.) *song, myth, legend*

> L. oda, odae, f. (ode, odes, f.) 노래, 송가(頌歌), 송시(頌詩)　　**E** *ode*

> ōideion, ōideiou, n. *a public building in Athens for musical performance*

> L. odeum, odei, n. 음악당　　**E** *odeum*

> melōidia, melōidias, f. (< melos *song* + ōidē *song*) *singing, chanting, choral song, music*

> L. melodia, melodiae, f. 선율　　**E** *melody*

> monōidia, monōidias, f. (< monos *alone* + ōidē *song*) *solo, lament*

> L. monodia, monodiae, f. 독창곡, 애가, 비가   **E** *monody*

> parōidia, parōidias, f. (< par(a)- *beside, along side of, beyond* + ōidē *song*) *parody*

> L. parodia, parodiae, f. 풍자적 변곡, 풍자적 시문   **E** *parody*

> prosōidia, prosōidias, f. (< pros- *towards, near, beside(s)* + ōidē *song*) *song sung to music, pronunciation of syllable*

> L. prosodia, prosodiae, f. 운율체계, 운율, 작시법   **E** *prosody*

> rhapsōidia, rhapsōidias, f. (< rhaptein *to sew, to stitch* + ōidē *song*) *the recitation of epic poetry*

> L. rhapsodia, rhapsodiae, f. 음송 서사시, 열광적이며 엉뚱한 시가; (음악) 광시곡   **E** *rhapsody*

> tragōidia, tragōidias, f. (< (*suggested*) *goatskin dress of the performers, representing satyrs; goat-song* < tragos *he-goat* + ōidē *song*) *tragedy*

> L. tragoedia, tragoediae, f. 비극   **E** *tragedy*

> aoidos, aoidou, m., f. ((*Attic*) ōidos, ōidou, m.) *singer, poet, enchanter*

> kōmōidia, kōmōidias, f. (< kōmos *merry-making* + aoidos *singer*) *comedy*

> L. comoedia, comoediae, f. 희극   **E** *comedy*

< IE. wed- *to speak*

akouein *to hear*

> akousis, akouseōs, f. *hearing*

> L. diplacusis, diplacusis, f. (< G. diploos *double*) 복청(複聽), 겹듣기   **E** *diplacusis*

> L. hyperacusis, hyperacusis, f. (< G. hyper- *over*) 청각과민   **E** *hyperacusis*

> L. hypacusis, hypacusis, f. (< G. hyp(o)- *under*) 청각장애, 난청   **E** *hypacusis (hypoacusis)*

> L. paracusis, paracusis, f. (< G. par(a)- *beside, along side of, beyond*) 청각이상   **E** *paracusis*

> L. presbyacusis, presbyacusis, f. (< G. presbys *old man, elder*) 노인성 난청   **E** *presbyacusis (presbycusis, presbyacusia)*

> akoustikos, akoustikē, akoustikon *pertaining to hearing*   **E** *acoustic*

< IE. kous- *to hear*   **E** *hear*

alexein *to protect*   **E** *alexin*

< IE. lek- *to ward off, to protect*

> G. Alexandros, Alexandrou, m. (< + IE. ner- *man*) *Alexander*

> L. Alexander, Alexandri, m. 알렉산더   **E** *Alexander*

arassein *to strike, to knock, to hammer, to dash*

> katarassein (< kat(a)- *down, mis-, according to, along, thoroughly* + arassein) *to dash down, to smash, to push back*

> kataraktēs, kataraktou, m. (katarraktēs, katarraktou, m.) *down-rushing, water-*
>> *fall, portcullis, (possibly) floodgate*
>>> L. cataracta, cataractae, f. (cataractes, cataractae, m.) 폭포, 내리닫이
>>>> 성문(城門), 수문(水門)
>>>>> **E** *cataract* (<(perhaps) 'the cataract obstructs vision, as the portcullis does a gateway')*

archein *to lead, to rule;* **archesthai** (*middle*) *to begin, to try*

> archos, archou, m. *leader, chief*

>> **E** *arch(i)-, archangel, archfiend, architect, archipelago* (< 'sea studded with islands' < 'the Aegean Sea' < 'the chief sea')

> monarchos, monarchou, m. (< monos *alone*) *monarch*

>> monarchēs, monarchou, m. *monarch*

>>> L. monarcha, monarchae, m. 군주 **E** *monarch*

>> monarchia, monarchias, f. *monarchy*

>>> L. monarchia, monarchiae, f. 군주정치, 군주국 **E** *monarchy*

> anarchia, anarchias, f. (< an- *not*) *state without a chief or head*

>> L. anarchia, anarchiae, f. 무정부상태 **E** *anarchy*

> -archēs, -archou, m. *ruling, ruler* **E** *-archy, patriarchy, ('patriarchy' >) matriarchy*

>> hierarchēs, hierarchou, m. (< hieros *sacred*) *steward or president of sacred*

>>> *rites, high priest*

>>> L. hierarcha, hierarchae, m. 제사장(祭司長), 고위 성직자 **E** *hierarch, hierarchical*

>>> hierarchia, hierarchias, f. *the power or rule of a hierarch*

>>>> L. hierarchia, hierarchiae, f. 천사의 계급(3급 9품), 천사단, 성직의
>>>> 위계(位階)제도, 계급제도; (생물) 분류체계 **E** *hierarchy*

> archē, archēs, f. *beginning, principle, power, rule,*

>> *magistracy* **E** *arch(e)- (archi-), archencephalon, archenteron, -arche, thelarche*

>> archaios, archaia, archaion *ancient,*

>>> *primitive* **E** *archae(o)- (arche(o)-), archaeology, Archaeozoic, archaeopteryx*

>>> L. Archaea, Archaeorum, n. (*neuter* pl.)

>>>> 고세균(古細菌) **E** *Archaea, (Archaea >) (neuter sing.) archaeon, archaean*

>>> archaikos, archaikē, archaikon *old-fashioned* **E** *archaic*

>>> archaizein *to copy the ancients (in languages, etc.)* **E** *archaize*

>> archeion, archeiou, n. *senate house, town hall*

>>> L. archium, archii, n. (archivum, archivi, n.) 기록보관소 **E** (pl.) *archives, archival*

>> archetypon, archetypou, n. (< + typos *blow, mold, die*) *archetype*

>>> L. archetypum, archetypi, n. 원형(原型), 본, 원본 **E** *archetype*

> L. menarche, menarches, f. (< G. mēn *month*) 초경(初經),
>> 첫월경 **E** *menarche, menarcheal (menarchial)*

blepein *to see, to look at*

> blepsis, blepseōs, f. *sight*

> parablepsis, parablepseōs, f. (< par(a)- *beside, along side of, beyond*) *looking askance at*

> parablepsia, parablepsiae, f. 이상시각, 착시　　　**E** *parablepsia*

boskein *to feed, to graze*

> botanē, botanēs, f. *plant, herb*

> botanikos, botanikē, botanikon *of plant, of herb*

> L. botanicus, botanica, botanicum 식물의, 식물학의　　**E** *botanic, (botanic >) botanical, (botanic >) botany, botanist*

> proboskis, proboskidos, f. (< pro- *before, in front* + boskein) (< *means of obtaining food*) *proboscis*

> L. proboscis, proboscidis, f. (개·돼지 등 코를 포함한) 내민 주둥이, 코끼리 코　**E** *proboscis*

< IE. gʷo- *to feed*

bryein *to swell with, to grow*

> embryon, embryou, n. (< em- (< en) *in* + bryein) *young animal, the fruit of the womb before birth*

> L. embryo, embryonis, m. 배(胚), 배아(胚芽), 자충(子蟲)　**E** *embryo, (pl.) embryos, embryonic, embryonal, embryoid, embryology*

brychein (brykein) (ebryxa *aorist root*) *to eat greedily, to grind teeth*

> brychē, brychēs, f. *grinding of teeth*　　　**E** *bruxism*

chezein *to defecate*

> L. *haematochezia, *haematocheziae, f. (< G. haima, haimatos, n. *blood*) 혈변배설　　　**E** *hematochezia*

< IE. ghed-, ghod- *hole, to defecate*　　**E** *(perhaps) gate (< 'opening'), gating, gateway*

didaskein *to teach, to instruct*

> didactos, didactē, didacton *taught, instructed*　　**E** *autodidact (< 'a self-taught person')*

> didactikos, didactikē, didactikon *skilled at teaching*　　**E** *didactic*

<IE. dens- *to use mental force*

dramein *to run*

> dromos, dromou, m. *running, race, race-course*

> L. dromos, dromi, m. (dromus, dromi, m.) 경주, 경주장

E *-drome, motordrome, aerodrome (drome), anadromous (< 'migrating up rivers from the sea to spawn'), catadromous (< 'migrating down rivers to the sea to spawn'), dromotropism (< 'affecting the conductivity of a nerve fiber')*

> hippodromos, hippodromou, m. (< hippos *horse*) *race-course for chariots*

> L. hippodromos, hippodromi, m. (hippodromus, hippodromi, m.) 이륜

마차 경주장, 경마장   **E** *hippodrome*

> prodromos, prodromou, m. (< pro- *before, in front*) *forerunner*

> L. prodromus, prodromi, m. 사자(使者), 선구자(先驅者),

전구증상(前驅症狀)   **E** *prodrome, prodromic (prodromal)*

> palindromos, palindromos, palindromon (< palin *back, backwards, again*)

running back again, recurring   **E** *palindrome, palindromic*

> syndromos, syndromos, syndromon (< syn- *with, together*) *running together,*

concurrent

> syndromē, syndromēs, f. *concourse*

> L. syndrome, syndromes, f. (< *concurrence of signs and symptoms*)

증후군(症候群)   **E** *syndrome, syndromic*

> dromas, dromados, m. *runner*

> L. dromedarius, dromedarii, m. 단봉낙타   **E** *dromedary*

< IE. der- *to run, to walk, to step*

  E *tread, treadmill, treadle, trade, trap* (< '*stair*'), *trap* (< '*snare*'), *entrap, trip, tramp, trample, trot*

elaunein *to drive* (< *to cause to go*), *to beat out* (metal)

> elasis, elaseōs, f. *driving, beating out*

> elastikos, elastikē, elastikon *that drives, propulsive, impulsive*

> L. elasticus, elastica, elasticum (< *originally describing a gas in the*

sense 'expanding spontaneously to fill the available space') 원래

대로 되돌아가게 하는, 신축성 있는, 융통성 있는, 탄력(彈力)의, 탄성의,

탄력성의   **E** *elastic, elasticity, elastin,* (*elastic* >) *elastance*

> elasmos, elasmou, m. *metal beaten out, metal plate*

> L. elasmobranchii, elasmobranchiorum, m. (pl.) (< + G. (pl.) branchia *gills*)

(상어 · 가오리 등) 판새류(板鰓類)   **E** *elasmobranch*

> elasma, elasmatos, n. *metal beaten out, metal plate*

> L. xanthelasma, xanthelasmatis, n. (< G. xanthos *yellow, red-yellow*) 황색

판종(黃色板腫)   **E** *xanthelasma* (< '*planar xanthoma*')

< IE. elə- *to go*

gargarizein *to gargle*

< IE. gard- *echoic root*

  E *gargle, gargoyle* (< '*waterspout of grotesque figure*' < '*throat*'), (*gargoyle* > '*gargoyle-like facies*' >) *gargoylism*

> Sp. garganta *throat, gullet*   **E** *Gargantua*

gemizein *to fill, to load*

> gemistos, gemistē, gemiston *full, laden*

E *gemistocyte*

glyphein *to carve, to engrave*

> glyphē, glyphēs, f. *carving, carved work*

E *glyph, dermatoglyph*

> hieroglyphikos, hieroglyphikos, hieroglyphikon (< hieros *sacred* + glyphē

carving) *hieroglyphic*

> L. hieroglyphicus, hieroglyphica, hieroglyphicum 신성(神聖) 문자의,

상형(象形) 문자의

E *hieroglyphic, (hieroglyphic >) hieroglyph*

> glyptēs, glyptou, m. *carver*

E *glyptic, glyptograph*

< IE. gleubh– *to tear apart, to cleave*

E *cleave, cleavage, cleft, clever (< 'skillful')*

graphein *to scratch, to draw, to write*

E *graphite*

> graphē, graphēs, f. *drawing, writing*

> graphikos, graphikē, graphikon *of drawing, of writing*

> L. graphicus, graphica, graphicum 새겨진, 그려진,

쓰인

E *graphic, (graphic formula >) graph*

> graphion, graphiou, n. (grapheion, grapheiou, n.) *stylus*

> L. graphium, graphii, n. 첨필(尖筆)

E *graft (< 'with reference to the tapered tip of the scion; the final –t is due to phonetic confusion'), engraft, autograft (< 'self'), isograft (< 'equal'), allograft (< 'other'), xenograft (< 'foreign'); It. graffito, (pl.) graffiti*

> –graphos, –graphou, m. *one who draws or writes*

–graphos, –graphē, –graphon *drawn, written*

E *–graph, glyptograph (< 'drawn by carving'), idiograph (< 'one's private mark or signature'), photograph, photomicrograph, microphotograph, monograph, polygraph; radiograph*

> paragraphos, paragraphou, m., f. (< par(a)– *beside, along side of, beyond*)

a short stroke marking a break in sense

> L. paragraphus, paragraphi, m., f. 절(節), 항(項)

E *paragraph*

> –graphia, –graphias, f. *drawing, writing*

E *–graphy, chromatography (< 'originally, showing colored bands of the separated plant pigments'), cymography (kymography) (< 'drawing in curves'), demography (< 'writing of people'), echocardiography (< 'recording of heart with reflected ultrasound'), tomography (< 'recording of cut section')*

> eikonographia, eikonographias, f. (< eikōn *image*) *the description*

or illustration of any subject by means of drawings or figures

> L. iconographia, iconographiae, f. 도상(圖像)

E *iconography*

> geōgraphia, geōgraphias, f. (< gē *earth*) *geography*

> L. geographia, geographiae, f. 지리, 지리학

E *geography*

> topographia, topographias, f. (< topos *place*) *topography*

> L. topographia, topographiae, f. 지형, 지세, 지지(地誌); 국소 해부학

E *topography*

> kalligraphia, kalligraphias, f. (< kallos *beauty*) *calligraphy*

> L. calligraphia, calligraphiae, f. 달필, 서예   **E** *calligraphy*

> kakographia, kakographias, f. (< kakos *bad*) *cacography*

> L. cacographia, cacographiae, f. 악필, 오기(誤記)   **E** *cacography*

> L. lithographia, lithographiae, f. (< G. lithos *stone*) 석판술, 석판인쇄   **E** *lithography*

> L. agraphia, agraphiae, f. (< G. a- *not*) 쓰기언어상실증, 실서증(失書症)   **E** *agraphia*

> gramma, grammatos, n. (< -ma *resultative noun suffix*) *thing written, letter of*

alphabet

E *-gram, cladogram* (< 'a dendrogram illustrating the supposed evolutionary relationships between clades'), *cryptogram* (< 'hidden letter'), *dactylogram* (< 'finger print'), *dendrogram* (< 'tree diagram'), *electrophoretogram (electropherogram)* (< 'written result of electrophoresis'), *histogram* (< 'graphical representation by columns which are set upright'), *hologram* (< 'wholly written'), *ideogram* (< 'written idea'), *idiogram* (< 'a diagrammatic representation of a chromosome complement, based on measurement of the chromosomes of a number of cells' < 'one's private mark'), *nomogram (nomograph)* (< 'a graphic table for computation' < 'law'), *phonogram* (< 'written sound'), (phonogram > (arbitrary inversion) >) *gramophone*, (gramophone >) *Grammy, sialogram* (< 'radiograph of salivary ducts'), *sphenogram* (< 'cuneiform letter'); *pictogram* (< 'written picture'), *scintigram* (< 'written scintillation')

> grammatikos, grammatikē, grammatikon *knowing how to read and write*

> L. grammaticus, grammatica, grammaticum 문법의

E (G. grammatikē technē > L. grammatica ars 'grammatical art' >) *grammar, glamour* (< 'magic, an occult learning' < 'Scottish variant of grammar')

> L. grammaticalis, grammaticale 문법의   **E** *grammatical*

> tetragrammatos, tetragrammatos, tetragrammaton (< tetr(a)- *four*) *four-lettered*

> tetragrammaton, tetragrammatou, n. *a word of four-letters;* (Tetragrammaton) *the Hebrew word written YHWH or JHVH as a symbol of the name of God*   **E** *tetragrammaton*

> L. gramma, grammatis, n. (< *what is drawn or written*) 그램(무게 단위, *weight of two oboli*), 작은 무게   **E** *gramme (gram, g)*

> grammē, grammēs, f. *stroke, line in writing, line*

> parallēlogrammon, parallēlogrammou, n. (< parallēlos *parallel* + grammē *line*) *parallelogram*

> L. parallelogrammum, parallelogrammi, n. 평행사변형   **E** *parallelogram*

> anagraphein (< an(a)- *up, upward; again, throughout; back, backward; against; according to, similar to*) *to write up, to write back, to write anew*

> L. anagramma, anagrammatis, n. 철자 순서를 바꾸어 만든 말   **E** *anagram*

> diagraphein (< di(a)- *through, thoroughly, apart*) *to mark out by lines, to draw, to draw out, to write in a register*

> diagramma, diagrammatos, n. *that which is marked out by lines, a geometrical figure, written list, register, the gamut or scale in music*

> L. diagramma, diagrammatis, n. 그림표, 도표(圖表), 도(圖)   **E** *diagram*

> epigraphein (< ep(i)- *upon*) *to write upon*

> epigraphē, epigraphēs, f. *the heading of a document of letter*

> L. epigraphe, epigraphes, f. 명(銘), 제명(題銘); 비명(碑銘), 비문(碑文)　**E** *epigraph*

> epigramma, epigrammatos, n. *a short poem ending in a witty or ingenious*
turn of thought, to which the rest of the composition is intended to lead up

> L. epigramma, epigrammatis, n. 경구(警句), 경구적 표현, (짧은) 풍자시　**E** *epigram*

> prographein (< pro– *before, in front*) *to write publicly*

> programma, programmatos, n. *order of the day, agenda, public written notice,*
proclamation, edict

> L. programma, programmatis, n. 공고문, 포고, 진행순서표, 계획표　**E** *program*

< IE. gerbh– *to scratch*　**E** *carve, crab, crawl*

hamartanein *to err, to fail, to sin*

> hamartia, hamartias, f. *error, fault, failure, guilt; the error or fault which entails*
the destruction of the tragic hero, with particular reference to Aristotle's Poetics　**E** *hamartia*

> L. hamartoma, hamartomatis, n. (< + G. –ōma *noun suffix denoting tumor*)
과오종(過誤腫)　**E** *hamartoma*

hepsein *to boil*

> kathepsein (< kath– (< kata) *down, mis–, according to, along, thoroughly* + hepsein)
to boil down, to digest　**E** *cathepsin*

heuriskein *to find*　**E** (heurēka (*first personal singular perfect*) '*I have found*' >) *eureka, heuristic*

< IE. werə– *to find*

iaptein *to assail*

> iambos, iambou, m. (< *the metric foot being first used, according to tradition, by*
the Greek satiric writers Archilochus and Hipponax) *iambus*

> L. iambus, iambi, m. 단장격(短長格), 약강격(弱强格)　**E** *iambus (iamb), iambic*

< *Of* non–IE. *origin*

kleiein *to praise, to tell, to celebrate*

> Kleiō, Kleious, f. (< *fame*) (*Greek mythology*) *the Muse of epic poetry and history;*
also a sea–nymph, sister of Beroe

> L. Clio, Clius, f. (그리스 신화) 역사를 주관하는 뮤즈　**E** *Clio*

< IE. kleu– *to hear*　**E** *listen, loud, leer (< 'side of face' < 'ear')*

> G. –klēs, –klou, m. (*earlier* –kleēs) '*fame*', *in Greek personal names*　**E** *–cles*

> G. Empedoklēs, Empedoklou, m. (< *having lasting fame* < empedos *on the*
ground, firmly set, lasting < em– (< en) *in* + pedon *ground*) *Empedocles*　**E** *Empedocles*

> G. Hēraklēs, Hēraklou, m. (< *having Hera's fame* < Hēra *Hera*) *Heracles*　**E** *Heracles*

> L. Hercules, Herculi, m. (Hercules, Herculis, m.) 헤라클레스　　**E** *Hercules*

> G. Periklēs, Periklou, m. (< *far-famed* < peri- *around, near, beyond, on account of*) *Pericles*　　**E** *Pericles*

> G. Sophoklēs, Sophokou, m. (< *famed for wisdom* < sophos *wise*) *Sophocles*　　**E** *Sophocles*

> G. Themistoklēs (< *famed in law and right* < themis, themistos, f. *custom, law, right*) *Themistocles*　　**E** *Themistocles*

> D. Laut, Laut(e)s, m. 소리, 목소리

> D. Ablaut, Ablaut(e)s, m. (< ab- *off* + Laut *sound*) 전모음(轉母音), 모음교체, 모음전환, 아블라우트(간모음의 규칙적 변화, 특히 동사의 강변화)　　**E** *ablaut*

> D. Umlaut, Umlaut(e)s, m. (< um- *about* + Laut *sound*) 변모음(變母音; ä, ö, ü, äu), 변음, 모음변이, 움라우트　　**E** *umlaut*

kryptein *to hide*

> kryptos, kryptē, krypton *hidden*

> **E** (*neuter* sing.) **krypton (Kr)** (< *'difficulty in isolating the element'*), **crypt(o)-, cryptogram** (< *'hidden letter'*), **cryptonym** (< *'hidden name'*), **cryptozoology, cryptogam, cryptogenic; encrypt, encryption, decrypt, decryption**

> kryptikos, kryptikē, kryptikon *hidden*

> L. crypticus, cryptica, crypticum 숨은　　**E** *cryptic*

> L. cryptorchismus, cryptorchismi, m. (cryptorchidismus, cryptorchidismi, m.) (< + G. orchis *testis* + -ismos *noun suffix*) 잠복고환증　　**E** *cryptorchism (cryptorchidism)*

> L. Cryptococcus, Cryptococci, m. (< *The organisms usually have a capsule and do not form a pseudomycelium.* < + G. kokkos *grain, berry*) (효모상 진균) 크립토콕쿠스속(屬)　　**E** *Cryptococcus*

> L. Cryptosporidium, Cryptosporidii, n. (< *hidden little spore* < + -sporidium < G. spora *spore* + -idion *diminutive suffix*) (포자충 胞子蟲) 크립토스포리듐속(屬), 와포자충속(窩胞子蟲屬)　　**E** *Cryptosporidium*

> kryptē, kryptēs, f. *crypt, vault*

> L. crypta, cryptae, f. 움, 토굴, 막힌 틈, 지하실　　**E** *crypt, grotto, grotesque*

> apokryptein (< ap(o)- *away from, from*) *to hide away*

> apokryphos, apokryphos, apokryphon *hidden, of unknown authorship, spurious*

> L. apocriphus, apocripha, apocriphum 외전(外典)의, 위경(僞經)의　　**E** (*neuter* pl.) (apocripha scripta *'hidden writings'* >) *Apocrypha*

< IE. krau- *to conceal, to hide*

lambanein (lēph- *root*) *to take, to seize, to assume*

> labē, labēs, f. *hand, hilt, hold*

> **E** **erythrolabe** (< *'red cone opsin'*), **chlorolabe** (< *'green cone opsin'*), **cyanolabe** (< *'blue cone opsin'*)

> lēpsis, lēpseōs, f. *taking, seizing, receiving*

> **E** *-lepsy* (< *'on the pattern of epilepsy'*), **narcolepsy, nympholepsy, psycholepsy, neurolepsy**

> lēmma, lēmmatos, n. *premise, assumption*

> L. lemma, lemmatis, n. 명제, 주제   **E** *lemma*

> dilēmma, dilēmmatos, n. (< *di- two*) *double proposition*

> L. dilemma, dilemmatis, n. 양도논법(兩刀論法), 진퇴양난,

궁지   **E** *dilemma, (dilemma >) trilemma*

> epilambanein (< *ep(i)- upon*) *to seize upon*

> epilēpsia, epilēpsias, f. *epilepsy*

> L. epilepsia, epilepsiae, f. 뇌전증(腦電症), 간질(癎疾), 전간(癲癇),

지랄병   **E** *epilepsy*

> epilēptikos, epilēptikos, epilēptikon *of epilepsy*

> L. epilepticus, epileptica, epilepticum 뇌전증의   **E** *epileptic, antiepileptic*

> analambanein (< *an(a)- up, upward; again, throughout; back, backward; against; according to, similar to*) *to take up*   **E** *analeptic*

> analēpsis, analēpseōs, f. *taking up*

> L. analepsia, analepsiae, f. 체력 회복, 강장(强壯), 각성(覺醒)   **E** *analepsy*

> katalambanein (< *kat(a)- down, mis-, according to, along, thoroughly*) *to seize down*   **E** *cataleptic*

> katalēpsis, katalēpseōs, f. *seizing down*

> L. catalepsia, catalepsiae, f. 강경증(强硬症)   **E** *catalepsy*

> syllambanein (< *syl-* (< *syn*) *with, together*) *to take together*

> syllabē, syllabēs, f. *syllable*

> L. syllaba, syllabae, f. (< *word element pronounced as a unit*)

음절   **E** *syllable, syllabic, syllabication (syllabification)*

> astrolabon, astrolabou, n. (< *astron star*) *taking the position of stars, celestial sphere*

> L. astrolabium, astrolabii, n. 천체 관측기   **E** *astrolabe*

< IE. (s)lag^w- *to seize*   **E** *latch*

lampein *to shine*   **E** *lamp, lantern*

> eklampein (< *ek- out of, away from*) *to shine forth*

> eklampsis, eklampseōs, f. *shining forth, sudden development*

> L. eclampsia, eclampsiae, f. (< *seizures seem to arrive as a flash of lightning out of the blue or flashes of light seen before the eyes*)

자간(子癎)   **E** *eclampsia, eclamptic, pre-eclampsia*

< IE. lap- *to light, to burn*

pauein *to stop, to check;* **pauesthai** (*middle, passive*) *to come to an end, to rest*

> pausis, pauseōs, f. *cessation*

> L. pauso, **pausavi**, pausatum, pausare 서다, 쉬다, 놓다

> **E** (*verb*) **pause, pose,** *(pose > 'meaning influenced by* componère *to put together'* >) **compose,** *(pose >)* **depose,** *(pose >)* **juxtapose;** *(compose >)* **decompose, decomposition**

> L. pausa, pausae, f. 쉼, 휴지(休止), 중단   **E** (*noun*) **pause,** *(pause >)* **diapause**

> L. menopausis, menopausis, f. (< G. mēn *month* + pausis)

폐경(閉經), 폐경기(閉經期)

> **E** **menopause, menopausal, premenopausal, perimenopausal, postmenopausal**

< IE. paus- *to leave, to desert, to cease, to stop*

pempein *to send*

> pompē, pompēs, f. *sending, procession, display*

> L. pompa, pompae, f. (화려하고 성대한) 행렬, 호화, 과시   **E** **pomp**

> L. pomposus, pomposa, pomposum 호화스런, 과시하는   **E** **pompous**

phagein (*aorist infinitive of* esthiein *to eat*) (< *to have a share of food*)

to eat   **E** **phag(o)-, phagocyte,** *(phagocyte >)* **phagocytize** *(phagocytose),* **phagosome**

> oisophagos, oisophagou, m. (< oisein (*future infinitive of* pherein *to carry*) + phagein *to eat*) *gullet*

> L. oesophagus, oesophagi, m. 식도(食道)

> **E** **oesophagus (esophagus), esophageal, oesophag(o)- (esophag(o)-), esophagogastric**

> anthrōpophagos, anthrōpophagos, anthrōpophagon (< anthrōpos *man* + phagein *to eat*) *man-eating*

> anthrōpophagos, anthrōpophagou, m. *man-eater*

> L. anthropophagus, anthropophagi, m.

식인종   **E** **anthropophagus,** (pl.) **anthropophagi, anthropophagous**

> anthrōpophagia, anthrōpophagias, f. *the eating of man, cannibalism*

> L. anthropophagia, anthropophagiae, f. 식인, 식인 풍습   **E** **anthropophagy**

> sarkophagos, sarkophagos, sarkophagon (< sarx *flesh* + phagein *to eat*) *flesh-eating*

> sarkophagos, sarkophagou, m. (< *a kind of stone reputed among the Greeks to have the property of consuming the flesh of dead bodies deposited in it and consequently used for coffins*) *sarcophagus*

> L. sarcophagus, sarcophagi, m. (조각 · 비문으로 장식한)

석관(石棺)   **E** **sarcophagus, sarcophagous**

> -phagos, -phagos, -phagon *-eating*

> L. -phagus, -phaga, -phagum 먹는   **E** **-phagous**

> -phagos, -phagou, m. *-eater*   **E** **-phage, bacteriophage (phage)**

> L. macrophagus, macrophagi, m. (< G. makros *long, large*) 대식(大食)

세포   **E** **macrophage**

> L. microphagus, microphagi, m. (< G. mikros *small*) 소식(小食)세포,

중성구   **E** **microphage**

> -phagia, -phagias, f. *-eating*   **E** *-phagia (-phagy), heterophagy, autophagy*

       > L. aerophagia, aerophagiae, f. (< G. aēr *air*) 공기연하증(嚥下症)   **E** *aerophagia*

       > L. polyphagia, polyphagiae, f. (< G. polys *much*) 다식증(多食症)   **E** *polyphagia*

       > L. dysphagia, dysphagiae, f. (< G. dys- *bad*) 삼킴곤란, 연하(嚥下)곤란,

          연하장애   **E** *dysphagia*

       > L. *odynophagia, *odynophagiae, f. (< G. odynē *pain*)

          연하통(嚥下痛)   **E** *odynophagia (odynphagia)*

     > L. phagocytosis, phagocytosis, f. (< *phagocyte* + G. -ōsis *condition*) 포식(胞食), 포식

       작용   **E** *phagocytosis, (phagocytosis >) phagocytose (phagocytize)*

  < IE. bhag- *to share out, apportion, also to get a share*

    > (*Sanskrit*) pagoda (< *blessed* < *good fortune*) 파고다   **E** *pagoda*

phthinein *to die away*

    > G. phthisis, phthiseōs, f. *decline, perishing, wasting, consumption*

       > L. phthisis, phthisis, f. 소멸, 소모; 황폐증, 쇠약, 위축, 노(癆); 결핵로(結核癆),

          결핵   **E** *phthisis, phthisic, phthisical*

          [용례] phthisis bulbi 안구위축   **E** *phthisis bulbi*

             (문법) phthisis 위축: 단수 주격

                bulbi 안구의: 단수 속격 < bulbus, bulbi, m.

       > L. myelophthisis, myelophthisis, f. (< G. myelos *bone marrow, spinal*

          marrow) 골수황폐증, 척수황폐증   **E** *myelophthisis*

       > L. *nephronophthisis, *nephronophthisis, f. (< *nephron, the structural*

          and functional unit of the kidney) 신장황폐증   **E** *nephronophthisis*

  < IE. dhg^{w}hei- *to perish, to die away*

prattein (*Attic*) (prassein (*non-Attic*)) *to pass through, to achieve, to do*

    > praktikos, praktikē, praktikon *fit for action, active, able*

       > L. practicus, practica, practicum 실행적, 실천적, 실제적   **E** *practical*

          > L. practizo, **practizavi**, practizatum, practizare (< practicare) (이론을)

             실행하다   **E** *practise (practice), malpractice*

       > praktikē, praktikēs, f. *practical (as opposed to theoretical) science*

          > L. practice, practices, f. 실행, 실제   **E** *practician, (practician >) practitioner*

       > chiropraktikos, chiropraktikos, chiropraktikon (< chir(o)- < cheir(o)- < cheir

          hand) *chiropractic*   **E** *chiropractic, chiropractor*

    > praktōr, praktōros, m. *doer*

    > praxis, praxeōs, f. (pragos, prageos, n.) *doing, action*

       > L. praxis, praxis, f. 실행, 실제, 행위, 행동, 동작   **E** *praxis*

       > apraxia, apraxias, f. (< a- *not* + praxis + -ia) *inaction*

          > L. apraxia, apraxiae, f. 행위상실증, 실행증(失行症)   **E** *apraxia*

> L. echopraxia, echopraxiae, f. (< G. ēchō *echo* + praxis + -ia) 동작모방(증)　**E** *echopraxia*

> L. dyspraxia, dyspraxiae, f. (< G. dys- *bad* + praxis + -ia) 통합 운동장애　**E** *dyspraxia*

> L. dyspragia, dyspragiae, f. (< G. dys- *bad* + pragos + -ia) 통증 기능장애　**E** *dyspragia*

> pragma, pragmatos, n. *thing done, deed, business*

> L. pragma, pragmatis, n. 실무, 사무　**E** *pragmatism*

> pragmatikos, pragmatikē, pragmatikon *relating to fact*

> L. pragmaticus, pragmatica, pragmaticum 실무적, 사무적,

실용주의적　**E** *pragmatic, pragmatics*

pseudein *to deceive*

> pseudēs, pseudēs, pseudes *false*

E *pseud(o)-, pseudocyst, pseudoaneurysm; pseudodiverticulum, pseudoscience, pseudo*

psychein *to breathe, to blow, to cool, to refresh*

> psychē, psychēs, f. *breath, spirit, soul, life;* (Psychē) (*Greek mythology*) *a Hellenistic personification of the soul as female, or as a butterfly*

> L. psyche, psychae, f. 심령, 마음, 정신　**E** *psyche, psych(o)-, psychiatry*

> L. Psyche, Psyches, f. (그리스 신화) 프시케　**E** *Psyche*

> psychikos, psychikē, psychikon *spiritual, of soul, of life*

> L. psychicus, psychica, psychicum 심령의, 마음의, 심리적인, 정신의　**E** *psychic*

> metempschychōsis, metempschychōseōs, f. (< met(a)- *between, along with, across, after* + em- (< en) *in* + psychē *soul* + -ōsis *condition*) *transmigration of the soul, passage of the soul from one body to another; especially (chiefly in Pythagoreanism and certain Eastern religions) the trans- migration of the soul of a human being or animal at or after death into a new body of the same or a different species*

> L. metempschychosis, metempschychosis, f. 영혼이체(靈魂移體),

윤회(輪回)　**E** *metempsychosis*

> L. psychologia, psychologiae, f. (< + G. -logia *study*) 심리학　**E** *psychology*

> L. psychosis, psychosis, f. (< + G. -ōsis *condition*) 정신병　**E** *psychosis*

> psychros, psychra, psychron *cold*　**E** *psychr(o)-, psychrophile, psychrotrophic*

< IE. bhes- *to breathe; probably imitative*

ptyssein *to fold, to fold up*

> ptychē, ptychēs, f. *fold, layer, plate (of metal or leather, used to form a shield)*　**E** *polyptychial, monoptychial*

> diptychos, diptychos, diptychon *two-folded*

> L. diptychum, diptychi, n. 둘로 접는 서판(書板, 그 안쪽에 밀초를 먹여

철필로 글을 썼음), 둘로 접는 책자　**E** *diptych, (diptych >) triptych*

> anaptyssein (< an(a)- *up, upward; again, throughout; back, backward; against;*

according to, similar to + ptyssein) *to unfold, to open, to develop*

> anaptyxis, anaptyxeōs, f. *unfolding, opening*

> L. anaptyxis, anaptyxis, f. (자음 사이의) 모음 삽입   **E** *anaptyxis*

seiein *to shake*

> seismos, seismou, m. *earthquake*   **E** *seism, seismic (seismal), seismograph (seismometer)*

< IE. twei- *to agitate, to shake, to toss*   **E** *whittle*

skēptein *to prop, to support, to lean upon a staff*

> skēptron, skēptrou, n. *stick, staff; scepter*

> L. sceptrum, sceptri, n. 왕장(王杖), 권장(權杖), 지휘봉; 왕권, 통치권 **E** *scepter (sceptre)*

stilbein *to shine, to glitter*

> stilbos, stilbē, stilbon *shining*

  E *stilbene, (stilbene derivative with estrogenic properties >) diethylstilbestrol (stilbestrol)*

strephein *to wind, to turn, to twist; (passive) to turn back, to attach oneself to*

> strophē, strophēs, f. *turning*

  E *strophe (< 'the movement of the chorus from right to left during which the choric ode was sung'), antistrophe*

> anastrophein (< an(a)- *up, upward; again, throughout; back, backward; against; according to, similar to* + strephein) *to turn back, to turn over, to return*

> anastrophē, anastrophès, f. *turning back*   **E** *anastrophe*

> apostrephein (< ap(o)- *away from, from* + strephein) *to turn away*

> apostrophos, apostrophou, m. *turning away, elision*

> L. apostrophos, apostrophi, m. (apostrophus, apostrophi, m.)

생략부호(´)   **E** *apostrophe*

> diastrephein (< di(a)- *through, thoroughly, apart* + strephein) *to turn apart*

> diastrophē, diastrophēs, f. *distortion, dislocation*   **E** *diastrophism*

> katastrephein (< kat(a)- *down, mis-, according to, along, thoroughly* + strephein) *to turn over, to overturn, to bring to an end*

> katastrophē, katastrophēs, f. *overturning, end, perdition*

> L. catastropha, catastrophae, f. (catastrophe, catastrophes, f.) 큰 재해, 파국; (연극) 대단원; (지질) 지각변동   **E** *catastrophe*

> *ekstrophia, *ekstrophias, f. (< ek- *out of, away from*) *turning inside out*

> L. *ecstrophia, *ecstrophiae, f. 외번(外飜), 뒤집힘증, 번짐증 **E** *(ecstrophy >) exstrophy*

> streptos, streptē, strepton *twisted, plaited, pliant, flexible*

> L. streptococcus, streptococci, m. (< G. streptos + kokkos *grain, berry*) 사슬 알균, 연쇄상구균(連鎖狀球菌)   **E** *streptococcus, (pl.) streptococci, streptococcal*

< (*European root*) streb(h)- *to wind, to turn*

> G. strobos, strobou, m. *twisting, whirling round* **E** *stroboscope*.

> G. strabos, strabē, strabon *squinting*

> G. strabizein *to squint*

> G. strabismos, strabismou, m. *squint*

> L. strabismus, strabismi, m. 사시(斜視) **E** *strabismus*

styphein *to contract, to have an astringent effect upon*

> stypsis, stypseōs, f. *application or use of styptics*

> L. stypsis, stypsis, f. 수렴(收斂), 수렴작용, 떫은 맛 **E** *stypsis*

> styptikos, styptikē, styptikon *astringent*

> L. stypticus, styptica, stypticum 수렴성의 **E** *styptic*

< IE. stewe- *to thicken, to contract*

> (*suggested*) G. styppē, styppēs, f. *the coarse fiber of flax or hemp, tow*

> L. stuppa, stuppae, f. (stupa, stupae, f.) 삼[麻] 부스러기,
찜질, 습포(濕布) **E** *stupe*, (*stuppare *'to stuff, to stop up'* >) *stop*

thalpein *to warm, to heat, to be warm*

> enthalpein (< en- *in*) *to warm in* **E** *enthalpy* (< *'heat contents for constant pressure'*)

thryptein *to crush small, to comminute*

E (pharmaka tōn en nephrois lithōn thryptika *'drugs comminutive of stones in the kidneys'* >) *lithotriptic*, (*lithotriptic* >) *lithotriptor*, (*lithotriptor* >) *lithotrity*, *lithotripsy* (< *'affected by* G. tripsis *'rubbing'*)

< IE. dhreu- *to fall, to flow, to drip, to droop* **E** *drizzle, dreary, drowse, drip, drop, droop*

tillein *to pluck, to pull out, to tear*

> tilos, tilou, m. *shred, fiber*

E (chrysos *'gold'* + tilos *'fiber'* > *'a golden fibrous variety of serpentine, a kind of asbestos, but the color varies from gray-white to golden yellow to green'* >) *chrysotile*

trechein *to run*

> trochos, trochou, m. *wheel, potter's wheel, disk; running race, racecourse*

> L. trochus, trochi, m. 바퀴, 굴렁쇠, 도르래 **E** *trochal, trochoid*, (*probably*) *truck*

> trochilia, trochilias, f. *system of pulleys, roller of a windlass*

> L. trochlea, trochleae, f. 활차(滑車), 도르래 **E** *trochlea, truckle*

> L. trochlearis, trochleare 활차의, 도르래의 **E** *trochlear*

> trochaios, trochaia, trochaion *running, tripping*

> L. trochaeus, trochaei, m. 장단격(長短格), 강약격(強弱格)   **E** *trochee*

> trochantēr, trochantēros, m. *trochanter*

> L. trochanter, trochanteris, m. (해부) 전자(轉子); (동물) 전절(轉節)   **E** *trochanter, trochanteric*

< IE. dhregh- *to run*

askein (askeein) *to exercise*

> askētēs, askētou, m. *monk, hermit*

> askētikos, askētikē, askētikon *pertaining to the exercise of extremely rigorous self-discipline*   **E** *ascetic*

dein (deein) *to bind*

E (deon, (gen.) deontos (*neuter present participle*) *'that which is binding, duty'* >) *deontology*

> desis, deseōs, f. *binding*

> L. arthrodesis, arthrodesis, f. (< G. arthron *joint*) 관절고정술(關節固定術), 관절유합술(關節癒合術)   **E** *arthrodesis*

> L. pleurodesis, pleurodesis, f. (< G. pleura *rib, side, flank*) 가슴막유착, 흉막유착, 늑막유착   **E** *pleurodesis*

> desmos, desmou, m. (desma, desmatos, n.) *fetter, band*

E *desmoid, desmosome, desmoglein, desmocollin, hemidesmosome, desmin, desmosine*

> L. *desmoplasia, *desmoplasiae, f. (< + G. plasis *formation*) 결합조직 증식증   **E** *desmoplasia*

> L. plasmodesma, plasmodesmatis, n. (< G. plasma *plasma*) (식물) 원형질 연락(原形質連絡), 원형질사(絲), 세포간교(細胞間橋)   **E** *plasmodesma,* (pl.) *plasmodesmata*

> syndein (syndeein) (< syn- *with, together* + dein (deein)) *to bind together*   **E** *syndecan*

> syndesis, syndeseōs, f. *binding together*

> L. spondylosyndesis, spondylosyndesis, f. (< G. spondylos *vertebra*) 척추고정술, 척추유합술   **E** *spondylosyndesis*

> syndesmos, syndesmou, m. *that which binds together, ligament*

> L. syndesmosis, syndesmosis, f. (< + G. -ōsis *condition*) 인대결합(靭帶結合)   **E** *syndesmosis*

< IE. de- *to bind*

euthēnein (euthēneein) (< eu- (< eus) *well* + IE. gwhen- *to swell*) *to thrive, to flourish*   **E** *euthenics*

hairein (haireein) *to seize, to take*

> hairesis, haireseōs, f. *taking, selection, school, sect; heresy*

> L. haeresis, haeresis, f. 학설, 학파; 이단   **E** *heresy*

> hairetikos, hairetikē, hairetikon *able to choose, factitious; heretic*   **E** *heretic*

> aphairein (< aph- (< apo) (*before* aspirate) *away from, from* + hairein) *to take away*

> aphairesis, aphaireseōs, f. *taking away, removal*

> L. aphaeresis, aphaeresis, f. (음성) 어두음(語頭音) 소실; 성분채집술

E *aphaeresis (apheresis, pheresis), plasmapheresis, leukapheresis, thrombocytapheresis*

> diairein (< di- (< dia) *through, thorough, apart* + hairein) *to take apart*

> diairesis, diaireseōs, f. *taking apart, separation*

> L. diaeresis, diaeresis, f. 음절분해, 분음(分音), 분음부호(¨) **E** *diaeresis (dieresis)*

> kathairein (< kath- (< kata) (*before* aspirate) *down, mis-, according to, along, thoroughly* + hairein) *to take down, to destroy*

> kathairesis, kathaireseōs, f. *destruction* **E** *hemocatheresis*

< IE. ser- *to seize*

krotein (kroteein) *to strike, to clap the hands*

> krotos, krotou, m. *striking, clapping, rattling noise, beat*

> dikrotos, dikrotos, dikroton (< di- *two*) *double-beating*

E *dicrotic, (anadicrotic >) anacrotic, (dicrotic >) monocrotic, (dicrotic >) polycrotic*

> krotalon, krotalou, n. *rattle, castanet*

> L. Crotalus, Crotali, m. 방울뱀속(屬) **E** Crotalus

∽ krotaphos, krotaphou, m. *side of the head, temple*

> krotaphios, krotaphia, krotaphion *of side of the head, of temple*

> krotaphion, krotaphiou, n. *a craniometric point at the tip of the great wing of the sphenoid*

> L. crotaphion, crotaphii, n. 크로타피온 **E** *crotaphion*

philein (phileein) *to love, to be fond of, to kiss* **E** *phil(o)-, philosophy, philanthropy, philharmonic*

> philos, philē, philon *loving, loved*

E *-phile (-phil), -philic, electrophile (< 'electron acceptor'), nucleophile (< 'electron donor to atomic nucleus'), halophile (< 'a salt-requiring microorganism'); chromatophil (chromophil) (< 'a cell or element that stains readily'), eosinophil (< 'a cell or element staining readily with eosin'), basophil (< 'a cell or element staining readily with basic dyes'), amphophil (< 'a cell or element staining readily with acidic or basic dyes'); neutrophil (< 'a cell or element staining readily with neutral dyes'), azurophilic (< 'staining readily with blue aniline dyes')*

> L. -philus, -phila, -philum 좋아하는

> L. Pamphilus, Pamphili, m. (< *loved by all* < + pam- (< pan-) *all*) 팜필루스 (Pamphilus seu de Amore '팜필루스 또는 사랑에 대하여' 연애시의 남주인공) **E** *pamphlet (< 'a booklet of* Pamphilus seu de Amore*')*

> philia, philias, f. *love, affection, friendship*

E *-philia, (*haima *'blood' >) haemophilia (hemophilia), (*pais *'child' >) paedophilia (pedophilia), (*xenos *'strange' >) xenophilia, (*phōs *'light' >) photophilia, (*skotos *'darkness' >) scotophilia*

> L. eosinophilia, eosinophiliae, f. (< *eosin*) 호산성(好酸性), 호산구증가(好酸球增加) **E** *eosinophilia*

> L. basophilia, basophiliae, f. (< *basic dye*) 호염기성(好鹽基性), 호염기구증가(好鹽基球增加) **E** *basophilia*

> L. neutrophilia, neutrophiliae, f. (< *neutral dye*) 호중성(好中性), 호중구증가(好中球增加), 중성구증가(中性球增加) **E** *neutrophilia*

> philēma, philēmatos, n. *kiss* **E** *philematology*

> philtron, philtrou, n. *love-charm, love-potion, charm, spell; dimple in the upper lip*
(< *The ancient Greeks used to believe that the philtrum was one of the most erogenous spots on the human body.*)

> L. philtrum, philtri, n. 미약(媚藥), 인중(人中) **E** *philtrum, philtre (philter)*

polein (poleein) *to wander*

> peripolein (peripoleein) (< peri- *around, near, beyond, on account of*) *to wander about*

> peripolēsis, peripolēseōs, f. *wandering about*

> L. peripolesis, peripolesis, f. *the movement of one cell around another; used to refer to the clustering of lymphocytes around macrophages in lymphoid tissue* **E** *peripolesis*

> L. emperipolesis, emperipolesis, f. (< G. em- (< en) *in*) *the movement of one cell within another* **E** *emperipolesis*

pōlein (pōleein) *to sell*

> pōlēs, pōlou, m. *seller, dealer* **E** *bibliopole*

> monopōlion, monopōliou, n. (< monos *alone*) *monopoly*

> L. monopolium, monopolii, n. 전매(專賣), 전매권 **E** *monopoly*

> L. oligopolium, oligopolii, n. (< oligos *few, little*) 소수에 의한 시장 독점, 과점(寡占) **E** *oligopoly*

< IE. pel- *to sell*

agapan (agapaein) *to greet with affection, to receive with friendship, to like, to love*

> agapē, agapēs, f. *brotherly love, charity* **E** *agape*

chalan (chalaein) *to loosen, to relax*

> chalasis, chalaseōs, f. *slackening, relaxation* **E** *cytochalasin*

> L. achalasia, achalasiae, f. (< G. a- *not* + chalasis + -ia) 이완(弛緩)못함증, 이완불능증 **E** *achalasia*

hōrakian (hōrakiaein) *to be giddy*

< IE. wor- *giddiness, faintness* **E** *weary*

kybernan (kybernaein) *to steer, to direct, to govern*

> kybernētēs, kybernētou, m. *steerman, governor*

> **E** *cybernetics (cyber)* (< *'the theory of control in machines or living organisms'*), *(cybernetics >) **cybernetic, cyber-**, (cybernetic organism >) **cyborg***

> L. guberno, **gubernavi**, gubernatum, gubernare 키를 잡다, 조종하다, 지도하다, 다스리다　　　　　　　　　　　　　　　　　　　　　　**E** *govern, government*

> L. gubernum, guberni, n. (다음 gubernaculum과 같음)

> L. gubernaculum, gubernaculi, n. (< + -culum *diminutive suffix*) 배의 키, 조종, 지휘, 통치, 정부　　　　　　　　　　　　　**E** *gubernaculum*

> L. gubernator, gubernatoris, m. (< *past participle*) 키잡이, 운전수, 조종자, 지도자, 통치자　　　　　　　　　　　　　　　　　　　　**E** *governor*

> L. gubernantia, gubernantiae, f. (< *present participle*) 통치　　**E** *governance*

skepan (skepaein) *to cover, to shelter*

> skepē, skepēs, f. *covering, shelter*

> L. sepalum, sepali, n. (< *influenced by 'petal'*) 꽃받침의 조각(귀), 악편(萼片)　　**E** *sepal*

phimoun (phimoein) *to muzzle, to gag; (passive) to be silent*

> phimōsis, phimōseōs, f. (< + -ōsis *condition*) *contraction of the prepuce, stopping up an orifice*

> L. phimosis, phimosis, f. 포경(包莖), 우멍거지　　　　　　　　**E** *phimosis*

> L. paraphimosis, paraphimosis, f. (< *retraction of a phimotic foreskin, causing constriction* < G. par(a)- *beside, along side of, beyond*) 감금 포경, 감돈(嵌頓)포경　　　　　　　　　　　　　　　　　**E** *paraphimosis*

> L. blepharophimosis, blepharophimosis, f. (< G. blepharon *eyelid*) 검열(瞼裂) 축소　　　　　　　　　　　　　　　　　　　　　　　　　**E** *blepharophimosis*

zēmioun (zēmioein) *to damage, to punish, to fine; (passive) to be hurt, to suffer damage*

> zēmia, zēmias, f. *damage, loss, penalty, punishment, fine*

> L. *haematozemia, *haematozemiae, f. (< *a gradual loss of blood* < G. haima, haimatos, n. *blood*) 실혈　　　　　　　　　　　　　　　**E** *hematozemia*

● ● ● **정형 mi 동사**

능동태 현재부정법이 –nai로, 능동태 직설법 현재 단수 일인칭이 –mi로 끝나는 동사. 능동태 직설법 현재 단수 및 복수 삼인칭과 현재분사 복수 여격의 (n)은 *'movable* (n)'이다.

didonai *to give*

능동태	부정법	현재				dido-nai	주다
	직설법	현재	단수	일인칭		didō-mi	나는 ~한다
				이인칭		didō-s	너는 ~한다
				삼인칭		didō-si(n)	그는 ~한다
			복수	일인칭		did-omen	우리는 ~한다
				이인칭		dido-te	너희는 ~한다
				삼인칭		dido-asi(n)	그들은 ~한다
	분 사	현재	단수	주 격		did-ous (m.) did-ousa (f.) did-on (n.)	
						~하는, ~하고 있는	
				속 격		did-ontos did-ousēs did-ontos	
중간태	부정법	현재				do-sthai	(주어가 주어에게) 주다
수동태	부정법	현재				dido-sthai	받다

einai *to be*

능동태	부정법	현재				ei-nai	이다, 있다
	직설법	현재	단수	일인칭		ei-mi	나는 ~이다, 있다
				이인칭		ei	너는 ~이다, 있다
				삼인칭		esti(n)	그는 ~이다, 있다
			복수	일인칭		esmen	우리는 ~이다, 있다
				이인칭		este	너희는 ~이다, 있다
				삼인칭		ei-si(n)	그들은 ~이다, 있다
	분 사	현재	단수	주 격		ōn (m.)	ousa (f.) on (n.)
						~인, ~있는	
				속 격		ontos	ousēs ontos
				여 격		onti	ousēi onti
				대 격		onta	ousan on
			복수	주 격		ontes	ousai onta
				속 격		ontōn	ousōn ontōn
				여 격		ousi(n)	ousais ousi(n)
				대 격		ontas	ousas onta

didonai (do- *root of* didonai) *to give*

< IE. do- *to give* (Vide DARE; *See* E. *date*)

einai *to be*

  < IE. es- *to be* (Vide ESSE: *See* E. *esse*)

keranynai *to mix*

  > krasis, kraseōs, f. *mixing, tempering*

   > L. crasis, crasis, f. 혼합, 체질, 기질   **E** *crasis*

   > eukrasia, eukrasias, f. (< eu- *well* + krasis + -ia *noun suffix*)

    good temperament (of body, air, etc.)

    > L. eucrasia, eucrasiae, f. 균형 잡힌 배합, 건강   **E** *eucrasia*

   > dyskrasia, dyskrasias, f. (< dys- *bad* + krasis + -ia *noun suffix*)

    bad temperament (of body, air, etc.)

    > L. dyscrasia, dyscrasiae, f. 악액질(惡液質); 질환, 병   **E** *dyscrasia*

   > synkrasis, synkraseōs, f. (< syn- *with, together*) *commixture, tempering*

    > idiosynkrasia, idiosynkrasias, f. (< idios *own, private, peculiar* + synkrasis

     + -ia *noun suffix*) *peculiarity of constitution or temperament*

     > L. *idiosyncrasia, *idiosyncrasiae, f. 특이체질, 특이습관,

      특이성   **E** *idiosyncrasy, idiosyncratic*

  > kratēr, kratēros, m. *mixing vessel, bowl, basin*

   > L. crater, crateris, m. 혼주기(混酒器), 그릇, 분화구; (Crater) (천문) 컵자리   **E** *crater*

   > (*perhaps*) L. gradalis, gradalis, m. 잔, 접시   **E** *grail*

  < IE. kerə- *to mix, to confuse, to cook*   **E** *uproar, rare* (< 'half-cooked')

sbennynai *to quench*

  > asbestos, asbestos, asbeston *unquenchable, endless*

   > asbestos, asbestou, m. *quicklime*

    > L. asbestos, asbesti, m. (*Applied by Dioscorides to quicklime ('unslaked').*
    Erroneously applied by Pliny to an incombustible fiber, which he
    believed to be vegetable, but which was really the amiantus of the
    Greeks. Since the identification of this, asbestos has been a more
    popular synonym for amiantus.) 석면(石綿)   **E** *asbestos*

     > L. asbestosis, asbestosis, f. (< + G. -ōsis *condition*) 석면증   **E** *asbestosis*

  < IE. (s)gʷes- *to be quenched*

● ● ●   ## 탈형동사

능동태 현재부정법이 -esthai(-eisthai, -asthai, -ousthai)로, 능동태 직설법 현재 단수 일인
칭이 -omai로 끝나는 동사.

gignesthai (ginesthai) *to be born, to become*

능동태	부정법	현재				gign-esthai	태어나다, 되다
	직설법	현재	단수		일인칭	gign-omai	나는 ~한다
					이인칭	gign-ēi	너는 ~한다
					삼인칭	gign-etai	그는 ~한다
			복수		일인칭	gign-ometha	우리는 ~한다
					이인칭	gign-esthe	너희는 ~한다
					삼인칭	gign-ontai	그들은 ~한다
	분 사	현재	단수		주 격	gign-omenos (m) gign-omenē (f.) gign-omenon (n.)	
							~하는, ~하고 있는
					속 격	gign-omenou gign-omenēs gign-omenou	

gignesthai (ginesthai) *to be born, to become*

　< IE. genə-, gen- *to give birth, to beget* (Vide GIGNĒRE; *See* E. *benign*)

drassesthai *to grasp, to seize*

　　　> drachmē, drachmēs, f. (< *probably, as much as one can hold in the hand*) *drachma*
　　　　(*an Attic weight and coin*)
　　　　　> L. drachma, drachmae, f. 드라크마(아티카의 무게 단위, 약 4.36 g; 아티카의 은화
　　　　　단위)　　　　　　　　　　　　　　　　　　　　　　　　　　　**E** *drachma*
　　< IE. (*perhaps*) dergh- *to grasp*　　　　　　　　　　**E** (*perhaps*) *targe, target*

erchesthai *to go, to come*

　　　　> proserchesthai (< pros- *towards, near, beside(s)*) *to approach, to visit*
　　　　　　> prosēlytos, prosēlytou, m. (< *one who has come over*) *newcomer, stranger;*
　　　　　　　proselyte
　　　　　　　　> L. proselytus, proselyti, m. 전향자, 개종자　　　　**E** *proselyte*
　　< IE. leudh- *to go*

machesthai *to fight*

　　　　> machē, machēs, f. *fight, battle, combat*
　　　　　　> -machia, -machias, f. *fighting, warfare*　　　　　　　**E** *-machy*
　　　　　　　> theomachia, theomachias, f. (< theos *god*) *A battle or strife among the*
　　　　　　　　gods, especially in reference to that narrated in Homer's Iliad **E** *theomachy*
　　< IE. magh- *to fight*
　　　　> G. Amazōn, Amazonos, f. (< *possibly borrowed from a hypothetical Iranian compound*
　　　　　ha-maz-an- (one) fighting together, warrior < *ha- with* < IE. sem- *one; also*
　　　　　adverbially 'as one', together with) (*Greek mythology*) *Amazones*

> L. Amazon, Amazonis, f. (그리스 신화) 흑해 동남해안 Thermodon 강변에 산다는
여전사, 아마조네스　　　　　　　　　　　　　**E** *Amazon*, (pl.) *Amazones*

phthengesthai *to utter*

> phthongos, phthongou, m. *voice, sound*

> diphthongos, diphthongou, m. (< di- *two*) *diphthong*

> L. diphthongus, diphthongi, m. 이중모음, 복모음　　　　**E** *diphthong*

iasthai *to heal, to cure*

> iatros, iatrou, m. *healer, physician*　　　　　　　**E** *iatr(o)-, iatrogenic*

> iatrikos, iatrikē, iatrikon *of healer, medical*

E *-iatric, -iatrics, bariatrics* (< 'treatment of weight'), *geriatrics* (< 'treatment of
the ailments that accompany growing older')

> L. paediatricus, paediatrica, paediatricum (< G. pais, paidos, m., f.
child) 소아 치료의　　　　　　　**E** *paediatric (pediatric), pediatrics*

> iatreia, iatreias, f. *healing, cure, remedy*　　　**E** *-iatry, psychiatry, podiatry*

orcheisthai *to dance*

> orchēstra, orchēstras, f. *the area in front of the stage in the ancient Greek theater
where the chorus sing and dance, the area in front of the stage in the ancient
Roman theater where the senators sat*

> orchestra, orchestrae, f. 악단석, 관현악단, 오케스트라　**E** *orchestra, orchestral, orchestrate*

전치사

　　전치사는 명사나 대명사 앞에 위치하여 형용사구나 부사구를 만든다. 전치사
뒤에 오는 명사나 대명사는 속격, 여격, 또는 대격의 어미변화를 해야 하며, 이
를 전치사의 격지배라고 한다.

　　전치사 중에는 두 가지 이상의 격을 지배하는 전치사가 있다. 뒤에 오는 명사
나 대명사의 격에 따라 뜻도 달라진다. 학술용어에서 그리스어 기원의 전치사는
다른 그리스어 기원의 낱말과 함께 여러 가지 합성어를 만든다. 이때 같은 전치
사라도 뜻이 다른 합성어를 만드는 것은, 합성어의 의미가 확장되었기 때문이기
도 하지만, 전치사가 뒤에 오는 명사나 대명사의 격에 따라 다른 뜻을 가지기
때문이기도 하다.

속격지배 전치사

anti (속격지배) ~에 대하여, ~ 대신에
> ant(i)-, anth- (*before* aspirate) *before, against, instead of*
< IE. ant- *front, forehead* (Vide ANTE: *See* E. *ante-*)

apo (속격지배) ~부터, ~ 떨어져서
> ap(o)- *away from, from*
< IE. apo-, ap- *off, away* (Vide AB: *See* E. *ab-*)

ex (자음 앞에서는 **ek**) (속격지배) ~에서부터
> ex-, ek- (*before* consonant) *out of, away from*
> exō (전치사, 속격지배; 부사) *outside, outwards*
> exō- *outside, outwards*
> ektos (부사) *outside, without*
> ekt(o)- *outside*
< IE. eghs *out* (Vide EX: *See* E. *ex-*)

pro (속격지배) ~ 앞서서, ~ 전에
> pro- *before, in front*
> pros (전치사) (속격지배) ~ 앞에, ~을 위하여; (여격지배) ~ 근처에;
(대격지배) ~ 쪽으로 향하여, ~와 함께
> pros- *towards, near, beside(s)*
< IE. per *basic meanings of 'forward', 'through'* (Vide PER: *See* E. *per-*)

여격지배 전치사

en (여격지배) ~ 안에, ~ 가운데
> en-, el- (*before* l), em- (*before* m, b, p, ph) *in*
< IE. en *in* (Vide IN: *See* E. *in-*)

syn (여격지배) ~와 함께
> syn-, syl- (*before* l), sym- (*before* m, b, p, ph), sy- (*before* s + consonant, z)
with, together

E *syn- (syl-, sym-, sy-), syndrome, syllable, symmetry, symbiosis, symptom, symphysis, systolic, syzygy*

< IE. ksun *preposition and preverb meaning 'with'*

> (*Russian*) soviet *council* E *soviet*

> (*Russian*) Sputnik (< put' *path, way*) *co-traveler* E *Sputnik*

대격지배 전치사

ana (대격지배) ~ 위로, ~ 가운데

> an(a)- *up, upward; again, throughout; back, backward; against; according to,*
> *similar to* E *an(a)-, anabolism, anode, anion*
> anō (*adverb*) *up, upwards, above,*
> *beyond* E (anō + meros *part* > 'an additional isomer' >) *anomer, anomeric*

< IE. an- *on* E *on, alike, acknowledge, aloft, amiss, onslaught,* D. *Anlage* (< 'laying on, for the first')

속격과 대격지배 전치사

dia (속격지배) ~ 통하여; (대격지배) ~ 때문에

> di(a)- *through, thoroughly, apart*

< IE. dwo- *two* (Vide DUO: *See* E. *duo*)

hyper (속격지배) ~ 대신에, ~에 대하여; (대격지배) ~ 위에, ~ 초월하여

> hyper- *over*

< IE. uper *over* (Vide SUPER: *See* E. *super-*)

hypo (속격지배) ~로 말미암아; (대격지배) ~ 아래, ~ 밑에

> hyp(o)- *under*

< IE. upo *up from under, over, under* (Vide SUB: *See* E. *sub-*)

kata (속격지배) ~ 아래로, ~에 대항하여; (대격지배) ~에 의해서, ~을 따라서

> kat(a)-, kath- (*before* aspirate) *down, mis-, according to, along,*
> *thoroughly* E *cat(a)- (cath-), catabolism, cathode, cation*
> kathizein (kata + -izein *-ize*) *to seat, to set, to sit*
> > kathisis, kathiseōs, f. *sitting*
> > > L. akathisia, akathisiae, f. (acathisia, acathisiae, f.) (< G. a- *not*)
> > > 좌불안석증 E *akathisia (acathisia)*

< IE. kat- *down*

peri (속격지배) ~에 대하여; (대격지배) ~ 주위에

> peri- *around, near, beyond, on account of*
< IE. per *basic meanings of 'forward', 'through'* (Vide PER; *See* E. *per-*)

속격, 여격, 대격지배 전치사

amphi (속격지배) ~ 주위에; (여격지배) ~ 주위에, ~ 때문에; (대격지배) ~ 주위에, ~ 동안에

> amphi- *on both sides, around*
< IE. ambhi, mbhi *around* (Vide AMBI-; *See* E. *amb(i)-*)
< IE. ant-bhi- *from both sides* < (*probably*) IE. ant- *front, forehead* (Vide ANTE; *See* E. *ante-*)

epi (속격지배) ~ 위에, ~ 때에; (여격지배) ~에 근거하여; (대격지배) ~에게

> ep(i)-, eph- (*before* aspirate) *upon*
< IE. epi, opi *near, at, against* (Vide OB; *See* E. *ob-*)

meta (속격지배) ~와 함께; (여격지배) ~와 함께; (대격지배) ~ 후에

> met(a)-, meth- (*before* aspirate) *between, along with, across, after*
< IE. me- *in the middle of* (Vide MEDIALIS; *See* E. *medial*)

para (속격지배) ~으로부터; (여격지배) ~ 옆에; (대격지배) ~ 옆에 나란히, ~을 따라서

> par(a)- *beside, along side of, beyond*
< IE. per *basic meanings of 'forward', 'through'* (Vide PER; *See* E. *per*)

pros (속격지배) ~ 앞에, ~을 위하여; (여격지배) ~ 근처에; (대격지배) ~ 쪽으로 향하여, ~와 함께

> pros- *towards, near, beside(s)*
< pro (전치사) ~ 앞서서, ~ 전에
< IE. per *basic meanings of 'forward', 'through'* (Vide PER; *See* E. *per*)

부사, 접속사

부사

학술용어의 이해에 필요한 부사는 극히 일부분이다.

tēle (*adverb*) *afar, far off*　**E** *telescope, telephone (phone), telegram, telepathy, telekinesis; television*
　< IE. kwel- *far (in space and time)*
　　> G. palaios, palaia, palaion *old, aged, ancient, antiquated,*
　　　obsolete　**E** *palae(o)- (pale(o)-), paleology, Paleozoic, Paleolithic, paleobiology*

접속사

학술용어의 이해에 필요한 접속사에는 영어의 접속사 *and*에 해당하는 kai가 있다. kai는 문장이나 낱말을 접속시켜 주며 숫자에도 이용된다.

kai *and*
　[용례] οφθαλμον αντι οφθαλμου και οδοντα αντι οδοντος (ophthalmon
　　　anti ophthalmou kai odonta anti odontos) (< *eye instead of eye
　　　and tooth instead of tooth*) 눈 대신에 눈을 그리고 이 대신에 이를
　　(문법) ophthalmon *eye*: 단수 대격 < ophthalmos, ophthalmou, m.
　　　　anti *instead of*: 전치사, 속격지배
　　　　ophthalmou *of eye*: 단수 속격 < ophthalmos, ophthalmou, m.
　　　　kai *and*: 접속사
　　　　odonta *tooth*: 단수 대격 < odous, odontos, m.
　　　　odontos *of tooth*: 단수 속격 < odous, odontos, m.
　> treiskaideka (< treis *three* + kai *and* + deka *ten*) *thirteen*　**E** *triskaidekaphobia*

용어
비교

Comparative Terminology

Terminologia Comparativa

용어 비교

비교하기 쉽도록 대비되는 접두사와 접미사들을 한데 모았다. 여기에는 다른 접두사와 대비되기 때문에 접두사처럼 쓰이는 자립형태소의 연결형을 포함시켰다. 생명과학 학술용어는 도형, 건축물, 의복, 지명, 동물, 식물, 원소 등 출처가 여기저기이므로 한데 모았다. 뜻이나 꼴의 비교가 필요한 낱말들도 한데 모았으며, 본디 영어 낱말과 라틴어·그리스어 기원의 영어 낱말로서 대조적으로 사용되나 어원이 다르기 때문에 흩어질 수밖에 없는 낱말들 역시 한데 모았다.

접사

의존형태소인 접사는 단독으로는 사용되지 못하나 다른 낱말의 앞 또는 뒤에 붙어 이런저런 파생어를 만든다.

영어로 명사 '불의'는 *injustice*이다. 접사를 붙여 파생어를 만들 때에도 언어의 순혈주의를 지켜야 한다는 원칙을 따랐다. 그러나 형용사 '옳지 못한'은 *unjust*로서 원칙을 따르지 않았다.

E. *injustice* < L. injustitia < L. in- *not* + L. justus *just*

E. †*injust* < L. injustus < L. in- *not* + L. justus *just*

E. *unjust* < E. un- '*not*' + E. *just* < L. justus *just*

E. *unnamed* < E. un- '*not*' + E. *name*

E. *innominate* < L. in- *not* + L. nomen *name*

E. *anonymous* < G. an- *not* + G. onyma *name*

†*injust* 같은 원칙이 죽고 *unjust* 같은 비원칙이 살아남는 예가 있기는 하다. 사람들의 입버릇 때문이다. 흔히 사용하는 낱말이 그렇다. 그래도 '무명의' 또는

'익명의'를 뜻하는 *unnamed, innominate, anonymous*에서 보듯, 파생어에서도 언어의 순혈주의는 지켜지고 있다. 학술용어에서는 특히 그러하다. 따라서 접사가 본디 영어인지, 라틴어 기원인지, 그리스어 기원인지, 접사의 국적을 눈여겨 보아 둘 필요가 있다. 이 말은 학술용어처럼 원칙을 따르는 낱말에서는 몇 안 되는 접사의 국적만으로도 뒤에 오는 여러 낱말의 국적을 알 수 있다는 말도 된다.

E. *un-* *not*　　　　　　　　　　　　　　　　　　　　　　　**E** *un-*
　　< IE. ne *not* (Vide NON: *See* E. *non-*)

L. in-, il- (*before* l), im- (*before* m, b, p), ir- (*before* r) *not*　　**E** *in- (il-, im-, ir-)*
　　< IE. ne *not* (Vide NON: *See* E. *non-*)

G. a-, an- (*before* bowel) *not*　　　　　　　　　　　　　　　**E** *a- (an-)*
　　< IE. ne *not* (Vide NON: *See* E. *non-*)

L. ne-, neg- *not*　　　　　　　　　　　　　　　　　　　　　**E** *ne-, neg-*
　　< IE. ne *not* (Vide NON: *See* E. *non-*)

L. non- *not*　　　　　　　　　　　　　　　　　　　　　　　**E** *non-*
　　< IE. ne *not* (Vide NON: *See* E. *non-*)

G. ne- *not*　　　　　　　　　　　　　　　　　　　　　　　**E** *ne-*
　　< IE. ne *not* (Vide NON: *See* E. *non-*)

L. bene- *well*　　　　　　　　　　　　　　　　　　　　　　**E** *bene-*
　　　　< L. bene (부사) 좋게, 잘
　　　< L. bonus, bona, bonum (< *useful, efficient, working*) 좋은
　　< IE. deu- *to do, to perform, to show favor, to revere* (Vide BONUS: *See* E. *bonus*)

L. male-, mal- *badly*　　　　　　　　　　　　　　　　　　**E** *male- (mal-)*
　　　　< L. male (부사) 나쁘게
　　　< L. malus, mala, malum 나쁜
　　< IE. mel- *false, bad, wrong* (Vide MALUS: *See* E. *dismal*)

G. eu– *well*   **E** *eu–*

        < G. eus, eus, eu *good, brave*

      < IE. (e)su– (< *being true, being good*) *good*

    < IE. es– *to be* (Vide ESSE: *See* E. *esse*)

G. dys– (*used as a prefix*) *bad*   **E** *dys–*

        < IE. dus– (< *a lack*) *bad, evil, mis–*

      < IE. deu– *to lack, to be wanting*   **E** *tire* (< 'to fall behind')

        > G. deuteros, deutera, deuteron (< *missing*) *next, second*

          > L. deuterium, deuterii, n. (< *the second of the three naturally occurring*

             hydrogen isotopes (protium, deuterium, and tritium)) 중수소

             (重水素) **E** *deuterium (^2H, D), (deuterium >* 'on the pattern of proton' *>) deuteron*

L. ambi–, amb– (*before* bowel) *on both sides,*

        around   **E** *amb(i)– (am–, an–), ambivalent, ambient, amputate, ancillary*

      < IE. ambhi, mbhi *around*

          E *by, but, be–,* ((*probably*) D. Beiwacht 'by-watch' >) *bivouac,* (D. um– 'about' +
          Laut 'sound' >) *umlaut, ombudsman*

        > G. amphi (*preposition, adverb*) *on both sides,*

          around   **E** *amphi–, amphiphilic* (< 'both hydrophilic and hydrophobic')

        > G. amphō (*dual pronoun*) *both*   **E** *ampho–*

          > G. amphoteros, amphotera, amphoteron (*comparative*) *both*

          E *amphoteric* (< 'both acidic and basic'), (*amphoteric >) amphotericin,*
          (*amphoteric + electrolyte >) ampholyte*

      < IE. ant–bhi– *from both sides*

    < (*probably*) IE. ant– *front, forehead* (Vide ANTE: *See* E. *ante–*)

L. re–, red– (*before* bowel *and* h) *back,*

        again   **E** *re– (red–), redundant, redintegrate, redeem, redemption (ransom)*

      < IE. wret– (*metathetical variant*) *to turn back*

    < IE. wer– *to turn, to bend, to wind* (Vide VERTĚRE: *See* E. *verse*)

L. semi– *half*   **E** *semi–*

      < L. semis 반(半)

    < IE. semi– *half, as first member of a compound* (Vide SEMIS: *See* E. *semi–*)

G. hemi– *half*   **E** *hemi–*

      < G. hēmisys, hēmiseia, hēmisy *half*

    < IE. semi– *half, as first member of a compound* (Vide SEMIS: *See* E. *semi–*)

F. demi- *half, incomplete*   E *demi-*

      < F. demi 절반의

     < L. dimidius, dimidia, dimidium (< di- (< dis-) *apart from, down, not* + medius

        mid) 절반의

    < L. medius, media, medium 가운데의

  < IE. medhyo- *middle* (Vide MEDIALIS: *See* E. *medial*)

L. se-, sed- *apart, without*   E *se- (sed-), select, separate, secret, sedition*

  < IE. s(w)e- *pronoun of the third person and reflexive (referring back to the subject of
the sentence), one's own; further appearing in various forms referring to the social
group as an entity, '(we our-) selves'.* (Vide SUI: *See* E. *suicide*)

L. dis-, dif- (*before* f), di- (*before* b, d, g, l, m, n, r, s, v) *apart from, down, not;
intensive*   E *dis- (dif-, di-), disinfect, difficult, digest, dilatate, direct, divert*

  < IE. dwo- *two* (Vide DUO: *See* E. *duo*)

L. -ulus, -ula, -ulum *diminutive suffix*   E *-ule, -ular*

  < IE. -lo- *secondary suffix, forming diminutives*

L. -ellus, -ella, -ellum *diminutive suffix*   E *-el*

  < IE. -lo- *secondary suffix, forming diminutives*

L. -alis, -ale (-aris, -are (*dissimilated form, after bases containing* l)) *adjective suffix*   E *-al, -ar*

    < L. -li- *adjective suffix*

  < IE. -lo- *secondary suffix, forming diminutives*

L. -ilis, -ile *adjective suffix meaning 'able'*   E *-ile*

    < L. -li- *adjective suffix*

  < IE. -lo- *secondary suffix, forming diminutives*

L. -bilis, -bile *adjective suffix meaning 'capable' or 'worth of being acted upon'*   E *-ble (-able, -ible)*

  < IE. -tro- (-tlo-, -dhro-, -dhlo-) *suffix forming nouns of instrument*

L. **linea**, lineae, f. (< linea fibra *flax fiber*) 선, 경계선, 소묘(素描)　　　**E** *line, linage, midline*

　　　[용례] linea alba 백색선　　　**E** *linea alba*

　　　　　　linea aspera 거친선　　　**E** *linea aspera*

　　　　　(문법) linea 선: 단수 주격

　　　　　　　alba 흰: 형용사, 여성형 단수 주격 < albus, alba, album

　　　　　　　aspera 거친, 험한: 형용사, 여성형 단수 주격

　　　　　　　　　< asper, aspera, asperum

　　　> L. linearis, lineare 선의,

　　　　　직선의　　　**E** *linear, collinear, curvilinear (curvilineal), rectilinear (rectilineal)*

　　　> L. linealis, lineale 선의, 직계의

　　　　　　E *lineal, curvilineal (curvilinear), rectilineal (rectilinear), matrilineal, patrilineal*

　　　> L. lineo, **lineavi**, lineatum, lineare 선을 긋다, (나란히) 줄지어 놓다,

　　　　　정렬시키다　　　**E** *align, alignment*

　　　　　> L. collineo, **collineavi**, collineatum, collineare (< col- (< cum)

　　　　　　　with, together + lineare *to draw lines*) 똑바로 맞추어 겨누다,

　　　　　　　적중시키다　　　**E** *(collineare > (erroneous reading) >) collimate*

　　　　　> L. delineo, **delineavi**, delineatum, delineare (< de- *apart from,*

　　　　　　　down, not; intensive + lineare *to draw lines*) 윤곽을 그리다,

　　　　　　　초벌 그림을 그리다　　　**E** *delineate*

　　　　　> L. *lineaticum, *lineatici, n. 가계(家系)　　　**E** *lineage*

　　　< L. lineus, linea, lineum 삼[亞麻]의, 삼으로 만든　　　**E** F. *lingerie*

< L. linum, lini, n. 삼[亞麻], 삼실, 삼베, 실, 끈, 줄, 밧줄　　　**E** *linseed, linen*

　　> L. linteum, lintei, n. 아마포, 수건, 린트　　　**E** *lint*

< IE. lino- *flax*

　　> G. **linon**, linou, n. *flax, linen, thread, line*

　　　　E *linoleic acid* (< *'found in linseed oil'*), *linolenic acid* (< *'more unsaturated linoleic acid'*)

　　> L. linitis, linitidis, f. (< *leather bottle stomach due to either malignancy or,*

　　　　occasionally, inflammation < *(originally) fibrosing inflammation of the*

　　　　filamentous network of areolar tissue of the gastric submucosa) 위벽염　　　**E** *linitis*

　　　[용례] linitis plastica 증식위벽염, 섬유증식위벽염　　　**E** *linitis plastica*

　　　　　(문법) linitis 위벽염: 단수 주격

　　　　　　　plastica 조직을 형성하는: 형용사, 여성형 단수 주격

　　　　　　　　< plasticus, plastica, plasticum

E. *ridge*
`E ridge`

< IE. (s)ker- *to turn, to bend* (Vide CURVUS: *See* E. *curve*)

E. *furrow*
`E furrow`

< IE. perk- *to dig out, to tear out*

E. *groove*
`E groove`

< IE. ghrebh- *to dig, to bury,*

to scratch`E grave (< 'to dig, to bury'), grave (< 'to scratch'), (grave >) engrave, grub`

L. crista, cristae, f. (닭의) 볏, 도가머리, 맨드라미, 투구의 깃털;

능(稜), 능선(稜線)`E crista, (pl.) cristae, crest, (perhaps) crease`

< IE. (s)ker- *to turn, to bend* (Vide CURVUS: *See* E. *curve*)

L. sulcus, sulci, m. 고랑
`E sulcus, (pl.) sulci`

> L. sulco, sulcavi, sulcatum, sulcare 고랑을 치다, 밭을 갈다

> L. sulcatus, sulcata, sulcatum (*past participle*) 고랑을 친, (가늘고 긴) 홈이 있는`E sulcate`

> L. persulcatus, persulcata, persulcatum (< per- *through, thoroughly*)

홈이 뚜렷한`E persulcate`

< IE. selk- *to pull, to draw*

> G. hēlkein *to drag*

> G. holkas, holkados, f. *a ship that is towed, hence a ship of burden,*

a trading vessel`E (suggested) hulk`

L. lira, lirae, f. 이랑(두둑과 고랑, (옛) 사래), 두둑, 고랑

< IE. leis- *track, furrow* (Vide DELIRARE: *See* E. *delirium*)

L. stria, striae, f. 도랑, 밭이랑, 좁은 폭의 띠 구조, 선조(線條), 조(條), 선(線)`E stria, (pl.) striae`

< (*European root*) streig- *to stroke, to rub, to press* (Vide STRINGĔRE: *See* E. *strain*)

G. lophos, lophou, m. *top of the head, crest, ridge, hill, tuft*
`E loph(o)-`

< IE. lobho- *top or back of the head*

E. *fold*
`E fold`

< IE. pel- *to fold* (Vide infra)

L. plica, plicae, f. (접어 만든, 접힌) 주름, 습벽(褶襞), 추벽(皺襞)

                                                                      E *plica*, (pl.) *plicae*
       < L. plico, plicavi (plicui), plicatum (plicitum), plicare 접다   **E** *plicate*
    < IE. plek- *to plait*   **E** *flax*
  < IE. pel- *to fold* (Vide PLICARE: *See* E. *plicate*)

L. ruga, rugae, f. (오글쪼글한) 주름, 추벽(皺襞); 찡그림, 슬픔, 엄격, (pl.) 늙음   **E** *ruga*, (pl.) *rugae*
    > L. rugosus, rugosa, rugosum 주름 많은, 주름투성이의   **E** *rugose (rugous)*
    > L. rugositas, rugositatis, f. 주름 많음, 주름투성이   **E** *rugosity*
      > L. rugo, rugavi, rugatum, rugare 주름지게 하다, 주름지다
        > L. corrugo, corrugavi, corrugatum, corrugare (< cor- (< cum) *with,*
         together + rugare *to wrinkle*) 주름지게 하다, 물결 모양으로 만들다   **E** *corrugate*
          > L. corrugator, corrugatoris, m. 주름근(筋)   **E** *corrugator*
  < IE. reuə- *to smash, to knock down, to tear out, to dig up,*
    to up-root   **E** *rag, ragweed* (< *'tattered appearance of the leaves')*, *rug, rough*
    > L. ruo, rui, rutum, ruĕre 들이닥치다, 무너지다
      > L. ruina, ruinae, f. 무너짐, 멸망, 폐허   **E** *ruin*
   > (*possibly*) L. rudis, rude 자연 그대로의, 첫경험의, 세련되지 않은, 미숙한, 버릇없는   **E** *rude*
      > L. rudimentum, rudimenti, n. 초보, 입문, 싹수,
      원기(原基)   **E** *rudiment,* (*rudiment* >) *rudimentary*
      > L. erudio, erudivi (erudii), eruditum, erudire (< e- *out of, away from* + rudis
      untrained) 교육하다   **E** *erudite*
        > L. eruditio, eruditionis, f. 교육, 학식, 박학   **E** *erudition*

G. helix, helikos, f. *winding, coil, spire, anything twisted*
      > L. helix, helicis, f. 나선(螺旋), 나선구조, 기둥머리의 소용돌이 장식, 아이비; 귀둘레,
      귓바퀴, 이륜(耳輪)   **E** *helix,* (pl.) *helices, helic(o)-*
      > L. *helicalis, *helicale 나선의, 나선 모양의   **E** *helical*
      > L. helicinus, helicina, helicinum 나선 모양의
         E *helicine* (< *'applied to certain small arteries of the penis and clitoris and*
         to the helix of the ear')
   < G. helissein *to turn round, to twist*
  < IE. wel- *to turn, to roll; with derivatives referring to curved, enclosing objects*
   (Vide VOLVĔRE: *See* E. *volute*)

G. speira, speiras, f. *winding, coil, spire*
    > L. spira, spirae, f. 와선(渦線), 나선(螺旋)   **E** *spire*
      > L. spiralis, spirale 나선형의   **E** *spiral*
      > L. Spirillum, Spirilli, n. (< + -illum *diminutive suffix*) (세균) 스피릴룸속(屬)   **E** Spirillum
      > L. Spirochaeta, Spirochaetae, f. (< + G. chaitē *long hair, mane*)
      (세균) 스피로키타속(屬)   **E** Spirochaeta, *spirochaete (spirochete), spirochetal*

> L. Leptospira, Leptospirae, f. (< G. leptos *cleaned of the husks, thin, slender,*
delicate) (세균) 렙토스피라속(屬)

E *Leptospira*

> G. speirēma, speirēmatos, n. *coil, convolution*

E *spireme*

> G. speiraia, speiraias, f. (< *used for garlands and wreaths*) *spiraea*

> L. spiraea, spiraeae, f. 조팝나무속(屬)의 장미과 식물,
조팝나무

E *spiraea (spirea), (acetylated spiraeic acid >) Aspirin®*

< IE. sper- *to turn, to twist*

> G. sparganon, sparganou, n. *swaddling band*

> L. sparganum, spargani, n. 스파르가눔, 고충(孤蟲)

E *sparganum, sparganosis*

G. sōlēn, sōlēnos, m. *pipe, channel, shell-fish*

> L. solen, solenis, m. (긴) 맛(조개)

E *solen, solenoid*

< IE. two- *tube*

> (*suggested*) G. syrinx, syringos, f. *tube, pipe, channel, fistula; water cavity*

> L. syrinx, syringis, f. 관(管), 갈대, 피리, 명관(鳴管), 지하통로, 샛길 **E** *syrinx, syring(o)-*

> L. syringa, syringae, f. 주사기, 라일락 (< *pipe-tree: the broad pith in*
the shoots easily hollowed out to make reed pipes and flutes in
early history)

E *syringe, Syringa*

> L. syringobulbia, syringobulbiae, f. (< G. syrinx *water cavity* + L.
bulbus *medulla oblongata*) 숨뇌구멍증, 연수공동증(延髓空洞症) **E** *syringobulbia*

> L. syringomyelia, syringomyeliae, f. (< G. syrinx *water cavity* + G.
myelos *spinal marrow*) 척수구멍증, 척수공동증(脊髓空洞症) **E** *syringomyelia*

L. globus, globi, m. 공, 구(球), 구체(球體), 구락부(俱樂部) **E** *globus, (pl.) globi, globe, (globe >) global*

> L. globosus, globosa, globosum 구형(球形)의 **E** *globose*

> L. globulus, globuli, m. (< + -ulus *diminutive suffix*) 소구(小球)

E *globule, globulin, euglobulin (< 'a fraction of serum globulin that is insoluble in pure*
water but soluble in saline solutions and is precipitated by half-saturation with
ammonium sulphate'), *pseudoglobulin* *(< 'a fraction of serum globulin that is soluble*
in pure water and in saline solutions of low ionic strength'), *cryoglobulin* *(< 'a serum*
globulin, invariably immunoglobulin, that precipitates at low temperature, e.g., 4℃, and
resolves at 37℃'), *immunoglobulin, (haematoglobulin >)* *hemoglobin, (hemoglobin >)*
globin, (hemoglobin >) *myoglobin, (hemoglobin >)* *haptoglobin, (oxygenated*
hemoglobin >) *oxyhemoglobin, (carbon monoxide >)* *carboxyhemoglobin, (G. meta*
> meth- 'across' > 'oxidation of ferrous to ferric state' >) *methemoglobin, (G. meta*
> meth- 'across' > 'oxidation of ferrous to ferric state' >) *metmyoglobin, globoside*
(< 'the substance with sugar residues forming globules under the microscope')

> L. globularis, globulare 소구의, 구형의 **E** *globular*

< IE. gel- *to make round, to clench as the fist, to grip, to cling to*

E *clod, clot, (clot >)* *clutter, cleat, cluster, cloud, clump, club, clubfoot, calf (<*
'fetus' < 'made round'), *calf* *(< 'the round part of the leg'),* *clench, cling, climb (<*
'to cling to, to grip'), *clamber, clamp, clam, claw, clew (clue) (< 'a ball of thread,*
used by Theseus as a guide out of the labyrinth'), *clue (clew)*

> (*probably*) L. galla, gallae, f. (< *spherical growth*) (식물) 몰식자(沒食子), 오배자
(五倍子), 충영(蟲纓), 나무혹, 벌레혹

> **E** *gall (< 'an excrescence produced on trees, especially the oak, by the action of various parasites, from fungi and bacteria to insects and mites; oak-galls are largely used in the manufacture of ink and tannin, as well as in dyeing and in medicine.'), gallic acid*

> G. ganglion, gangliou, n. *swelling, tumor, node*

> L. ganglion, ganglii, n. 신경절(神經節), 결절종(結節腫)

> **E** *ganglion,* (pl.) *ganglia, ganglionic, aganglionic, preganglionic, postganglionic, ganglioside(s) (< 'first isolated from ganglion cells of brain')*

> L. paraganglion, paraganglii, n. (< *a ganglion beside the sympathetic ganglia* < G. par(a)- *beside, along side of, beyond*) 곁신경절,
부신경절(副神經節)　　　　　　　**E** *paraganglion,* (pl.) *paraganglia*

> G. gloutos, gloutou, m. *rump, buttock*

> L. gluteus, glutei, m. 볼기근, 둔근(臀筋)　　　　**E** *gluteus (muscle), gluteal*

G. sphaira, sphairas, f. *ball, globe*

> L. sphaera, sphaerae, f. (sphera, spherae, f.) 둥근 물체, 공, 구(球), 천구(天球); 영역,
권(圈)　　　　**E** *sphere, spher(o)-, spherocyte, -sphere, biosphere, microsphere*

> L. sphaerula, sphaerulae, f. (spherula, spherulae, f.) (< + -ula *diminutive suffix*) 작은 공　　　　　　　　　　　　　　**E** *spherule*

> G. sphairikos, sphairikē, sphairikon *spheric*

> L. sphaericus, sphaerica, sphaericum (sphericus, spherica, sphericum) 구의,
구형의, 천구의　　　　　　　　　　　　　**E** *spherical*

> G. hēmisphairion, hēmisphairiou, n. (< hemi- *half* + sphaira + -ion *diminutive suffix*)
a half sphere

> L. hemisphaerium, hemisphaerii, n. 반구(半球)　　**E** *hemisphere, hemispheric*

> L. atmosphaera, atmosphaerae, f. (< G. atmos *vapor* + sphaira) 대기(大氣), 기압,
분위기　　　　　　　　　　　　　**E** *atmosphere, atmospheric*

> G. sphairoeidēs, sphairoeidēs, sphairoeides (< + eidos *shape*) *ball-shaped*

> L. sphaeroides, (gen.) sphaeroidis 구형의, 둥근　　　　**E** *spheroid*

G. kōnos, kōnou, m. (< *sharp-pointed object*) *cone, conical object*

> L. conus, coni, m. 원추(圓錐), 원추형(圓錐形), 원추체(圓錐體), 원뿔, 투구 꼭대기,
솔방울　　　**E** *cone, conization (< 'removal of a cone of tissue'), conoid; coniform*

> L. *keratoconus, *keratoconi, m. (< G. kerat(o)- *cornea* < G. keras, keratos, n.
horn) 원추각막　　　　　　　　　　　**E** *keratoconus*

> L. conifer, conifera, coniferum (< conus *cone* + -fer (< ferre *to carry, to bear*)
carrying, bearing) 솔방울이 달리는, 구과(毬果) 식물의　　**E** *conifer*

> G. kōnikos, kōnikē, kōnikon *of a cone*

> L. conicus, conica, conicum 원뿔꼴의   **E** *conic (conical)*

   < IE. ko- *to sharpen, to whet*   **E** *hone*

건축

L. vallum, valli, n. 방책(方柵), 누벽(壘壁), 방어진지   **E** *wall, vallum*

      > L. intervallum, intervalli, n. (< *space between palisades or ramparts* < inter-
         between, among + vallum *rampart*) 간격, 기간, 범위   **E** *interval*

      > L. circumvallo, circumvallavi, circumvallatum, circumvallare (< circum- *around*
         + vallum *rampart*) (성벽·참호로) 주위를 둘러싸다   **E** *circumvallate*

    < L. vallus, valli, m. 말뚝, 울타리

   < IE. walso- *post*

L. murus, muri, m. 성벽(城壁), 돌담, 성(城), 보루, 보호

> **E** *intramural, transmural, muramic acid* (< *'an amino sugar in the cell walls of bacteria and bacterial spores')*, *(muramic acid >muramide >)* **muramidase** *(lysozyme),* **murein(s)** *(peptidoglycan(s))*

    > L. muralis, murale 성벽의, 담의   **E** *mural*

    > L. immuro, immuravi, immuratum, immurare (< im- (< in) *in, on, into, toward*) 가두다,
      한정하다   **E** *immure*

  < IE. mei- *to fix; to build fences or fortifications*

    > L. munio, munivi (munii), munitum, munire 성벽을 쌓다, 방비하다

      > L. munitio, munitionis, f. 방비, 방비품, 군수품

      > **E** *munition,* (F, la munition *'the munition'* > *(altered by wrong division)* >) **ammunition**

    > L. praemunio, praemunivi, praemunitum, praemunire (< prae- *before, beyond*)
      앞쪽에 보루를 구축하다, 방비하다   **E** *premunitive*

      > L. praemunitio, praemunitionis, f. 방비, 예방, 방어물; (*infection immunity:*
         state of relative immunity to severe or symptomatic infection by a
         pathogen resulting from the continued presence of small numbers
         of the same pathogen in the body) 감염면역, 상관면역(相關免疫)   **E** *premunition*

G. teichos, teichous, n. *wall, fortification, fortress,*
   castle   **E** *teich(o)-, teichoic acid* (< *'found in the walls of Gram-positive bacteria')*

L. paries, parietis, m. (집의) 바람벽, 벽

    > L. parietalis, parietale 바람벽의, 벽의, 측벽(側壁)의; 체벽(體壁)의, 두정부(頭頂部)의,

마루의 　　　　　　　　　　　　　　　　　　　　　　　　　　　　　　 **E** *parietal*

L. saeptum, saepti, n. (septum, septi, n.) 울타리, 칸막이 벽, 격벽, 사이벽,

　　　중격(中隔) 　　　　　　　　　　　　　　　　　 **E** *septum,* (pl.) *septa,* *(septum >)* *septal*

　　　> L. saeptatus, saeptata, saeptatum (septatus, septata, septatum) 사이벽이

　　　　　있는, 격벽이 있는 　　　　　　　　　　　　　　　　 **E** *septate, multiseptate*

　　　　　> L. saeptulum, saeptluli, n. (septulum, septluli, n.) (< + -ulum

　　　　　　　diminutive suffix) 작은 사이벽, 소중격(小中隔) 　　**E** *septulum,* (pl.) *septula*

　　　< L. saepio, saepsi (saepivi, saepii), saeptum, saepire 울타리로 둘러막다

　　< L. saepes, saepis, f. 울타리

< IE. saip- *hedge fence*

L. arcus, arcus, m. 활, 궁(弓), 고리, 무지개, 아치, 홍예문(虹霓門), 만곡(灣曲) 　**E** *archer, arc, arch, arcade*

　　　[용례] lamina arcus vertebrae 척추뼈(의) 고리(의) 판, 추궁판(椎弓板)

　　　　(문법) lamina 판: 단수 주격 < lamina, laminae, f. 판, 층

　　　　　arcus 고리의: 단수 속격

　　　　　vertebrae 척추뼈의: 단수 속격 < vertebra, vertebrae, f.

　　　> L. arcuo, **arcuavi**, arcuatum, arcuare 활 모양으로 휘게 하다, 활 모양으로 휘다 　**E** *arcuate*

< IE. arku- *bow and arrow (uncertain which, perhaps both as a unit)* 　　　　　　**E** *arrow*

L. fornix, fornicis, m. (< *vaulted brick oven*) 둥근 천장, 원개(圓蓋), 반원형 지붕이 있는 통로,

　　　유곽(遊廓); 천장, 구석, 뇌활 　　　　　　　　　 **E** *fornix,* *(fornix >)* *fornical, subfornical*

　　　> L. fornicatus, fornicata, fornicatum 둥근 천장을 한 　　　　 **E** *(adjective)* *fornicate*

　　　> L. fornicor, fornicatus sum, fornicari 매음하다, (미혼으로) 사통(私通)하다 　**E** *(verb)* *fornicate*

< IE. gʷher- *to heat, warm*

　　　E *burn, heartburn (< 'burning sensation in the lower part of the chest'), brimstone (< 'burning stone, sulfur'), brand (< 'piece of burning wood, sword'), brandish, brandy (< 'to burn, to distill')*

　　　> L. fornus, forni, m. (furnus, furni, m.) 빵 굽는 가마, 화덕

　　　　　> L. fornax, fornacis, f. 화덕, 가마, 노(爐), 아궁이; (Fornax) (로마 신화) 아궁이의

　　　　　　　여신 　　　　　　　　　　　　　　　　　　　　　 **E** *furnace, Fornax*

　　　> L. forceps, forcipis, m., f. (< formus *hot* + -ceps *taking* < capĕre *to take*) 부집게,

　　　　집게, 족집게, 집게발, 겸자(鉗子), 학익진(鶴翼陣) 　　　　 **E** *forceps,* *(forceps >)* *forcipate*

　　　> G. thermos, thermē, thermon *warm, hot*

　　　　　> G. thermē, thermēs, f. *warmth, heat*

　　　　　E *therm(o)-, thermic, thermal, thermodynamics, thermometer, thermoplastic, thermostat, thermophile, diathermy; thermolabile, thermostable*

　　　　　> L. hyperthermia, hyperthermiae, f. (< G. hyper- *over*) 고열,

　　　　　　　고열요법 　　　　　　　　　　　　　　　　 **E** *hyperthermia (hyperthermy)*

　　　　　> L. hypothermia, hypothermiae, f. (< G. hyp(o)- *under*) 체온저하 　**E** *hypothermia*

　　　> L. Thermus, Thermi, m. 호열균속(好熱菌屬)

[용례] Thermus aquaticus 호열균

(문법) Thermus 호열균속(屬): 단수 주격

    aquaticus 물속에서 사는: 형용사, 남성형 단수 주격

    < aquaticus, aquatica, aquaticum

E Thermus aquaticus

L. **trabs, trabis,** f. 대들보[梁], 통나무, 통나무집   **E** *architrave*

> L. trabicula, trabiculae, f. (trabecula, trabeculae, f.) (< + -cula *diminutive suffix*)

    작은 들보, 서까래; 잔기둥, 소주(小柱), 주(柱)

>   **E** *trabecula,* (pl.) *trabeculae,* *(trabecula >)* *trabecular,* *(trabecula >)* *trabeculate,* *(trabeculate >)* *trabeculation*

> L. taberna, tabernae, f. (< *traberna) 오막살이집, 초막; 가계, 주점   **E** *tavern*

>   > L. tabernaculum, tabernaculi, n. (< + -culum *diminutive suffix*) 막사   **E** *tabernacle*

< IE. treb- *beamed structure, building, dwelling*

L. **columna, columnae,** f. (둥근) 기둥, 원주(圓柱), 주(柱); (신문·잡지의)

    특별 기고란   **E** *column, columnist, colonel, colonnade*

> L. columnaris, columnare 원주형의   **E** *columnar*

> L. columnella, columnellae, f. (columella, columellae, f.) (< + -ella *diminutive*

    suffix) 작은 기둥, 소주(小柱), 축주(軸柱), 코기둥   **E** *columnella (columella)*

< IE. kel- *to be prominent, hill*   **E** *hill, (hill + -ock > 'little hill' >) hillock, holm*

> L. columen, columinis, n. 꼭대기, 정점, 절정

> > (*contracted*) L. culmen, culminis, n. 꼭대기, 정점, 절정   **E** *culmen*

>   > L. culmino, culminavi, culminatum, culminare 남중(南中)하다, 절정에

        이르다, 완결시키다, ~으로 끝나다   **E** *culminate*

> L. collis, collis, m. 언덕, 야산

>   > L. colliculus, colliculi, m. (< + -cullus *diminutive suffix*) 작은 언덕, 둔덕,

      소구(小丘)   **E** *colliculus,* (pl.) *colliculi*

> L. celsus, celsa, celsum 우뚝 솟은

∽ L. cello, –, celsum, cellĕre 우뚝 솟다

>   > L. excello, **excellui**, excelsum, excellĕre (< ex- *out of, away from* + cellĕre

    to project) 두드러지다, 뛰어나다   **E** *excel, excellent*

>   > L. excelsus, excelsa, excelsum (*past participle*) 뛰어난

>   > L. excelsior, excelsior, excelsius ((gen.) excelsioris) (< + -ior

        comparative suffix) 더 뛰어난   **E** *excelsior*

>   > L. excelentia, excelentiae, f. 탁월; (Excelentia) 각하(閣下)   **E** *excellence, excellency*

L. **porta, portae,** f. 배의 하역구, 성문, 대문, 현관문, 문(門)   **E** *port, portal*

< IE. per- *to lead, to pass-over; a verbal root belonging to the group of* IE. per *forward,*

    through (Vide PORTARE: *See* E. *portable*)

G. pylē, pylēs, f. *gate, entrance, mountain-pass*

> G. pylis, pylidos, f. *little gate*

> L. Dipylidium, Dipylidii, n. (< *proglottids of the adult have genital pores on both sides < two little gates < G.* di- *two* + pylid- + -ion *diminutive suffix*) (조충 條蟲) 디필리듐속(屬)　　　　　　　**E** Dipylidium

> G. pylōros, pylōrou, m., f. (pylouros, pylourou, m.) (< + ouros, ourou, m. *watcher, warder*) *gatekeeper, porter*

> L. pylorus, pylori, m. 날문(-門), 유문(幽門)　　　　**E** *pylorus*

> L. pyloricus, pylorica, pyloricum 날문의, 유문의　　**E** *pyloric*

> G. dipylos, dipylos, dipylon (< di- *two*) *double-gated*　　**E** *Dipylon* (< 'the double gateway in Athens on the north-west side of the city')

L. valva, valvae, f. (< *leaf of a door < that which turns*) 두 짝으로 된 접는 문의 한 짝, 쌍 문의 한 짝; 판(瓣), 판막(瓣膜)　　　　　　　　　　**E** *valve*

> L. valvula, valvulae, f. (< + -ula *diminutive suffix*) 소판(小瓣), 판막　**E** *valvular*

< IE. wel- *to turn, to roll; with derivatives referring to curved, enclosing objects* (Vide VOLVĔRE: *See* E. *volute*)

L. fenestra, fenestrae, f. 창(窓)　　　　　　**E** *fenestra,* (pl.) *fenestrae*

> L. fenestro, fenestravi, fenestratum, fenestrare 창을 내다, 창문을 달다　　　　　　　　**E** *fenestrate, fenestrated, fenestration*

< (*probably*) (*Etruscan*) *fnestra *window*

L. vestibulum, vestibuli, n. 현관, 입구, 전정(前庭), 어귀　　　　　　**E** *vestibulum (vestibule),* (*vestibule* >) *vestibular, vestibulocochlear*

L. atrium, atrii, n. (< *the open central court, from which the enclosed rooms led off, in the type of a large Roman house known as a domus < perhaps originally the place where the smoke from the hearth escaped through a hole in the roof*) 중정(中庭), 안뜰, 경매장의 큰 방, 방(房), 심방(心房)　　　**E** *atrium,* (pl.) *atria,* (*atrium* >) *atrial, atrioventricular*

< IE. ater- *fire*

> L. ater, atra, atrum (< *blackened by fire*) 거무칙칙한, 검은

> L. atrox, (gen.) atrocis 포악한　　　　　　**E** *atrocious*

> L. atrocitas, atrocitatis, f. 포악　　　　**E** *atrocity*

> (*Persian*) zar *gold*　　　　　　　**E** *zircon, zirconium (Zr)*

> (*possibly*) (*Sanskrit*) atharva *priest*　　　　**E** *Atharvaveda*

L. focus, foci, m. 벽로(壁爐), 화로(火爐), 가정; 중심부, 초점(焦點), 병소(病巢), 병터, 국소(局所)　　　**E** *focus* (< ' *burning point of a lens or mirror'*), (pl.) *foci, foyer, fusillade*

> L. focalis, focale 화로의; 중심부의, 초점의, 병소의, 병터의, 국소의,

국소적　　　**E** (focalia (*neuter* pl.) >) *fuel; focal, unifocal, bifocal, multifocal, confocal*

< IE. bhok- *to flame, to burn*

G. kamara, kamaras, f. *vault, chamber*

> L. camara, camarae, f. 반원형 천장이 있는 방, 방, 반원형 천장

E (camera obscura *'dark chamber'* >) *camera, unicameral, bicameral, chamber, chamberlain,* (Sp. camarada *'chamberful'* > *'chamber-mate'* >) *comrade*

< IE. kam-, kam-er- *to arch, to bend*

> (*suggested*) G. kaminos, kaminou, f. *furnace, kiln*

> L. caminus, camini, m. 아궁이, 화덕, 가마　　　　　　**E** *chimney*

G. thalamos, thalmou, m. *inner chamber, bedroom, bridal chamber*

> L. thalamus, thalami, m. (< *a part of the brain at which a nerve originates or appears*

to originate; now specifically the optic thalamus out of which the optic nerve

rises) 안방, 침실, 신방(新房), (부부의) 침상(寢床); (해부) 시상(視床)　　**E** *thalamus, thalamic*

> L. epithalamus, epithalami, m. (< G. ep(i)- *upon*)

시상상부(視床上部)　　　　　　　**E** *epithalamus, epithalamic*

> L. hypothalamus, hypothalami, m. (< G. hyp(o)- *under*)

시상하부(視床下部)　　　　　　**E** *hypothalamus, hypothalamic*

< IE. dhel- *cavity, hollow*　　　　　　　　　　　　**E** *dale, dell*

> D. Tal, Tals (Tales), n. (Thal, Thals (Thales), n.) 계곡

> D. Joachimstal (Joachimsthal) (< *St. Joachim's valley*) 보헤미아 지방의 지명

> D. Taler, Talers, m. (Thaler, Thalers, m.) Joachimstal의 은으로 주조한

화폐; 은화, 경화, 돈　　　　　　　　**E** *dollar*

> D. Neandertaler, Neandertalers, m. (< *Neander valley*)

네안데르탈인　　　　　　　　　**E** *Neandertal (Neanderthal)*

> D. Delle, Delle, f. 얕게 오목 패인 곳, 물이 없는 얕은 골짜기　　**E** *delle,* (pl.) *dellen*

의복

L. toga, togae, f. 로마시민의 겉옷, 로마 시민권　　　　**E** *toga, togavirus* (< *'enveloped virus'*)

< IE. (s)teg- *to cover* (Vide TEGĔRE: See E. *tectum*)

L. tunica, tunicae, f. (< *cituna) 로마인의 속옷, 소매가 짧은 속두루마기; 층, 막　　**E** *tunica, tunic*

< *Of Phoenician origin, akin to* (*Hebrew*) kuttonet, kətonet

> G. chitōn, chitōnos, m. *tunic*

> E *chiton,* (chitonin > 'the major constituent in the exoskeleton of arthropods and the cell walls of fungi' >) *chitin, chitinous, chitosan* (< 'a polysaccharide obtained by deacetylation of chitin')

< (*Central Semitic*) kuttan, kittan *linen garment*

< (*Akkadian*) kitu, kitaum *flax, linen*

< (*Sumerian*) gada, gida *flax, linen*

L. pallium, pallii, n. 그리스인의 himation을 로마인이 걸쳤을 때의 명칭, 외투(큰 4각 천), 휘장; 연체동물의 외투막, 겉질, 피질(皮質)　　E *pallium, pall*

> L. neopallium, neopallii, n. (< G. neos *new* + L. pallium *cloak*)

　신(新)피질　　E *neopallium* (neocortex)

> L. archipallium, archipallii, n. (< G. archē *beginning* + L. pallium *cloak*)

　원시(原始)피질　　E *archipallium* (archicortex)

> L. palaeopallium, palaeopallii, n. (< G. palaios *old, ancient* + L. pallium *cloak*)

　고(古)피질　　E *palaeopallium* (paleopallium) (paleocortex)

> L. pallio, palliavi, palliatum, palliare 가리다, 겉꾸미다, (일시적으로) 완화 시키다　　E *palliate, palliative*

∽ L. palla, pallae, f. 로마인의 길고 넓은 부인용 외투 (큰 4각 천), 관을 덮는 검은 보

G. himation, himatiou, n. (< + -ion *diminutive suffix*) *the outer garment worn by the ancient Greeks: an oblong piece of cloth thrown over the left shoulder, and fastened either over or under the right*　　E *himation*

< G. hima, himatos, n. (heima, heimatos, n.) *garment, cover*

< G. hennynai *to clothe*

< IE. wes- *to clothe* (Vide VESTIS: *See* E. *vest*)

G. peplos, peplou, m. *garment, robe, cloak, long dress*

E *peplos* (< 'viral envelope'), (peplos + meros 'part' > 'a knob-like projection on the viral envelope' >) *peplomer*

> L. peplus, pepli, m. (peplum, pepli, n.). 겉옷, 예복　　E *peplus (peplum)*

G. chlamys, chlamydos, f. *cloak (draped around the shoulder), military cloak*

> L. chlamys, chlamydis, f. 짧은 외투,

　그리스식 군복　　E *chlamydospore* (< 'Each spore... has its own protective envelope.')

> L. Chlamydia, Chlamydiae, f. (< *the cytoplasmic inclusions 'draped' around the infected cell's nucleus*) (세균) 클라미디아속(屬)　　E Chlamydia, *chlamydial*

지명

L. **Latium, Latii,** n. 라티움(로마 동남쪽에 있던 이탈리아 원주민의 지방, 라틴어의 발상지)

> L. Latinus, Latina, Latinum 라티움의, 라틴인의, 라틴어의   **E** *Latin*

> L. Latinitas, Latinitatis, f. 라티어법   **E** *Latinity*

> L. Latinizo, -, -, Latinizare (Latino, -, -, Latinare) 라틴어로 번역하다,
라틴어화하다   **E** *Latinize, Latinate*

L. **Graecia, Graeciae,** f. 그리스   **E** *Greece, Grecian*

< L. Graecus, Graeca, Graecum 그리스의, 그리스인의,
그리스어의   **E** *Greek, Graeco- (Greco-)*

< G. Graikos, Graikē, Graikon *of Graes; originally used by Illyrians for the Dorians*
in Epirus, later applied by Italians to all Hellenes

> G. graikizein *to speak Greek*   **E** *Grecize*

< G. Graes *native name of the people of Epirus*

L. **Africa, Africae,** f. 아프리카   **E** *Africa*

> L. Africanus, Africana, Africanum 아프리카의, 아프리카인의   **E** *African*

< L. Afer, Afri, m. 북아프리카의 옛민족 이름 (현대 Berber족의 선조)   **E** *Afr(o)-*

L. **America, Americae,** f. 아메리카   **E** *America, americium (Am)*

> L. Americanus, Americana, Americanum 아메리카의,
아메리카인의   **E** *American, Afro-American (Aframerican)*

< L. Americus Vespucius **Amerigo Vespucci** (1451-1512), *Italian explorer and cartographer*

L. **Corea, Coreae,** f. 한국   **E** *Korea*

> L. Coreanus, Coreana, Coreanum 한국의, 한국인의   **E** *Korean*

∞ L. Koreanus, Koreana, Koreanum (*not conformed*) 한국의, 한국인의

∞ L. Koreensis, Koreense (*not conformed*) 한국의, 한국 출신의

< (*Korean*) Korai (Koryu) 고려 (918-1392)

> L. Koraiensis, Koraiense 한국의, 한국 출신의

[용례] Aster koraiensis 벌개미취

(문법) Aster 국화과 식물의 속명(屬名): 단수 주격 < Aster, Asteris, m.
koraiensis 한국의, 한국산의: 형용사, 남·여성형 단수 주격

L. **Europa, Europae,** f. 유럽   **E** *Europe, Euro, Eur(o)-, europium (Eu)*

> L. Europaeus, Europaea, Europaeum 유럽의, 유럽인의   **E** *European*

< G. Eurōpē, Eurōpēs, f. *Europe*

L. Attica, Atticae, f. 아티카 **E** *Attica*

    < G. Attikē, Attikēs, f. *a triangular promontory of eastern Greece, of which Athens is the*
        capital

        > G. Attikos, Attikē, Attikon *of Attic*

           > L. Atticus, Attica, Atticum 아티카의   **E** *Attic, attic (< 'an Attic style')*

L. Aegyptus, Aegypti, f. (Aegyptos, Aegypti, f.) 이집트   **E** *Egypt*

    > L. Aegyptius, Aegyptia, Aegyptium 이집트의, 이집트인의, 이집트어의

        E *Egyptian, (Egyptian >) Gypsy (Gipsy) (< 'a member of a wandering race (by themselves*
        called Romany), of Hindu origin, which was thought to have come from Egypt')

    < G. Aigyptos, Aigyptou, m. *Egypt*

        > G. Aigyptikos, Aigyptikē, Aigyptikon *of Egypt*

           > L. Aegypticus, Aegyptica, Aegypticum 이집트의

    > (*Arabic*) al-gibt (al-gubt) *Copts*

        > L. Coptus, Copti, m. 콥트 사람, 콥트 교도   **E** *Copt, Coptic*

L. Arabia, Arabiae, f. 아라비아   **E** *Arabia, Arabian*

        < L. Arabius, Arabia, Arabium 아랍인의, 아랍의

        < L. Arabs, Arabis, m. 아랍인, 아랍   **E** *Arab, arabesque*

           > L. Arabis, Arabidis, f. (< *growing on sandy or stony places*) (식물)

           장대속(屬)   **E** *Arabis*

               > L. Arabidopsis, Arabidopsis, f. (< *resembling the genus* Arabis

                    < G. opsis, opseōs, f. *seeing*) (식물) 애기장대속(屬)   **E** *Arabidopsis*

    < G. Araps, Arabos, m. *an Arab*

        > G. Arabikos, Arabikē, Arabikon *Arabic*

           > L. Arabicus, Arabica, Arabicum 아랍의

        E *Arabic;* (gummi Arabicum *'gum arabic'* >) *arabin,* (arabin >) *arabinose,*
        (arabinose > (formed arbitrarily by rearrangement of some of the
        letters) >) ribose, (ribose >) deoxyribose, (ribose >) ribulose

  < (*Arabic*) arab *the indigenous name of the people*

L. Asia, Asiae, f. 아시아   **E** *Asia, Euro-Asian (Eurasian)*

        > L. Asianus, Asiana, Asianum 아시아의   **E** *Asian*

    < G. Asia, Asias, f.

        > G. Asiatikos, Asiatikē, Asiatikon *of Asia*

           > L. Asiaticus, Asiatica, Asiaticum 아시아의   **E** *Asiatic*

  < (*suggested*) (*Akkadian*) asu *to rise (of the sun), to go out*

L. Hispania, Hispaniae, f. 스페인
E *Spain, Spanish, Spaniard*, Sp. *España*

> L. Hispanus, Hispana, Hispanum 스페인의

> L. Hispaniensis, Hispaniense 스페인의, 스페인 출신의

< G. Hispania, Hispanias, f. *Spain*

> G. Hispanikos, Hispanikē, Hispanikon *of Spain*

> L. Hispanicus, Hispanica, Hispanicum 스페인의
E *Hispanic*

L. India, Indiae, f. 인도
E *India, Indian*

> L. Indus, Inda, Indum 인도의

< G. India, Indias, f. *India*

> G. Indikos, Indikē, Indikon *of India*

> L. Indicus, Indica, Indicum 인도의

> E (indicum (*neuter* sing.) *'Indian substance'* >) *indigo*, (*indigo blue* + oleum *'oil'* >) *indole*, (indole + methyl + acetic + -in >) *indo-methacin*

< G. Indos *the river Indus*

< (*Sanskrit*) sindhu *river, the river Indus*

L. Persia, Persiae, f. 페르시아
E *Persia, Persian*

> L. Perseus, Persea, Perseum 페르시아의

< G. Persis, Persidos, f. *Persia*

> G. Persikos, Persikē, Persikon *Persian*

> L. Persicus, Persica, Persicum 페르시아의

[용례] Persicum malum (< G. Persikon malon) 복숭아
E *peach*
(문법) Persicum (< G. Persikon) 페르시아의: 형용사,
중성형 단수 주격
malum (< G. malon) 사과: 단수 주격
< malum, mali, n. (< G. malon, malou, n.)

> L. lycopersicon, lycopersici, n. (< *an Egyptian plant with a strong-smelling yellowish juice* < (*suggested*) *referring to the poisonous or toxic properties* < G. lykos *wolf* + Persikon malon *peach*) 리코페르시콘속(屬)의 가지과 식물

[용례] Lycopersicon esculentum 토마토
E *lycopene*
(문법) Lycopersicon 속명(屬名): 단수 주격
esculentum 식용에 알맞은: 형용사, 중성형 단수 주격
< esculentus, esculenta, esculentum

< (*Old Persian*) parsa

L. Germania, Germaniae, f. 게르만족의 나라, 독일
E *Germany*

> L. Germanus, Germana, Germanum 독일의   **E** *German, germanium (Ge)*

> L. Germanicus, Germanica, Germanicum 게르만족 나라의, 게르만족의, 독일의   **E** *Germanic*

L. Japonia, Japoniae, f. 일본

> L. Japonensis, Japonense 일본의, 일본 출신의

> L. Japonicus, Japonica, Japonicum 일본의

< (*Chinese*) Jih-pŭn 日本   **E** *Japan, japan, Japanese*

< (*Japanese*) 日本 にっぽん

L. Sina, Sinae, f. 중국   **E** *Sino-*

> L. Sinensis, Sinense 중국의, 중국 출신의

> L. Sinicus, Sinica, Sinicum 중국의

< (*Arabic*) Sin *China*

< (*Chinese*) Qin (Chin) 진(秦, 221-206 B.C.E.)   **E** *(probably) China, chinaware, (chinaware >) china*

> L. Chinensis, Chînense (< *on the pattern of* L. sinensis < E. *china*) 중국의,
중국 출신의

L. Paris, Paris, f. (< Lutetia Parisiorum *midwater-dwelling of the Parisians*) 파리   **E** *Paris*

> L. Parisiensis, Parisiense 파리의, 파리 출신의   **E** *Parisian, F. Parisien, F. Parisienne*

< L. Parisii, Parisiorum, m. 세느강 주위 골(*Gaul*) 부족의 이름

L. Seoul, f. (불변화 명사) 서울

> L. Seoulensis, Seoulense 서울의, 서울 출신의

< (*Korean*) 서울

동물

L. fauna, faunae, f. (< *adopted by Linnaeus as term parallel to flora*) 동물상(相)   **E** *fauna*

< L. Fauna, Faunae, f. (로마 신화) Faunus의 누이이며 아내

< L. Faunus, Fauni, m. (로마 신화) Saturnus의 손자, Picus의 아들, Latinus의
아버지, Latium의 왕, 농산물과 가축의 수호신이 됨   **E** *faun*

< (*probably*) IE. dhaunos *wolf, strangler*

< IE. dhau- *to strangle*

L. bos, bovis, m., f. 소, 황소   **E** *beef*

> L. bovinus, bovina, bovinum 소의   **E** *bovine*

> L. buculus, buculi, m. (< + -culus *diminutive suffix*) 어린 황소　E *(bugle-horn >)* **bugle**

< IE. gᵂou- *ox, bull, cow*　E **cow**

　> L. buccina, buccinae, f. (소)뿔나팔

　　> L. buccino, **buccinavi**, buccinatum, buccinare 나팔 불다

　　　> L. buccinator, buccinatoris, m. 볼근, 협근(頬筋)　E *buccinator*

> G. **bous, boos, m., f.** *ox, bull, cow*

　> G. boubalos, boubalou, m. *antelope,*

　　wild ox　E **buffalo,** *(buffalo > 'leather of whitish yellow color' >)* **buff,** *(buff >)* **buffy**

　> G. boutyron, boutyrou, n. (< bous + tyros, tyrou, m. *cheese / but perhaps of*
　　Scythian or other barbarous origin) *butter*

　　> L. butyrum, butyri, n. 버터, 우락(牛酪)　E *butter, butyric acid, butterfly*

　> G. boulimia, boulimias, f. (< bous + limos, limou, m. *hunger, famine*) *great*
　　hunger

　　> L. bulimia, bulimiae, f. 폭식(증)　E *bulimia*

　> G. Boukephalos, Boukephalou, m. (< *ox-headed* < bous + -kephalos *-headed*)
　　the name of Alexander the Great's celebrated charger

　　> L. Bucephalus, Bucephali, m. 알렉산더 대왕의 애마　E *Bucephalus*

　> L. buphthalmos, buphthalmi, m. (buphthalmus, buphthalmi, m.) (< *ox eye:*
　　enlargement of the eyeball owing to increased intra-ocular pressure <
　　G. bous + ophthalmos *eye*) 우안(牛眼), 소눈증　E *buphthalmos (buphthalmus)*

L. **vacca, vaccae, f.** 암소　E Sp. *vaquero*

　> L. vaccinus, vaccina, vaccinum 암소의

　　> L. vaccinia, vacciniae, f. 우두(牛痘)　E *vaccinia*

　　　> L. vacciniformis, vacciniforme (< forma *form*) 우두 모양의　E *vacciniform*

　　> L. vaccina, vaccinae, f. (< *early use of the cowpox virus against smallpox*)
　　　우두종(牛痘種), 백신　E *vaccine, (vaccine >)* **vaccinate,** *(vaccinate >)* **vaccination**

< IE. wak- *cow*

G. **tauros, taurou, m.** *bull,*

　　　ox　E **taurine** *(< 'obtained from ox-bile'),* **taurocholic acid** *(< 'obtained from ox-bile')*

　> L. taurus, tauri, m. 황소; (Taurus)

　　(천문) 황소자리　E *Taurus, toreador (< 'bull-fighter'),* **torero** *(< 'bull-fighter')*

　　> G. Minōtauros, Minōtaurou, m. (< Minōs *Minos*) *(Greek mythology) Minotaur*

　　　> L. Minotaurus, Minotauri, m. (그리스 신화) 미노타우루스　E *Minotaur*

　< IE. tauro- *bull*

< IE. sta- *to stand* (Vide STARE: *See* E. *stay*)

L. **vitulus, vituli, m.** 송아지, 동물의 새끼

　> L. vitellus, vitelli, m. (< + -ellus *diminutive suffix*) 송아지, 귀염둥이; 계란 노른자위,

난황(卵黃)　　　　　　　　　　　　**E** *veal, vellum;* (vitellus ovi *'yolk of egg'* >) *vitellin*

> L. vitellinus, vitellina, vitellinum 난황(卵黃)의　　　　　　　　**E** *vitelline*

< IE. wet- *year*

> L. vetus, (gen.) veteris 나이든, 늙은, 묵은, 옛, 낡은

　　> L. veteranus, veterana, veteranum 옛, 보병의　　　　　　　**E** *veteran*

　　> L. veterinus, veterina, veterinum (일할 수 있을 만큼) 나이든, 짐바리 짐승의

　　　　> L. veterinarius, veterinaria, veterinarium 짐바리 짐승의,

　　　　　　수의사의　　　　　　　　　　　**E** *veterinary, veterinarian*

　　> L. invetero, **inveteravi**, inveteratum, inveterare (< in- *in, on, into, toward* +

　　　　vetus *old*) 오래 가게 하다, 묵히다　　　　　　　**E** *inveterate*

L. equus, equi, m. 말

　　　　> L. equinus, equina, equinum 말의　　　　　　　　　　**E** *equine*

　　　　> L. eques, equitis, m. 기수, 기병, 기사

　　　　　　> L. equester, equestris, equestre 기수의, 기병의, 기사의　**E** *equestrian*

< IE. ekwo- *horse*

> G. hippos, hippou, m., f. *horse*　**E** *hippuric acid* (< *'acid found in the urine of horses'*)

　　> G. hippodromos, hippodromou, m. (< + dromos, dromou, m. *race-course*)

　　　　race-course for chariots

　　　　　> L. hippodromos, hippodromi, m. (hippodromus, hippodromi, m.) 이륜

　　　　　　마차 경주장, 경마장　　　　　　　　　　**E** *hippodrome*

　　> G. hippokampos, hippokampou, m. (< + kampos, kampou, m. *sea monster*)

　　　　sea horse

　　　　　> L. hippocampus, hippocampi, m. 해마(海馬)　**E** *hippocampus, hippocampal*

　　> G. hippopotamos, hippopotamou, m. (< + potamos, potamou, m. *river*) *river*

　　　　horse

　　　　　> L. hippopotamus, hippopotami, m. 하마(河馬)　　**E** *hippopotamus*

　　> G. Hippokratēs, Hippokratous, m. (< *one superior in horses* < + kratos, kratous,

　　　　n. *power*) *Hippocrates*

　　　　　> L. Hippocrates, Hippocratis, m. 히포크라테스　　**E** *Hippocrates*

　　> G. Hippokrēnē, Hippokrēnēs, f. (< Hippou krēnē *fountain of the Horse, so*

　　　　called because it was fabled to have been produced by a stroke of Pegasus'

　　　　hoof) *Name of a fountain on Mount Helicon, sacred to the Muses; hence*

　　　　used allusively in reference to poetic or literary inspiration

　　　　　> L. Hippocrene, Hippocrenes, f. 헬리콘산의 샘, 뮤즈의 영천(靈泉), 시적

　　　　　　영감　　　　　　　　　　　　　**E** *Hippocrene*

　　> G. philippos, philippos, philippon (< philein (phileein) *to love*) *fond of horses*

　　　　> G. Philippos, Philippou, m. (*personal name*) *Philip*

　　　　　> L. Philippus, Philippi, m. (남자 이름)

　　　　　　필립　　　　　　　　**E** *Philip,* (King Philip II of Spain >) *Philippines*

L. caballus, caballi, m. 짐 끄는 말   E *cavalier, chevalier*

    > L. caballarius, caballarii, n. 마부   E *cavalry*

    > L. caballico, −, −, caballicare 말타고 가다   E *cavalcade*

  < *Of Asiatic origin*

L. asinus, acini, m. (acina, acinae, f.) 당나귀   E *ass, easel*

    > L. asininus, asinina, asininum 당나귀의   E *asinine*

  < (*probably*) *Of Semitic origin*

    > G. onos, onou, m., f. *ass*

L. mulus, muli, m. (mula, mulae, f.) 노새   E *mule*

  < (*probably*) *Of* non-IE. *origin*

L. porcus, porci, m. 돼지   E *pork,* (porcus *'hog'* + spina *'thorn'* > *'spinous hog'* >) *porcupine*

    > L. porcinus, porcina, porcinum 돼지의   E *porcine*

    > L. porculus, porculi, m. (< + −ulus *diminutive suffix*) 새끼돼지

    > L. porcella, porcellae, f. (< + −ella *diminutive suffix*) 새끼돼지

         E *porcelain (< 'cowrie shell' < 'the curved shape of the cowrie shell, probably on account of the resemblance of the fissure of its shell to a vulva (it is unclear whether the reference is specifically to the vulva of a sow)')*

  < IE. porko- *young pig*   E *farrow*

L. sus, suis, m., f. 돼지

      > L. suculus, suculi, m. (sucula, suculae, f.) (< + −ulus (−ula) *diminutive suffix*)

         새끼돼지   E *soil (< 'muddy wallow for wild boar')*

      > L. suile, suilis, n. 돼지우리

    < IE. su- *pig*   E *swine, sow, hog, socket (< 'plowshare')*

        > G. hys, hyos, m., f. *sow, pig*

            > G. hyoskyamos, hyoskyamou, m. (< *pig's bean* < + kyamos, kyamou, m.

               bean) *henbane*

                > L. Hyoscyamus, Hyoscyami, m. (가지과의 유독성 식물)

                 사리풀속(屬)   E *hyoscyamine,* (hyoscyamine >) *hyoscine*

             > G. hyaina, hyainēs, f. (< *hog-like mane*) *hyena*

               > L. hyaena, hyaenae, f. 하이에나   E *hyaena (hyena)*

    < (*probably*) IE. seuə- *to give birth*   E *son*

L. scrofa, scrofae, f. (scropha, scrophae, f.) (< *rooter, digger*) 씨암돼지   E *screw*

    > (*supposed to be subject to the disease*) L. scrofulae, scrofularum, f. (scrophulae,

       scrophularum, f.) (pl.) (< + −ula *diminutive suffix*) 결핵성 경부 림프절염,

피부샘병　　　　　　　　　　　　　　　　　　　　　　　　　　　**E** *scrofula*

　　< IE. (s)ker- *to cut*

　< IE. sek- *to cut* (Vide SECARE; *See* E. *secant*)

L. hybrida, hybridae, m., f. (hibrida, hibridae, m., f.) 집돼지 암컷과 멧돼지 수컷의

　　튀기, 잡종, 혼혈아　　　　　　　　　　　　**E** *hybrid, hybridize, hybridization*

　　> L. *hybridoma, *hybridomatis, n. (< + G. -ōma *noun suffix denoting tumor*) 잡종

　　세포종, 하이브리도마　　　　　　　　　　　　　　　　　　**E** *hybridoma*

　< (*probably*) *Of* non-IE. *origin*

L. hircus, hirci, m. 염소, 산양, 노린내, 호색한

　　> L. hircinus, hircina, hircinum 염소의, 산양의, 노린내 나는　　　　**E** *hircine*

　< (*probably*) IE. ghers- *to bristle* (Vide HORRĒRE; *See* E. *horror*)

G. aix, aigos, m., f. *goat*

　　> G. aigokerōs, aigokerōtos, m. (< + keras, keratos, n. *horn*) *goat-horned, Capricorn*

　　> (*suggested*) G. aigis, aigidos, f. (*Greek mythology*) *goatskin breastplate of Zeus or*
　　　　Athena, shield of Zeus or Athena

　　　　> L. aegis, aegidis, f. (그리스 신화) 제우스신의 방패, 아테나 여신의 방패; 방패,
　　　　　　보호　　　　　　　　　　　　　　　　　　　　**E** *aegis (egis)*

　< IE. aig- *goat*

L. caper, capri, m. 숫염소, 산양, 땀내, 암내

　　E *capric acid* (< *'goat-like smell'*), (capric acid >) *caproic acid, chevron* (< *'pair of rafters, perhaps from the angular shape of a goat's hind legs'*)

　　> L. capra, caprae, f. 암염소, 산양

　　　　E (It. capriola (*diminutive*) *'carriage's bouncing motion like goat's leap'* >) *cabriolet (cab)*

　　> L. caprinus, caprina, caprinum 염소의, 산양의　　　　　　　　**E** *caprine*

　　> L. Capricornus, Capricorni, m. (< + cornu *horn*) (천문) 산양좌　**E** *Capricorn*

　< IE. kap-ro- *he-goat, buck*

G. tragos, tragou, m. *he-goat*

　　　> G. tragōidia, tragōidias, f. (< (*suggested*) *goatskin dress of the performers,*
　　　　representing satyrs; goat-song < tragos + ōidē *song*) *tragedy*

　　　　> L. tragoedia, tragoediae, f. 비극　　　　　　　　　　　**E** *tragedy*

　　　> G. tragikos, tragikē, tragikon (< *of he-goat, but in sense associated with*
　　　　tragedy) *tragic*

　　　　> L. tragicus, tragica, tragicum 비극의　　　　　　　　　　**E** *tragic*

　　> L. tragus, tragi, m. 귀구슬　　　**E** *tragus* (< *'hair tuft like a goat's beard'*), *intertragic*

> L. antitragus, antitragi, m. (< G. ant(i)- *before, against, instead of*)

맞구슬, 대주(對珠)

E *antitragus*

< IE. treg- *to gnaw*

< IE. terə- *to rub, to turn* (Vide TERĒRE; *See* E. *trite*)

G. **chimaira, chimairas, f.** (< *female animal one year (winter) old*) *she-goat; a fire-spouting monster with lion's head, serpent's tail, and goat's body*

> L. chimaera, chimaerae, f. (chimera, chimerae, f.)

키메라

E *chimaera (chimera), chimeric, chimerism*

< IE. ghei- *winter, snow* (Vide HIEMS; *See* E. *hiemal*)

L. **ovis, ovis, f.** 양

> L. ovinus, ovina, ovinum 양의

E *ovine*

< IE. owi- *sheep*

E *ewe*

L. **agnus, agni, m.** (한 살 미만의) 어린 양

< IE. agʷh-no- *lamb*

E *yean*

> G. **amnos, amnou, m., f.** *lamb*

> G. amnion, amniou, n. (< + -ion *diminutive suffix*) *lamb, bowl in which the blood of victims was caught, membrane around a fetus*

> L. amnion, amnii, n. 양막(羊膜)

E *amnion, amniotic, amni(o)-, amniocentesis, amnioscope, (amnion > (variant) amnios >) hydramnios (< 'excess of amniotic fluid'), oligohydramnios*

L. **lepus, leporis, m.** 산토끼, 토끼

> L. leporinus, leporina, leporinum 산토끼의, 토끼의

E *leporine*

< *Of Iberian-Balearic origin*

G. **lagōs, lagō, m.** (lagōos, lagōou, m.) (< *with drooping ears*) *hare*

E *lagophthalmos (lagophthalmus) (< 'being unable to close the eyes, as the hare was supposed to')*

< IE. (s)leg- *to be slack, to be languid* (Vide LAXARE; *See* E. *laxative*)

+ IE. ous- *ear* (Vide AURIS; *See* E. *aural*)

L. **canis, canis, m., f.** ((gen. pl.) canum) 개

> L. caninus, canina, caninum 개의

E *kennel*

E *canine*

> L. canarius, canaria, canarium 개의

E *(Canaria Insula 'Isle of Dogs; the island noted in Roman times for large dogs' >) canary*

< IE. kwon- *dog*

E *hound, dachshund*

> G. kyōn, kynos, m., f. *dog*

> G. kynikos, kynikē, kynikon *dog-like;* (Kynikos) *of the sect of philosophers called Cynics*

> L. cynicus, cynica, cynicum 개의, 개 같은; (Cynicus) 견유학파(犬儒學派)의, 냉소적인　　　　　　　　　　　　**E** *cynic, cynical*

> G. kynanchē, kynanchēs, f. (< *dog-choking* < kyōn + anchein *to throttle, to strangle*) *peritonsillar abscess*

> L. quinancia, quinanciae, f. 편도주위 농양, 편도주위 고름집　　**E** *quinsy*

L. catus, cati, m. (cattus, catti, m.) 고양이　　　　**E** *cat, cattish,* F. *chat, kitten,* D. *Katze*

< (*probably*) *Of Afro-Asiatic origin*

L. feles, felis, f. (felis, felis, f.) 고양이

> L. felinus, felina, felinum 고양이의, 고양이 성질의　　　　　　　　**E** *feline*

L. lupus, lupi, m. 늑대; (*skin lesions, originally ulcerative, from eating into the substances* >)

루푸스, 낭창(狼瘡)　　　　　　　　　　　　　　　**E** Sp. *lobo; lupus*

[용례] lupus vulgaris 보통 루푸스　　　　　　　　　　**E** *lupus vulgaris*

lupus erythematosus 홍반(紅斑) 루푸스　　　　　　**E** *lupus erythematosus*

(문법) lupus 루푸스: 단수 주격

vulgaris 보통의: 형용사, 남·여성형 단수 주격

< vulgaris, vulgare 서민적, 일반적, 보통의, 통속적, 저속한

erythematosus 홍반의: 형용사, 남성형 단수 주격

< erythematosus, erythematosa, erythematosum 홍반(紅斑)의

> L. lupinus, lupina, lupinum 늑대의　　　　　　　　　　　　**E** *lupine*

< IE. lupo- (*taboo variant*) *wolf*

< IE. wlkʷo- *wolf*

E *wolf, werewolf,* ((Germanic) wolf *'wolf'* + (Germanic) ram *'dirt, soot'* > *'probably a pejorative term referring to the ore's inferiority to tin, with which it occurred'* >) *wolfram,* (wolfram >) *wolframium (W)*

> IE. lukʷo- (*taboo variant*) *wolf*

> G. lykos, lykou, m. *wolf*　　　　　　　　　　　　　　　**E** *lyc(o)-*

> G. lykanthrōpos, lykanthrōpou, m. (< + anthrōpos *man*) *wolf-man, werewolf*

> L. lycanthropus, lycanthropi, m. 늑대인간, 낭광(狼狂)병자　**E** *lycanthrope*

> G. lykanthrōpia, lykanthrōpias, f. *lycanthropy*

> L. lycanthropia, lycanthropiae, f. 수화망상(獸化妄想)　**E** *lycanthropy*

> L. lycopersicon, lycopersici, n. (< G. lykos + Persikon malon *peach*)

리코페르시콘속(屬)의 식물　　**E** (Lycopersicon esculentum *'tomato'* >) *lycopene*

> G. lyssa, lyssēs, f. (< *wolfness*) *rage, fury, madness, rabies*
>> L. lyssa, lyssae, f. 광견병, 공수병(恐水病)　　　**E** *lyssa, lyssavirus; lyssophobia*

L. vulpes, vulpis, f. 여우
> L. vulpinus, vulpina, vulpinum 여우의　　　**E** *vulpine*
< IE. wlp-e- *fox*
> IE. əlopek- (*taboo variant*) *fox*
>> G. alōpēx, alōpekos, f. *fox*
>>> G. alōpekia, alōpekias, f. *fox-mange* > *baldness*
>>>> L. alopecia, alopeciae, f. 탈모증　　　**E** *alopecia*

[용례] alopecia areata 원형탈모증　　　**E** *alopecia areata*
(문법) alopecia 탈모증: 단수 주격
areata 구역지어 생기는, 원형으로 생기는: 형용사,
여성형 단수 주격 < areatus, areata, areatum

L. simia, simiae, f. 꼬리 없는 원숭이, 유인원, 원숭이　　　**E** *simian*
< (*probably*) G. simos, simē, simon *flat-nosed*
< (*probably*) IE. swei- *to bend, to turn*　　　**E** *swap, swift (< 'turning quickly'), (possibly) switch*

G. pithēkos, pithēkou, m. *ape, monkey*　　　**E** *pithecoid*
> L. pithecus, pitheci, m. 유인원(類人猿), 원숭이
>> L. Australopithecus, Australopitheci, m. (< *southern ape* < australis
southern + pithecus *ape*) (원인 猿人) 오스트랄로피테쿠스속(屬)　　　**E** Australopithecus
< (*suggested*) IE. bhidhi- *dreadful*
< IE. bhoi- *to be afraid*
> L. foedus, foeda, foedum 소름끼치는, 더러운, 흉한

L. ursus, ursi, m. 곰　　　**E** *ursodeoxycholic acid*
> L. ursa, ursae, f. 암곰; (Ursa) (천문) 곰자리

[용례] Ursa Major (< *Big Bear*) 큰곰자리　　　**E** *Ursa Major*
Ursa Minor (< *Little Bear*) 작은곰자리　　　**E** *Ursa Minor*
(문법) ursa 곰자리: 단수 주격
major 더 큰: 형용사 magnus의 비교급, 남·여성형 단수 주격
< major, major, majus ((gen.) majoris)
minor 더 작은: 형용사 parvus의 비교급, 남·여성형 단수 주격
< minor, minor, minus ((gen.) minoris)
> L. ursinus, ursina, ursinum 곰의　　　**E** *ursine*
< IE. rtko- *bear*　　　**E** *Arthur (< 'bear-man')*

> G. arktos, arktou, m., f. *bear;* (Arktos) *the constellation Ursa Major*

    > L. Arctos, Arcti, f. (Arctus, Arcti, f.) (천문) 곰자리, 북극, 북쪽

    > G. Arktikos, Arktikē, Arktikon *of the Bear, northern*

        > L. Arcticus, Arctica, Arcticum 곰자리의, 북극의, 북쪽의   E *Arctic*

        > G. Antarktikos, Antarktikos, Antarktikon (< ant(i)- *before, against,*

            instead of) *opposite to the north*

            > G. Antarcticus, Antarctica, Antarcticum 남극의, 남쪽의   E *Antarctic*

    > G. Arktouros, Arktourou, m. (< *from its situation at the tail of the Bear* <

        Arktos + ouros, ourou, m. *watcher, warder*) *the Bear guardian*

        > L. Arcturus, Arcturi, m. (천문) 목동자리, 대각성(大角星)   E *Arcturus*

G. leōn, leontos, m. *lion*

    > L. leo, leonis, m. 사자   E *lion*

        > L. leoninus, leonina, leoninum 사자의   E *leonine*

    > G. chamaileōn, chamaileontos, m. (< *ground lion* < chamai *on the ground, dwarf*

        + leōn) *chameleon*

        > L. chamaeleon, chamaeleontis, m. 카멜레온   E *chamaeleon (chameleon)*

  < (*probably*) *Of non-IE. origin*

G. pardos, pardou, m. *pard*

        > L. pardus, pardi, m. (parda, pardae, f.) 표범

        > G. leopardos, leopardou, m. (< *supposed to be a hybrid between lion and*

            pard < leōn *lion* + pardos) *leopard*

            > L. leopardus, leopardi, m. 표범   E *leopard*

    < G. pardalis, pardaleōs, m. *pard*

  < (*probably*) *Of Old Iranian origin*

G. elephas, elephantos, m. *elephant, ivory*

        > L. elephantus, elephanti, m. 코끼리   E *elephant*

        > L. elephantiasis, elephantiasis, f. (< + G. -iasis *suffering from*) 코끼리피부병,

        상피증(象皮症)   E *elephantiasis*

  < (*probably*) *Of Hamitic origin*

L. rattus, ratti, m. 쥐

    < E. *rat*   E *rat*

  < IE. red- *to scrape, to scratch, to gnaw* (Vide RADĔRE: *See* E. *razor*)

L. mus, muris, m. ((gen. pl.) murium) 쥐, 생쥐

> L. murinus, murina, murinum 쥐의, 생쥐의　　　　　　　　　　　　　　　　**E** *murine*

< IE. mus- *mouse; also a muscle, from the resemblance of a flexing muscle to the movements of a mouse* (Vide MUSCULUS: See E. *muscle*)

> G. mys, myos, m. *mouse; muscle*

L. **aquila, aquilae,** f. 독수리; 로마 군단의 독수리 군기, 독수리 군단; (Aquila) (천문) 독수리자리　　**E** *Aquila*

> L. aquilinus, aquilina, aquilinum 독수리의, 독수리 같은　　　　　　　　**E** *aquiline*

L. **gallus, galli,** m. 수탉

> L. gallina, gallinae, f. 암탉

> L. gallinaceus, gallinacea, gallinaceum 닭의, 가금(家禽)의　　　　　　**E** *gallinaceous*

< IE. gal- *to call, to shout*　　　　　　　　　　　　　　　　　**E** *call, recall, clatter*

L. **anser, anseris,** m. (< *hanser) 거위, 기러기

> L. anserinus, anserina, anserinum 거위의, 기러기의　　　　　　　**E** *anserine*

[용례] cutis anserina 닭살　　　　　　　　　　　　　　　　　**E** *cutis anserina*

(문법) cutis 피부: 단수 주격 < cutis, cutis, f.

anserina 거위의: 여성형 단수 주격

< IE. ghans- *goose*　　　　　　　　　　　　　　　　　**E** *goose, gosling, gander*

> G. chēn, chēnos, m., f. *goose* **E** *chenodeoxycholic acid* (< *'found in the bile of goose'*)

L. **pica, picae,** f. 까치

E *((probably) 'Magot + pie' >)* **magpie,** *(magpie > '(probably) baked dish of ingredients compared to objects randomly collected by a magpie' >)* **pie, piebald** (< *'magpie's black and white plumage'*), **piebaldism**

> L. pica, picae, f. (< *craving for strange food; on account of the magpie's feeding on miscellaneous foodstuffs*) 이식증(異食症), 이미증(異味症), 무분별탐식증　**E** *pica*

< IE. (s)peik- *bird's name, magpie, woodpecker*

> L. picus, pici, m. 딱따구리

L. **corvus, corvi,** m. 까마귀　　　　　　　　**E** *(corvus marinus 'sea raven' >)* **cormorant**

> L. corvinus, corvina, corvinum 까마귀의　　　　　　　　　　**E** *corvine*

< IE. ker- (*echoic root*) *base of various derivatives indicating loud noises or birds*　　　　　　**E** *cricket, screak, screech, scream, raven, retch, ring*

> L. crepo, **crepui,** crepitum, crepare 삐꺽 소리가 나다, 삐꺽 소리를 내다　**E** *crevice, crevasse*

> L. crepitus, crepitus, m. 소음, 잡음, 비빔소리, 마찰음　　　　　**E** *crepitus*

> L. crepito, **crepitavi,** crepitatum, crepitare (*frequentative*) 탁탁거리는 소리가 나다, 털비빔소리가 나다, 마찰음이 나다　　　　　　　　**E** *crepitate, crepitant*

> L. discrepo, discrepui (discrepavi), discrepitum, discrepare (< dis- *apart from, down, not* + crepare *to creak*) 소리가 맞지 않다, 다르다, 의견이 구구하다   **E** *discrepant*

> L. discrepantia, discrepantiae, f. 불일치   **E** *discrepancy*

> G. korōnē, korōnēs, f. *crow, raven*   **E** *coronoid (< 'shaped like a crow's beak')*

> G. korax, korakos, m. *raven*   **E** *coracoid (< 'shaped like a raven's beak')*

> L. coracidium, coracidii, n. (< *with hooklets like beaks of small ravens* < + G. -idion *diminutive suffix*) 섬모유충   **E** *coracidium*

L. cuculus, cuculi, m. 뻐꾸기, 두견새

< *Of mimicry origin*   **E** *cuckoo*

> G. kokkyx, kokkygos, m. *cuckoo*

> L. coccyx, coccygis, m. 뻐꾸기; (os coccygis *cuckoo bone, because in man it was supposed to resemble the bill of the cuckoo* >) 꼬리뼈, 미골(尾骨)   **E** *coccyx*

> L. coccygeus, coccygea, coccygeum 꼬리뼈의, 미골의   **E** *coccygeal*

L. grus, gruis, f. 두루미, 학

> **E** *((Anglo-Norman) pe de grue 'foot of crane' > 'the clawlike, three-branched mark used in genealogy to show succession' >)* **pedigree**

< IE. gerə- *to cry hoarsely; also the name of the crane*

> **E** *crane, cranberry, cranesbill, crow, croak, crack, cracker, crackle, croup (< 'hoarse croaking')*

> G. geranos, geranou, f. *crane*

> G. geranion, geraniou, n. (< + -ion *diminutive suffix*) *stork's bill, cranesbill, geranium (< cranesbill-shaped fruit)*

> L. geranium, geranii, n. 쥐손이풀, 이질풀

> **E** *geranium, geraniol (< 'a monoterpenoid alcohol obtained from geranium leaves'), (geraniol >)* **geranyl**

L. strouthos, strouthou, m. *sparrow, ostrich*

> L. struthio, struthionis, m. 타조   **E** *(avis 'bird' + struthio >)* **ostrich**

< (*probably*) IE. trozdo- *thrush*   **E** *thrush, throstle*

> L. turdus, turdi, m. (조류) 티티새; (어류) 놀래기   **E** *(suggested)* **sturdy**

G. ikteros, ikterou, m. *a yellow bird, jaundice*

> L. icterus, icteri, m. 노란색 깃털을 갖는 꾀꼬리과 또는 지빠귀과의 새 이름(그리스 사람들은 황달 환자가 이 새를 보면 낫는다고 생각함), 황달(黃疸)   **E** *icterus*

> L. kernicterus, kernicteri, m. (< *nuclear icterus* < D. Kern *kernel, nucleus*)

핵(核)황달   **E** *kernicterus*

> G. ikterikos, ikterikē, ikterikon *jaundiced*

> L. ictericus, icterica, ictericum 황달의, 황달 든   **E** *icteric, (icteric >) anicteric*

G. iynx, iyngos, f. *wryneck*

> L. iynx, iyngis, f. (jynx, jyngis, f.) 개미잡이 딱따구리

E *iynx (jinx)* (< 'a bird made use of in witchcraft, in black magic; hence, a charm, a spell')

G. psittakos, psittakou, m. *parrot*

> L. psittacus, psittaci, m. 앵무새   **E** *psittacine*

> L. psittacosis, psittacosis, f. (< + G. -ōsis *condition*) 앵무새병   **E** *psittacosis*

< (*probably*) *Of Oriental origin*

E. *snake*   **E** *snake*

< IE. sneg- *to creep, creeping thing*   **E** *snail, sneak*

L. serpens, serpentis, m., f. 뱀

> L. serpentinus, serpentina, serpentinum 뱀의, 뱀 같은   **E** *serpentine*

[용례] Rauwolfia serpentina

snakeroot   **E** (Rauwolfia serpentina > 'contracted' >) *reserpine*

(문법) Rauwolfia 속명(屬名): 단수 주격 < Rauwolfia, Rauwolfiae, f.

라우볼피아속(屬)의 협죽도과 식물 < Leonhard Rauwolf

(1535-1596), *German physician and botanist*

serpentina 뱀 같은: 형용사, 여성형 단수 주격

< L. serpo, **serpsi**, serptum, serpĕre 기다

> L. serpigo, serpiginis, f. 사행상(蛇行狀) 피부질환   **E** *serpiginous*

< IE. serp- *to crawl, to creep*

> G. herpein *to creep*

> G. herpeton, herpetou, n. *creeping animal, reptile, living being*   **E** *herpetology*

> G. herpēs, herpētos, m. *shingles*

> L. herpes, herpetis, m. 포진(疱疹), 헤르페스   **E** *herpes, herpetic, herpesvirus*

[용례] herpes simplex 단순포진, 단순헤르페스   **E** *herpes simplex*

(문법) herpes 포진, 헤르페스: 단수 주격

simplex 단순한: 형용사, 남·여·중성형 단수 주격

< simplex, (gen.) simplicis

G. ophis, opheōs, m. *snake, serpent*   **E** *ophiology, ophiolatry*

< IE. eghi- *snake*

> G. echidna, echidnēs, f. *adder, viper;* (Echidna) *(Greek mythology) a mythical creature which gave birth to the Hydra*

    > L. echidna, echidnae, f. 독사; (Echidna) (그리스 신화) Lerna의 물뱀; 바늘두더쥐   **E** *echidna*

> G. echinos, echinou, m. (*snake eater* >) *hedgehog,*

   (*hedgehog* >) *sea urchin*   **E** *echin(o)-* (< *spines, spiny'*), *echinocyte* (< 'burr cell')

    > L. Echinococcus, Echinococci, m. (< *spiny berry* < + G. kokkos *grain, berry*)

       (조충) 에키노코쿠스속(屬); 극구충(棘球蟲), 포충(胞蟲), 포낭충(胞囊蟲)   **E** Echinococcus

    > L. Echinostoma, Echinostomatis, n. (< *spiny mouth* < + G. stoma *mouth*) (흡충)

       극구흡충속(棘口吸蟲屬)   **E** Echinostoma

L. lacertus, lacerti, m. (lacerta, lacertae, f.) 도마뱀   **E** *lizard*

G. sauros, saurou, m. (saura, sauras, f.) *lizard*

    > L. saurus, sauri, m. (saura, saurae, f.) 도마뱀   **E** *saur(o)-, -saurus (-saur)*

G. salamandra, salamandras, f. *a lizard-like animal supposed to live in, or to be able to endure, fire*

    > L. salamandra, salamandrae, f. 불도마뱀, 불 속에서 사는 요정, 도롱뇽, 영원(蠑螈)   **E** *salamander*

L. rana, ranae, f. 개구리

    > L. ranula, ranulae, f. (< + -ula *diminutive suffix*) 작은 개구리, 올챙이;

       두꺼비종(腫)   **E** *ranula, ranular*

L. bufo, bufonis, m. 두꺼비   **E** *bufotoxin*

  < (*Germanic*) gʷebh- *hypothetical base of some Germanic words associated with the notion of sliminess, and related to Latin and Slavic words for frog*

L. hirudo, hirudinis, f. 거머리   **E** *hirudin*

L. locusta, locustae, f. 메뚜기   **E** *locust,* (locusta > (corrupted) >) *lobster*

L. apis, apis, f. 벌 [蜂]   **E** *apiculture*

    > L. apianus, apiana, apianum 벌의   **E** *apian*

L. musca, muscae, f. 파리

  E (musca > Sp. mosquito 'little gnat' >) *mosquito, musket* (< 'a male sparrowhawk that looks as if speckled with flies'), *musketeer*

> L. muscarius, muscaria, muscarium

파리의　　　　　　　　**E** (Amanita muscaria *'fly agaric'* >) *muscarine*, *(muscarine* >) *muscarinic*

> L. muscarium, muscarii, n. 파리채, 총채

< IE. mu- (*imitative root*) *gnat, fly*　　　　　**E** *midge, (midge (diminutive)* >) *midget*

> G. myia, myias, f. *fly*

> L. myiasis, myiasis, f. (< G. myia + -iasis *suffering from*) 구더기증　　**E** *myiasis*

G. kōnōps, kōnōpos, m. *mosquito, gnat*

> G. kōnōpeion, kōnōpeiou, n. *mosquito curtain*

> L. conopeum, conopei, n. 모기장, 천개(天蓋), 닫집　　**E** *canopy*

L. aedes, aedis, m. 에데스모기, 숲모기　　**E** *aedes*

< G. aēdēs, aēdēs, aēdes (< a- *not*) *unpleasant*

< G. hēdys, hēdeia, hēdy *sweet, pleasant*

< IE. swad- *sweet, pleasant* (Vide SUADĒRE: *See* E. *suasion*)

L. anopheles, anophelis, m. 아노펠레스모기, 학질모기, 얼룩날개모기　　**E** *anopheles, anopheline*

< G. anōphelēs, anōphelēs, anōpheles (< an- *not*) *unprofitable, useless, hurtful*

< G. ophelos, ophelou, n. *profit, advantage, usefulness*

< IE. obhel- *to avail*

L. culex, culicis, m. 모기, 각다귀, 등에; 집모기　　**E** *culex,* (culex >) *culicine*

< IE. ku- *sharp, pointed* (Vide CUNEUS: *See* E. *cuneate*)

L. pulex, pulicis, m. 벼룩　　**E** *puce* (< *'flea-color'*)

> L. pulicinus, pulicina, pulicinum 벼룩의　　**E** *pulicine*

< IE. plou- *flea*　　**E** *flea*

> G. psylla, psyllēs, f. *flea*

> G. psyllion, psylliou, n. (< *the resemblance of the seeds to fleas* < + -ion *diminutive suffix*) *psyllium*

> L. psyllium, psyllii, n. 질경이 씨, 질경이　　**E** *psyllium*

> L. Psylla, Psyllae, f. 나무이(*jumping plant louse*) 속(屬)　　**E** Psylla

E. *louse*　　**E** *louse*

< IE. lus- *louse*

L. pediculus, pediculi, m. (< + -culus *diminutive suffix*) 이[蝨]　　**E** *pediculus*

> L. pedicularis, pediculare 이의, 이투성이의   **E** *pedicular*

> L. pediculosus, pediculosa, pediculosum 이가 꾀는, 이가 기생하는   **E** *pediculous*

> L. pediculosis, pediculosis, f. (< + G. -ōsis *condition*) 이 [蝨] 감염증   **E** *pediculosis*

< L. pedis, pedis, m., f. (< *foul-smelling insect*) 이 [蝨]

< (*perhaps*) IE. pezd- *to fart*   **E** *feist*

> L. pedo, pepedi, peditum, pedēre 방귀 뀌다, 실례하다   **E** *petard*

G. phtheir, phtheiros, m. (< *Ancient authors believed that lice were generated spontaneously in decaying flesh*) *louse*

> L. phthirus, phthiri, m. 사면발이, 모슬(毛蝨)   **E** *phthirus*

> G. phtheirian *to be infested with lice*

> G. phtheiriasis, phtheiriaseōs, f. *infestation with lice*

> L. phthiriasis, phthiriasis, f. 사면발이증   **E** *phthiriasis*

< G. phtheirein *to destroy*

< (*perhaps*) IE. dhgʷher- *to flow, to move forcefully, with derivatives referring to ruin and destruction*

L. formica, formicae, f. 개미, 의(蟻)

E *formic acid* (< '*natural occurrence in ants*'), *formaldehyde (Formalin®), formyl,* (formica + -vorous '*devouring*' >) *formicivorous*

> L. formicarium, formicarii, n. 개미집, 개미 언덕   **E** *formicary*

> L. formico, formicavi, formicatum, formicare 개미가 피부를 기어가는 것 같은 가려움을 느끼다, 의주감(蟻走感)을 느끼다

> L. formicatio, formicationis, f. 개미 기는 느낌, 의주감, 스멀거림   **E** *formication*

< IE. morwi- *ant*   **E** *pismire* (< '*urinous smell of an anthill*')

> G. myrmēx, myrmēkos, m. *ant*   **E** *myrmec(o)-, myrmecology*

G. arachnē, arachnēs, f. *spider;* (Arachnē) (*Greek mythology*) *A great mortal weaver. She boasted that her skill was greater than that of Athena the goddess of crafts, which resulted in a contest between her and the goddess. In the end the goddess turned Arachne into a spider.*   **E** *Arachne, arachn(o)-, arachnophobia, arachnodactyly*

> G. arachnoeidēs, arachnoeidēs, arachnoeides (< + eidos *shape*) *cobweb-like*

> L. arachnoideus, arachnoidea, arachnoideum 거미줄 같은

E (arachnoidea mater '*cobweb-like mother*' >) *arachnoid, arachnoidal, subarachnoid*

> L. Arachnida, Arachnidorum, n. (pl.) (거미·전갈·진드기 등) 거미목(目)   **E** *arachnid, arachnidism* (araneism) (< '*spider envenomation*')

∞ L. aranea, araneae, f. 거미, 거미줄   **E** *araneism* (arachnidism) (< '*spider envenomation*')

L. tarantula, tarantulae, f. (< + -ula *diminutive suffix*) (< *a large wolf-spider of Southern*

Europe, named from Taranto where it is commonly found, whose bite is slightly poisonous, and was fabled to cause tarantism) 타란토거미

> **E** *tarantula*

< It. Taranto *a seaport in southern Italy*

> **E** *tarantism* (< *'a hysterical malady, characterized by an extreme impulse to dance, which prevailed as an epidemic in southern Italy from the 15th to the 17th century, popularly attributed to the bite or 'sting' of the tarantula'),* **tarantella** (< *'a rapid whirling southern Italian dance popular with the peasantry since the fifteenth century, when it was supposed to be the sovereign remedy for tarantism')*

G. skorpios, skorpiou, m. *scorpion*

> L. scorpio, scorpionis, m. (< scorpius, scorpii, m.) 전갈(全蠍); (Scorpio) 전갈자리

> **E** *scorpion*

L. blatta, blattae, f. 좀벌레, 진디

> L. blattella, blattellae, f. (< + -ella *diminutive suffix*) 바퀴

> **E** *blattella*

L. acarus, acari, m. (좀진드기 *mite*와 참진드기 *tick*을 포함)

진드기

> **E** *acarus*, (pl.) *acari, acarian, acarophobia*

< G. (*ancient Greek*) akari *mite*

< G. akarēs, akarēs, akares (< a- *not*) *too short for cutting, minute*

< G. keirein (kar- *aorist stem*) *to cut*

< IE. (*probably*) (s)ker- *to cut*

< IE. sek- *to cut* (Vide SECARE: *See* E. *secant*)

L. Ixodes, Ixodis, m. (진드기) 참진드기속(屬)

> **E** Ixodes, *ixodiasis*

< G. ixōdēs, ixōdēs, ixōdes (< + -ōdēs *like, resembling*) *birdlime-like, sticky*

< G. ixos, ixou, m. *mistletoe, birdlime*

< IE. weis- *to flow* (Vide VIRUS: *See* E. *virus*)

L. coccum, cocci, m. 낟알, 씨, 장과; 연지벌레(중남미산), 연지벌레 암컷으로 만든 붉은 염료, 심홍색

> L. coccineus, coccinea, coccineum 심홍색의

> **E** *cochineal*

< G. kokkos, kokkou, m. *kernel, grain, berry; scarlet berry* (< *the insect bodies were mistaken for grains or berries*) (Vide COCCUS: *See* E. *coccus*)

> L. coccus, cocci, m. 낟알, 씨, 장과(漿果); 알균, 구균(球菌)

> **E** *coccus*, (pl.) *cocci*

L. kermes, kermis, m. 연지벌레(지중해지방산), 연지벌레 암컷으로 만든 붉은 염료, 심홍색

> **E** *carmine, mucicarmine, crimson*

< (*Arabic*) qirmiz *kermes*

L. lacca, laccae, f. 연지벌레(인도·동남아시아산, 락 깍지진디), 연지벌레 암컷으로 만든 붉은 염료

      < (*Portuguese*) laca (lacca) *lac*   **E** *lac, lacquer*

    < (*Hindi*) lakh *lac*

  < (*Sanskrit*) laksha *lac*

G. kastōr, kastoros, m. (< *Castor as protector of women from diseases; oil substance from the sexual glands of the beaver was used for treating women's diseases*) *beaver*

    > L. castor, castoris, m. 해리(海狸), 바다삵, 해리의 가죽; (castoreum) 해리향(海狸香)

        E *castor, (castor > 'the seed oil from* Ricinus communis, *thought to have medicinal properties similar to the castor' >)* **castor oil**

    < G. Kastōr, Kastoros, m. (< *originally, he who excels*) (*Greek mythology*) *Castor, the mortal twin of the Dioscuri, protector of women from diseases*

G. phōkē, phōkēs, f. *seal*

    > L. phoca, phocae, f. (phoce, phoces, f.) 바다표범

      > L. phocomelia, phocomeliae, f. (< + G. melos *limb*) 바다표범발증, 해표상지증

      (海豹狀肢症)   **E** *phocomelia*

L. squalus, squali, m. 상어의 일종; 물개   **E** *squalene (< 'discovered first in shark liver oil')*

  < IE. (s)kʷal-o- *big fish*   **E** *whale*

L. pristis, pristis, f. (pistris, pistricis, f.) 바다괴물; 고래, 상어

      E *pristane (< 'an alkane obtained from shark liver oil')*, **pristanic acid** *(< 'a fatty acid obtained from shark liver oil')*

L. cancer, cancri, m. (cancer, canceris, m.) 게; (*meaning from a translation of* G. karkinōma (*Aulus Cornelius Celsus*) >) 암(癌); (Cancer) (천문) 게자리, 거해궁(巨蟹宮)   **E** *cancer*

  < IE. kar-, ker- *hard* (Vide CANCER: *See* E. *cancer*)

    > G. karkinos, karkinou, m. *crab*

      > G. karkinōma, karkinōmatos, n. (< (*suggested*) *the swollen veins surrounding the part affected bear a resemblance to the limbs of a crab* (*Galen of Pergamon*) < karkinos + -ōma *noun suffix denoting tumor*) *carcinoma*

        > L. carcinoma, carcinomatis, n. 암(癌),

          암종(癌腫)   **E** *carcinoma,* (pl.) *carcinomata (carcinomas)*

G. konchē, konchēs, f. (konchylē, konchylēs, f.) *mussel, shell, shell-like cavity*

    > L. concha, conchae, f. 조가비, 조가비 모양의 나팔; 여자의 음부; (코)선반,

      갑개(甲介)   **E** *concha,* (pl.) *conchae, conchoidal, conch, conchology*

> G. konchylion, konchyliou, n. (< + -ion *diminutive suffix*) *cockle*

> L. conchylium, conchylii, n. 새조개류

E *cockle*

< IE. ko(n)kho- *mussel, shellfish*

> G. **kochlos, kochlou, m.** *mussel, shellfish (used for dyeing purple), land snail*

> L. cochlea, cochleae, f. 달팽이, ·나선형, 와우(蝸牛)

E *cochlea*

> L. *cochlearis, *cochleare 달팽이의, 나선형의,
와우의

E *cochlear, vestibulocochlear*

G. **korallion, koralliou, n.** *coral*

> L. corallium, corallii, n. (붉은) 산호(珊瑚)

E *coral*

< (*perhaps*) *Of Semitic origin, meaning pebble or small stone used for casting lots*

식물

L. **Flora, Florae, f.** (로마 신화) 꽃의 여신; (flora) 식물상(相), 세균총(叢)

E *Flora, flora*

< L. flos, floris, m. 꽃

< IE. bhle- *to thrive, to bloom* (Vide FLOS: *See* E. *floral*)

G. **amygdalē, amygdalēs, f.** *almond*

> L. amygdala, amygdalae, f. 아몬드, 파단행(巴旦杏),
편도(扁桃)

E *amygdala,* (pl.) *amygdalae, amygdaloid, amygdalin*

> L. amandola, amandolae, f. (*Medieval Latin*) 아몬드

E *almond*

> D. Mandel, Mandel, f. *almond*

E *mandelic acid* (< *'found in amygdalin'*), *vanillylmandelic acid (vanilmandelic acid) (VMA)* (< *'structurally related to vanillin and mandelic acid'*)

G. **balaustion, balaustiou, n.** *the blossom of the wild pomegranate*

> L. balaustium, balaustii, n. 야생 석류꽃

E *baluster* (< *'the resemblance of a baluster to the double-curving calyx-tube of this flower'*), *balustrade,* (baluster > (corrupted) >) *banister*

L. **citrus, citri, f.** 구연수(枸櫞樹), 감귤류(柑橘類)의 식물,
감귤류

E *citric, citric acid* (< *'isolated from juice of* Citrus limon*'*), *citrate*

> L. citrullus, citrulli, m. (< + -ullus *diminutive suffix*)

수박　　　　　　　　　　　　　**E** *citrulline (< 'originally isolated from watermelon')*

∽ G. kedros, kedrou, f. *cedar tree*

> L. cedrus, cedri, f. 삼(杉)나무, 백향목(栢香木)　　　　**E** *cedar*

< *Of Semitic origin*

L. coffea, coffeae, f. 커피나무, 커피

< (*Turkish*) kahveh *coffee*　　　　　　　　　　　　**E** *coffee*

> It. caffe *coffee*　　　　**E** *(Mexican Spanish)* **cafeteria** *(< 'coffee shop')*

> F. café *coffee, coffee house*　　　　　　**E** *café, caffeine*

< (*Arabic*) qahwah *coffee*

L. cornus, corni, f. 산딸나무, 산수유나무, 창(槍)　　　　**E** *cornel*

< IE. ker– *a kind of cherry*

> (*probably*) G. kerasos, kerasou, m. *cherry tree,*

cherry　　　　　　　**E** *(cherise > (interpreted as a plural) >) **cherry***

G. elaia, elaias, f. (< *elaiwa) *olive tree, olive*

> L. oliva, olivae, f. (> olea, oleae, f.) 올리브 나무, 올리브 열매　　**E** *olive*

> L. olivarius, olivaria, olivarium 올리브의　　　　　**E** *olivary*

> G. elaion, elaiou, n. *olive oil*

> **E** *elaioplast, elaidic acid (< 'trans isomer of oleic acid'), (D. Wasser 'water' + elaion + -ine >) **Vaseline**®*

> L. olivum, olivi, n. (> oleum, olei, n.) 올리브 기름, 기름

> **E** *oil, oleic acid, linoleic acid (< 'found in linseed oil'), linolenic acid (< 'more unsaturated linoleic acid'), -ol, -ole, (linum 'flax' + oleum 'oil' > 'made by coating canvas with oxidized linseed oil' >) **linoleum***

> L. petroleum, petrolei, n. (< *mineral oil formed by the decomposition of organic matter and present in some rock formations (sometimes seeping out on to the ground)* < petra (< G. petra) *rock* + oleum (< G. elaion) *oil*) 석유(石油)

> **E** *petroleum, petrol (< 'a light fuel oil made by distilling petroleum'), petrolatum (< 'petroleum jelly such as Vaseline®')*

< *Of Mediterranean origin*

L. fagus, fagi, f. (fagus, fagus, f.) (< *esculent oak* < *tree with edible fruit*) 너도밤나무

< IE. bhago– *beech tree*

> **E** *beech (< 'esculent oak' < 'tree with edible fruit'), (probably) book (< 'beechwood tablets carved with runes'), buckwheat*

L. ficus, fici, f. (ficus, ficus, f.) 무화과나무, 무화과   E *fig, ficin (< 'obtained from the sap of fig')*

   < *Of* non-IE. *origin*

       > G. sykon, sykou, n. *fig*

          > G. sykophantēs, sykophantou, m. *(< (perhaps) with reference to making the insulting gesture of the 'fig' (sticking the thumb between two fingers) to informers < + G. phainein to show) an informer against the unlawful exportation of figs, a class of informers in ancient Athens*

            > L. sycophanta, sycophantae, m. 무화과 수출법 위반자를 고발하는 자, 고발인, 아첨꾼   E *sycophant*

          > G. sykōsis, sykōseōs, f. *(< + -ōsis condition) any skin disease resembling a fig*

            > L. sycosis, sycosis, f. *(< a fig-shaped, eruptive skin disease characterized by inflammation of the hair-follicles, especially of the beard)* 털 종기증, 모창(毛瘡)   E *sycosis*

L. fraxinus, fraxini, f. 물푸레나무, 물푸레나무로 만든 창   E *fraxinus*

   < IE. bherəg- *to shine; bright, white*   E *bright, birch (< 'white tree')*

   ∽ IE. bherək- *to shine, to glitter*

     E *braid (< 'to move jerkily' < 'to shimmer'), upbraid (< 'to bring forth as a ground for censure' < 'to move up quickly'), bridle (< 'referring to the movement of a horse's head'), debride (< 'to remove the bridle'), debridement*

L. fuchsia, fuchsiae, f. 퓨셔(바늘꽃과의 관상용 식물);

     적자색   E *fuchsine (< 'from the resemblance of the color to the flower')*

   < Leonard Fuchs (1501-1566), *German physician and botanist*

L. guaiacum, guaiaci, n. 구아약, 유창목지(癒瘡木脂)   E *guaiac*

     < *Spanish South American vernacular name guaiac or guayaco for* Guaiacum officinale

G. kinnamōmon, kinnamōmou, n. *cinnamon*

     > L. cinnamomum, cinnamomi, n. 육계(肉桂), 계피(桂皮), 계수나무   E *cinnamon*

   < *Of Semitic origin, perhaps based on Malay*

L. laurus, lauri, f. 월계수, 월계수 잎(가지),

     월계관   E *laurel, lauric acid (< 'obtained from the laurel berries'), lauryl*

     > L. laureus, laurea, laureum 월계수의

         > L. laurea, laureae, f. 월계수, 월계관

            > L. laureatus, laureata, laureatum 월계수 잎으로 장식한, 월계관을 쓴   E *laureate*

   < *Of* non-IE. *origin*

> G. daphnē, daphnēs, f. *laurel, bay tree;* (Daphnē) (*Greek mythology*) *a nymph fabled to have been metamorphosed into a laurel*
>> L. daphne, daphnes, f. 월계수; (Daphne) (그리스 신화) 다프네   **E** *Daphne*

G. lōtos, lōtou, m. (< *the name of several dissimilar plants; it is not known whether the word in the various applications is etymologically identical*) *lotus-tree and fruit; water-lily, Indian lotus; clover*
> L. lotus, loti, f. 로터스; 수련(睡蓮), 연(蓮); 벌노랑이   **E** *lotus*
< *Of Semitic origin*

L. malus, mali, f. 사과나무
> < L. malum, mali, n. 사과나무, 사과   **E** *malic acid* (< '*first isolated from apple juice*'), *malate*
>> < G. (*Doric*) malon, malou, n., (*Attic*) mēlon, mēlou, n. *apple*   **E** *malonic acid* (< '*prepared from malic acid via oxidation*'), *malonate*
>>> > G. mēlopepōn, mēlopepōnos, m. (< *melon eaten when ripe* < + pepōn *ripe*) *melon*   **E** *melon*
< (*perhaps*) *Of Mediterranean origin*

L. morus, mori, f. 뽕나무
> > L. morum, mori, n. 뽕, 오디   **E** (morum + *berry* >) *mulberry*
>> > L. morula, morulae, f. (< morum *mulberry* + -ula *diminutive suffix*) 상실배 (桑實胚), 오디배   **E** *morula*, (*morula* >) *morular*, (*morula* >) *morulation*
< IE. moro- *blackberry, mulberry*

L. hopea, hopeae, f. (*dammar resin*을 생산하는)
   호페아나무   **E** *hopane* (< '*a triterpene discovered in varnish from hopea tree*'), *hopanoid(s)*
< John Hope (1725-1786), *Scottish physician and botanist*

L. pinus, pini, f. 소나무   **E** *pine* (< '*yielding a resin*')
> L. pinea, pineae, f. 솔방울
>> L. pinealis, pineale 솔방울 모양의   **E** (glandula pinealis '*pineal gland*' >) *pineal*
< IE. peiə- *to be fat, to swell* (Vide PINUS: *See* E. *pine*)

L. pirus, piri, f. (pyrus, pyri, f.) 배나무
> < L. pirum, piri, n. (pyrum, pyri, n.) 배   **E** *pear*
>> > L. piriformis, piriforme (pyriformis, pyriforme) 배 모양의, 조롱박 모양의   **E** *piriform (pyriform)*

< *Of Mediterranean origin*

L. pomus, pomi, f. 과실나무, 사과나무

    < L. pomum, pomi, n. 과실, 사과

        E *pomade* (< *'originally perfumed with apple pulp')*, (pomum granatum *'apple with many seeds'* >) **pomegranate, pomiculture** (< *'fruit gardening'),* (*diminutive*) **pommel**

        > L. Pomona, Pomonae, f. (로마 신화) 과일과 과수의 여신   **E** *Pomona*

L. prunus, pruni, f. 오얏(자두)나무

      < L. prunum, pruni, n. 오얏(자두)   **E** *plum, prune*

    < G. proumnon, proumnou, n. *plum*

  < *Of Asiatic origin*

L. quercus, quercus, f. (quercus, querci, f.) 참나무, 도토리; 참나무 잎으로 엮은 관(冠),

    참나무로 만든 배·창·술잔   **E** *cork*

    > L. quercetum, querceti, n.

      참나무 숲   **E** *quercetin* (< *'a flavonoid obtained from* quercus *in* quercetum*')*

  < IE. perk^{w}u- *oak*   **E** *fir*

L. rosa, rosae, f. 장미   **E** *rose, rosy, rosette*

    > L. roseus, rosea, roseum 장미의, 장밋빛의

        > L. roseola, roseolae, f. (< + -ola *diminutive suffix*) 장미진(疹) **E** *roseola, roseoliform*

    > L. rosaceus, rosacea, rosaceum 장미의,

      장밋빛의   **E** (acne rosacea *'rosaceous acne'* >) *rosacea*

    > L. rosarius, rosaria, rosarium 장미의

        > L. rosarium, rosarii, n. 장미원, 묵주(默珠), 염주(念珠)   **E** *rosary*

  < (*Of unknown origin*) wrod- *rose*

      > G. rhodon, rhodou, n. *rose*

        E *rhod(o)-, rhodium (Rh)* (< *'rose color of a dilute solution of its salts'),* **rhodamine(s)** (< *'rose-colorerd amine dyes'),* **rhodopsin** (< *'visual purple, scotopsin with retinal')*

    > (*suggested*) G. rhous, rhois, m., f. (< *bright red autumn leaves*) *sumach*

      > L. rhus, rhois, m., f. 옻나무   **E** *rhus*

L. salix, salicis, f. 버드나무

    E *salicin* (< *'obtained from the bark of* salix*'),* (*salicin* >) **salicylic acid, salicylate, acetyl-salicylic acid**

  < IE. sal- *dirty, gray*   **E** *sallow*

    > L. saliva, salivae, f. 침, 타액 (Vide SALIVA: *See* E. *saliva*)

L. sorbus, sorbi, f. 마가목

> L. sorbum, sorbi, n. 마가목 열매

> **E** **sorbic acid** (< *'found in the berries of the mountain-ash'),* (sorbum + *-ite* + *-ol* >
> *'found in the berries of the mountain-ash'* >) **sorbitol**

G. styrax, styrakos, m., f. *styrax tree*

> L. styrax, styracis, f. (storax, storacis, f.) 때죽나무과(科)의 나무, 소합향(蘇合香)나무,
> 소합향수지(樹脂)

> **E** **styrax, styrene** (< *'unsaturated hydrocarbon, originally obtained from the styrax tree,*
> *now recovered as a by-product of petroleum'),* **polystyrene,** *(polystyrene foam >)*
> **Styrofoam**®

[용례] Styrax benzoin (*benzoin tree,* (*corrupted*) *benjamin tree, Sumatra snowball*)
　　　　안식향의 때죽나무과 나무
　　(문법) styrax 때죽나무과 나무: 단수 주격
　　　　　benzoin 안식향의: 불변화 명사, 속격으로 쓰임
　　　　　　　< benzoin, f. (불변화) 안식향(安息香)
　　　　　　　　< (*Arabic*) luban jawi *incense of Java (probably confused with*
　　　　　　　　　　Sumatra) obtained from the Styrax benzoin

< *Of Semitic origin*
　　> (*Hebrew*) tsori *terebinth resin from* Styrax officinalis

G. terebinthos, terebinthou, f. *terebinth*

> L. terebinthus, terebinthi, f. 테레빈 나무 (Pistacia terebinthus *terebinth*), 테레빈 수지
> (樹脂, *turpentine*)　　　　　　　　　　　　　　　　　　　　**E** *terebinth*
> > L. terebinthinus, terebinthina, terebinthinum 테레빈 나무의, 테레빈 수지의

> **E** **terebinthine,** (terebinthina resina *'terebinthine resin'* >) **turpentine,** *(turpentine >)*
> **terpene(s),** *('terpenes of two isoprene units'* >) **monoterpene(s),** (sesqui- *'one*
> *and a half* > *'terpenes of three isoprene units'* >) **sesquiterpene(s),** *('terpenes of*
> *four isoprene units'* >) **diterpene(s),** (sester- *'two and a half* > *'terpenes of five*
> *isoprene units'* >) **sesterterpene(s),** *('terpenes of six isoprene units'* > **triterpene(s)**

< (*probably*) *Of* non-IE. *origin*

L. thea, theae, f. 차(茶)나무, 차　　　　　　　**E** *theophylline* (< *'an alkaloid found in tea leaves'*)
　　　< (*Dutch*) thee *tea*
　< (*Chinese*) ch'a (茶) 차　　　　　　　　　　　　　　　　　　　**E** *tea*

L. ulex, ulicis, m. 가시금작화 (로즈매리와 비슷한 관목의 콩과 식물)

[용례] Ulex europaeus 유럽산 가시금작화　　　　　　　　　　**E** Ulex europaeus
　　(문법) ulex 가시금작화: 단수 주격
　　　　　europaeus 유럽의: 형용사, 남성형 단수 주격
　　　　　　　< Europaeus, Europaea, Europaeum

<Europa, Europae, f. 유럽

L. viscum, visci, n. (viscus, visci, m) 겨우살이; 겨우살이 열매에서 채취하는
새잡이 끈끈이   **E** *viscid, viscose (viscous), viscosity*
  < IE. weis- *to flow* (Vide VIRUS: *See* E. *virus*)

G. absinthion, absinthiou, n. *wormwood*
    > L. absinthium, absinthii, n. 쓴쑥(Artemisia absinthium)   **E** *absinth (absinthe)*
  < *Of* non-IE. *origin*

G. akoniton, akonitou, n. *aconite*
    > L. aconitum, aconiti, n. 바곳

> **E** *aconite, aconitine (< 'the essential principle of aconite, an extremely poisonous alkaloid'), aconitic acid (< 'discovered in leaves and tubers of Aconitum napellus'), aconitate, aconitase*

G. anison, anisou, n. *anise (an umbelliferous plant* Pimpinella anisum, *a native of the Levant, cultivated for its aromatic and carminative seeds)*
    > L. anisum, anisi, n. 아니스, 아니스 열매   **E** *anise, aniseed, anis-*

G. asparagos, asparagou, m. *asparagus*
    > L. asparagus, asparagi, m. 아스파라거스

> **E** *asparagus, asparagine (Asn, N) (< 'first isolated from asparagus juice'), aspartic acid (Asp, D) (< 'formed arbitrarily, with regard mainly to euphony, on asparagus; produced by the action of alkalis or acids on asparagine'), aspartate, (aspartyl-phenylalanine-1-methyl ester >) aspartame, (cysteine-dependent aspartate-directed proteases >) caspase(s)*

  < (*suggested*) IE. spergh- *to move, to hasten, to spring*   **E** *spring, offspring*

G. asphodelos, asphodelou, m. *asphodel*
    > L. asphodelus, asphodeli, m. 무릇난, 시들지 않는 꽃; 수선화   **E** *asphodel, daffodil*

L. fumaria, fumariae, f. 괴불주머니와 비슷한 보라색 꽃이 피는 양꽃주머니과의
식물   **E** *fumaric acid, fumarate*
  < L. fumus, fumi, m. 연기, 김, 증기   **E** *(noun) fume*
  < IE. dheu-, dheuə- *The base of a wide variety of derivatives meaning 'to rise in a cloud', as dust, vapor, or smoke, and related to semantic notions of breath, various color adjectives, and forms denoting defective perception or wits.* (Vide FUMUS: *See* E. *fume*)

L. gentiana, gentianae, f. 용담(龍膽)

> **E** (*dried rhizome and roots of* Gentiana lutea >) ***gentian,*** *(gentian >)* ***gentisic acid, homogentisic acid; gentian violet*** *(< 'referred to its colour, being like that of the petals of a gentian flower; not made from gentians')*

   < L. Gentius, Gentii, m. Illyria의 왕(fl. 181-168 B.C.E.)

< *Of Illyrian origin*

G. hyakinthos, hyakinthou, m. *hyacinth, hyacinthine gem;* (Hyakinthos) (*Greek mythology*)

   a beautiful boy whom the god Apollo loved but killed accidentally with a discus. From his blood Apollo caused the hyacinth to spring up.

     > L. hyacinthus, hyacinthi, m. 히아신스, 히아신스석(石); (Hyacinthus) (그리스 신화)

       히아킨토스   **E** *hyacinth, Hyacinthus*

   < (*probably*) *Of Mediterranean origin*

     > L. vaccinium, vaccinii, n. 월귤(越橘)나무   **E** *vaccinium*

G. kanna, kannas, f. *reed*

     > L. canna, cannae, f. 갈대,

       갈대피리   **E** *canna, cane, cannon* (< *'large tube'*), *canyon* (< *'tube'*)

       > L. cannula, cannulae, f. (< + -ulla *diminutive suffix*) 관(管), 도랑, 수로,

         삽입관   **E** *cannula, cannulation*

       > L. canalis, canalis, m. 관(管), 도랑, 수로, 통로, 길   **E** *canal, channel*

         > L. canaliculus, canaliculi, m. (< + -ulus *diminutive suffix*) 소관(小管),

           세관(細管), 작은 수로   **E** *canaliculus,* (pl.) *canaliculi*

           > L. canalicularis, canaliculare 작은 관의, 작은 수로의   **E** *canalicular*

    > G. kaneon, kaneou, n. (kaneion, kaneiou, n.) *reed basket*

      > G. kanēphoros, kanēphoros, kanēphoron (< + -phoros, -phoros, -phoron *carrying,*

       bearing) *basket-carrying*

        E *canephorus* (< *'one of the maidens who carried on their heads baskets containing the sacred things used at the feasts of Demeter, Bacchus, and Athena')*

    > G. kanōn, kanonos, m. *rod, rule, standard*

      > L. canon, canonis, m. 규범, 법규, 정전(正典)   **E** *canon*

      > G. kanonikos, kanonikē, kanonikon *canonic*

       > L. canonicus, canonica, canonicum 규범에 맞는, 법규에 맞는, 정전의 **E** *canonic*

        > L. canonicalis, canonicale 규범에 맞는, 법규에 맞는, 정전의 **E** *canonical*

   < *Of Semitic origin*

G. kannabis, kannabios, f. *hemp, garment of hemp*

     > L. cannabis, cannabis, f. 삼[麻], 대마(大麻)

E *cannabis,* (cannabis resin >) **cannabin,** (cannabin >) **cannabinol,** (a hydrogenated derivative of cannabinol that is the active principle in cannabis >) **tetrahydro-cannabinol (THC),** (cannabinol >) **cannabinoid(s)**

> L. *cannabaceus, *cannabacea, *cannabaceum 삼의, 삼으로 만든

> **E** *canvas* (< 'made of hemp'), **canvass** (< 'to seek support for' < 'to toss in a canvas sheet')

< IE. kannabis *hemp*　　　　　　　　　　　　　　　　　　　　　　　　**E** *hemp*

E. *hashish*　　　　　　　　　　　　　　　　　　　　　　　　　　**E** *hashish*

< (*Arabic*) hashish (< *dry herb, hay*) *the dry leaves of hemp powdered, the intoxicant thence prepared*

> (*Arabic*) hashishash (hashishiyy) *hashish-eater who used to intoxicate oneself with hashish or hemp when preparing to dispatch a king or public man*

> L. assassinus, assassini, m. 암살자, 자객　　　　　　　**E** *assassin*

> L. assassino, assassinavi, assassinatum, assassinare 암살하다　　**E** *assassinate*

G. kolchikon, kolchikou, n. *meadow-saffron*

> L. colchicum, colchici, n. 콜치쿰

E *colchicine* (< 'an alkaloid found in all parts of the Colchicum autumnale and inhibiting microtubule polymerization by binding to tubulin')

< G. Kolchikos, Kolchikē, Kolchikon *of Colchis, Colchian*

< G. Kolchis, Kolchidos, f. *Colchis, ancient country south of the Caucasus Mountains, east of the Black Sea, in what is now Georgia*

L. lilium, lilii, n. 백합(百合), 백합화, 나리, 나리꽃　　　　　　　**E** *lily*

< *Of* non-IE. *origin*

> G. leirion, leiriou, n. (lirion, liriou, n.) *lily*　　　　　　**E** *liri(o)-*

L. malva, malvae, f. 아욱, 접시꽃　　　　　　**E** *mallow, mauve, mauveine*

> L. malvaceus, malvacea, malvaceum 아욱의　　　　　　**E** *malvaceous*

< *Of* non-IE. *origin*

> G. malachē, malachēs, f. *mallow*

E *malachite* (< 'perhaps from the similarity in color between the mineral and the leaves of the mallow plant'), **malachite green** (< 'dye of malachite's green color')

L. mentha, menthae, f. (menta, mentae, f.) 박하(薄荷)

E *menthol,* (menthol >) **mentholated,** (menthol >) **Mentholatum®, mint, spearmint** (< (probably) 'from the appearance of the flowers on the stem'), **peppermint** (< 'pungent mint')

< *Of* non-IE. *origin*

> G. minthē, minthēs, f. *mint*

L. nelumbo, nelumbonis, f. 연(蓮)   **E** *nelumbo*
    < (*Sinhalese*) nelumbu *Indian lotus*
  < (*Sanskrit*) nalina *Indian lotus*

L. nicotiana, nicotianae, f. (< herba nicotiana *herb of Nicot*) 담배속(屬)의 식물, 담배

> **E** *nicotine, (nicotine >) nicotinic, nicotinic acid (niacin), (nicotinic acid + -in >) niacin (nicotinic acid), (the amide of nicotinic acid >) nicotinamide*

    < L. nicotianus, nicotiana, nicotianum *of herb of Nicot*
    < Jean Nicot (1530-1604), *French ambassador in Lisbon and lexicographer, who introduced tobacco into France in 1560*

G. oxalis, oxalidos, f. (< *acid foliage*) *sorrel*
        > L. oxalis, oxalidis, f. 괭이밥   **E** *oxalis, oxalic acid, oxalate*
        < G. oxys, oxeia, oxy *sharp, sour, quick*
    < IE. ak- *sharp* (Vide ACUTUS: *See* E. *acute*)

L. papaver, papaveris, n. 아편(阿片), 앵속(罌粟), 양귀비(楊貴妃)   **E** *poppy, papaverine*
    < (*suggested*) IE. pap- *to swell* (Vide PAPILLA: *See* E. *papilla*)

L. opium, opii, n. 아편(阿片), 앵속(罌粟), 양귀비(楊貴妃)   **E** *opium, opioid*
        > L. opiatum, opiati, n. 아편제제(阿片製劑)   **E** *opiate*
        < G. opos, opou, m. *juice of plants, juice of fig-tree*
    < IE. s(w)okʷo- *resin, juice*

G. mēkōn, mēkōnos, f. *poppy*   **E** *mecon(o)-*
        > L. mecon, meconis, f. 아편(阿片), 앵속(罌粟), 양귀비(楊貴妃)
        > G. mēkōnion, mēkōniou, n. (< + -ion *diminutive suffix*) *poppy juice, feces of a new-born* (< *dark green color, resembling that of poppy juice*)
            > L. meconium, meconii, n. 아편, 배내똥, 태변(胎便)   **E** *meconium*
    < IE. mak(en)- *poppy*

L. ricinus, ricini, m. (진드기 > 진드기를 닮은 씨앗 >) 아주까리,
        덜 익은 오디 **E** *ricin (< 'a protein toxin that is extracted from castor bean (Ricinus communis)')*

G. rhytē, rhytēs, f. *rue*

> L. ruta, rutae, f. 루타(운향과(芸香科)의 쓴 약초, 향신료로 쓰였음);
쓰라림, 신랄　　　　　　　　　**E** *rue, rutin* (< *a glycoside obtained from* Ruta graveolens*)*

G. strychnos, strychnou, f. *nightshade*

> L. strychnos, strychni, f. 가지과(科)의 식물　　　　　　　　　**E** *strychnine*

L. valeriana, valerianae, f. 쥐오줌풀

E *valeric acid, (valeric acid >)* **valine** *(Val, V), (2-propylvaleric acid >)* **valproic acid***, (β , δ -dihydroxy-β -methylvaleric acid >)* **mevalonic acid**

< L. Valeria, Valeriae, f. *ancient name of a province of low Pannonia in Italy where the plants were grown*

or Valerius, Valerii, m. *personal name*

G. oryza, oryzēs, f. *rice*

> L. oryza, oryzae, f. 벼, 쌀　　　　　　　　　**E** *rice*
< (*probably*) *Of Oriental origin*

L. hordeum, hordei, n. 보리

> L. hordeolum, hordeoli, n. (< + -olum *diminutive suffix*) 다래끼, 맥립종(麥粒腫)　**E** *hordeolum*
< IE. (*probably*) ghers- *to bristle* (Vide HORRĒRE: *See* E. *horror*)

L. legumen, leguminis, n. 콩류　　　　　　　　　**E** *legume, leguminous*
< IE. leg- *to collect; with derivatives meaning 'to speak'* (Vide LEGĒRE: *See* E. *lecture*)

G. pison, pisou, n. (pisos, pisou, m.) *pea*

> L. pisum, pisi, n. 완두(豌豆), 콩, 팥　　　　**E** *(pease > (interpreted as a plural) >)* **pea**
> L. pisiformis, pisiforme 콩 모양의, 두상(豆狀)의　　　　　　　　　**E** *pisiform*

L. lens, lentis, f. 렌즈콩, 제비콩, 불콩, 편두(扁斗); (볼록) 렌즈, 수정체

E *lens,* (pl.) *lenses, lentiform* (< *'having the form of a lentil or of a lens'*), **retrolental** (< *'behind the lens of the eye'*)

> L. lenticula, lenticulae, f. (< + -cula *diminutive suffix*) 작은 렌즈콩, 제비콩, 불콩, 편두(扁斗); 렌즈콩 모양으로 생긴 것(보석), 주근깨, 기미　　　**E** *lentil*
> L. lenticularis, lenticulare 렌즈콩 모양의, (볼록) 렌즈 모양의, 수정체의, 렌즈핵(*lenticular nucleus*)의　　　　　　　　　**E** *lenticular*
> L. lenticella, lenticellae, f. (< + -cella *diminutive suffix*) (식물) 껍질눈, 피목(皮目)　**E** *lenticel*
> L. lentigo, lentiginis, f. 렌즈콩 모양의 반점, 검정사마귀,

흑색점(黑色點)   **E** *lentigo,* (pl.) *lentigines, lentiginous*

[용례] lentigo senilis (< *senile lentigo*) 노인성 흑점   **E** *lentigo senilis*

lentigo maligna (< *malignant lentigo*) 악성 흑점   **E** *lentigo maligna*

(문법) lentigo 흑색점: 단수 주격

senilis 노인의: 형용사, 남·여성형 단수 주격 < senilis, senile

maligna 악성의: 형용사, 여성형 단수 주격

< malignus, maligna, malignum

∽ (*suggested*) G. lathyros, lathyrou, m. *a kind of vetch*

\> L. lathyrus, lathyri, m. 갯완두속(屬)의 콩과 식물   **E** *lathyrism*

L. faba, fabae, f. 콩, 잠두(蠶豆)

\> L. fabella, fabellae, f. (< + -ella *diminutive suffix*) 작은 콩; 비복근두종자골(腓腹筋頭

種子骨)   **E** *fabella*

\> It. fava *broad bean, fava bean*   **E** *favism*

< IE. bha-bha- *broad bean*   **E** *bean*

\> G. phakos, phakou, m. *lentil, lentil-shaped*

objects   **E** *phac(o)- (phak(o)-), phacoemulsification, -phakia*

\> L. aphakia, aphakiae, f. (< G. a- *not*) 무수정체(증)   **E** *aphakia, aphakic*

\> L. phacoma, phacomatis, n. (phakoma, phakomatis, n.) (< *lentil-shaped*

hamartoma < + G. -ōma *noun suffix denoting tumor*) 모반(母斑), 모종(母腫),

수정체종(水晶體腫)   **E** *phacoma (phakoma), phacomatosis (phakomatosis)*

G. arachis, arachidos, f. *peanut*

\> L. arachis, arachidis, f. 땅콩

E *(arachid- + -ic > 'obtained from the peanut oil' >)* **arachidic acid** *(eicosanoic acid, icosanoic acid), (arachid- + -one (< G. -ōne 'feminine patronymic suffix') + -ic > 'the polyunsaturated counterpart to the saturated arachidic acid' >)* **arachidonic acid**

L. cucumis, cucumeris, m. 오이   **E** *cucumber*

< (*perhaps*) *Of Mediterranean origin*

L. cucurbita, cucurbitae, f. 호박, 호리병박, 졸대가리; (의학) 흡각(吸角), 흡종(吸鐘) **E** *cucurbit, gourd*

< (*perhaps*) *Of Mediterranean origin*

L. allium, allii, n. (alium, alii, n.) 마늘 **E** *alliin, (alliin >)* **allicin, allyl** *(< 'first obtained from garlic')*

< (*probably*) *Of Italic origin*

\> G. allas, allantos, m. *sausage* (Vide ALLAS; See E. *allantiasis*)

\> L. allantois, allantois, f. 요막(尿膜), 요낭(尿囊)

L. Capsicum, Capsici, n. (< *podlike fruit*) 고추속(屬)　**E** *capsicum, (capsicine > (altered) >) capsaicin*

    < (*perhaps*) L. capsa, capsae, f. 상자

  < IE. kap- *to grasp* (Vide CAPĔRE; *See* E. *caption*)

L. curcuma, curcumae, f. (< *so named because the color of the spices resembles that of*
    saffron) (Curcuma longa *turmeric*) 울금(鬱金), 심황(~黃); (Curcuma aromatica *wild*
    turmeric) 강황(薑黃)　**E** *curcumin*

    < (*Arabic*) kurkum *saffron, turmeric*

  < (*Sanskrit*) kunkuman *crocus, saffron*

    > G. krokos, krokou, m. *crocus, saffron*

      > L. crocus, croci, m. 사프란(Crocus sativus)　**E** *crocus*

L. piper, piperis, n. 후추나무, 후추; 신랄(한 말)

  E *pepper, peppermint* (< '*pungent mint*'), ***piperine*** (< '*an alkaloid obtained from pepper
  plants, especially black pepper and white pepper*')

    > L. piperatus, piperata, piperatum 후추 친, 후추가 들어간

    > L. piperitis, piperitis, f. (piperitis, piperitidis, f.) 고추

    > (*Serbo-Croatian*) paprika (< papr- (< papar < L. piper) *pepper* + -(i)ka *diminutive
       suffix*) *paprika*

      > (*Hungarian*) paprika *paprika*　**E** *paprika*

  < *Of Indo-Aryan origin*

    > G. (*ancient Greek*) peperi *pepper*

    > (*Sanskrit*) pippali *peppercorn, long pepper*

L. safranum, safrani, n. 사프란(Crocus sativus), 그 암술　**E** *saffron, safranine(s) (safranin(s))*

  < (*Arabic*) za 'faran *yellow*

L. zingiber, zingiberis, n. 새앙, 생강(生薑)　**E** *ginger*

    < G. zingiberis *ginger*

  < *Of Dravidian origin*

G. amanitai, amanitōn, f. (pl.) *a sort of fungi, mentioned by Dioscorides*

    > L. amanita, amanitae, f. 아마니타속(屬)의 버섯

      [용례] Amanita muscaria (< *fly agaric*) 무스카리아 버섯　**E** *muscarine, muscarinic*
      Amanita phalloides
        팔로이드 버섯　**E** *amanitin (amanitine), phalloidin (phalloidine), phallacidin*
      (문법) amanita 아마니타속 버섯: 단수 주격
        muscaria 파리의 (파리 잡는): 형용사, 여성형 단수 주격

< muscarius, muscaria, muscarium

phalloides 음경같이 생긴: 형용사, 남·여·중성형 단수 주격

< phalloides, (gen.) phalloidis

G. agarikon, agarikou, n. (< *said by Dioscorides to be named from Agaria in Sarmatia, the ancient region in Europe comprising much of Poland and Russia*) *the tree fungus used for tinder, touchwood*

> L. agaricum, agarici, n. 주름버섯, 서양송이 　　　　　　　　　　　　 **E** *agaric*

원소

L. elementum, elementi, n. 원소(元素), 기본 요소, 4대 요소(불·물·공기·흙); 원리, 기초, 초보　　**E** *element, (picture element >) pixel, (pixel >) pixelate, (volume element >) voxel*

> elementarius, elementaria, elementarium 기본 원리의, 기초적, 초보의　　　**E** *elementary*

E. *gold*　　　　　　　　　　　　　　　　　　　　　　　　　　　　　　　　　**E** *gold*

< IE. ghel- *to shine; with derivatives referring to colors, bright materials, gold (probably 'yellow metal'), and bile or gall* (Vide FULVUS; *See* E. *fulvous*)

L. aurum, auri, n. 금, 금화　　　**E** *aurum (Au),* Sp. *El Dorado (< 'the gilded'), auriasis (chrysiasis)*

> L. aureus, aurea, aureum 금으로 만든, 도금한, 금빛의, 싯누런

　　> L. aureolus, aureola, aureolum (< + -olus *diminutive suffix*) 금빛의, 금으로 장식한　　　　　　　　　　　**E** *(aureola corona 'golden crown' >) aureole*

　　> L. aureatus, aureata, aureatum 금으로 장식한　　　　　　　　**E** *aureate*

> L. aurifer, aurifera, auriferum (< aurum *gold* + -fer (< ferre *to carry, to bear*) *carrying, bearing*) 금이 나는, 금을 함유한　　　　　　　　　**E** *auriferous*

> L. auripigmentum, auripigmenti, n. (< aurum *gold* + pigmentum *pigment*) 석웅황 (石雄黃) (황색 안료용 비소화합물)　　　　　　　　　　　　　　**E** *orpiment*

< IE. aus- *to shine (said especially of the dawn), gold*　**E** *east, eastern, Easter,* (Österreich >) *Austria*

> L. auster, austri, m. (< *shift in meaning from 'east' probably due to false assumption concerning direction of axis of Italy*) 남풍, 남쪽　　　**E** *Auster, Austr(o)-*

　　> L. australis, australe 남풍의, 남쪽의　　　**E** *austral, (terra australis 'southern land' >) Australia*

　　　　> L. Australopithecus, Australopitheci, m. (< *southern ape* < australis *southern* + G. pithēkos *ape*) (원인 猿人)

오스트랄로피테쿠스속(屬)　　　　　　　　　　　　　**E** Australopithecus

> L. aurora, aurorae, f. 동트기, 여명, 서광, 동쪽, 오로라 (< *the appearance of dawn or approaching sunrise*); (Aurora) (로마 신화) 새벽의 여신　　　**E** *aurora, Aurora*

> G. ēōs, ēous, f. (heōs, heō, f.) *dawn, daybreak, morning, east;* (Ēōs) (*Greek mythology*) *goddess of the dawn*

　　E *eo-, eosin* (< *'the morning red'*), *eosinophil* (< *'a cell or element staining readily with eosin'*), *Eos*

G. chrysos, chrysou, m. *gold, gold coin, gold vessel*　　　　**E** *chrys(o)-*

> G. chrysallis, chrysallidos, f. *the gold-colored chrysalis of butterflies*

　> L. chrysallis, chrysallidis, f. (chrysalis, chrysalidis, f.) (나비) 번데기　　　**E** *chrysalis,* (pl.) *chrysalides (chrysales), chrysalid*

> G. chrysanthemon, chrysanthemou, n. (< chrysos + anthemon *flower*) *the corn-marigold*

　> L. chrysanthemum, chrysanthemi, n. 국화(菊花)　　　**E** *chrysanthemum*

> L. *chrysiasis, *chrysiasis, f. (< G. chrysos + -iasis *suffering from*) (조직 내) 금 침착증, 금피증(金皮症)　　　**E** *chrysiasis (auriasis)*

< (*Semitic root*) hrs *to be(come) yellow, gold(en)*

E. *silver*　　　　　　　　　　　　　　　　　　　　　　　**E** *silver*

< *Of Asiatic origin*

L. argentum, argenti, n. 은, 은화

　E *argentum (Ag), argentaffin* (< *'stained black by ammoniacal silver in the absence of a reducing agent'*)

> L. argentinus, argentina, argentinum 은의, 은 같은　　　**E** *argentine,* Sp. *Argentina*

> L. argentaria, argentariae, f. 은광, 은행

< IE. arg- *to shine, white, the shining or white metal, silver* (Vide infra)

> L. arguo, argui, argutum, arguĕre 밝히다, 증명하다　　　**E** *argue*

　> L. argumentum, argumenti, n. 논증, 논의, 변론　　　**E** *argument*

G. argyros, argyrou, m. *silver, money*

　E *argyr(o)-, argyria (argyrosis, argyriasis, argyrism)* (< *'silver poisoning'*), *argyrophil* (< *'stained black by ammoniacal silver in the presence of a reducing agent'*)

> L. hydrargyrum, hydrargyri, n. (< G. hydōr, hydōratos, n. *water* + argyros) 수은(水銀)

　E *hydrargyrum (Hg), hydrargyria (hydrargyrosis, hydrargyriasis, hydrargyrism)* (< *'mercurial poisoning'*)

< IE. arg- *to shine, white, the shining or white metal, silver* (Vide supra)

> G. arginoeis, arginoessa, arginoen *shining, bright,*

white　　　　**E** *(perhaps)* **arginine (Arg, R)** *(< 'its first discovered salts were silvery')*

L. cuprum, cupri, n. 구리　　　　**E** *cuprum (Cu), cuprous (Cu⁺), cupric (Cu⁺⁺), copper*

　　　< L. cyprum, cypri, n. (< *Cyprium aes Cyprian metal* < aes, aeris, n.
　　　　　metal (Vide AERUGINOSUS: *See* E. *era*)) 구리

　　　　< L. Cyprius, Cypria, Cyprium 사이프러스(키프로스)의　　　　**E** *Cyprian*
　　　　　< L. Cyprus, Cypri, f. 사이프러스(키프로스)　　　　**E** *Cyprus*
　　　　　< G. Kypros, Kyprou, f. *Cyprus (known as Aphrodite's birthplace)*
　　　　　　> G. Kypris, Kypridos, f. *Aphrodite*
　　　　　　　> L. cypripedium, cypripedii, n. (< *Venus' shoe, lady's slipper; in reference*
　　　　　　　　to the inflated pouch formed by the labellum) < G. Kypris + pedilon,
　　　　　　　　pedilou, n. *slipper*) 개불알꽃　　　　**E** *cypripedium*

G. chalkos, chalkou, m. *copper, copper coin, bronze, brass*　　　　**E** *chalc(o)- (chalk(o)-), chalcography*

E. *iron* (< *holy metal*)　　　　**E** *iron*

　　　< IE. eis- *in words denoting passion* (Vide IRASCI: *See* E. *irate*)

L. ferrum, ferri, n. 철, 쇠, 철제 기구

> **E** *ferrum (Fe), ferrous (Fe⁺⁺), ferric (Fe⁺⁺⁺), ferrated (< 'charged-with iron'), ferritin (< 'iron-apoferritin complex'), apoferritin (< 'ferritin without iron'), transferrin (< 'a protein to bind and transport iron'), lactoferrin (< 'a protein found in milk and other secretions, whose iron-binding properties have a bactericidal effect')*

　　> L. ferrugo, ferruginis, f. 쇠의 녹, 암갈색, 질투
　　　> L. ferrugineus, ferruginea, ferrugineum 녹슨 쇳빛의, 암갈색의, 쇠비린내 나는,
　　　　　철분이 함유된　　　　**E** *ferruginous*
　　< *(possibly) Borrowed (via Etruscan) from the same obscure source as brass*　　　　**E** *brass, brazen*

G. sidēros, sidērou, m. *iron, steel, iron tool*

> **E** *sideroblast (< 'a nucleated red blood cell containing ferritin granules'), hemosiderin (< 'intracellular storage complex of iron, often formed after hemorrhage')*

　　> L. siderosis, siderosis, f. (< *iron deposition* < + G. -ōsis *condition*) 철침착증, 철증　**E** *siderosis*
　　　> L. haemosiderosis, haemosiderosis, f. (< *deposition of hemosiderin without*
　　　　associated tissue damage < G. haima *blood*) 혈철소증(血鐵素症), 헤모
　　　　시데린증　　　　**E** *hemosiderosis*

E. *lead*　　　　**E** *lead*

L. plumbum, plumbi, n. 납, 납으로 만든 물건, 납덩어리를 단 채찍

E *plumbum (Pb), plumbous (Pb⁺⁺), plumbic (Pb⁺⁺⁺⁺), plumbism* (*< 'lead poisoning'*), *plumb, plumbless, plummet,* (*plumbicare '*to throw a leaded line*' >) *plunge*

> L. plumbarius, plumbarii, f. 연공(鉛工), 연관공(鉛管工)　　　　　　**E** *plumber*

< *Of Mediterranean origin, probably borrowed from the same unidentified source as* G. molybdos

G. molybdos, molybdou, m. *lead*　　　　　　　　　　　**E** *molybdenum (Mo)*

< *Of Mediterranean origin, probably borrowed from the same unidentified source as* L. plumbum

E. *brimstone* (< *burning stone*)　　　　　　　　　　　　**E** *brimstone*

< IE. gʷher– *to heat, to warm* (Vide FORNIX; *See* E. *fornix*)

+ IE. stai– *stone* (Vide STEAR; *See* E. *stone*)

L. sulphur, sulphuris, n. (sulfur, sulfuris, n.) 유황

E *sulphur (sulfur, S), sulfurous (S⁺⁺⁺⁺), sulfuric (S⁺⁺⁺⁺⁺⁺), sulfite (SO₃⁻⁻), sulfate (SO₄⁻⁻), sulf(o)–, sulfide(s)*

> L. sulphureus, sulphurea, sulphureum (sulfureus, sulfurea, sulfureum) 유황의,

　　　유황을 칠한　　　　　　　　　　**E** *sulphureous (sulfureous)*

< (*probably*) *Of Mediterranean origin*

G. theion, theiou, n. *brimstone, sulfur*

E *thi(o)–* (< '*a name for sulphur*'), *thiamine (thiamin) (vitamin B₁)* (< '*sulfur-containing amine*', '*sulfur-containing vitamin*'), *thiol–* (< '*a name for the group SH or SR (R for alkyl) in combination*'), *thion–* (< '*a name for sulphur taking the place of oxygen in a compound and joined by two bonds to carbon, with exceptions*'), *(methyl + thion– + –ine >) methionine (Met, M)*

< IE. dheu–, dheuə– *the base of a wide variety of derivatives meaning 'to rise in a cloud', as dust, vapor, or smoke, and related to semantic notions of breath, various color adjectives, and forms denoting defective perception or wits* (Vide FUMUS; *See* E. *fume*)

E. *sodium* (< *caustic soda (NaOH)* + *–ium*)　　　　　　**E** *sodium*

　　　　< L. soda *sodium carbonate (Na₂CO₃); separated into caustic soda (NaOH)*
　　　　　　and carbon dioxide (CO₂)

　　　< (*Arabic*) suwwad *saltwort*

　　< (*Arabic root*) swd *to be black, to become black*

L. natrium, natrii, n. (< F. natron + –ium)

　　　　　　나트륨　　　**E** *natrium (Na); hypernatremia, hyponatremia, natriuresis, natriuretic*

　　　　< F. natron *sodium carbonate (Na₂CO₃)*

　　　< G. nitron *nitre (niter) (originally sodium carbonate (Na₂CO₃), later sodium nitrate (NaNO₃) or potassium nitrate (KNO₃))*

> F. nitre *nitre (niter)*

> **E** *nitr(o)–, nitrous, nitric, nitrite (NO_2^-), nitrate (NO_3^-), nitrify (< 'to convert (ammonia) into a nitrite or nitrate')*

> F. nitrogene *nitrogen*　　　　　　　　　　　　　　　**E** *nitrogen (N)*

< (*Egyptian*) ntr *nitre (niter)*

E. *potassium* (< *caustic potash (KOH)* + –ium)

포타슘　**E** *potassium, hyperpotassemia (hyperkalemia), hypopotassemia (hypokalemia)*

< E. potash (< *obtained by leaching wood ashes and evaporating the leach in a pot) potassium carbonate (K_2CO_3); separated into caustic potash (KOH) and carbon dioxide (CO_2)*　　　**E** *potash*

< E. pot

> **E** *pot, pottage (< 'food cooked in a pot'), (pottage >) porridge, potpourri (< 'rotten pot')*

< *Of pre-Celtic origin*

L. kalium, kalii, n. 칼륨

> **E** *kalium (K), hyperkalemia (hyperpotassemia), hypokalemia (hypopotassemia)*

< F. alcali *alkali*

< (*Arabic*) al-qaliy *the 'calcined ashes' of the plants* Salsola *and* Salicornia

> **E** *alkali, alkaline, alkalinity, alkaloid(s) (< 'nitrogenous basic substances found in plants'), (alkali + G. kapton (neuter present participle of kaptein 'to swallow greedily') >) alkapton (< 'darkened on the addition of alkali'), alkaptonuria*

> L. alkalosis, alkalosis, f. (< *alkali* + G. –ōsis *condition*) 알칼리증(症)　**E** *alkalosis*

< (*Arabic*) qalay *to fry, to roast in a pan*

< (*Semitic*) qly *to burn, to roast*

L. aluminium, aluminii, n. 알루미늄　　　　　　**E** *aluminium (aluminum, Al)*

< L. alumen, aluminis, n. 명반(明礬)　　　　　　　　　　　　　　**E** *alum*

> L. alumina, aluminae, f. 반토(礬土)　　　　　　　　　　　　**E** *alumina*

< IE. alu– *bitter, beer, alum*　　　　　　　　　　　　　　　　　**E** *ale*

L. antimonium, antimonii, n. 안티몬　　　　　　　　　　　**E** *antimony*

< (*suggested*) (*Arabic*) al ithmid *antimony*

< G. stimmi *powdered antimony used to paint the eyelids*

> L. stimmi, stimmis, n. (stibi, stibis, n., stibium, stibii, n.) 안티몬, 안티몬 분(粉), 눈썹 그리는 검정색 화장품　　　　　　　　　**E** *stibium (Sb)*

< (*Egyptian*) sdmt *mixture used to protect the eyes from flies*

L. borax, boracis, m. 붕사(硼砂)　　　　　　　　　　**E** *borax, boron (B)*

< (*Arabic*) buraq *borax*

< (*Probably*) (*Persian*) burah *borax*

L. ytterbium, ytterbii, n. (희토류 원소) 이테르븀 | E ytterbium (Yb) |

    < (*Swedish*) Ytterby *a village in the Stockholm archipelago*

      > L. yttrium, yttrii, n. (희토류 원소) 이트륨 | E yttrium (Y) |

      > L. terbium, terbii, n. (희토류 원소) 테르븀 | E terbium (Tb) |

      > L. erbium, erbii, n. (희토류 원소) 에르븀 | E erbium (Er) |

뜻의 비교

L. primordium, primordii, n. (< primus *first* + ordiri *to begin* + -ium *noun suffix*) 시작,

    최초, 원본, 원기(原基) | E primordium, (pl.) primordia |

      > L. primordialis, primodiale 최초의, 원시의 | E primordial |

    < L. ordior, orsus sum, ordiri 베틀에 날을 날다, 베를 짜기 시작하다, 짜다, 시작하다

  < (*Italic root of uncertain origin*) ord- *to arrange, arrangement* (Vide ORDO; *See* E. *order*)

D. Anlage, Anlage, f. (< *laying on, for the first*) 기초, 원기(原基) | E anlage |

    < IE. an- *on* (Vide ANA; *See* E. *an(a)-*)

    + IE. legh- *to lie, to lay* (Vide LECTUS; *See* E. *litter*)

L. rudimentum, rudimenti, n. 초보, 입문, 싹수 | E rudiment, (rudiment >) rudimentary |

    < L. rudis, rude 자연 그대로의, 첫경험의, 세련되지 않은, 미숙한, 버릇없는 | E rude |

  < (*possibly*) IE. reuə- *to smash, to knock down, to tear out, to dig up, to up-root*

    (Vide RUGA; *See* E. *ruga*)

L. vestigium, vestigii, n. 발자국, 흔적 | E vestige, (vestigium >) vestigial |

    > L. vestigo, vestigavi, vestigatum, vestigare 발자취를 뒤따르다, 구석구석 찾다

      > L. investigo, investigavi, investigatum, investigare (< in- *in, on, into, toward*)

        추적하다, 조사하다 | E investigate |

L. resina, resinae, f. (< *plant exudates of terpene-based compounds, e.g., from pine and fir*)

    나무의 진, 수지(樹脂) | E resin, rosin, oleoresin (< 'essential oil and resin') |

    < G. rhētinē, rhētinēs, f. *resin*

< *Of* non-IE. *origin*

L. latex, laticis, m. (< *plant exudates of polyisoprenes, e.g., from rubber tree; any dispersion*
　　　　in water of polymer particles) 유동성 액체(흐르는 물·음료·술·젖 등), 유액(乳液), 유탁액
　　　　(乳濁液), 라텍스　　　　　　　　　　　　　　　　　　　　　　　　　　　E *latex*
　　　　　< G. latax, latagos, m. *drop, wine lees*
　　< IE. lat- *wet, moist*

L. gummi, n. (cummi, n.) (불변화); (gummis, gummis, f.) (< *plant exudates of poly-*
　　　　saccharides, e.g., from gum arabic tree) 고무　　　　　　　E *gum,* (*Dutch*) *gom*

　　　　　　[용례] gummi Arabicum (< *gum arabic*) 아라비아 고무
　　　　　　　　　gummi elasticum (< *gum elastic*) 탄성 고무, 고무
　　　　　　　　(문법) gummi 고무: 단수 주격
　　　　　　　　　　Arabicum 아랍의: 형용사, 중성형 단수 주격
　　　　　　　　　　　< Arabicus, Arabica, Arabicum
　　　　　　　　　　elasticum 탄성의: 형용사, 중성형 단수 주격
　　　　　　　　　　　< elasticus, elastica, elasticum

　　　　　　　> L. gumma, gummatis, n. 고무, 고무종(腫)　　E *gumma,* (pl.) *gummata, gummatous*
　　　　　< G. kommi, kommidos, n. (kommi, kommeōs, n.) *plant gum*
　　< (*Egyptian*) gmyt *plant gum*

L. balsamum, balsami, n. (< *fragrant plant exudates, e.g., from frankincense and myrrh*)
　　　　　발삼 수지(樹脂), 발삼 향유; 발삼 나무(발삼을 분비하는 각종 나무, 특히 Commiphora
　　　　　속), 발삼 전나무
　　　　　　E *balsam, balm, embalm,* (*tolu balsam exported from Santiago de Tolu in Columbia >*)
　　　　　　toluene
　　　　　　> L. balsaminus, balsamina, balsaminum 발삼의, 발삼 성분의
　　　　　< G. balsamon, balsamou, n. *balsam*
　　< *Of Semitic origin*

L. alveolus, alveoli, m. (< + -olus *diminutive suffix*) 작은 통, 꽈리, 포(胞), 허파꽈리, 폐포
　　　　　(肺胞), 조(槽), 치조(齒槽)　　　　　　　　　　　　　　E *alveolus,* (pl.) *alveoli*
　　　　　　> L. alveolaris, alveolare 꽈리의, 폐포의, 치조의　　E *alveolar, palatoalveolar*
　　　　　< L. alveus, alvei, m. 파인 곳, 물통, 목욕통, 벌집　　　E *alveus*
　　　　< L. alvus, alvi, f. 배, 아랫배, 위, 배설물, 벌집, 선창
　　< IE. aulo- *hole, cavity*
　　　　> G. aulos, aulou, m. *hollow tube, pipe, flute*　　　　　E *hydraulic*
　　　　　> G. choraulēs, choraulou, m. (< choros *dance* + aulos *fluit*) *fluit player who*
　　　　　　accompanied the dance

> L. choraules, choraulae, m. 합창 반주의 플루트 주자　　　　　　　　E *carol*

L. foveola, foveolae, f. (< + -ola *diminutive suffix*) 작은 오목,
　　　소와(小窩)　　　　　　　　　　　　　　　　　　　　　E *foveola, (foveola >) foveolar*
　　　< L. fovea, foveae, f. 구덩이, 함정, 오목, 와(窩)　　　　　　E *fovea, (fovea >) foveal*

L. caveola, caveolae, f. (< + -ola *diminutive suffix*)
　　　소포(小胞)　　　　　　　　　　　　　　E *caveola, (pl.) caveolae, (caveola >) caveolar*
　　　< L. cavea, caveae, f. 새장, 우리, 움집, 실(室)　E *cage, ((Dutch) de kooi 'the cage' >) decoy*
　< IE. keuə- *to swell; vault, hole* (Vide CAVUS; *See* E. *cave*)

L. acinus, acini, m. (*a berry which grows in clusters, as grapes, currants, etc.; sometimes*
　　　applied to the whole cluster) 포도알 > 포도상선(葡萄狀腺) > 샘꽈리, 세엽(細葉), 소엽
　　　(小葉), 선방(腺房), 선포(腺胞)　　　E *acinus, (pl.) acini, acinar (acinose (acinous), acinic)*

L. folliculus, folliculi, m. (< + -culus *diminutive suffix*) (작은) 주머니, 소포(小胞), 난포(卵胞),
　　　여포(濾胞), 낭(囊)　　　　　　　　　　　　　　　　　　E *follicle, follicular*
　　　< L. follis, follis, m. 가죽주머니, 가죽공, 풀무　　　　　　E *folly, fool*
　< IE. bhel- *to blow, to swell; with derivatives referring to various round objects and to the*
　　notion of tumescent masculinity (Vide FOLLIS; *See* E. *folly*)

L. ascus, asci, m. (식물) 자낭(子囊), 주머니세포　　E *ascus, (pl.) asci, asc(o)-, ascospore*
　　　< G. askos, askou, m. *hide, leather bag, wineskin, bladder, belly*
　　　　　> G. askitēs, askitēs, askites *of wineskin, wineskin-like*

　　　　　　　　[용례] askitēs hydrōps (*abdominal dropsy*) 복수(腹水), 뱃물
　　　　　　　　[문법] askitēs *wineskin-like*: 형용사, 남·여성형 단수 주격
　　　　　　　　　　　hydrōps *edema*: 단수 주격 < hydrōps, hydrōpos, f.

　　　　　　> L. ascites, ascitis, m. (< G. askitēs hydrōps) 복수(腹水), 뱃물　E *ascites, ascitic*
　　　　　> G. askidion, askidiou, n. (< + -idion *diminutive suffix*) *small ascus*
　　　　　　> L. ascidium, ascidii, n. (동물) 병(瓶) 모양의 기관　　　E *ascidium, (pl.) ascidia*

L. saccus, sacci, m. 거칠고 투박한 천, 껄껄한 짐승털로 짠 천; 그 천으로 소매 없이 만든 자루
　　　모양의 옷 (참회·고행·슬픔의 표시로 입었음); (위의 천으로 만든) 자루, 낭(囊),
　　　포(胞)　　　　　　E *sac, sack, knapsack, rucksac, F. cul-de-sac (< 'bottom of a sac')*
　　　> L. sacculus, sacculi, m. (< + -ulus *diminutive suffix*) 작은 자루, 둥근 주머니,
　　　　　소낭(小囊)　　　　　E *saccule, (sacculus >) saccular, (sacculus >) sacculation*
　　　　　> L. saccellus, saccelli, m. (< + -ellus *diminutive suffix*) 작은 자루,

주머니   **E** *satchel*

    < G. sakkos, sakkou, m. (sakos, sakou, m.) *sack-cloth, mourning dress, bag, sack*

  < (*Semitic root*) sqq- *sack-cloth, grain sack*

     > (*Hebrew*) saq *sack*

L. utriculus, utriculi, m. (< + -culus *diminutive suffix*) 작은 가죽부대, 타원낭,

        소실(小室)   **E** *utricle*, (utriculus >) *utricular*

      < L. uter, uteris, m. (물·포도주를 담는) 가죽부대

    < (*probably*) (*Via Etruscan*) G. hydōr, hydōratos, n. *water*

  < IE. wed- *water, wet* (Vide UNDA: *See* E. *undulate*)

L. cisterna, cisternae, f. 물통, 수조(水槽),

       조(槽)   **E** *cisterna (cistern)*, (pl.) *cisternae (cisterns)*, (*cisterna* >) *cisternal*

      [용례] cisterna magna 큰수조, 소뇌숨뇌수조   **E** *cisterna magna*

        (문법) cisterna 수조: 단수 주격

          magna 큰: 형용사, 여성형 단수 주격 < magnus, magna, magnum

     < L. cista, cistae, f. (고리버들의 작은 가지로 만든) 바구니, 궤, 함   **E** *cist, chest*

    < G. kistē, kistēs, f. *chest, box, basket*

  < IE. kista *woven container*

E. *bladder* (< *something blown up*)   **E** *bladder*

   < IE. bhle- *to blow* (Vide FLARE: *See* E. *flatus*)

L. vesica, vesicae, f. (< *perhaps taboo deformation*) 가죽주머니, 방광(膀胱), 낭(囊), 수포(水胞),

       물집   **E** *vesica, vesic(o)-*

      [용례] vesica urinaria 방광(膀胱)

        vesica biliaris (vesica fellea) 담낭(膽囊)

       (문법) vesica 가죽주머니: 단수 주격

         urinaria 오줌의: 형용사, 여성형 단수 주격

           < urinarius, urinaria, urinarium

         biliaris 담즙의: 형용사, 남·여성형 단수 주격 < biliaris, biliare

         fellea 담즙의: 형용사, 여성형 단수 주격 < felleus, fellea, felleum

    > L. vesicalis, vesicale 낭의, 방광의   **E** *vesical*

    > L. vesicula, vesiculae, f. (< + -ula *diminutive suffix*) 작은 가죽주머니, 작은 방광,

       소낭(小囊), 소포(小胞), 수포(水胞), 잔물집   **E** *vesicle, vesicular, multivesicular, vesiculate*

    > L. vesico, vesicavi, —, vesicare 물집이 생기다   **E** *vesicate, vesicant, vesication*

  < IE. udero- *abdomen, womb, stomach; with distantly similar forms* (*perhaps taboo deformations*)

   in various languages (Vide UTERUS: *See* E. *uterus*)

L. cystis, cystidis, f. 주머니, 낭(囊), 낭포(囊胞), 낭종(囊腫), 방광(膀胱)

> **E** cyst, cyst(o)-, -cyst, pseudocyst, encyst, encystation (encystment), excyst, excystation (excystment), cystoscope

> L. urocystis, urocystidis, f. (cystis urinaria) 방광

> **E** cystine (< 'found in a rare kind of urinary calculus'), (cystine >) cysteine (Cys, C)

> L. cholecystis, cholecystidis, f. (cystis biliaria, cystis fellea) 담낭　　**E** cholecyst(o)-

> L. Pneumocystis, Pneumocystidis, f. (< cyst-forming fungus within the lungs

< G. pneumōn lung) (진균) 폐포자충속(屬)

E Pneumocystis

< G. kystis, kystidos, f. bellows > bag, bladder

> G. *kystikos, *kystikē, *kystikon of bag, of bladder

> L. cysticus, cystica, cysticum 낭(囊)의

E cystic, polycystic

< IE. kwes- to pant, to wheeze

E wheeze

> L. queror, questus sum, queri 불평하다, 원망하다

> L. querela, querelae, f. (querella, querellae, f.) 불평, 원망, 소송

E quarrel

> L. querulus, querula, querulum 불평하는, 원망하는

E querulous

L. rumen, ruminis, n. 인후, 식도; 혹위(유위 瘤胃, 전위 前胃, 반추동물의 제1위)　　**E** rumen

> L. rumino, ruminavi, ruminatum, ruminare 새김질하다, 반추(反芻)하다,

되새기다

E ruminate, ruminant

< IE. reusmen throat, rumination

< IE. reu- to belch

L. reticulum, reticuli, n. (< + -culum diminutive suffix) 작은 그물, 세망(細網); 벌집위(봉소상

위 蜂巢狀胃, 반추동물의 제2위)

E reticulum, reticule (reticle)

< L. rete, retis, n. 그물 [網]

E rete, retiform

< IE. erə- to separate (Vide RETE: See E. rete)

L. omasum, omasi, n. 겹주름위(중판위 重瓣胃, 반추동물의 제3위)　　**E** omasum

< Of Gaulish origin

L. abomasum, abomasi, n. (< ab- off, away from + omasum bullock's tripe) 주름위(추위 皺胃,

반추동물의 제4위)

E abomasum

L. virus, viri, n. (복수 없음) 즙, 악취, 독기

> **E** virus, (pl.) viruses, (virus >) viral, viricide (virucide); virion (< 'a complete, infective form that a virus has outside a host cell, with a core and a capsid; called also a viral particle'), viroid, virology; (Hantan (Hantaan) River >) Hantavirus, (Norwalk Town >) norovirus

> L. virulentus, virulenta, virulentum 유독한, 유해한

E virulent

> L. virulentia, virulentiae, f. 악취　　　　　　　　　　　　　**E** *virulence*

< IE. weis- *to flow*　　　　　　　　　　　　　**E** *ooze (< 'mire, mud')*

　　> L. viscum, visci, n. (viscus, visci, m.) 겨우살이; 겨우살이 열매에서 채취하는 새잡이

　　　　끈끈이

　　　　> L. viscidus, viscida, viscidum 끈적끈적한　　　　　　　**E** *viscid*

　　　　> L. viscosus, viscosa, viscosum 끈적끈적한　　　　**E** *viscose (viscous)*

　　　　　　> L. viscositas, viscositatis, f. 점성(粘性), 점도(粘度)　　　**E** *viscosity*

　　> (*suggested*) G. ixos, ixou, m. *mistletoe, birdlime*

　　　　> G. ixōdēs, ixōdēs, ixōdes (< + -ōdēs *like, resembling*) *birdlime-like, sticky*

　　　　　　> L. Ixodes, Ixodis, m. (진드기) 참진드기속(屬)　　　**E** *Ixodes, ixodiasis*

L. chlamydia, chlamydiae, f. (< *the cytoplasmic inclusions 'draped' around the infected*

　　　cell's nucleus) 클라미디아　　　　　**E** *chlamydia, (chlamydia >) chlamydial*

　　< L. chlamys, chlamydis, f. 짧은 외투, 그리스식

　　　　군복　　　**E** *chlamydospore (< 'Each spore... has its own protective envelope.')*

　　< G. chlamys, chlamydos, f. *cloak (draped around the shoulder), military cloak*

L. rickettsia, rickettsiae, f. 리케차　　　　　**E** *rickettsia, (rickettsia >) rickettsial*

　　< Howard Taylor Ricketts (1871-1910), *American pathologist*

L. mycoplasma, mycoplasmatis, n. (< *fungus-like growth pattern of* M. mycoides)

　　　미코플라스마　　　　　**E** *mycoplasma, (mycoplasma >) mycoplasmal*

　　　> L. ureaplasma, ureaplasmatis, n. (< *able to metabolize urea*)

　　　　우레아플라스마　　　　　**E** *ureaplasma*

　　< G. plasma, plasmatos, n. *something molded, something formed, figure, image,*

　　　fiction, forgery

　　< IE. pelə- *flat, to spread* (Vide PLANUS; *See* E. *plane*)

L. bacterium, bacterii, n. 세균

　　　E *bacterium,* (pl.) *bacteria, (bacterium >) bacterial, bacteriostatic; bactericidal*

　　　> L. -bacter, -bacteris, m. -세균　　　　　**E** *-bacter*

　　　　> L. Helicobacter, Helicobacteris, m. (< G. helix, helikos, f. *winding,*

　　　　　spire, coil, anything twisted) (세균) 헬리코박터속(屬)　　**E** Helicobacter

　　　> L. bacteraemia, bacteraemiae, f. (< + G. haima, haimatos, n. *blood* +

　　　　-ia *noun suffix*) 세균혈증　　　　　**E** *bacteraemia (bacteremia)*

　　< G. baktērion, baktēriou, n. (< + -ion *diminutive suffix*) *small staff,*

　　　bacterium　　　　　**E** *bacterioid (bacteroid)*

　　　> L. bacteroides, (gen.) bacteroidis (< *bacterium-like* < + G. eidos *shape*)

　　　　박테로이드의

> L. bacteroides, bacteroidis, m.

박테로이드   **E** *bacteroides, bacteroid* (*bacterioid*)

< G. baktēria, baktērias, f. (baktron, baktrou, n.) *staff, stick*

< IE. bak- *staff used for support*   **E** *peg*

> L. baculus, baculi, m. (baculum, baculi, n.) 지팡이,

막대기   **E** *baculum, baculine, baculiform,* F. *baguette, debacle* (< *'to free'* < *'to unbar'*)

> L. bacillus, bacilli, m. (< + -illus *diminutive suffix*) 작은 막대기, 막대균, 간균

(桿菌), 바실러스; (Bacillus) (세균) 바실러스속(屬)   **E** *bacillus,* (pl.) *bacilli*

> L. bacillarius, bacillaria, bacillarium 작은 막대기의, 막대균의   **E** *bacillary*

> L. bacilliformis, bacilliforme 작은 막대기 모양의, 막대균 모양의   **E** *bacilliform*

> L. imbecillus, imbecilla, imbecillum (< *without a supporting staff* <

im- (< in-) *not*) 약한, 저능의   **E** *imbecile*

> L. bacillum, bacilli, n. (< + -illum *diminutive suffix*) 작은 막대기

L. fungus, fungi, m. 버섯, 곰팡이, 진균(眞菌)   **E** *fungus,* (pl.) *fungi, fungicidal, fungistatic, fungiform*

> L. fungalis, fungale 버섯의, 곰팡이의, 진균의   **E** *fungal* (*fungous*)

> L. fungosus, fungosa, fungosum 버섯의, 곰팡이의, 진균의   **E** *fungous* (*fungal*)

> L. fungoides, (gen.) fungoidis (< + G. eidos *shape*) 버섯 모양의, 곰팡이 모양의   **E** *fungoid*

[용례] mycosis fungoides 균상식육종(菌狀息肉腫), 용상진균증

(茸狀眞菌症)   **E** *mycosis fungoides*

(문법) mycosis 진균증: 단수 주격 < mycosis, mycosis, f.

fungoides: 형용사, 남·여·중성형 단수 주격

< G. (*Attic*) sphongos, sphongou, m. ((*non-Attic*) spongos, spongou, m.) *sponge*

> G. spongia, spongias, f. *sponge*

> L. spongia, spongiae, f. 갯솜, 해면(海綿), 스펀지   **E** *sponge, spongy; spongiform*

> L. spongiosus, spongiosa, spongiosum 해면 같은, 구멍이 숭굴

숭굴한

E (substantia spongiosa ossium *'spongy substance of the bones'* >)
spongiosa

L. nunc (< *nunce < IE. nu- *now* + IE. ke- (*deictic particle*) *this, here* (< IE. ko- *stem of*

demonstrative pronoun meaning 'this'; Vide cis: *See* E. *he*))

지금   **E** (quid nunc? *'what now?'* > *'a person who constantly asks 'What now?'* >) *quidnunc*

< IE. nu- *now* (*related to* IE. newo- *new*)   **E** *now*

> G. nyn *now*

L. hodie (< hoc die *on this day*) (부사) 오늘

L. cras (부사) 내일

> L. crastinus, crastina, crastinum 내일의

> L. procrastino, **procrastinavi**, procrastinatum, procrastinare (< pro- *before, for, forward, instead of*) 내일로 미루다, 연기하다, 지체하다   **E** *procrastinate*

L. crepusculum, crepusculi, n. 땅거미, 박명(薄明)   **E** *crepuscule, crepuscular*

L. mane, n. (불변화 명사) 아침; (부사) 아침에

G. ēōs, ēous, f. (heōs, heō, f.) *dawn, daybreak, morning, east;* (Ēos) (*Greek mythology*) *goddess of the dawn*   **E** *eo-, Eos*
  < IE. aus- *to shine (said especially of the dawn), gold* (Vide AURUM; *See* E. *aurum*)

L. vesper, vesperi, m. (vesper, vesperis, m.) 저녁, 저녁식사, 서쪽; (Vesper) (천문) 금성, 개밥바라기   **E** *vesper*
  > L. vespertinus, vespertina, vespertinum 저녁의, 저녁에 일어나는   **E** *vespertine*
  < IE. wes-pero- *evening, night*   **E** *west*
    > G. hesperos, hesperou, m. *evening, west*
      > L. Hesperus, Hesperi, m. 금성, 개밥바라기   **E** *Hesperus*
      > G. hesperios, hesperia, hesperion *of the evening, western*
        > L. Hesperia, Hesperiae, f. 서쪽 나라 (그리스에서는 이탈리아를, 이탈리아 에서는 스페인을 가리킴)   **E** *Hesperia*

L. nox, noctis, f. 밤[夜]; (Nox) (로마 신화) 밤의 여신   **E** *nocturia (nycturia)*
  > L. nocturnus, nocturna, nocturnum 밤의, 밤에 일어나는   **E** *nocturn*
    > L. nocturnalis, nocturnale 밤의   **E** *nocturnal*
  > L. aequinoctium, aequinoctii, n. (< aequus *equal* + nox *night*) 주야 평분시(平分時), 춘·추분   **E** *equinox*
  < IE. nek^w^t- *night*   **E** *night*
    > G. nyx, nyktos, f. *night;* (Nyx) (*Greek mythology*) *the goddess of night (daughter of* Chaos*)*   **E** (nyx + alaos *'blind'* + ōps *'eye'* >) *nyctalopia, nycturia (nocturia)*
    > L. niger, nigra, nigrum *black* (Vide NIGER; *See* E. *negro*)

L. ver, veris, n. 봄
    > L. vernalis, vernale 봄의, 청춘의   **E** *vernal, vernalization*
  < IE. wesr- *spring*

L. aestas, aestatis, f. 여름
  < IE. ai- *to burn*   **E** *anneal* (< *'to alter by heating'* < *'to set on fire'*)

> L. aestus, aestus, m. 더위, 끓어오름, 격정, 바다 물결의 출렁댐, 조수(潮水)

    > L. aestivus, aestiva, aestivum 여름의

        > L. aestivalis, aestivale 여름의   **E** *aestival (estival)*

        > L. aestivo, **aestivavi**, aestivatum, aestivare 여름을 지내다, 피서하다, (동물)

            하면(夏眠)하다   **E** *aestivate (estivate)*

            > L. *aestivatio, *aestivationis, f. 여름나기, 하면   **E** *aestivation (estivation)*

    > L. aestuarium, aestuarii, n. 해안에 부딪는 파도, (바닷물이 들락날락하는) 해변

        늪지대, 개펄, 강어귀, 하구(河口), 기수역(汽水域)   **E** *estuary*

> L. Aetna, Aetnae, f. (< *the fiery one*) 에트나 화산   **E** *Etna*

> L. aedes, aedis, f. (< *hearth*) 집, 건물

    > L. aedifico, aedificavi, aedificatum, aedificare (< aedes *dwelling* + -ficare

        (< facĕre) *to make*) 짓다, 건축하다   **E** *edify (< 'to build up morally')*

        > L. aedificium, aedificii, n. 저택, 건축물   **E** *edifice*

> G. aithein *to kindle, to burn, to shine*

    > G. aithēr, aitheros, m., f. *the upper air, clear sky*

        > L. aether, aetheris, m. (acc. aethera) 에테르(대기권을 덮고 있는 상공의

            영기(靈氣), 불로 되어 있으며 천체의 양식으로 생각했음), 천공, 신들의

            거처, 순수한 공기

            E *aether (ether), (ether + -anus 'adjective suffix' >)* **ethane,** *(ethane + -ol >)* **ethanol,** *(ether + -yl >)* **ethyl,** *(ethyl + -ene >)* **ethylene,** *(acid + ether >)* **ester**

        > G. aitherios, aitheria, aitherion *of the upper air, of clear sky*

            > L. aetherius, aetheria, aetherium (aethereus, aetherea, aethereum)

            에테르의, 하늘의, 공기의   **E** *etherial (ethereal)*

L. **autumnus, autumni, m.** 가을   **E** *autumn*

    > L. autumnalis, autumnale 가을의   **E** *autumnal*

  < (*probably*) *Of Etruscan origin*

L. **hiems, hiemis, f.** (hyems, hyemis, f.) 겨울, 한 해, 1년

    > L. hiemalis, hiemale (hyemalis, hyemale) 겨울의   **E** *hiemal*

    > L. hibernus, hiberna, hibernum 겨울의

        > L. hiberno, **hibernavi**, hibernatum, hibernare 겨울나다, 동면(冬眠)하다   **E** *hibernate*

            > L. hibernatio, hibernationis, f. 겨울나기, 동면   **E** *hibernation*

  < IE. ghei- *winter, snow*

    > G. **cheimōn, cheimōnos, m.** *winter*

    > G. chiōn, chionos, f. *snow*   **E** *chion(o)- (chio-)*

    > G. chimaira, chimairas, f. (< *female animal one year (winter) old*) *she-goat; a fire-spouting monster with lion's head, serpent's tail, and goat's body*

        > L. chimaera, chimaerae, f. (chimera, chimerae, f.)

키메라

> (*Sanskrit*) himah *snow*

> (*Sanskrit*) Himalayah (< + alayah *abode* < IE. (s)lei- *slimy* (Vide LAEVIS: *See*

E. *levigate*))

> E chimaera (chimera), chimeric, chimerism

> E Himalayas

꼴의 비교

G. brōmos, brōmou, m. *bad smell, stink*

> E bromidrosis (bromhidrosis), bromopnoea (bromopnea), bromine (Br) (< *'a strong or rank odor'*), bromide(s)

G. brōma, brōmatos, n. *food*

> E bromatology

< IE. g^{w}erə- *to swallow* (Vide GLUTIRE: *See* E. *glut*)

G. hydōr, hydatos, n. *water*

> E hydr(o)- (< *'water or hydrogen'*)

< IE. wed- *water, wet* (Vide UNDA: *See* E. *undulate*)

G. hygros, hygra, hygron *wet*

> E hygr(o)-

< IE. weg^w- *wet* (Vide HUMOR: *See* E. *humor*)

G. hidrōs, hidrōtos, m. *sweat, perspiration*

> E hidr(o)-

< IE. sweid- *sweat, to sweat* (Vide SUDARE: *See* E. *sudation*)

G. lēmma, lēmmatos, n. *premise, assumption*

> E lemma, dilemma, (dilemma >) trilemma

< G. lambanein (lēph- *root*) *to take, to seize, to assume*

< IE. (s)lag^w- *to seize* (Vide LAMBANEIN: *See* E. *dilemma*)

G. lemma, lemmatos, n. *husk*

> E plasmalemma, sarcolemma, oolemma

< G. lepein *to peel off*

< IE. leup-, lep- *to peel off, to break off, to scale* (Vide LIBER: *See* E. *library*)

G. eilēma, eilēmatos, n. *coil,*

covering

> E neurolemma (neurilemma) (< *'by association of* G. lemma *'husk'*)

< G. eilein *to turn, to roll, to squeeze*

< IE. wel- *to turn, to roll; with derivatives referring to curved, enclosing objects*
(Vide VOLVĒRE: *See* E. *volute*)

L. laesio, laesionis, f. 손상, 환부, 병변, 병소(病巢), 병터   **E** *lesion, intralesional*

    < L. laedo, laesi, laesum, laedĕre 치다, 상하게 하다 (Vide LAEDĒRE: *See* E. *lesion*)

L. legio, legionis, f. 군단, 떼   **E** *legion*

    < L. lego, legi, lectum, legĕre 모으다, 뽑다, 읽다

   < IE. leg- *to collect; with derivatives meaning 'to speak'* (Vide LEGĒRE: *See* E. *legion*)

L. regio, regionis, f. (로마 본토 이외의) 통치지역, 지방(地方), 부위   **E** *region*

     > L. regionalis, regionale 지역의, 지방의, 부위의   **E** *regional*

    < L. rego, rexi, rectum, regĕre 올바로 이끌다, 다스리다

   < IE. reg- *to move in a straight line* (Vide REGĒRE: *See* E. *regent*)

L. mens, mentis, f. 정신   **E** *mental*

   < IE. men- *to think* (Vide MEMINISSE: *See* E. *comment*)

L. mentum, menti, n. 턱   **E** *mental, (mental >) submental*

    < IE. men- *to project* (Vide MONS: *See* E. *mount*)

G. oulē, oulēs, f. *scar*   **E** *ul(o)- (ule-), ulectomy, ulegyria*

    < IE. welə- *to strike, to wound* (Vide VULNUS: *See* E. *vulnerary*)

G. oula, oulōn, n. (pl.) ((sing.) oulon, oulou, n.) *gums*   **E** *ul(o)-, ulectomy*

     > G. epoulis, epoulidos, f. (< ep(i)- *upon* + oulon *gum*) *epulis*

      > L. epulis, epulidis, f. 잇몸종, 치은종(齒齦腫)   **E** *epulis, (pl.) epulides*

L. pila, pilae, f. (< *probably a knot of hair*) (가지고 노는) 공, 공 모양의 것

     E *piles (< 'hemorrhoids'), pellet (< 'small ball'), platoon (< 'small detachment of soldiers' < 'small ball')*

     > L. pilula, pilulae, f. (< + -ula *diminutive suffix*) 작은 공, 작고 동그란 열매,
      알약   **E** *pill (< 'small ball')*

   < (*probably*) IE. pilo- *hair* (Vide PILUS: *See* E. *pilus*)

L. pila, pilae, f. 쌓아올린 것, 더미, 덩어리, 방파제,

받침대, 지주, 기둥　　　　　　　　　　　　　　　　**E** *pile* (< *'pillar, pier'*), *pillar, piloti*

　> L. pilo, pilavi, pilatum, pilare 짓누르다, 압축하다, 깊이 박다

　　> L. compilo, compilavi, compilatum, compilare (< com- (< cum) *with, together;*

　　　　intensive + pilare *to press*) 한데 묶어서 가져가다, 탈취하다　**E** *compile, compiler*

　　　　> L. compilatio, compilationis, f. 탈취, 자료 수집, 편집, 편찬, 편집물,

　　　　　편찬물　　　　　　　　　　　　　　　　　　　　**E** *compilation*

L. pilum, pili, n. 공이, 절굿공이, 유봉(乳棒), 말뚝, (로마 보병의) 투창　　**E** *pile* (< *'javelin, stake'*)

　< IE. peis- *to crush*

　　> L. pinso, pinsi (pinsui), pinsum (pinsitum, pistum), pinsĕre 빻다, 찧다, 가루로 만들다,

　　　매질하다

　　　> L. pistillum, pistilli, n. (pistillus, pistilli, m.) 공이, 절굿공이;

　　　　암술　　　　　　　　　　　　　　　　**E** *pestle, pistil,* (*pistil* >) *pistillate*

　　　> L. pisto, pistavi, pistatum, pistare (*frequentative*) 공이질하다　　**E** *piston*

L. pilus, pili, m. 털[毛], 섬모, 털끝만큼의 것

　　E *pilus,* (pl.) *pili, pilin, pile* (< *'hair'*), *piliform, pilomotor* (< *'on the pattern of vasomotor'*),
　　caterpillar (<(*perhaps*) *'hairy cat'*), *pelage* (< *'mammal's fur'*)

　> L. pilaris, pilare 털의　　　　　　　　　　　　　　　　　　　**E** *pilar*

　> L. pilosus, pilosa, pilosum 털이 많은, (부드러운) 털로 뒤덮인　　**E** *pilose*

　> L. pilo, pilavi, pilatum, pilare 털이 나다, 털을 뽑다, 강탈하다　**E** *peel, peeling, pluck*

　　> L. depilo, depilavi, depilatum, depilare (< de- *apart from, down, not*) 털을

　　　제거하다　　　　　　　　　　　　　　　　　　　　　**E** *depilation*

　< IE. pilo- *hair* (Vide PILA; *See* E. *pellet*)

　　> G. pilos, pilou, m. *wool made into felt, felt,*

　　　felt cap　　　　　　　　　**E** *pilocarpine* (< *'felt cap-shaped fruit'*)

　　　> G. pilein *to make wool into felt*

　　　　> G. pilema, pilematos, n. *felt*

　　　　　E ((*probably*) neuropilema >) *neuropil* (< *'feltwork of cytoplasmic processes*
　　　　　of nerve cells and of neuroglial cells')

L. reticulum, reticuli, n. (< + -culum *diminutive suffix*) 작은 그물, 세망(細網); 벌집위(봉소상

　　위 蜂巢狀胃, 반추동물의 제2위)　　　　　　　**E** *reticulum, reticule (reticle)*

　　< L. rete, retis, n. 그물[網]　　　　　　　　　　**E** *rete, retiform*

　< IE. erə- *to separate* (Vide RETE; *See* E. *rete*)

L. retinaculum, retinaculi, n. (< retinēre *to hold back, to retain* + -culum *noun suffix*)

　　　붙들어 매는 끈, 지대(支帶), 지지구(支持鉤)　　　　　　**E** *retinaculum*

　　　< L. retineo, retinui, retentum, retinēre (< re- *back, again* + tenēre *to hold*

붙잡다, 머물러 있게 하다　　　　　　　　　　　　　E *retain, retention, retinue, rein*

　　< L. teneo, **tenui**, tentum, tenēre 잡다, 지키다, 소유하다, 깨닫다

< IE. ten- *to stretch* (Vide TENĒRE: *See* E. *tenet*)

G. **tainia, tainias, f.** *head-band, ribbon, tape*

　　　　> L. taenia, taeniae, f. (tenia, teniae, f.) 머리띠, 띠, 붕대; 촌충(寸蟲),

　　　　　조충(條蟲)　　　　　　　　　E *taenia (tenia), (pl.) taeniae (teniae), -tene*

　　　　　　[용례] taenia coli, (pl.) taeniae coli 결장띠, 잘록창자띠　E *taenia coli, (pl.) taeniae coli*
　　　　　　　　(문법) taenia 띠: 단수 주격
　　　　　　　　　　　taeniae 띠들: 복수 주격
　　　　　　　　　　　coli 결장의, 잘록창자의: 단수 속격 < colon, coli, n.

　　　　　　[용례] Taenia saginata (< *well-fed tapeworm*) 무구조충(無鉤條蟲)　E Taenia saginata
　　　　　　　　　　Taenia solium (< *throned tapeworm, having a scolex with hooks*)
　　　　　　　　　　　유구조충(有鉤條蟲)　　　　　　　　　E Taenia solium
　　　　　　　　(문법) taenia 띠: 단수 주격
　　　　　　　　　　　saginata 살찐: 형용사, 여성형 단수 주격
　　　　　　　　　　　　< saginatus, saginata, saginatum
　　　　　　　　　　　solium 왕좌: 단수 주격, 동격의 꾸밈말로 사용
　　　　　　　　　　　　< solium, solii, n.

　　　　< G. teinein *to stretch*

　　< IE. ten- *to stretch* (Vide TENĒRE: *See* E. *tenet*)

L. **tinea, tineae, f.** 좀, 좀벌레; 버짐, 선(癬), 백선(白癬), 백선증, 피부곰팡이증　　　　E *tinea*

　　　　[용례] tinea capitis 머리백선증, 두부(頭部)백선　　　　　　　E *tinea capitis*
　　　　　　　tinea faciei 얼굴백선증, 얼굴피부곰팡이증, 안면(顔面)백선　　E *tinea faciei*
　　　　　　　tinea barbae 수염백선증, 백선성모창(白癬性毛瘡), 수선(鬚癬)　E *tinea barbae*
　　　　　　　tinea corporis 몸백선증, 몸피부곰팡이증, 체부(體部)백선, 구간(軀幹)백선　E *tinea corporis*
　　　　　　　tinea cruris 샅백선증, 완(頑)백선, 고부(股部)백선　　　　E *tinea cruris*
　　　　　　　tinea manus, tinea manuum 수부(手部)백선　　　E *tinea manus, tinea manuum*
　　　　　　　tinea pedis 발백선증, 발피부곰팡이증, 무좀, 족부(足部)백선　E *tinea pedis*
　　　　　　　tinea unguium (*onychomycosis*) 손발톱백선증, 손발톱피부곰팡이증,
　　　　　　　　조갑(爪甲)백선　　　　　　　　　　　　　E *tinea unguium*
　　　　　　　tinea versicolor (pityriasis versicolor) 어루러기　E *tinea versicolor, pityriasis versicolor*
　　　　　　(문법) tinea 백선증: 단수 주격
　　　　　　　　　capitis 머리의: 단수 속격 < caput, capitis, n.
　　　　　　　　　faciei 얼굴의: 단수 속격 < facies, faciei, f.
　　　　　　　　　barbae 수염의: 단수 속격 < barba, barbae, f.
　　　　　　　　　corporis 몸의: 단수 속격 < corpus, corporis, n.
　　　　　　　　　cruris 샅의: 단수 속격
　　　　　　　　　　< crus, cruris, n. 아랫다리, 다리, 각(脚), 다리 같은 구조, 샅

manus 손의: 단수 속격 < manus, manus, f.

manuum 손들의: 복수 속격 < manus, manus, f.

pedis 발의: 단수 속격 < pes, pedis, m.

unguium 손톱·발톱들의: 복수 속격 < unguis, unguis, m.

pityriasis 잔비늘증, 비강진(粃糠疹): 단수 주격 < pityriasis, pityriasis, f.

versicolor 변색하는, 얼룩덜룩한: 형용사, 남·여·중성형 단수 주격

　　< versicolor, (gen.) versicoloris

L. viscum, visci, n. (viscus, visci, m.) 겨우살이; 겨우살이 열매에서 채취하는

　　새잡이 끈끈이　　　　　　　　　　　**E** *viscid, viscose (viscous), viscosity*

　< IE. weis- *to flow* (Vide VIRUS: *See* E. *virus*)

L. viscus, visceris, n. 내장　　　　　　　　　**E** *viscus, (pl.) viscera*

　> L. visceralis, viscerale 내장의　　　　　　　**E** *visceral*

　> L. eviscero, evisceravi, evisceratum, eviscerare (< e- *out of, away from* + (pl.) viscera

　　internal organs) 내장을 들어내다　　　　　　**E** *eviscerate*

본디 영어 낱말과 라틴어·그리스어 기원의 영어 낱말 비교

　　하나의 인도·유럽어 말뿌리에서 비롯된 동족어 무리 낱말들은 한군데로 모아
지나, 말뿌리가 다른 낱말들은 흩어진다. 이 부분에서는 말뿌리는 다르나 뜻이
같아 사용상 무리를 이루는 본디 영어 낱말과, 그에 대응하는 라틴어 및 그리스
어 기원의 영어 낱말들을 모아 놓았다. 본디 영어 낱말이 없는 경우에는 본디
낱말처럼 사용되는 차용어를 제시하였다.

E. *health*　　　　　　　　　　　　　　　　　**E** *health, healthy*

　< IE. kailo- *whole, uninjured, of good omen*

　　E *whole, wholesome, unwholesome, hale, hail, heal, holy, holiday, hallow, (All-Hallow-Even*
　　'Eve of All Saints' >) Halloween

L. sanitas, sanitatis, f. 건강　　　　　　　　　　**E** *sanity*

　> L. *sanitarius, *sanitaria, *sanitarium 건강의, 위생의 **E** *sanitary, (sanitary >) sanitation*

　　> L. sanitarium, sanitarii, n. 요양소　　　**E** *sanitarium (sanatorium)*

< L. sanus, sana, sanum 건강한, 건전한, 제정신의　　　　　　　　　　`E sane`

    > L. sano, **sanavi**, sanatum, sanare 건강해지게 하다　　　　`E sanative`

        > L. sanatorius, sanatoria, sanatorium 요양의　　　　`E sanatory`

            > L. sanatorium, sanatorii, n. 요양소　　`E sanatorium (sanitarium)`

        > L. insanus, insana, insanum (< in- *not*) 정신이상의　　`E insane`

            > L. insanitas, insanitatis, f. 정신이상　　　`E insanity`

G. **hygieia, hygieias, f.** (hygeia, hygeias, f.) *health, soundness of body;* (Hygieia) (*Greek mythology*) *goddess of health, daughter of Asclepius*　　`E Hygeia (Hygieia)`

    < G. hygiēs, hygiēs, hygies (< + IE. gʷeiə-, gʷei- *to live*) *healthy*

        > G. hygieinos, hygieinē, hygieinon *healthful*　`E hygiene, hygienic, hygienics`

  < IE. aiw-, ayu- *vital force, life, long life, eternity; also endowed with the acme of vital force, young* (Vide JUVENIS; *See* E. *juvenile*)

    > (*Sanskrit*) ayuh *life, health*

        > (*Sanskrit*) Ayurveda (< + veda *knowledge, sacred knowledge, sacred book*) *the traditional Hindu system of medicine*　　`E Ayurveda`

E. *body*　　　　　　　　　　　　　　　　　　`E body`

L. **corpus, corporis,** n. 몸, 체(體), 몸통, 전집(全集)　`E corpus, corps, corpse, corsage, corset`

    [용례] corpus spongiosum 요도해면체(尿道海綿體)　　`E corpus spongiosum`

    (문법) corpus 체(體): 단수 주격

        spongiosum 해면 같은, 구멍이 숭굴숭굴한: 형용사, 중성형 단수 주격

            < spongiosus, spongiosa, spongiosum

    [용례] corpora cavernosa (pl.) 해면체(海綿體)　　`E (pl.) corpora cavernosa`

    (문법) corpora 체(體): 복수 주격

        cavernosa 굴이 많은, 움푹하게 파인: 형용사, 중성형 복수 주격

            < cavernosus, cavernosa, cavernosum

  > L. corpusculum, corpusculi, n. (< + -culum *diminutive suffix*) (인간의 보잘 것 없는) 육체, 소체(小體), 미립자　　`E corpuscle (corpuscule), corpuscular`

  > L. corporalis, corporale (인간의) 몸의, 몸통의　　`E corporal`

  > L. corporeus, corporea, corporeum (영혼에 대한) 육체의, 물질적인, 형체가 있는　　`E corporeal; extracorporeal`

  > L. corpulentus, corpulenta, corpulentum (병적으로) 살찐　`E corpulent`

  > L. corporo, **corporavi**, corporatum, corporare 육체를 갖추게 하다, 형체를 만들다, 가입시키다　　`E corporate`

    > L. corporatio, corporationis, f. 조합, 단체　　`E corporation`

    > L. incorporo, **incorporavi**, incorporatum, incorporare (< in- *in, on, into, toward* + corporare *to form into a body*) 육체를 갖추게 하다, 가입시키다, 합체하다, 합일화하다, 결합시키다　　`E incorporate`

> L. incorporatio, incorporationis, f. 합체, 합일화, 결합, 융합, 통합,
편입　　　　　　　　　　　　　　　　　　　　　　　　**E** *incorporation*
< IE. kʷrep- *body, form, appearance*　　　　　　　　**E** *midriff* (< 'mid-belly')

G. sōma, sōmatos, n. *body*
> L. soma, somatis, n. 몸, 체(體), 신체(身體), 몸통, 구간(軀幹), 체간(體幹),
세포체(細胞體)　　　　　　　　　　　　　　　　**E** *soma,* (pl.) *somata*
< IE. teuə-, teu- *to swell* (Vide TUMOR; *See* E. *tumor*)

E. *vertebra,* (pl.) *vertebrae* (Vide infra)

L. vertebra, vertebrae, f. (< *the hinge of the body*< + -bra *instrumental suffix*) 등마루뼈,
척추(脊椎)뼈, 추골(椎骨)　　　　　　　　　　　　**E** *vertebra,* (pl.) *vertebrae*
< L. verto, verti, versum, vertĕre 돌리다, 돌다, 바꾸다
< IE. wer- *to turn* (Vide VERTĔRE; *See* E. *verse*)

G. spondylos, spondylou, m. *vertebra*

> **E** *spondyl(o)-,* (+ -itis > 'inflammation of the vertebra' >) *spondylitis,* (+ -olisthesis >
'dislocation of the vertebra' >) *spondylolisthesis,* (+ -cace (< G. kakē 'badness' < G.
kakos 'bad') > 'tuberculosis of the vertebra' >) *spondylocace*

< IE. sp(h)e(n)d- *to jerk, to dangle*

E. *backbone*　　　　　　　　　　　　　　　　　　　　　**E** *backbone*

L. spina, spinae, f. 가시, 등마루(척추 脊椎, 척주 脊柱)　　　**E** *spine, spiny*
> L. spinosus, spinosa, spinosum 가시 많은, 가시의, 뾰족한, 까다로운　　**E** *spinous*
> L. spinalis, spinale 등마루의, 척추의; 척수(脊髓)의　　　　　　**E** *spinal*
< IE. spei- *sharp point* (Vide SPINA; *See* E. *spine*)

G. rhachis, rhacheōs, f. *backbone*

> **E** *rhachi(o)-,* (rhachi(o)- > (modified) >) *rachi(o)-,* (+ -schisis > 'congenital fissure of the
backbone' >) *rachischisis,* (+ -itis > 'inflammatory disease of the vertebral column' >)
rachitis, (rachitis > 'disorder due to impaired mineralization of bone matrix in children,
mostly by vitamin D deficiency' >) *rickets, antirachitic* (< 'against rickets')

< IE. wragh- *thorn, point*

E. *rib* (< *covering of the chest cavity*)　　　　**E** *rib, spareribs* (< 'ribs on a spear')
< IE. rebh- *to roof over*　　　　　　　　　　　　　　　　　　　**E** *reef*

L. costa, costae, f. 갈비, 늑골(肋骨), 엽맥(葉脈), 옆구리
    > L. costalis, costale 갈비의, 갈비뼈의, 늑골의
  < IE. kost- **bone** (Vide COSTA: *See* E. *coast*)

E *coast*
E *costal*

G. pleura, pleuras, f. *rib, side, flank*
    > L. pleura, pleurae, f. 가슴막, 흉막(胸膜), 늑막(肋膜)
      > L. pleuralis, pleurale 가슴막의, 흉막의, 늑막의
  < (*suggested*) IE. plat- (pletə-) *to be flat, to spread* (Vide PLEURA: *See* E. *pleura*)

E *pleura*
E *pleural*

E. *cartilage*
    < L. cartilago, cartilaginis, f. 연골 (Vide infra)

L. cartilago, cartilaginis, f. 연골
    > L. cartilaginosus, cartilaginosa, cartilaginosum 연골이 많은, 연골질의
  < IE. kert- *to entwine*
    > L. cratis, cratis, f. 발[簾], 격자, 난간, 고리짝, 나뭇단,
      적쇠
      > L. craticula, craticulae, f. (< + -cula *diminutive suffix*) 적쇠; 눈금
    > L. crassus, crassa, crassum 두터운, 투박한, 살찐, 우둔한
      > L. crassitudo, crassitudinis, f. 두터움, 투박, 우둔
      > L. crassula, crassulae, f. (< + -ula *diminutive suffix*) (다육식물) 돌나무속(屬)
      식물
        > L. Crassulaceae, Crassulacearum, f. (pl.) (< + -aceae *a suffix for*
        taxonomic family) 돌나무과(科) 식물

E *cartilage*
E *cartilaginous*
E *hurdle* (< '*wickerwork frame, frame*')
E *crate, grate, grating, gridiron,* (*gridiron* >) *grid, grill*
E *graticule*
E *crass, grease*
E *crassitude*
E *crassula*
E Crassulaceae, *crassulacean*

G. chondros, chondrou, m. *grain, lump, cartilage*

> E *chondr(o)-, chondral, chondroid, chondroblast, chondrocyte, chondroclast,* (*chondr(o)-* + -ite (< G. -itēs '*adjective suffix*') + -in > '*a sulfated glycosaminoglycan isolated from cartilage*') >) *chondroitin sulfate*

  > G. chondrion, chondriou, n. (< + -ion *diminutive suffix*) *granule*
    > G. mitochondrion, mitochondriou, n. (< mitos *thread*) *mitochondrion*
      > L. mitochondrion, mitochondrii, n. 사립체(絲粒體),
      미토콘드리아
  > G. chondrios, chondria, chondrion *of cartilage*
    > G. (*neuter* sing.) hypochondrion, hypochondriou, n. (< hyp(o)- *under*)
    hypochondrium
      > L. hypochondrium, hypochondrii, n. 갈비아래부위, 늑하부(肋下部),
      계륵부(季肋部)
    > G. (*neuter* pl.) hypochondria, hypochondriōn, n. *those parts of the*

E *chondri(o)-*
E *mitochondrion,* (pl.) *mitochondria, mitochondrial*
E *hypochondrium, hypochondriac*

human abdomen which lie immediately under the ribs and on each side of the epigastric region; the viscera (the liver, gall-bladder, spleen, etc.) situated in the hypochondria formerly supposed to be the seat of melancholy and 'vapors'

> L. hypochondria, hypochondriae, f. 건강염려증, 심기증(心氣症)

> E *hypochondria (hypochondriasis), hypochondriac, hypochondriacal, (hypochondria >) hypochondriasis (hypochondria)*

> L. perichondrium, perichondrii, n. (< *on the pattern of* periosteum < G. peri- *around, near, beyond, on account of*)

연골막(軟骨膜)

E *perichondrium, perichondrial*

< (*suggested*) IE. ghrendh- *to grind*

E *grind, gristle*

< IE. gher- *to scrape, to scratch* (Vide CHROMA; *See* E. *chromatic*)

E. *flesh* (< *piece of meat torn off*)

E *flesh*

< (*perhaps*) IE. ple-(i)k-, plek- *to tear*

E *flay (< 'to strip the skin from'), fleck (< 'piece of skin or flesh, spot, stain')*

L. caro, carnis, f. (< *piece of meat*) 고기, 살, 육신

E *carnal*

< IE. (s)ker- *to cut* (Vide SECARE; *See* E. *secant*)

G. sarx, sarkos, f. (< *piece of meat*) *flesh*

E *sarcophagus (< 'a kind of stone reputed among the Greeks to have the property of consuming the flesh of dead bodies deposited in it, and consequently used for coffins'), sarcoplasm, sarcoplasmic, sarcolemma, sarcomere (< 'the contractile unit of myofibrils in striated muscle'), sarcopenia (< 'flesh deficiency')*

> G. sarkazein *to tear flesh, to gnash the teeth, to speak bitterly*

E *sarcastic*

> G. sarkasmos, sarkasmou, m. *a sharp, bitter, or cutting expression or remark; a bitter gibe or taunt*

> L. sarcasmus, sarcasmi, m. 비꼼, 빈정댐, 야유, 풍자

E *sarcasm*

> G. sarkōma, sarkōmatos, n. (< + -ōma *noun suffix denoting tumor*) sarcoma

> L. sarcoma, sarcomatis, n. 육종(肉腫)

E *sarcoma, (pl.) sarcomata (sarcomas), sarcomatous, sarcoid (< 'sarcoma-like')*

> G. sarcoidēs, sarcoidēs, sarcoides, (< + eidos *shape*) *flesh-like*

> L. sarcoidosis, sarcoidosis, f. (< + G. -ōsis *condition*)

사르코이드증

E *sarcoidosis, sarcoid (< 'sarcoidosis')*

> L. Sarcoptes, Sarcoptis, f. (< G. sarx, sarkos, f. *flesh* + koptein *to strike, to cut off*) (진드기) 옴진드기속(屬)

E Sarcoptes, *sarcoptic*

> L. anasarca, anasarcae, f. (< *excessive flesh, figuratively* < G. an(a)- *up, upward; again, throughout; back, backward; against; according to, similar*

to + sarx) 전신부종   **E** *anasarca*

< IE. twerk- *to cut*

G. kreas, kreōs, n. (< *raw flesh*) *flesh,*

    meat   **E** *creatine* (< *'discovered first in the juice of flesh'*), *(creatine* >) *creatinine*

< IE. kreuǝ- *raw flesh* (Vide CRUDUS: *See* E. *crude*)

E. *skin*   **E** *skin*

    < IE. sek- *to cut* (Vide SECARE: *See* E. *secant*)

L. integumentum, integumemti, n. 덮개, 옷, 피부   **E** *integument, integumentary*

    < IE. (s)teg- *to cover* (Vide TEGĚRE: *See* E. *tectum*)

L. cutis, cutis, f. 껍질, 가죽, 살갗, 피부   **E** *cutin,* (per cutem *'through the skin'* >) *percutaneous*

    > L. cuticula, cuticulae, f. (< cutis *skin* + -cula *diminutive suffix*) 표피,

       겉껍질   **E** *cuticula (cuticle), cuticular*

    > L. cutaneus, cutanea, cutaneum 피부의   **E** *cutaneous*

    > L. subcutis, subcutis, f. (< sub- *under, up from under* + cutis *skin*) 피하, 피하조직

       > L. subcutaneus, subcutanea, subcutaneum 피하의, 피부 밑의   **E** *subcutaneous*

   < IE. (s)keu- *to cover,*

     to conceal   **E** *sky* (< *'cloud'*), *scum, skimmer, (skimmer* >) *skim, hide, hoard, huddle, hut, hose*

    > L. obscurus, obscura, obscurum (< L. ob- *before, toward(s), over, against, away* +

       IE. (s)keu-) 어두운, 희미한, 분명하지 않은

       E *obscure,* (clarus + obscurus *'clear and obscure'* > *'of light and shade'* >) It. *chiaroscuro*

       > L. obscuritas, obscuritatis, f. 어둠, 애매, 무명   **E** *obscurity*

    > L. custos, custodis, m., f. 경비원, 수호자   **E** *custody, custodian*

    > L. cunnus, cunni, m. (< *vulva* < *sheath*) 여자의 음부, 여자

       > L. cunnilingus, cunnilingi, m. (< lingĕre *to lick*) 외음핥기   **E** *cunnilingus*

    > L. culus, culi, m. 엉덩이, 항문,

       뒤쪽   **E** *recoil* (< *'back again'*), F. *cul-de-sac* (< *'bottom of a sac'*)

    > (*probably*) L. cucullus, cuculli, m. (cuculla, cucullae, f.) (외투나 망토에 달린) 두건,

       고깔   **E** *cucullate, cowl*

    > G. kytos, kytous, n. *hollow vessel, urn; skin; shield, cuirass*

       E *cyt(o)-, -cyte, -cytic, cytology, cytosine (C)* (< *'obtained by hydrolysis of cellular nucleic acids'*), *cytidine (C)*

       > L. syncytium, syncytii, n. (< G. syn- *with, together*) 융합체,

         합포체(合胞體)   **E** *syncytium,* (pl.) *syncytia, syncytial*

       > L. -cytosis, -cytosis, f. (< G. kytos + -ōsis *condition*) 세포의 상태를 가리키는

         합성어 성분   **E** *-cytosis, endocytosis, exocytosis*

L. corium, corii, n. (< *piece of hide*) (짐승의) 가죽, 가죽 갑옷, 모피, 껍질, 진피(眞皮)　**E** *corium (dermis)*

      < IE. (s)ker- *to cut*

   < IE. sek- *to cut* (Vide SECARE: *See* E. *secant*)

L. pellis, pellis, f. (양·여우·밍크·족제비 등 모피로 쓰이는 동물의 무두질하지 않은) 날가죽,
    모피, 피부　**E** *peltry, (peltry >) pelt*

    > L. pellicula, pelliculae, f. (< + -cula *diminutive suffix*) 얇은 가죽, (지방막·균막
       등 액체 표면의) 박막(薄膜), 더껑이　**E** *pellicle*

    > It. pellagra (< *skin disease (dermatitis due to niacin deficiency)* < L. pellis *skin*
       + G. agra *seizing*) 펠라그라　**E** *pellagra*

  < IE. pel- *skin, hide*　**E** *fell, film*

    > G. pella, peltēs, f. *skin*

      > (*suggested*) G. erysipelas, erysipelatos, n. (< *erysis *reddening* + pella *skin*)
        erysipelas

        > L. erysipelas, erysipelatis, n. 단독(丹毒), 얕은연조직염(軟組織炎)　**E** *erysipelas*

    > G. peltē, peltēs, f. *light shield made of hide*

      > L. pelta, peltae, f. 작은 방패, 반달 모양의 방패

        > L. peltatus, peltata, peltatum 작은 방패로 무장한　**E** *peltate*

G. derma, dermatos, n. *skin, hide*

      > L. derma, dermatis, n. 피부(皮膚)

        E *dermic (dermal)* (< *'of skin'*), *intradermal, dermat(o)- (derm(o)-, derma-),
        dermatology, dermatan sulfate* (< *'a sulfated glycosaminoglycan isolated from
        the skin'*), *dermatome, dermoid; -derm* (< *'skin or germ layer'*), *blastoderm,
        ectoderm, mesoderm, endoderm (entoderm), neuroectoderm*

        > L. erythroderma, erythrodermatis, n. (< G. erythros *red* + derma) 홍색
         피부증　**E** *erythroderma*

        > L. pachyderma, pachydermatis, n. (< G. pachys *thick* + derma) 경피증
         (硬皮症), 피부비후증　**E** *pachyderma*

        > L. poikiloderma, poikilodermatis, n. (< *skin of mottled pigmentation*
         < G. poikilos *variegated* + derma) 다형(多形)피부증　**E** *poikiloderma*

        > L. xeroderma, xerodermatis, n. (< G. xēros *dry* + derma) 건피증
         (乾皮症)　**E** *xeroderma*

          [용례] xeroderma pigmentosum 색소성 건피증　**E** *xeroderma pigmentosum*
            (문법) xeroderma: 단수 주격
              pigmentosum 색깔이 많은 (< 색소가 많은):
                 형용사, 중성형 단수 주격
               < pigmentosus, pigmentosa, pigmentosum

       > L. epidermis, epidermidis, f. (< G. ep(i)- *upon* + derma)
        표피(表皮), 상피(上皮)　**E** *epidermis, epidermic (epidermal), epidermoid*

> L. dermis, dermis, f. 진피(眞皮)　　　**E** *dermis (corium), dermic (dermal)* (< *'of dermis'*)

> L. hypodermis, hypodermis, f. (< G. hyp(o)- *under* + derma)

피하조직(皮下組織), 피부밑조직　　　**E** *hypodermis, hypodermic (hypodermal)*

< G. derein *to flay*

> G. dartos, dartē, darton *flayed*

> L. dartos, darti, m. (< *the layer of connective and smooth muscle tissues immediately beneath the skin of the scrotum*) 음낭근

(陰囊筋, musculus dartos), 음낭막(陰囊膜, tunica dartos)　　　**E** *dartos*

< IE. der- *to split, to peel, to flay; with derivatives referring to skin and leather*

E *tear* (< *'to split'*), *tart* (< *'sharp, severe'*), *(suggested)* *trend* (< *'to turn in a specified direction'* < *'split-off piece of a tree trunk, as a disk or wheel'*)

> (*possibly*) IE. drop- *cloth*

> L. drappus, drappi, m. 옷　　　**E** *drape, drapery*

E. *hair*

E *hair*

< (*possibly*) IE. ker(s)- *to bristle*

L. pilus, pili, m. 털[毛], 섬모, 털끝만큼의 것

E *pilus*, (pl.) *pili, pile* (< *'hair'*), *piliform, pilomotor* (< *'on the pattern of vasomotor'*), *caterpillar* (< *(perhaps) 'hairy cat'*), *pelage* (< *'mammal's fur'*)

[용례] arrector pili, (pl.) arrectores pilorum 털세움근　　　**E** *arrector pili*, (pl.) *arrectores pilorum*

(문법) arrector 세움근: 단수 주격 < arrector, arrectoris, m.

< arrigo, arrexi, arrectum, arrigĕre 일으켜 세우다

pili 털의: 단수 속격

arrectores 세움근들: 복수 주격

pilorum 털들의: 복수 속격

> L. pilaris, pilare 털의　　　**E** *pilar*

> L. pilosus, pilosa, pilosum 털이 많은, (부드러운) 털로 뒤덮인　　　**E** *pilose*

> L. pilo, pilavi, pilatum, pilare 털이 나다, 털을 뽑다, 강탈하다　　　**E** *peel, peeling*

> L. depilo, depilavi, depilatum, depilare (< de- *apart from, down, not*) 털을

제거하다　　　**E** *depilation*

< IE. pilo- *hair*

> G. pilos, pilou, m. *wool made into felt, felt, felt cap*

E *pilocarpine* (< *'felt cap-shaped fruit'*)

> G. pilein *to make wool into felt*

> G. pilema, pilematos, n. *felt*

E (*(probably) neuropilema* >) *neuropil* (< *'feltwork of cytoplasmic processes of nerve cells and of neuroglial cells'*)

> L. pileus, pilei, m. (주로 양털을 축융(縮絨)하여 만든 고깔 모양의) 모전(毛氈) 모자,

(버섯·해파리의) 갓　　　　　　　　　　　　　　　　　　**E** *pileus*

> (*probably*) L. pila, pilae, f. (< *probably a knot of hair*) (가지고 노는) 공, 공 모양의 것

　　　E *piles* (< '*hemorrhoids*'), *pellet* (< '*small ball*'), *platoon* (< '*small detachment of soldiers*' < '*small ball*')

　　> L. pilula, pilulae, f. (< + -ula *diminutive suffix*) 작은 공, 작고 동그란 열매;

　　　알약　　　　　　　　　　　　　　　　　　　**E** *pill* (< '*small ball*')

L. capillus, capilli, m.

　　머리털　　**E** (dis- '*apart from, down, not*' + capillus '*hair*' > '*disordered hair*' >) *disheveled*

　> L. capillaris, capillare 머리털의, 머리털 같은; 모세관의,

　　　모세혈관의　　　　　　　　　　　　**E** *capillary*, (*capillary* >) *capillarity*

　　　> L. choriocapillaris, choriocapillare (< chorion *fetal membrane; highly vascularized tissue*) 맥락막 모세혈관의

　　　　[용례] lamina choriocapillaris 맥락막

　　　　　모세혈관층　　　　　　　　**E** *lamina choriocapillaris (choriocapillaris)*

　　　　　(문법) lamina 층: 단수 주격 < lamina, laminae, f. 판, 층

　　　　　choriocapillaris: 형용사, 남·여성형 단수 주격

　　< (*suggested*) L. caput, capitis, n. 머리

　< IE. kaput- *head* (Vide CAPUT: *See* E. *cape*)

L. villus, villi, m. 털 묶음, 양의 긴 털, 융모(絨毛)　**E** *villus*, (pl.) *villi, velvet*, (*Portuguese*) *veludo*

　> L. villosus, villosa, villosum 융모가 많은, 융모로 뒤덮인　　**E** *villose (villous)*

　> L. microvillus, microvilli, m. (< G. mikros *small, little, short*) 미세

　　융모　　　　　　　　　　　　　**E** *microvillus*, (pl.) *microvilli, microvillous*

< IE. wel- *to tear, to pull*

　> L. vello, velli (vulsi), vulsum, vellĕre 잡아 빼다, 잡아 뽑다

　　> L. avello, avelli (avulsi), avulsum, avellĕre (< a- (< ab) *off, away from* + vellĕre *to pluck*) 찢어내다, 빼내다　　　　　　　　　**E** *avulsive*

　　　> L. avulsio, avulsionis, f. 찢김, 견열(牽裂)　　　　　**E** *avulsion*

　　> L. convello, convelli (convulsi), convulsum, convellĕre (< com- (< cum) *with, together; intensive* + vellĕre *to pluck*) 뽑다, (여기저기를 격렬하게) 잡아 당기다, (심하고 급하게) 비틀다

　　　　E *convulse, convulsive;* (*French present participle* >) *convulsant, anticonvulsant*

　　　> L. convulsio, convulsionis, f. 경련(痙攣), 발작(發作)　　**E** *convulsion*

　　> L. revello, revelli (revulsi), revulsum, revellĕre (< re- *back, again* + vellĕre *to pluck*) 뽑아내다,

　　　제거하다　　　**E** †*revulse, revulsive;* (*French present participle* >) *revulsant*

　　　> L. revulsio, revulsionis, f. 심한 반동, 급변, 회수, 유도요법　　**E** *revulsion*

　> (*probably*) L. vultur, vulturis, m. 독수리, 매, 난폭한 자　　**E** *vulture*

∞ (*probably*) IE. welǝ- *wool* (Vide VELLUS: *See* E. *vellus*)

∞ (*probably*) IE. welə- *to strike, to wound* (Vide VULNUS; *See* E. *vulnerary*)

G. thrix, trichos, f. *hair, wool, bristle*　　　　　**E** *trich(o)-, -thrix, -trichous,* (*perhaps*) *tress*

　　> G. trichoun (trichoein) *to cover with hair;* (*passive*) *to be hairy*

　　　　> G. trichōsis, trichōseōs, f. (< + -ōsis *condition*) *growth of hair*

　　　　　　> L. trichosis, trichosis, f. 모발발육이상

　　　　　　E *trichosis, -trichosis, hypertrichosis, hypotrichosis, atrichosis* (*atrichia*)

　　> G. trichian (trichiaein) *to be hairy*

　　　　> G. trichiasis, trichiaseōs, f. (< + -iasis *suffering from*) *trichiasis*

　　　　　　> L. trichiasis, trichiasis, f. 첩모난생(睫毛亂生, *a condition of ingrowing*

　　　　　　　　hairs about an orifice, or ingrowing eyelashes); 모섬유뇨(毛纖維尿,

　　　　　　　　the appearance of hairlike filaments in the urine)　　**E** *trichiasis*

　　> L. -trichia, -trichiae, f. (< G. -ia *noun suffix*) ~모증(~毛症), 모~(毛~)

　　　　> L. atrichia, atrichiae, f. (< G. a- *not*) 무모증(無毛症)　　**E** *atrichia* (*atrichosis*)

　　> L. monilethrix, moniletrichis, f. (< L. monile *necklace*) 염주털(증),

　　　　연주모증(連珠毛症)　　**E** *monilethrix*

　　> G. trichinos, trichinē, trichinon *of hair*

　　　　> L. Trichina, Trichinae, f. (모충 毛蟲) 트리키나속(屬)

　　　　　　(트리키넬라속)　　**E** *Trichina* (*Trichinella*), *trichinosis* (*trichinellosis*)

　　　　　　> L. Trichinella, Trichinellae, f. (< + -ella *diminutive suffix*) (모충 毛蟲)

　　　　　　　　트리키넬라속(屬) (트리키나속)　**E** *Trichinella* (*Trichina*), *trichinellosis* (*trichinosis*)

　　　　　　　　[용례] Trichinella spiralis 선모충(旋毛蟲)　　**E** *Trichinella spiralis*

　　　　　　　　(문법) trichinella 모충: 단수 주격

　　　　　　　　　　spiralis 나선형의: 형용사, 남·여성형 단수 주격

　　　　　　　　　　　　< spiralis, spirale

　　　　> L. Trichomonas, Trichomonadis, f. (< + G. monas *unit*) (편모충 鞭毛蟲)

　　　　　　트리코모나스속(屬)　　**E** *Trichomonas, trichomoniasis*

　　　　> L. Trichuris, Trichuridis, f. (< + G. oura *tail*) (선충 線蟲) 편충속(鞭蟲屬),

　　　　　　트리쿠리스속(屬)　　**E** *Trichuris, trichuriasis*

　　　　> L. Trichophyton, Trichophyti, n. (< *hair-plant which luxuriates on the beard* <

　　　　　　+ G. phyton *plant*) (불완전 진균) 백선균속(白癬菌屬)　**E** *Trichophyton, trichophyte*

　　< (*suggested*) IE. dhrigh-, dhreikh- *hair, bristle*

G. komē, komēs, f. *hair of the head, foliage*

　　> L. coma, comae, f. 머리채, (동물의) 갈기, (식물) 더부룩이 우거진 잎, 빗살　　**E** *coma*

　　　　> L. comatus, comata, comatum 머리숱 많은, 털 많은, 잎이 우거진　　**E** *comate*

　　　　> L. comosus, comosa, comosum 머리숱 많은, 털 많은, 잎이 우거진　　**E** *comose*

　　> G. komētēs, komētou, m. *long-haired one, comet*

　　　　> L. cometes, cometae, m. (cometa, cometae, m.) 혜성, 꼬리별　　**E** *comet*

G. chaitē, chaitēs, f. *long hair, mane*

> L. Spirochaeta, Spirochaetae, f. (< G. speira *winding, coil, spire*)

(세균) 스피로키타속(屬)　　　　| **E** Spirochaeta, *spirochaete (spirochete), spirochetal* |

< (*suggested*) IE. ghait-, ghait-s- *long hair*

E. *wool*

< IE. welə- *wool* (Vide infra)

L. vellus, velleris, n. 털가죽, 모피, 양털송이; 솜털, 연모(軟毛)　　| **E** *vellus* |

< IE. welə- *wool*　　| **E** *wool, flannel* |

> L. lana, lanae, f. 양털, (동물의) 털, 모직물, (식물의) 솜털, 새털구름

| **E** (lana *'wool'* + oleum *'oil'* + -in > *'extracted from sheep's wool'* >) *lanolin*, (lana *'wool'* + sterol > *'a sterol present in wool fat'* >) *lanosterol* |

> L. lanatus, lanata, lanatum 털로 덮인　　| **E** *lanate* |

> L. lanosus, lanosa, lanosum 털이 많은　　| **E** *lanose* |

> L. lanifer, lanifera, laniferum (< lana *wool* + -fer (< ferre *to carry, to bear*)

carrying, *bearing*) 털이 나는　　| **E** *laniferous* |

> L. lanugo, lanuginis, f. (동식물의) 솜털, 배냇솜털　　| **E** *lanugo* |

> (*possibly*) G. oulos, oulē, oulon *woolly, curly, matted*　　| **E** *ulotrichous* |

∽ (*probably*) IE. wel- *to tear, to pull* (Vide VILLUS: *See* E. *villus*)

∽ (*probably*) IE. welə- *to strike, to wound* (Vide VULNUS: *See* E. *vulnerary*)

G. erion, eriou, n. (eirion, eiriou, n.) *wool*　　| **E** *eri(o)-* |

E. *eyelid*　　| **E** *eyelid* |

< IE. ok^w- *to see* (Vide OCULUS: *See* E. *oculus*)

+ IE. klei- *to lean* (Vide CLINARE: *See* E. *decline*)

L. palpebra, palpebrae, f. (< *that which shakes or moves quickly*) 눈꺼풀,

안검(眼瞼)　　| **E** *palpebra, (pl.) palpebrae* |

< L. palpo, palpavi, palpatum, palpare 어루만지다, 쓰다듬다, 다독거리다

< IE. pal- *to touch, to feel, to shake* (Vide PALPARE: *See* E. *palpate*)

G. blepharon, blepharou, n. *eyelid*

| **E** *blephar(o)-* (< *'eyelid or cilium/flagellum'*); *blepharal, blepharoplasty* (< *'plastic surgery of the eyelids'*), *blepharospasm, blepharoptosis, blepharophimosis; blepharoplast* (< *'basal body forming cilium/flagellum'*) |

> L. symblepharon, symblephari, n. (< *an adhesion between the tarsal conjunctiva*

and the bulbar conjunctiva < G. sym- (< syn) *with, together*) 결막붙음증, 검구
유착(瞼球癒着)
E *symblepharon*

E. *pupil* (Vide infra)

　　< L. pupilla, pupillae, f. 어린 소녀, 작은 인형; 동공(瞳孔)

L. pupilla, pupillae, f. (< + -illa *diminutive suffix*) (< *on account of the small reflected
　　image seen when looking into someone's pupil*) 어린 소녀, 작은 인형;
　　동공(瞳孔)
E *pupil*, (pupilla >) *pupillary*

　　　　< L. pupa, pupae, f. 소녀, 인형; 번데기,
　　　　　용(蛹)
E *pupa*, (pupa >) *pupal*, (pupa >) *pupate, puppy, puppet*

　　< (*possibly*) IE. pau-, pou- *little, few* (Vide PUER: *See* E. *puerile*)

　　or (*possibly*) IE. pu-, phu- *to blow, to swell; echoic of blowing out cheeks, puffing*
　　　　(Vide PUSTULA: *See* E. *pustule*)

　　　　　> L. pupus, pupi, m. 소년

　　　　　　　> L. pupillus, pupilli, m. (< + -illus *diminutive suffix*) 어린 소년
E *pupil*

G. korē, korēs, f. (kourē, kourēs, f.) *girl, daughter, doll; pupil (of eyeball)*

　　　> L. isocoria, isocoriae, f. (< G. isos *equal* + korē *pupil* + -ia *noun suffix*) 양안동공
　　　동등
E *isocoria*

　　　　> L. anisocoria, anisocoriae, f. (< G. anisos *unequal* < an- *not* + isos *equal*)
　　　　　동공부등
E *anisocoria*

　　　　> L. *leukocoria, *leukocoriae, f. (*leukokoria, *leukokoriae, f.) (< G. leukos *white* +
　　　　　korē *pupil* + -ia *noun suffix*) 백색동공
E *leukocoria (leukokoria)*

　　< IE. ker- *to grow* (Vide CRESCĒRE: *See* E. *crescent*)

　　　　> G. koros, korou, m. (kouros, kourou, m.) *boy, son*

E. *nose*

　　< IE. nas- *nose* (Vide infra)

L. nasus, nasi, m. 코

E *nas(o)-, nasopharynx, nasogastric, nasolacrimal, nasolabial*, F. *pince-nez* (< 'pinch-nose')

　　> L. nasalis, nasale 코의

E *nasal; paranasal* (< 'located beside the nose; specifically, of the sinuses situated
　　beside the nose')

　　> L. nasion, nasii, n. (< + G. -ion *diminutive suffix*) 코뿌리점, 비근점(鼻根點)　　**E** *nasion*

< IE. nas- *nose*　　**E** *nose, nozzle, nostril* (< 'nose hole' < 'boring through the nose')

　　> L. naris, naris, f. 콧구멍
E *naris*, (pl.) *nares*

G. rhis, rhinos, f. *nose,* (pl.) *nostrils*

> **E** *rhin(o)-, rhinoceros, rhinology, rhinovirus, rhinal, entorhinal* (< *'interior to the rhinal sulcus'*)

< (*suggested*) IE. ser- *to stream* (Vide SERUM: *See* E. *serum*)

E. *mouth*   **E** *mouth*

< IE. men- *to project* (Vide MONS: *See* E. *mount*)

L. os, oris, n. 입[口]

> **E** (per os *'by way of the mouth'* >) **peroral,** (ad os *'to the mouth'* >) **adoral,** (ab + *oral 'away from the mouth'* >) **aboral,** (ore rotundo *'with rounded mouth'* >) **orotund**

[용례] nil per os (NPO) (< *nothing peroral*) 금식(禁食)   **E** *NPO*
(문법) nil 무(無): 불변화 명사 < nil, n. < nihill, n.
per 통하여: 전치사, 대격지배
os 입을: 단수 대격

> L. oralis, orale 입의, 입으로 하는, 구두(口頭)의   **E** *oral*
> L. osculum, osculi, n. 작은 입, 입맞춤   **E** *osculum*
>> L. osculor, osculatus sum, osculari 입맞추다, 접촉하다   **E** *osculate, osculation*
>> L. osculo, -, -, osculare 문합(吻合)시키다,
연결시키다   **E** *inosculate* (< *'on the pattern of* G. anastomoun'), *inosculation*
> L. oscillum, oscilli, n. (< os *mouth* + -cillum *diminutive suffix*) 또는 (< os *mouth* +
cillare *to swing*) 콩 중앙부의 옴폭 파인 곳, Bacchus나 Saturnus에 대한 미신 행위로
나무에 걸던 가면상; (가면상의 움직임 > (*suggested*) >) 그네,
진동   **E** *oscillate; oscilloscope, oscillograph*
> L. ostium, ostii, n. 입구, 구(口), 구멍   **E** *ostium,* (pl.) *ostia*
>> L. ostiarius, ostiaria, ostiarium 입구의, 문(門)의
>>> L. ostiarius, ostiarii, m. 문지기, 안내원   **E** *ostiary, usher*
> L. ora, orae, f. 둘레, 가장자리, 경계

[용례] ora serrata 톱니둘레, 거상연(鋸狀緣)   **E** *ora serrata*
(문법) ora 둘레: 단수 주격
serrata 톱니 자국의: 형용사, 여성형 단수 주격
< serratus, serrata, serratum
< serro, serravi, serratum, serrare 톱으로 켜다, 자르다

> L. orificium, orificii, n. (< os *mouth* + facĕre *to make*) 작은 입구, 구멍   **E** *orifice*
> L. oscito, oscitavi, oscitatum, oscitare (oscitor, oscitatus sum, oscitari) (< os *mouth*
+ citare *to rouse*) 입을 크게 벌리다, 하품하다   **E** *oscitation*
< IE. os- *mouth*

G. stoma, stomatos, n. *mouth*

> L. stoma, stomatis, n. 입[口], 입구(入口), 기공(氣孔)

> **E** *stoma,* (pl.) *stomata (stomas), stomat(o)-, -stomy* (< 'An opening is made into the indicated internal organ or a permanent connection is made between the internal organs indicated.')

> L. Ancylostoma, Ancylostomatis, n. (< *crooked mouth* < G. ankylos *crooked*)

(선충 線蟲) 구충속(鉤蟲屬)　　　　　　　　　　　　　　　**E** Ancylostoma

> L. Echinostoma, Echinostomatis, n. (< *spiny mouth* < G. echinos *hedgehog*)

(흡충 吸蟲) 극구흡충속(棘口吸蟲屬)　　　　　　　　　　**E** Echinostoma

> L. Distoma, Distomatis, n. (< *two suckers* < G. di- *two*) (흡충 吸蟲) 이구흡충속

(二口吸蟲屬), 디스토마속(屬)　　　　　　　　　　　**E** (obsolete) Distoma

> L. -stomia, -stomiae, f. *mouth exhibiting (such) a condition*　　**E** -stomia (-stomy)

> L. ozostomia, ozostomiae, f. (< G. ozein *to smell*) 입냄새증, 구취증(口臭症)　**E** ozostomia

> L. xerostomia, xerostomiae, f. (< G. xēros *dry*) 입안마름증, 구강건조증　**E** xerostomia

> G. anastomoun (anastomoein) (< an(a)- *up, upward; again, throughout; back, backward;*

against; according to, similar to) *to furnish with a mouth or outlet*

> G. anastomōsis, anastomōseōs, f. (< + -ōsis *condition*) *anastomosis*

> L. anastomosis, anastomosis, f. 문합(吻合), 문합술, 연결,

교통(交通)　**E** *anastomosis,* (pl.) *anastomoses, (anastomosis >) anastomose*

> G. stomachos, stomachou, m. *stomach*

> L. stomachus, stomachi, m. 위(胃)　　　　　　　　　　**E** *stomach*

> L. stomachalis, stomachale 위의　　　　　　　　　　**E** *stomachal*

> G. stomachikos, stomachikē, stomachikon *of the stomach, good for the stomach*

> L. stomachicus, stomachica, stomachicum 위의,

위에 좋은　　　　　　**E** *stomachic, (stomachic >) stomachical*

< IE. stom-en- *denoting orifices and body parts with orifices*

E. *lip*

< IE. leb- *to lick, lip* (Vide infra)

L. labium, labii, n. 입술, 구순(口脣), 음순(陰脣); (동물) 아랫입술, (식물) 아래 순판

(脣瓣)　　　　　　　　　　　　　　　　　　　　　　**E** *labium,* (pl.) *labia*

> L. labialis, labiale 입술의, 구순의, 음순의, 순음(脣音)의　　**E** *labial, bilabial*

> L. labiatus, labiata, labiatum 입술이 있는, 입술 모양의　　**E** *labiate*

< IE. leb- *to lick, lip*　　　　　　　　　　　　　　　　　**E** *lip*

> L. labrum, labri, n. 입술, 테두리, (그릇의) 아가리; (동물) 윗입술　**E** *labrum,* (pl.) *labra; labret*

> L. labellum, labelli, n. (< + -ellum *diminutive suffix*) 작은 입술, 귀여운 입술;

(동물·식물) 순판(脣瓣)　　　　　　　　　　　**E** *labellum,* (pl.) *labella*

G. cheilos, cheileos, n. *lip, rim*　　　　　**E** *cheil(o)- (chil(o)-), cheiloplasty (chiloplasty)*

< IE. ghel-una- *jaw*　　　　　　　　　　　　　　　　　**E** *gill*

E. *gum*

    < IE. gheu– *to gape, to yawn* (Vide HIARE; *See* E. *hiatus*)

E *gum*

L. gingiva, gingivae, f. 잇몸, 치은(齒齦)

    > L. gingivalis, gingivale 잇몸의, 치은의

    < IE. geng– *lump, ball*

E *gingiva*
E *gingival*
E *kink*

G. oula, oulōn, n. (pl.) ((sing.) oulon, oulou, n.) *gums*

    > G. epoulis, epoulidos, f. (< ep(i)– *upon* + oulon *gum*) *epulis*

      > L. epulis, epulidis, f. 잇몸종, 치은종(齒齦腫)

E *ul(o)–, ulectomy*
E *epulis*, (pl.) *epulides*

E. *tongue*

    < IE. dnghu– *tongue* (Vide infra)

L. lingua, linguae, f. 혀, 소리, 언어

E *language, langue, linguistic, linguistics; linguocentric, metalanguage (< 'a language or set of terms used for the description or analysis of another language'), paralanguage (< 'the non-phonemic component of speech')*

    > L. lingualis, linguale 혀의, 언어의; (음성) 설음의   **E** *lingual, multilingual (polyglot)*

      > L. sublingualis, sublinguale (< sub– *under, up from under* + lingualis

          of tongue) 혀 밑의   **E** *sublingual*

    > L. bilinguis, bilingue (< bi– *two*) 2개 국어를 사용하는   **E** *bilingual (diglot)*

    > L. lingula, lingulae, f. (< + –ula *diminutive suffix*) 작은 혀,

        혀돌기   **E** *lingula, (lingula >) lingular*

    > L. ligula, ligulae, f. (< + –ula *diminutive suffix; by-form of* lingula) 작은 혀,

        작은 혀 모양의 구조   **E** *ligula, ligule*

    < (*Archaic Latin*) dingua 혀

    < IE. dnghu– *tongue*   **E** *tongue*

G. glōssa, glōssēs, f. (*non-Attic*) *tongue, speech, language*

    > L. glossa, glossae, f. 혀, 어휘, 용어 해설   **E** *glossa, (glossa >) glossal, gloss(o)–*

      > L. glossarium, glossarii, n. 용어 해설, 용어 사전   **E** *glossary*

      > L. hypoglossus, hypoglossi, m. (< G. hyp(o)– *under*)

        혀밑신경   **E** (hypoglossus >) *hypoglossal*

    < IE. glogh– *thorn, point*

G. glōtta, glōttēs, f. (*Attic*) *tongue, speech, language*   **E** *diglot (bilingual), polyglot (multilingual)*

    > L. glottis, glottidis, f. (< *the vocal apparatus consisting of the vocal folds and the*

opening between them) 성문(聲門), 성대문(聲帶門)　　　　　**E** *glottis, glottic, glottal, glottalize*

　　> L. epiglottis, epiglottidis, f. (< G. ep(i)- *upon*) 후두덮개,

　　　　후두개(喉頭蓋)　　　　　**E** *epiglottis, epiglottic*

　> G. *proglōttis, *proglōttidos, f. (< G. pro- *before, in front*) *tip of the tongue*

　　　> L. proglottis, proglottidis, f. (< *from its shape*) (촌충) 마디, 편절(片節),

　　　　체절(體節)　　　　　**E** *proglottid*

< IE. glogh- *thorn, point* (Vide sufra)

E. *chin*

< IE. genu- *jawbone, chin* (Vide infra)

L. mentum, menti, n. 턱　　　　　**E** *mental, submental*

< IE. men- *to project* (Vide MONS: *See* E. *mount*)

G. gnathos, gnathou, f. *jaw, mouth*

E *gnathic, gnath(o)-, -gnathia, -gnathous, prognathia, prognathous, prognathism, macrognathia, micrognathia*

< IE. genu- *jawbone, chin*　　　　　**E** *chin*

　> G. genys, genyos, f. *chin, jaw, axe*

　　> G. geneion, geneiou, n. *chin, lower jaw, beard*　　　　　**E** *genial, geni(o)-*

E. *neck*　　　　　**E** *neck*

L. collum, colli, n. (< *that on which the head turns*) 목

E *collar, collarette,* (*accollare (< ad *'to, toward, at, according to'* + collum *'neck'*) *'to embrace about the neck'* > *accollata (*past participle*) >) *accolade*

> L. torticollis, torticollis, f. (< tortus *crooked, twisted* + collum *neck*) 기운목, 사경

　(斜頸)　　　　　**E** *torticollis*

< IE. kʷel-, kʷelə- *to turn, to be around, to dwell* (Vide COLÈRE: *See* E. *colony*)

L. cervix, cervicis, f. 목, 경부(頸部)　　　　　**E** *cervix*

　> L. *cervicalis, *cervicale 목의, 경부의　　　　　**E** *cervical*

< IE. ker- *horn, head; with derivatives referring to horned animals, horn-shaped objects, and projecting parts* (Vide CORNU: *See* E. *unicorn*)

G. trachēlos, trachēlou, m. *neck, throat*　　　　　**E** *trachel(o)-*

E. *breast*　　　　　**E** *breast*

< IE. bhreus- *to swell.*　　　　　**E** *browse* (< *'young shoot eaten by animals'*)

L. mamma, mammae, f. 엄마, 젖, 유방(乳房)　　　　　　　　　　　E *mamma*, (pl.) *mammae*
    < IE. ma- *mother; a linguistic near-universal found in many of the world's languages, often*
        in reduplicated form (Vide MATER: *See* E. *maternal*)

G. mastos, mastou, m. *breast*　　　　　　　　　　　　　　　E *mastalgia (mastodynia)*
    > G. mastoidēs, mastoidēs, mastoides (< + eidos *shape*) *breast-shaped*
      > L. mastoideus, mastoidea, mastoideum 유방 같은, 꼭지돌기(*mastoid process*)의　E *mastoid*
        > L. sternocleidomastoideus, sternocleidomastoidea, sternocleidomastoideum
          (< G. sternon, sternou, n. *breastbone* + kleis, kleidos, f. *collar bone*)
          흉쇄유돌(胸鎖乳突)의, 목빗근의　　　　　　　　　　　E *sternocleidomastoid*
    > L. Mastodon, Mastodontis, m. (< *nipple-shaped protrusions on the crowns of its*
      molars < + G. odous, odontos, m. *tooth*) (대형 화석 코끼리) 마스토돈속(屬)　E *mastodon*
    > L. gynaecomastia, gynaecomastiae, f. (< G. gynē, gynaikos, f. *woman*) 여성형
      유방증　　　　　　　　　　　　　　　　E *gynaecomastia (gynecomastia)*
    < IE. mad- *moist, wet, dripping (with fat, sap); also refers various qualities of food*

> E *meat, mate* (< *'he with whom one shares one's food'*), *mast* (< *'the nuts of forest trees*
> *accumulated on the ground, used especially as food for swine'*), *mastocyte* (*mast cell*) (<
> *'fattening cell'* < *'filled with metachromatic granules misunderstood to nourish the*
> *surrounding tissue'*)

E. *basin*　　　　　　　　　　　　　　　　　　　　　　　　　E *basin*

L. pelvis, pelvis, f. 세숫대야, 반(盤), 골반(骨盤), 신우(腎盂)　　　E *pelvis*, (*pelvis* >) *pelvic*
    < IE. pelə- *to fill; with derivatives referring to abundance and multitude* (Vide PLĒRE:
    See E. *complete*)

G. pyelos, pyelou, f. *trough, basin*　　　　　　　　　　　　　E *pyel(o)-*
    < IE. pleu- *to flow* (Vide PULMO: *See* E. *pulmonary*)

E. *anus*
    < L. anus, ani, m. 가락지, 항문(肛門) (Vide infra)

L. anus, ani, m. 가락지, 항문(肛門)　　　　　　　　　　　　　E *anus*
    > L. analis, anale 항문의　　　　　　　　　　　　　　　E *anal*
    > L. annulus, annuli, m. (anulus, anuli, m.) (< + -ulus *diminutive suffix*) 작은 가락지,
      고리, 환(環), 윤(輪)　　　　　　　　　　　　　　　E *annulus (anulus)*
      > L. annularis, annulare 고리 모양의, 환상(環狀)의, 윤상(輪狀)의　E *annular (anular)*
      > L. annulatus, annulata, annulatum 가락지 낀, 고리가 있는, 윤행(輪行)하는　E *annulate*
      > L. annellus, annelli, m. (< + -ellus *diminutive suffix*) 작은 가락지　E *annelid*
    > L. anilingus, anilingi, m. (< lingĕre *to lick*) 항문핥기　　　E *anilingus*

< IE. ano- *ring*

G. prōktos, prōktou, m. *anus, anus and rectum*　　　　　　E *proct(o)-, proctology, proctoscope*

　　< IE. prokto- *anus*

E. *testis*

　　< L. testis, testis, m. 불알, 고환(睾丸) (Vide infra)

L. testis, testis, m. 불알, 고환　　　　　　　　　　　　　　　E *testis*, (pl.) *testes*

　　> L. testiculus, testiculi, m. (< + -culus *diminutive suffix*) 불알, 고환　　E *testicle, testicular*

　　< IE. trei- *three* (Vide IE. trei- *three*; See E. *three*)

G. orchis, orcheōs, m. (orchis, orchios, m.) *testis*

> E *orchi(o)-, orchiopexy (orchiorrhaphy), orchid(o)- (<'mistaken stem'), cryptorchism (cryptorchidism), orchic (orchidic); orchis (<'the shape of the (frequently paired) tubers in many species), orchid*

　　< IE. ergh- *to mount* (Vide ORBIS; See E. *orb*)

G. didymoi, didymōn, m. (pl.) *testes*

　　　　　　　　> L. epididymis, epididymidis, f. (< ep(i)- *upon*)

　　　　　　　　　부고환(副睾丸)　　　　　　E *epididymis*, (pl.) *epididymides, epididym(o)-*

　　　　　　　　< G. didymos, didymē, didymon (< *reduplication of* dyo *two*) *double, twofold,*

　　　　　　　　　　twin

　　　　　　< G. dyo, dyo, dyo *two*

< IE. dwo- *two* (Vide IE. dwo- *two*; See E. *two*)

E. *vagina*

　　< L. vagina, vaginae, f. 칼집, 초(鞘), 질(膣) (Vide infra)

L. vagina, vaginae, f. (< *sheath 'probably made of split pieces of wood'*) 칼집, 초(鞘), 질(膣)　E *vagina*

　　> L. vaginalis, vaginale 초(鞘)의, 질(膣)의　　　　　　　　　　　　　　　　　E *vaginal*

　　　　[용례] tunica vaginalis 초막　　　　　　　　　　　　　　　E *tunica vaginalis*

　　　　　　(문법) tunica 막: 단수 주격 < tunica, tunicae, f. 층, 막

　　　　　　　　vaginalis 초의: 형용사, 남·여성형 단수 주격

　　　　[용례] portio vaginalis (cervicis) (*ectocervix, exocervix*) (자궁경)질부(子宮頸膣部),

　　　　　　질부분　　　　　　　　　　　　　　　　　　　　　　　　E *portio vaginalis*

　　　　　　(문법) portio 부분: 단수 주격 < portio, portionis, f. 부분, 몫, 비율

vaginalis 질(膣)의: 형용사, 남·여성형 단수 주격

cervicis 목의: 단수 속격 < cervix, cervicis, f. 목, 경부(頸部)

> L. vaginismus, vaginismi, m. 질경련(膣痙攣)   **E** *vaginismus*

> L. evagino, **evaginavi**, evaginatum, evaginare (< e- *out of, away from* + vagina
sheath) 칼을 칼집에서 빼다, 팽출(膨出)하다, 외번(外飜)하다   **E** *evaginate*

> L. invagino, **invaginavi**, invaginatum, invaginare (< in- *in, on, into, toward* + vagina
sheath) 칼을 칼집에 넣다, 함입(陷入)하다   **E** *invaginate*

> Sp. vaina *sheath*

> Sp. vanilla (< *little pod* < (*diminutive*) *little sheath*) *vanilla*

> L. vanilla, vanillae, f. (열대 아메리카산 난초과 식물) 바닐라

E *vanilla, vanillin, vanillic acid, vanillylmandelic acid (vanilmandelic acid)*
(VMA) (< '*structurally related to vanillin and mandelic acid*')

< IE. wag- *to break, to split, to bite*

G. kolpos, kolpou, m. *bosom, womb, fold of a garment, bay, hollow, depth,*
vagina   **E** *gulf, engulf, colposcopy, colpitis, colpopexy*

< IE. kwelp- *to arch*   **E** *overwhelm*

E. *back*   **E** *back*

L. dorsum, dorsi, n. 등, 뒤, 등쪽, 배부(背部)   **E** *dorsum, dorsal, dorsad, dorsiflexion, endorse*

G. nōton, nōtou, n. (nōtos, nōtou, m.) *back*   **E** *notochord, notomelia*

< IE. not- *buttock, back* (Vide NATIS: *See* E. *natal*)

E. *tail*   **E** *tail*

< IE. dek- *referring to such things as a fringe, lock of hair,*
horsetail   **E** *(perhaps) tag* (< '*pendent piece*'), *(perhaps) tack*

L. cauda, caudae, f. 꼬리

E *caudad, coward* (< '*probably, an animal turning tail in flight or drawing the tail between*
the hinder legs'), It. *coda, queue (cue), curlicue; (bicaudal-like* >) *bicoid*

[용례] cauda equina 말꼬리, 마미(馬尾), 말총   **E** *cauda equina*

(문법) cauda 꼬리: 단수 주격

equina 말의: 형용사, 여성형 단수 주격

< equinus, equina, equinum < equus, equi, m. 말

> L. caudalis, caudale 꼬리의   **E** *caudal*

> L. caudatus, caudata, caudatum 꼬리가 있는   **E** *caudate*

G. oura, ouras, f. *tail, rear*　　　　　　　　　　　　　　　　　　E ur(o)-, (an- *'not'* > *'tailless'* >) *anurous (anourous)*

　　> G. kynosoura, kynosouras, f. (< *dog's tail* < kyōn *dog* + oura *tail*) Ursa minor

　　　　> L. Cynosura, Cynosurae, f. (Ursa minor) (천체) 작은곰자리, 소웅좌(小熊座)　　E *Cynosure*

　　　　　　> L. Cynosuris, (gen.) Cynosuridis (*adjective*) 작은곰자리의

　　> G. skiouros, skiourou, m. (< *shadow tailed* < skia *shadow* + oura *tail*) squirrel

　　　　> L. sciurus, sciuri, m. 다람쥐　　　　　　　　　　　E Sciurus, *(sciurus* >) *squirrel*

　　> L. Trichuris, Trichuridis, f. (< G. thrix, trichos, f. *hair, wool, bristle* + oura *tail*)

　　　　(선충 線蟲) 편충속(鞭蟲屬), 트리쿠리스속(屬)　　　　　　E Trichuris, *trichuriasis*

　　　　[용례] Trichuris trichiura 편충(鞭蟲)　　　　　　　　　　E *Trichuris trichiura*

　　　　　　(문법) Trichuris 편충속(鞭蟲屬): 단수 주격

　　　　　　　　trichiura 실꼬리를 한: 형용사, 여성형 단수 주격 (Vide infra)

　　> L. -urus, -ura, -urum ~ 꼬리를 한

　　　　> L. trichiurus, trichiura, trichiurum (< G. thrix, trichos, f. *hair, wool, bristle* +

　　　　　　oura *tail*) 실꼬리를 한

　< IE. ors- *buttocks, backside*

G. kerkos, kerkou, f. *tail*

> E *cercoid* (< *'larva with a tail-like structure'*), (pro- *'before, in front'* > *'early cercoid'* >) *procercoid*, (plērēs *'full, filled with, complete'* > *'completed cercoid'* >) *plerocercoid*

　　> L. cercaria, cercariae, f. (< *larva with a tail*) 꼬리유충(幼蟲), 꼬리애벌레,

　　　　유미유충(有尾幼蟲)　　　　　　　　　　　　　　　　　　E *cercaria*

　　　　> L. mesocercaria, mesocercariae, f. (< G. mes(o)- *middle*)

　　　　　　무낭(無囊)유충　　　　　　　　　　　　　　　　　E *mesocercaria*

　　　　> L. metacercaria, metacercariae, f. (< G. met(a)- *between, along with, across,*

　　　　　　after) 피낭(被囊)유충　　　　　　　　　　　　　E *metacercaria*

　　> L. cysticercus, cysticerci, f. (< G. kystis *bladder, bag*) 낭미충

　　　　(囊尾蟲)　　　　　　　　　　　　　　　　　E *cysticercus, cysticercosis*

　　> L. Onchocerca, Onchocercae, f. (< G. onkos *barb, grabble-hook*) (사상충 絲狀蟲)

　　　　옹코서카속(屬)　　　　　　　　　　　　　E Onchocerca, *onchocerciasis*

E. *hand*　　　　　　　　　　　　　　　　　　　　　　　　　　E *hand*

　< (*suggested*) IE. kent- *to seize*

L. manus, manus, f. 손

> E *manage* (< *'to handle (a horse)'*), (*manage* >) *manager*, (*manager* >) *managerial*, (manus + cura *'care'* >) *manicure*, (manu facĕre *'to make by hand'* >) *manufacture*, (manu operari *'to work by hand'* >) *maneuver (manoeuvre)*, (manu operari *'to cultivate'* >) *manure*, F. *manchette* (< *'ornamental sleeve'*)

　　> L. manualis, manuale 손의, 손에 들 만한, 소책자의, 교범(教範)의　　　E *manual*

< IE. man– *hand* (Vide MANUS: *See* E. *manage*)

G. cheir, cheiros, f. *hand*   **E** *chir(o)-, chiral, (chiral >) chirality*

> G. Cheirōn, Cheirōnos, m. (*Greek mythology*) *the wisest of all centaurs, famous for his knowledge of medicine: he is the teacher of Asclepius, Achilles, and Hercules*

> L. Chiron, Chironis, m. (Chiro, Chironis, m.) (그리스 신화) 키론   **E** *Chiron (Cheiron)*

> G. cheirourgia, cheirourgias, f. (< cheir + –ourgia *working* < ergon *work*) *manual labor, craft*   **E** *surgery*

> G. encheiridion, encheiridiou, n. (< en– *in* + cheir + –idion *diminutive suffix*) *handbook, manual*   **E** *enchiridion*

< IE. ghes– *hand*

> L. praesto (< *at hand* < (*perhaps*) < IE. prai– < IE. per *basic meanings of 'forward', 'through'* + IE. ghes–) 가까이에, 준비된 상태에   **E** It. *presto* (< *'quick, quickly'*)*, prestidigitation* (< *'quick fingering'*)

E. *finger*   **E** *finger*

< IE. penk^we *five* (Vide IE. penk^we; *See* E. *five*)

E. *toe*   **E** *toe*

< (*possibly*) IE. deik–, deig– *to show, to pronounce solemnly; also in derivatives referring to the directing of words or objects* (Vide DICĔRE: *See* E. *dictum*)

L. digitus, digiti, m. (< *pointer, indicator*) 손가락, 발가락   **E** *digit*

> L. digitalis, digitale 손가락의, 손가락만 한   **E** *digital,* (digitalis herba *'thimble'* >) *digitalis, (digitalis + toxin >) digoxin*

> L. digitatus, digitata, digitatum 손가락이 있는, 발가락이 있는, 손가락 모양의   **E** *digitate, (digitate >) interdigitate*

< (*possibly*) IE. deik–, deig– *to show, to pronounce solemnly; also in derivatives referring to the directing of words or objects* (Vide DICĔRE: *See* E. *dictum*)

G. daktylos, daktylou, m. *finger, toe; date; a metric foot of dactyl*

E *dactyl(o)-, dactylogram* (< *'finger print'*)*, -dactyl, -dactyly, syndactyly, polydactyly, arachnodactyly*

> L. dactylus, dactyli, m. (동물) 손가락, 발가락; 대추야자 열매; 장단단격(長短短格), 강약약격(強弱弱格)   **E** *date, dactyl* (< *'a metrical foot suggesting the three joints of a finger'*)

E. *ham*   **E** *ham, hamstring, Spam*® (< *'spiced ham'*)*, (Spam*® *>) spam*

< IE. konə mo– *shin, leg, bone* (Vide KNĒMĒ: *See* E. *gastrocnemius*)

L. popules, poplitis, m. 오금, 무릎

> L. popliteus, poplitea, popliteum 오금의, 무릎의   **E** *popliteal*

G. knēmē, knēmēs, f. *shin-bone, leg*

> G. gastroknēmia, gastroknēmias, f. (gastēr *belly* + knēmē *leg*) *calf*

> L. gastrocnemius, gastrocnemii, m. 장딴지근   **E** *gastrocnemius (muscle)*

< IE. konə mo- *shin, leg, bone*

E. *calf*   **E** *calf*

< IE. gel- *to make round, to clench as the fist, to grip, to cling to* (Vide GLOBUS: *See* E. *globus*)

L. sura, surae, f. 장딴지, 종아리

> L. suralis, surale 장딴지의, 종아리의   **E** *sural*

E. *brain*   **E** *brain*

< IE. mregh-m(n)o- *brain*

> G. bregma, bregmatos, n. *the front part of the head*

> L. bregma, bregmatis, n. (< *the point on the surface of the skull at the junction of the coronal and sagittal sutures*) 정수리점, 브레그마   **E** *bregma, bregmatic*

L. cerebrum, cerebri, n. 대뇌(大腦)   **E** *cerebrum, cerebral, cerebr(i)- (cerebro-)*

> L. cerebellum, cerebelli, n. (< + -ellum *diminutive suffix*)

소뇌(小腦)   **E** *cerebellum, cerebellar, cerebell(i)- (cerebello-)*

< IE. ker- *horn, head; with derivatives referring to horned animals, horn-shaped objects, and projecting parts* (Vide CORNU: *See* E. *unicorn*)

G. enkephalos, enkephalou, m. (< *what is within the head* < en- *in* + -kephalos)

brain   **E** *encephal(o)-, -encephaly, encephalitis, enkephalin*

< G. -kephalos, -kephalos, -kephalon -*head*

> L. cephalon, cephali, n. 머리, 두부(頭部)   **E** *cephalon*

> G. enkephalon, enkephalou, n. (< *what is within the head* < en- *in* + -kephalon) *brain*

> L. encephalon, encephali, n. 뇌(腦)   **E** *encephalon*

> L. archencephalon, archencephali, n. (< G. archē *beginning*) 원뇌(原腦)   **E** *archencephalon*

> L. prosencephalon, prosencephali, n. (< G. pros- *towards, near, beside(s)*) 앞뇌   **E** *prosencephalon (forebrain)*

> L. telencephalon, telencephali, n. (< G. tēle *afar, far off*) 끝뇌, 종뇌(終腦)   **E** *telencephalon*

> L. diencephalon, diencephali, n. (< G. di(a)- *through,*
thoroughly, apart) 사이뇌, 간뇌(間腦)　　　**E** *diencephalon*

> L. mesencephalon, mesencephali, n. (< G. mesos *middle*)
중간뇌(中間腦)　　　**E** *mesencephalon (midbrain)*

> L. rhombencephalon, rhombencephali, n. (< G. rhombos
rhombus) 마름뇌, 능형뇌(菱形腦)　**E** *rhombencephalon (hindbrain)*

> L. metencephalon, metencephali, n. (< G. met(a)- *between,*
along with, across, after) 뒤뇌　　　**E** *metencephalon*

> L. myelencephalon, myelencephali, n. (< G. myelos *spinal*
marrow) 숨뇌, 연수(延髓)　　　**E** *myelencephalon*

> G. anenkephalos, anenkephalos, anenkephalon (< an- *not* + en- *in* +
-kephalos) *brainless*

> L. anencephalus, anencephali, m. 무뇌체, 뇌없는아이　**E** *anencephalus*

> L. anencephalia, anencephaliae, f. 무뇌증　　**E** *anencephaly*

> G. hydrokephalon, hydrokephalou, n. (< hydōr, hydōratos, n. *water*)
hydrocephalus

> L. hydrocephalus, hydrocephali, m. 수두증(水頭症)　**E** *hydrocephalus*

[용례] hydrocephalus ex vacuo (뇌실질의 위축 때문에 생긴)
공간 수두증, 무강(無腔) 수두증　**E** *hydrocephalus ex vacuo*
(문법) hydrocephalus 수두증: 단수 주격
ex ~으로부터: 전치사, 탈격지배
vacuo 공간: 단수 탈격 < vacuum, vacui, n.

< G. kephalē, kephalēs, f. *head*

E *cephal(o)-, -cephaly, dyscephaly (< 'malformation of the cranium and bones of the*
face'), cephalization (< 'centralization of the nervous system, sensory organs, etc.
in or near the head'); cephalad (< + -ad 'toward')

> G. kephalikos, kephalikē, kephalikon *of head*

> L. cephalicus, cephalica, cephalicum 머리의　　　**E** *cephalic, -cephalic*

[용례] vena cephalica (< *cephalic vein* < *the opening of this vein*
was anciently supposed to relieve disorders of the head;
translation error of (Arabic) al-kifal *the outer*) 노쪽피부정맥,
요측피부정맥(橈側皮靜脈)　　　**E** *cephalic vein*
(문법) vena 정맥: 단수 주격 < vena, venae, f. 맥, 혈관, 정맥
cephalica 머리의: 형용사, 여성형 단수 주격

> L. brachiocephalicus, brachiocephalica, brachiocephalicum (<
of both arm and head < G. brachiōn *arm, upper arm*) 팔과
머리의　　　**E** *brachiocephalic*

< IE. ghebh-el- *head*　　　**E** *gable*

E. *kidney*　　　**E** *kidney*

L. ren, renis, m. 허리, 콩팥, 신장(腎臟)　　　　　　　　　　　　　　　**E** *renin*

> **L. renalis, renale** 콩팥의, 신장의　　　　　　　　　　　　　　　**E** *renal*

> **L. suprarenalis, suprarenale** (< **supra-** *above*) 콩팥 위의, 부신(副腎)의　　**E** *suprarenal*

> **L. *adrenalis, *adrenale** (< **ad-** *to, toward, at, according to*) 콩팥 쪽의, 부신
(副腎)의

E *adrenal, adrenaline,* (normal adrenaline without methyl substituents >)
noradrenaline, adrenocortical, adrenocorticotropin (corticotropin)

> **L. reniformis, reniforme** 콩팥 모양의　　　　　　　　　　　　　**E** *reniform*

G. nephros, nephrou, m. *kidney*

E *pronephros,* (pl.) *pronephroi, mesonephros,* (pl.) *mesonephroi, metanephros,* (pl.)
metanephroi, -nephric, pronephric, mesonephric, metanephric, nephr(o)-, nephron (<
'the structural and functional unit of the kidney'), *nephrite* (< 'supposed efficacy in
treating kidney disease'), *epinephrine* (< 'secreted by the gland located upon the
kidney'), (normal epinephrine without methyl substituents >) *norepinephrine,* (metabolite
of epinephrine >) *metanephrine*

> **L. nephritis, nephritidis,** f. (< + **-itis** *noun suffix denoting inflammation*) 콩팥염,
신장염　　　　　　　　　　　　　　　　　　　　　　　**E** *nephritis, nephritic*

> **L. nephrosis, nephrosis,** f. (< + **G. -ōsis** *condition*) 콩팥증, 신장증　**E** *nephrosis, nephrotic*

> **L. hydronephrosis, hydronephrosis,** f. (< **G. hydros** *water*) 물콩팥증,
수신증(水腎症)　　　　　　　　　　　　　　　　　　　**E** *hydronephrosis*

< **IE. neg^wh-ro-** *kidney*

E. *spleen*

< **G. splēn, splēnos,** m. *spleen* (Vide infra)

L. lien, lienis, m. 비(脾), 비장(脾臟), 지라　　　　　　　　**E** (lien >) *lienal*

G. splēn, splēnos, m. *spleen*

> **L. splen, splenis,** m. 비(脾), 비장(脾臟), 지라 **E** *spleen, hypersplenism, polysplenia, asplenia*

> **L. splenulus, splenuli,** m. (< + **-ulus** *diminutive suffix*) 부비장(副脾臟),
덧지라　　　　　　　　　　　　　　　　　　　　　　　　**E** *splenulus*

> **G. splēnikos, splēnikē, splēnikon** *splenic*

> **L. splenicus, splenica, splenicum** 비장의, 지라의　　　　　**E** *splenic*

> **G. splēnion, splēniou,** n. (< *from its shape* < + **-ion** *diminutive suffix*) *compress,
bandage*

> **L. splenium, splenii,** n. 습포(濕布), 붕대(繃帶), 대상구조(帶狀構造), 팽대(膨大)　**E** *splenium*

> **L. splenius, splenia, splenium** 대상구조의, 판상(板狀)의　　　**E** *splenius (muscle)*

< **IE. spelgh-** *spleen, milt*

> **G. splanchnon, splanchnou,** n. (*usually* pl.) *internal organs, inwards*　　**E** *splanchn(o)-*

> G. splanchnikos, splanchnikē, splanchnikon *splanchnic*

> L. splanchnicus, splanchnica, splanchnicum 내장의

E *splanchnic*

E. *womb*

E *womb*

L. uterus, uteri, m. 자궁 < 배[腹]

E *uterus*

    < IE. udero- *abdomen, womb, stomach: with distantly similar forms (perhaps taboo deformations) in various languages* (Vide UTERUS: *See* E. *uterus*)

G. hystera, hysteras, f. *womb*

E *hyster(o)-*

    < IE. udero- *abdomen, womb, stomach: with distantly similar forms (perhaps taboo deformations) in various languages* (Vide UTERUS: *See* E. *uterus*)

G. delphys, delphynos, f. *womb*

E *didelphys (didelphia)*

> L. didelphia, didelphiae, f. (< G. di- *two* + delphys + -ia *noun suffix*) 이자궁(二子宮), 중복자궁

E *didelphia (didelphys)*

> G. delphis, delphinos, m. (< *womb-shaped*) *dolphin*

> L. delphinus, delphini, m. (delphin, delphinis, m.) 돌고래

E *dolphin*

    < IE. gʷelbh- *womb*

> G. adelphos, adelphou, m. (< *of the same womb*) *brother*

> G. philadelphia, philadelphias, f. (< philein (phileein) *to love* + adelphos + -ia *noun suffix*) *brotherly love*

E *Philadelphia*

> L. thoracodelphus, thoracodelphi, m. (< *a double monster with one head, two arms, and four legs, the bodies being joined above the navel* < G. thōrax *chest* + adelphos) 가슴결합체

E *thoracodelphus*

G. mētra, mētras, f. *womb*

E *metr(o)-, -metrium*

    < G. mētēr, mētros, f. *mother*

    < IE. mater- *mother* (*based ultimately on the baby-talk form* ma-, *with the kinship term suffix* -ter-) (Vide MATER: *See* E. *maternal*)

E. *vessel*

    < L. vascellum, vascelli, n. 작은 그릇, 관, 맥관, 혈관 (Vide infra)

L. vas, vasis, n. (복수 속격은 vasum이나 실제로는 vasorum을 씀) 그릇; 관, 맥관, 혈관

> E *vase, vas(o)-, vasoconstrictor, vasodilatator, vasomotor, vasopressor, vasopressin, extravasation, intravasation*

[용례] vasa vasorum (pl.) 맥관벽혈관

E (pl.) *vasa vasorum*

vasa nervorum (pl.) 신경혈관

E (pl.) *vasa nervorum*

vasa recta (pl.) 직혈관(直血管)

E (pl.) *vasa recta*

(문법) vasa 혈관들: 복수 주격

vasorum 혈관들의: 복수 속격

nervorum 신경들의: 복수 속격 < nervus, nervi, m.

recta 곧은: 형용사, 중성형 복수 주격 < rectus, recta, rectum

> L. vasculum, vasculi, n. (< + -culum *diminutive suffix*) 작은 그릇, 관, 맥관, 혈관

E *vascul(o)-, vasculogenesis* (< 'the de novo development of a vascular system'), *intravascular, extravascular, intervascular*

> L. vascellum, vascelli, n. (< + -ellum *diminutive suffix*) 작은 그릇, 관, 맥관, 혈관

E *vessel*

> L. vascularis, vasculare 관의, 맥관의, 혈관의

E *vascular, vasculature* (< 'on the pattern of musculature'), *vascularity, vascularize, vascularization; avascular*

> L. vasculitis, vasculitidis, f. (< + -itis *noun suffix denoting inflammation*) 맥관염, 혈관염

E *vasculitis,* (pl.) *vasculitides*

G. angeion, angeiou, n. (< + -ion *diminutive suffix*) *container, receptacle, urn; vessel*

E *angi(o)-, angiology, angiogenesis* (< 'the formation of blood vessels from pre-existing ones'), *angiopoiesis* (< 'the process of vessel formation'), *angioplasty; angiotensin*

> L. angiitis, angiitidis, f. (< + -itis *noun suffix denoting inflammation*) 맥관염, 혈관염

E *angiitis,* (pl.) *angiitides*

> L. lymphangiitis, lymphangiitidis, f. (< lympha *lymph*)

림프관염

E *lymphangiitis,* (pl.) *lymphangiitides*

> L. mesangium, mesangii, n. (< G. mesos *middle* + angeion *vessel*) 토리사이질, 사구체간질, 사구체맥관막, 혈관사이막

E *mesangium, (mesangium >) mesangial*

> L. sporangium, sporangii, n. (< G. spora *spore* + angeion *vessel*) 홀씨주머니, 포자낭(胞子囊)

E *sporangium,* (pl.) *sporangia, sporangiospore, sporangiophore*

< G. angos, angeos, n. *chest, box*

E. *vein*

< L. vena, venae, f. 맥, 혈관, 정맥 (Vide infra)

L. vena, venae, f. 맥, 혈관, 정맥

E *vein, ven(i)- (veno-), venipuncture (venepuncture), venisection (venesection)* (phlebotomy), (vena >) *venation* (< 'arrangement of veins')

[용례] vena cava 대정맥

E *vena cava (cava),* (pl.) *venae cavae, caval*

vena cava superior 위대정맥, 상대정맥

vena cava inferior 아래대정맥, 하대정맥

(문법) vena 정맥: 단수 주격

　　　　cava 움푹한, 동굴의: 형용사, 여성형 단수 주격 < cavus, cava, cavum

　　　　superior 더 위의: 형용사 비교급, 남·여성형 단수 주격

　　　　　< superior, superior, superius

　　　　inferior 더 아래의: 형용사 비교급, 남·여성형 단수 주격

　　　　　< inferior, inferior, inferius

> L. venosus, venosa, venosum 맥이 많은, 정맥의　　　　　　　**E** *venous, intravenous*

> L. venula, venulae, f. (< + -ula *diminutive suffix*) 세정맥　　**E** *venule, venular*

G. phleps, phlebos, f. *vein*　　　　　　　　　　　　　　　　**E** *phleb(o)-*

　> G. phlebotomia, phlebotomias, f. (< + tomē *cutting* < temnein *to cut*) *incision of a*

　　　vein, as for the letting of blood; needle puncture of a vein for the drawing of blood

　　　> L. phlebotomia, phlebotomiae, f. 정맥절개술, 사혈(瀉血), 방혈(放血);

　　　　　정맥천자(靜脈穿刺)　　　　　　　　　　**E** *phlebotomy (venisection, venesection)*

　> G. phlebotomos, phlebotomou, m. (< + tomos *piece cut off, slice, section* < temnein

　　　to cut) lancet used for phlebotomy

　　　> L. phlebotomus, phlebotomi, m. 정맥절개(천자)용 란셋; (Phlebotomus) (파리)

　　　　　플레보토무스속(屬)　　　　　　　　**E** *Phlebotomus (< 'bloodsucking sandflies')*

　> L. phlebitis, phlebitidis, f. (< + -itis *noun suffix denoting inflammation*)

　　　정맥염　　　　　　　　　　　　　**E** *phlebitis, (pl.) phlebitides, -phlebitis*

　　　> L. pylephlebitis, pylephlebitidis, f. (< *inflammation of the portal vein* < G.

　　　　　pylē *gate*) 문맥염　　　　　　　　　　　　　　**E** *pylephlebitis*

　　　> L. thrombophlebitis, thrombophlebitidis, f. (< G. thrombos *blood clot*) 혈전

　　　　　정맥염　　　　　　　　　　　　　　　　　　　**E** *thrombophlebitis*

　> L. phlebothrombosis, phlebothrombosis, f. (< G. thrombōsis *thrombosis*)

　　　정맥혈전증　　　　　　　　　　　　　　　　　**E** *phlebothrombosis*

< IE. bhle- *to blow* (Vide FLARE; *See* E. *flatus*)

E. *marrow*　　　　　　　　　　　　　　　　　　　　　　　**E** *marrow*

　< IE. mozgo- *marrow*

L. medulla, medullae, f. (< (*perhaps*) *influenced by* medius *middle*) 골수(骨髓); 수(髓),

　　　수질(髓質), 속질, 골; 알짜, 진수(眞髓)

　　　E *medulla, medulloblast (< 'an undifferentiated cell of the embryonic neural tube (medullary*
　　　tube, cerebromedullary tube) that may develop into either a neuroblast or a glioblast')

　　[용례] medulla ossium (*bone marrow*) 골수(骨髓)

　　　　　medulla spinalis (*spinal marrow, spinal cord*) 척수(脊髓), 등골

　　　　　medulla oblongata 연수(延髓), 숨뇌　　　　　　　　**E** *medulla oblongata*

(문법) medulla 수(髓): 단수 주격

　　　　ossium 뼈들의: 복수 속격 < os, ossis, n.

　　　　spinalis 등마루의, 척추의, 척수의: 형용사, 남·여성형 단수 주격

　　　　　< spinalis, spinale < spina, spinae, f. 가시, 등마루

　　　　oblongata 길쭉한, 장방형의, 연(延): 형용사, 여성형 단수 주격

　　　　　< oblongatus, oblongata, oblongatum (< ob- *before, toward(s),*

　　　　　　　over, against, away + longus *long*)

　> L. medullaris, medullare 골수(骨髓)의; 수(髓)의, 수질(髓質)의, 속질의;

　　　　진수(眞髓)의　　　　E *medullary, intramedullary, extramedullary, juxtamedullary*

　　　　[용례] conus medullaris 척수원추, 척수원뿔　　　E *conus medullaris*

　　　　　(문법) conus 원추: 단수 주격 < conus, coni, m.

　　　　　　　medullaris 수(髓)의: 남·여성형 단수 주격

< IE. (s)mer- *grease, fat*　　　　　　　　　　　　　　E *smear*

　> (*suggested*) G. myron, myrou, n. *fragrant oil, unguent*

　　> G. myristikos, myristikē, myristikon *fragrant*　E (Nux myristica *'nutmeg'* >) *myristic acid*

G. myelos, myelou, m. *bone marrow; spinal marrow* (< *the spinal cord seen within the*
　　spinal column's vertebral canal resembles the bone marrow within the medullary
　　cavities of long bones)

　　E *myel(o)-;* (*'bone marrow'* >) *myeloblast, myelocyte, myeloid;* (*'spinal marrow'* >)
　　myelin (< *'peripheral nerve marrow apparently identical to what could be found in
　　the spinal cord'*), *myelinate, demyelinate, unmyelinated, myelinize, -myelia*

　> L. myelitis, myelitidis, f. (< G. myelos *bone marrow, spinal marrow* + -itis
　　　noun suffix denoting inflammation) 골수염(骨髓炎);
　　　척수염(脊髓炎)　　　　E *myelitis; osteomyelitis; encephalomyelitis, poliomyelitis*

　> L. myelophthisis, myelophthisis, f. (< G. myelos *bone marrow, spinal marrow*
　　　+ phthisis *wasting*) 골수로(骨髓癆); 척수로(脊髓癆)　　E *myelophthisis*

　> L. myeloma, myelomatis, n. (< G. myelos *bone marrow* + -ōma *noun suffix*
　　　denoting tumor) 골수종(骨髓腫)　　　　　E *myeloma*

　> L. myelencephalon, myelencephali, n. (< G. myelos *spinal marrow* + en-
　　　kephalon *brain*) 숨뇌, 연수(延髓)　　　E *myelencephalon*

　> L. hydromyelia, hydromyeliae, f. (< *dilatation of the central canal of the*
　　　spinal cord < G. hydōr *water* + myelos *spinal marrow*) 물척수증, 수척수증
　　　(水脊髓症)　　　　E *hydromyelia*

　> L. syringomyelia, syringomyeliae, f. (< G. syrinx *water cavity* + myelos *spinal*
　　　marrow) 척수구멍증, 척수공동증(脊髓空洞症)　　E *syringomyelia*

　< G. (*probably*) myōn, myōnos, m. *muscle, cluster of muscles*

< IE. mus- *mouse; also a muscle, from the resemblance of a flexing muscle to the movements*
　of a mouse (Vide MUSCULUS; *See* E. *muscle*)

E. *fat*　　　　　　　　　　　　　　　　　　　　　　　E *fat*

< IE. peiə- *to be fat, to swell* (Vide PINUS: *See* E. *pine*)

> G. piōn, piōn, pion *fat, plump; fertile; rich*

> **E** (pro- *'before, in front'* + piōn >) ***propionic acid*** (< *'being the first in the order of the carboxylic acid series to form fatty compounds; formic (methanoic) and acetic (ethanoic) acids, which precede it in the series, lack this property'*), ***propane, propyl, propylene,*** *(iso- + pr(opyl)ene* >) ***isoprene, isoprenoid***

L. adeps, adipis, m., f. 지방(脂肪),

비계   **E** ***adip(o)-,*** (adeps *'fat'* + cera *'wax'* >) ***adipocere; adipocyte*** (*adipose cell*)

> L. adiposus, adiposa, adiposum 지방이 많은, 지방의   **E** *adipose*

< IE. leip- *to stick, to adhere; fat*

> **E** *life* (< *'continuance'*), *live, alive, liver* (< *'formerly thought to be the organ producing blood, a source of life'*), *leave* (< *'to have remaining'*), ***delay, relay***

> G. lipos, lipou, n. *fat, oil*

> **E** ***lip(o)-, lipid(s), lipase, phospholipid(s)*** (< *'any lipid containing a phosphate group'*), ***glycolipid(s)*** (< *'any lipid containing a carbohydrate or carbohydrate derivative, especially a sugar'*), ***lipopolysaccharide(s), lipoprotein(s), lipofuscin, lipoblast, lipocyte*** (*fat cell, adipose cell (adipocyte)*), ***lipophilic, liposome, lipoid(s), lipoic acid***

> G. aleiphein *to anoint with oil*

> G. aleiphar, aleiphatos, n. *anointing-oil*

> **E** *aliphatic* (< *'organic compounds in which carbon atoms form open chains, not aromatic rings'*)

L. sebum, sebi, n. 수지(獸脂), 비계, 피지(皮脂), 피부기름   **E** *sebum, suet*

> L. sebaceus, sebacea, sebaceum 피지의, 피부기름의   **E** *sebaceous*

> L. seborrhoea, seborrhoeae, f. (< L. sebum *suet, grease* + rhoia *flow*) 지루(脂漏),

기름흐름   **E** *seborrhoea (seborrhea), seborrheic*

< IE. seib- *to pour out, to sieve, to drip, to trickle*

> **E** ***seep, soap*** (< *'originally a reddish hair dye used by Germanic warriors to give a frightening appearance'* < *'dripping'*), ***sieve, sift***

> L. sapo, saponis, m. (< *dripping*) 비누

> **E** ***saponin(s)*** (< *'steroid glycosides obtained from plants, which are usually toxic (especially to fish), and are characterized by the property of soap-like foaming in aqueous solution'*)

> L. saponifico, **saponificavi**, saponificatum, saponificare 비누로 만들다,

비누화하다   **E** *saponify, saponification*

L. lardum, lardi, n. (lardum, laridi, n.) (돼지) 비계, 라드   **E** *lard*

> L. lardaceus, lardacea, lardaceum (돼지) 비계의, 라드의   **E** *lardaceous*

< IE. lai- *fat* (Vide LARGUS: *See* E. *large*)

G. stear, steatos, m. *solid fat, suet, tallow*　**E** *steat(o)- (stear(o)-), stearic acid* (< *'found in tallow'*)

  > L. steatosis, steatosis, f. (< *abnormal accumulation of fat within parenchymal*

     cells < + G. -ōsis *condition*) 지방증(脂肪症)　**E** *steatosis*

  > L. steatoma, steatomatis, n. (< + G. -ōma *noun suffix denoting tumor*) 지방종(脂肪腫),

    피지낭종(皮脂囊腫)　**E** *steatoma*

     > L. cholesteatoma, cholesteatomatis, n. (< *fatty tumor principally composed*

      of crystals of cholesterol < *cholesterol*) 진주종(眞珠腫)　**E** *cholesteatoma*

  > L. steatorrhoea, steatorrhoeae, f. (< + G. rhoia *flow*)

    지방변증(脂肪便症)　**E** *steatorrhoea (steatorrhea), steatorrheal*

 < IE. stai- *stone; to become thick, to compress,*

    to stiffen　**E** *stone, brimstone* (< *'burning stone'*), (Swedish) *tungsten* (< *'heavy stone'*)

  > L. stiria, stiriae, f. 고드름

    > L. stilla, stillae, f. (< + -illa *diminutive suffix*) 물방울

      > L. stillo, stillavi, stillatum, stillare 방울방울 떨어지다, 방울져 떨어지게 하다

        > L. distillo, distillavi, distillatum, distillare (< di- (< dis-) *apart from,*

         down, not) 방울져 떨어지다, 방울져 떨어지게 하다,

         증류하다　**E** *distil (distill), distillate, distillation*

        > L. instillo, instillavi, instillatum, instillare (< in- *in, on, into,*

         toward) 한 방울씩 주입하다, 서서히 가르쳐 주다, 암시하다,

         속삭이다　**E** *instil (instill), instillation*

E. *wax*　**E** *wax*

 < IE. wokso- *wax* (< (*perhaps*) *that which grows*) (Vide VELLUM: *See* E. *vellum*)

L. cera, cerae, f. 밀랍(蜜蠟), 밀초[蜜燭], 밀랍목판

  E (cera + amide > *'N-acylsphingosine'* >) *ceramide(s)*, (adeps *'fat'* + cera *'wax'* >) *adipocere, ceroid* (< *'wax-like'*)

  > L. cereus, cerea, cereum 밀랍의, 밀초 빛의, 밀초같이 나긋나긋한

    [용례] Bacillus cereus (< *wax-like colonies on blood agar*) 바실루스

      세레우스　**E** Bacillus cereus

     (문법) Bacillus 바실루스속(屬): 단수 주격

        < bacillus, bacilli, m. 작은 막대기, 막대균, 간균(桿菌),

         바실루스; (Bacillus) (세균) 바실루스속(屬)

        < baculus, baculi, m. (baculum, baculi, n.) 지팡이, 막대기

      cereus 밀초 빛의: 형용사, 남성형 단수 주격

    > L. cerumen, ceruminis, n. 귀지, 이구(耳垢)　**E** *cerumen, ceruminal (ceruminous)*

 < G. kēros, kērou, m.

    wax　**E** *kerosene* (< *'denotes the crude mineral oil from which kerosene is obtained'*)

    > G. kērion, kēriou, n. (< + -ion *diminutive suffix*) *honeycomb*

      > L. kerion, kerii, n. (< *a pustular folliculitis of the scalp*) 백선종창(白癬

      腫瘡), 독창(禿瘡)　**E** *kerion*

L. olivum, olivi, n. (> oleum, olei, n.) 올리브 기름, 기름

> **E** *oil, oleic acid, linoleic acid* (< 'found in linseed oil'), *linolenic acid* (< 'more unsaturated linoleic acid'), *-ol, -ole,* (linum 'flax' + oleum 'oil' > 'made by coating canvas with oxidized linseed oil' >) *linoleum*

> L. petroleum, petrolei, n. (< *mineral oil formed by the decomposition of organic matter and present in some rock formations (sometimes seeping out on to the ground)* < petra (< G. petra) *rock* + oleum (< G. elaion) *oil*) 석유(石油)

> **E** *petroleum, petrol* (< 'a light fuel oil made by distilling petroleum'), *petrolatum* (< 'petroleum jelly such as Vaseline®')

< G. elaion, elaiou, n. *olive oil*

> **E** *elaioplast, elaidic acid* (< 'trans isomer of oleic acid'), (D. Wasser 'water' + elaion + -ine >) *Vaseline®*

< G. elaia, elaias, f. (< *elaiwa) *olive tree, olive*

> L. oliva, olivae, f. (> olea, oleae, f.) 올리브 나무, 올리브 열매　　**E** *olive*

> L. olivarius, olivaria, olivarium 올리브의　　**E** *olivary*

< *Of Mediterranean origin*

L. unguentum, unguenti, n. 기름, 향료, 연고, 고약　　**E** *unguent, ointment*

< L. unguo, unxi, unctum, unguěre (ungo, unxi, unctum, ungěre) 기름을 바르다, 향료를 바르다

> L. unctio, unctionis, f. 기름 바름, 도유(塗油), 연고, 고약, 운동연습　　**E** *unction*

> L. unctum, uncti, n. 바르는 기름

> L. unctuosus, unctuosa, unctuosum 기름 바른, 기름기 있는, 기름 같은, 겉으로의　　**E** *unctuous*

> L. inunguo, inunxi, inunctum, inunguěre (inungo, inunxi, inunctum, inungěre) (< in- *in, on, into, toward* + unguěre *to smear, to anoint*) ~ 위에 기름을 바르다　　**E** *anoint, inunction*

< IE. ong^w- *to salve, to anoint*

G. chrisma, chrismatos, n. (chrima, chrimatos, n.) *unguent, oil*

> L. chrisma, chrismatis, n. 기름, 기름 바름, 도유(塗油), 성유(聖油)　　**E** *chrism, cream*

< G. chriein *to anoint*

> G. christos, christē, christon *anointed*

> G. Christos, Christou, m. (< (*Hebrew*) masiah *messiah, anointed*) *the Anointed One, the Christ*

> L. Christus, Christi, m. 그리스도　　**E** *Christ*

> L. christianus, christiana, christianum 그리스도의, 그리스도교의

> **E** *Christian, cretin* (< 'wretched, innocent victim'), *cretinism*

< IE. ghrei- *to rub*

E *grisly* (< 'to grate on the mind')

E. *water*

    < IE. wed- *water, wet* (Vide UNDA: *See* E. *undulate*)

E *water*

L. aqua, aquae, f. 물

    < IE. akʷa- *water* (Vide AQUA: *See* E. *aqueous*)

E *aqua-*

G. hydōr, hydatos, n. *water*

    < IE. wed- *water, wet* (Vide UNDA: *See* E. *undulate*)

E *hydr(o)-* (< 'water or hydrogen')

E. *blood*

    < IE. bhle- *to thrive, to bloom* (Vide FLOS: *See* E. *floral*)

E *blood*

L. sanguis, sanguinis, m. 피 [血]

    > L. sanguineus, sanguinea, sanguineum 피의, 핏빛의,

      피비린내 나는

E *sanguin(o)- (sangui-)*

E *sanguineous (sanguine), serosanguineous*

        > L. consanguineus, consanguinea, consanguineum (< con- (< cum) *with,*

           together + sangineus *of blood*) 같은 핏줄의,

           혈연관계의

E *consanguineous (consanguine, consanguineal)*

           > L. consanguinitas, consanguinitatis, f. 혈족, 친족

E *consanguinity*

    > L. sanguinarius sanguinaria, sanguinarium 피에 관한, 피 흘리는, 피투성이의, 피에

      굶주린

E *sanguinary*

    > L. exsanguino, exsanguinavi, exsanguinatum, exsanguinare (< ex- *out of, away from*

      + sanguis *blood*) 피를 빼내다, 피가 빠지다

E *exsanguination*

    > L. *sanguicolus, *sanguicola, *sanguicolum (< sanguis *blood* + -colus *inhabiting*)

      혈액에서 사는, 혈액 속에서 기생하는

E *sanguicolous*

    > L. *sanguivorus, *sanguivora, *sanguivorum (< sanguis *blood* + -vorus *devouring*)

      흡혈성의

E *sanguivorous*

G. haima, haimatos, n. *blood*

E *haemat(o)- (hemat(o)-),* (krites *'judge'* >) *haematocrit (hematocrit)* (< 'a centrifuge used to estimate the volume occupied by the red blood cells in a sample of blood; the value obtained, expressed as a percentage of the volume of the sample'), (haematoglobulin >) *haemoglobin (hemoglobin),* (haemoglobin (hemoglobin) >) *haem (heme), haematin (hematin), haem(o)- (hem(o)-), -aemia (-emia), -aemic (-emic)*

    > G. haimorrhagia, haimorrhagias, f. (< + -rrhagia < -rrhag- *stem of* rhēgnynai *to*

      break, to burst) hemorrhage

        > L. haemorrhagia, haemorrhagiae, f. 출혈(出血)

E *haemorrhage (hemorrhage)*

> G. haimorrhagikos, haimorrhagikos, haimorrhagikon *of hemorrhage*

> L. haemorrhagicus, haemorrhagica, haemorrhagicum (hemorrhagicus, hemorrhagica, hemorrhagicum) 출혈의   **E** *haemorrhagic (hemorrhagic)*

[용례] corpus hemorrhagicum 출혈체   **E** *corpus hemorrhagicum*
(문법) corpus 몸, 체(體): 단수 주격 < corpus, corporis, n.
hemorrhagicum 출혈의: 형용사, 중성형 단수 주격

> G. haimatoun (haimatoein) *to turn into blood*

> G. *haimatoma, *haimatomatos, n. (< + -ōma *noun suffix denoting tumor*)
a bloody tumor, a bloody fungus, a swelling containing blood

> L. haematoma, haematomatis, n. 혈종
(血腫)   **E** *haematoma (hematoma)* (< 'blood within tissue'), *hematomatous*

> G. haimorrhois, haimorrhoidos, f. (< + -rrhoos (< rhein (rheein) *to flow*) *stream*)
blood discharging

> L. haemorrhoida, haemorrhoidae, f.
치핵(痔核)   **E** *haemorrhoid (hemorrhoid), hemorrhoidal*

> G. hyphaimos, hyphaimos, hyphaimon (< hyph- (< hypo) *under* + haima) *suffused
with blood, bloodshot, especially
of the eyes*   **E** *hyphema* (< 'hemorrhage within the anterior chamber of the eye')

> G. haimas, haimados, f. *blood stream*   **E** *hemadostenosis* (< 'narrowing of a blood vessel')

> G. anaimia, anaimias, f. (< an- *not* + haima + -ia *noun suffix*) *anemia*

> L. anaemia, anaemiae, f. (anemia, anemiae, f.) 빈혈(貧血)   **E** *anaemia (anemia), anemic*

> L. polycythaemia, polycythaemiae, f. (polycythemia, polycythemiae, f.) (< G. polys
many + kytos *hollow vessel* + haima + -ia)
적혈구증가증   **E** *polycythaemia (polycythemia), polycythemic*

[용례] polycythemia vera 진성(眞性) 적혈구증가증   **E** *polycythemia vera*
(문법) polycythemia 적혈구증가증: 단수 주격
vera 참된: 형용사, 여성형 단수 주격 < verus, vera, verum

> L. erythraemia, erythraemiae, f. (< G. erythros *red* + haima + -ia) 진성(眞性) 적혈구
증가증(*polycythemia vera*)   **E** *erythraemia (erythremia)*

> L. leukaemia, leukaemiae, f. (< G. leukos *white* + haima + -ia)
백혈병(白血病)   **E** *leukaemia (leukemia), leukemic, leukemoid*

> L. hyperaemia, hyperaemiae, f. (< G. hyper- *over* + haima + -ia)
충혈(充血)   **E** *hyperaemia (hyperemia), hyperemic*

> L. hypervolaemia, hypervolaemiae, f. (< G. hyper- *over* + *volume* + haima + -ia)
혈액량증가   **E** *hypervolaemia (hypervolemia), hypervolemic*

> L. hypovolaemia, hypovolaemiae, f. (< G. hyp(o)- *under* + *volume* + haima + -ia)
혈액량감가   **E** *hypovolaemia (hypovolemia), hypovolemic*

> L. hyperglycaemia, hyperglycaemiae, f. (< G. hyper- *over* + glykys *sweet* + haima
+ -ia) 고혈당(증)   **E** *hyperglycaemia (hyperglycemia), hyperglycemic*

> L. hypoglycaemia, hypoglycaemiae, f. (< G. hyp(o)- *under* + glykys *sweet* + haima

+ -ia) 저혈당(증)

E *hypoglycaemia (hypoglycemia), hypoglycemic*

> L. haemophilia, haemophiliae, f. (< *bleeding tendency* < + G. philia *affection*)

혈우병(血友病)

E *haemophilia (hemophilia), hemophilic, hemophiliac*

> L. Haemophilus, Haemophili, m. (< *requiring growth factors present in blood* < +

G. philos *affecting*) (세균) 헤모필루스속(屬)

E Haemophilus

[용례] Haemophilus influenzae 인플루엔자균

E Haemophilus influenzae

(문법) Haemophilus 헤모필루스속: 단수 주격

influenzae 인플루엔자의: 단수 속격 < influenza, influenzae, f.

< IE. sai- *thick fluid*

E. *gall*

E *gall*

< IE. ghel- *to shine; with derivatives referring to colors, bright materials, gold (probably 'yellow metal'), and bile or gall* (Vide FULVUS; See E. *fulvous*)

L. bilis, bilis, f. 쓸개즙, 담즙

E *bile, bilirubin (< 'a reddish pigment occurring in bile'), biliverdin (< 'a green pigment occurring in bile'), urobilinogen, stercobilinogen*

> L. biliosus, biliosa, biliosum 쓸개즙이 많은, 쓸개즙의, 담즙의, 담즙 이상에서 생기는 **E** *bilious*

> L. biliaris, biliare 쓸개즙의, 담즙의 **E** *biliary*

< IE. bistli-s *bile*

L. fel, fellis, n. 쓸개즙, 담즙, 쓸개

> L. felleus, fellea, felleum 쓸개즙의, 담즙의

G. cholē, cholēs, f. *bile, gall*

E *chol(o)- (chole-)*

< IE. ghel- *to shine; with derivatives referring to colors, bright materials, gold (probably 'yellow metal'), and bile or gall* (Vide FULVUS; See E. *fulvous*)

E. *spittle*

E *spittle*

< IE. sp(y)eu- *to spit, to spew* (Vide SPUTUM; See E. *sputum*)

L. saliva, salivae, f. 침, 타액

E *saliva*

> L. salivarius, salivaria, salivarium 침의, 침샘의 **E** *salivary*

> L. salivo, -, salivatum, salivare 침을 흘리다 **E** *salivate*

< IE. sal- *dirty, gray* **E** *sallow*

> IE. sal(i)k- *willow*

> L. salix, salicis, f. 버드나무 (Vide SALIX; See E. *salicin*)

G. sialon, sialou, n. *spittle, saliva*

E *sial(o)-, sialism (ptyalism), sialic acid(s)* (< 'isolated from the salivary glands of cattle; an N-acyl derivative of neuraminic acid'), *sialogram* (< 'radiograph of salivary ducts')

   < IE. sp(y)eu- *to spit, to spew* (Vide SPUTUM: *See* E. *sputum*)

      > G. ptyein *to spit*

         > G. ptysis, ptyseōs, f. *spitting*   **E** *-ptysis* (< 'expectoration')

         > G. ptyalon, ptyalou, n. *spittle,*

             saliva   **E** *ptyal(o)-, ptyalism (sialism), ptyalin (salivary amylase)*

E. *dung*   **E** *dung*

   < IE. dhengh-, dhngh- *to cover, to lie upon*

E. *stool* (< *a wooden seat, the place of evacuation, the matter evacuated*)   **E** *stool*

   < IE. sta- *to stand, with derivatives meaning 'place or thing that is standing'* (Vide STARE: *See* E. *stay*)

L. **faex, faecis, f.** 찌꺼기, 앙금, 재강, 지게미, 버캐, 젓갈; 똥, 대변(大便),

   분변(糞便) **E** *(pl.)* *faeces (feces);* (faex 'dregs' + G. lithos 'stone' >) *fecalith (stercolith, coprolith)*

   > L. faecalis, faecale 찌꺼기의; 대변의   **E** *faecal (fecal)*

   > L. faecula, faeculae, f. (< + -ula *diminutive suffix*) 지게미, 술찌끼, 주석(酒石),

       젓갈   **E** *faecula (fecula)*

      > L. faeculentus, faeculenta, faeculentum 찌꺼기가 많은, 불순한   **E** *faeculent (feculent)*

   > L. defaeco, **defaecavi**, defaecatum, defaecare (< de- *apart from, down, not* + faex

       dregs) 깨끗이 하다, 똥 싸다   **E** *defaecate (defecate)*

      > L. defaecatio, defaecationis, f. 정화, 순화, 배변   **E** *defaecation (defecation)*

L. **stercus, stercoris, n.** 똥, 거름, 두엄, 찌꺼기,

   톱밥   **E** *sterc(o)-;* (stercus 'dung' + G. lithos 'stone' >) *stercolith (fecalith, coprolith)*

   > L. stercoralis, stercorale 똥의, 거름의   **E** *stercoral (stercoraceous)*

   > L. stercoraceus, stercoracea, stercoraceum 똥의, 거름의   **E** *stercoraceous (stercoral)*

   < IE. sker- *excrement, dung*   **E** *dreck*

      > G. skōr, skatos, n. *dung*

          E *scat(o)- (skat(o)-), scatology, scatacratia* (< 'fecal incontinence'), *skatole (scatol)* (< 'produced from tryptophan in the mammalian digestive tract')

        > G. skōria, skōrias, f. *slag, dross*

           > L. scoria, scoriae, f. 쇠똥; 광재(鑛滓), 화산암의 암재(岩滓)   **E** *scoria*

G. **kopros, koprou, f.** *dung*

       E *copr(o)-, coprophagous, coprolalia,* (kopros + lithos 'stone' >) *coprolith (fecalith, stercolith)*

   > L. encopresis, encopresis, f. (< *incontinence of feces not due to organic defect or*

illness < G. en- *in*) 대변찔끔, 유분증(遺糞症)   **E** *encopresis*

  < IE. kek^w- *excrement*

(*Quechua*) huanu *dung*

    > Sp. huano *the excrement of seabirds, used as fertilizer*

      E *guano, guanine (G) (< 'obtained abundantly from guano, forming a constituent of the excrement of birds'), guanosine (G), guanidine (< 'isolated by the degradation of guanine')*

E. *yolk*   **E** *yolk*

   < IE. ghel- *to shine; with derivatives referring to colors, bright materials, gold (probably 'yellow metal'), and bile or gall* (Vide FULVUS; *See* E. *fulvous*)

L. vitellus, vitelli, m. (< + -ellus *diminutive suffix*) 송아지, 귀염둥이; 계란 노른자위,

     난황(卵黃)   **E** *veal, vellum;* (vitellus ovi *'yolk of egg'* >) *vitellin*

       > L. vitellinus, vitellina, vitellinum 난황(卵黃)의   **E** *vitelline*

    < L. vitulus, vituli, m. 송아지, 동물의 새끼

  < IE. wet- *year* (Vide VITULUS; *See* E. *veal*)

G. lekithos, lekithou, m. *egg yolk*

      E *lecith(o)-, lecithin(s) (< 'isolated from egg yolk; phosphatidylcholine and related phospholipids, sometimes used as a synonym for pure phosphatidylcholine')*

  < (*probably*) *Of* non-IE. *origin*

E. *fever*

     < L. febris, febris, f. 열, 열병

   < IE. dheg^wh- *to burn, to warm* (Vide infra)

L. febris, febris, f. 열, 열병   **E** *fever, feverish, febrifuge*

     > L. febrilis, febrile 열의, 열성(熱性)의, 열병의   **E** *febrile*

  < IE. dheg^wh- *to burn, to warm*

     > L. foveo, fovi, fotum, fovēre 따뜻하게 하다, 품다

       > L. fomentum, fomenti, n. (< *fovimetum) 불쏘시개, 찜질   **E** *foment, fomentation*

       > L. fomes, fomitis, m. 불씨, 불쏘시개, 도화선; 매개물, 계기

         E *fomes,* (pl.) *fomites, (fomites > (incorrect back-formation for* sing.*) >) fomite (fomes)*

G. pyr, pyros, n. *fire; fever*

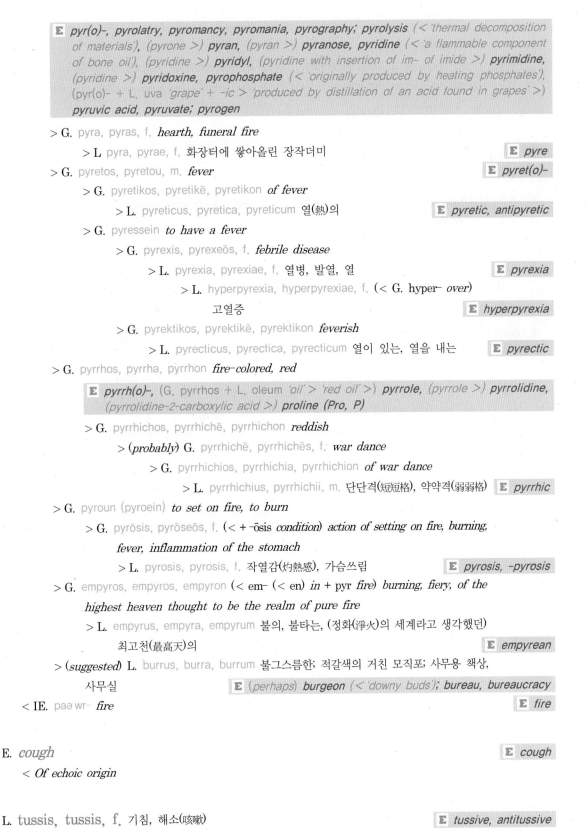

E *pyr(o)-, pyrolatry, pyromancy, pyromania, pyrography; pyrolysis (< 'thermal decomposition of materials'), (pyrone >) pyran, (pyran >) pyranose, pyridine (< 'a flammable component of bone oil'), (pyridine >) pyridyl, (pyridine with insertion of im- of imide >) pyrimidine, (pyridine >) pyridoxine, pyrophosphate (< 'originally produced by heating phosphates'), (pyr(o)- + L. uva 'grape' + -ic > 'produced by distillation of an acid found in grapes' >) pyruvic acid, pyruvate; pyrogen*

> G. pyra, pyras, f. *hearth, funeral fire*

> L pyra, pyrae, f. 화장터에 쌓아올린 장작더미 　　**E** *pyre*

> G. pyretos, pyretou, m. *fever* 　　**E** *pyret(o)-*

> G. pyretikos, pyretikē, pyretikon *of fever*

> L. pyreticus, pyretica, pyreticum 열(熱)의 　　**E** *pyretic, antipyretic*

> G. pyressein *to have a fever*

> G. pyrexis, pyrexeōs, f. *febrile disease*

> L. pyrexia, pyrexiae, f. 열병, 발열, 열 　　**E** *pyrexia*

> L. hyperpyrexia, hyperpyrexiae, f. (< G. hyper- *over*)

고열증 　　**E** *hyperpyrexia*

> G. pyrektikos, pyrektikē, pyrektikon *feverish*

> L. pyrecticus, pyrectica, pyrecticum 열이 있는, 열을 내는 　　**E** *pyrectic*

> G. pyrrhos, pyrrha, pyrrhon *fire-colored, red*

E *pyrrh(o)-, (G. pyrrhos + L. oleum 'oil' > 'red oil' >) pyrrole, (pyrrole >) pyrrolidine, (pyrrolidine-2-carboxylic acid >) proline (Pro, P)*

> G. pyrrhichos, pyrrhichē, pyrrhichon *reddish*

> (*probably*) G. pyrrhichē, pyrrhichēs, f. *war dance*

> G. pyrrhichios, pyrrhichia, pyrrhichion *of war dance*

> L. pyrrhichius, pyrrhichii, m. 단단격(短短格), 약약격(弱弱格) 　**E** *pyrrhic*

> G. pyroun (pyroein) *to set on fire, to burn*

> G. pyrōsis, pyrōseōs, f. (< + -ōsis *condition*) *action of setting on fire, burning, fever, inflammation of the stomach*

> L. pyrosis, pyrosis, f. 작열감(灼熱感), 가슴쓰림 　　**E** *pyrosis, -pyrosis*

> G. empyros, empyros, empyron (< em- (< en) *in* + pyr *fire*) *burning, fiery, of the highest heaven thought to be the realm of pure fire*

> L. empyrus, empyra, empyrum 불의, 불타는, (정화(淨火)의 세계라고 생각했던)

최고천(最高天)의 　　**E** *empyrean*

> (*suggested*) L. burrus, burra, burrum 불그스름한; 적갈색의 거친 모직포; 사무용 책상,

사무실 　　**E** *(perhaps) burgeon (< 'downy buds'); bureau, bureaucracy*

< IE. paəwr- *fire* 　　**E** *fire*

E. *cough* 　　**E** *cough*

< *Of echoic origin*

L. tussis, tussis, f. 기침, 해소(咳嗽) 　　**E** *tussive, antitussive*

> L. pertussis, pertussis, f. (< per- *through, thoroughly* + tussis *cough*)
백일해(百日咳)

E *pertussis*

< IE. (s)teu- *to push, to stick, to knock, to beat; with derivatives referring to projecting objects, fragments, and certain related expressive notions and qualities* (Vide TUNDĒRE: *See* E. *contusion*)

G. bēx, bēchos, m., f. *cough*

E *bechic*

E. *ache* (< (perhaps) *to cause mental pain*)

E *ache, headache, earache, toothache, stomachache*

< IE. ag-es- *fault, guilt*

E. *sore*

E *sore, bedsore*

< IE. sai- *suffering*

E *sorry* (< *'suffering mentally, sad'*)

E. *pain*

E *pain, painful, painless, painkiller, painstaking*

< L. poena, poenae, f. 벌(罰)

E *penology, pine, (pine >) repine*

> L. punio, punivi (punii), punitum, punire 벌하다 **E** *punish, punishment, punitive*

> L. poenalis, poenale 형(刑)의, 형벌의

E *penal*

> L. poenalitas, poenalitatis, f. 형벌, 처벌

E *penalty*

> L. impunis, impune (< im- (< in-) *not*) (형사상) 면책의

> L. impunitas, impunitatis, f. (형사상) 면책

E *impunity*

> L. subpoena, subpoenae, f. (< sub poena *under a penalty, being the first words of the writ*) (불응시 벌칙이 따르는) 소환장

E *subpoena*

< G. poinē, poinēs, f. *ransom, requital, vengeance, penalty, punishment*

< IE. kʷei- *to pay, to atone, to compensate*

L. dolor, doloris, m. 아픔, 고통, 통증

E *dolor (dolour),* F. *douloureux*

< L. doleo, dolui, dolitum, dolēre 아프다, 괴로워하다

> L. dolens, (gen.) dolentis (*present participle*) 아픈, 괴로운

E *dolent*

> L. indolens, (gen.) indolentis (< in- *not*) 무통성의, 나태한

E *indolent*

< IE. del(ə)- *to split, to carve, to cut* (Vide DOLOR: *See* E. *dolor*)

G. algos, algeos, n. *pain, sorrow, grief*

E *alg(o)-, -algia, arthralgia, cephalalgia, gastralgia, mastalgia, metralgia, myalgia, neuralgia, odontalgia, otalgia, pleuralgia, podalgia, spondylalgia, thoracalgia*

> L. algophobia, algophobiae, f. (< + G. -phobia *fear*) 통증공포증 **E** *algophobia*

> L. nostalgia, nostalgiae, f. (< G. nostos *return home* + algos *pain* + -ia *noun suffix*) 향수(鄕愁)

E *nostalgia*

> L. causalgia, causalgiae, f. (< *burning pain* < G. kausos *heat* + algos + -ia)

작열통(灼熱痛)   **E** *causalgia (thermalgia), causalgic*

> L. *thermalgia, *thermalgiae, f. (< *burning pain* < G. thermē *heat* + algos +

-ia) 작열통(灼熱痛)   **E** *thermalgia (causalgia)*

> L. *synalgia, *synalgiae, f. (< G. syn- *with, together* + algos + -ia)

연관통증   **E** *synalgia (< 'referred pain')*

> L. *pantalgia, *pantalgiae, f. (< G. pant(o)- *all* + algos + -ia) 전신통증   **E** *pantalgia*

> L. *analgia, *analgiae, f. (< G. an- *not* + algos + -ia) 진통(鎭痛),

무통증   **E** *analgia (analgesia), analgic (analgetic, analgesic)*

< G. algein (algeein) *to suffer, to feel pain, to be troubled or sad, to grieve*

> G. algēsis, algēseōs, f. *pain, grief, sorrow*

> G. analgēsia, analgēsias, f. (< an- *not* + algēsis + -ia) *painlessness,*
lack of feeling

> L. analgesia, analgesiae, f. 진통(鎭痛),

무통증   **E** *analgesia, analgetic (analgesic) (analgic)*

> L. hyperalgesia, hyperalgesiae, f. (< G. hyper- *over* + algēsis + -ia)

통각과민   **E** *hyperalgesia*

> L. *thermalgesia, *thermalgesiae, f. (< *a dysesthesia in which the*
application of heat produces pain < G. thermē *heat* + algēsis + -ia)

열통증   **E** *thermalgesia, hyperthermalgesia*

G. odynē, odynēs, f. *gnawing care* > *pain, grief*

> **E** *odyn(o)-, -odynia, arthrodynia, cephalodynia, gastrodynia, mastodynia, metrodynia, myodynia, neurodynia, odontodynia, otodynia, pleurodynia, pododynia, spondylodynia, thoracodynia*

> G. anōdynos, anōdynos, anōdynon (< an- *not* + odynē) *painless, easing pain*

> L. anodynus, anodyna, anodynum 고통 없는, 진통의   **E** *anodyne*

> L. *odynophagia, *odynophagiae, f. (< + G. -phagia *eating*)

연하통(嚥下痛)   **E** *odynophagia (odynphagia)*

< G. odynan (odynaein) *to cause pain;* (*passive*) *to feel pain, to suffer*

< IE. ed- *to eat; original meaning 'to bite'* (Vide EDĚRE: *See* E. *edible*)

E. *death*   **E** *death*

< IE. dheu-, dheuə- *to die*   **E** *dead, die, dwindle*

L. mors, mortis, f. 죽음, 주검; (Mors) (로마 신화) 죽음의 신   **E** *Mors, mortal, immortal*

< IE. mer- *to rub away, to harm* (Vide MORI: *See* E. *mortal*)

G. thanatos, thanatou, m. *death, murder, execution;* (Thanatos) (*Greek mythology*) *the god*
of death   **E** *Thanatos, thanatology*

> G. athanasia, athanasias, f. (< a- *not* + thanatos) *immortality*

> L. athanasia, athanasiae, f. 불사, 불멸

> **E** *athanasia (athanasy),* *(athanasia >)* *tansy* *(< 'probably referring to the long persistence of the flowers')*

> G. euthanasia, euthanasias, f. (< eu- *well* + thanatos) *easy death, happy death, mercy killing*

> L. euthanasia, euthanasiae, f. 고통 없는 죽음, 안락사(安樂死) **E** *euthanasia, euthanize*

< IE. dhwenə- *to disappear, to die*

E. *mask*

E *mask*

< It. maschera *mask*

E *masque, masquerade, mascara*

< (*possibly*) (*Arabic*) maskhara *clown, buffoonery*

> L. masca, mascae, f. 마스크, 여자 마술사

E *mascot*

E. persona, personae, f. (광대의) 탈, 역할, 인격, 인물; (문법) 인칭

E *persona,* (pl.) *personae, person, parson, personate, impersonate* *(< 'on the pattern of incorporate'),* *personify*

> L. personalis, personale 사람의, 개인의, 사사로운, 인격의; (문법) 인칭의

E *personal, personnel* *(< 'contrasted with material'),* *personalize, depersonalization, personalism*

> L. personalitas, personalitatis, f. 인격, 인성, 개성 **E** *personality*

< (*probably*) (*Etruscan*) phersu *mask*

G. prosōpon, prosōpou, n. (< pros *towards, near, beside(s)* + ōps *eye, face*) *face, appearance, mask (worn by actors), person*

E *prosop(o)-*

< IE. per *basic meanings of 'forward', 'through'* (Vide PER: *See* E. *per-*)

+ IE. okʷ- *to see* (Vide OCULUS: *See* E. *oculus*)

E. *cheese*

< L. caseus, casei, m. 치즈, 건락(乾酪) (Vide infra)

L. caseus, casei, m. 치즈, 건락(乾酪)

E *cheese, casein; caseate* *(< 'to undergo caseous necrosis'),* *caseation* *(< 'caseous necrosis')*

> L. caseosus, caseosa, caseosum 치즈가 많은, 치즈의, 치즈 같은 **E** *caseous*

< IE. kwat- *to ferment, to be sour*

G. tyros, tyrou, m. (< *swelling, coagulating*) *cheese* **E** *tyrosine (Tyr, Y)* *(< 'first discovered in casein')*

< IE. teuə-, teu- *to swell* (Vide TUMOR: *See* E. *tumor*)

E. *sausage* (< *salted*)　　　　　　　　　　　　　　　　　　　　　　　　　　　　　　　　　　　E *sausage*

　　　　　　< L. salio, salii, salitum (salsum), salire 소금 치다, 짜게 하다, 소금에 절이다

　　　　< L. sal, salis, m., n. 소금

　　< IE. sal- *salt* (Vide SAL; *See* E. *sal*)

L. botulus, botuli, m. 창자,

　　　순대　　　　　　　　E *bowel, disembowel,* (botulus + -in 'chemical suffix' >) *botulin, botulism*

　　> L. botulinus, botulina, botulinum 창자의, 순대의

　　　　[용례] Clostridium botulinum 클로스트리듐 보툴리눔

　　　　　　　　E *Clostridium botulinum,* (Clostridium botulinum >) *botulinum,* (botulinum toxin
　　　　　　　　>) *Botox®*

　　　　　　(문법) Clostridium (세균) 클로스트리듐속(屬): 단수 주격
　　　　　　　　< Clostridium, Clostridii, n.
　　　　　　botulinum 순대의: 형용사, 중성형 단수 주격

　　< IE. gʷet- *intestine*

G. allas, allantos, m. *sausage*　　　　E *allantiasis* (< 'botulism from sausages containing botulin')

　　> G. allantoeidēs, allantoeidēs, allantoeides (< + eidos *shape*) *sausage-shaped*　　E *allantoid*

　　　　> (*factitious*) L. allantois, allantois, f. (< *an initially sausage-shaped ventral
　　　　　　diverticulum of the hindgut of embryos of reptiles, birds, and mammals.
　　　　　　In reptiles and birds, it expands to a large sac for storing urine and,
　　　　　　after fusing with the chorion which lines the shell, provides for gas
　　　　　　exchange. The allantois is prominent in some mammals (carnivores,
　　　　　　ungulates); in others, including humans, it is vestigial except that its
　　　　　　blood vessels give rise to those of the umbilical cord*) 요막(尿膜), 요낭(尿囊)

　　　　　　E *allantois, allantoic, allantoin* (< 'the nitrogenous constituent of the allantoic
　　　　　　fluid'), (allantoin + oxalic acid + -an >) *alloxan*

　　< (*probably*) *Of Italic origin*

　　　　> L. allium, allii, n. (alium, alii, n.)

　　　　　마늘　　　　　　　　E *alliin,* (alliin >) *allicin, allyl* (< 'first obtained from garlic')

E. *thread*　　　　　　　　　　　　　　　　　　　　　　　　　　　　　　　　　　　　　　　E *thread*

　　< IE. terə- *to rub, to turn* (Vide TERĒRE; *See* E. *trite*)

L. filum, fili, n. 실

　　　　E *file* (< 'a string or wire, on which papers and documents are strung'), *fillet, filiform,
　　　　filovirus* (< 'thread-like structure'), (filum 'thread' + granum 'grain' >) *filigree, profile* (< 'to
　　　　draw forth in lines'); *filopodia*

　　[용례] filum terminale 종말끈, 종사(終絲)　　　　　　　　　　　　　　　　E *filum terminale*

(문법) filum 실: 단수 주격

terminale 경계선에 있는, 마지막의: 형용사, 중성형 단수 주격

< terminalis, terminale

> L. filo, −, −, filare 실 뽑다, 잣다

> L. filamentum, filamenti, n. 섬조(纖條), 수술의 화사(花絲), 잔섬유,

미세섬유 ・ **E** *filament, filamentous*

> L. filaria, filariae, f. 사상충(絲狀蟲) ・ **E** *filaria, filarial, filariasis*

> L. microfilaria, microfilariae, f. 미세사상충 ・ **E** *microfilaria*

> L. Dirofilaria, Dirofilariae, f. (< dirus *dreadful*) (사상충 絲狀蟲) 디로필라리아속(屬),

개사상충속(屬) ・ **E** *Dirofilaria, dirofilariasis*

< IE. gʷhi- *thread, tendon*

> L. (*possibly*) fibra, fibrae, f. 가는 줄, 섬유(纖維)

E *fiber (fibre), fibroblast, fibronectin, fibrinogen, fibrin, fibrinous, fibrinolysis, fibroin; fiberscope, fibrinoid*

> L. fibrosus, fibrosa, fibrosum 섬유가 많은, 섬유 모양의,

섬유성의 ・ **E** *fibrous, (adjective) fibrose*

> L. fibrosis, fibrosis, f. (< + G. -ōsis *condition*) 섬유증,

섬유화 ・ **E** *fibrosis, (fibrosis >) (verb) fibrose*

> L. fibrilla, fibrillae, f. (< + -illa *diminutive suffix*) 가는 섬유, 원섬유(原纖維)

E *fibrilla (fibril), fibrillar (fibrillary), fibrillin, fibrillate, fibrillation (< 'being fibrillar', 'uncoordinated contraction of muscle fibers'), defibrillation*

G. nēma, nēmatos, n. *thread* ・ **E** *nemat(o)-, nem(o)- (nema-), -nema (-neme)*

< IE. (s)ne- *to spin, to sew* (Vide NERVUS; *See* E. *nerve*)

G. mitos, mitou, m. *thread*

> L. mitosis, mitosis, f. (< + G. -ōsis *condition*) 유사(有絲)분열

E *mitosis, mitotic, endomitosis (endopolyploidy) (< 'division of chromosomes in a nucleus without subsequent division of the nucleus'), mitogen, mitomycin (< 'inhibition of DNA synthesis')*

> G. mitochondrion, mitochondriou, n. (< + chondrion, chondriou, n. *granule* < chondros, chondrou, m. *grain, lump, cartilage* + -ion, -iou, n. *diminutive suffix*)

> L. mitochondrion, mitochondrii, n. 사립체(絲粒體),

미토콘드리아 ・ **E** *mitochondrion, (pl.) mitochondria, mitochondrial*

< IE. mei- *to tie*

> G. mitra, mitras, f. *girdle, head-dress*

> L. mitra, mitrae, f. 고대 페르시아인의 챙 없는 모자, 주교관, 승모(僧帽) ・ **E** *mitre (miter)*

> L. mitralis, mitrale 주교관 모양의, 승모 모양의, 승모판(僧帽瓣)의 ・ **E** *mitral*

> (*Persian*) Mithras (< *contractual partner*) (페르시아 신화) 미트라 (빛과 진리의 신,

후에는 태양의 신; 조로아스터교에서는 선신과 악신의 중재자) ・ **E** *Mithras*

> G. Mithridatēs, Mithridatou, m. (< *gift of Mithras*) *the name of Mithridates VI, king of Pontus (134-63 B.C.E.), who was said to have rendered himself proof against poisons by administration of gradually increasing non-lethal doses*　　　**E** *mithridatism*

> (*Sanskrit*) Mitrah (< *contractual partner*) (바라문교) 미트라 (Veda에 나오는 정의와 우애의 신)　　　**E** *Mitra*

> (*Russian*) mir *world, peace*　　　**E** *mir*

E. *band*　　　**E** *band*

< IE. bhendh- *to bind*

> **E** *bind, woodbine, (band >) bandage, (band >) bond, ribbon, bundle, bend* (< *to put in bonds, to tension a bow by means of string*)

L. fascia, fasciae, f. 끈, 띠, 강보(襁褓), 붕대, 판(板), 막(膜), 근막(筋膜)　　　**E** *fascia*

[용례] fascia adherens 부착판　　　**E** *fascia adherens*

(문법) fascia 판: 단수 주격

adherens 부착하고 있는: 현재분사, 남·여·중성형 단수 주격

< adherens, (gen.) adherentis

< adhereo, adhesi, adhesum, adherēre 부착하다

> L. fascialis, fasciale 근막(筋膜)의　　　**E** *fascial*

> L. fasciola, fasciolae, f. (< + -ola *diminutive suffix*) 작은 띠, 작은 막; (Fasciola) 파시올라속(屬)　　　**E** *fasciola,* (pl.) *fasciolae;* Fasciola

> L. fasciolaris, fasciolare 작은 띠의, 작은 막의　　　**E** *fasciolar*

> L. fascio, fasciavi, fascitum, fasciare 끈으로 묶다, 기저귀로 싸다　　　**E** *fasciate*

< IE. bhasko- *band, bundle*

> L. fascis, fascis, m. 다발, 단, 속(束); (pl.) 고대 로마의 권표(權標)　　　**E** (pl.) *fasces, fascin,* It. *fascio, fascism*

> L. fasciculus, fasciculi, m. (< + -culus *diminutive suffix*) 작은 다발, 소속(小束), 속(束)

> **E** *fasciculus (fascicle),* (pl.) *fasciculi (fascicles), fascicular* (< *'of a fascicle'*), *fasciculation* (< *'being fasciculate', 'uncoordinated contraction of muscle fascicles'*)

> L. fasciculatus, fasciculata, fasciculatum 다발을 이룬, 다발 모양을 하고 있는, 속상(束狀)의　　　**E** *fasciculate*

G. tainia, tainias, f. *head-band, ribbon, tape*

> L. taenia, taeniae, f. (tenia, teniae, f.) 머리띠, 띠, 붕대; 촌충(寸蟲), 조충(條蟲)　　　**E** *taenia (tenia),* (pl.) *taeniae (teniae), -tene*

< IE. ten- *to stretch* (Vide TENĒRE; *See* E. *tenet*)

E. *spindle*　　　**E** *spindle*

< IE. (s)pen- *to draw, to stretch, to spin* (Vide PENDĒRE: *See* E. *poise*)

L. fusus, fusi, m. (fusum, fusi, n.) 물레 가락,

　　방추(紡錘)　　　　　　　　**E** *('detonating')* **fuse,** *('safety')* **fuse, fuselage** *(< 'its spindle-like shape')*

　　> L. fusiformis, fusiforme 방추형(紡錘形)의　　　　　　　**E** *fusiform*

　　> L. Fusarium, Fusarii, n. (< *fusiform macroconidia*)

　　　　(진균) 푸사륨속(屬)　　　　　　**E** Fusarium, *fusarial, fusariosis*

G. klōstēr, klōstēros, m. *spindle*

　　　　> G. klōstridion, klōstridiou, n. (< *small spindle-shaped because of the presence*

　　　　　of an endospore <+ -idion *diminutive suffix*) *clostridium*

　　　　　　> L. Clostridium, Clostridii, n. (세균) 클로스트리듐속(屬)　**E** Clostridium, *clostridial*

　　　　　　　> L. Clostridioides, Clostridioidis, n. (< *clostridium-like micro-*

　　　　　　　　organism < + G. eidos *shape*) (세균)

　　　　　　　　클로스트리디오이데스속(屬)　　　　　**E** Clostridioides

　　　　　　　[용례] Clostridioides difficile (< *difficult to isolate*)

　　　　　　　　　클로스트리디오이데스 디피실레　　**E** Clostridioides difficile

　　　　　　　　(문법) Clostridioides 클로스트리디오이데스속(屬): 단수 주격

　　　　　　　　difficile 어려운: 형용사, 중성형 단수 주격

　　　< G. klōthein *to spin*

　　　　> G. klōthō, klōthous, f. *spinner;* (Klōthō) (*Greek mythology*) *the youngest of*

　　　　　the three Fates, who spins the thread of life

　　　　　> L. Clotho, Clothus, f. (그리스 신화) 운명을 맡은 세 여신 중 가장 어린

　　　　　　여신(사람의 출생을 맡음)　　　　　　**E** *Clotho*

　< IE. klo- *to spin*

E. *box*　　　　　　　　　　　　　　　　　　　**E** *box*

　　　　< (*probably*) L. buxus, buxi, f. 회양목

　　< G. pyxos, pyxou, f. *boxwood*

　　　> G. pyxis, pyxidos, f. *box*

　　　　> L. pyxis, pyxidis, f. 상자, 함(函), 갑(匣)　　　**E** *pyxis, pyx*

　　　　> G. pyxidion, pyxidiou, n. (< + -idion *diminutive suffix*) *small box*

　　　　　> L. pyxidium, pyxidii, n. (식물) 개과(蓋果), 포자낭　**E** *pyxidium*

L. capsa, capsae, f. 상자

E *case, encase, caisson, cash* (< *'cash box'*), *lowercase* (< *'small-letter type kept in the lower case'*), *uppercase* (< *'capital-letter type kept in the upper case'*), *capsid* (< *'protein shell that protects the nucleic acid of a virus'*), *capsomere* (< *'morphological unit of the viral capsid'*), (*diminutive of* F. cassee >) *cassette,* (*suggested*) *casket*

> L. capsula, capsulae, f. (< + -ula *diminutive suffix*) 작은 상자, 캡슐,

피낭(被囊), 피막(皮膜)　　　　　　　　　　　**E** *capsule,* (capsula >) *encapsulate, encapsulation*

> L. capsularis, capsulare 꼬투리 모양 삭과(蒴果)의, 캡슐의, 피낭(被囊)의,

피막(被膜)의　　　　　　　　　　　　　　　　　　　**E** *capsular*

< IE. kap- *to grasp* (Vide CAPĔRE: See E. *caption*)

G. thekē, thekēs, f. *repository, receptacle, box, chest, tomb, coffin,*

sheath　　　　　　　　　　　　　**E** *bibliotheca, apothecary, boutique, discotheque*

> L. theca, thecae, f. 막(膜), 초(鞘), 난포막(卵胞膜), 건초(腱鞘), 경막(硬膜), 수막(髓膜)　**E** *theca*

< IE. dhe- *to put, to set* (Vide FACĔRE: See E. *facsimile*)

E. *wedge*　　　　　　　　　　　　　　　　　　　　　　　**E** *wedge*

< IE. wog^wh-ni- *plowshare, wedge* (Vide VOMER: See E. *vomer*)

L. cuneus, cunei, m. 쐐기

E *coin* (< 'die for stamping money or medals; the die had the form or action of a wedge'), *coinage*

> L. cuneiformis, cuneiforme 쐐기 모양의, 설상(楔狀)의, 설형(楔形)의　　**E** *cuneiform*

> L. cuneo, cuneavi, cuneatum, cuneare 쐐기를 박다, 쐐기 모양으로 만들다

> L. cuneatus, cuneata, cuneatum 쐐기 모양을 한, 설형의　　　　**E** *cuneate*

< IE. ku- *sharp, pointed*

> L. culex, culicis, m. 모기, 각다귀, 등에; 집모기　　　　**E** *culex,* (culex >) *culicine*

G. sphēn, sphēnos, f. *wedge*　　　**E** *sphen(o)-, sphenic, sphenogram* (< 'cuneiform letter')

> G. sphēnoidēs, sphēnoidēs, sphēnoides (< + eidos *shape*) *wedge-shaped*

> L. sphenoides, (gen.) sphenoidis 쐐기 모양의;

(해부) 쐐기뼈의, 나비뼈의, 접형골(蝶形骨)의　　　　　　**E** *sphenoid*

> L. sphenoidalis, sphenoidale 쐐기뼈의, 나비뼈의, 접형골의　　**E** *sphenoidal*

< IE. spe- *long, flat piece of wood*　　　　**E** *spoon, spade* (< 'digging tool')

> G. spathē, spathēs, f. *broad blade*

> L. spatha, spathae, f. 길쭉한 주걱, 길쭉한 쌍날칼, 불염포(佛焰苞)

E *spathe, spade* (< 'sword, used as a mark on playing-cards'), *spay* (< 'to cut with a sword the ovaries of a female animal')

> L. spathula, spathulae, f. (spatula, spatulae, f.) (< + -ula *diminutive*

suffix) 작은 주걱, 다루개　　　　　　　　　　　　**E** *spatula*

E. *sickle*　　　　　　　　　　　　　　　　　　　　　　　**E** *sickle*

< L. secula, seculae, f. (Campania 지방의 낱말) 낫

< IE. sek- *to cut* (Vide SECARE: See E. *secant*)

L. falx, falcis, f. 낫, 겸(鎌)

E *falx, falchion*

[용례] falx cerebri 대뇌낫

E *falx cerebri*

falx cerebelli 소뇌낫

E *falx cerebelli*

(문법) falx 낫: 단수 주격

cerebri 대뇌의: 단수 속격 < cerebrum, cerebri, n.

cerebelli 소뇌의: 단수 속격 < cerebellum, cerebelli, n.

> L. falcatus, falcata, falcatum 낫 모양을 한, 낫으로 무장한

E *falcate*

> L. falciformis, falciforme (< + forma *form*) 낫 모양의

E *falciform*

> L. falciparus, falcipara, falciparum (< + -parus *bearing*) (Plasmodium falciparum)
낫 모양의 생식모세포(*gametocyte*)를 만드는

> (*probably*) L. falco, falconis, m. (< *resemblance of the hooked talons to a reaping-hook*) (동물) 매

E *falcon*

< *Of* non-IE. *origin*

G. drepanon, drepanou, n. (drepanē, drepanēs, f.) *sickle, scythe, curved sword, scimitar*

E *drepan(o)-, drepanocyte (sickle cell)*

E. *sword*

E *sword*

< IE. swer- *to cut, to pierce*

L. ensis, ensis, f. 검

E *ensiform*

< IE. nsi- *sword*

L. gladius, gladii, m. 검

E *gladiator*

< IE. kel- *to strike, to cut; with derivatives referring to something broken or cut off, piece of wood, twig* (Vide GLADIUS: *See* E. *gladiolus*)

G. xiphos, xiphous, n. *sword*

E *xiphoid*

E. *whip*

E *whip, whiplash*

< IE. weip- *to turn, to vacillate, to tremble ecstatically* (Vide VIBRARE: *See* E. *vibrate*)

E. *lash*

E *lash, eyelash*

< (*probably*) Imitative

L. flagellum, flagelli, n. (< + -ellum *diminutive suffix*) 작은 채찍, 도리깨, 편모(鞭毛)

E *flagellum*, (pl.) *flagella*, (flagellum >) *flagellin*, (flagellum >) *flagellar*, (*adjective*) (flagellum >) *flagellate, flail*

> L. flagello, flagellavi, flagellatum, flagellare 채찍질하다,

　　　　　도리깨질하다 　　　　　　　　　　　**E** *(verb)* ***flagellate, flagellant,*** *(possibly)* ***flog***

　　< L. flagrum, flagri, n. 채찍, 도리깨

　< IE. bhlag- *to strike* 　　　　　　　　　　**E** *(probably)* ***bat*** *(< 'leather-flutterer')*

G. mastix, mastigos, f. *whip; scourge, plague*

> 　　　**E** ***mastig(o)-, mastigote*** *(< 'having a flagellum')*, ***-mastigote, amastigote*** *(< 'not having a flagellum')*

　　> L. Mastigophora, Mastigophorum, n. (pl.) (< + G. –phoros, –phoros, –phoron *carrying, bearing*) (원충) 편모충아문(鞭毛蟲亞門) 　　　　　**E** Mastigophora

E. *sand*

　　< IE. bhes- *to rub* (Vide infra)

L. arena, arenae, f. (harena, harenae, f.) 모래, 모래땅, 원형극장

> 　　　**E** ***arena, arenicolous*** *(< 'sand-inhabiting')*, ***arenavirus*** *(< 'fine granules seen in the virion by electron microscopy')*

　　> L. arenaceus, arenacea, arenaceum 모래의, 모래땅의, 사질(沙質)의 　　　**E** *arenaceous*

　　　　[용례] corpora arenacea (pl.) 사질체(沙質體) 　　　　　**E** *(pl.) corpora arenacea*

　　　　　　(문법) corpora 몸, 체(體): 복수 주격 < corpus, corporis, n.

　　　　　　　arenacea 사질의: 형용사, 중성형 복수 주격

G. psammos, psammou, f. *sand* 　　　　　　　　　　　　**E** *psammite*

　　> L. psammoma, psammomatis, n. (< + G. –ōma *noun suffix denoting tumor*) 모래종(腫), 사종(沙腫), 사종체(沙腫體) 　　　　　**E** *psammoma, psammomatous*

　　< IE. bhes- *to rub* 　　　　　　　　　　　　　　　　**E** *sand*

　　> L. sabulum, sabuli, n. 굵은 모래, 모래

　　　　> L. sabulosus, sabulosa, sabulosum 모래가 많은, 모래와 같은; 침전물이 많은 　**E** *sabulous*

E. *glass* 　　　　　　　　　　　　　　　　　　　　**E** *glass*

　　< IE. ghel- *to shine; with derivatives referring to colors, bright materials, gold (probably 'yellow metal'), and bile or gall* (Vide FULVUS; See E. *fulvous*)

L. vitrum, vitri, n. 유리(琉璃), 초자(硝子) 　　　　　　　　**E** *vitreous, in vitro*

　　< IE. weid- *to see, to know* (Vide VIDĒRE; See E. *video*)

G. hyalos, hyalou, m. *glass, crystal*

> 　　　**E** ***hyal(o)-, hyaluronan (hyaluronic acid)*** *(< 'a nonsulfated glycosaminoglycan isolated first from the vitreous or hyaloid body of the eye, with a high uronic acid content')*, *(hyaluronic acid > hyaluronid- >)* ***hyaluronidase, hyalomere*** *(< 'glassy part of platelet')*

> G. hyalinos, hyalinē, hyalinon *of glass, of crystal*

   > L. hyalinus, hyalina, hyalinum 유리의, 투명한

      E *(noun)* **hyalin** (< *'translucent substance'*), *(adjective)* **hyaline** (< *'translucent'*), **hyalinize**

> G. hyaloeidēs, hyaloeidēs, hyaloeides (< + eidos *shape*) *glassy*

   > L. hyaloides, (gen.) hyaloidis 유리 같은, 투명한, 유리질의   **E** *hyaloid*

< *(suggeted)* *Of Egyptian origin*

E. *island*   **E** *island*

   < IE. ak^{w}a- *water* (Vide AQUA; *See* E. *aqueous*)

   + IE. lendh- *open land*   **E** *land, landscape, lawn*

L. insula, insulae, f. 섬   **E** *insulin* (< *'produced by the islets of Langerhans in the pancreas'*), *isle, islet*

   > L. insularis, insulare 섬의   **E** *insular*

   > L. insulatus, insulata, insulatum 섬에 옮겨진, 격리된,

      고립된   **E** *insulate, insulation, insulator, isolate, isolation*

   > L. paeninsula, paeninsulae, f. (peninsula, peninsulae, f.) (< paene (pene) *almost*

      + insula *island*) 반도(半島)   **E** *peninsula, peninsular*

G. nēsos, nēsou, f. *island, peninsula*   **E** *Indonesia, Melanesia, Micronesia, Polynesia*

     > G. nēsidion, nēsidiou, n. (< nēsos + -idion *diminutive suffix*) 작은 섬 **E** *nesidioblast*

   < G. nein (neein) *to swim*   **E** *neuston*

  < IE. (s)na-, (s)nau- *to swim, to flow, to let flow, to suckle* (Vide NUTRIRE; *See* E. *nourish*)

E. *dry*   **E** *dry*

   < *(Germanic root)* dreug- dry   **E** *drought, drain, drainage*

L. siccus, sicca, siccum 마른, 건조한

    > L. sicco, siccavi, siccatum, siccare 말리다   **E** *siccative*

     > L. desicco, desiccavi, desiccatum, desiccare (< de- *apart from, down, not;*

      intensive) 바짝 말리다   **E** *desiccate, desiccant, desiccator*

      > L. exsicco, exsiccavi, exsiccatum, exsiccare (< ex- *out of, away from; in-*

      tensive) 바짝 말리다, (잔을) 비우다, 쭉 마셔버리다   **E** *exsiccate*

  < IE. seik^w- *to flow out*

G. xēros, xēra, xēron *dry*   **E** *xer(o)-, xerography, xeroderma, xerophthalmia, xerostomia*

    > G. xērion, xēriou, n. *powder for drying wounds*   **E** *((Arabic) al-iksir 'the desiccant' >) elixir*

    > G. xērōsis, xērōseōs, f. (< + -ōsis *condition*) *dryness*

     > L. xerosis, xerosis, f. 건조증   **E** *xerosis, xerotic*

< IE. ksero- *dry*

> L. serenus, serena, serenum (바람이) 건조한, 맑은, (바다가) 잔잔한, (마음이)
차분한 **E** *serene, serenade*

> L. serenitas, serenitatis, f. 청명, 청징(清澄), 평온 **E** *serenity*

E. *bird* **E** *bird*

L. avis, avis, f. 새 **E** (avis >) *avian,* (avis >) *aviation*

> L. auspex, auspicis, m., f. (< *inspector of birds* < avispex, avispicis, m., f. < avis +
–spex, –spicis, m. *observer*) 새점쟁이, 가호자 **E** *auspex*

> L. auspicium, auspicii, n. 새점, 조짐, (일의 상서로운) 시작,
가호 **E** *auspice,* (auspicium >) *auspicious*

> L. auca, aucae, f. 새, 기러기 **E** (It.) *ocarina* (< *'little goose, with reference to its shape'*)

< IE. awi- *bird*

> IE. owyo-, oyyo- *egg* (Vide OVUM: *See* E. *ovum*)

G. ornis, ornithos, m., f. *bird; fowl, cock, hen; bird of augury; augury*

E *ornith(o)-, ornithomancy, ornithology, ornithine* (< *'an amino acid isolated from birds'*
excrement')

> L. ornithosis, ornithosis, f. (< + G. –ōsis *condition*) 비둘기병, 오르니토시스 **E** *ornithosis*

< IE. or- *bird*

E. *spur* **E** *spur*

< IE. sperə- *ankle* **E** *spurn* (< *'to kick'*), *spoor* (< *'track of an animal'*)

F. ergot (닭 등의) 며느리발톱, (개 등의) 뒷발톱; (건축) 꼭지; 맥각(麥角), 맥각병

E *ergot* (< *'resembling a cock's spur'*), *ergotism, ergosterol* (< *'a sterol isolated initially from*
ergot'), *ergotamine, lysergic acid* (< *'obtained by hydrolysis of ergot alkaloids'*), *lysergic*
acid diethylamide (LSD)

L. calcar, calcaris, n. 박차(拍車), 며느리발톱, 조거(鳥距); 자극 **E** *calcar*

> L. calcarinus, calcarina, calcarinum 며느리발톱의, 조거(鳥距)의, 며느리발톱
모양의 **E** *calcarine*

< L. calx, calcis, f., m. 발꿈치

< IE. (s)kel- *crooked, with derivatives referring to a bent or curved part of the body, such*
as a heel or a leg (Vide CALX: *See* E. *calcaneus*)

G. kentron, kentrou, n. *prick, sting, goad, spur, pain*

> L. centrum, centri, n. (< *that point of the compass around which the other describes the circle*) 중심

        E *centr(o)- (centr(i)-)*

< IE. kent- *to prick, to jab* (Vide CENTRUM: *See* E. *centre*)

E. *fish*

< IE. peisk- *fish* (Vide infra)

L. piscis, piscis, m. 물고기; ((pl.) Pisces) (동물) 어강(魚綱), (천문) 물고기자리, 쌍어궁(雙魚宮)

        E (pl.) Pisces, *pisciculture, piscivorous*

> L. piscinus, piscina, piscinum 물고기의   **E** *piscine*

> L. piscor, piscatus sum, piscari 물고기를 잡다   **E** *piscatory*

< IE. peisk- *fish*   **E** *fish*

G. ichthys, ichthyos, m. *fish*   **E** *ichthy(o)-, ichthyology*

> L. ichthyosis, ichthyosis, f. (< G. ichthys + -ōsis *condition*) 비늘증, 어린선(魚鱗癬)   **E** *ichthyosis*

> L. Ichthyosaurus, Ichthyosauri, m. (< G. ichthys + sauros *lizard*)

     어룡속(魚龍屬)   **E** *ichthyosaurus (ichthyosaur)*

< IE. dhghu- *fish*

E. *seed*

< IE. se- *to sow* (Vide infra)

L. semen, seminis, n. 씨[種], 싹수, 발단, 정액(精液)   **E** *semen*

> L. seminalis, seminale 씨의, 정액의   **E** *seminal*

> L. seminarius, seminaria, seminarium 종자의, 묘포의

    > L. seminarium, seminarii, n. 묘포, 못자리, 온상, 양성소, 연구반, 연구실   **E** *seminary, seminar*

> L. seminifer, seminifera, seminiferum (< semen *seed* + -fer (< ferre *to carry, to bear*) *carrying, bearing*) 씨를 내는(맺는), 정액을 내는, 수정(輸精)의 **E** *seminiferous*

> L. semino, seminavi, seminatum, seminare 씨 뿌리다

    > L. dissemino, disseminavi, disseminatum, disseminare (< dis- *apart from, down, not* + seminare *to sow*) 파종하다, 살포하다, 퍼뜨리다 **E** *disseminate*

        > L. disseminatio, disseminationis, f. 파종, 살포, 전염   **E** *dissemination*

    > L. insemino, inseminavi, inseminatum, inseminare (< in- *in, on, into, toward* + seminare *to sow*) 씨 뿌리다, 심다   **E** *inseminate*

        > L. inseminatio, inseminationis, f. 정액주입, 수정(授精)   **E** *insemination*

< L. sero, sevi, satum, serĕre 씨 뿌리다

> L. satio, sationis, f. 파종   **E** *season* (< *'time of sowing'*), (*season* >) *seasonal*

> L. sativus, sativa, sativum 재배의, 재배하는, 재배한

> (*perhaps*) L. Saturnus, Saturni, m. (로마 신화) 농경의 신; (천문) 토성;
(saturnus) (연금술) 납

> **E** *Saturn, Saturnian,* (G. hēmera Kronou *'day of Kronos',* L. dies Saturni *'day of Saturnus'* >) *Saturday; saturnism* (< *'lead poisoning'*), *saturnine*

< IE. se– *to sow*　　　　　　　　　　　　　　　　　　　　　**E** *seed, sow*

G. sperma, spermatos, n. (< *that which is scattered*) *seed*

> L. sperma, spermatis, n. 정액(精液); 정자(精子)

> **E** *sperm, spermatic, spermatogenesis, spermatogonium, spermatocyte, spermatid, spermatozoon (zoosperm); spermicide*

> L. azoospermia, azoospermiae, f. (< G. a– *not* + zōe *life* + sperma + –ia)
무정자증(無精子症)　　　　　　　　　　　　　　**E** *azoospermia*

> L. oligospermia, oligospermiae, f. (< G. oligos *few, little* + sperma +
–ia) (*originally*) *reduction in the quantity of ejaculated semen (now
rare or disused); (later) reduction in the number of spermatozoa
in the semen*) 정자부족증　　　　　　　　　　**E** *oligospermia*

> L. *dyszoospermia, *dyszoospermiae, f. (< G. dys– *bad* + zōe *life* + sperma
+ –ia) 정자형성장애　　　　　　　　　　　　　**E** *dyszoospermia*

> G. polyspermia, polyspermias, f. (< polys *many* + sperma + –ia) *abundance
of seed*　　　　　**E** *polyspermy* (< *'penetration of an ovum by more than one sperm'*)

> G. spermeion, spermeiou, n. (< + –ion *diminutive suffix*) *sperm*

> L. spermium, spermii, n. 정자(精子)　**E** *spermi(o)–, spermiogenesis, spermiation*

> G. –spermos, –spermos, –spermon *of seed*

> L. angiospermus, angiospermi, m. (< G. angeion *vessel*) 속씨식물,
피자(被子)식물　　　　　　　　　　　　　　　　**E** *angiosperm*

> L. gymnospermus, gymnospermi, m. (< G. gymnos *naked*) 겉씨식물,
나자(裸子)식물　　　　　　　　　　　　　　　　**E** *gymnosperm*

< G. speirein *to sow, to scatter, to spread; (passive) to be scattered*

> G. spora, sporas, f. (sporos, sporou, m.) *sowing, scattering, seed, offspring;
spore*　　　　　　　　　**E** *spor(o)–, sporocyst, sporophyte, sporozoite, –spore*

> L. spora, sporae, f. 홑씨, 포자(胞子), 아포(芽胞)　　　　**E** *spore*

> L. sporula, sporulae, f. (< + –ula *diminutive suffix*) 작은 홑씨,
소포자(小胞子)

> **E** *sporule,* (*sporule* >) *sporular,* (*sporule* >) *sporulate,* (*sporulate* >)
sporulation

> L. sporangium, sporangii, n. (< G. spora *spore* + angeion *vessel*) 홑씨
주머니, 포자낭　**E** *sporangium,* (pl.) *sporangia, sporangiospore, sporangiophore*

> L. Microsporum, Microspori, n. (< G. mikros *small*) 소포자균(小胞子菌)
속(屬)　　　　　　　　　　　　　　　　　　　　**E** Microsporum

> G. diaspora, diasporas, f. (< di(a)– *through, thoroughly, apart*) *dispersion*

> L. diaspora, diasporae, f. 사방으로 흩어짐　　**E** *Diaspora, diaspore*

> G. sporadikos, sporadikē, sporadikon *scattered, dispersed*

> L. sporadicus, sporadica, sporadicum 산재(散在)하는, 산발적으로

일어나는   **E** *sporadic, sporadicity*

< IE. sper- *to strew*   **E** *spray, spread, sprawl, sprout*

L. gonium, gonii, n. 생식원세포(生殖原細胞)   **E** *gonium,* (pl.) *gonia*

> L. oogonium, oogonii, n. (< G. ōion *egg*) 난조세포(卵祖細胞), 난원세포

(卵原細胞)   **E** *oogonium,* (pl.) *oogonia*

> L. spermatogonium, spermatogonii, n. (< G. sperma, spermatos, n. *seed*)

정조세포(精祖細胞), 정원세포(精原細胞)   **E** *spermatogonium,* (pl.) *spermatogonia*

< G. gonē, gonēs, f. ((*ancient Greek*) gonos) *begetting, birth, origin; offspring,*

seed

< G. gignesthai *to be born*

< IE. genə-, gen- *to give birth, to beget; with derivatives referring to aspects and results*

of procreation and to familial and tribal groups (Vide GIGNĔRE: *See* E. *genital*)

E. *bud*   **E** *bud*

< IE. beu-, bheu- *probably imitative root, appearing in words loosely associated with the*

notion 'to swell' (Vide BULLA: *See* E. *bulla*)

E. *shoot*   **E** *shoot*

< IE. skeud- *to shoot, to chase, to throw* **E** *shot, shut* (< *'by pushing a crossbar'*), *shout, shuttle, sheet*

E. *sprout*   **E** *sprout*

< IE. sper- *to strew* (Vide SPERMA: *See* E. *sperm*)

L. germen, germinis, n. 종자(種子), 싹[芽], 배아(胚芽), 미생물   **E** *germ, germinal, germinate*

< IE. genə-, gen- *to give birth, to beget; with derivatives referring to aspects and results*

of procreation and to familial and tribal groups (Vide GIGNĔRE: *See* E. *genital*)

G. blastos, blastou, m. (blastē, blastēs, f.) *sprout, origin*

> **E** *blast* (< *'a primitive or formative element, layer, or cell'*), *-blast;* (*'a formative layer'* >) *blast(o)-, blastomere, blastoderm, blastocoele, blastocyst, trophoblast* (< *'an extra-embryonic layer which supplies nutrition to the embryo'*), *epiblast* (< *'the upper layer of the bilaminar embryonic disk'*), *hypoblast* (< *'the lower layer of the bilaminar embryonic disk'*), *mesoblast* (< *'mesoderm, especially in the early undifferentiated stages; also, a cell of the mesoblast'*); (*'a formative cell'* >) *gonadoblast, myeloblast, erythroblast, megakaryoblast, lymphoblast*

> G. blastanein (*stem* blaste-, blasta-) *to sprout, to bud*

> G. blastēma, blastēmatos, n. (< + -ma *resultative noun suffix*) *bud*

> L. blastema, blastematis, n. 발생모체, 싹

> **E** *blastema* (< 'a group of primitive or formative cells'), **blastemic (blastemal),** **mesoblastema** (< 'the cells comprising the mesoblast')

> L. blastula, blastulae, f. (< + -ula *diminutive suffix*) 포배(胞胚),
주머니배　　　　　　　　**E** *blastula (blastosphere),* (blastula >) **blastulation**

> L. blastoma, blastomatis, n. (< + G. -ōma *noun suffix denoting tumor*) 배세포종
(胚細胞腫), 모세포종(母細胞腫)　　　　　　　　**E** *blastoma, -blastoma*

G. thallos, thallou, m. *young shoot, sprouting twig, olive-branch, foliage*

> L. thallus, thalli, m. 푸른 가지, 도금양 나뭇가지; 엽상체(葉狀體)

> **E** *thallus,* (pl.) *thalli, thallophyte* (< 'a plant the vegetative body of which is thallus, including algae, fungi, and lichens'), **thallium (Tl)** (< 'green line in the spectrum')

< G. thallein *to bloom, to shoot, to sprout*

< IE. dhal- *to bloom*

E. *grass*　　　　　　　　**E** *grass*

< IE. ghre- *to grow, to become green*

> **E** *grow, growth, ingrowth, outgrowth, green, grass, graze,* (IE. ghre- > 'a role as a growth hormone-releasing peptide' >) *ghrelin*

L. herba, herbae, f. 풀[草]　　　　　　　　**E** *herb, herbicide*

> L. herbaceus, herbacea, herbaceum 풀의, 풀색의　　　　　　　　**E** *herbaceous*

> L. herbalis, herbale 풀에 관한　　　　　　　　**E** *herbal, herbalist*

> L. herbarium, herbarii, n. 식물 표본실　　　　　　　　**E** *herbarium*

> L. arbor, arboris, f. (< *tree* < *shady place formed by trees* < *herb garden*)
나무, 수목 (Vide ARBOR: See E. *arbor*)

> L. herbivorus, herbivora, herbivorum (< + -vorus *devouring*) 초식의　　　　**E** *herbivorous*

< (*suggested*) IE. ghre- *to grow, to become green* (Vide supra)

G. poa, poas, f. *grass, fodder*

> L. Poa, Poae, f. (벼과) 포아풀속(屬)　　　　　　　　**E** Poa

E. *tree*　　　　　　　　**E** *tree*

< IE. deru-, dreu- *to be firm, solid, steadfast; hence specialized senses 'tree', 'wood', and derivatives referring to objects made of wood* (Vide DURUS: See E. *endure*)

L. arbor, arboris, f. (< *tree* < *shady place formed by trees* < *herb garden*) 나무, 수목

E *arbor (arbour)*, (arbor > *'to make tree-like, to give the appearance of a tree'* >) *arborize*
> L. arboreus, arborea, arboreum 나무의   **E** *arboreal*
> L. aboresco, –, –, arborescĕre (< arbor *tree* + –escĕre *suffix of inceptive*
    *(inchoative) verb)*나무가 되다, 나무로 자라다   **E** *arborescent*
    > L. arboretum, arboreti, n. 수목원, 식물원   **E** *arboretum*
  < L. herbarium, herbarii, n. 식물 표본실 (Vide HERBA: *See* E. *herb*)

G. dendron, dendrou, n. *tree*

E *dendr(o)-, dendroid, dendrocyte, oligodendroglia (oligodendrocyte), -dendron; dendriform*
> G. dendritēs, dendritēs, dendrites *of a tree*   **E** *dendrite, (dendrite >) dendritic*
> G. rhododendron, rhododendrou, n. (< rhodon *rose* + dendron) *rhododendron*
    > L. rhododendron, rhododendri, n. 진달래속(屬)의 식물   **E** *rhododendron*
  < IE. deru–, dreu– *to be firm, solid, steadfast; hence specialized senses 'tree', 'wood', and*
    derivatives referring to objects made of wood (Vide DURUS: *See* E. *endure*)

E. *wood*   **E** *wood*
  < IE. widhu– *tree, wood*

L. buscus, busci, m. (boscus, bosci, m.) 목재

E (in- *'in, on, into, toward'* + boscus *'wood'* >) **inboscare 'to place in a wood or among the bushes'* >) *ambush*

< (*Germanic*) busk– *bush*

E *bush, bouquet* (< *'clump of trees'*), (F. haut *'high'* + bois *'wood'* > F. hautbois *'wooden instrument with high notes'* >) *oboe*

L. lignum, ligni, n. (< *that which is gathered*) 목재, 장작   **E** *lignin, (lignum >) lignify*
    > L. ligneus, lignea, ligneum 목재의   **E** *ligneous*
  < IE. leg– *to collect; with derivatives meaning 'to speak'* (Vide LEGĔRE: *See* E. *lecture*)

G. xylon, xylou, n. *wood, timber*

E *xyl(o)-, xylography, xylophone, xylem, xylose* (< *'a sugar first isolated from wood'*), *(xylose + -ite + -ol > 'a sugar alcohol derived from xylose'* >) *xylitol, xylene (xylol)* (< *'obtained from wood-spirit'*)

    > L. –xylum, –xyli, n. ~나무   **E** *–xylum*

    [용례] Haematoxylum campechianum (*Campeachy wood, bloodwood tree,*
        logwood) 캄페체 지방의 피나무 (헤마톡실린의 원자재)   **E** *hematoxylin*
      (문법) haematoxylum 피나무: 단수 주격 < haematoxylum, haematoxyli, n.
        (< G. haima, haimatos, n. *blood* + -xylum *–wood*)
      campechianum 캄페체 지방의: 형용사, 중성형 단수 주격

< Campechianus, Campechiana, Campechianum

< (*Mexican*) Campeche (멕시코) 캄페체 지방

> L. xylophagus, xylophaga, xylophagum (< + G. –phagos *eating*) 나무를 좀먹는　**E** *xylophagous*

< (*suggested*) IE. (k)selwa- *forest, wood*

> (*suggested*) L. silva, silvae, f. (sylva, sylvae, f.) 숲, 나무　**E** *silviculture (sylviculture)*

> L. silvester, silvestris, silvestre (silvestris, silvestre) 숲의, 시골의

> L. silvaticus, silvatica, silvaticum 숲의, 야생의, 야만의　**E** *savage*

E. *thorn*　**E** *thorn*

< IE. (s)ter-n- *name of thorny plants*

< IE. ster- *stiff* (Vide TORPOR; *See* E. *torpor*)

E. *prickle*　**E** *prickle*

L. spina, spinae, f. 가시, 등마루(척추 脊椎, 척주 脊柱)　**E** *spine, spiny*

> L. spinosus, spinosa, spinosum 가시 많은, 가시의, 뾰족한, 까다로운　**E** *spinous*

> L. spinalis, spinale 등마루의, 척추의; 척수(脊髓)의　**E** *spinal*

< IE. spei- *sharp point* (Vide SPINA; *See* E. *spine*)

G. akantha, akanthēs, f. *thorn, thistle*

E *acanthus, acanth(o)-, acanthocyte, acanthosis, acantholysis, -acanth, coelacanth, tragacanth*

< G. akē, akēs, f. *point*

< IE. ak- *sharp* (Vide ACUTUS; *See* E. *acute*)

E. *amber*　**E** *amber*

< (*Arabic*) 'anbar *ambergris*

L. succinum, succini, n. 호박

(琥珀)　**E** *succinic acid* (< '*obtained by dry distillation of amber* (succinum)'), *succinate*

G. ēlectron, ēlectrou, n. (< *shining one*) *amber*

E *electric* (< '*electrostatic phenomena caused by rubbing amber*'), *electrical, electricity, electr(o)-, (electric + -on 'a termination of Greek neuter nouns and adjectives' >) electron, (electron >) electronic, (electron >) -tron*

∽ G. Elektra, Elektras, f. (< *shining one*) *Electra, the daughter of Agamemnon and Clytemnestra (She persuaded her brother Orestes to kill Clytemnestra and Aegisthus (their mother's lover) in revenge for the murder of Agamemnon.)*　**E** *Electra*

E. *leaf*　**E** *leaf*

< IE. leup-, lep- *to peel off, to break off, to scale* (Vide LIBER; *See* E. *library*)

L. folium, folii, n. 잎; (종이의) 낱장

> **E** *folio,* (portare *'to carry'* > *'briefcase for carrying loose papers'* >) ***portfolio,
> foil, foliage,*** (trifolium *'three-leaved'* >) ***trefoil,*** (quinquefolium *'five-leaved'* >)
> ***cinquefoil, folic acid*** (< *'abundant in green leaves'*)

> L. foliaceus, foliacea, foliaceum 잎의, 잎으로 된, 잎 모양을 한   **E** *foliaceous*
> L. -folius, -folia, -folium ~잎의, ~잎으로 된, ~잎 모양을 한
> L. foliatus, foliata, foliatum 잎이 있는, 잎으로 덮인, 잎 모양을 한   **E** *foliate*
> L. defolio, **defoliavi,** defoliatum, defoliare (< de- *apart from, down, not*
>   + folium *leaf*) 잎을 지게 하다, 잎이 지다   **E** *defoliate, defoliant*
> L. exfolio, **exfoliavi,** exfoliatum, exfoliare (< ex- *out of, away from* +
>   folium *leaf*) 벗겨내다, 박리(剝離)하다, 벗겨지다, (얇은 조각이 되어)
>   탈락하다, 박탈(剝脫)하다, 낙설(落屑)되다   **E** *exfoliate, exfoliative*

   < IE. bhol-yo- *leaf*

> G. phyllon, phyllou, n. *leaf*

> > **E** *phyll(o)-, phylloid, -phyll (-phyl), chlorophyll (chlorophyl)* (< *'the
> > coloring matter of the green leaves'*), *xanthophyll (xanthophyl)* (<
> > *'the coloring matter of the yellow leaves in autumn, a constituent or
> > derivative of chlorophyll'*), (Podophyllum *'duck's-foot leaved'* >)
> > *podophyllin* (< *'a resin found in the rhizome'*), *theophylline* (< *'an
> > alkaloid found in tea leaves'*)

> > G. phyllōdēs, phyllōdēs, phyllōdes (< + -ōdēs *-shaped, -like,*
> > *resembling*) *leaf-like*   **E** *phyllodes*
> > > L. phyllodium, phyllodii, n. (식물) 헛잎, 가엽(假葉)   **E** *phyllode*

   < IE. bhel- *to thrive, to bloom*

  < IE. bhel- *to blow, to swell* (Vide FOLLIS; *See* E. *folly*)

E. *flower*

   < L. flos, floris, m. 꽃 (Vide infra)

L. flos, floris, m. 꽃; (pl. flores) 승화약(昇華藥)   **E** *flower, floret, florist, florigen, flour*

> L. floralis, florale 꽃의   **E** *floral*
> L. Flora, Florae, f. (로마 신화) 꽃의 여신; (flora) 식물상(相), 세균총(叢)   **E** *Flora, flora*
> > L. Floralis, Florale (로마 신화) 꽃의 여신의; (floralis) 식물상의,
> > 세균총의   **E** *floral*
> L. -florus, -flora, -florum ~꽃의, ~꽃을 피우는, ~꽃이 피는
> L. floreo, florui, -, florēre 꽃이 피다

> > **E** *(third personal singular, perfect indicative, active 'he/she flourished'* >)
> > *floruit (fl.), flourish, Florence*

> L. floridus, florida, floridum 꽃이 핀, 꽃이 만발한, 화려한   **E** *florid, Florida*

> L. floresco, florui, −, florescĕre (< florēre *to bloom* + -escĕre

    suffix of inceptive (inchoative) verb) 개화하다   **E** *florescence*

    > L. effloresco, efflorui, −, efflorescĕre (< ef- (< ex) *out of,*

        away from; intensive) 만발하다; (화학) 풍해(風解)하다;

        (의학) 발진(發疹)하다   **E** *effloresce*

< IE. bhle- *to thrive, to bloom*

    E *blow (< 'to flower'), bloom, blossom, blood (< 'to swell, to gush, to spurt'),*
    bloody, bleed, bless (< 'to treat or hallow with blood'), blade (< 'leaf')

< IE. bhel- *to thrive, to bloom*

< IE. bhel- *to blow, to swell* (Vide FOLLIS: *See* E. *folly*)

G. anthos, anthous, n. *flower,*

   blossom   **E** *anthocyanin(s) (< 'blue, violet, or red flavonoid pigments in flowers')*

> G. anthemon, anthemou, n. *flower*

  > G. chrysanthemon, chrysanthemou, n. (< chrysos *gold*) *the corn-marigold*

    > L. chrysanthemum, chrysanthemi, n. 국화(菊花)   **E** *·chrysanthemum*

> G. anthēros, anthēra, anthēron *flowery, blooming*

  > G. anthēra, anthēras, f. *pollen-bearing organ, medicine extracted from flowers*

    > L. anthera, antherae, f. (수술 끝의) 꽃밥, 약(葯)   **E** *anther*

> G. anthein (antheein) *to blossom*

  > G. exanthēma, exanthēmatos, n. (< *an efflorescence* < ex- *out of, away from* +

    anthein (antheein) + -ma *resultative noun suffix*) *skin eruption*

    > L. exanthema, exanthematis, n. 발진(發疹), 피진(皮疹)

       E *exanthema (exanthem),* (pl.) *exanthemata (exanthemas), exanthematous*

  > G. enanthēma, enanthēmatos, n. (< en- *in* + anthein (antheein) + -ma *re-*

    sultative noun suffix) *mucosal eruption*

    > L. enanthema, enanthematis, n.

      점막진(粘膜疹)   **E** *enanthema (enanthem),* (pl.) *enanthemata (enanthemas)*

  > G. -anthēs, -anthēs, -anthes *flowering, flowered*

    > L. -anthes, -anthis, f. ~꽃

> G. anthologia, anthologias, f. (< + logia *collection*) *collection of poems*

  > L. anthologia, anthologiae, f. 시선집(詩選集), 작품집   **E** *anthology*

> L. Anthozoa, Anthozoorum, n. (pl.) (< + G. zōia (pl.) < zōion *animal*) (강장동물

  腔腸動物) 화충강(花蟲綱)   **E** *Anthozoa, anthozoan*

< IE. andh- *bloom*

E. *nut*

< IE. kneu- *nut* (Vide infra)

L. nux, nucis, f. 견과(堅果)
E *nougat, nucleus, nucleolus*
    < IE. kneu- *nut* (Vide NUCLEUS: *See* E. *nucleus*)   **E** *nut*

G. karyon, karyou, n. *nut*   **E** *procaryote (prokaryote), eucaryote (eukaryote)*
    < IE. kar-, ker- *hard* (Vide CANCER: *See* E. *cancer*)

E. *grape* (< *hooked; something hooked*)   **E** *grape*
    < IE. g(e)r- *curving, crooked; hypothetical Indo-European base for a variety of Germanic*
    words with initial kr-

> **E** (*Words meaning 'to bend, to curl; bent, crooked, hooked; something bent or hooked'*)
> *grapple, crumple, cramp, cripple, creep, creepy, cringle, cringe, crinkle, creek, crook,*
> *crouch, encroach, crutch, curl, crank, gooseberry;* (*Words meaning 'a round mass,*
> *collection; a round object, vessel, container'*) *crumb, crumble, group, crock* (< *'pot'*),
> (*crock* >) *crockery, crib, cradle, cart, crop, croft*

L. uva, uvae, f. 포도알, 포도송이   **E** *pyruvic acid* (< *'produced by distillation of an acid found in grapes'*)
    > L. uvula, uvulae, f. (< + -ula *diminutive suffix*) 작은 포도송이; 수(垂); 목젖,
        구개수(口蓋垂)   **E** *uvula*
        > L. uvularis, uvulare 목젖의   **E** *uvular*
    > L. uvea, uveae, f. (< *resembling a reddish-blue grape when the corneoscleral coat*
        has been dissected away) 포도막(葡萄膜)   **E** *uvea*
        > L. *uvealis, *uveale 포도막의   **E** *uveal*
    < IE. og- *fruit, berry*   **E** *acorn*

L. racemus, racemi, m. 포도송이; (포도처럼) 송아리로 맺힌 과실, 총상화서(總狀花序); 포도,
    포도즙   **E** *racemic acid* (< *'originally referring to tartaric acid obtained from grape juice'*), *raisin*
    > L. racemosus, racemosa, racemosum (포도)송이가 많은, 송이 모양으로 된,
        총상화서의   **E** *racemose*
    < *Of Mediterranean origin*
        > G. rhax, rhagos, f. *berry, grape*
            > G. rhagion, rhagiou, n. (< + -ion *diminutive suffix*) *little berry,*
            little grape **E** *rhagiocrine* (< *'secretory granules resembling small bunch of grapes'*)

G. botrys, botryos, m. *bunch of grapes*   **E** *botry(o)-; botryose*
    > G. botryoeidēs, botryoeidēs, botryoeides (< + eidos *shape*) *botryoid*
        > L. botryoides, (gen.) botryoidis 포도송이 모양의   **E** *botryoid (botryoidal)*

G. staphylē, staphylēs, f. *bunch of grapes; uvula, palate*
    > G. staphylinos, staphylinē, staphylinon *of bunch of grapes; of uvula, of palate* **E** *staphyline*

> L. staphylococcus, staphylococci, m. (< *cocci forming groups resembling bunches of grapes* < G. kokkos *grain, berry*) 포도알균, 포도상구균(葡萄狀球菌) **E** *staphylococcus, (pl.) staphylococci, staphylococcal*

> L. staphyloma, staphylomatis, n. (< *a protrusion of the uveal tissue through a weakened area in the corneoscleral layer* < + G. -ōma *noun suffix denoting tumor*) 포도종(葡萄腫) **E** *staphyloma*

< IE. stebh-, steb-, stabh- *post, stem; to support, to place firmly on, to fasten*

E *staff, distaff, stave, staple, step* (< *'a treading firmly on, foothold'*), ((probably) step >) *instep, stamp, stampede, stump*

> G. stephanos, stephanou, m. *crown, wreath* **E** *stephan(o)-*

> G. stemma, stemmatos, n. *wreath*

> L. stemma, stemmatis, n. 화관; (*the wreaths were placed on ancestral images* >) 족보 **E** *stemma, stemmatics*

E. *seaweed* **E** *seaweed*

E. *agar-agar* *a gelatinous substance extracted from East-Indian seaweeds, especially from the Ceylon moss Gracilaria lichenoides; used in China for soups and the manufacture of transparent silk and paper; adopted in bacteriology as a solidifying agent in culture media and in molecular biology as an electrophoretic matrix*

< (*Malayan*) agar-agar (< *jelly*) 한천(寒天)

E *agar-agar, (agar-agar > (shortened) >) agar* (< *'jelly extracted from seaweed'*), *agarose* (< *'polysaccharide extracted from agar'*)

L. alga, algae, f. 해조(海藻), 조류(藻類), 말[藻]무리; 하찮은 물건 **E** *alga, (pl.) algae, algology*

< (*probably*) IE. el-, ol- *to be moldy, to be putrid*

G. phykos, phykeos, n. *seaweed; rouge* **E** *phyc(o)-, phycology*

> L. fucus, fuci, m. 모자반(갈조류); 자홍색, 분(粉), 꾸밈, 겉꾸밈 **E** *fucose* (< *'a hexose rich in fucus'*)

< *Of Semitic origin*

제5부

학명

Scientific Names

Nomina Scientifica

학명

생명과학에서는 헤아릴 수 없이 많은 종(種)이 학명을 내세우며 등장한다. 그러나 학명은 그 명명법이 잘 알려져 있지 않고 어원론적으로 분석되어 있지 않아 이해하기 쉽지 않게 되어 있다.

다른 학술용어와 마찬가지로 학명을 명명하는 규칙과 어원을 알면 종의 이름은 사람의 본 이름보다도 더 쉽고 친숙해진다. 사람과 그 사람의 본 이름 사이에는 개인적 바람 말고는 아무 관계 없지만, 종과 종의 이름 사이에는 떼려야 뗄 수 없는 관계가 있기 때문이다. 종의 특성을 안다는 것은 종의 이름을 안다는 것이 되고, 그 역도 성립한다.

종과 아종

미노스왕(G. Minōs)의 왕비 파시파에(G. Pasiphaē)와 하얀 황소(G. tauros) 사이에서 태어났다는 미노타우로스(G. Minōtauros)는 신화 속의 반인반수이며 생물학적으로는 불가능한 존재이다. 사람(Homo sapiens)과 소(Bos taurus)는 종이 달라 그 사이에서는 새끼가 태어날 수 없기 때문이다.

호랑이 수컷과 사자 암컷 사이에서 태어난 타이건(*tigon*), 호랑이 암컷과 사자 수컷 사이에서 태어난 라이거(*liger*), 숫말과 암나귀 사이에서 태어난 버새(*hinny*), 암말과 숫나귀 사이에서 태어난 노새(*mule*)처럼 다른 종 사이에서 태어나는 새끼가 없는 것은 아니다. 이는 호랑이(Panthera tigris)와 사자(Panthera leo)가 다르긴 해도 가까운 사이의 종이고 말(Equus caballus)과 당나귀(Equus asinus)가 다르긴 해도 가까운 사이의 종이기 때문이다. 그러나 가깝긴 해도 엄연히 다른 종이므로 타이건, 라이거, 버새, 노새는 불임성이 커 다음 세대를 낳을 수 없다. 종이 다르면 아예 새끼를 낳지 못하거나 낳는다 하더라도 생식력이 없는 새끼를 낳는 것이 고작인 것이다. 유전학 용어로는 유전자 풀(*gene pool*)이 다르다고 표현한다. 정리하자면, 종이 같다는 것은 유전자 풀이 같기 때문에 자연스레 짝짓기가 이루어지고 그 결과 생식력을 가진 새끼가 태어남으로써 세대를 계속 이어갈 수 있다는 것을 뜻한다. (이런 이유로 지구상에 살고 있는 지금 사람들은 모두 하나의 종에 속한다. 멀든 가깝든 지금 사람들은 모두 친인척인 것이며 튀기니 혼혈아니 하는 표현은 생물학적으로 불가한 표현이다.)

이처럼 종을 구분하는 첫 번째 기준은 세대의 연속성이다. 그러나 세대의 연속성을 지켜보지 않아도, 대개의 경우, 같은 종인지 아닌지를 바로 알 수 있다. 종이 다르면 형태가 다르기 때문이다. (종을 가리키는 라틴어 species의 본디 뜻은 '외형'이며 '바라보다'라는 동사 specěre에서 비롯하였다.) 형태의 차이가 모호한 경우에는 성격이나 유전정보가 들어 있는 핵산의 염기서열이 얼마나 같고 다른가를 보고서 판정한다. 짝짓기를 하지 않는 생물이거나 화석생물인 경우에도 세대의 연속성, 형태와 내용, 핵산의 염기서열을 보고서 같은 종인지 다른 종인지 결정한다.

종은 진화가 일어나는 단위 집단이기도 하다. 하나의 종 안에서 유전자 변화가 쌓여 원래의 종과는 조금 다른 유전자 풀과 내용과 형태를 갖는 무리가 생기면 이 무리를 원래의 종 밑에(L. sub *under*) 생긴 아종(亞種, L. subspecies)이라고 한다. subspecies를 동물 분류에서는 ssp.로, 식물과 미생물 분류에서는 subsp.로 줄여 표기한다. 원래의 종과 아종 간의 짝짓기는, 다른 종 간의 짝짓기보다야 덜 하지만, 다소 제한적이다.

종의 이름 – 이명법

사람을 다른 동물과 구분하여 우리말로는 사람 또는 인간이라고 하고, 영어로는 *man*이라고 하며, 라틴어로는 vir 또는 homo, 그리스어로는 anēr 또는 anthrōpos라고 한다. 중국어로는 rén(人) 또는 rénjiān(人間), 일본어로는 ひと(人) 또는 にんげん(人間)이라고 한다. 이처럼 모든 언어는 나름대로 종을 가리키는 이름을 가지고 있으니 그 이름은 통속명 또는 보통명이다.

학술용어에서 종의 이름은 유일해야 하고 체계적이어야 하며 모든 사람이 받아들일 수 있어야 한다. 그런 점에서 언어마다 다른 통속명을 학술명, 즉 학명으로 채택하기에는 문제점이 너무 많다.

Homo sapiens라는 종의 이름은 오로지 현생인류라는 한 가지 종만을 가리키며, 멸종된 Homo neanderthalensis, Homo heidelbergensis, Homo erectus, Homo habilis 등과는 같은 속(屬)에 속하나 종(種)이 다르고, 현존 유인원인 침팬지(Pan troglodytes), 보노보(Pan paniscus), 고릴라(Gorilla gorilla)와는 속(屬)마저 다르다는 것을 보여주어 체계적이다. 또한 전 세계적으로 통용된다. 학술용어로 써야 하는 학명은 Homo sapiens인 것이다.

Homo sapiens 현생인류

　　　L. homo 사람: 남성 명사, 단수 주격
　　　　　　　< L. homo, hominis, m. 사람
　　　　　< IE. dhghem- *earth, earthling* (Vide HOMO: *See* E. *homo*)
　　　L. sapiens 지혜로운: 현재분사, 남·여·중성형 단수 주격
　　　　　　　< L. sapiens, (gen.) sapientis 맛을 아는, 지혜로운
　　　　　< L. sapio, sapivi (sapii, sapui), –, sapĕre 맛있다, 맛을 알다, 알다,
　　　　　　　지혜롭다
　　　　　< IE. sep–, sap– *to taste, to perceive* (Vide SAPĔRE: *See* E. *sage*)

Homo sapiens에서 보듯, 학명으로서 종(種, L. species)의 이름은 종이 속하는 속(屬, L. genus)의 이름인 속명(屬名, *generic name*) 하나와 속명을 수식함으로써 종(種)을 특징짓는 꾸밈말(*epithet*) 하나, 즉 두(L. bi- *two*) 이름(L. nomen *name*)으로 만들도록 국제 규약 상 정해놓고 있다. 이명법(二名法, *binomial nomenclature*)이라고 한다.

　　　종의 이름 (이명법)　　속명(屬名)　　Homo
　　　　　　　　　　　　　　꾸밈말　　　sapiens: 속명 Homo를 수식

이명법을 사용하여 식물과 동물을 체계적으로 분류한 사람은 스웨덴의 의사이자 식물학자인 린네(Carl von Linné, 1707~1778)이다. 린네는 그의 저술명인 라틴어 이름 카롤루스 린내우스(Carolus Linnaeus)로도 알려져 있다. Homo sapiens도 린네가 명명한 학명이다.

린네는 어렸을 때부터 목사인 아버지로부터 식물에 대해 배워 여덟 살 때에는 '어린 식물학자'라는 말을 들을 정도이었다. 룬드대학과 웁살라대학에서 공부하였고 웁살라대학에서 의학사 학위를 받았다. 웁살라에서 원로 식물학자 첼시우스(Olof Celsius)를 만나 많은 영향을 받았으며, 1730년 웁살라대학의 식물학 강사가 되었고, 2년 뒤 웁살라과학협회의 지원 아래 스칸디나비아 북단에 있는 라플란드 지역을 탐사하였다. 1735년 네덜란드에 체재하였으며 그 해에 〈Systema Naturae 자연의 체계〉를, 1737년에는 〈Flora Lapponica 라플란드의 식물상〉을 발간하였다. 열한 쪽짜리 〈자연의 체계〉에서 린네는 처음으로 종의 이름을 이명법(二名法)으로 명명하여 분류학의 체계를 세웠고 현대 분류학의 아버지라고 일컬어지게 되었다.

[예] 땅꽈리 (다른 이름: 때꽈리, 애기땅꽈리, 좀꼬아리, 덩굴꼬아리, 덩굴꽈리)

그 당시 통용되던 땅꽈리 이름: Physalis annua ramosissima, ramis angulosis glabris, foliis dentato-serratis (가장자리가 치아와 톱니처럼 생긴 잎과, 털이 없고 각이 있는 가지를 가지며, 가지가 무성한 한해살이 꽈리)

〈자연의 체계〉에서 땅꽈리 이름: Physalis angulata (각진 꽈리)

린네는 1738년 귀국하여 스톡홀름에서 잠시 개원의 생활을 하였으며, 1741년 웁살라대학의 의학교수가 되었고 다음해 식물학교수로 자리를 옮겼다. 〈자연의 체계〉의 개정판 외에도 1753년에는 〈Species Plantarum 식물의 종〉을 발간하였으며 식물뿐 아니라 동물과 광물의 분류에 관한 저술을 남겼다. 1757년 스웨덴 국왕으로부터 작위를 받았다. 1774년 뇌졸중으로 쓰러졌고 4년 뒤인 1778년 사망하였다. 그의 사후 1788년 영국의 J. E. 스미스(James Edward Smith)가 린네를 기념해 런던에 린네학회(*The Linnean Society of London*)를 설립하였으며, 학회는 린네가 수집한 표본과 장서를 구입해 보존해 오고 있다. 국제회의에서 식물은 린네가 1753년 발간한 〈식물의 종〉에 따라, 동물은 1758년 발간한 〈자연의 체계〉 제10판에 따라 학명을 이명법으로 정하기로 결정해 오늘까지 이어진다.

아종의 이름 - 삼명법

린네가 현생인류를 Homo sapiens라고 명명한 것은 현생인류와 침팬지를 구분하기 위해서였다. 린네가 명명한 유인원 침팬지의 학명은 Homo troglodytes 이었다. (린네는 '만물의 영장'인 현생인류와 침팬지 같은 유인원을 Homo라는 같은 속에 분류함으로써 웁살라교회 당국으로부터 '믿음이 없는 자'로 비난받기도 하였다.)

Homo troglodytes 침팬지

    L. homo 사람: 남성 명사, 단수 주격
           < L. homo, hominis, m. 사람
       < IE. dhghem- *earth, earthling* (Vide HOMO: *See* E. *homo*)
    L. troglodytes 동굴에서 사는: 형용사, 남·여·중성형 단수 주격
            < L. troglodytes, (gen.) troglodytis 동굴에서 사는
         < G. trōglodytēs, trōglodytēs, trōglodytes *cave-entering, cave-dwelling*
       < G. trōglē, trōglēs, f. *hole, cave*
         + G. dyein *to enter, to put on* (Vide EPENDYMA: *See* E. *ependyma*)

'믿음이 있는 자'들은 침팬지의 학명을 그리스 신화에 나오는 '염소의 머리와 다리를 가졌으며 일곱 개 대롱으로 만든 피리를 불고 다닌 반인반수(半人半獸)' 판의 이름을 따 Pan troglodytes라고 하였다. 현재는 사람과 침팬지의 차이가 속(屬)의 차이를 충분히 넘어선다고 보기 때문에 침팬지의 학명으로는 Pan troglodytes가 인정받고 있다.

Pan troglodytes 침팬지

    L. Pan 판: 남성 명사, 단수 주격
           < L. Pan, Panis, m. (Pan, Panos, m.) 판 (가축과 목동의 신, 숲의 신)
        < G. Pan, Panos, m. (원뜻은 사육사) 판 (Vide PAN: *See* E. *pan*)
    L. troglodytes 동굴에서 사는: 형용사, 남·여·중성형 단수 주격 (Vide supra)

1856년 독일 뒤셀도르프 근처 네안더(D. Neander) 계곡(D. Thal)에 있는 한 채석장에서 고대인(古代人)의 것으로 판명된 뼈가 발견되었다. 멸종된 이 고대 인종의 학명은 Homo neanderthalensis가 된다.

Homo neanderthalensis 네안데르탈인

L. homo 사람: 남성 명사, 단수 주격

    < L. homo, hominis, m. 사람

   < IE. dhghem- *earth, earthling* (Vide HOMO: *See* E. *homo*)

L. neanderthalensis 네안더 계곡의: 형용사, 남·여성형 단수 주격

    < L. Neanderthalensis, Neanderthalense 네안더 계곡의

  < D. Neander (< Joachim Neander (1650-1680), *German theologian*) 네안더

  + D. Thal 계곡 (Vide THALAMUS: *See* E. *thalamus*)

  + L. -ensis, -ense 장소, 기원, 소속의 형용사를 만드는 라틴어 접미사

    (Vide -(D)ENSIS: *See* E. -*ese*)

네안데르탈인의 골격은 현생인류의 골격과는 분명 다르지만 다른 어떤 영장류의 골격보다도 현생인류의 골격에 더 닮아 있어서 한때는 네안데르탈인을 현생인류의 아종으로 분류하던 때가 있었다. 그 때의 학명은 Homo sapiens (ssp.) neanderthalensis, 또는 (ssp.)를 뺀 Homo sapiens neanderthalensis이었다. 속명(屬名) Homo와 속명을 수식함으로써 종(種)을 특징짓는 꾸밈말 sapiens 뒤에다 속명을 한 번 더 수식함으로써 아종(亞種)을 특징짓는 덧꾸밈말 neanderthalensis를 덧붙여 세(L. tri- *three*) 개의 이름으로 만든 것이다. 삼명법(三名法, *trinomial nomenclature*)이라고 한다. 삼명법에 의한 현생인류의 학명은 Homo sapiens sapiens가 된다. '멍청해도 현명한' 사람이라는 뜻이다.

종의 이름 (삼명법)   속명(屬名)   Homo

                꾸밈말   sapiens: 속명 Homo를 수식

                덧꾸밈말   sapiens: 속명 Homo를 수식

네안데르탈인을 현생인류와 다른 종으로 볼 것인지 아니면 현생인류의 아종으로 볼 것인지 (또는 현생인류를 네안데르탈인의 아종으로 볼 것인지) 논란 속에 최근 네안데르탈인의 골격 안에 남아 있는 사립체의 핵산을 뽑아 현생인류와 비교해보았더니 종이 달랐다. 그래서 네안데르탈인의 학명은 다시 Homo neanderthalensis가 되었고, 현생인류는 아종이 없는 단일종 Homo sapiens로 남게 되었다.

1997년 에디오피아의 아파르(Afar) 지방에서 세 개의 오래된 두개골이 발견되었다. 네안데르탈인의 두개골보다도 더 현생인류에 가까운 두개골이었다. 학명은 Homo sapiens idaltu이다. idaltu란 아파르 지방어로 연장자란 뜻이며, 현생인류의 아프리카 기원설('*out of Africa*')에 따라 그리 이름하였다. 이것이 사

실로 인정된다면 그 때부터 Homo sapiens라는 종은 현생인류라는 Homo sapiens sapiens와 그 조상이라고 주장되는 멸종된 Homo sapiens idaltu의 두 아종을 가지게 될 것이다.

생명과학에 등장하는 종의 이름은, 그러나, 대부분 이명법에 의한 이름이다. 아종을 아우르는 삼명법 이름은 어쩌다 한 번 꼴로 만나게 된다.

학명의 가변성

종을 결정하는 기준은 세대의 연속성, 형태와 내용의 차이, 핵산 염기서열의 차이이다. 이 중 가장 이론적인 것은 세대의 연속성이고 가장 결정적인 것은 핵산의 염기서열이다. 그러나 가장 실제적인 것은 형태와 내용이며 그 중에서도 일차적인 것은 형태이다. 지금 통용되는 종의 분류와 이름도 대부분 형태적 차이에 의한 분류와 이름이다.

종의 분류와 이름이 일차적으로 형태적 차이에 따라 정해졌기 때문에 핵산의 염기서열이 밝혀지면서 분류와 이름이 바뀌는 경우가, 드물지만, 있다. 극단적으로 말하자면 지금 통용되는 종의 분류와 이름은 유전자 풀의 염기서열이 모두 밝혀진 몇 안 되는 종을 제외하고는 그럴 것이라는 가정 하에 이루어진 가설로서 바뀔 수 있는 것이다. 면역능이 떨어진 사람에서 폐렴을 일으키는 폐포자충이, 핵산 분석 결과, 오랫동안 알고 있었던 Pneumocystis carinii와는 다른 포자충으로 밝혀져 Pneumocystis jirovecii라는 새 이름을 갖게 된 것이 그 예이다.

Pneumocystis jirovecii (Pneumocystis jiroveci) 이로베치 폐포자충

L. Pneumocystis 폐포자충속(屬): 여성 명사, 단수 주격
< L. Pneumocystis, Pneumocystidis, f. (< *cyst-forming fungus within the lungs*) (진균) 폐포자충속(屬)
< G. pneumōn, pneumonos, m. *lung*
< IE. pleu- *to flow* (Vide PULMO; *See* E. *pulmonic*)
+ G. kystis, kystidos, f. *bladder, bag < bellows*
< IE. kwes- *to pant, to wheeze* (Vide CYSTIS; *See* E. *cyst*)
L. jirovecii (jiroveci): 남성 명사, 단수 속격 (*International Code of Botanical Nomenclature*는 jirovecii를 표준으로 한다. Jirovec 이름이 자음으로 끝나기 때문이다.)
< L. Jirovecius, Jirovecii, m. (Jirovecus, Jiroveci, m.) 이로베치
< Otto Jirovec (1910–1972), *Czech parasitologist*

명명법의 국제 규약

명명은 조류·진균류·식물의 경우 국제조류·진균류·식물명명규약(*International Code of Nomenclature for algae, fungi, and plants*)을, 재배식물의 경우 국제재배식물명명규약(*International Code of Nomenclature for Cultivated Plants*)을, 동물의 경우 국제동물명명규약(*International Code of Zoological Nomenclature*)을, 세균과 고세균의 경우 국제원핵생물명명규약(*International Code of Nomenclature of Prokaryotes*)을 따라 명명한다. 세부 사항에 관한 규정은 규약에 따라 다르나 모두 린네의 이명법을 원칙으로 하기 때문에 중심 내용이 같다.

종의 이름

종의 이름은 종이 속하는 속명(屬名)과, 속명을 수식함으로써 종을 특징짓는 꾸밈말의 두 낱말로 만든다. 두 낱말은 모두 라틴어나 라틴어화한 그리스어 낱말로서 라틴어 문법을 따라야 하며, 짧고 발음하기 좋고 듣기 좋아야 한다. 라틴어나 라틴어화한 그리스어 낱말이 아닌 제3언어의 낱말은 가능한 한 사용하지 않으며 꼭 사용해야 할 경우에도 라틴어화하는 것을 원칙으로 한다. 속명의 첫 글자는 대문자로 쓴다. 의미 전달이 분명한 경우에는 H. sapiens처럼 속명을 머리글자 하나로 줄여 쓸 수 있으나 꾸밈말 하나만을 쓸 수는 없다.

라틴어 학명의 예

Homo sapiens 현생인류

    L. homo 사람: 남성 명사, 단수 주격
        < L. homo, hominis, m. 사람
      < IE. dhghem- *earth, earthling* (Vide HOMO: *See* E. *homo*)
    L. sapiens 지혜로운: 현재분사, 남·여·중성형 단수 주격
        < L. sapiens, (gen.) sapientis 맛을 아는, 지혜로운
        < L. sapio, sapivi (sapii, sapui), –, sapĕre 맛있다, 맛을 알다, 알다, 지혜롭다

< IE. sep-, sap- *to taste, to perceive* (Vide SAPĔRE: *See* E. *sage*)

라틴어화한 그리스어 학명의 예

Entamoeba histolytica 이질(痢疾) 아메바

L. Entamoeba (체내 기생성) 아메바속(屬): 여성 명사, 단수 주격

　　　< L. Entamoeba, Entamoebae, f. (체내 기생성) 아메바속(屬)

　　< G. entos *within, inside*

< IE. en *in* (Vide IN: *See* E. *in-*)

　+ G. amoibē, amoibēs, f. *change*

< IE. mei- *to change, to go, to move* (Vide MUTARE: *See* E. *mutate*)

L. histolytica 조직을 녹이는: 형용사, 여성형 단수 주격

　　　< L. histolyticus, histolytica, histolyticum 조직을 녹이는

　　< G. histos, histou, m. *tissue*

< IE. sta- *to stand* (Vide STARE: *See* E. *stay*)

　+ G. lyein *to loosen, to release, to dissolve*

< IE. leu- *to loosen, to divide, to cut* (Vide SOLVĔRE: *See* E. *solve*)

　+ G. -tikos, -tikē, -tikon *adjective suffix*

라틴어화한 제 3 언어 학명의 예

Homo neanderthalensis 네안데르탈인

L. homo 사람: 남성 명사, 단수 주격

　　　< L. homo, hominis, m. 사람

　　< IE. dhghem- *earth, earthling* (Vide HOMO: *See* E. *homo*)

L. neanderthalensis 네안더 계곡의: 형용사, 남·여성형 단수 주격

　　　< L. Neanderthalensis, Neanderthalense 네안더 계곡의

　　< D. Neander (< Joachim Neander (1650–1680), *German theologian*) 네안더

　　+ D. Thal 계곡 (Vide THALAMUS: *See* E. *thalamus*)

　　+ L. -ensis, -ense 장소, 기원, 소속의 형용사를 만드는 라틴어 접미사

　　　　(Vide -(I)ENSIS: *See* E. *-ese*)

속명

　　속명은 명사 또는 명사적 용법의 형용사이어야 하며 순수한 형용사나 그 외 품사는 속명이 될 수 없다. 속명의 성은 본디 낱말의 성에 따라서, 또는 라틴어화 하면서 붙인 어미에 따라서 남성, 여성, 중성 중 하나가 되며 수는 단수, 격은

주격이 된다.

형용사의 명사적 용법에 의한 속명의 예

Anopheles sinensis 중국얼룩날개모기

L. anopheles 얼룩날개모기: 남성 명사, 단수 주격

    < L. anopheles, anophelis, m. (형용사의 명사적 용법)

       아노펠레스모기, 학질모기, 얼룩날개모기

    < G. anōphelēs, anōphelēs, anōpheles (< an- *not*)

       unprofitable, useless, hurtful

    < G. ophelos, ophelou, n. *profit, advantage, usefulness*

    < IE. obhel- *to avail* (Vide ANOPHELES; *See* E. *anopheles*)

L. sinensis 중국의, 중국 출신의: 형용사, 남·여성형 단수 주격

    < L. Sinensis, Sinense 중국의, 중국 출신의

    < L. Sina, Sinae, f. 중국

    < (*Arabic*) Sin *China*

    < (*Chinese*) Qin (Chin) 진(秦, 221–206 B.C.E.) (Vide SINA; *See* E. *China*)

속명으로서 사람 이름

사람 이름을 속명으로 사용할 때에는, 남녀 관계없이, 라틴어 명사 제1변화의 단수 주격 어미 –a를 붙이고 여성 명사로 취급한다. 이름이 –a 이외의 모음으로 끝나면 –a만을 붙이고 –a 모음으로 끝나면 발음의 편의상 –e–를 끼워 넣은 후 –a를 붙인다. 자음으로 끝나면 연결 모음 –i–를 끼워 넣은 후 –a를 붙이나 발음이 불편하지 않으면 연결 모음 없이 –a만을 붙인다. 여성형 지소 접미사를 붙일 수도 있다. 이미 라틴어화한 이름의 경우에는 라틴어 어미를 떼어낸 다음, 같은 방식을 따른다.

사람 이름에 여성형 어미를 붙여 속명으로 사용한 학명의 예

Serratia marcescens (< *rapid deterioration of the pigment*) 세라티아 마르체센스균

L. Serratia 세라티아속(屬): 여성 명사, 단수 주격

    < L. Serratia, Serratiae, f. (세균) 세라티아속(屬)

    < Serafino Serrati (18c.), *Italian physicist, developer of steamboat*

L. marcescens 시드는: 현재분사, 남·여·중성형 단수 주격

    < L. marcescens, (gen.) marcescentis 시드는, 쇠약해지는

    < L. marcesco, marcui, –, marcescĕre 시들다, 이울다, 쇠약해지다

Yersinia pestis 페스트균

L. Yersinia 예르시니아속(屬): 여성 명사, 단수 주격

    < L. Yersinia, Yersiniae, f. (세균) 예르시니아속(屬)

    < Alexandre Emile Jean Yersin (1863–1943), *Swiss–French bacteriologist*

L. pestis 페스트의: 여성 명사, 단수 속격

    < L. pestis, pestis, f. 전염병, 흑사병, 페스트, 멸망, 불행 (Vide PESTIS; *See* E. *pest*)

Naegleria fowleri 파울러 자유아메바

L. Naegleria 자유아메바속(屬): 여성 명사, 단수 주격

    < L. Naegleria, Naegleriae, f. (원충) 자유아메바속(屬)

    < F. P. O. Nägler (Nagler) (20c), *Australian bacteriologist*

L. fowleri 파울러의: 남성 명사, 단수 속격

    < L. Fowlerus, Fowleri, m. 파울러

    < Malcolm Fowler (20c), *Australian pathologist who first isolated the organism from a patient with amebic meningoencephalitis*

Euphorbia splendens 꽃기린

L. Euphorbia 버들옷속(屬): 여성 명사, 단수 주격

    < L. Euphorbia, Euphorbiae, f. (식물) 버들옷속(屬)

    < L. Euphorbus, Euphorbi, m. (Euphorbos, Euphorbi, m.) (< G. eu- *well, good* + phorbē, phorbēs, f. *food, fodder, victuals, forage*) *First century Greek court physician to Juba II, king of Mauritania*

L. splendens 화려한: 현재분사, 남·여·중성형 단수 주격

    < L. splendens, (gen.) splendentis 빛나는, 화려한

    < L. splendeo, splendui, –, splendēre 빛나다, 화려하다

    < IE. splend- *to shine, to glow* (Vide SPLENDĒRE; *See* E. *splendid*)

사람 이름에 여성형 지소 접미사를 붙여 속명으로 사용한 학명의 예

Salmonella typhi 장티푸스균

Salmonella enteritidis 식중독 살모넬라균

L. Salmonella 살모넬라속(屬): 여성 명사, 단수 주격

    < L. Salmonella, Salmonellae, f. (< + -ella *feminine diminutive suffix*) (세균) 살모넬라속(屬)

    < Daniel Elmer Salmon (1850–1914), *American pathologist*

L. typhi 티푸스의: 남성 명사, 단수 속격

    < L. typhus, typhi, m. 티푸스

< G. typhos, typhou, m. *smoke, steam, stupor*

< G. typhein *to smoke*

< IE. dheu-, dheuə- *to rise in a cloud* (Vide FUMUS; *See* E. *fume*)

L. enteritidis 장염의: 여성 명사, 단수 속격

< L. enteritis, enteritidis, f. (< + -itis *noun suffix denoting inflammation*) 장염

< G. enteron, enterou, n. *gut*

< IE. en *in* (Vide IN; *See* E. *in-*)

Bordetella pertussis 백일해균(百日咳菌)

L. Bordetella 보르데텔라속(屬): 여성 명사, 단수 주격

< L. Bordetella, Bordetellae, f. (< + -ella *feminine diminutive suffix*) (세균) 보르데텔라속(屬)

< Jules Jean Baptiste Vincent Bordet (1870–1961), *Belgian bacteriologist and immunologist*

L. pertussis 백일해의: 여성 명사, 단수 속격

< L. pertussis, pertussis, f. (< per- *through, thorough* + tussis *cough*) 백일해(百日咳)

< L. tussis, tussis, f. 기침, 해소(咳嗽)

< IE. (s)teu- *to push, to stick, to knock, to beat* (Vide TUNDĔRE; *See* E. *contusion*)

Klebsiella pneumoniae 폐렴막대균

L. Klebsiella 클렙시엘라속(屬): 여성 명사, 단수 주격

< L. Klebsiella, Klebsiellae, f. (< + -i- *combining vowel* + -ella *feminine diminutive suffix*) (세균) 클렙시엘라속(屬)

< Theodor Albrecht Edwin Klebs (1834–1913), *German bacteriologist*

L. pneumoniae 폐렴의: 여성 명사, 단수 속격

< L. pneumonia, pneumoniae, f. 폐렴

< G. pneumonia, pneumonias, f. *pneumonia*

< G. pneumōn, pneumonos, m. *lung*

< IE. pleu- *to flow* (Vide PULMO; *See* E. *pulmonic*)

꾸밈말

속명을 꾸미는 꾸밈말은 단수 주격 형용사, 단수 주격 분사, 또는 단수나 복수의 속격 명사를 원칙으로 한다. 권장하는 꾸밈말은 형용사이다. 형용사나 분사는 속명의 성을 따라야 한다. 속명과 동격어의 의미로 단수 주격 명사를 사용할 수

있다.

형용사를 꾸밈말로 사용한 학명의 예

Mimosa pudica 미모사, 함수초(含羞草)

L. mimosa 미모사, 함수초(含羞草): 여성 명사, 단수 주격

< L. mimosa, mimosae, f. 미모사

< G. mimos, mimou, m. *imitator, actor* (Vide MIMICUS; See E. *mimic*)

L. pudica 부끄러워하는: 형용사, 여성형 단수 주격

< L. pudicus, pudica, pudicum 부끄러워하는, 정숙한, 순결한

< L. pudeo, pudui, puditum, pudēre 부끄러워하다, 부끄럽게 하다

< IE. (s)peud- *to push, to repulse* (Vide PUDENDUM; See E. *pudendum*)

Culex tritaeniorhynchus (< *proboscis with three ochreous bands*) 작은빨간집모기

L. culex: 남성 명사, 단수 주격

< L. culex, culicis, m. 모기, 각다귀, 등에; 집모기

< IE. ku- *sharp, pointed* (Vide CUNEUS; See E. *cuneate*)

L. tritaeniorhynchus 세 개의 띠무늬가 있는 주둥이의: 형용사, 남성형 단수 주격

< L. tritaeniorhynchus, tritaeniorhyncha, tritaeniorhynchum

of proboscis with three (ochreous) bands

< G. treis, treis, tria *three*

< IE. trei- *three* (Vide TRES; See E. *tri-*)

+ G. tainia, tainias, f. *head-band, ribbon*

< IE. ten- *to stretch* (Vide TENĒRE; See E. *tenet*)

+ G. rhynchos, rhynchou, m. *snout, bill, beak*

< IE. srenk- *to snore* (Vide RHONCHUS; See E. *rhonchus*)

Clostridium botulinum 클로스트리듐 보툴리눔

L. Clostridium 클로스트리듐속(屬): 중성 명사, 단수 주격

< L. Clostridium, Clostridii, n. (세균) 클로스트리듐속(屬)

< G. klōstridion, klōstridiou, n. (< + -idion *diminutive suffix*)

clostridium

< G. klōstēr, klōstēros, m. *spindle*

< G. klōthein *to spin*

< IE. klo- *to spin* (Vide CLOSTRIDIUM; See E. *clostridial*)

L. botulinum 순대의: 형용사, 중성형 단수 주격

< L. botulinus, botulina, botulinum 창자의, 순대의

< L. botulus, botuli, m. 창자, 순대

< IE. g^wet- *intestine* (Vide BOTULUS; See E. *bowel*)

Enterococcus faecalis 분변(糞便) 장알균

L. Enterococcus 엔테로코쿠스속(屬), 장알균속(屬): 남성 명사, 단수 주격

    < L. Enterococcus, Enterococci, m. (세균) 엔테로코쿠스속(屬),
장알균속(屬)

    < G. enteron, enterou, n. *gut*

    < IE. en *in* (Vide EN: *See* E. *in-*)

    + G. kokkos, kokkou, m. *kernel, grain, berry*

L. faecalis 분변(糞便)의: 형용사, 남·여성형 단수 주격

    < L. faecalis, faecale 찌꺼기의; 대변의, 분변의

    < L. faex, faecis, f. 찌꺼기; 대변(大便), 분변(糞便) (Vide FAEX: *See* E. *faeces*)

Trichomonas vaginalis 질편모충(膣鞭毛蟲), 질트리코모나스

L. Trichomonas 트리코모나스속(屬): 여성 명사, 단수 주격

    < L. Trichomonas, Trichomonadis, f. (편모충 鞭毛蟲) 트리코모나스속(屬)

    < G. thrix, trichos, f. *hair, wool, bristle*

    < (*suggested*) IE. dhrigh-, dhreikh- *hair, bristle* (Vide TRICHOSIS: *See* E. *trichosis*)

    + G. monas, monados, f. *unit*

    < IE. men- *small, isolated* (Vide MONAS: *See* E. *monad*)

L. vaginalis 질(膣)의: 형용사, 남·여성형 단수 주격

    < L. vaginalis, vaginale 질(膣)의

    < L. vagina, vaginae, f. (< *sheath 'probably made of split pieces of wood'*)
칼집, 초, 질(膣)

    < IE. wag- *to break, to split, to bite* (Vide VAGINA: *See* E. *vagina*)

Mycobacterium intracellulare 마이코박테륨 인트라셀룰라레

L. mycobacterium 마이코박테륨: 중성 명사, 단수 주격

    < L. mycobacterium, mycobacterii, n. (< *moldlike growth on the
surface of liquid media*) (세균) 마이코박테륨

    < G. mykēs, mykētos, m. *mushroom*

    < IE. meug- *slimy, slippery; with derivatives referring to various wet or slimy
substances and conditions* (Vide MUCUS: *See* E. *mucus*)

    + G. baktērion, baktēriou, n. *small staff, bacterium*

    < IE. bak- *staff used for support* (Vide BACTERIUM: *See* E. *bacterium*)

L. intracellulare 세포 안의: 형용사, 중성형 단수 주격

    < L. intracellularis, intracellulare (< intra- *inside*) 세포 안의

    < L. cellula, cellulae, f. (< + -ula *diminutive suffix*) 작은 방; 세포

    < L. cella, cellae, f. 광

    < IE. kel- *to cover, to conceal, to save* (Vide CELLULA: *See* E. *cell*)

Plasmodium falciparum (< *crescentic gametocyte*) 열대열원충

Plasmodium ovale (< *oval trophozoite*) 난형열원충

Plasmodium vivax (< *ameboid trophozoite*) 삼일열원충

L. Plasmodium 말라리아원충속(原蟲屬): 중성 명사, 단수 주격

  < L. Plasmodium, Plasmodii, n. (< G. plasm(o)- + G. -ōdēs
    like, resembling + L. -ium *noun suffix*) 말라리아원충속
    (原蟲屬), 열원충속(熱原蟲屬)

  < G. plasma, plasmatos, n. *something molded, something formed,*
    figure, image, fiction, forgery

  < G. plassein (< *to shape, to spread out*) *to mold, to form*

  < IE. pelə- *flat, to spread* (Vide PLANUS: *See* E. *plane*)

L. falciparum 낫 모양의 생식모세포를 만드는: 형용사, 중성형 단수 주격

  < L. falciparus, falcipara, falciparum (< + -parus, -para, -parum
    bearing) 낫 모양의 생식모세포를 만드는

  < L. falx, falcis, f. 낫, 겸(鎌)

  < *Of* non-IE. *origin* (Vide FALX: *See* E. *falx*)

L. ovale 난형의: 형용사, 중성형 단수 주격

  < L. ovalis, ovale 난형의, 난원형의

  < L. ovum, ovi, n. 알

  < IE. owyo-, oyyo- *egg* (Vide OVUM: *See* E. *ovum*)

L. vivax 활기 있는: 형용사, 남·여·중성형 단수 주격

  < L. vivax, (gen.) vivacis 활기 있는, 오래 사는

  < L. vivo, vixi, victum, vivĕre 살다

  < IE. gʷeiə-, gʷei- *to live* (Vide VIVĔRE: *See* E. *vivarium*)

분사를 꾸밈말로 사용한 학명의 예

Candida albicans 칸디다 알비칸스

L. Candida 칸디다속(屬): 여성 명사, 단수 주격

  < L. Candida, Candidae, f. (불완전 진균) 칸디다속(屬)

  < L. candidus, candida, candidum 흰, 순결한, 꾸밈없는

  < L. candeo, candui, -, candēre 불에 달궈져 빛을 내다, 백열(白熱)을 내다,
    하얗다

  < IE. kand-, kend- *to shine* (Vide CANDĒRE: *See* E. *candent*)

L. albicans 하얀: 현재분사, 남·여·중성형 단수 주격

  < L. albicans, (gen.) albicantis 하얀, 하얗게 되는

  < L. albico, albicavi, albicatum, albicare 하얗다, 하얗게 되다

< IE. albho- *white* (Vide ALBUS: *See* E. *albino*)

Caenorhabditis elegans (< *new rod-shaped organism with elegant sinusoidal movement*) 예쁜꼬마선충

L. Caenorhabditis 꼬마선충속(屬): 여성 명사, 단수 주격
    < L. Caenorhabditis, Caenorhabditis, f. 꼬마선충속(屬)
    < G. kainos, kainē, kainon *new, strange*
    < IE. ken- *fresh, new, young* (Vide RECENS: *See* E. *recent*)
    + G. rhabdos, rhabdou, f. *rod*
    < IE. wer- *to turn, to bend, to wind* (Vide VERTÈRE: *See* E. *verse*)
L. elegans 우아한: 현재분사, 남·여·중성형 단수 주격
    < L. elegans, (gen.) elegantis (< *elegare) 뛰어난, 우아한
    < L. eligo, elegi, electum, eligĕre (< e- *out of, away from* + legĕre *to choose*) 뽑아내다, 선출하다
    < L. lego, legi, lectum, legĕre 모으다, 뽑다, 읽다
    < IE. leg- *to collect; with derivatives meaning 'to speak'* (Vide LEGÈRE: *See* E. *lecture*)

Clostridium perfringens 클로스트리듐 퍼프린젠스

L. Clostridium 클로스트리듐속(屬): 중성 명사, 단수 주격
    < L. Clostridium, Clostridii, n. (세균) 클로스트리듐속(屬)
    < G. klōstridion, klōstridiou, n. (< +-idion *diminutive suffix*) *clostridium*
    < G. klōstēr, klōstēros, m. *spindle*
    < G. klōthein *to spin*
    < IE. klo- *to spin* (Vide CLOSTRIDIUM: *See* E. *clostridial*)
L. perfringens 깨트리는: perfringĕre의 현재분사, 남·여·중성형 단수 주격
    < L. perfringens, (gen.) perfringentis 깨트리는
    < L. perfringo, perfregi, perfractum, perfringĕre (< per- *through, thoroughly* + frangĕre *to break*) 깨트리다
    < L. frango, fregi, fractum, frangĕre 분지르다, 깨트리다
    < IE. bhreg- *to break* (Vide FRANGÈRE: *See* E. *fractal*)

명사 단수 속격을 꾸밈말로 사용한 학명의 예

Corynebacterium diphtheriae 디프테리아균

L. Corynebacterium 코리네박테륨속(屬): 중성 명사, 단수 주격
    < L. Corynebacterium, Corynebacterii, n. (< *non-spore-forming, Gram-positive, mostly non-motile rods that are often swollen*

at one end) (세균) 코리네박테륨속(屬)

< G. korynē, korynēs, f. *club, mace*

< IE. ker- *horn, head* (Vide CORNU: *See* E. *unicorn*)

\+ G. baktērion, baktēriou, n. *small staff, bacterium*

< IE. bak- *staff used for support* (Vide BACTERIUM: *See* E. *bacterium*)

L. diphtheriae 디프테리아의: 여성 명사, 단수 속격

< L. diphtheria, diphtheriae, f. (< *formation of false mem-brane* < G. diphthera + -ia *noun suffix*) 디프테리아

< G. diphthera, diphtheras, f. *prepared hide, leather (used to write on)*

< G. dephein *to tan hides*

< IE. deph- *to stamp* (Vide LITERA: *See* E. *letter*)

Mycobacterium leprae 나병균, 한센병균

L. mycobacterium 마이코박테륨: 중성 명사, 단수 주격

< L. mycobacterium, mycobacterii, n. (< *moldlike growth on the surface of liquid media*) (세균) 마이코박테륨

< G. mykēs, mykētos, m. *mushroom*

< IE. meug- *slimy, slippery; with derivatives referring to various wet or slimy substances and conditions* (Vide MUCUS: *See* E. *mucus*)

\+ G. baktērion, baktēriou, n. *small staff, bacterium*

< IE. bak- *staff used for support* (Vide BACTERIUM: *See* E. *bacterium*)

L. leprae 나병의, 한센병의: 여성 명사, 단수 속격

< L. lepra, leprae, f. 나병, 한센병

< G. lepra, lepras, f. *leprosy*

< G. lepros, lepra, lepron *scaly, rough*

< G. lepis, lepidos, f. *scale, shell*

< G. lepein *to peel off*

< IE. leup-, lep- *to peel off, to break off, scale* (Vide LIBER: *See* E. *library*)

Plasmodium malariae 사일열원충

L. Plasmodium 말라리아원충속(原蟲屬): 중성 명사, 단수 주격

< L. Plasmodium, Plasmodii, n. (< G. plasm(o)- + G. -ōdēs *like, resembling* + L. -ium *noun suffix*) 말라리아원충속(原蟲屬), 열원충속(熱原蟲屬)

< G. plasma, plasmatos, n. *something molded, something formed, figure, image, fiction, forgery*

< G. plassein (< *to shape, to spread out*) *to mold, to form*

< IE. pelə- *flat, to spread* (Vide PLANUS: *See* E. *plane*)

L. malariae 말라리아의: 여성 명사, 단수 속격

< L. malaria, malariae, f. 말라리아, 학질(瘧疾), 학(瘧)

< It. mala aria *bad air*

< L. malus, mala, malum 나쁜

< IE. mel- *false, bad, wrong* (Vide MALUS: *See* E. *male-*)

+ G. aēr, aeros, m., f. *air, mist*

< IE. we- *to blow* (Vide AËR: *See* E. *air*)

Saccharomyces cerevisiae *bakers' yeast, brewers' yeast, wine yeast*

L. saccharomyces 사카로미세스, 효모균: 남성 명사, 단수 주격

< L. saccharomyces, saccharomycetis, m. 사카로미세스

< G. sakcharon, sakcharou, n. *sugar*

< (*Persian*) sakar *sugar*

< (*Sanskrit*) sarkara *sugar, akin to* sarkarah *pebble* (Vide SACCHARUM:
See E. *sugar*)

+ G. mykēs, mykētos, m. *mushroom*

< IE. meug- *slimy, slippery* (Vide MUCUS: *See* E. *mucus*)

L. cerevisiae 맥주의: 여성 명사, 단수 속격

< L. cerevisia, cerevisiae, f. (cervisia, cervisiae, f.) 맥주

< L. Ceres, Cereris, f. (로마 신화) 농업의 여신, 곡물의 여신

< IE. ker- *to grow* (Vide CRESCĚRE: *See* E. *crescent*)

Schizosaccharomyces pombe *fission yeast*

L. schizosaccharomyces 분열사카로미세스, 분열효모균: 남성 명사, 단수 주격

< L. schizosaccharomyces, schizosaccharomycetis, m.
분열사카로미세스

< G. schizein *to split*

< IE. skei- *to cut, to split* (Vide SECARE: *See* E. *secant*)

+ G. sakcharon, sakcharou, n. *sugar*

< (*Sanskrit*) sarkara *sugar, akin to* sarkarah *pebble* (Vide SACCHARUM:
See E. *sugar*)

+ G. mykēs, mykētos, m. *mushroom*

< IE. meug- *slimy, slippery* (Vide MUCUS: *See* E. *mucus*)

L. pombe 맥주의: 불변화 명사 (단수 속격의 뜻으로 사용)

< (*Swahili*) pombe *beer*

Clostridium tetani 클로스트리듐 테타니

L. Clostridium 클로스트리듐속(屬): 중성 명사, 단수 주격

< L. Clostridium, Clostridii, n. (세균) 클로스트리듐속(屬)

< G. klōstridion, klōstridiou, n. (< + -idion *diminutive suffix*)
clostridium

< G. klōstēr, klōstēros, m. *spindle*

< G. klōthein *to spin*

     < IE. klo- *to spin* (Vide CLOSTRIDIUM: *See* E. *clostridial*)

L. tetani 테타너스의: 남성명사, 단수 속격

        < L. tetanus, tetani, m. 파상풍(破傷風), 강축(强縮), 테타너스

      < G. tetanos, tetanē, tetanon *stretched, rigid*

      < G. teinein *to stretch, to strain*

     < IE. ten- *to stretch* (Vide TETANUS: *See* E. *tetanus*)

Helicobacter pylori 날문 헬리코박터, 위나선균, 위염균

L. Helicobacter 헬리코박터속(屬): 남성 명사, 단수 주격

     < L. Helicobacter, Helicobacteris, m. (세균) 헬리코박터속(屬)

    < G. helix, helikos, f. *winding, spire, coil, anything twisted*

   < IE. wel- *to turn, to roll* (Vide VOLVĔRE: *See* E. *volute*)

    + G. baktērion, baktēriou, n. *small staff, bacterium*

   < IE. bak- *staff used for support* (Vide BACTERIUM: *See* E. *bacterium*)

L. pylori 날문의, 유문의: 남성 명사, 단수 속격

      < L. pylorus, pylori, m. 날문(-門), 유문(幽門)

     < G. pylōros, pylōrou, m., f. (pylouros, pylourou, m.)

      gatekeeper, porter

    < G. pylē, pylēs, f. *gate* (Vide PYLORUS: *See* E. *pylorus*)

    + G. ouros, ourou, m. *watcher, warder*

   < IE. wer- *to perceive, to watch out for* (Vide VERERI: *See* E. *revere*)

Toxoplasma gondii 톡소포자충

L. Toxoplasma 톡소플라스마속(屬), 톡소포자충: 중성 명사, 단수 주격

      < L. Toxoplasma, Toxoplasmatis, n. (< *bow-shaped*) (포자충 胞子蟲)

      톡소플라스마속(屬)

    < G. toxon, toxou, n. (< *those which fly*) *bow;* (pl. toxa) *bow and arrows*

   < IE. tek^w- *to run, to flee* (Vide TOXICUM: *See* E. *toxic*)

    + G. plasma, plasmatos, n. *something formed*

   < IE. pelə- *flat, to spread* (Vide PLANUS: *See* E. *plane*)

L. gondii 곤디의: 남성 명사, 단수 속격

     < L. gondius, gondii, f. 곤디

    < (*Maghrebi Arabic*) gondi *rat*

Neisseria meningitidis 수막염균(髓膜炎菌)

L. Neisseria 나이세리아속(屬): 여성 명사, 단수 주격

     < L. Neisseria, Neisseriae, f. (세균) 나이세리아속(屬)

    < Alfred Ludwig Sigesmund Neisser (1855–1916), *German physician*

L. meningitidis 수막염의: 여성 명사, 단수 속격

< L. meningitis, meningitidis, f. (< + -itis *noun suffix denoting inflammation*) 수막염(髓膜炎)

< G. mēninx, mēningos, f. *membrane (of the brain)*

< IE. mems- *flesh, meat* (Vide MEMBRANA: *See* E. *membrane*)

Chlamydia trachomatis 클라미디아 트라코마티스

L. Chlamydia 클라미디아(屬): 여성 명사, 단수 주격

< L. Chlamydia, Chlamydiae, f. (< *the intracytoplasmic inclusions 'draped' around the infected cell's nucleus*) (세균) 클라미디아(屬)

< L. chlamys, chlamydis, f. 짧은 외투, 그리스식 군복

< G. chlamys, chlamydos, f. *cloak (draped around the shoulder), miliary cloak* (Vide CHLAMYDIA: *See* E. *chlamydia*)

L. trachomatis 트라코마의: 중성 명사, 단수 속격

< L. trachoma, trachomatis, n. 트라코마

< G. trachōma, trachōmatos, n. *roughness, rough tumor*

< G. trachys, tracheia, trachy *rough*

< IE. dher- *to make muddy, darkness* (Vide TRACHYS: *See* E. *trachoma*)

Mycobacterium tuberculosis 결핵균

Mycobacterium bovis 소결핵균

L. mycobacterium 마이코박테륨: 중성 명사, 단수 주격

< L. mycobacterium, mycobacterii, n. (< *moldlike growth on the surface of liquid media*) (세균) 마이코박테륨

< G. mykēs, mykētos, m. *mushroom*

< IE. meug- *slimy, slippery; with derivatives referring to various wet or slimy substances and conditions* (Vide MUCUS: *See* E. *mucus*)

+ G. baktērion, baktēriou, n. *small staff, bacterium*

< IE. bak- *staff used for support* (Vide BACTERIUM: *See* E. *bacterium*)

L. tuberculosis 결핵의: 여성 명사, 단수 속격

< L. tuberculosis, tuberculosis, f. 결핵(結核)

< L. tuberculum, tuberculi, n. 구근(球根), 융기(隆起), 결절(結節); 종기(腫氣), 결핵(結核)

< L. tuber, tuberis, n. 혹, 종기; 매듭, 나무의 옹이, 괴경(塊莖)

< L. tumeo, -, -, tumēre 부풀다, 붓다, 화나다, 오만하다

< IE. teuə -, teu- *to swell* (Vide TUMOR: *See* E. *tumor*)

L. bovis 소의: 남·여성 명사, 단수 속격

< L. bos, bovis, m., f. 소

< IE. gʷou- *ox, bull, cow* (Vide BOS: *See* E. *beef*)

Toxocara canis 개회충

Toxocara cati 고양이회충

L. Toxocara 톡소카라속(屬): 여성 명사, 단수 주격

    < L. Toxocara, Toxocarae, f. (< *arrow-shaped*) (선충 線蟲)
    톡소카라속(屬)

    < G. toxon, toxou, n. (< *those which fly*) *bow;* (pl. toxa) *bow and arrows*

< IE. tek^w– *to run, to flee* (Vide TOXICUM; *See* E. *toxic*)

    + G. kara, karatos, n. *head*

< IE. ker– *horn, head* (Vide CORNU; *See* E. *unicorn*)

L. canis 개의: 남·여성 명사, 단수 속격

    < L. canis, canis, m., f. 개

    < IE. kwon– *dog* (Vide CANIS; *See* E. *canine*)

L. cati 고양이의: 남성 명사, 단수 속격

    < L. catus, cati, m. (cattus, catti, m.) 고양이

    < IE. (*probably*) *Of Afro-Asiatic origin* (Vide CATUS; *See* E. *cat*)

Brucella abortus 소유산균(流産菌), 우유산균(牛流産菌)

L. Brucella 부르셀라속(屬): 여성 명사, 단수 주격

    < L. Brucella, Brucellae, f. (< + –ella *feminine diminutive suffix*)
    (세균) 부르셀라속(屬)

    < Sir David Bruce (1855–1931), *Scottish physician*

L. abortus 유산의: 남성 명사, 단수 속격

    < L. abortus, abortus, m. 유산, 낙태;
    유산아(流産兒), 낙태아(落胎兒)

    < L. aborior, abortus sum, aboriri (< ab– *off, away from* + oriri
    to arise) 좌절하다, 수포가 되다, 유산(流産)하다

    < L. orior, ortus sum, oriri 돋다, 나다, 출현하다

    < IE. er– *to move, to set in motion* (Vide ORIRI; *See* E. *orient*)

Sarcoptes scabiei 옴진드기

L. Sarcoptes 옴진드기속(屬): 여성 명사, 단수 주격

    < L. Sarcoptes, Sarcoptis, f. (진드기) 옴진드기속(屬)

    < G. sarx, sarkos, f. *flesh*

    < IE. twerk– *to cut* (Vide SARCASMUS; *See* E. *sarcasm*)

    + G. koptein *to strike, to cut off*

    < IE. kop– *to beat, to strike* (Vide COMMA; *See* E. *comma*)

L. scabiei 옴의, 개선의: 여성 명사, 단수 속격

    < L. scabies, scabiei, f. 옴, 개선(疥癬)

    < L. scabo, scabi, –, scaběre 긁다

< IE. (s)kep– *base of words with various technical meanings such as 'to cut with a sharp tool', 'to scrape', 'to hack'* (Vide SCABIES; *See* E. *scabies*)

명사 복수 속격을 무리[類]의 꾸밈말로 사용한 학명의 예

Enterococcus faecium 분변류(糞便類) 장알균

L. Enterococcus 엔테로코쿠스속(屬), 장알균속(屬): 남성 명사, 단수 주격

    < L. Enterococcus, Enterococci, m. (세균) 엔테로코쿠스속(屬), 장알균속(屬)

    < G. enteron, enterou, n. *gut*

< IE. en *in* (Vide EN; *See* E. *in-*)

    + G. kokkos, kokkou, m. *kernel, grain, berry*

L. faecium (< faecum) 대변(大便)들의, 분변류(糞便類)의: 여성 명사, 복수 속격

    < L. faex, faecis, f. 찌꺼기; 대변(大便), 분변(糞便)

        (Vide FAEX; *See* E. *faeces*)

Mycobacterium avium 마이코박테륨 아비움, 조류(鳥類) 결핵균

L. mycobacterium 마이코박테륨: 중성 명사, 단수 주격

    < L. mycobacterium, mycobacterii, n. (< *moldlike growth on the surface of liquid media*) (세균) 마이코박테륨

    < G. mykēs, mykētos, m. *mushroom*

< IE. meug– *slimy, slippery; with derivatives referring to various wet or slimy substances and conditions* (Vide MUCUS; *See* E. *mucus*)

    + G. baktērion, baktēriou, n. *small staff, bacterium*

< IE. bak– *staff used for support* (Vide BACTERIUM; *See* E. *bacterium*)

L. avium 새들의, 조류(鳥類)의: 여성 명사, 복수 속격

    < L. avis, avis, f. 새

    < IE. awi– *bird* (Vide AVIS; *See* E. *avian*)

명사 주격을 동격의 꾸밈말로 사용한 학명의 예

Panthera leo 사자

L. Panthera 표범속(屬): 여성 명사, 단수 주격

    < L. panther. patheris, m. 표범; panthera, pantherae, f. 암표범

    < G. panthēr, panthēros, m. *panther, leopard*

    < (*probably*) *Of Oriental origin*

L. leo 사자: 남성 명사, 단수 주격

    < L. leo, leonis, m. 사자

< G. leōn, leontos, m. *lion*

< (*probably*) *Of* non-IE. *origin* (Vide LEO: *See* E. *lion*)

Atropa belladonna 아트로파 벨라돈나

L. Atropa 아트로파속(屬): 여성 명사, 단수 주격

     < L. Atropa, Atropae, f. (가지과의 유독성 식물) 아트로파속(屬)

     < G. Atropos, Atropou, f. (< -a *not*) (*Greek mythology*) *one of the three Fates who severs the thread of life*

     < G. trepein *to turn, to turn away*

     < IE. trep- *to turn* (Vide TROPICUS: *See* E. *tropic*)

L. belladonna 벨라도나: 여성 명사, 단수 주격

     < L. belladonna, belladonnae, f. (< *perhaps from the use of its juice to add brilliance to the eyes by dilating the pupils*) 벨라도나 (가지과의 유독성 식물)

     < It. bella donna (< L. bella domina) *fair lady*

     < L. bellus, bella, bellum *beautiful*

     < IE. deu- *to do, to perform, to show favor, to revere* (Vide BONUS: *See* E. *bonus*)

     + L. domina, dominae, f. *lady*

     < IE. dem- *house, household* (Vide DOMINUS: *See* E. *domina*)

Drosophila melanogaster 초파리

L. Drosophila 초파리속(屬): 여성 명사, 단수 주격

     < L. Drosophila, Drosophilae, f. 초파리속(屬); (drosophila) 초파리

     < G. drosos, drosou, f. *dew*

     < IE. ros- *dew* (Vide ROS: *See* E. *rosemary*)

     + G. philos, philē, philon *loved, loving* (Vide PHILTRUM: *See* E. *philtrum*)

L. melanogaster 검은 배를 가진 생물: 여성 명사, 단수 주격

     < L. melanogaster, melanogastris, f. 검은 배를 가진 생물

     < G. melas, melaina, melan *dark, dusky, gloomy, black*

     < IE. mel- *of a darkish color* (Vide MELASMA: *See* E. *melasma*)

     + G. gastēr, gastros, f. *belly, womb, sausage*

     < IE. gras- *to devour* (Vide GASTER: *See* E. *gastrin*)

Nicotiana tabacum (식물) 담배

L. nicotiana (식물) 담배: 여성 명사, 단수 주격

     < L. nicotiana, nicotianae, f. (< herba nicotiana *herb of Nicot*) 담배속(屬)의 식물, 담배

     < L. Nicotianus, Nicotiana, Nicotianum *of Nicot*

     < Jean Nicot (1530–1604), *French ambassador in Lisbon and lexicographer,*

who introduced tobacco into France in 1560

L. tabacum 담배: 중성 명사, 단수 주격

< L. tabacum, tabaci, n. 담배, 연초

< Sp. tabaco *tobacco*

< (*American Indian*)

꾸밈말로서 장소 이름

장소의 이름을 꾸밈말로 사용할 때에는 라틴어 형용사가 있는 경우 단수 주격의 형용사를 사용한다. 라틴어 명사의 속격을 사용할 수 있다.

새로운 라틴어 형용사를 만들어 사용할 때에는 장소 이름에 접미사 −ensis (m.), −ensis (f.), −ense (n.)를 붙여 제3변화 제2식 형용사를 만들고 단수 주격을 사용한다.

장소의 라틴어 형용사를 꾸밈말로 사용한 학명의 예

Rubus coreanus 복분자 딸기

L. rubus 나무딸기: 남성 명사, 단수 주격

< L. rubus, rubi, m. 나무딸기, 가시덤불

< IE. reudh− *red, ruddy* (Vide RUBER: *See* E. *rubric*)

L. coreanus 한국의: 형용사, 남성형 단수 주격

< L. Coreanus, Coreana, Coreanum 한국의

< L. Corea, Coreae, f. 한국

< (*Korean*) Korai (Koryu) 고려(918−1392) (Vide COREA: *See* E. *Korea*)

Haematoxylum campechianum 캄페체 지방의 피나무 (헤마톡실린의 원자재)

L. haematoxylum *bloodwood*: 중성 명사, 단수 주격

< L. haematoxylum, haematoxyli, n. 피나무

< G. haima, haimatos, n. *blood*

< IE. sai− *thick fluid* (Vide HAEMORRHAGIA: *See* E. *haemorrhage*)

+ G. xylon, xylou, n. *wood, timber*

< (*suggested*) IE. (k)selwa− *forest, wood* (Vide XYLOPHAGUS: *See* E. *xylophagous*)

L. campechianum 캄페체 지방의: 형용사, 중성형 단수 주격

< L. Campechianus, Campechiana, Campechianum 캄페체 지방의

< (*Mexican*) Campeche (멕시코) 캄페체 지방

Brucella melitensis 몰타열균(Malta 熱菌)

  L. Brucella 부르셀라속(屬): 여성 명사, 단수 주격
      < L. Brucella, Brucellae, f. (< + -ella *feminine diminutive suffix*)
        (세균) 부르셀라속(屬)
     < Sir David Bruce (1855–1931), *Scottish physician*
  L. melitensis 몰타 섬의: 형용사, 남·여성형 단수 주격
        < L. Melitensis, Melitense 몰타 섬의
      < L. Melita, Melitae, f. (Melite, Melites, f.) 몰타 섬
     < G. Melitē, Melitēs, f. (지중해의) 몰타(*Malta*) 섬
    < (*perhaps*) *Of* pre-IE. *origin*

Clonorchis sinensis 간흡충

  L. Clonorchis 간흡충속(屬): 여성 명사, 단수 주격
      < L. Clonorchis, Clonorchis, f. (흡충) 간흡충속(屬); (clonorchis)
       간디스토마
     < G. klōn, klōnos, m. *twig, shoot, sprout*
    < IE. kel- *to strike, to cut; with derivatives referring to something broken or*
      cut off, piece of wood, twig (Vide GLADIUS: *See* E. *gladiator*)
    + G. orchis, orcheōs, m. (orchis, orchios, m.) *testis*
    < (*perhaps*) IE. ergh- *to mount* (Vide ORBIS: *See* E. *orb*)
  L. sinensis 중국의, 중국 출신의: 형용사, 남·여성형 단수 주격
        < L. Sinensis, Sinense 중국의, 중국 출신의
      < L. Sina, Sinae, f. 중국
     < (*Arabic*) Sin *China*
    < (*Chinese*) Qin (Chin) 진(秦, 221–206 B.C.E.) (Vide SINA: *See* E. *China*)

장소의 라틴어 명사 단수 속격을 꾸밈말로 사용한 학명의 예

Aedes aegypti 이집트숲모기

  L. aedes 숲모기: 남성 명사, 단수 주격
       < L. aedes, aedis, m. (형용사의 명사적 용법) 에데스모기, 숲모기
      < G. aēdēs, aēdēs, aēdes (< a- *not*) *unpleasant*
     < G. hēdys, hēdeia, hēdy *sweet, pleasant*
    < IE. swad- *sweet, pleasant* (Vide SUADĒRE: *See* E. *suasion*)
  L. aegypti 이집트의: 여성 명사, 단수 속격
      < L. Aegyptus, Aegypti, f. (Aegyptos, Aegypti, f.) 이집트
     < G. Aigyptos, Aigyptou, m. *Egypt* (Vide AEGYPTUS: *See* E. *Egypt*)

꾸밈말로서 사람 이름

사람 이름을 꾸밈말로 사용할 때에는 마땅한 라틴어 형용사가 있는 경우 단수 주격의 형용사를 사용한다. 이름 명사의 속격을 사용할 수도 있다.

새롭게 라틴어 이름을 만들어 사용할 때에는, 여성 이름이거나 남성 이름이라도 -a로 끝나면 제1변화 여성명사(-a, -ae, f.)로 만들고, 그렇지 않으면 제2변화 제1식 남성명사(-us, -i, m.)로 만들어 속격을 사용한다. 발음의 편의상 어미 앞에 연결 모음 -e- 또는 -i-를 끼워 넣을 수 있다.

사람 이름의 라틴어 형용사를 꾸밈말로 사용한 학명의 예

Arabidopsis thaliana 애기장대

L. arabidopsis 애기장대속(屬): 여성 명사, 단수 주격

  < L. Arabidopsis, Arabidopsis, f. (< *resembling the genus*
    Arabis < Arabis + G. opsis, opseōs, f. *seeing*)
    (식물) 애기장대속(屬)

   < L. Arabis, Arabidis, f. (< *growing on sandy or stony places*)
    (식물) 장대속(屬)

  < L. Arabs, Arabis, m. 아랍인, 아랍 (Vide ARABS; *See* E. *Arab*)

 < G. Araps, Arabos, m. *an Arab*

L. thaliana 탈(Thal)의: 형용사, 여성형 단수 주격

  < L. Thalianus, Thaliana, Thalianum 탈(Thal)의

 < Johannes Thal (1542–1583), *German botanist*

Giardia lamblia 람블 편모충

L. Giardia 편모충속(屬): 여성 명사, 단수 주격

  < L. Giardia, Giardiae, f. (원충) 편모충속(屬), 지아르디아속(屬)

 < Alfred Mathieu Giard (1846–1908), *French biologist*

L. lamblia 람블의: 형용사, 여성형 단수 주격

  < L. Lamblius, Lamblia, Lamblium 람블의

 < Vilem Dusan Lambl (1824–1895), *Czech physician*

사람 이름의 라틴어 명사 단수 속격을 꾸밈말로 사용한 학명의 예

Bartonella henselae 헨젤 바르토넬라균

L. Bartonella 바르토넬라속(屬): 여성 명사, 단수 주격

< L. Bartonella, Bartonellae, f. (< + -ella *feminine diminutive suffix*)

(세균) 바르토넬라속(屬)

< Alberto Barton (1870–1950), *Argentine–born Peruvian bacteriologist*

L. henselae 헨젤의: 여성 명사, 단수 속격

< L. Hensela, Henselae, f. 헨젤

< Diane Marie Hensel (b. 1953), *American microbiology technologist*

Shigella sonnei 손네 이질균, 손네균

L. Shigella 시겔라속(屬), 이질균속(屬): 여성 명사, 단수 주격

< L. Shigella, Shigellae, f. (< + -ella *feminine diminutive suffix*)

(세균) 시겔라속(屬), 이질균속(屬)

< Kiyoshi Shiga (1871–1957), *Japanese bacteriologist*

L. sonnei 손네의: 남성 명사, 단수 속격

< L. Sonneus, Sonnei, m. 손네

< Carl Olaf Sonne (1882–1948), *Danish bacteriologist*

Actinomyces israelii 이스라엘 방선균

L. actinomyces: 남성 명사, 단수 주격

< L. actinomyces, actinomycetis, m. (세균) 방선균(放線菌), 바큇살균

< G. aktis, aktinos, f. *ray, light* (Vide ACTINOMYCES: *See* E. *actinomyces*)

+ G. mykēs, mykētos, m. *mushroom*

< IE. meug- *slimy, slippery* (Vide MUCUS: *See* E. *mucus*)

L. israelii 이스라엘(사람 이름)의: 남성 명사, 단수 속격

< L. Israelius, Israelii, m. 이스라엘(사람 이름)

< James Adolf Israel (1848–1926), *German surgeon*

Rickettsia prowazekii 프로바제크 리케차

Rickettsia rickettsii 리케츠 리케차

L. Rickettsia 리케차속(屬): 여성 명사, 단수 주격

< L. Rickettsia, Rickettsiae, f. (리케차) 리케차속(屬)

< Howard Taylor Ricketts (1871–1910), *American pathologist*

L. prowazekii 프로바제크의: 남성 명사, 단수 속격

< L. Prowazekius, Prowazekii, m. 프로바제크

< Stanislaus Josef Matthias von Prowazek (1875–1915), *Czech protozoologist*

L. rickettsii 리케츠의: 남성 명사, 단수 속격

< L. Rickettsius, Rickettsii, m. 리케츠

< Howard Taylor Ricketts (1871–1910), *American pathologist*

Leishmania donovani 도노반 리슈만편모충, 내장 리슈만편모충

    L. Leishmania 리슈만편모충속(屬): 여성 명사, 단수 주격
               < L. Leishmania, Leishmaniae, f. (원충) 리슈만편모충속(屬)
             < Sir William Boog Leishman (1865–1926), *English army surgeon*
    L. donovani 도노반의: 남성 명사, 단수 속격
               < L. Donovanus, Donovani, m. 도노반
             < Charles Donovan (1863–1951), *Irish physician in India*

Paragonimus westermani 폐흡충

    L. Paragonimus 폐흡충속(屬): 남성 명사, 단수 주격
                   < L. Paragonimus, Paragonimi, m. (< G. par(a)– *beside,*
                      along side of, beyond) (흡충) 폐흡충속(屬)
                < G. gonimos, gonimos, gonimon *productive, fertile, vigorous*
              < G. gonē, gonēs, f. ((*ancient Greek*) gonos) *begetting, birth,*
              origin; offspring, seed
             < G. gignesthai (ginesthai) (gen– *root*) *to be born, to become*
           < IE. genə–, gen– *to give birth, to beget* (Vide GIGNÈRE; *See* E. *genital*)
    L. westermani 베스터만의: 남성 명사, 단수 속격
             < L. Westermanus, Westermani, m. 베스터만
           < Pieter Westerman (1859–1925), *Amsterdam zookeeper who noted the*
           trematode in a Bengal tiger

삼명법

    삼명법에 의한 학명도 이명법의 규칙을 그대로 따른다. 종을 특징짓는 꾸밈말처럼 아종을 특징짓는 덧꾸밈말 역시 속명을 수식하며 라틴어나 라틴어화한 단수 주격 형용사, 단수 주격 분사, 또는 속격 명사를 원칙으로 한다. 식물명의 경우, 아종 밑에 변종(E. *variety*, L. varietas)이나 품종(E. *form*, L. forma)이 있을 수 있기 때문에 아종임을 밝히기 위해 subsp.를 써준다. 동물명의 경우, 아종까지만 분류하므로 ssp.를 써주지 않는다.

Oryza sativa (*subsp.*) indica 재배종 벼, 인도형 아종

Oryza sativa (*subsp.*) japonica 재배종 벼, 일본형 아종

    L. oryza 벼: 여성 명사, 단수 주격
               < L. oryza, oryzae, f. 벼, 쌀

< G. oryza, oryzēs, f. *rice*

< (*probably*) *Of Oriental origin*

L. sativa 재배하는: 형용사, 여성형 단수 주격

    < L. sativus, sativa, sativum 재배의, 재배하는, 재배한

    < L. sero, sevi, satum, serĕre 씨 뿌리다

< IE. se- *to sow* (Vide SEMEN; *See* E. *semen*)

L. indica 인도의: 형용사, 여성형 단수 주격

    < L. Indicus, Indica, Indicum 인도의

    < G. Indikos, Iṅdikē, Indikon *of India*

    < G. India, Indias, f. *India*

< (*Sanskrit*) sindhu *river, the river Indus* (Vide INDIA; *See* E. *India*)

L. japonica 일본의: 형용사, 여성형 단수 주격

    < L. Japonicus, Japonica, Japonicum 일본의

    < L. Japonia, Japoniae, f. 일본

    < (*Chinese*) Jih-pǔn (日本)

< (*Japanese*) 日本 (にっぽん) (Vide JAPONIA; *See* E. *Japan*)

Pediculus humanus corporis 몸니, 옷엣니

Pediculus humanus capitis 머릿니

L. pediculus 이[蝨]: 남성 명사, 단수 주격

    < L. pediculus, pediculi, m. (< + -culus *diminutive suffix*) 이[蝨]

    < L. pedis, pedis, m., f. (< *foul-smelling insect*) 이[蝨]

< IE. (*perhaps*) pezd- *to fart* (Vide PEDICULUS; *See* E. *pediculus*)

L. humanus 사람의: 형용사, 남성형 단수 주격

    < L. humanus, humana, humanum 사람의, 사람다운

< IE. dhghem- *earth, earthling* (Vide HOMO; *See* E. *homo*)

L. corporis 몸의: 중성 명사, 단수 속격

    < L. corpus, corporis, n. 몸, 체(體)

< IE. k^{w}rep- *body, form, appearance* (Vide CORPUS; *See* E. *corpus*)

L. capitis 머리의: 중성 명사, 단수 속격

    < L. caput, capitis, n. 머리

< IE. kaput- *head* (Vide CAPUT; *See* E. *cape*)

부록

라틴어 품사 변화표

명사 변화

제1변화

cellula, cellulae, f. 세포

	단 수	복 수	
주격	cellul-a	cellul-ae	~이, ~가, ~은, ~는, ~께서
속격	cellul-ae	cellul-arum	~의
여격	cellul-ae	cellul-is	~게, ~에게, ~께, ~한테
대격	cellul-am	cellul-as	~을, ~를
탈격	cellul-a	cellul-is	~에서, ~로부터, ~으로부터
호격	cellul-a	cellul-ae	~여, ~이여

제2변화 제1식

nucleus, nuclei, m. 핵

	단 수	복 수	
주격	nucle-us	nucle-i	~이, ~가, ~은, ~는, ~께서
속격	nucle-i	nucle-orum	~의
여격	nucle-o	nucle-is	~게, ~에게, ~께, ~한테
대격	nucle-um	nucle-os	~을, ~를
탈격	nucle-o	nucle-is	~에서, ~로부터, ~으로부터
호격	nucle-e	nucle-i	~여, ~이여

제2식

faber, fabri, m. 목수

	단 수	복 수	
주격	faber	fabr-i	~이, ~가, ~은, ~는, ~께서
속격	fabr-i	fabr-orum	~의
여격	fabr-o	fabr-is	~게, ~에게, ~께, ~한테
대격	fabr-um	fabr-os	~을, ~를
탈격	fabr-o	fabr-is	~에서, ~로부터, ~으로부터
호격	faber	fabr-i	~여, ~이여

제2변화　제3식

ovum, ovi, n. 알

	단 수	복 수	
주격	ov-um	ov-a	~이, ~가, ~은, ~는, ~께서
속격	ov-i	ov-orum	~의
여격	ov-o	ov-is	~게, ~에게, ~께, ~한테
대격	ov-um	ov-a	~을, ~를
탈격	ov-o	ov-is	~에서, ~로부터, ~으로부터
호격	ov-um	ov-a	~여, ~이여

제3변화　제1식 a

homo, hominis, m. 사람

	단 수	복 수	
주격	homo	homin-es	~이, ~가, ~은, ~는, ~께서
속격	homin-is	homin-um	~의
여격	homin-i	homin-ibus	~게, ~에게, ~께, ~한테
대격	homin-em	homin-es	~을, ~를
탈격	homin-e	homin-ibus	~에서, ~로부터, ~으로부터
호격	homo	homin-es	~여, ~이여

제1식 b

caput, capitis, n. 머리

	단 수	복 수	
주격	caput	capit-a	~이, ~가, ~은, ~는, ~께서
속격	capit-is	capit-um	~의
여격	capit-i	capit-ibus	~게, ~에게, ~께, ~한테
대격	caput	capit-a	~을, ~를
탈격	capit-e	capit-ibus	~에서, ~로부터, ~으로부터
호격	caput	capit-a	~여, ~이여

제2식 a

dens, dentis, m. 이, 치아

	단 수	복 수	
주격	dens	dent-es	~이, ~가, ~은, ~는, ~께서
속격	dent-is	dent-ium	~의
여격	dent-i	dent-ibus	~게, ~에게, ~께, ~한테
대격	dent-em	dent-es	~을, ~를
탈격	dent-e	dent-ibus	~에서, ~로부터, ~으로부터
호격	dens	dent-es	~여, ~이여

제3변화　제2식 b

cor, cordis, n. 심장, 마음

	단 수	복 수	
주격	cor	cord-a	~이, ~가, ~은, ~는, ~께서
속격	cord-is	cord-ium	~의
여격	cord-i	cord-ibus	~게, ~에게, ~께, ~한테
대격	cor	cord-a	~을, ~를
탈격	cord-e	cord-ibus	~에서, ~로부터, ~으로부터
호격	cor	cord-a	~여, ~이여

제2식 c

auris, auris, f. 귀

	단 수	복 수	
주격	aur-is	aur-es	~이, ~가, ~은, ~는, ~께서
속격	aur-is	aur-ium	~의
여격	aur-i	aur-ibus	~게, ~에게, ~께, ~한테
대격	aur-em	aur-es	~을, ~를
탈격	aur-e	aur-ibus	~에서, ~로부터, ~으로부터
호격	aur-is	aur-es	~여, ~이여

제3식

mare, maris, n. 바다

	단 수	복 수	
주격	mar-e	mar-ia	~이, ~가, ~은, ~는, ~께서
속격	mar-is	mar-ium	~의
여격	mar-i	mar-ibus	~게, ~에게, ~께, ~한테
대격	mar-e	mar-ia	~을, ~를
탈격	mar-i	mar-ibus	~에서, ~로부터, ~으로부터
호격	mar-e	mar-ia	~여, ~이여

제4변화　제1식

manus, manus, f. 손

	단 수	복 수	
주격	man-us	man-us	~이, ~가, ~은, ~는, ~께서
속격	man-us	man-uum	~의
여격	man-ui	man-ibus	~게, ~에게, ~께, ~한테
대격	man-um	man-us	~을, ~를
탈격	man-u	man-ibus	~에서, ~로부터, ~으로부터
호격	man-us	man-us	~여, ~이여

제 4 변화 제 2 식

cornu, cornus, n. 뿔

	단 수	복 수	
주격	corn-u	corn-ua	~이, ~가, ~은, ~는, ~께서
속격	corn-us	corn-uum	~의
여격	corn-u	corn-ibus	~게, ~에게, ~께, ~한테
대격	corn-u	corn-ua	~을, ~를
탈격	corn-u	corn-ibus	~에서, ~로부터, ~으로부터
호격	corn-u	corn-ua	~여, ~이여

제 5 변화

dies, diei, m. 날; f. 날짜

	단 수	복 수	
주격	di-es	di-es	~이, ~가, ~은, ~는, ~께서
속격	di-ei	di-erum	~의
여격	di-ei	di-ebus	~게, ~에게, ~께, ~한테
대격	di-em	di-es	~을, ~를
탈격	di-e	di-ebus	~에서, ~로부터, ~으로부터
호격	di-es	di-es	~여, ~이여

대명사 변화

인칭대명사 제 1 인칭

	단 수		복 수	
주격	ego	나는, 내가	nos	우리는, 우리가
속격	mei	나에게 대한, 나를	nostri	우리에게 대한, 우리를
			nostrum	우리 중의
여격	mihi	나에게	nobis	우리에게
대격	me	나를	nos	우리를
탈격	me	나로	nobis	우리로

제 2 인칭

	단 수		복 수	
주격	tu	너는, 네가	vos	너희는, 너희가
속격	tui	너에게 대한, 너를	vestri	너희에게 대한, 너희를
			vestrum	너희 중의
여격	tibi	너에게	vobis	너희에게
대격	te	너를	vos	너희를
탈격	te	너로	vobis	너희로

제 3 인칭 (재귀대명사)

	단 수		복 수	
주격	–		–	
속격	sui	자신에게 대한, 자신을	sui	자신들에게 대한, 자신들을
여격	sibi	자신에게	sibi	자신들에게
대격	se	자신을	se	자신들을
탈격	se	자신으로	se	자신들로

소유대명사

	단 수		복 수	
일인칭	meus, mea, meum	나의	noster, nostra, nostrum	우리의
이인칭	tuus, tua, tuum	너의	vester, vestra, vestrum	너희의
삼인칭	suus, sua, suum	자기의	suus, sua, suum	자기들의

지시대명사

is (m.), **ea** (f.), **id** (n.) 그 사람, 그 남자; 그 여자; 그것; 그, 저

	단 수			복 수		
	남성	여성	중성	남성	여성	중성
주격	is	ea	id	ii (ei)	eae	ea
속격	ejus	ejus	ejus	eorum	earum	eorum
여격	ei	ei	ei	iis (eis)	iis (eis)	iis (eis)
대격	eum	eam	id	eos	eas	ea
탈격	eo	ea	eo	iis (eis)	iis (eis)	iis (eis)

hic (m.), **haec** (f.), **hoc** (n.) 이 사람, 이 남자; 이 여자; 이것; 이

	단 수			복 수		
	남성	여성	중성	남성	여성	중성
주격	hic	haec	hoc	hi	hae	haec
속격	hujus	hujus	hujus	horum	harum	horum
여격	huic	huic	huic	his	his	his
대격	hunc	hanc	hoc	hos	has	haec
탈격	hoc	hac	hoc	his	his	his

관계대명사

qui (m.), quae (f.), quod (n.)

	단 수			복 수		
	남성	여성	중성	남성	여성	중성
주격	qui	quae	quod	qui	quae	quae
속격	cujus	cujus	cujus	quorum	quarum	quorum
여격	cui	cui	cui	quibus	quibus	quibus
대격	quem	quam	quod	quos	quas	quae
탈격	quo	qua	quo	quibus	quibus	quibus

대명사적 형용사

alius (m.), alia (f.), aliud (n.) 다른 사람, 다른 남자; 다른 여자; 다른 것

	단 수			복 수		
	남성	여성	중성	남성	여성	중성
주격	alius	alia	aliud	alii	aliae	alia
속격	alterius (alius)	alterius (alius)	alterius (alius)	aliorum	aliarum	aliorum
여격	alii	alii	alii	aliis	aliis	aliis
대격	alium	aliam	aliud	alios	alias	alia
탈격	alio	alia	alio	aliis	aliis	aliis

형용사 변화

제 1 · 2 변화 제 1 식

bonus, bona, bonum 좋은

	단 수			복 수		
	남성	여성	중성	남성	여성	중성
주격	bon-us	bon-a	bon-um	bon-i	bon-ae	bon-a
속격	bon-i	bon-ae	bon-i	bon-orum	bon-arum	bon-orum
여격	bon-o	bon-ae	bon-o	bon-is	bon-is	bon-is
대격	bon-um	bon-am	bon-um	bon-os	bon-as	bon-a
탈격	bon-o	bon-a	bon-o	bon-is	bon-is	bon-is
호격	bon-e	bon-a	bon-um	bon-i	bon-ae	bon-a

제 2 식

niger, nigra, nigrum 검은

	단 수			복 수		
	남성	여성	중성	남성	여성	중성
주격	niger	nigr-a	nigr-um	nigr-i	nigr-ae	nigr-a
속격	nigr-i	nigr-ae	nigr-i	nigr-orum	nigr-arum	nigr-orum
여격	nigr-o	nigr-ae	nigr-o	nigr-is	nigr-is	nigr-is
대격	nigr-um	nigr-am	nigr-um	nigr-os	nigr-as	nigr-a
탈격	nigr-o	nigr-a	nigr-o	nigr-is	nigr-is	nigr-is
호격	niger	nigr-a	nigr-um	nigr-i	nigr-ae	nigr-a

제 3 변화   제 1 식

acer, acris, acre 신, 날카로운, 혹독한

	단 수			복 수		
	남성	여성	중성	남성	여성	중성
주격	acer	acr-is	acr-e	acr-es	acr-es	acr-ia
속격	acr-is	acr-is	acr-is	acr-ium	acr-ium	acr-ium
여격	acr-i	acr-i	acr-i	acr-ibus	acr-ibus	acr-ibus
대격	acr-em	acr-em	acr-e	acr-es	acr-es	acr-ia
탈격	acr-i	acr-i	acr-i	acr-ibus	acr-ibus	acr-ibus
호격	acer	acr-is	acr-e	acr-es	acr-es	acr-ia

제 3 변화   제 2 식

omnis, omne 모든

	단 수			복 수		
	남성	여성	중성	남성	여성	중성
주격	omn-is	omn-is	omn-e	omn-es	omn-es	omn-ia
속격	omn-is	omn-is	omn-is	omn-ium	omn-ium	omn-ium
여격	omn-i	omn-i	omn-i	omn-ibus	omn-ibus	omn-ibus
대격	omn-em	omn-em	omn-e	omn-es	omn-es	omn-ia
탈격	omn-i	omn-i	omn-i	omn-ibus	omn-ibus	omn-ibus
호격	omn-is	omn-is	omn-e	omn-es	omn-es	omn-ia

제3식

potens, (gen.) potentis 힘 있는, 능력 있는

	단 수			복 수		
	남성	여성	중성	남성	여성	중성
주격	potens	potens	potens	potent-es	potent-es	potent-ia
속격	potent-is	potent-is	potent-is	potent-ium	potent-ium	potent-ium
여격	potent-i	potent-i	potent-i	potent-ibus	potent-ibus	potent-ibus
대격	potent-em	potent-em	potens	potent-es	potent-es	potent-ia
탈격	potent-i	potent-i	potent-i	potent-ibus	potent-ibus	potent-ibus
호격	potens	potens	potens	potent-es	potent-es	potent-ia

제3식 예외

vetus, (gen.) veteris 나이든, 늙은, 묵은, 옛, 낡은

	단 수			복 수		
	남성	여성	중성	남성	여성	중성
주격	vetus	vetus	vetus	veter-es	veter-es	veter-a
속격	veter-is	veter-is	veter-is	veter-um	veter-um	veter-um
여격	veter-i	veter-i	veter-i	veter-ibus	veter-ibus	veter-ibus
대격	veter-em	veter-em	vetus	veter-es	veter-es	veter-a
탈격	veter-e	veter-e	veter-e	veter-ibus	veter-ibus	veter-ibus
호격	vetus	vetus	vetus	veter-es	veter-es	veter-a

동사변화

정형 제1변화

amo, amavi, amatum, amare 사랑하다

능동태	부정법	현재				
					am-are	사랑하다
	직설법	현재	단수	일인칭	am-o	나는 ~한다
				이인칭	am-as	너는 ~한다
				삼인칭	am-at	그는 ~한다
			복수	일인칭	am-amus	우리는 ~한다
				이인칭	am-atis	너희는 ~한다
				삼인칭	am-ant	그들은 ~한다
		과거	단수	일인칭	am-abam	나는 ~하였다
		미래	단수	일인칭	am-abo	나는 ~하겠다
		완료	단수	일인칭	amav-i	나는 ~하였다

	가정법	현재	단수	일인칭	am-em	나는 ~하리라
	명령법	현재	단수	이인칭	am-a	너는 ~하라
			복수	이인칭	am-ate	너희는 ~하라
	분 사	현재			amans, (gen.) amant-is	~하는, ~하고 있는
	목적분사				amat-um	~하러, ~하기 위하여
수동태	부정법	현재			am-ari	사랑받다
	분 사	미래			amand-us, amand-a, amand-um	~받아야 할
		과거			amat-us, amat-a, amat-um	~받은, ~받고서

정형 제 2 변화   habeo, habui, habitum, habēre 가지다

능동태	부정법	현재			hab-ēre	가지다
	직설법	현재	단수	일인칭	hab-eo	나는 ~한다
				이인칭	hab-es	너는 ~한다
				삼인칭	hab-et	그는 ~한다
			복수	일인칭	hab-emus	우리는 ~한다
				이인칭	hab-etis	너희는 ~한다
				삼인칭	hab-ent	그들은 ~한다
		과거	단수	일인칭	hab-ebam	나는 ~하였다
		미래	단수	일인칭	hab-ebo	나는 ~하겠다
		완료	단수	일인칭	habu-i	나는 ~하였다
	가정법	현재	단수	일인칭	hab-eam	나는 ~하리라
	명령법	현재	단수	이인칭	hab-e	너는 ~하라
			복수	이인칭	hab-ete	너희는 ~하라
	분 사	현재			habens, (gen.) habent-is	~하는, ~하고 있는
	목적분사				habit-um	~하러, ~하기 위하여
수동태	부정법	현재			hab-eri	가지게 되다
	분 사	미래			habend-us, habend-a, habend-um	~받아야 할
		과거			habit-us, habit-a, habit-um	~받은, ~받고서

정형 제 3 변화 A 식   lego, legi, lectum, legĕre 모으다, 뽑다, 읽다

능동태	부정법	현재			leg-ĕre	모으다, 뽑다, 읽다
	직설법	현재	단수	일인칭	leg-o	나는 ~한다
				이인칭	leg-is	너는 ~한다
				삼인칭	leg-it	그는 ~한다

			복수	일인칭	leg-imus	우리는 ～한다
				이인칭	leg-itis	너희는 ～한다
				삼인칭	leg-unt	그들은 ～한다
		과거	단수	일인칭	leg-ebam	나는 ～하였다
		미래	단수	일인칭	leg-am	나는 ～하겠다
		완료	단수	일인칭	leg-i	나는 ～하였다
	가정법	현재	단수	일인칭	leg-am	나는 ～하리라
	명령법	현재	단수	이인칭	leg-e	너는 ～하라
			복수	이인칭	leg-ite	너희는 ～하라
	분 사	현재			legens, (gen.) legent-is	～하는, ～하고 있는
	목적분사				lect-um	～하러, ～하기 위하여
수동태	부정법	현재			leg-i	모아지다, 읽히다
	분 사	미래			legend-us, legend-a, legend-um	～받아야 할
		과거			lect-us, lect-a, lect-um	～받은, ～받고서

정형 제 3 변화 B 식   capio, cepi, captum, capĕre 잡다, 붙잡다, 획득하다

능동태	부정법	현재			cap-ĕre	붙잡다
	직설법	현재	단수	일인칭	cap-io	나는 ～한다
				이인칭	cap-is	너는 ～한다
				삼인칭	cap-it	그는 ～한다
			복수	일인칭	cap-imus	우리는 ～한다
				이인칭	cap-itis	너희는 ～한다
				삼인칭	cap-iunt	그들은 ～한다
		과거	단수	일인칭	cap-iebam	나는 ～하였다
		미래	단수	일인칭	cap-iam	나는 ～하겠다
		완료	단수	일인칭	cep-i	나는 ～하였다
	가정법	현재	단수	일인칭	cap-iam	나는 ～하리라
	명령법	현재	단수	이인칭	cap-e	너는 ～하라
			복수	이인칭	cap-ite	너희는 ～하라
	분 사	현재			capiens, (gen.) capient-is	～하는, ～하고 있는
	목적분사				capt-um	～하러, ～하기 위하여
수동태	부정법	현재			cap-i	붙잡히다
	분 사	미래			capiend-us, capiend-a, capiend-um	～받아야 할
		과거			capt-us, capt-a, capt-um	～받은, ～받고서

정형 제4변화

audio, audivi (audii), auditum, audire 듣다

능동태	부정법	현재			aud-ire	듣다
	직설법	현재	단수	일인칭	aud-io	나는 ~한다
				이인칭	aud-is	너는 ~한다
				삼인칭	aud-it	그는 ~한다
			복수	일인칭	aud-imus	우리는 ~한다
				이인칭	aud-itis	너희는 ~한다
				삼인칭	aud-iunt	그들은 ~한다
		과거	단수	일인칭	aud-iebam	나는 ~하였다
		미래	단수	일인칭	aud-iam	나는 ~하겠다
		완료	단수	일인칭	audiv-i	나는 ~하였다
	가정법	현재	단수	일인칭	aud-iam	나는 ~하리라
	명령법	현재	단수	이인칭	aud-i	너는 ~하라
			복수	이인칭	aud-ite	너희는 ~하라
	분 사	현재			audiens, (gen.) audient-is	~하는, ~하고 있는
	목적분사				audit-um	~하러, ~하기 위하여
수동태	부정법	현재			aud-iri	들리다
	분 사	미래			audiend-us, audiend-a, audiend-um	~받아야 할
		과거			audit-us, audit-a, audit-um	~받은, ~받고서

탈형 제1변화

imitor, imitatus sum, imitari 모방하다, 본받다

	부정법	현재			imit-ari	모방하다
	직설법	현재	단수	일인칭	imit-or	나는 ~한다
				이인칭	imit-aris	너는 ~한다
				삼인칭	imit-atur	그는 ~한다
			복수	일인칭	imit-amur	우리는 ~한다
				이인칭	imit-amini	너희는 ~한다
				삼인칭	imit-antur	그들은 ~한다
		과거	단수	일인칭	imit-abar	나는 ~하였다
		미래	단수	일인칭	imit-abor	나는 ~하겠다
		완료	단수	일인칭	imitat-us, -a, -um sum	나는 ~하였다
	가정법	현재	단수	일인칭	imit-er	나는 ~하리라
	명령법	현재	단수	이인칭	imit-are	너는 ~하라
			복수	이인칭	imit-amini	너희는 ~하라
	분 사	현재			imitans, (gen.) imitant-is	~하는, ~하고 있는
		과거			imitat-us, imitat-a, imitat-um	~한
	수동형	미래분사			imitand-us, imitand-a, imitand-um	~받아야 할

탈형 제 2 변화

tueor, tuitus (tutus) sum, tueri 지켜보다, 주시하다, 보살피다

부정법	현재			tu-eri	지켜보다, 보살피다
직설법	현재	단수	일인칭	tu-eor	나는 ~한다
			이인칭	tu-eris	너는 ~한다
			삼인칭	tu-etur	그는 ~한다
		복수	일인칭	tu-emur	우리는 ~한다
			이인칭	tu-emini	너희는 ~한다
			삼인칭	tu-entur	그들은 ~한다
	과거	단수	일인칭	tu-ebar	나는 ~하였다
	미래	단수	일인칭	tu-ebor	나는 ~하겠다
	완료	단수	일인칭	tuit-us (tut-us), -a, -um sum	나는 ~하였다
가정법	현재	단수	일인칭	tu-ear	나는 ~하리라
명령법	현재	단수	이인칭	tu-ēre	너는 ~하라
		복수	이인칭	tu-emini	너희는 ~하라
분 사	현재			tuens, (gen.) tuent-is	~하는, ~하고 있는
	과거			tuit-us, tuit-a, tuit-um (tut-us, -a, -um)	~한
수동형	미래분사			tuend-us, tuend-a, tuend-um	~받아야 할

탈형 제 3 변화 A 식

loquor, locutus sum, loqui 말하다

부정법	현재			loqu-i	말하다
직설법	현재	단수	일인칭	loqu-or	나는 ~한다
			이인칭	loqu-eris	너는 ~한다
			삼인칭	loqu-itur	그는 ~한다
		복수	일인칭	loqu-imur	우리는 ~한다
			이인칭	loqu-imini	너희는 ~한다
			삼인칭	loqu-untur	그들은 ~한다
	과거	단수	일인칭	loqu-ebar	나는 ~하였다
	미래	단수	일인칭	loqu-ar	나는 ~하겠다
	완료	단수	일인칭	locut-us, -a, -um sum	나는 ~하였다
가정법	현재	단수	일인칭	loqu-ar	나는 ~하리라
명령법	현재	단수	이인칭	loqu-ĕre	너는 ~하라
		복수	이인칭	loqu-imini	너희는 ~하라
분 사	현재			loquens, (gen.) loquent-is	~하는, ~하고 있는
	과거			locut-us, locut-a, locut-um	~한
수동형	미래분사			loquend-us, loquend-a, loquend-um	~받아야 할

탈형 제3변화 B식   patior, passus sum, pati 당하다, 견디다, 참다, 고통받다, 내버려 두다

부정법	현재			pat-i	참다, 고통받다
직설법	현재	단수	일인칭	pat-ior	나는 ~한다
			이인칭	pat-eris	너는 ~한다
			삼인칭	pat-itur	그는 ~한다
		복수	일인칭	pat-imur	우리는 ~한다
			이인칭	pat-imini	너희는 ~한다
			삼인칭	pat-iuntur	그들은 ~한다
	과거	단수	일인칭	pat-iebar	나는 ~하였다
	미래	단수	일인칭	pat-iar	나는 ~하겠다
	완료	단수	일인칭	pass-us, -a, -um sum	나는 ~하였다
가정법	현재	단수	일인칭	pat-iar	나는 ~하리라
명령법	현재	단수	이인칭	pat-ĕre	너는 ~하라
		복수	이인칭	pat-imini	너희는 ~하라
분 사	현재			patiens, (gen.) patient-is	~하는, ~하고 있는
	과거			pass-us, pass-a, pass-um	~한
수동형	미래분사			patiend-us, patiend-a, patiend-um	~받아야 할

탈형 제4변화   orior, ortus sum, oriri 돋다, 나다, 출현하다

부정법	현재			or-iri	돋다
직설법	현재	단수	일인칭	or-ior	나는 ~한다
			이인칭	or-iris	너는 ~한다
			삼인칭	or-itur	그는 ~한다
		복수	일인칭	or-imur	우리는 ~한다
			이인칭	or-imini	너희는 ~한다
			삼인칭	or-iuntur	그들은 ~한다
	과거	단수	일인칭	or-iebar	나는 ~하였다
	미래	단수	일인칭	or-iar	나는 ~하겠다
	완료	단수	일인칭	ort-us, -a, -um sum	나는 ~하였다
가정법	현재	단수	일인칭	or-iar	나는 ~하리라
명령법	현재	단수	이인칭	or-ire	너는 ~하라
		복수	이인칭	or-imini	너희는 ~하라
분 사	현재			oriens, (gen.) orient-is	~하는, ~하고 있는
	과거			ort-us, ort-a, ort-um	~한
수동형	미래분사			oriend-us, oriend-a, oriend-um	~받아야 할

불규칙 동사의 변화

sum, fui, -, esse ~이다, 있다

능동태	부정법	현재			esse	~이다, 있다
	직설법	현재	단수	일인칭	sum	나는 ~이다, 있다
				이인칭	es	너는 ~이다, 있다
				삼인칭	est	그는 ~이다, 있다
			복수	일인칭	sumus	우리는 ~이다, 있다
				이인칭	estis	너희는 ~이다, 있다
				삼인칭	sunt	그들은 ~이다, 있다
		과거	단수	일인칭	er-am	나는 ~이었다, 있었다
		미래	단수	일인칭	er-o	나는 ~이겠다, 있겠다
		완료	단수	일인칭	fu-i	나는 ~이었다, 있었다
	가정법	현재	단수	일인칭	sim	나는 ~이리라, 있으리라
	명령법	현재	단수	이인칭	es	너는 ~이어라, 있어라
			복수	이인칭	es-te	너희는 ~이어라, 있어라
	분 사	현재			없음	
		미래			futur-us, futur-a, futur-um	~일, 있을
	목적분사				없음	
수동태					없음	

possum, potui, -, posse 할 수 있다, 가능성 있다

능동태	부정법	현재			posse	할 수 있다, 가능성 있다
	직설법	현재	단수	일인칭	pos-sum	나는 ~ 있다
				이인칭	pot-es	너는 ~ 있다
				삼인칭	pot-est	그는 ~ 있다
			복수	일인칭	pos-sumus	우리는 ~ 있다
				이인칭	pot-estis	너희는 ~ 있다
				삼인칭	pos-sunt	그들은 ~ 있다
		과거	단수	일인칭	pot-eram	나는 ~ 있었다
		미래	단수	일인칭	pot-ero	나는 ~ 있겠다
		완료	단수	일인칭	potu-i	나는 ~ 있었다
	가정법	현재	단수	일인칭	pos-sim	나는 ~ 있으리라
	명령법	현재	단수	이인칭	없음	
			복수	이인칭	없음	
	분 사	현재			potens, (gen.) potent-is	~ 있는
	목적분사				없음	
수동태					없음	

능동태	부정법	현재			ire	가다
	직설법	현재	단수	일인칭	e-o	나는 간다
				이인칭	i-s	너는 간다
				삼인칭	i-t	그는 간다
			복수	일인칭	i-mus	우리는 간다
				이인칭	i-tis	너희는 간다
				삼인칭	e-unt	그들은 간다
		과거	단수	일인칭	i-bam	나는 갔다
		미래	단수	일인칭	i-bo	나는 가겠다
		완료	단수	일인칭	i-i	나는 갔다
	가정법	현재	단수	일인칭	e-am	나는 가리라
	명령법	현재	단수	이인칭	i	너는 가라
			복수	이인칭	i-te	너희는 가라
	분 사	현재			iens, (gen.) eunt-is	가는, 가고 있는
	목적분사				it-um	가러, 가기 위하여
수동태					관용적 비인칭 수동태 외에는 없음	

능동태	부정법	현재			ferre	가져가다, 견디다
	직설법	현재	단수	일인칭	fer-o	나는 ~한다
				이인칭	fer-s	너는 ~한다
				삼인칭	fer-t	그는 ~한다
			복수	일인칭	fer-imus	우리는 ~한다
				이인칭	fer-tis	너희는 ~한다
				삼인칭	fer-unt	그들은 ~한다
		과거	단수	일인칭	fer-ebam	나는 ~하였다
		미래	단수	일인칭	fer-am	나는 ~하겠다
		완료	단수	일인칭	tul-i	나는 ~하였다
	가정법	현재	단수	일인칭	ferr-em	나는 ~하리라
	명령법	현재	단수	이인칭	fer	너는 ~하라
			복수	이인칭	fer-te	너희는 ~하라
	분 사	현재			ferens, (gen.) ferent-is	~하는, ~하고 있는
	목적분사				lat-um	~하러, ~하기 위하여
수동태	분 사	미래			ferend-us, ferend-a, ferend-um	~받아야 할
		과거			lat-us, lat-a, lat-um	~받은, ~받고서

능동태	부정법	현재				velle	원하다
	직설법	현재	단수	일인칭		vol-o	나는 ~한다
				이인칭		vi-s	너는 ~한다
				삼인칭		vul-t	그는 ~한다
			복수	일인칭		vol-umus	우리는 ~한다
				이인칭		vul-tis	너희는 ~한다
				삼인칭		vol-unt	그들은 ~한다
		과거	단수	일인칭		vol-ebam	나는 ~하였다
		미래	단수	일인칭		vol-am	나는 ~하겠다
		완료	단수	일인칭		vol-ui	나는 ~하였다
	가정법	현재	단수	일인칭		vel-im	나는 ~하리라
	명령법					없음	
	분 사	현재				volens, (gen.) volent-is	~하는, ~하고 있는
	목적분사					없음	
수동태						없음	

그리스어 품사 변화표

명사 변화

제1변화　**제1식**　　　　　　　　hōra, hōras, f. *year, season, period, time, hour*

	단 수	복 수	
주격	hōr-a	hōr-ai	~이, ~가, ~은, ~는, ~께서
속격	hōr-as	hōr-ōn	~의
여격	hōr-ai	hōr-ais	~게, ~에게, ~께, ~한테
대격	hōr-an	hōr-as	~을, ~를
호격	hōr-a	hōr-ai	~여, ~이여

제2식　　　　　　　　　　　　　doxa, doxēs, f. *opinion, glory*

	단 수	복 수	
주격	dox-a	dox-ai	~이, ~가, ~은, ~는, ~께서
속격	dox-ēs	dox-ōn	~의
여격	dox-ēi	dox-ais	~게, ~에게, ~께, ~한테
대격	dox-an	dox-as	~을, ~를
호격	dox-a	dox-ai	~여, ~이여

제3식　　　　　　　　　　　　　graphē, graphēs, f. *drawing, writing*

	단 수	복 수	
주격	graph-ē	graph-ai	~이, ~가, ~은, ~는, ~께서
속격	graph-ēs	graph-ōn	~의
여격	graph-ēi	graph-ais	~게, ~에게, ~께, ~한테
대격	graph-ēn	graph-as	~을, ~를
호격	graph-ē	graph-ai	~여, ~이여

제1변화	제4식		poiētēs, poiētou, m. *maker, creator, poet*
	단 수	복 수	
주격	poiēt-ēs	poiēt-ai	~이, ~가, ~은, ~는, ~께서
속격	poiēt-ou	poiēt-ōn	~의
여격	poiēt-ēi	poiēt-ais	~게, ~에게, ~께, ~한테
대격	poiēt-ēn	poiēt-as	~을, ~를
호격	poiēt-a	poiēt-ai	~여, ~이여

제5식			neanias, neaniou, m. *young man, youth*
	단 수	복 수	
주격	neani-as	neani-ai	~이, ~가, ~은, ~는, ~께서
속격	neani-ou	neani-ōn	~의
여격	neani-ai	neani-ais	~게, ~에게, ~께, ~한테
대격	neani-an	neani-as	~을, ~를
호격	neani-a	neani-ai	~여, ~이여

제2변화	제1식	logos, logou, m. *word, speech, discourse, reason, account, ratio, proportion*	
	단 수	복 수	
주격	log-os	log-oi	~이, ~가, ~은, ~는, ~께서
속격	log-ou	log-ōn	~의
여격	log-ōi	log-ois	~게, ~에게, ~께, ~한테
대격	log-on	log-ous	~을, ~를
호격	log-e	log-oi	~여, ~이여

제2식			dōron, dōrou, n. *gift*
	단 수	복 수	
주격	dōr-on	dōr-a	~이, ~가, ~은, ~는, ~께서
속격	dōr-ou	dōr-ōn	~의
여격	dōr-ōi	dōr-ois	~게, ~에게, ~께, ~한테
대격	dōr-on	dōr-a	~을, ~를
호격	dōr-on	dōr-a	~여, ~이여

제3변화　제1식 a

geron, gerontos, m. *oldness, old man*

	단 수	복 수	
주격	gerōn	geront-es	~이, ~가, ~은, ~는, ~께서
속격	geront-os	geront-ōn	~의
여격	geront-i	gerou-si(n)	~게, ~에게, ~께, ~한테
대격	geront-a	geront-as	~을, ~를
호격	gerōn	geront-es	~여, ~이여

제1식 b

onoma, onomatos, n. *name*

	단 수	복 수	
주격	onoma	onomat-a	~이, ~가, ~은, ~는, ~께서
속격	onomat-os	onomat-ōn	~의
여격	onomat-i	onoma-si(n)	~게, ~에게, ~께, ~한테
대격	onoma	onomat-a	~을, ~를
호격	onoma	onomat-a	~여, ~이여

제2식

anēr, andros, m. *man, male*

	단 수	복 수	
주격	anēr	andr-es	~이, ~가, ~은, ~는, ~께서
속격	andr-os	andr-ōn	~의
여격	andr-i	andr-a-si(n)	~게, ~에게, ~께, ~한테
대격	andr-a	andr-as	~을, ~를
호격	anēr	andr-es	~여, ~이여

제3식

genos, genous, n. (genes- *original stem*) *race, family, kind, sex, gnder*

	단 수	복 수	
주격	gen-os	gen-ē	~이, ~가, ~은, ~는, ~께서
속격	gen-ous	gen-ōn	~의
여격	gen-ei	gen-e-si(n)	~게, ~에게, ~께, ~한테
대격	gen-os	gen-ē	~을, ~를
호격	gen-os	gen-ē	~여, ~이여

제 3 변화　　제 4 식 　　　　　　　　　　　　　　　polis, poleōs, f. (poli- *original stem*) *city, state*

	단 수	복 수	
주격	poli-s	pol-eis	~이, ~가, ~은, ~는, ~께서
속격	pol-eōs	pol-eōn	~의
여격	pol-ei	pol-e-si(n)	~계, ~에게, ~께, ~한데
대격	poli-n	pol-eis	~을, ~를
호격	poli	pol-eis	~여, ~이여

정관사

ho (m.), hē (f.), to (n.) *the*

	단 수			복 수		
	남성	여성	중성	남성	여성	중성
주격	ho	hē	to	hoi	hai	ta
속격	tou	tēs	tou	tōn	tōn	tōn
여격	tōi	tēi	tōi	tois	tais	tois
대격	ton	tēn	to	tous	tas	ta
호격	(−)	(−)	(−)	(−)	(−)	(−)

형용사변화

제 1·2 변화

katharos, kathara, katharon *clean, pure*

	단 수			복 수		
	남성	여성	중성	남성	여성	중성
주격	kathar-os	kathar-a	kathar-on	kathar-oi	kathar-ai	kathar-a
속격	kathar-ou	kathar-as	kathar-ou	kathar-ōn	kathar-ōn	kathar-ōn
여격	kathar-ōi	kathar-ai	kathar-ōi	kathar-ois	kathar-ais	kathar-ois
대격	kathar-on	kathar-an	kathar-on	kathar-ous	kathar-as	kathar-a
호격	kathar-e	kathar-a	kathar-on	kathar-oi	kathar-ai	kathar-a

dynamikos, dynamikē, dynamikon *powerful*

	단 수			복 수		
	남성	여성	중성	남성	여성	중성
주격	dynamik-os	dynamik-ē	dynamik-on	dynamik-oi	dynamik-ai	dynamik-a
속격	dynamik-ou	dynamik-ēs	dynamik-ou	dynamik-ōn	dynamik-ōn	dynamik-ōn
여격	dynamik-ōi	dynamik-ēi	dynamik-ōi	dynamik-ois	dynamik-ais	dynamik-ois
대격	dynamik-on	dynamik-ēn	dynamik-on	dynamik-ous	dynamik-as	dynamik-a
호격	dynamik-e	dynamik-ē	dynamik-on	dynamik-oi	dynamik-ai	dynamik-a

제 2 변화

atomos, atomos, atomon *uncut, indivisible*

	단 수			복 수		
	남성	여성	중성	남성	여성	중성
주격	atom-os	atom-os	atom-on	atom-oi	atom-oi	atom-a
속격	atom-ou	atom-ou	atom-ou	atom-ōn	atom-ōn	atom-ōn
여격	atom-ōi	atom-ōi	atom-ōi	atom-ois	atom-ois	atom-ois
대격	atom-on	atom-on	atom-on	atom-ous	atom-ous	atom-a
호격	atom-e	atom-e	atom-on	atom-oi	atom-oi	atom-a

제 3 변화

hygiēs, hygiēs, hygies *healthy*

	단 수			복 수		
	남성	여성	중성	남성	여성	중성
주격	hygi-ēs	hygi-ēs	hygi-es	hygi-eis	hygi-eis	hygi-ē
속격	hygi-ous	hygi-ous	hygi-ous	hygi-ōn	hygi-ōn	hygi-ōn
여격	hygi-ei	hygi-ei	hygi-ei	hygi-e-si(n)	hygi-e-si(n)	hygi-e-si(n)
대격	hygi-ē	hygi-ē	hygi-es	hygi-eis	hygi-eis	hygi-ē
호격	hygi-ēs	hygi-ēs	hygi-es	hygi-eis	hygi-eis	hygi-ē

piōn, piōn, pion *fat, plump, fertile, rich*

	단 수			복 수		
	남성	여성	중성	남성	여성	중성
주격	piōn	piōn	pion	pion-es	pion-es	pion-a
속격	pion-os	pion-os	pion-os	pion-ōn	pion-ōn	pion-ōn
여격	pion-i	pion-i	pion-i	pio-si(n)	pio-si(n)	pio-si(n)
대격	pion-a	pion-a	pion	pion-as	pion-as	pion-a
호격	piōn	piōn	pion	pion-es	pion-es	pion-a

제 1·3 변화

pas, pasa, pan *all*

	단 수			복 수		
	남성	여성	중성	남성	여성	중성
주격	pas	pas-a	pan	pant-es	pas-ai	pant-a
속격	pant-os	pas-ēs	pant-os	pant-ōn	pas-ōn	pant-ōn
여격	pant-i	pas-ēi	pant-i	pa-si(n)	pas-ais	pa-si(n)
대격	pant-a	pas-an	pan	pant-as	pas-as	pant-a
호격	(—)	(—)	(—)	(—)	(—)	(—)

동사변화

정형 ō 동사

lyein *to loosen, to release, to dissolve*

능동태	부정법	현재			ly-ein	풀어주다		
	직설법	현재	단수	일인칭	ly-ō	나는 ~한다		
				이인칭	ly-eis	너는 ~한다		
				삼인칭	ly-ei	그는 ~한다		
			복수	일인칭	ly-omen	우리는 ~한다		
				이인칭	ly-ete	너희는 ~한다		
				삼인칭	ly-ousi(n)	그들은 ~한다		
	분 사	현재	단수	주 격	ly-ōn (m.)	ly-ousa (f.)	ly-on (n.)	
						~하는, ~하고 있는		
				속 격	ly-ontos	ly-ousēs	ly-ontos	
중간태	부정법	현재			ly-esthai	(주어가 주어에게) 풀어주다		
수동태	부정법	현재			ly-esthai	풀리우다		

정형 mi 동사

didonai *to give*

능동태	부정법	현재			dido-nai	주다		
	직설법	현재	단수	일인칭	didō-mi	나는 ~한다		
				이인칭	didō-s	너는 ~한다		
				삼인칭	didō-si(n)	그는 ~한다		
			복수	일인칭	did-omen	우리는 ~한다		
				이인칭	dido-te	너희는 ~한다		
				삼인칭	dido-asi(n)	그들은 ~한다		
	분 사	현재	단수	주 격	did-ous (m.)	did-ousa (f.)	did-on (n.)	
						(~하는, ~하고 있는)		
				속 격	did-ontos	did-ousēs	did-ontos	
중간태	부정법	현재			do-sthai	(주어가 주어에게) 주다		
수동태	부정법	현재			dido-sthai	받다		

능동태	부정법	현재				ei-nai	이다, 있다	
	직설법	현재	단수	일인칭		ei-mi	나는 ~이다, 있다	
				이인칭		ei	너는 ~이다, 있다	
				삼인칭		esti(n)	그는 ~이다, 있다	
			복수	일인칭		esmen	우리는 ~이다, 있다	
				이인칭		este	너희는 ~이다, 있다	
				삼인칭		ei-si(n)	그들은 ~이다, 있다	
	분 사	현재	단수	주 격		ōn (m.)	ousa (f.) ~인, ~있는	on (n.)
				속 격		ontos	ousēs	ontos
				여 격		onti	ousēi	onti
				대 격		onta	ousan	on
			복수	주 격		ontes	ousai	onta
				속 격		ontōn	ousōn	ontōn
				여 격		ousi	ousais	ousi
				대 격		ontas	ousas	onta

탈형 동사

능동태	부정법	현재				gign-esthai	태어나다, 되다	
	직설법	현재	단수	일인칭		gign-omai	나는 ~한다	
				이인칭		gign-ēi	너는 ~한다	
				삼인칭		gign-etai	그는 ~한다	
			복수	일인칭		gign-ometha	우리는 ~한다	
				이인칭		gign-esthe	너희는 ~한다	
				삼인칭		gign-ontai	그들은 ~한다	
	분 사	현재	단수	주 격		gign-omenos (m)	gign-omenē (f.)	gign-omenon (n.)
				속 격		gign-omenou	gign-omenēs	gign-omenou
							~하는, ~하고 있는	

참고 자료

사전

표준국어대사전 (온라인 판: stdict.korean.go.kr). 국립국어원

슈프림 영한사전. 민중서관, 2001

영한대사전. 시사영어사, 1991

YBM English-Korean Dictionary. 시사영어사, 2000

동아 프라임 독한사전. 동아출판사, 1987

엣센스 불한사전. 민중서림, 1987

동아 프라임 일한사전. 두산출판, 1996

라틴-한글 사전. 가톨릭대학교 고전라틴어연구소. 가톨릭대학교출판부, 1995

영한-한영 과학기술용어집. 한국과학기술한림원. 도서출판 아카데미아, 1998

의학용어집 (제6판, 온라인 판: term.kma.org). 대한의사협회 의학용어위원회. 2020

The American Heritage Dictionary of the English Language (5th ed). Massachusetts: Houghton Mifflin, 2012

Oxford Dictionary of English (2nd ed). Oxford: Oxford University Press, 2003

The Oxford English Dictionary (2nd ed). Oxford: Oxford University Press, 1989

Webster's New World College Dictionary (4th ed). California: IDG Books Worldwide, 2001

Webster's Third New International Dictionary of the English Language (3rd ed). Massachusetts: G & C Merriam, 1971

Epitomē tou Megalou Lexikou tēs Hellēnikēs Glossēs. Lindell HG, Scott R. Athēna: Ekdoseis Pelekanos, 2007

Pocket Oxford Classical Greek Dictionary. Morwood J, Taylor J (ed). Oxford: Oxford University Press, 2002

The Merck Index. Merck Research Laboratories (12th ed). New Jersey: Whitehouse Station, 1996

Dorland's Illustrated Medical Dictionary (28th ed). Pennsylvania: WB Saunders, 1994

Online Etymology Dictionary (On-line dictionary: etymonline.com). Harper D. 2001-2023

Wiktionary (On-line dictionary: wiktionary.org). Wikimedia Foundation

어원론

영어의 역사. 이동국, 손창용. 한국방송통신대학교출판부, 2017

A Dictionary of Literary Symbols. Ferber M. Cambridge: Cambridge University Press, 1999

A Dictionary of Medical Derivations: The Real Meaning of Medical Terms. Casselman W. New York: Parthenon Publishing, 1998

Chambers Dictionary of Etymology. Barnhart RK (ed). Edinburgh: Chambers Harrap Publishers Ltd, 1988

Dictionary of Word Origins. Ayto J. London: Bloomsbury, 1990

Greek and Latin in Scientific Terminology (1st ed). Nybakken OE. Iowa: Iowa State University Press, 1959

Indo-European Language and Culture: An Introduction. Forston IV, BW. Massachusetts: Blackwell Publishing, 2004

Morphology (2nd ed). Katamba F, Stonham J. New York: Palgrave Macmillan, 2006

NTC's Dictionary of Latin and Greek Origins. Moore B, Moore M. Illinois: NTC Publishing Group, 1997

The American Heritage Dictionary of Indo-European Roots (3rd ed). Watkins C. Massachusetts: Houghton Mifflin, 2011

The Cambridge Illustrated History of Medicine. Porter R (ed). Cambridge: Cambridge University Press, 1996

The Concise Oxford Dictionary of English Etymology. Hoad TF (ed). Oxford: Oxford University Press, 1996

The Origins and Development of the English Language (6th ed). Algeo J. Boston: Wadsworth, 2010

The Pronunciation of English (2nd ed). Kreidler CW. Oxford: Blackwell, 2004

The Oxford Introduction to Proto-Indo-European and the Proto-Indo-European World. Mallory JP, Adams DQ. New York: Oxford University Press, 2006

학명

국가표준식물목록 (온라인 판: nature.go.kr/kpni). 국가수목유전자원목록위원회, 국립수목원

CRC World Dictionary of Plant Names. Quattrocchi U. Vols. I-IV, Florida: CRC Press, 2000

International Code of Nomenclature for algae, fungi, and plants (Shenzhen Code, On-line version: iapt-taxon.org/nomen/main.php). 2018

International Code of Nomenclature for Cultivated Plants (9th ed). International Society for Horticultural Science, 2016

International Code of Zoological Nomenclature (4th ed, On-line version: code.iczn.org). 1999

International Code of Nomenclature of Prokaryotes. International Journal of Systematic and Evolutuinary Microbiology 69(1A): S1-S111, 2019

영어
색인

A

acceptance 587

access 496

accessible 496

accession 496

accessional 496

accessory (accessary) 496

accident 493

accidental 493

acclaim 410

acclimate (acclimatize) 412

acclimation (acclimatation,
  acclimatization) 412

acclivity 412

accolade 501, 872

accommodate 616

accommodation 616

accommodative 616

accompany 239

accomplice 429

accomplish 466

accord 233

accost 235

account 434

accredit 233

accrete 579

accretion 579

accrual 579

accrue 579

acculturation 500

accumbent 413

accumulate 303

accumulative 303

accuracy 102

accurate 102

accusative (acc.) 194

accuse 194

accustom 286

—aceous 373

acerbic 340

acetabular 341

acetabulum 341

acetal 341

acetate 341

acetic acid 341

acet(o)— 341

acetobacter 341

acetone 341

acetyl 341

acetylcholine 350

acetylsalicylic acid 830

achalasia 778

ache 894

achieve 207

achlorhydria 117, 349

acholia 350

acholic 350

acholous 350

achromatic 218

acid 341

acidic 341

acidify 341, 592

acidity 341

acidophil 341

acidophilic 341

acidosis 341

acinar (acinose (acinous), acinic)
  846

acinetobacter 456

acinus 846

acknowledge 584, 785

acme 342

acne 342

acneic 342

acneiform (acneform) 342

aconitase 832

aconitate 832

aconite 832

aconitic acid 832

aconitine 832

acorn 914

acoustic 762

acquaint 583

acquaintance 583

acquest 540

acquiesce 196

acquiescence 196

acquiescent 196

acquire 540, 658

acquisition 540

acquit 196

acral 342

acre 491

acrid 322, 340

acrimony 340

acr(o)— 342

acrobat 609

acrocentric 173

acrochordon 122

acromegaly 298

acromial 135

acromion 135

acronym 210

acrophobia 342, 729

acropolis 342, 722

acrosome 185, 342

across 306

acrostic 707

act 487

actin 487

actinic 718

actinin 487

actinium (Ac) 718

actinomyces 718

Actinomyces israelii 945

actinotherapy 692

action 487

activate 487

active 369, 487

activity 369, 487

actor 276, 487

actress 276, 487

actual 487

actuality 487

actuarial 487

actuary 487

acuity 340

acumen 340

acupoint 340, 578

acupuncture 340, 579

acute 340

acyanotic 746

acyl 696

ad— (ac—, af—, ag—, al—, an—, ap—,
  ar—, as—, at—, a—) 658

—ad 659

adage 647

adagio 596

Adam 266

adamant 648

adamantine 648

adapt 491

adaptation 492

adaptive 491

adaptor (adapter) 491

add 416, 658
addendum 416
addicament 416
addict 504
addiction 504
addition 416
additional 416
additive 416
address 542
adduce 507
adducent 507
adduct^1 507
adduct^2 508
adduction 507
adductor 507
−ade 378
adenine (A) 209
adenitis 209
aden(o)− 209
adenocarcinoma 209
adenohypophyseal 249
adenohypophysis 249
adenoid 209, 481
adenoma 209
adenomatous 209
adenosine (A) 209
adenovirus 209
adept 492
adequacy 302
adequate 302
adhere 460
adherent 460
adhesion 460
adhesive 460
ad hoc 289
adieu 265
adios 265
adip(o)− 885
adipocere 885, 886
adipocyte 885
adipose 885
aditus (adit) 635
adjacent 596
adjective 595
adjoin 525
adjoint 525
adjourn 264
adjunct 525

adjunction 525
adjure 212
adjust 525
adjuvant 421
ad libitum (ad libit., ad lib.) 461
ad litteram 658
adluminal 201
administrate 358
administrative 358
admire 310
admission 528
admit 528
admix 463
admixture 463
admonish 645
admonition 645
adnexa 529
adnexal 529
ado 592, 659
adolesce 581
adolescence 581
adolescent 581
adopt 425
adoption 425
adoral 869
adore 425
adorn 179
adornment 179
adrenal 880
adrenaline 880
adrenergic 174
adrenocortical 880
adrenocorticotropic (corticotropic)
  343
adrenocorticotropin (corticotropin)
  343, 880
adrenoleukodystrophy 345
adsorb 470
adsorption 470
adult 581
adulterate 290
adultery 290
advance 659
advantage 659
advent 608
adventitia 365, 608
adventitial 365, 608
adventitious 608

adventure 608
adverb 164
adverbial 164
adversarial 566
adversary 566
adverse 566
adversity 566
advert 566
advertent 566
advertize (advertise) 566
advice 479
advise 479
advocate 200
aedes 471, 822
Aedes aegypti 943
aegis (egis) 813
−aemia (−emia) 888
−aemic (−emic) 888
aeon (eon) 245
aerate 202
aeration 202
aeri− (aer(o)−^{1}) 202
aerial 202
aer(o)−^{1} (aeri−) 202
aer(o)−^{2} 203
aerobe 203, 570
aerobic 203, 570
aerobics 203
aerodrome (drome) 764
aerophagia (aerophagy) 203, 772
aerosol 202
aeruginous 282, 352
Aesculapius (Asclepius) 701
−aesthesia (−esthesia) 602
aesthetic (esthetic) 602
aestival (estival) 852
aestivate (estivate) 852
aestivation (estivation) 852
aether (ether) 852
aetiology (etiology) 690
affable 611
affair 590, 658
affect^1 590
affect^2 590
affectation 590
affection 590
affectionate 590
affective 590

alimentation 581
alimony 581
aliphatic 885
aliquot 290, 293
alive 885
alkali 843
alkaline 843
alkalinity 843
alkaloid 481
alkaloid(s) 843
alkalosis 843
alkane 696
alkapton 843
alkaptonuria 843
alkene 696
alkyl 696
alkyne 696
allantiasis 897
allantoic 897
allantoid 897
allantoin 897
allantois 897
allay 135
allegate 484
allegation 484
allege 488
alleged 488
allegedly 488
allegory 653
allegro 256
allele (allelomorph) 739
allelic 739
allel(o)− 739
allelomorph (allele) 739
allergen 739
allergic 174
allergy 174, 739
alleviate 325
alley 408
alliance 423
allicin 837, 897
alligator 289
alliin 837, 897
alliterate 107
alliteration 107
all(o)− 290, 739
alloantibody 659
alloantigen 659

allocate 136
allocation 136
allocortex 438
allogeneic 523
allograft 766
allomorphism 104
allopathy 720
allophone 613
allosteric 183
allot 499
allotransplantation 313
allotrope 344
allotropy 344
allotype 562
allow 197
allowable 197
allowance 197
alloxan 897
alloy 423
allude 527
allusion 527
ally 423, 658
allyl 837, 897
almagest 298
almamater 581
almond 826
aloe 126
aloft 159, 785
alone 381
along 346, 659
alopecia 816
alopecia areata 816
already 434
altar 256
alter 290
alteration 290
alterative 290
altercate 290
altercation 290
alternate 290
alternation 290
alternative 290
altitude 582
alto 582
altruism 290
altruistic 290
alum 843
alumina 843

aluminium (aluminum, Al) 843
alumni 582
alveolar 845
alveolus 845
alveus 845
always 564
am 632
amacrine 206
amalgamate 335
amalgam 335
amanitin (amanitine) 838
amantadine 648
amaranth 626
amass 108
amastigote 903
amateur 408
amatory 408
amaurosis 734
amaurotic 735
Amazon 783
ambassador 490
amber 911
amb(i)− (am−, an−) 793
ambidexter 332
ambidexterity 332
ambient 635, 793
ambiguity 488
ambiguous 488
ambit 635
ambition 635
ambitious 635
ambivalence 582
ambivalent 582, 793
amblyopia 143, 335
ambrosia 626
ambulance 408
ambulate 408
ambulation 408
ambulatory 409
ambush 910
ameba (amoeba) 425
amebic 425
ameboid 425, 481
ameliorate 299
ameloblast 335
amenable 224
amend 166
amenity 408

ancylostomiasis 128
and 670
andante 408
androecium (andrecium) 120
androgen(s) 716
androgenesis 522, 716
androgyny 715
android 481, 716
Andromeda 716
-ane 376
-anean 376
anecdote 417, 740
anemia (anaemia) 889
anemic 889
anemometer 420
anemone 421
anencephalus 879
anencephaly 879
-aneous 373
anergy 175
aneroid 310
anesthesia (anaesthesia) 602
anesthesiology 602
anesthetic 602
aneuploid 430
aneuploidy 430
aneurysm 743
aneurysmal 743
angel 150
anger 491
angiitides 882
angiitis 882
angina 491
angina pectoris 491
anginal 491
angi(o)- 882
angiogenesis 882
angiology 882
angioplasty 882
angiopoiesis 698, 882
angiopoietic 698
angiopoietin 698
angiosperm 907
angiotensin 473, 882
angle¹ 128
angle² 128
Anglican 128
Anglicize 128

Anglo- 128
Angst 491
anguish 491
angular 128
anhedonia 471
anhidrosis (anidrosis) 448
anhydride(s) 117
anhydrous 117
anicteric 820
anidrosis (anhidrosis) 448
anil 465
anile 258
aniline 465
anilingus 205, 873
anility 258
anima 420
animal 255, 420
animalcule 420
animate 420
animation 420
animism 420
animosity 420
anion 637
anion 785
anionic 637
anis- 832
anisakiasis 342
Anisakis 342
anise 832
aniseed 832
aniseikonia (anisoeiconia,
   anisoiconia) 718
anis(o)- 738
anisocoria 581, 868
anisometric 738
anisometropia 143
anisopia 143
anisotropic 343, 738
ankle 128
ankyl(o)- (ancyl(o)-) 128
ankylose 128
ankylosis 128
ankyrin 128
anlage 135, 844
Anlage 785
annals 129
anneal 851
annelid 873

annex 529
annihilate 675
anniversary 129, 565
Anno Domini (A.D.) 130
annotate 584
annotation 584
announce 651, 658
announcement 651
annoy 647
annoyance 647
annual 129
annuity 129
annul 381, 674
annular (anular) 873
annulate 873
annulus (anulus) 873
annunciation 651
anode 709, 785
anodyne 895
anoikis 120
anoint 887
anomalous 738
anomaly 738
anomer 463, 785
anomeric 785
anomia 210
anomy (anomie) 141
anonymity 210
anonymous 210
anopheles 822
Anopheles sinensis 928
anopheline 822
anorectic 544
anorexia 544
anorexia nervosa 544
anosmia 182
anourous (anurous) 876
anovulatory 164
anoxia 342
anoxic 342
anserine 818
antacid 341, 659
antagonism 489
antagonist 489
antagonize 489
antarctic 659
Antarctic 817
ante- (anti-) 659

antebrachial (antibrachial) 347, 659

antebrachium (antibrachium) 347

antecede 495

antecedent 495

ante cibum (a.c.) 659

antecubital 413

antegrade (anterograde) 625

antemeridian 264, 659

ante meridiem (a.m.) 659

antemortem 659

antenatal (prenatal) 520

antenna 475

antennapedia 475

antepartal 427

antepartum 427

antepenult 290, 624

antepenultimate 290, 624

anteprandial (preprandial) 509

anterior 360, 659

anterograde (antegrade) 625

anteversion 566

antevert 566

anth- (ant(i)-) 659

anthelix (antihelix) 573, 659

anthelminthic (anthelmintic) 573, 659

anthem 613

anther 913

anthocyanin(s) 745, 913

anthology 485, 913

Anthozoa 913

anthozoan 913

anthracene 204

anthracosis 204

anthrax 204

anthrop(o)- 142, 716

anthropoid 481, 716

anthropology 716

anthropometry 716

anthropophagi 771

anthropophagous 771

anthropophagus 771

anthropophagy 716, 771

anthropophobia 716, 729

anti- (ante-) 659

ant(i)- (anth-) 659

antibiosis 571

antibiotic 571, 659

antibody 659

antibrachial (antebrachial) 347, 659

antibrachium (antebrachium) 347

anticipant 588

anticipate 588, 659

anticipation 588

anticipatory 588

anticlimax 412

anticoagulant 488

anticodon 194

anticonvulsant 865

antidepressant 539

antidiuretic 118

antidote 417, 725

antiemetic 574

antiepileptic 770

antigen(s) 522, 659

antigenic 522

antigenicity 522

antihelix (anthelix) 573, 659

antimicrobial 659

antimony 843

antinomic 141

antioxidant 342

antiparallel 739

antiperiodic 709

antiperistalsis 137

antiphon 613

antipodal 188, 189

antipode 189

antipodean 189

antipodes 189

antipyretic 893

antiquate 659

antique 659

antirachitic 859

antiseptic 748

antisocial 622

antistrophe 774

antithesis 252

antithetically 252

antithrombin(s) 345

antithrombotic 345

antitoxin 711

antitragus 557, 814

antitussive 562, 893

antitype 562

antivenin 374

antler 142

antonym 210

antral 172

antrum 172

anucleate 127

anular (annular) 873

anulus (annulus) 873

anuria 119

anurous (anourous) 876

anus 873

anvil 531

anxiety 491

anxiolytic 491

anxious 491

any 381

aorist 726

aorta 121

aortic 121

apart 227

apartheid 227

apartment 228

apathetic 720

apathy 720

apatite 224

aperient 605

aperistalsis 137

aperitif 605

aperture 605, 667

apex 492

aph- (ap(o)-) 667

aphaeresis (apheresis, pheresis) 667, 777

aphakia 837

aphakic 837

aphasia 612

apheresis (aphaeresis, pheresis) 667, 777

aphesis 596

aphetic 596

aphonia (aphony) 613

aphorism 726

aphrodisiac 694

Aphrodite 694

aphtha 492

aphthoid 492

aphthous 492

apian 821

apical 492

apiculture 500, 821

aplanatic 312
aplasia 311
apneic 219
apnoea (apnea) 219
ap(o)− (aph−) 667
apocalypse 98
apocope 220
apocrine 498
Apocrypha 769
Apodemus 701
apoenzyme 213
apoferritin 841
apologize 486
apology 486, 667
apomixis 463
aponeurosis 140
aponeurotic 140
aponia 534
apophasis 612
apophyge 594
apoplectic 576
apoplexy 576
apoprotein(s) 665
apoptosis 536
aporia 431
apostasy 446
a posteriori 666
apostle 136
apostolic 136
apostrophe 774
apothecary 593, 901
apotropaic 344
appall (appal) 354
apparatus 426
apparel 228
apparent 466
apparition 466
appeal 531
appear 466, 658
appearance 466
appease 577
appellant 531
appellation 531
appellee 531
append 532
appendage 532
appendiceal 532
appendicle 532

appendicular 532
appendix 532
appendix vermiformis 568
apperceive 587
apperception 587
appetite 534
appetizer 534
applanation 311
applaud 537
applause 537
applausive 537
appliance 429
applicable 429
applicant 429
application 429
apply 429
appoint 578
appointment 578
apport 430
appose 537
apposite 537
apposition 537
appositional 537
appraisal 168
appraise 168
appreciate 168
apprehend 524
apprentice 524
approach 664
appropriate 665
approval 251, 664
approve 251, 664
approximant 664
approximate 664
apraxia 772
apricot 502
April 694
a priori 666
apron 108
apse 492
apsis 492
apt 491
apteryx 535
aptitude 491
aqua− 99, 888
aquaculture 99, 500
aquaporin 99, 432
aquarelle 99

aquarium 99
Aquarius 99
aquatic 99
aqueduct 99, 507
aqueous 99
Aquila 818
aquiline 818
−ar 375, 794
Arab 807
arabesque 807
Arabia 807
Arabian 807
Arabic 807
Arabidopsis 807
Arabidopsis thaliana 944
arabin 807
arabinose 807
Arabis 807
arable 409
arachidic acid 837
arachidonic acid 837
Arachne 823
arachnid 823
arachnidism 823
arachn(o)− 823
arachnodactyly 823, 877
arachnoid 481, 823
arachnoidal 823
arachnoidea mater 361
arachnophobia 729, 823
aramid 217
araneism 823
arbiter 375
arbitrary 375
arbor (arbour) 910
arboreal 910
arborescent 910
arboretum 910
arborize 910
arbovirus 227
arc 801
arcade 801
arcane 453
arch 801
Archaea 763
archaean 763
archae(o)− (arche(o)−) 763
archaeocortex (archeocortex,

archicortex) 438
archaeology 763
archaeon 763
archaeopteryx 535, 763
Archaeozoic 763
archaic 763
archaize 763
archangel 151, 763
arch(e)− (archi−) 763
−arche 763
archencephalon 763, 878
archenteron 670, 763
arche(o)− (archae(o)−) 763
archeocortex (archaeocortex,
　archicortex) 438
archer 801
archetype 563, 763
archfiend 624, 763
arch(i)− 763
archi− (arch(e)−) 763
archicortex (archaeocortex,
　archeocortex) 438
archipallium 805
archipelago 314, 763
architect 558, 763
architectonic 558
architecture 558
architrave 802
archival 763
archives 763
−archy 763
Arctic 817
Arcturus 617, 817
arcuate 801
−ard 161
ardent 453
ardor (ardour) 453
arduous 302
are^1 270
are^2 628
area 270
areal 270
areflexia 514
arena 903
arenaceous 903
arenavirus 903
arenicolous 500, 903
areola 270

areolar 270
Areopagus 578
argentaffin 513, 840
Argentina 840
argentine 840
argentum (Ag) 840
arginine (Arg, R) 841
argon (Ar) 175
argonaut 122
argue 840
argument 840
argyria (argyrosis, argyriasis,
　argyrism) 840
argyr(o)− 840
argyrophil 840
aria 202
arid 453
aright 543
arise 628
aristocracy 227
Aristoteles 227
arithmetic 617
ark 453
arm^1 226
arm^2 226
Armada 226
armadillo 226
armament 226
armamentaria 226
armamentarium 226
armature 226
armillary 226
armistice 226, 443
armor (armour) 226
arms 226
army 226
aroma 217
aromatase 217
aromatherapy 692
aromatic 217
aromatize 217
arrange 305
array 434
arrayal 434
arrears 569
arrector 542
arrector pili 864
arrest 445

arrhen(o)− 741
arrhythmia 156
arrive 113, 658
arrogant 543
arrogate 543
arrow 801
arsenic (As) 350
arsenical 350
arson 453
arsonist 453
art 225
artefact (artifact) 225
artefactual (artifactual) 225
Artemis 714
artemisia 714
artemisinin 714
arterial 121
arteriolar 121
arteriole 121, 270
arteriolosclerosis 177
arteriosclerosis 177
arteriovenous 121
arteritis 121
artery 121
arthralgia 226, 894
arthr(o)− 226
arthrodesis 226, 776
arthrodynia 895
arthrology 226
arthropod 227
Arthropoda 227
−arthrosis 226
arthrospore 226
Arthur 816
article 226
articular 226
articulate 226
articulation 226
artifact (artefact) 225
artifactual (artefactual) 225
artifice 225
artificial 226
artillery 491
artiodactyl 226
artisan 225
artist 225
−ary 279, 375
aryl 696

arytenoid 281
asbestos 781
asbestosis 781
ascariasis 205
ascarid 205
ascaris 205
Ascaris lumbricoides 329
ascend 546, 658
ascendent (ascendant) 546
ascension 546
ascent 546
ascertain 497
ascetic 776
ascidium 846
ascites 846
ascitic 846
Asclepius (Aesculapius) 701
asc(o)− 846
ascorbic acid 437
ascospore 846
ascribe 439
ascribe 658
ascus 846
−ase 446
asepsis 748
aseptic 748
asexual 435
Asgard 134
ash 454
ashen 454
Asia 807
Asian 807
Asiatic 807
aside 315
asinine 812
−asis (−iasis) 728
asparagine (Asn, N) 832
asparagus 832
aspartame 832
aspartic acid (Asp, D) 832
aspect 599, 658
asperate 338
aspergillus 548
Aspergillus flavus 548
asperity 338
asperse 548
asphalt 170
asphodel 832

asphyxia 729
asphyxial 729
asphyxiant 729
asphyxiate 729
asphyxiation 729
aspirant 441
aspirate 441
aspiration 441
aspirator 441
aspire 441
Aspirin® 798
asplenia 880
ass 812
assail 606
assassin 834
assassinate 834
assault 606
assay 487
assemblage 382
assemble 382
assembly 382
assent 607
assert 546
assertion 546
assess 468
asset 327
assiduous 468
assign 622
assimilate 382
assimilation 382
assist 443
assistance 443
assistant 443
assize 468
associate 622, 658
association 623
associative 622
assonance 146
assonant 146
assort 547
assuage 471
assuasive 471
assume 510
assumption 510
assumptive 510
assure 103
astatic 446
astatine (At) 446

aster 115
−aster 274
asterion 115
asterisk 115, 724
asterixis 183
asteroid 115, 481
asthenia 124
−asthenia 124
asthenic 124
asthma 220
asthmatic 220
astigmatic 549
astigmatism 549
astonish 449
astound 449
astragal 235
astragalus 235
astral 115
astray 315
astringent 550, 658
astrocyte 115
astrolabe 770
astrology 115
astronaut (cosmonaut) 115, 121
astronomy 115, 142
astrovirus 115
astute 119
asunder 669
asylum 173
asymmetric 630
asymptomatic 536
asynapsis 492
asynchronism 343
asynchronous 343
asynchrony 343
asynclitism 412
asystole (asystolia) 137
asystolic 137
at 659
ataraxia (ataraxy) 744
atavism 129
atavistic 129
ataxia 252
ataxic 252
−ate 378
atelectasis 477, 501
atelectatic 477, 501
athanasia (athanasy) 896

Atharvaveda 482, 803
atheism 167
Athena (Athene) 693
Athenian 693
Athens 693
atherogenesis 695
atherogenic 695
atheroma 695
atheromatous 695
atherosclerosis 177, 695
atherosclerotic 695
athetosis 252
athlete 699
athwart 479
athymic 155
atlantal 449
atlantes 449
Atlantic 449
atlantoaxial 236, 449
atlas 449
Atlas 449
atman 149
atmosphere 149, 799
atmospheric 149, 799
atom 171, 740
atomic 171, 740
atone 659
atonic 476
atonicity 476
atony 476
atopic 155
atopy 155
atraumatic 557
atresia 557
atretic 557
atria 803
atrial 803
atrichia 866
atrichosis 866
atrioventricular 803
atrium 803
atrocious 803
atrocity 803
Atropa 344
Atropa belladonna 941
atrophic 345
atrophy 345
atropine 344

Atropos 344
attach 549
attack 549
attain 554
attainable 554
attempt 474
attend 474
attendance 474
attendant 474
attender 474
attention 474
attentive 474
attenuate 474
attenuation 474
attenuator 474
attest 385
attic 807
Attic 807
Attica 807
attitude 491
atto− 388
attorney 557
attract 560, 658
attractant 560
attraction 560
attractive 560
attribute 385
attrite 556
attrition 556
attune 476
atypia 562
atypical 562
atypism 562
auction 454
audacious 455
audacity 455
audible 602
audience 601
audient 601
audile 601
audio 601
audi(o)− 601
audiogram 601
audiometer 601
audiovisual 601
audit 601
audition 601
auditor 601

auditorium 601
auditory 601
Aufklärung 410
auger 148
augment 454
augmentation 454
augur 454
augury 454
august 454
August 454
Augustus 454
aunt 408
aura 203
aural¹ 203
aural² 236
aureate 839
aureole 839
auriasis 839
auricle 236
auricular 236
auriferous 839
aurora 840
Aurora 840
aurotherapy 692
aurum (Au) 839
auscultate 236
auscultation 236
auspex 599, 905
auspice 599, 905
auspicious 599, 905
Auster 839
austere 317
austerity 317
austral 839
Australia 839
Australopithecus 816, 840
Austria 839
Austr(o)− 839
autacoid 721
autarky 453
autecism (autoecism) 120
authentic 732
author 454
authority 454
authorize 454
autism 732
autistic 732
aut(o)− 731

autoantibody 659

autoantigen 659

autochthonous 178

autoclave 500

autocrat 162

autocrine 498

autodidact 764

autoecism (autecism) 120

autogenous 522

autograft 766

autoimmune 424

autokinesis 457

autologous 485

autolysis 247

automata 646

automate 646

automatic 646

automaticity 646

automation 646

automatism 646

automaton 646

automobile 464

autonomic 141

autonomous 141

autonomy 141

autophagy 772

autopsy 144

autosome 185, 731

autotransplantation 313

autotrophic 345

autumn 852

autumnal 852

auxiliary 454

auxin 454

avail 582

available 582

avant-garde 659

avarice 454

avaricious 454

avascular 882

avatar 661

avenge 505

avenue 608

averse 566

aversion 566

avert 566

avertible 566

avian 905

aviation 905

avid 454

avidin 454

avidity 454

avoid 450

avow 200

avulsion 667, 865

avulsive 865

avuncular 129

awake 649

award 617

aware 617

away 564

awkward 667

awry 567

axial 236

axil 237

axilla 237

axillary 237

axiology 490

axiom 490

axiomatic 490

axis 236

axle 237

axon 237

axonal 237

axoneme 140, 237

axoplasm 237

Ayurveda 245, 482, 858

azalea 454

azide 571

azo 571

az(o)- 571

azoospermia 907

azotaemia (azotemia) 571

azote 571

azotobacter 571

azure 164

azurophilic 164, 777

azygos (azygous) 526

azygospore 526

B

babble 740

bacillary 850

bacilliform 850

bacillus 850

Bacillus anthracis 204

Bacillus cereus 886

Bacillus subtilis 558

back 875

backbone 859

backward 567

-bacter 849

bacteraemia (bacteremia) 849

bacterial 849

bactericidal 495, 849

bacterioid 364, 849

bacteriophage (phage) 771

bacteriostasis 446

bacteriostatic 446, 849

bacterium 849

bacteroid (bacterioid) 364, 481, 850

bacteroides 364, 850

baculiform 850

baculine 850

baculum 850

baguette 850

bail 651

bailout 651

bait 276

balance 383

balanic 225

balanitis 225

balan(o)- 225

balanoposthitis 225, 697

Balantidium 725

balcony 232

balk (baulk) 232

ball^1 153

ball^2 238

ballad 153

below 135
belvedere 297
bench 575
bend 899
bene— 297, 792
benediction 504
benefaction 297, 590
benefic 591
benefice 591
beneficiary 592
benefit 590
benevolent 297, 644
benign 297, 519
benignancy 297
benignant 297
benthos 742
benumb 141
benzene 267
bereave 545
beriberi 100
berry 248
—berry 248
berth 640
beryl 151
berylliosis 151
beryllium (Be) 151
beseech 328
beset 469
bestial 100
bestiality 100
bestiary 100
bestow 445
betoken 506
betray 416
betroth 334
between 384
bevel 409
beverage 433
beyond 288
bezoar 239, 511
bi— (bin—) 383
biannual 129
bias 438
biathlon 699
bib 433
bibber 433
Bible 724
Biblical 724

biblio— 724
bibliography 724
bibliopole 778
bibliotheca 593, 724, 901
bibliotherapy 692
bibulous 433
bicameral 804
bicarbonate 180
biceps 208
biceps brachii (muscle) 208
biceps femoris (muscle) 208
bicipital 208
bicoid 875
biconcave 303
biconcavity 303
biconvex 564
biconvexity 564
bicornuate 260
bicuspid 196
bicycle 501
bid 728
b.i.d. 381
bidirectional 542
biennale 129
biennial 129
bier 640
bifid 276
bifocal 804
biform 103
bifurcate 105
bigeminal 307
bigeminum 307
bigeminy 307
bigot 517
bigotry 517
bilabial 870
bilaminar 106
bilateral 309
bile 890
biliary 890
bilingual 871
bilious 890
bilirubin 319, 890
biliverdin 352, 890
bill 100
billet 100
billion 390
billow 238

bilobate 620
bilocular 135
bimanual 257
bin— (bi—) 383
binary 380, 383
bind 899
binocular 142, 383
binomen 210
binomial 210
binominal 210
bi(o)— 570
biobank 570
biochemistry 517, 570
biochip 570
bioclean 570
biodegradable 570
biofeedback 570
biofuel 570
biology 570
biome 570
biopsy 144
—biosis 570
biosphere 799
biosynthesis 253
biota 570
biotic 570
—biotic 570
biotin 570
biotope (biotop) 155, 570
biotron 570
biowarfare 570
bipartite 228
biphasic 247
bipolar 501
birch 828
bird 905
birefringent 575
birth 640
birthmark 195, 640
bis— 383
biscuit 383, 502
bisect 434
bisexual 435
bishop 600
bit[1] 276
bit[2] 383
bite 276
bitter 276

bracteal 100

bracteate 100

bracteolate 100

bracteole 100

brady— 742

bradycardia 233, 742

bradycardiac 233

bradykinin 456, 742

bradypnoea (bradypnea) 219, 742

bradyzoite 571

braid 828

brain 217, 878

braise 459

brake 575

branchia 604

branchial 604

branchi(o)— 604

brand 801

brandish 801

brandy 801

brass 841

brassiere 347

brave 740

brawn 459

brawny 459

brazen 841

breach 575

bread 459

break 575

breakthrough 575

breast 872

breech 100

breeches 100

breed 459

bregma 217, 878

bregmatic 217, 878

breve 346

brevity 346

brew 459

brewery 459

brick 575

bridegroom 178

bridle 828

brief 346

brigade 324

brigand 324

bright 828

brilliant 151

brimstone 801, 842, 886

bring 640

briquette (briquet) 575

bristle 377

brittle 419

broach 302

broccoli 302

brochure 302

broker 302

bromatology 604, 853

bromatotherapy (bromatherapy) 692

bromide(s) 853

bromidrosis (bromhidrosis) 448, 853

bromine (Br) 853

bromopnoea (bromopnea) 853

bronchial 604

bronchiectasis (bronchiectasia) 477

bronchiectatic 477

bronchiolar 604

bronchiole 604

bronchiolus 604

bronchogenic 604

bronchus 604

brontosaurus (brontosaur) 259

brooch 302

brood 459

broth 459

brothel 419

brother 244

brown 353

browse 872

Brucella abortus 939

Brucella melitensis 943

bruise 419

bruit 183

—brum (—bra) 279

brunescent 353

brutal 325

brutalism 325

brute 325

bruxism 764

bubo 100

bubonic 100

bubonulus 100

buccal 100

buccinator 810

Bucephalus 810

buckle 100

buckwheat 827

bud 100, 908

Buddha 728

buddhism 728

buddhist 728

budge 100

budget 238

buff 810

buffalo 810

buffy 810

bufotoxin 821

bug 100

bugle 810

build 250

bulb 151

bulbar 151

bulbospinal 114, 151

bulbous 151

bulge 238

bulimia 810

bulk 238

bulky 238

bull 238

bulla 100

bullet 100

bulletin 100

bullion 100

bullock 238

bullous 100

bully 244

—bulum (—bula, —ble) 279

bulwark 174, 238

—bund 371

bundle 899

buoy 248

buoyancy (buoyance) 248

buoyant 248

buphthalmos (buphthalmus) 144, 810

burden 640

bureau 893

bureaucracy 893

—burg 337

burgeon 893

burglar 337

burgle 337

burn 801

bursa 122

bursary 122

C

cardiomegaly 233

care 603

careen 161

career 504

caress 278

caret 411

cargo 504

caricature 504

caries 265

carina 161

carinate 161

cariogenic 265

carious 265

carminative 277

carmine 824

carnal 437, 861

carneous 373, 437

carnitine 437

carnival 325, 437

carnivorous 437, 604

carol 134, 846

carotene (carotin) 261

carotenoid(s) 261

carotid 261

carp 495

—carp 495

carpal 129

carpel 495

carpenter 504

carpet 495

carphology 485

carp(o)— 495

—carpous 495

carpus 129

carriage 504

carrier 504

carrion 437

carrot 261

carry 504

carryall 504

cart 914

cartel 125

Cartesian 129

cartilage 860

cartilaginous 860

carton 125

cartoon 125

cartridge 125

caruncle 437

carve 768

cary(o)— (kary(o)—) 162

cascade 493

case[1] 493

case[2] 586, 900

caseate 896

caseation 896

casein 896

caseous 896

cash 586, 900

cashier 411

casino 101

casket 586, 900

caspase(s) 832

cassation 411

cassette 586, 900

caste 411

castellan 411

castellated 411

castigate 411

castle 411

castor 825

castor oil 825

castrate 411

castration 411

casual 493

casualty 493

cat 815

cat(a)— (cath—) 785

catabolic 153

catabolism 153, 785

catabolite 153

catabolize 153

cataclysm 102

catadromous 764

catafalque 103

catagen 522

catalase 247

catalepsy 770

cataleptic 770

catalysis 247

catalyst 247

catalytic 247

catalyze 247

catamenia 630

cataphora (cataphor) 641

cataplasm 312

cataplexy 576

catapult 426

cataract 763

catarrh 157

catarrhal 157

catastrophe 774

catatonia 476

catch 586

catechin(s) 263

catechism 723

catechol 263

catecholamine 263

catechu 263

categorize 653

category 653

catenate 101

catenin 101

cater 586

caterpillar 855, 864

catgut 517

cath— (cat(a)—) 785

catharsis 734

cathartic 734

cathedra 470

cathedral 470

cathepsin 768

catheter 596

catheterize 596

cathode 709, 785

catholic 338

cation 638, 785

cationic 638

cattish 815

cattle 208

caudad 659, 875

cauda equina 875

caudal 875

caudate 875

cauldron (caldron) 183

caul(i)— 99

cauliflower 99

caulis 99

caul(o)— 99

causal 194

causalgia 727, 895

causalgic 727, 895

causation 194

causative 194

cause 194

caustic 727

cauterize 726

cautery 726

caution 455

cautious 455

cava (vena cava) 882

caval 882

cavalcade 812

cavalier 812

cavalry 812

cave 302

caveat 455

caveola 303, 846

caveolar 303, 846

caveolin 303

cavern 303

cavernous 303

caviar 164

caviare 164

cavitary 302

cavitation 302

cavity 302

cease 495

cecal 333, 367

cecum (caecum) 333, 367

cedar 827

cede 495

celandine 718

−cele¹ 696

−cele² (−coele, −coel) 303

celeb 322

celebrate 322

celebration 322

celebrity 322

celerity 322, 340

celestial 353

celiac (coeliac) 303

cell 97, 269

cellar 97

Cellophane® 97, 248

cellular 97

cellularity 97

cellulite 97

cellulitis 97

cellulose 97

cel(o)− (coel(o)−) 303

celom (coelom) 303

celomic (coelomic) 303

cement 494

cementicle 494

cementum 494

cemetery 237

−cene 328

cen(o)− (caen(o)−, cain(o)−) 328

cenotaph 707, 736

Cenozoic (Caenozoic, Cainozoic) 328

censor 456

censure 456

census 455

cent 390

centaur 703

centenarian 390

centenary 390

centesimal 390

centesis 173

−centesis 173

cent(i)− 390

centigrade 624

centipede 188

central 173

centre (center) 173

centr(i)− 173, 906

centric 173

−centric 173

centrifugal 173, 594

centrifuge 594

centriole 173

centripetal 173, 535

centr(o)− 173, 906

centromere 173, 463

centrosome 173

centrum 173

centum 390

century 390

cephalad 659, 879

cephalalgia 894

cephalic 879

−cephalic 879

cephalic vein 879

cephalization 879

cephal(o)− 879

cephalodynia 895

cephalon 878

cephalopod 189

cephalotoxin 189

−cephaly 879

ceramic 180

ceramide(s) 886

Cerberus 150

cercaria 876

cerclage 305

cercoid 876

cereal 581

cerebellar 261, 878

cerebell(i)− (cerebello−) 261, 878

cerebellum 261, 878

cerebral 261, 878

cerebrate 261

cerebration 261

cerebr(i)− (cerebro−) 261, 878

cerebroside(s) 261

cerebrum 261, 878

ceremony 101

Ceres 581

cerium (Ce) 581

ceroid 481, 886

certain 497

certainty 497

certificate 497

certify 497

certitude 497

cerulean 352

ceruloplasmin 352

cerumen 886

ceruminal (ceruminous) 886

cervical 261, 872

cervine 261

cervix 261, 872

cervix uteri 148

cesarean (caesarean) 186

cesium (caesium, Cs) 353

cessation 495

cestode 173, 481

cestus 173

chain 101

chair 470

chalaza 693

chalazion 693

chalc(o)− (chalk(o)−) 841

chalcography 841

chalice 205

chalk 230

chalk(o)− (chalc(o)−) 841

challenge 101
chamaeleon (chameleon) 178, 817
chamber 804
chamberlain 804
champagne 414
champion (champ) 415
chance 493
chancellor 163
chancre 161
chancroid 161, 481
chandelier 455
change 414
channel 833
chant 649
chaos 421
chaotic 421
chaotropic 343
chap 180
chapel 209
chaperon (chaperone) 209
chaplain 209
chapman 180
chapter 208
character 219
characteristic 219
characterize 219
charge 504
chariot 504
charisma 221
charismatic 221
charity 278
charm 649
charnel 437
chart 125
charter 125
chary 603
chase 586
chasm 421
chaste 411
chasten 411
chastise 411
chastity 411
chat 815
chateau 411
chattel 208
chauffeur 184
cheap 180
cheer 261

cheese 896
chef 207
cheil(o)− (chil(o)−) 870
cheiloplasty (chiloplasty) 870
Cheiron (Chiron) 877
chelate 421
Chelidonium 718
chemi− (chem(o)−) 517
chemical 517
chemist 517
chemistry 517
chem(o)− (chemi−) 517
chemoattractant 560
chemodectoma 458
chemokine 456
chemotactic 251
chemotaxis 251
chemotherapy 692
chemotroph 345
chemotropism 344
chenodeoxycholic acid 350, 818
cherish 278
cherry 827
cherubism 266
chest 847
−chester 411
chevalier 812
chevron 813
chiaroscuro 862
chiasma (chiasm) 221
chiasmatic (chiasmal) 221
chiasmus 221
chickenpox 100
chief 207
chieftain 207
chilblain 238, 262
chill 262
chil(o)− (cheil(o)−) 870
chiloplasty (cheiloplasty) 870
chimaera (chimera) 814, 853
chime 414
chimeric 814, 853
chimerism 814, 853
chimney 804
chin 872
china 809
China 809
chinaware 809

chion(o)− (chio−) 852
chiral 877
chirality 877
chir(o)− 877
Chiron (Cheiron) 877
chiropractic 772
chiropractor 727, 772
chisel 494
chitin 805
chitinous 805
chiton 805
chitosan 805
chlamydia 849
Chlamydia 805
chlamydial 805, 849
Chlamydia trachomatis 938
chlamydospore 805, 849
chloasma 349
chlorella 349
chlorhydric acid (hydrochloric acid,
    HCl) 117, 349
chloride 349
chlorinate 349
chlorine (Cl) 349
chlor(o)− 349
chlorolabe 769
chloroma 349
chlorophyll (chlorophyl) 349, 912
chloroplast 312, 349
chloroquine 165
chlorosis 349
chlorotic 349
choana 517
choice 420
choir 134
cholagogue 350
cholecalciferol 230, 350, 638
cholecyst(o)− 350, 848
choledochal 458
choledoch(o)− 350, 458
cholelithiasis 704
cholera 350
choleraic 350
cholestasis 446
cholestatic 446
cholesteatoma 350, 886
cholesterol 183, 350
cholesterolosis (cholesterosis) 350

cholic 350
cholic acid 350
choline 350
cholinergic 174
chol(o)– (chole–) 350, 890
chondral 860
chondri(o)– 860
chondr(o)– 860
chondroblast 860
chondroclast 134, 860
chondrocyte 860
chondroid 481, 860
chondroitin sulfate 860
choose 420
choral 134
chord (cord) 122
Chordata 122
chordate 122
chorda tendinea 373
chorea 134
choreatic 134
choreic 134
choreiform 134
choreographer 134
choreomania 134, 729
chorion 123
chorion frondosum 123
chorionic 123
chorion laeve 123
choripetalous 196
choristoma 196
chorography 196
choroid (chorioid) 364, 481
choroidal (chorioidal) 364
choroidea (chorioidea) 364
chorus 134
chrism 887
Christ 887
Christian 887
Christopher 642
chromaffin 218, 513
chromate 218
chromatic 218
–chromatic 218
chromatid 218
chromatin 218
chromat(o)– (chrom(o)–) 218
chromatography 218, 766

chromatophil (chromophil) 218, 777
chromatophore 218, 642
chrome 218
–chromia 218
chromic (Cr^{+++}) 218
–chromic 218
chromium (Cr) 218
chrom(o)– (chromat(o)–) 218
chromogen 218
chromophil (chromatophil) 218, 777
chromophobe 218
chromophore 218, 642
chromoplast 312
chromosome 185, 218
chromothripsis 556
chromous (Cr^{++}) 218
chronic 342
chronicity 342
chronicle 342
chron(o)– 342
chronological 343
chronology 343
chronometry 342
chronotropic 342
–chronous 343
chrysalid 840
chrysalis 840
chrysanthemum 840, 913
chrysiasis 840
chrys(o)– 840
chrysotherapy 692
chrysotile 775
church 304
chute 493
chyle 517
chylemia 517
chylocele 696
chylomicron 517, 743
chylous 517
chyluria 517
chyme 517
chymification 517
chymotrypsin 517, 556
ciao 146
cicatricial 197
cicatrix 197
cicatrize 197
–cide 495

ciliary^1 98
ciliary^2 98
ciliary body 98
ciliate 98
ciliated 98
cilium 98
cinch 279
cine– 457
cinematograph (cinema, cine) 457
cinematography 457
cinemicrography 457
cinerary 191
cinereous 191, 353
cingulate 279
cingule 279
cingulum 279
cinnamon 828
cinquefoil 387, 912
cipher (cypher) 101
circa (ca., c.) 306
circa– 306, 660
circadian 264, 306
circinate 306
circle 305
circuit 635
circuitous 635
circuitry 635
circuity 635
circular 305
circulate 305
circulation 305
circulatory 305
circulus 305
circum– 306, 660
circumcise 494
circumcision 494
circumduct 507
circumduction 507
circumference 639
circumferential 639
circumflex 514
circumlocution 618
circumnavigate 488
circumscribe 439
circumscription 439
circumspect 599
circumspection 599
circumspective 599

Clostridium botulinum 897, 931
Clostridium perfringens 934
Clostridium tetani 936
closure 499
clot 798
Clotho 725, 900
cloud 798
clove 499
cloy 499
club 798
clubfoot 798
clue 798
clump 798
cluster 798
clutter 798
clysis 101
clyster 102
coacervate 128
coagulant 488
coagulate 488, 667
coagulation 488
coagulopathy 488
coagulum 488
coalesce 581
coalescence 581
coalescent 581
coalition 581
coarctation 226
coarse 503
coast 235, 860
coaxial 236
cobalamin 202
cocaine 166
coccal 151
−coccal 151
Coccidioides 152
Coccidioides immitis 325
coccidioidomycosis 152
coccidiosis 151
coccus 151, 824
−coccus 151
coccygeal 819
coccyx 819
cochineal 151, 824
cochlea 826
cochlear 826
cockle 826
cockney 164

cocoon 151
coction 502
coda 875
code 194
codeine 303
codify 194
codominant 131
codon 194
coefficient 590
coelacanth 303, 341, 911
−coele (−cele², −coel) 303
coelenterate 303
coeliac (celiac) 303
coel(o)− (cel(o)−) 303
coelom (celom) 303
coelomic (celomic) 303
coenzyme 213
coerce 453
cofactor 589
coffee 827
coffer 703
coffin 703
cogent 488
cogitate 487
cognate 521, 667
cognition 583
cognitive 583
cognizance 583
cognize 583
cohabit 452, 667
cohabitant 452
cohere 460
coherence 460
coherent 460
cohesion 460
cohesive 460
cohort 134
coil 483
coin 901
coinage 901
coincide 493
coincidence 494
coincident 493
coincidental 493
coital 636
coitus 636
colander 166
colchicine 834

cold 262
coleoptera 98
coleoptile 98
coleorhiza 98
coleus 99
colic 176
colicin 176
colicky 176
coliform 103, 176
colistin 176
collaborate 620
collage 693
collagen 693
collapse 620
collar 501, 872
collarette 501, 872
collate 639
collateral 309, 667
colleague 484
collect 483
collectible (collectable) 483
collection 483
collective 483
college 484
collegium 484
colliculus 802
collide 526
colligate 423
colligative 423
collimate 795
collinear 795
collision 526
collocate 136
collocation 136
collodion 481, 693
colloid 481, 693
colloidal 693
colloquial 618
colloquium 618
colloquy 618
collude 527
collutory 422
collyrium 724
coloboma 134
colobus monkey 133
colon¹ 176
colon² 230
colonel 802

cymbidium 414

cymography (kymography) 303, 766

cymose 303

cynic 815

cynical 815

Cynosure 876

cypher (cipher) 101

Cyprian 841

cypripedium 190, 841

Cyprus 841

cyst 848

—cyst 848

cysteine (Cys, C) 848

cystic 848

cysticercosis 876

cysticercus 876

cystine 848

cyst(o)— 848

cystocele 696

cystoscope 848

—cyte 862

—cytic 862

cytidine (C) 862

cyt(o)— 862

cytochalasin 778

cytochrome(s) 218

cytokine 456

cytokinesis 457

cytokinin 456

cytology 862

cytomegalovirus (CMV) 298

cytoplasm 311

cytosine (C) 862

—cytosis 862

cytoskeletal 177

cytoskeleton 177

cytosol 547

cytotoxic 711

cytotrophoblast 345

D

dachshund 814

dacry(o)— 106

dacryocyst 106

dacryon 106

dactyl 877

—dactyl 877

dactyl(o)— 877

dactylogram 767, 877

—dactyly 877

daemon (demon, daimon) 702

daffodil 832

daft 159

dainty 458

dairy 513

daisy 142

dale 804

damage 166

dame 131

damn 166

damsel 131

dandelion 222

danger 131

Daphne 829

dare 656

Darius 336

dark 744

darn 166

dartos 864

dasyure 299

data 415

date¹ 415

date² 877

dative (dat.) 415

datum 415

daub 348

daunt 648

de— 668

deacon 610

dead 192, 895

deaf 132

deal 702

dean 389

death 192, 895

debacle 850

debase 302

debate 492

debauch 232

debilitate 337

debility 337

debit 453

debride 668, 828

debridement 668, 828

debris 419

debt 453

debug 668

debut 419

dec(a)— 389

decad 389, 752

decade 389, 752

decadent 493

decalcomania 229

Decalogue (Decalog) 389, 485

Decameron 389, 691

decant 414

decapacitate 586

decapacitation 586

decapitate 209

decapod 189

decathlon 699

decay 493

decease 496

deceased 496

decedent 496

deceit 587

deceive 587

decelerate 322

December 389

decency 457

decendent (decendant) 546

decent 457

deception 587

deceptive 587

decerebrate 261

deci— 389

decide 494

decidua 493

decidua basalis 493

decidua capsularis 493

decidual 493

decidua parietalis 493

deciduate 493

deciduous 493

decimal 389

delirium tremens 650

deliver 321

delivery 321

dell 804

delle 804

dellen 804

Delphi 701

Delphic (Delphian) 701

deltoid 481, 750

delude 527

deluge 422

delusion 527

delusive 527

demagogic 490

demagogue 490, 701

demagogy 490

demand 258, 416

demarcate 195

demarcation 195

demasculinize 301

demean[1] 224

demean[2] 423

dement 645

dementia 645

demerit 463

Demeter 243

demi− 326, 794

demifacet 326, 589

demigod 326, 517

demilitarize 376

demilune 201, 326

demimondaine 326, 376

demise 528

demission 528

demit 528

dem(o)− 701

demobilize 464

democracy 162, 701

demography 701, 766

demolish 272

demolition 272

demon (daemon, daimon) 702

demoniac 702

demonic 702

demonstrate 645

demote 464

demotion 464

demur 110

demure 309

demyelinate 140, 884

denarius 389

denary 380, 389

denature 520

dendriform 103, 334, 910

dendrite 334, 749, 910

dendritic 334, 749, 910

dendr(o)− 334, 910

dendrocyte 334, 910

dendrogram 767

dendroid 334, 481, 910

−dendron 334, 910

denervate 140

denial 674

denigrate 319

denizen 671

denominate 210

denominative 210

denominator 210

denotation 584

denote 584

denouement 529

denounce (denunciate) 651

de novo 362, 668

dens 222

dense 299

density 299

dental 223

dentate 223

denticle 223

denticulate 223

dentifrice 419

dentigerous 518

dentin 222

dentinal 222

dentist 222

dentistry 222

dentition 223

denture 222

denudate 310

denude 310

denunciate (denounce) 651

denunciation 651

deny 674

deodar 334

deodorant 182

deontology 776

deoxygenate 342

deoxyribose 807

depart 228

department 228

departure 228

depend 532

dependence 532

dependency 532

dependent 532

depersonalization 896

depict 578

depigmentation 578

depilation 855, 864

deplane 668

deplenish 467

deplete 466

depletion 466

deplore 375

deploy 429

depolarization 501

deponent 537

deport 431

depose 771

deposit 537

depositary 537

deposition 537

depository 538

depot 537

depravation 315

deprave 314

depravity 314

deprecate 432

depreciate 169

depredate 524

depress 539

depressant 539

depression 539

depressor 539

deprivation 665

deprive 665

depth 717

deputation 434

depute 434

deputy 434

derange 305

dereism 265

dereistic 265

derelict 527

di- 384
di(a)- 384
diabetes 126, 609, 726
diabetes insipidus 126
diabetes mellitus 126
diabetic 126, 609
diabetogenic 126, 609
diabolic 153
diabolism 153
diabolize 153
diachronic 343
diacritic 498
Diadochi 458
diadochokinesia 457, 458
diaeresis (dieresis) 777
diagnose 245
diagnosis 245
diagnostic 245
diagnostician 245
diagonal 263
diagram 767
diakinesis 457
dial 264
dialect 486
dialectic 487
dialogue (dialog) 487
dialysate 247
dialysis 247
dialyze 247
diamagnetic 691
diameter 629
diamond 648
Diana 265
Dianthus 265
diapason 742
diapause 771
diapedesis 190
diaper 338
diaphanous 248
diaphoresis 643
diaphragm 603
diaphragma sellae 468
diaphragmatic 603
diaphyseal 249
diaphysis 249
diarrheal 156
diarrhoea (diarrhea) 156
diarthrosis 226

diary 264
Diaspora 907
diaspore 907
diastase 446
diastasis 446
diastema (diastem) 447
diaster (amphiaster) 115
diastole 136
diastolic 136
diastrophism 774
diataxia 252
diathermy 801
diathesis 252
diathetic 252
diatom 171
diatomaceous 171
diaz(o)- 571
dice 415
dichotomous 384
dichotomy 171, 384
dichroic 218
dichromat 218
dicotyledon (dicot) 130
dicrotic 777
dictate 504
dictator 504
diction 504
dictionary 504
dictum 504
dicty(o)- 506
dictyosome 506
didactic 764
didelphia 881
didelphys 881
die^1 192, 895
die^2 415
diecious (dioecious, dioicous) 120
diencephalon 879
dieresis (diaeresis) 777
diestrus (dioestrus) 619
diet 690
dietary 690
dietetic 690
dietetics 690
diethylstilbestrol (stilbestrol) 774
differ 639
difference 639
different 639

differentiable 639
differential 639
differentiate 639
differentiation 639
difficile 589
difficult 383, 589, 794
difficulty 589
diffidence 511
diffident 511
diffract 574
diffraction 574
diffuse 516
diffusion 516
dig 512
digastric 231
digest 519, 794
digestion 519
digestive 519
digit 506, 877
digital 506, 877
digitalis 506, 877
digitate 506, 877
digitigrade 625
digitoxin 506
diglot 871
dignitary 458
dignity 458
digoxigenin 506
digoxin 506, 877
digress 625
dike 512
dilapidate 159
dilatate (dilate) 308, 794
dilatation (dilation) 309
dilatator (dilator) 309
dilator pupillae (muscle) 309
dilatory 640
dilemma 770, 853
dilettante 306
diligence 483
diligent 483
diluent 422
dilute 422
dilution 422
dime 389
dimension 629
dimensional 629
dimensionless 629

disparage 228

disparate 427

disparity 228

dispel 530

dispensable 533

dispensary 533

dispensation 532

dispensatory 533

dispense 532

disperse 548

dispersion 548

displace 313

display 429

disport 430

disposable 538

disposal 538

dispose 538

disposition 538

disproof 251, 664

disproportion 228

disproportional 228

disproportionate 228

disprove 251, 664

disputation 434

dispute 434

disquiet 196

disregard 617

disrupt 544

disruption 544

disruptive 544

disrupture 544

dissect 435

dissection 435

dissemble 382

disseminate 906

dissemination 906

dissension 608

dissent 608

dissertate 547

dissertation 547

dissever 427

dissidence 469

dissident 468

dissimilar 382

dissimilate 382

dissimilation 382

dissimulate 382

dissipate 415

diss(o)— (ditt(o)—) 384

dissociate 623

dissociation 623

dissociative 623

dissolution 547

dissolve 547

dissonance 147

dissonant 147

dissuade 471

distaff 915

distal 444

distance 444

distant 444

distemper 216

distend 474

distensible 474

distention (distension) 474

distil (distill) 886

distillate 886

distillation 886

distinct 548

distinctive 548

distinguish 548

Distoma 870

disto—occlusion (distoclusion) 499

distort 478

distortion 478

distract 560

distrain 550

distraught 560

distress 550

distribute 385

district 550

disturb 116

disturbance 116

ditch 512

diterpene(s) 831

ditto 504

ditt(o)— (diss(o)—) 384

diuresis 118

diuretic 118

diurnal 264

diva 264

divalent 582

dive 717

diverge 568

divergence 568

divergent 568

diverse 566

diversion 566

diversity 566

divert 566, 794

diverticular 566

diverticulum 566

Dives 265

divest 240

divide 506

dividend 506

divine 264

divinity 265

divisible 506

division 506

divisor 506

divorce 566

divulge 150

dizygotic 526

dizziness 132

dizzy 132

do 592

docent 457

docile 457

docosahexaenoic acid (DHA) 390

doctor 457

doctrine 457

document 457

documentary 457

documentation 457

dodec(a)— 389

dodecahedron 470

doff 592

dogma 459

dogmatic 459

dolce 323

doleful 186

dolent 186, 894

dolich(o)— 346

dolichocephalic 346

dolichocranial 346

dolichol 346

dollar 804

dolor (dolour) 186, 894

dolphin 881

—dom 592

domain 131

dome 131

domestic 131

dural 334
dura mater 361
duration 417
during 417
dusk 132
dust 132
duty 453
dwarf 197
dwarfism 197
dwell 132
dwindle 192, 895
dyad 384, 752
dynamic 735
dynamics 735
dynamism 735
dynamite 735
dynam(o)− 735
dynast 735
dynasty 736
dyne 735
dynein 735
dys− 793
dysaesthesia (dysesthesia) 602
dysarthria 227
dysautonomia 141
dysbasia 609

dyscalculia 230
dyscephaly 879
dyscrasia 781
dysdiadochokinesia 457, 458
dysenteric 671
dysentery 671
dysesthesia (dysaesthesia) 602
dysesthetic 602
dysfunction 619
dysgenesis 523
dysgeusia 420
dysharmony 227
dysidrosis (dyshidrosis) 448
dyskeratosis 261
dyskinesia 457
dyslexia 485
dysmenorrhoea (dysmenorrhea) 630
dysmorphic 104
dysmorphogenesis 105
dysmorphosis 105
dysostosis 235
dyspareunia 695
dyspepsia 503
dyspeptic 503
dysphagia 772
dysphasia 612

dysphemism 612
dysphonia 613
dysphoria 643
dysphoric 643
dysplasia 311
dyspneic 219
dyspnoea (dyspnea) 219
dyspragia 773
dyspraxia 773
dysraphism 569
dysregulation 542
dysrhaphism 569
dysrhythmia 156
dysstasia 446
dyssynergy 175
dysthymia 132
dystocia 708
dystonia 476
dystonic 476
dystopia 156
dystrophic 345
dystrophin 345
dystrophy 345
dysuria 119
dyszoospermia 907

E

eager 322, 340
ear¹ 236
ear² 340
earache 894
earnest 628
ease 596
easel 812
east 839
Easter 839
eastern 839
easy 596
eat 509
eaves 673
eavesdrop 673
ebb 667
ebony 708
ebriety 306
ebullient 100

ebullition 100
eccentric 173, 669
ecchymosed 517
ecchymosis 517
ecclesia 411
Ecclesiastes 411
ecclesiastical 411
eccrine 498
ecesis 120
ECG (electrocardiogram) 233
echelon 546
echidna 821
echin(o)− 821
Echinococcus 821
echinocyte 821
Echinostoma 821, 870
echo 722
echo− 722

echocardiography 722, 766
echogenic 722
echoic 722
echolalia 691
echopraxia 773
eclampsia 770
eclamptic 770
eclectic 486
eclecticism 486
eclipse 527
eclipsis 527
ecliptic (ecliptical) 527
eclosion 499
ecology (oecology) 120
economic 120
economical 120
economy 120, 142
ecstasy 446, 669

epenthetic 253
ephapse 492
ephaptic 492
ephedrine 470
ephelis 205
ephemera 691
ephemeral 662, 691
ep(i)- (eph-) 662
epiblast 908
epic 200
epicanthic 414
epicanthus 414
epicardial 233
epicardium 233
epicenter 173
epicondyle 152
epidemic 701
epidemicity 701
epidemiology 701
epidermic (epidermal) 863
epidermis 863
epidermoid 863
epididymis 384, 874
epididym(o)- 384, 874
epidural 334
epigastric 231
epigastrium 231
epigeal 695
epigenesis 523
epiglottic 872
epiglottis 872
epigram 768
epigraph 768
epilepsy 770
epileptic 770
epilogue (epilog) 485, 662
epimer 463
Epimetheus 722
epimysial 139
epimysium 139
epinephrine 880
epineurial 140
epineurium 140
epiphany 248
epiphenomenon 248
epiphora 641
epiphyseal 249
epiphysis 249

epiphyte 250
epiploic 430
epiploon 430
episclera 177
episcleral 177
episcopal 600
episi(o)- 710
episiorrhaphy 569, 710
episiotomy 710
episode 671, 709
episome 185
epispadias 534
epistasis 446
epistaxis 652
episteme 447
epistle 136
epistolary 136
epitaph 707
epitendineum 475
epithalamic 804
epithalamus 804
epithelial 300
epithelialize 300
epithelioid 300, 481
epithelium 300
epithet 253
epitome 171
epitomize 171
epitope 155
epoch 124
eponychium 240
eponym 210, 662
epos 200
epoxide(s) 342
epoxy 342
epulis 854, 871
equable 302
equal 301
equalitarian (egalitarian) 301
equality 301
equalize 301
equanimity 420
equate 302
equation 302
equator 302
equatorial 302
equestrian 811
equi- 301

equidistance 444
equidistant 444
equilateral 309
equilibrate 107
equilibrium 107
equine 811
equinox 851
equipoise 531
equiponderate 531
equisetum 376
equity 302
equivalence 583
equivalent 583
equivocal 200
equivocate 200
era 352
eradicable 198
eradicate 198
erase 541
eraser 541
erasion 541
erasure 541
erbium (Er) 844
erect 543
erectile 543
erection 543
eremite 257
erg 174
ergastoplasm 174
-ergic 174
ergo 543
ergocalciferol 230, 638
ergonomics 174
ergosterol 905
ergot 905
ergotamine 905
ergotism 905
eri(o)- 867
erode 541
Eros 713
erose 541
erosion 541
erosive 541
erotic 713
erotica 713
erotism 713
erotogenous 713
erotomania 713, 729

err 417
erratic 417
erratum 417
erroneous 417
error 417
eructation 434
erudite 797
erudition 797
erupt 544
eruption 544
eruptive 544
erysipelas 320, 863
erythema 320
erythema multiforme 372
erythematous 320
erythraemia (erythremia) 320, 889
erythr(o)− 320
erythroblast 320, 908
erythroblastosis fetalis 320
erythrocyte 320
erythroderma 863
erythrolabe 769
erythroplakia 314, 320
erythropoiesis 698
erythropoietic 698
erythropoietin (hematopoietin,
  hemopoietin) 320, 698
erythrose 320
escalate 546
escalator 546
escape 209
eschar 691
escharotic 691
Escherichia coli 176
esculent 508
escutcheon 436
−ese 376
eso− 671
esophageal 771
esophag(o)− (oesophag(o)−) 771
esophagogastric 771
esophagus (oesophagus) 771
esophoria 643
esoteric 671
esotropia 344, 671
Espana 808
especial 598
Esperanto 204

espionage 600
espouse 471
espresso 539
esprit 441
esquire 436
essay 487
esse 631
essence 632
essential 632
establish 443
estate 442
esteem 408
ester 341, 852
esterase 341
Esther 115
−esthesia (−aesthesia) 602
esthetic (aesthetic) 602
estimate 408
estival (aestival) 852
estivate (aestivate) 852
estivation (aestivation) 852
estradiol 619
estrane 619
estrange 669
estriol 619
estrogen(s) (oestrogen(s)) 619
estrous (oestrous) 619
estrus (oestrus) 619
estuary 852
et alibi (et al.) 290
et alii (et al.) 290
etat 442
et cetera (etc.) 660
etch 509
etching 509
eternal 245
ethane 852
ethanol 194, 852
ether (aether) 852
etherial (ethereal) 852
ethical 286
ethics 286
ethmoid 481, 730
ethmoidal 730
ethnic 286
ethnicity 286
ethnocentric 173, 286
ethnology 286

ethnos 286
ethology 286
ethos 286
ethyl 696, 852
ethylene 696, 852
etiolate 651
etiology (aetiology) 690
etiquette 549
Etna 852
etude 562
etymologic (etymological) 633
etymology 633
etymon 633
eu− 633, 793
eucalyptus 98
eucaryote (eukaryote) 162, 914
Eucharist 221
euchromatin 218
eucrasia 781
eudaemonics (eudemonics) 702
eugenics 522
Euglena 696
euglenoid 696
euglobulin 798
eukaryote (eucaryote) 162, 914
eulogize 486
eulogy 486
eumelanin 746
eunuch 124, 695
eunuchism 124
eunuchoid 124, 695
eupepsia 503
eupeptic 503
euphemism 612
euphemize 612
euphonic 613
euphony 613
Euphorbia splendens 929
euphoria 642
euphoriant 642
euphoric 642
euphorigenic 642
euploid 430
euploidy 430
eureka 768
eurhythmia 156
Euro 806
Eur(o)− 806

exist 443

existence 443

existent 443

existential 443

existentialism 443

exit 636

exo— 669

exocarp 495

exocervix (ectocervix) 261

exocrine 498

exocytosis 669, 862

exodontics 223, 669

exodus 709

exogenous 522

exon 539

exonerate 214

exophoria 643

exophthalmos (exophthalmus) 144

exophytic 250

exorbitant 238

exorcism 374

exorcist 374

exorcize (exorcise) 374

exoskeleton 177

exosmosis 254

exostosis 235

exoteric 669

exotic 669

exotoxin 669

exotropia 344, 669

expand 576

expanse 576

expansion 576

expatriate 242

expect 599

expectancy 599

expectant 599

expectation 599

expectorant 216

expectorate 216

expedient 187

expedite 187

expedition 187

expeditious 187

expel 530

expellent (expellant) 530

expend 533

expenditure 533

expense 533

expensive 533

experience 628

experiment 628

experimental 628

expert 628

expertise 628

expiate 315

expiration 441

expiratory 441

expire 441

expiry 441

explain 311

explanation 311

explanatory 311

expletive 466

explicate 429

explicit 429

explode 537

exploit 429

exploration 375

exploratory 375

explore 375

explosion 537

explosive 537

exponent 538

exponential 538

export 431

expose 538

exposition (expo) 538

expository 538

expostulate 432

exposure 538

expound 538

express 539

expression 539

expressive 539

expressivity 539

expulsion 530

expulsive 530

expunction 579

expunge 579

exquisite 540

exsanguination 888

exscind 436

exsert 547

exsiccate 904

exstrophy 669, 774

extant 444

extemporaneous 216

extemporary 216

extempore 216

extemporize 216

extend 474

extensible 474

extensile 474

extension 474

extensive 474

extensor 474

extensor digitorum longus (muscle) 138

extent 474

extenuate 474

exterior 358, 669

exterminate 147

extern 301

external 301, 669

externalize 301

extinct 548

extinguish 548

extirpate 183

extirpation 183

extol 449

extorsion 479

extort 478

extortion 478

extra— 661, 669

extracellular 97

extracorporeal 858

extract 560

extractant 560

extraction 560

extractor 560

extracurricular 503

extradite 416

extradition 416

extradural 334

extramarital 301

extramedullary 884

extraneous 669

extraocular 142

extraordinary 179

extrapolate 531

extraterrestrial 116, 377

extrauterine 148

extravagant 315

extravasation 881
extravascular 882
extreme 358, 669
extremity 669
extricable 558
extrinsic 621
extro— 661, 669
extrorse 565
extroversion 565

extrovert 565, 669
extrude 561
extrusion 561
extubation 268
exuberant 118
exudate 448
exudation 448
exude 448
exult 606

exuviae 241
ex vivo 363
eye 142
eyeball 142, 238
eyebrow 142
eyelash 142, 902
eyelid 142, 412, 867

F

F_1 300
F_2 300
fabella 837
fable 611
fabric 159
fabricate 159
fabrication 159
fabulous 611
face 589
facet 589
facetiae 307
facetious 307
facial 590
—facient 589
facies 589
facies hippocratica 589
facile 589
facilitate 589
facility 589
facsimile 362, 382, 589
fact 589
faction 589
—faction 589
factitious 589
factor 589
factorial 589
factory 589
factotum 331, 589
factual 589
factum 589
facture 589
facultative 589
faculty 589
faecal (fecal) 891
faeces (feces) 891

faecula (fecula) 891
faeculent (feculent) 891
fagot (faggot) 706
fail 369
failure 369
faint 513
fair 167
fairy 611
faith 511
falcate 902
falchion 902
falciform 103, 902
falcon 902
fallacious 369
fallacy 369
false 369
falsehood 369
falsific 592
falsification 369, 592
falsify 369, 592
falter 430
falx 902
falx cerebelli 902
falx cerebri 902
fame 612
familial 593
familiar 593
familiarity 593
family 593
famine 241
famish 241
famous 612
fan 149
fanatic (fan) 167
fancy 248

fang 577
fantastic 248
fantasy (phantasy) 248
fantom (phantom) 248
far 663
farce 603
fare 431
farewell 431
farina 377
farinaceous 377
farm 335
farmer 335
farnesol 341
farnesyl 341
farnesylate 341
farrow 812
fart 714
fasces 899
fascia 899
fascia adherens 899
fascial 899
fasciate 899
fascicle (fasciculus) 899
fascicular 899
fasciculate 899
fasciculation 899
fasciculus (fascicle) 899
fascin 899
fascinate 167
fascio 899
fasciola 899
Fasciola 899
fasciolar 899
fascism 899
fashion 589

fiber (fibre) 898
fiberscope 898
fibrilla (fibril) 898
fibrillar (fibrillary) 898
fibrillate 898
fibrillation 898
fibrillin 898
fibrin 898
fibrinogen 898
fibrinoid 481, 898
fibrinolysis 898
fibrinous 898
fibroblast 898
fibroin 898
fibronectin 529, 898
fibrose 898
fibrosis 898
fibrous 377, 898
fibula 512
fibular 512
−fic 591
−fication 592
ficin 828
fiction 513
fictitious 513
−fid 276
fidelity 511
fiducial 511
fiduciary 511
fief 263
field 311
fiend 624
fierce 307
fifteen 387
fifth 387
fifty 387
fig 828
fight 187
figment 513
figurative 513
figure 513
figurine 513
filament 898
filamentous 898
filaria 898
filarial 898
filariasis 898
file[1] 578

file[2] 897
filial 300
filibuster 419
filicide 300, 495
filiform 103, 897
filigree 270, 897
fill 467
fillet 897
filly 160
film 863
filopodia 188, 897
filovirus 897
fils 300
filter 531
filterable (filtrable) 531
filth 213
filtrate 531
filtration 531
filum terminale 897
fimbria 103
fimbriate 103
fimbrin 103
final 512
finance 512
financial 512
find 224
fine 512
finger 387, 877
finish 512
finite 512
fiord (fjord) 431
fir 830
fire 893
firm 335
firmament 335
first 663
fiscal 131
fish 906
fissi− 276
fissile 276
fission 276
fissure 276
fist 387
fistula 103
fistular 103
fistulous 103
five 387
fix 511

fixation 511
fixative 511
fjord (fiord) 431
flabellate 418
flabellum 418
flaccid 307
flaccidity 307
flagellant 903
flagellar 902
flagellate 902, 903
flagellin 902
flagellum 902
flagrant 350
flail 902
flair 419
flake 313
flamboyant 350
flame 350
flamingo 350
flammable 350
flannel 867
flat 312
flatter 312
flatulence 418
flatulent 418
flatus 418
flavin(s) 350
flavivirus 350
flavonoid(s) 350, 481
flavoprotein(s) 350
flavor (flavour) 418
flaw 313
flawless 313
flax 429, 797
flay 861
flea 822
fleck 861
fledge 180
flee 180
fleece 112
fleet 180
flesh 861
flex 513
flexibility 514
flexible 514
flexile 514
flexion 513
flexiplace 514

forgive 453
forgo 196
fork 105
forlorn 548, 663
form 103, 104
─form 103, 372
formal 103
formaldehyde (Formalin®) 823
format 104
formation 104
formative 104
forme fruste 103
former 663
formic acid 823
formicary 823
formication 823
formicivorous 604, 823
formidable 653
Formosa 103
formula 103
formulary 103
formulate 103
formyl 823
Fornax 801
fornical 801
fornicate 801
fornix 801
forsake 328
fort 337
forte 355
forth 663
fortification 337
fortify 337
fortis 337
fortissimo 355
fortitude 337
fortnight 387
fortress 337
fortuitous 640
Fortuna 640
fortunate 640
fortune 640
forty 387
forum 376
forward 567
fossa 593
fossa ovalis 593
fossil 593

fossorial 593
fossula 593
foster 239
foul 213
found 133
foundation 133
foundling 224
fount (font²) 516
fountain 223
four 387
fourchette 105
fourteen 387
fourth 387
fovea 846
foveal 846
foveola 846
foveolar 846
fowl 180
foyer 803
fractal 574
fraction 574
fractional 574
fractionate 574
fracture 574
fragile 336, 574
fragility 336, 574
fragment 574
fragmental 574
fragmentary 574
fragmentation 574
fragrance 419
fragrant 419
frail 336, 574
frailty 336, 574
frambesia (framboesia) 248
frame 663
France 307
franchise 307
francium (Fr) 307
frangible 574
frank 307
Frank 307
frankincense 307, 455
frantic 718
fraternal 244
fraternity 244
fraud 197
fraudulent 197

fraxinus 828
fray 419
freckle 548
free 419
freebooter 419
freemason 109
freeze 275
fremitus 259
French 307
frenetic (phrenetic) 718
frenulum 336
frenum 336
frenzy 718
frequency 603
frequent 603
frequentative 603
fret 509
fretful 509
friability 419
friable 419
friar 244
fricative 419
friction 419
frictional 419
Friday 419
friend 419
Frigg 419
frigid 370
frigidity 370
fringe 103
frivolous 419
frizz 516
frizzle 516
fro 663
from 663
frond 225
frondose 225
front 225
frontal 225
frontier 225
frontispiece 599
frost 275
frostbite 275
fructification 260
fructose 259
frugal 260
frugality 260
frugivorous 260, 604

G

gnosis 245, 728
—gnosis 245
gnotobiotic 246
go 196
god 517
goiter (goitre) 217
goitrogen 217
goitrous 217
gold 349, 839
gom 845
gomphosis 105
—gon 263
gonad 523
gonadal 523
gonadoblast 908
gonadocorticoid(s) 438, 523
gonadotrope 343, 523
gonadotropic 343
gonadotropin(s) 343, 523
—gonal 263
goniometer 263
gonion 263
gonioscope 263
gonitis 263
gonium 523, 908
gonococcus 156, 523
gonorrheal 156
gonorrhoea (gonorrhea) 156, 523
gonotyl 185
—gony 523
goodbye 517
goose 818
gooseberry 914
gorge 604
gorgeous 604
Gorgon 736
gosling 818
gossip 285, 517
gourd 837
gout 105
gouty 105
govern 779
governance 779
government 779
governor 779
gown 105
grace 308
graceful 308

gracile 348
gracilis (muscle) 348
gracility 348
gracious 308
gradation 624
grade 624
gradient 624
grading 624
gradual 624
graduate 625
Graeae 712
Graeco— (Greco—) 806
graffito 766
graft 766
grail 781
grain 270
—gram 767
gramineous 231
graminivorous 231, 604
grammar 767
grammatical 767
gramme (gram, g) 767
Grammy 767
gramophone 767
granary 270
grand 324
grand mal 297
grandeur 324
grandiloquence 324
grandiose 324
grandiosity 324
granite 270
grant 233
granular 269
granulation 269
granule 269
granulocyte 269
granulocytosis 269
granuloma 269
granuloma inguinale 269
granulomatous 269
granulomere 269, 463
granulosa 269
granum 270
grape 914
graph 766
—graph 766
graphic 766

graphite 766
—graphy 766
grapple 914
grass 909
grate 860
grateful 308
graticule 860
gratify 308, 592
grating 860
gratis 308
gratitude 308
gratuitous 308
gratuity 308
grave^1 324
grave^2 796
grave^3 796
gravel 218
gravid 324
gravida (G.) 324
gravidity 324
gravitate 324
gravitation 324
graviton 324
gravity (g) 324
gray (grey) 353
graze 909
grease 348, 860
great 218
Grecian 806
Grecize 806
Greco— (Graeco—) 806
Greece 806
greedy 221
Greek 806
green 909
gregarious 653
grenade 270
gressorial 624
grey (gray) 353
greyhound 353
grid 860
gridiron 860
grief 324
grieve 324
grill 860
grind 219, 861
griseofulvin 349, 353
griseous 353

H

hal(o)— 193
halobiont 193, 632
halogen(s) 193, 522
halophile 777
halophilic 193
halothane 193
halt 322
halve 545
ham 877
hamartia 768
hamartoma 768
hamate 369
hammer 340
hamstring 877
hamulus 369
hand 876
handicap 209
handkerchief 207, 606
hang 610
hanker 610
Hantavirus 848
haploid 430
haploidy 430
haplotype 383
hapten 492
haptic 492
haptics 492
haptoglobin 492, 798
harbinger 337
harbor 337
hard 161
hardness 161
hardy 161
hare 353
harlequin 520
harmonica 227
harmony 227
harness 705
harpoon 545
hart 260
haruspex 123, 599
harvest 495
hashish 834
hat 196
hatchet 220
hatred 617
haughty 582
haul 410

haulm 130
haunt 259
haustellum 281
haustorium 281
haustral 280
haustrum 280
have 588
haven 588
hawk 588
hay 194
hazmat 243
he 660
head 209
headache 894
heal 857
health 857
healthy 857
hear 762
hearse 461
heart 233
heartburn 801
hearten 233
heartful 233
hearth 180
heartless 233
hearty 233
heave 588
heavy 588
hebdomad 388, 752
Hebe 696
hebephrenia 696, 718
hebephreniac 696
hebephrenic 696, 718
hebetate 278
hebetic 696
hebetude 278
hecatomb 383, 390
hectare 270
hectic 124
hect(o)— 390
hederaceous 524
hedge 166
hedonic 471
hedonism 471
hedonophobia 471, 729
—hedral 470
—hedron 470
heed 196

hegemony 329
heir 195
—helcosis 654
Helen 574
helianthus 193
helicab 573
helical 573, 797
helicase 573
helicine 573, 797
helic(o)— 573, 797
Helicobacter 849
Helicobacter pylori 937
helicoid 573
helicopter 535, 573
helicotrema 557
heli(o)— 193
Helios 193
heliotaxis 193
heliotrope 193
heliotropic 343
heliotropism 193
helium (He) 193
helix 573, 797
hell 97
Hellenic 717
Hellenism 717
Hellenize (hellenize) 717
helmet 97
helminth 254, 573
helminthiasis 254, 573
helminthology 573
hemadostenosis 889
hemagglutinate 654
hemagglutination 654
hemagglutinin 654
hemarthrosis 226
hematemesis (haematemesis) 574
hematin (haematin) 888
hemat(o)— (haemat(o)—) 888
hematocele 696
hematochezia 764
hematocrit (haematocrit) 498, 888
hematoma (haematoma) 889
hematomatous 889
hematopoiesis (haematopoiesis, hemopoiesis) 698
hematopoietic (hemopoietic) 698
hematopoietin (hemopoietin,

hexad 388, 752

hexagon 263

hexagonal 263

hexahedron 470

hexavalent 582

hiatal 421

hiatus 421

hibernate 852

hibernation 852

hide 862

hidr(o)− 448, 853

hidrosis 448

−hidrosis 448

hiemal 852

hierarch 763

hierarchical 763

hierarchy 619, 763

hier(o)− 619

hierocracy 619

hieroglyph 619, 766

hieroglyphic 766

hilar 167

hilarious 614

hilarity 614

Hilda 133

hill 802

hillock 802

hilt 133

hilum 167

hilus 167

him 660

Himalayas 339, 853

himation 241, 805

Hinayana 196, 638

hindbrain 217

hindgut 517

hinge 610

hip 414

hippocampal 811

hippocampus 811

hippocras 162

Hippocrates 162, 811

Hippocratic 162

Hippocratic Corpus 162

Hippocrene 811

hippodrome 765, 811

hippopotamus 536, 811

hippuric acid 811

hircine 460, 813

hirsute 460

hirsutism 460

hirudin 821

his 660

Hispanic 808

histamine 447

histidine (His, H) 447

histi(o)− 447

histiocyte 447

histiocytic 447

hist(o)− 447

histogram 447, 767

histology 447

histolytic 318

histone 447

Histoplasma 312

historian 482

historic 482

historical 482

historicity 482

history 482

histrionic 180

hither 660

hoard 862

hodometer (odometer) 708

hoe 194

hog 812

hold 322

hole 97

holiday 857

holism 338

holistic 338

hollow 97

holm 802

hol(o)− 338

holocaust 338, 727

holocrine 498

holoenzyme 213

hologram 338, 767

holster 97

holy 857

homage 178

home 259

home(o)− (homoe(o)−, homoi(o)−) 738

homeobox 738

homeodomain 738

homeopathy (homoeopathy) 720

homeosis (homoeosis) 738

homeostasis (homoeostasis) 446, 738

homeostatic 446, 738

homeothermic (homoeothermic) 738

homeotic 738

homicide 178, 495

homily 738

hominid 178

homo 178

hom(o)− 738

homoe(o)− (home(o)−, homoi(o)−) 738

homoeopathy (homeopathy) 720

homoeosis (homeosis) 738

homoeostasis (homeostasis) 446, 738

homoeothermic (homeothermic) 738

Homo faber 159

homogenate 522, 738

homogeneity 522, 738

homogeneous 522, 738

homogenize 522, 738

homogentisic acid 833

homologous 486, 738

homologue (homolog) 486, 738

homology 486, 738

Homo ludens 527

Homo neanderthalensis 927

homonym 210, 211, 738

homonymous 211

Homo sapiens 926

homosexual (homo) 435, 738

homotype 562

homotypic 562

homozygosity 526

homozygote 526

homunculus 178, 271

hone 800

honest 192

honesty 192

honor (honour) 192

honorable 192

honorarium 192

honorary 192

honorific 192

hood 196

hoof 220

hop 414

imbibe 433, 670

imbibition 433

imbricate 186

imbue 186

imide(s) 202

imine(s) 202

imino 202

imitable 195, 610

imitate 195, 610

immaculate 108

immanent 462

immature 309

immaturity 309

immeasurable 629

immediacy 326

immediate 326

immense 629

immensity 629

immerge (immerse) 528

immersion 528

immigrant 424

immigrate 424

imminent 224, 670

immitigable 325, 488

immobile 464

immobility 464

immobilize 464

immoderate 340, 616

immodest 616

immolate 109

immortal 626, 895

immortality 626

immortalize 626

immotile 464

immune 424

immunity 425

immunize 424

immuno— 424

immunocompetence 424, 534

immunocompetent 424, 534

immunocompromised 424, 529

immunodeficiency 424

immunoglobulin (Ig) 424, 798

immunoincompetence 534

immunoprecipitation 209

immunotherapy 692

immure 800

immutable 423

impact 577

impair 190

impairment 190

impale 577

impalpable 426

impar 229

impart 228

impartial 227

impassable 576

impasse 576

impatience 624

impatiens 624

impatient 624

impeach 187

impeccable 190

impecunious 263

impedance 187

impede 187

impel 530

impellent 530

impend 532

imperative 427

imperfect 591

imperforate 418

imperial 427

imperious 427

impermeability 424

impermeable 424

impermeant 424

impersonate 896

impertinent 473

imperturbable 116

impervious 564

impetiginous 281, 534

impetigo 281, 534

impetuous 534

impetus 534

impinge 577

implacable 314

implant 312

implantation 312

implement 466

implementation 466

implicate 429

implicit 429

implode 537

implore 375

implosion 537

imply 429

import 431

importance 431

important 431

importunate 431

importune 431

impose 538

imposition 538

impost 538

impostor (imposter) 538

imposture 538

impotence (impotency) 634

impotent 634

impoverish 161, 428

imprecate 433

impregnable 524

impregnate 521

impregnation 521

impress 539

impression 539

impressive 539

imprint 539, 670

impromptu 509

improve 632, 664

improvement 632

improvise 480

impudence 275

impudent 275

impugn 579

impulse 530

impulsion 530

impulsive 530

impunity 894

imputation 434

impute 434

in 670

in—^{1} (il—^{1}, im—^{1}, ir—^{1}) 670

in—^{2} (il—^{2}, im—^{2}, ir—^{2}) 675, 792

inability 452

inaction 487

inactivate 487

inactive 487

inactivity 487

inadequacy 302

inadequate 302

inadvertent 566

inalienable (unalienable) 290

inane 327

interact 487
interaction 487
interactive 487
inter alia 661
inter alios 661
intercalary 410
intercalate 410
intercede 496
intercellular 97
intercept 587
intercession 496
interchange 414
intercommissural 528
intercostal 236
intercourse 503
intercurrent 503
interdental 223
interdependent 532
interdict 505
interdigitate 506, 877
interest 632
interface 589
interfere 418
interference 418
interferon 418
interfuse 516
interim 672
interior 360, 672
interject 595
interjection 595
interleukin(s) 201
interlobar 620
interlobular 620
interlock 655
interlocution 618
interlocutor 618
interlude 527
intermediary 326, 332
intermediate 326, 332
interminable 147
intermingle 109
intermission 528
intermit 528
intermittent 528
intern 301, 672
internal 301, 672
internalize 301, 672
international 521

internecine 465
interneuron 140, 652
internment 301, 672
internuncial 652
interosseous 235
interphase 247
interpolate 531
interpose 538
interposition 538
interpret 169
interpretation 169
interpreter 169
interregnum 542
interrogate 543
interrogative 543
interrupt 544
interruption 544
interruptive 544
inter se 285
intersect 435
intersex 435
interspace 204
intersperse 548
interstice 443
interstitial 443
interstitium 443
intertragic 557, 813
intertriginous 281
intertrigo 281
intertwine 384
interval 800
intervascular 882
intervene 608
intervention 608
interventional 608
interventricular 148
interview 479
intestinal 363, 671
intestine 363, 671
intima 360, 365, 672
intimacy 672
intimal 365
intimate 672
intimation 672
intimidate 370
intimidation 370
into 670
intolerable 449

intolerance 449
intonation 476
intone 476
intorsion 479
intort 479
in toto 331
intoxicate 711
intoxication 711
intra- 661, 671
intracellular 97
intracranial 262
intractable 559
intradermal 863
intradural 334
intraepithelial 300
intragenic 671
intralesional 526, 854
intraluminal 201
intramedullary 884
intramural 800
intramuscular 139
intransigent 488
intransitive 637
intraocular 142
intraoperative 214
intraosseous 235
intrapartal 427
intrapartum 427
intraperitoneal 477
intrathecal 592
intrauterine 148
intravasation 881
intravascular 882
intravenous 883
intraventricular 148
intrepid 277
intricacy 558
intricate 558
intrigue 558
intrinsic 621
intro- 672
introduce 508
introduction 508
introductory 508
introgression 625
introitus 637
intromission 528
intromit 528

intromittent 528
intron 671
introrse 565
introspect 600
introspective 600
introversion 565
introvert 565, 672
intrude 561
intrusion 561
intubate 268
intubation 268
intuition 614
intuitional 614
intuitive 614
intumescent 184
intussuscept 588
intussusception 588, 671
intussusceptum 588
intussuscipiens 588
inulin 574
inunction 887
inundate 117
inure (enure) 214
in utero 148
invade 563
invaginate 875
invalid 583
invalidate 583
invaluable 582
invariant 316
invasion 563
invasive 563
invent 608
invention 608
inventory 608
inverse 567
inversion 567
invert 567
invertase 567
invertebrate 565
inverter 567
invertor 567
invest 241
investigate 844
investment 241
inveterate 811
invigorant 649
invigorate 649

invincible 569
inviolable 197
invisible 479
invitation 197
invite 197
in vitro 480, 903
in vivo 363
invocation 200
invoice 564
invoke 200
involucrin 572
involucrum 572
involuntary 644
involute 572
involution 572
involutional 572
involve 572
involvement 572
inward 567
iodide 353
iodinate 353
iodine (I) 353, 481
iod(o)− 353
iodopsin(s) 144, 353
ion 637
−ion 276
ionic 637
ionize 637
ionized 637
ionophore 637, 642
ionotropic 343
iontophoresis 637, 641
−ious 373
ipsi− 290
ipsilateral 309
irascible 619
irate 619
ire 619
Ireland (Eire) 149
iridesce 579
iridescence 579
iridescent 205, 579
iridial 205
iridium (Ir) 205
iridocorneal 205
iris 205
Iris 205
irk 174

irksome 174
iron 619, 841
ironic 164
irony 164
irradiate 199, 670
irradiation 199
irradicable 198
irrational 617
irreal 265
irrefragable 575
irregular 542
irrelevant 325
irresistible 443
irresolute 548
irresponsible 471
irreversible 567
irrevocable 200
irrigate 421
irrigation 421
irritability 628
irritable 628
irritant 628
irritate 628
irritation 628
irrupt 545
irruption 545
irruptive 545
is 632
ischaemia (ischemia) 124
ischemic 124
ischiadic 174
ischial 173
ischium 173
ischuria 119
iseikonia (isoeiconia, isoiconia) 718
−isk 724
island 99, 904
isle 904
islet 904
−ism 730
is(o)− 738
isoantibody 659
isoantigen 659
isobar 325, 738
isochronism 343
isochronous 343
isochrony 343
isocoria 581, 868

J

K

kail (kale) 99
kainite 328
Kaiser 186
kale (kail) 99
kaleidoscope 480, 736
kalium (K) 843
kallikrein 304, 736
Kama 278
Kamasutra 278, 553
karat (carat) 261
karma 716
kary(o)- (cary(o)-) 162
karyokinesis 457
karyolysis 162, 247
karyoplast 162
karyopyknosis 162, 737
karyorrhexis 162, 479
karyosome 162
karyotype 162
Katze 815
keel 603
keen 584
keloid 421
ken 584
kennel 814
kenning 584
keratan sulfate 261
keratin 261
keratinize 261
keratin(o)- 261
keratinocyte 261
keratitis 261
kerat(o)- 261
keratoconus 799
keratocyte 261
keratohyalin 261
keratohyaline 261
keratolysis 261

keratomalacia 335
keratomileusis 697
keratoplasty 261
keratosis 261
keratotomy 261
kerchief 207, 606
kerion 886
Kern 270
kernel 270
kernicterus 270, 820
kerosene 886
ketal 341
keto 341
ket(o)- 341
ketone 341
ketosis 341
kettle 130
kidney 879
kill 154
kiln 502
kilo- 390
kin 520
kinaesthesia (kinesthesia) 602
kinase 456
kind 520
kindergarten 134
kindred 520, 617
kine- (kin(o)-) 456
-kine 456
kinematics 457
-kinesia 457
kinesics 456
kinesin 456
kinesiology 456
kinesis 456
-kinesis 456
kinesitherapy 692
kinesthesia (kinaesthesia) 602

kinesthetic 602
kinetic 456
kinetics 456
kinetochore 196, 456
kinetophore 456
kinetoplast 456
king 520
kingdom 520
kinin 456
kink 871
kin(o)- (kine-) 456
kinocilium 98
kinship 520
kitchen 502
kitten 815
-klasis 134
Klebsiella pneumoniae 930
kleptomania (cleptomania) 99, 729
knapsack 846
knee 263
kneel 263
know 584
knowledge 584
koilocyte 303
koilonychia 240, 303
Koine 667
Korea 806
Korean 806
kosmotropic 343
kraurosis 735
Krieg 324
krypton (Kr) 769
kurtosis 305
kylix 205
kymography (cymography) 303, 766
kyphosis 414
Kyrie 304

L

label 620
labellum 870
labial 870

labiate 870
labile 620
lability 620

labiodental 223
labium 870
labium majus 357

labium minus 357
labor (labour) 620
laboratory 620
laborious 620
labret 870
labrum 870
labyrinth 704
labyrinthine 704
lac 825
lace 306
lacerate 347
laceration 348
lachrymal (lacrimal) 106
laciniate 348
laconic 717
lacquer 825
lacrimal (lachrymal) 106
lacrimation 106
lacrimator 106
lactam 234
lactate¹ 234
lactate² 234
lactation 234
lacteal 234
lactic 234
lactic acid 234
lactiferous 234, 638
lactifluous 515
lactim 234
lact(o)– 234
lactobacillus 234
lactoferrin 841
lactone 234
lactose 234
lactotrope 343
lactotropic 343
lactotropin (prolactin) 234, 343
lactulose 234
lacuna 106
lacunar 106
lacustrine 106
ladder 412
lady 513
laev(o)– (lev(o)–) 332
Lager 135
lagoon 106
lagophthalmos (lagophthalmus) 145,
   655, 814

lair 135
laity 704
lake 106
–lalia 691
lambdoid 481
lamella 106
lamellar 106
lamellate 106
lamellipodia 106, 188
lament 657
lamentable 657
lamentation 657
lamin 106
lamina 106
lamina choriocapillaris
   (choriocapillaris) 865
lamina cribrosa 106
lamina densa 301
lamina propria 137
laminar 106
lamina rara externa 301
lamina rara interna 301
laminaria 106
laminate 106
lamination 106
laminectomy 106
laminin 106
lamp 770
lanate 867
Lancaster 411
lance 106
lanceolar 106
lanceolate 106
lancet 106
lanciform 106
lancinate 348
land 904
landmark 195
landscape 266, 904
language 871
langue 871
languid 655
languish 655
languor 655
laniferous 638, 867
La Niña 289
lanolin 867
lanose 867

lanosterol 867
lantern 770
lanthanum (La) 461
lanugo 282, 867
lap 620
laparoscope 160
laparotomy 160
lapel 620
lapidary 159
lapse 619, 620
lar 106
larceny 180
lard 308, 885
lardaceous 308, 885
large 308
largo 308
lariat 289, 491
larva 106
larval 106
larva migrans 424
larvicide 106, 495
laryngeal 231
laryng(o)– 231
laryngopharynx (hypopharynx) 419
laryngoscope 600
larynx 231
lascivious 309
LASEK 697
laser 201
lash 902
LASIK 697
lassitude 337
lasso 306
last¹ 337
last² 650
latch 770
late 337
latebra 461
latency 461
latent 461
later 337
–later 180
laterad 309, 659
lateral 309, 327
–lateral 309, 327
laterality 309
lateralize 309
laterite 309

liposome 885
liquefacient 462
liquefaction 462
liquefy 462
liquescent 462
liquid 462
liquidate 462
liquor 462
liquorice (licorice) 198, 323
lira 107
liri(o)— 834
lissencephaly (agyria) 154, 744
liss(o)— 744
lissive 744
list 309
listen 768
listless 309
—lite 704
literacy 107
literal 107
literally 107
literary 107
literate 107
literatim 107
literature 107
literatus 107
—lith 704
lithe 340
lithiasic 704
lithiasis 704
—lithiasis 704
lithium (Li) 704
lith(o)— 704
lithography 767
litholapaxy 160, 704
lithotomy 171, 704
lithotripsy 704, 775
lithotriptic 704, 775
lithotriptor 704, 775
lithotrity 704, 775
litigate 488
litmus 138
litotes 339
litre (liter) 107
litter 135
littermate 135
littoral 422
liturgy 174, 704

live 885
livedo 354
liver 885
livery 321
livid 353
lividity 353
livor mortis 353
lizard 821
loan 527
lobar 620
lobate 620
lobation 620
lobby 159
lobe 620
lobo 815
lobster 821
lobular 620
lobulate 620
lobulation 620
lobule 620
local 135
locale 135
locality 135
localize 135
locate 135
location 135
loch 106
lochia 135
lock 655
locomotion 135
locomotor 135
locoregional 135
locular 135
loculate 135
loculus (locule) 135
locus 135
locus caeruleus (locus coeruleus,
    locus ceruleus) 353
locust 821
locution 618
lodge 159
loft 159
logarithm (log) 617
logic 485
logical 485
—logism 486
logistic 485
logistics 159

logotherapy 692
—logue (—log) 485
—logy 486
loin 137
lone 381
lonely 381
long 346
longevity 245, 346
longevous 346
longitude 346
longitudinal 346
loose 548
loosen 548
loot 545
loph(o)— 796
loquacious 618
loquacity 618
lord 617
lordosis 737
lore 650
lorica 573
loricrin 573
lorn 548
lose 548
loss 548
lost 548
lot 499
lotion 422
lotus 829
loud 768
louse 822
love 461
low^1 135
low^2 410
lower 135
lowercase 586, 900
loyal 484
loyalty 484
lubricant 656
lubricate 656
lubricious 656
lucent 200, 656
lucid 200, 354
Lucifer 201
luciferase 201
luciferin 201
lucrative 168
lucre 168

ludicrous 527

lues 548

luetic 548

lugubrious 462

lukewarm 184

lumbaginous 137, 281

lumbago 137, 281

lumbar 137

lumbrical 330

lumbrical muscles 138

lumbricoid 329

lumbus 137

lumen 201

luminal 201

luminesce 201, 579, 657

luminescence 201, 579, 657

luminescent 201, 579, 657

luminol 201

luminophore 201, 642

lump 621

lumpectomy 621

lunar 201

lunate 201

lunatic 201

lung 325

lunge 346

lunula 201

lupine 815

lupus 815

lupus erythematosus 815

lupus vulgaris 815

lush 655

lust 309

lustrate 201

lustre (luster) 201

lustrum 201

lute 351

luteal 351

lutein 351

luteinize 351

luteolysis 351

luteotropic 351

luteotropin 351

luteous 351

lux 200

luxate 655

luxation (dislocation) 655

luxuriant 655

luxuriate 655

luxurious 655

luxury 655

lyase 247

lycanthrope 815

lycanthropy 815

lyc(o)- 815

lycopene 808, 815

lye 422

lymph 108

lymphadenitis 209

lymphangiitis 882

lymphatic 108

lymphedema (lymphoedema) 108

lymph(o)- 108

lymphoblast 108, 908

lymphocyte 108

lymphoedema (lymphedema) 108

lymphogranuloma 269

lymphogranuloma venereum 269

lymphoid 108, 481

lymphoma 108

lymphopenia 534

lyophilic 247

lyophilize 247

lyre 121

lyric 121

lyrical 121

lysate 247

lysergic acid 905

lysergic acid diethylamide (LSD) 905

lysin 247

lysine (Lys, K) 247

lysis 247

lysosome 185

lysozyme 213

lyssa 816

lyssavirus 816

lyssophobia 729, 816

lytic 247

-lytic 247

M

-m (-sm) 730

-ma (-m, -sm) 730

macerate 109

machinate 122

machine 122

machinery 122

macho 301

-machy 782

macr(o)- 743

macrogamete 702

macroglia 654

macrognathia 872

macromolecule 271

macron 743

macrophage 771

macroscopic 600

macula (macule) 108

macula adherens 460

macula lutea (retinae) 256

macular 108

maculate 108

mad 423

madame 131

Madame 284

mademoiselle 131

madonna 131

Madonna 284

maestro 298

maggot 722

magic 122

magician 122

magisterial 298

magistral 298

magistrate 298

magma 109

magnanimity 420

magnanimous 420

magnate 298

magnesium (Mg) 692

magnet 691

magnetic 691

magnetism 691

medulla oblongata 883
medullary 884
medulloblast 883
Medusa 616
meek 137
meg(a)— 298
megacolon 176
megakaryoblast 908
megakaryocyte 162
megalith 298, 704
megal(o)— 298
megaloblast 298
—megaly 298
mei(o)— (mio—, mi—) 358
meiosis (miosis[1]) 358
meiotic (miotic[1]) 358
melaena (melena) 746
melancholy 350, 746
Melanesia 605, 904
melanin(s) 746
melan(o)— 746
melanocyte 746
melanophore 642
melanosome 185, 746
melasma 746
melatonin 476
melena (melaena) 746
—melia 719
meliorate 299
meliorism 299, 356
melittin 234
melliferous 234, 638
mellifluous 515
mellow 109
melodrama 719
melody 720, 761
melon 829
melt 335
—melus 719
member 362
membranaceous 362
membrane 362
membranous (membraneous) 362
meme 705
memo 329
memorable 329
memoranda 329
memorandum 329

memorial 329
memory 329
memos 329
—men 277
menace 224
menage 462
menagerie 462
menarche 630, 763
menarcheal (menarchial) 630, 763
mend 166
mendacious 166
mendacity 166
mendicant 166
menhir 315
meningeal 363
meningismus (meningism) 363
meningitic 206, 363
meningitis 206, 363
mening(o)— 363
meningocele 696
meninx 363
meniscus 630, 724
menopausal 630, 771
menopause 630, 771
menorrhagia 479, 630
menorrhalgia 630
menorrhoea (menorrhea) 630
mensal[1] 362
mensal[2] 630
menses 630
Menshevik 358
menstrual 630
menstruate 630
menstruation 630
mensural 629
—ment 277
mental[1] 224, 854, 872
mental[2] 645, 854
mentality 645
menthol 834
mentholated 834
Mentholatum® 834
mention 645
mentor 646
Mentor 646
menu 357
—mer 463
mercapt(o)— 231, 586

mercenary 230
merchandise 230
merchant 230
mercurial 231
mercuric (Hg+) 231
mercurous (Hg++) 231
mercury 231
Mercury 231
mercy 230
—mere 463
merge 528
meridian 264, 326
meridional 264
meristem 463
meristematic 463
merit 462
meritocracy 462
mermaid 255
mer(o)— 463
merocrine 498
merogony 523
meront 463, 632
merozoite (schizozoite) 463, 571
merry 346
mesa 362
mesangial 882
mesangium 327, 882
mesaxon 237, 327
mesencephalon 879
mesenchyma (mesenchyme) 327, 518
mesenchymal 518
mesenteric 671
mesentery 327, 671
mesiad 327, 659
mesial 327
mes(o)— 327
mesoappendix 327, 532
mesoblast 908
mesoblastema 909
mesocarp 495
mesocercaria 876
mesocolon 176, 327
mesoderm 327, 863
mesometrium 243, 327
meson 327
mesonephric 880
mesonephros 880
Mesopotamia 327, 536

model 615
modeling 615
moderate 339, 616
moderato 616
moderator 340, 616
modern 615
modest 616
modesty 616
modification 616
modify 592, 616
modiolus 615
modular 615
modulate 615
module 615
modulus 615
modus 615
moiety 326
Moirai 463
moist 137
moisture 137
moisturize 137
molal 271
molality 271
molar^1 109
molar^2 109
molar^3 271
molarity 271
mold^1 (mould^1) 137
mold^2 (mould^2) 615
moldy (mouldy) 137
mole^1 109
mole^2 221
mole^3 271
molecular 271
molecule 271
molest 271
molestation 272
molimen 272
mollification 334
mollify 334
mollusc (mollusk) 334
molluscum 334
molt (moult) 423
molybdenum (Mo) 842
moment 464
momentary 464
momentous 464
momentum 464

monad 737, 752
monarch 763
monarchy 763
monastery 737
Monday 630
monecious (monoecious) 120
monetary 110
money 110
moneyed (monied) 110
mongrel 109
monied (moneyed) 110
monilethrix 256, 866
monilial 256
moniliform 103, 256
moniliosis (moniliasis) 256
monition 645
monitor 645
monk 737
mon(o)− 737
monoceros 261
monoclonality 134
monocotyledon (monocot) 130
monocrotic 777
monocular 142
monocyte 737
monody 762
monoecious (monecious) 120
monogamy 702
monograph 766
monogyny 715
monolith 704
monologue (monolog) 485
monomer 463
monomorium 463
monomorphic (monomorphous) 104
mononucleosis 737
monophasic 247
monophyletic 250
monopoly 778
monopsony 662
monoptychial 773
monosaccharide(s) 175
monosomy 185
monoterpene(s) 831
monotheism 167
monotreme 557
monovalent 582
monozygotic 526

monsieur 244
Monsieur 284
mons pubis (mons veneris) 223
monster 645
monstrosity 645
monstrous 645
mons veneris (mons pubis) 223
montage 224
montane 224
month 630
monument 645
−mony 278
mood^1 192
mood^2 615
moon 630
moor 423
mora 110
moral 192
moratorium 110
moratory 110
morbid 371, 626
morbidity 371, 626
morbilliform 103, 273, 626
mordant 626
mordent 626
mores 192
moribund 371, 626
moron 735
moronic 735
morphea 104
morpheme 104
morphine 105
morphogenesis (morphogeny) 105
morphogenic 104
morphogeny (morphogenesis) 104
morphology 104
Mors 626, 895
morsel 626
mortal 626, 895
mortality 626
mortar 626
mortgage 168, 626
mortify 626
mortuary 626
morula 829
morular 829
morulation 829
mosaic 647

mycelial 138
mycelium 138
—myces 138
—mycete 138
—mycetin 138
mycet(o)— 138
—mycin 138
myc(o)— 138
mycobacterial 138
mycobacterium 138
Mycobacterium avium 940
Mycobacterium bovis 938
Mycobacterium intracellulare 932
Mycobacterium leprae 935
Mycobacterium tuberculosis 938
mycology 138
mycoplasma 849
Mycoplasma pneumoniae 181
mycoplasmal 849
mycosis 138
—mycosis 138
mycosis fungoides 850
mycotic 138
—mycotic 138
mydriasis 254
mydriatic 254
myelencephalon 879, 884
—myelia 140, 884
myelin 140, 884
myelinate 140, 884
myelinize 140, 884

myelitis 884
myel(o)— 140, 884
myeloblast 140, 884, 908
myelocele 696
myelocyte 140, 884
myeloid 140, 481, 884
myeloma 884
myelophthisis 772, 884
myenteric 671
myiasis 822
myl(o)— 109
mylohyoid 750
my(o)— 139
myoblast 139
myocardial 233
myocardium 233
myoclonus 323
myocyte 139
myodynia 895
myofiber 139
myofibril 139
myoglobin 798
myoid 139, 481
myometrial 243
myometrium 243
myopia 143, 333
myosin 139
myosis (miosis^2) 254, 333
myosotis 139, 236
myotatic 477
myotic (miotic^2) 254, 333

myotome 171
myotonia 476
myotonic 476
myriad 735, 752
myring(o)— 363
myringoplasty 363
myristic acid 884
myrmec(o)— 823
myrmecology 823
myrrh 110
myrtle 110
myself 284
mysophobia 138, 729
mystagogic 490
mystagogue 490
mystagogy 490
mystery 333
mystic 333
mystical 333
myth 705
mythical 705
mythology 705
mythopoeia 699
mythopoeic 699, 705
myx(o)— 137
myxoedema (myxedema) 138
myxoid 137, 481
myxoma 137
myxovirus 137

N

Naegleria fowleri 929
naevus (nevus) 521
naiad 605
nail 240
naive 520
naivety 520
naked 310
name 210
nanism 111
nano 111
nan(o)— 111
napalm 111, 311
naphtha 111

naphthalene 111
napkin 108
narcissism 697
narcissus 697
narc(o)— 696
narcolepsy 696, 770
narcosis 697
narcotic 697
narcotism 697
naris 868
narration 584
narrative 584
narrator 584

narrow 697
nasal 868
nascent 520
nasion 868
nas(o)— 868
nasogastric 868
nasolabial 868
nasolacrimal 868
nasopharynx 419, 868
natal^1 240
natal^2 520
natant 605
natation 605

neurolemma (neurilemma) 573, 853
neurolepsy 770
neuromelanin 746
neuromuscular 139
neuron 140
neuronal 140
neuropeptide(s) 502
neuropil 855, 864
neuropore 431
Neurose 140
neurosis 140
neurotic 140
neurotize 140
neurotmesis 171
neurotrophic 345
neurotropic 343
neurula 140
neurulation 140
neuston 605, 904
neuter (n.) 675
neutral 675
neutrality 675
neutralization 675
neutralize 675
neutron 675
neutropenia 534
neutrophil 675, 777
neutrophilia 778
never 245, 675
nevoid 521
nevus (naevus) 521
new 310
newborn 640
nexin 529
nexus 529
niacin 835
Nibelung 111
nice 436
niche 470
nickname 454
Nicotiana tabacum 941
nicotinamide 835
nicotine 835
nicotinic 835
nicotinic acid 835
nictate 648
nictitate 648
nidation 470

nidus 470
niece 191
Niflheim 111
night 851
nightingale 718
nightmare 626
nihil 675
nihilism 675
Nike 697
nil 675
nimble 141
nimbus 111
nine 389
nineteen 389
ninety 389
ninth 389
nirvana 203
nitrate (NO_3-) 843
nitric 843
nitrify 843
nitrite (NO_2-) 843
nitr(o)− 843
nitrogen (N) 522, 843
nitroglycerin 324
nitrous 843
no 245, 675
No. 141
noble 584
noblesse oblige 584
nocebo 465
nocent 465
nociceptive 465
nociceptor 465
nocturia (nycturia) 119, 851
nocturn 851
nocturnal 851
nodal 529
node 529
nodose 529
nodosity 529
nodular 529
nodule 529
nodulose 529
Noël 520
noise 121
noisome 647
nomad 142
nombril 148

nomenclature 210, 410
nominal 210
nominate 210
nominative (nom.) 210
nominee 210
nomo− 141
nomogenesis 141
nomogram (nomograph) 141, 767
−nomy 141
non− 674, 792
non(a)− 389
nonagenarian 388
nonan 389
nonce 381
nondescript 439
nondisjunction 525
none 381, 675
nonfiction 674
nongovernmental 674
nongranular 269
nonionized 637
nonmotile 464
nonparametric 630
nonplus 467
nonproliferation 674
nonprotein 674
nonsense 674
nonsmoker 674
nonstop 674
nonunion 381
noon 389
noose 529
nor 675
noradrenaline 880
norepinephrine 880
norm 246
normal 246
normalcy 246
normality 246
normalize 246
normochromic 218
normoskeocytosis 735
normotension 473
normotensive 473
norovirus 848
nose 868
nosencephaly 709
nos(o)− 709

O

oenophilist 172

oesophag(o)- (esophag(o)-) 771

oesophagus (esophagus) 771

oestrogen(s) (estrogen(s)) 619

oestrous (estrous) 619

oestrus (estrus) 619

of 667

off 667

offend 510

offense (offence) 510

offensive 510

offer 640, 662

office 214

officer 214

official 214

officiate 214

officinal 214

officious 214

offset 469

offspring 832

often (oft) 673

-oid 481, 750

oil 827, 887

ointment 887

-ol¹ 194

-ol² 827, 887

old 582

-ole 827, 887

olecranon 117, 262

oleic acid 827, 887

oleoresin 844

olfaction 182

olfactory 182

olig(o)- 738

oligodendroglia
  (oligodendrocyte) 334, 654, 910

oligohydramnios 814

oligomenorrhea 630

oligomer 463

oligopoly 778

oligosaccharide(s) 175

oligospermia 907

oliguria 119

olisthe (olisthy) 339

-olisthesis 339

olivary 827, 887

olive 827, 887

Olympia 706

Olympiad 706

Olympic 706

Olympus 706

-oma 731

omasum 848

ombudsman 728, 793

omega 298

omelet 106

omen 211

omental 241

omentum 241

omicron 743

ominous 211

omission 528

omit 528, 662

omni- 323, 331

omnibus (bus) 323, 362

omnipotence 634

omnipotent 634

omniscient 436

omnium-gatherum 323

omnivorous 604

om(o)- 135

omohyoid 750

omphal(o)- 148

omphalocele 148, 696

omphalos 148

omphaloscepsis (omphaloskepsis)
  148, 600

on 785

-on 749

once 381

Onchocerca 128, 876

onchocerciasis 128, 876

onc(o)- 705

oncocyte 705

oncogene 522, 705

oncogenesis 522, 705

oncology 705

oncotic 705

oncovirus 705

one 381

-one 341

onerous 214

onion 381

onlay 135

onomatomania 210, 729

onomatopoeia 210, 699

onomatopoeic 699

onset 469

onslaught 785

-ont 632, 758

ont(o)- 632, 758

ontogeny 522, 632, 758

ontology 632, 758

onus 214

onychia 240

onych(o)- 240

onycholysis 240

onychomycosis 240

onyx 240

oo- 164

oocyte 164

oogenesis 164

oogonium 164, 523, 908

oolemma 160, 164, 853

oolemmal 160

oophorectomy 164, 642

oophoritis 164, 642

oophor(o)- 642

oospore 164

ootid 164

ooze 849

opacification 354

opacity 354

opal 674

opalesce 579

opalescence 579, 674

opalescent 579

opaque 354

open 673

opera 214

operant 214

operate 214

operation 214

operative 214

operator 214

opercular 606

operculate 606

operculum 606

operetta 214

operon 214

ophiolatry 180, 820

ophiology 820

ophthalmia 144

-ophthalmia 144

ophthalmic 144

ophthalm(o)— 144

ophthalmocopia 704

ophthalmology 144

—ophthalmos (—ophthalmus) 144

—opia 142

opiate 835

—opic 142

opinion 425

opinionated 425

opioid 481, 835

Opis 214

opisth(o)— 662

opisthorchiasis 238

Opisthorchis 238, 662

opisthotonos (opisthotonus) 477, 662

opium 835

opponent 538

opportune 431

opportunism 431

opportunistic 431, 662

opportunity 431

opposable 538

oppose 538

opposite 538

opposition 538

oppress 539

oppression 539

oppugn 579

—ops 142

—opsia 144

opsin(s) 144

—opsis 144

opsonin 663

opsonization 663

opsonize 663

—opsy 144

opt 425

optic 144

—optic 144

optical 144

optics 144

optimal 215

optimism 215, 356

optimize 215

optimum 215, 356

option 425

opulent 214

opus 214

opuscule 214

—or 276

oracle 425

oracular 425

oral 869

ora serrata 869

oration 425

orator 425

oratorio 425

oratory 425

orb 238

orbicular 238

orbicularis oculi (muscle) 138

orbicularis oris (muscle) 138

orbit 238

orbital 238

orchard 134

orchestra 783

orchestral 783

orchestrate 783

orchic (orchidic) 238, 874

orchid 239, 874

orchid(o)— 238, 874

orchi(o)— 238, 874

orchiopexy (orchiorrhaphy) 238, 569,
  577, 874

orchiorrhaphy (orchiopexy) 238, 569,
  577, 874

orchis 239, 874

ordain 179

ordeal 702, 747

order 179

ordinal 179

ordinance 179

ordinary 179

ordinate 179

ordnance 179

ore 352

organ 174

organellar 174

organelle 174

organic 174

organism 174

organization 174

organize 174

organizer 174

organomegaly 298

orgasm 730

orgasmic 730

orgiastic 174

orgy 174

orient 627

oriental 627

orientate 627

orientation 627

orienteering 627

orifice 869

origin 627

original 628

originate 627

ornament 179

ornamental 179

ornamentation 179

ornate 179

ornithine 905

ornith(o)— 905

ornithology 905

ornithomancy 905

ornithosis 905

oro— 628

oropharynx 419

orotic acid 169

orotund 869

orphan 737

orpiment 839

orth(o)— 302

orthochromic 218

orthodontics 223, 302

orthodox 302, 459, 693

orthogonal 263

orthomyxovirus 137

orthopaedics (orthopedics) 161, 302

orthophoria 643

orthopneic 219

orthopnoea (orthopnea) 219

—ory 279, 375

Oryza sativa (subsp.) indica 946

Oryza sativa (subsp.) japonica 946

os 234

oscillate 869

oscillograph 869

oscilloscope 869

oscine 649

oscitation 869

os coxae 234

pantothenic acid 742

pantry 239

papa 242

papacy 242

papal 242

papaverine 274, 835

paper 374

papery 374

papilionaceous 426

papilla 273

papillary 273

papilloedema (papilledema) 273

papilloma 273

pappus 242

paprika 838

papular 274

papule 274

papyraceous 374

papyrus 374

par 228

para 427

par(a)— 666

—para 427

parabiosis 570

parabiotic 570

parable 153

parablepsia 764

parabola 153

parabolic 153

paracentesis 173

parachromatopsia 144

parachute 426, 493

paracortex 438

paracrine 498

paracrystalline 304

paracusis 762

parade 426

paradigm 506

paradise 513, 666

paradox 459, 693

paradoxical 459

paraesthesia (paresthesia) 602

paraffin 161, 513

parafollicular 237

paraganglion 799

paragon 342

paragonimiasis 523

Paragonimus 523

Paragonimus westermani 946

paragraph 766

parakeratosis 261

paralanguage 666, 871

parallaxis (parallax) 739

parallel 739

parallelogram 767

paralogism 486

Paralympian 666

Paralympics 666

paralysis 247

paralysis agitans 487

paralytic 247

paralyze 247

paramagnetic 691

paramecium 743

paramedian 326

paramedical 615

paramedics 274, 615

paramenia 630

parameter 630

parametrial 243

parametric 630

parametrium 243

paramnesia 646

paramount 223, 663

paramyoclonus 323

paramyxovirus 137

paranasal 868

paraneoplastic 311

paranoia 705

paranoiac 705

paranoid 705

paraparesis 597

parapet 215

paraphasia 612

paraphernalia 641

paraphimosis 779

paraphonia 613

paraphrase 719

paraphrenia 718

paraphrenic 718

paraplegia 576

paraquat 386

parasite 706

parasitic 706

parasiticide 495, 706

parasitism 706

parasitize 706

parasitology 706

parasol 193, 426

parasympathetic 720

parasympatholytic 720

parasympathomimetic 705, 720

paratenic 475

parathormone 318

parathyroid 318, 377

paratope 155

paratyphoid 132

parcel 228

parchment 749

pardon 415

pare 426

paregoric 653

pareidolia 481

parenchyma (parenchyme) 518

parenchymal 518

parenchymatous 518

parent 427

parentage 427

parental 427

parenteral 670

parenthesis 253, 670

parenthetically 253

paresis 597

paresthesia (paraesthesia) 602

paresthetic 602

paretic 597

parietal 801

pari passu 228

Paris 809

parish 120

Parisian 809

Parisien 809

Parisienne 809

parity^1 228

parity^2 428

—parity 428

parlance 153

parliament 153

parlor (parlour) 153

parochial 120

parody 762

parole 153

paronychia (perionychia) 240

parosmia 183

-pede 187
pedestal 136, 187
pedestrian 187
ped(i)- 187
pediatric (paediatric) 161, 783
pediatrician 161
pediatrics 161, 783
pedicel 187, 272
pedicle 187
pedicular 823
pediculosis 823
pediculous 823
pediculus 822
Pediculus humanus capitis 947
Pediculus humanus corporis 947
pedicure 102, 187
pedigree 187, 819
ped(o)-[1] 190
ped(o)-[2] (paed(o)-) 161
pedophilia (paedophilia) 161, 777
peduncle 187
pedunculate 187
peel 855, 864
peeling 855, 864
peer[1] 228
peer[2] 466
peg 850
pejorate 190, 356
pejoration 190
pejorative 190
pelage 855, 864
pelagic 314
peliosis 354
pellagra 490, 863
pellet 854, 865
pellicle 863
pellucid 200, 663
Peloponnesus 354
Pelops 354
pelt[1] 530
pelt[2] 863
peltate 863
peltry 863
pelvic 467, 873
pelvis 467, 873
pemphigoid 481, 713
pemphigus 713
pen 535

penal 894
penalty 894
penance 624
pencil 239, 273
pend 532
pendant 532
pendent 532
pendulous 532
pendulum 532
pen(e)- (paen(e)-) 624
penetrance 656
penetrant 656
penetrate 656, 672
penetration 656
-penia 534
-penic 534
penicillamine 239
penicillar 239
penicilliary 239
penicillin 239
penicillium 239
Penicillium chrysogenum 239
penile 239
peninsula 624, 904
peninsular 904
penis 239
penitence 624
penitent 624
penna 535
pennant 532, 535
pennate 535
pennon 535
penology 894
pensée 531
pensile 532
pension 531
pensive 531
pent(a)- 387
pentad 387, 752
pentagon 263
pentagonal 263
pentalogy 485
pentathlon 699
pentavalent 582
Pentecost 389
penthouse 532
penult 290, 624
penultimate 290, 624

penumbra 273, 624
people 145
peplomer 805
peplos 805
peplus (peplum) 805
pepo 503
pepper 838
peppermint 834, 838
pepsin 503
peptic 502
peptidase 502
peptide(s) 502
peptidoglycan(s) 323
peptize 502
peptone 502
per- (pel-) 663
perambulate 409
per capita 663
perceive 587
percent 390
percentage 390
percentile 390
percept 587
perceptible 587
perception 587
perceptive 587
perceptual 587
percolate 166
percuss 597
percussion 597
percutaneous 862
perdition 416
perdurable 417
perdure 417
peregrine 491
peremptory 509
perennial 129
perfect 591, 663
perfection 591
perfidious 511
perfidy 511, 663
perforate 418
perforation 418
perform 663
performance 663
perfume 131
perfunctory 619, 663
perfusate 516

pilot 190

piloti 855

pilus 855, 864

pimiento (pimento) 578

pince-nez 868

pine¹ 149, 829

pine² 894

pineal 149, 829

pinealocyte 149

pineapple 149

pinguecula 149

pinguid 149

pinna 535

pinnacle 535

pinnate 535

pinniped 535

pinochle 142, 383

pinocytosis 433

pint 578

pinta 578

pinto 578

Pinus densiflora 372

pioneer 187

pious 315

pip 149

pipe 428

piperine 838

pipette 428

piracy 629

pirate 629

piriform (pyriform) 103, 829

piscatory 906

Pisces 906

pisciculture 500, 906

piscine 906

piscivorous 604, 906

pisiform 103, 836

pismire 823

pistil 855

pistillate 855

piston 855

pit 434

pitch 199

pitchblende 199, 350

pithecoid 816

pituicyte 149

pituitary 149

pity 315

pityriasis 254

pityriasis versicolor 856

pivot 578

pivotal 578

pixel 839

pixelate 839

placable 314

placate 314

place 313

placebo 314

placenta 314

placenta accreta 580

placenta increta 580

placental 314

placenta membranacea 362

placenta percreta 580

placenta previa 564

placentation 314

placid 314

placode 314, 481

placoid 314, 481

plagiarism 313

plagi(o)- 314

plague 575

plain 310

plaint 575

plaintiff 575

plait 428

plan 310

planar 310

plane 310

planet 312

plane-tree 313

plangent 575

plan(i)- (plano-) 310

plank 313

plankton 576

plano- (plan(i)-) 310

plant 312

plantain 313

plantar 312

plantarflexion 312, 513

plantation 312

plantigrade 625

planula 310

-plasia 311

plasma 311

plasma- (plasm(o)-) 311

-plasma (-plasm) 311

plasmalemma 160, 311, 853

plasmalemmal 160

plasmapheresis 777

-plasmic 311

plasmid 311

plasmin 311

plasm(o)- (plasma-) 311

plasmocyte (plasmacyte, plasma cell) 311

plasmodesma 776

plasmodesmata 776

plasmodium 312, 481

Plasmodium falciparum 933

Plasmodium malariae 935

Plasmodium ovale 933

Plasmodium vivax 933

-plast 312

plaster 312

plastic 312

-plastic 311

plasticity 312

plasticizer 312

plastid 312

plastoquinone 165

-plasty 312

platanus 313

plate 313

plateau 313

platelet 313

platform 103, 313

platinum (Pt) 313

platitude 313

Plato (Platon) 313

Platonic 313

platoon 854, 865

platter 313

platy- 313

platybasia 313, 609

platyhelminth 313, 573

platysma 313

plaudits 537

plausible 537

play 461

plaza 313

-ple 430

plea 314

plead 314

posse 634

possess 469, 634

possession 469, 634

possessive 469, 634

possibility 634

possible 634

post¹ 443

post² 537

post— 660, 667

post cibum (p.c.) 659

postcoital 636

poster 443

posterior 359, 667

posterity 667

postern 667

postganglionic 799

posthetomy 697

posthumous 359, 667

postmenopausal 630, 771

postmeridian 264, 659

post meridiem (p.m.) 659

postmortem 660

postnatal 520

postoperative 214

postpartal 427

postpartum 427

postpone 538

postpose 538

postposition 538

postprandial 509, 665

postpubertal 161

postscript (P.S.) 439

postsynaptic 492

postulate 432

postural 537

posture 537

pot 843

potable 433

potamology 536

potash 454, 843

potassium 454, 843

potency (potence) 634

potent 328, 634

potential 634

potentiality 634

potion 433

potomania 433, 729

potpourri 213, 843

pottage 843

pouch 100

pouchitis 100

poudrage 211

poultice 211

poultry 161

pounce 578

pound 531

poverty 161, 428

powder 211, 634

pox 100

poxvirus 100

practical 772

practician 772

practise (practice) 772

practitioner 772

praedial 168

pragmatic 773

pragmatics 773

pragmatism 773

prairie 315

praise 168

Prakrit 716

prandial 509, 665

pravity 314

praxis 772

pray 432

pre— 663

preach 505

preamble 409

preantepenult 290

precancerous 161

precarious 432

precaution 455

precautious 455

precede 496

precedent 496

precept 587

preceptor 587

precession 496

precinct 279

precious 168

precipice 209

precipitant 209

precipitate 209

precipitation 209

precipitin 209

precipitous 209

precise 494

precision 495

preclude 499

preclusion 499

preclusive 499

precocious 502

precocity 502

precordial 232

precordium 232

precursor 503

predator 524

predecessor 496

predestinate 445

predestination 445

predicament 505

predicate 505

predicative 505

predict 505, 663

predictable 505

predictive 505

predilection 483

predispose 538

predisposition 538

predominant 131

predominate 131

pre—eclampsia 770

preempt 509

preemption 509

preemptive 509

preface 611

prefatory 611

prefect 591

prefecture 591

prefer 640

preferable 640

preference 640

preferential 640

prefix 512

preganglionic 799

pregnable 524

pregnancy 521

prehensile 524

prehension 524

prehistoric 482

preictal 524

prejudice 212, 504

prekallikrein 304, 736

prelibation 422

probe 251, 664
problem 153
problematic 153
proboscis 764
procaryote (prokaryote) 162, 914
procedure 496
proceed 496
proceedings 496
procercoid 876
procerus (muscle) 579
process 496
procession 496
processor 496
proclaim 410
proclamation 410
proclisis 413
proclitic 412
proclivity 412
procoagulant 488
procrastinate 851
procreate 580
procrustean 699
Procrustes 699
proct(o)- 874
proctodeum 708
proctology 874
proctor 103
proctoscope 874
procuracy 102
procurator 102
procure 102, 663
prodigal 488, 663
prodigious 647
prodigy 647, 663
prodrome 765
prodromic (prodromal) 765
produce 508
producer 508
product 508
production 508
productive 508
proenzyme 213
proestrus (pro-oestrus) 619
profane 167
profanity 167
profess 611
profession 611
professional 611

professor 611
proffer 640
proficiency 591
proficient 591
profile 897
profit 591
profluent 515
profound 133, 333
profundity 133, 333
profuse 516
profusion 516
progenitor 520
progeny 520
progeria 712
progestational 518
progesterone 518
progestogen(s) (progestin(s)) 518
proglottid 872
prognathia 872
prognathism 872
prognathous 872
prognose 246
prognosis 246
prognostic 246
prognosticate 246
prograde 625
program 768
progravid 324
progress 625
progression 625
progressive 625
prohibit 453
prohibition 453
project 595
projectile 595
projection 595
projective 595
projector 595
prokaryote (procaryote) 162, 914
prolactin (lactotropin) 234, 343
prolapse 620
prolapsus 620
prolapsus uteri 620
proletarian 582
proletariat 582
proliferate 582
proliferation 582
proliferative 582

proliferous 582, 638
prolific 582, 592
proline (Pro, P) 893
prolix 462
prolixity 462
prologue (prolog) 485, 665
prolong 346
prolongate 346
promenade 224
Prometheus 722
prominence 224
prominent 224
promiscuous 463
promise 529
promontorium 224
promontory 224
promote 464
promotion 464
promotor 464
prompt 509
promptitude 509
promulgate 150
pronate 663
pronation 663
pronator 663
prone 663
pronephric 880
pronephros 880
pronoun 210, 663
pronounce 652
pronucleus 663
pronunciation 652
pro-oestrus (proestrus) 619
proof 251, 664
propaganda 577
propagate 577
propagation 577
propane 149, 885
propel 531
propellent (propellant) 531
propeller 531
propensity 532
proper 665
properdin 416
property 665
prophase 247
prophecy 612
prophesy 612

Q

quaternity 380, 386

quay 166

queen 715

queer 479

quell 154

quercetin 830

querulous 848

query 540

quest 540

question 540

questionnaire 540

queue (cue²) 875

quick 570

quicksilver 570

quidnunc 292, 850

quiescent 196

quiet 196

quietude 196

quilt 102

quincentenary 387

quindecennial 387

quinic acid 165

quinine 165

quinoline 165

quinone(s) 165

quinquagenarian 387

quinqu(e)− 387

quinquevalent 582

quinsy 491, 815

quintan 387

quintessence 387, 632

quintet 387

quintile 387

quintuple 387

quintuplicate 387

quit 196

quite 196

quiver 570

quorum 291

quota 293

quotation 293

quote 293

quotidian 293

quotient 293

R

rabid 597

rabies 597

race 417

racemic acid 914

racemose 914

rachi(o)− 859

rachischisis 437, 859

rachitis 859

rack 543

radar 198

radial 198

radian 198

radiant 198

radiate 198

radiation 198

radiator 198

radical 197

radicle 197

radicular 197

radio 198

radio− 198

radi(o)− 198

radioactive 198

radiodensity 198, 299

radiograph 198, 766

radioisotope 198

radiology 198

radiolucent 198, 200, 656

radiopaque 198, 354

radioresistant 198

radiosensitive 198

radiotherapy 692

radish 197

radium (Ra) 198

radius 198

radix 197

radon (Rn) 198

raffinose 512

rag 797

rage 597

ragweed 797

raid 434

rail 542

rain 421

raise 628

raisin 914

rake 543

rally 423

ramify 198, 592

ramose 198

ramp 306

rampant 306

rampart 426

ramulose 198

ramulus 198

ramus 198

ramus communicans 368

ranch 305

rancid 370

rancidify 370

rancidity 370

rancor (rancour) 370

random 145

randomize 145

range 305

rank¹ 305

rank² 543

rankle 713

ransom (redemption) 510, 793

ranula 821

ranular 821

rapacious 598

rape 597

raphe 569

rapid 598

rapport 430

rapprochement 664

rapt 597

raptor 598

rapture 598

rare¹ 256, 299

rare² 781

rarefaction 257, 299

rarefy 257, 299

rarity 257, 299

rascal 541

rash 541

respiratory 441
respire 441
respite 600
resplendent 470
respond 471
response 471
responsible 471
rest 445
restaurant 446
restitute 444
restitution 444
restive 445
restoration 446
restorative 446
restore 446
restrain 550
restraint 550
restrict 550
restriction 550
restrictive 550
result 607
resultant 607
resultative 607
resume 510
résumé 510
resumption 510
resumptive 510
resupinate 673
resurge 543
resurgent 543
resurrection 543
resuscitate 456
resuscitator 456
retail 115
retain 473, 856
retaliate 449
retard 340
retardant 340
retardation 340
retch 818
rete 256, 848, 855
retention 473, 856
rete ovarii 256
rete testis 256
reticent 472
reticular 256
reticulate 256
reticule (reticle) 256, 848, 855

reticulin 256
reticulocyte 256
reticulum 256, 848, 855
retiform 103, 256, 848, 855
retina 256
retinaculum 473, 855
retinal[1] 256
retinal[2] 256
retinoic acid 256
retinoid(s) 256, 481
retinol 256
retinoscope 600
retinue 473, 856
retort 479
retortion 479
retract 560
retractable 560
retractile 560
retraction 560
retractor 560
retreat 560
retribute 385
retrieval 344
retrieve 344
retrimentum 556
retro– 569
retroactive 487
retrobulbar 151
retrocede 496
retrocession 496
retrograde 625
retrogress 625
retrogression 625
retrogressive 625
retrolental 836
retromolar 109
retroperitoneal 477
retroperitoneum 477
retrorse 567
retrospect 600
retrospective 600
retroversion 567
retrovert 567
retrovirus 567
retrude 561
retrusion 561
retrusive 561
return 557

retuse 561
revamp 187
reveal 172
revel 165
revelation 172
revenant 608
revenge 505
revenue 609
reverberant 568
reverberate 568
revere 617
reverence 617
reverend (Rev.) 617
reverent 617
reversal 567
reverse 567
reversible 567
reversion 567
revert 567
revertase 567
review 479
revise 480
revision 480
revival 570
revive 570
revocable 200
revoke 200
revolution 572
revolutionary 572
revolve 572
revolver 572
revulsant 865
revulse 865
revulsion 865
revulsive 865
reward 617
Rex 193, 542
Rhabditis 568
rhabd(o)– 568
rhabdomancy 568
rhabdomy(o)– 568
rhabdovirus 568
rhachi(o)– 859
rhagades 479
rhagas 479
rhagiocrine 914
rhaphe 569
rhapsody 568, 762

rhectic 479
rhegma 479
rhegmatogenous 479
Rhein 145
rheo- 156
rheostat 156
rheotactic 251
rheotaxis 251
rhesus (Rh) 150
rhetoric 164
rhetorical 164
rheum 156
rheumatic 156
rheumatism 156
rheumatoid 156, 481
rhexis 479
rhigosis 337
rhinal 169, 869
Rhine 145
rhin(o)- 169, 869
rhinoceros 169, 261, 869
rhinolalia 691
rhinology 169, 869
rhinophyma 250
rhinorrheal 157
rhinorrhoea (rhinorrhea) 157
rhinoscope 600
rhinovirus 169, 869
rhiz(o)- 198
rhizobium 198
rhizoma (rhizome) 198
rhizophagous 198
Rhizopus 189, 198
rhizotomy 171, 198
rhodium (Rh) 830
rhod(o)- 830
rhododendron 334, 910
rhodopsin 144, 830
rhombencephalon 879
rhombic 568
rhomboid 481, 568
rhombus 568
rhonchal (rhonchial) 154
rhonchus 154
rhopal(o)- 568
rhus 830
rhyme 617
rhynch(o)- 155

-rhynchus 155
rhythm 156
rhythmic 156
rhythmical 156
rib 859
ribbon 899
riboflavin 350
ribose 807
ribosome 185
ribozyme 213
ribulose 807
rice 836
rich 543
ricin 835
rickets 859
rickettsia 849
rickettsial 849
Rickettsia prowazekii 945
Rickettsia rickettsii 945
riddle 617
ride 434
ridge 305, 796
ridicule 468
ridiculous 468
rife 113
rifle 113
rift 113
rig 102
right 543
rigid 336
rigidity 336
rigor 336
rigor mortis 336
rigorous 336
Rigveda 482
rima 113
rima glottidis 113
rimose 113
rimple 306
ring^1 305
ring^2 818
rink 305
riot 183
rip 545
ripe 113
ripen 113
rise 628
Risorgimento 543

risorius (muscle) 468
rite 617
ritual 617
rival 145
rivalry 145
rive 113
river 113
rivulet 145
road 434
roam 628
rob 545
robe 545
roborant 320
robot 737
robust 320
rodent 541
rodenticide 495, 541
rodeo 347
rogation 543
rogatory 543
rogue 543
role 347
roll 347
Roma (Rome) 113
Roman 113
Romance 113
romance 113
Romanize 113
romantic 113
romanticism 113
rookie 580
room 214
root 198
rootlet 198
rope 113
rosacea 830
rosaniline 465
rosary 830
rose 830
rosemary 192, 255
roseola 830
roseoliform 830
rosette 830
rosin 844
rostellum 273, 541
rostrad 541, 659
rostral 541
rostrum 541

rosy 830
rotary 347
rotate 347
rotation 347
rotator 347
rotatory 347
rotavirus 347
rotor 347
rotund 347
rotunda 347
rouge 320
rough 797
rouleau 347
roulette 347
round 347
rout 544
route 544
routine 544
rover 545
row[1] 113
row[2] 240
rowan 320
rowen 197
royal 542
royalty 542
−rrhagia (−rrhage) 479

−rrhagic 479
−(r)rhaphy 569
−rrhexis 479
rub 545
rubber 545
rubefacient 320
rubella 320
rubeola 320
rubeosis 320
rubescent 320
rubidium (Rb) 320
rubor 184, 320
rubral 319
rubric 320
rubricate 320
Rubus coreanus 942
ruby 320
rucksack 305, 846
ructus 183
rudder 240
ruddy 320
rude 797, 844
rudiment 797, 844
rudimentary 797, 844
rue[1] 699
rue[2] 836

rug 797
ruga 797
rugitus 183
rugose (rugous) 797
rugosity 797
ruin 797
rule 542
rumen 848
ruminant 848
ruminate 848
rummage 214
rumor (rumour) 183
run 145
runny 145
rupestrine 545
rupicolous 500, 545
rupture 544
rural 214
russet 320
Russophobia 729
rust 320
rustic 214
rut 183
ruth 699
ruthless 699
rutin 836

S

sabulous 903
sac 846
saccharide(s) 175
saccharin 175
saccharine 175
sacchar(o)− 175
saccharomyces 138
Saccharomyces cerevisiae 936
saccular 846
sacculation 846
saccule 846
sack 846
sacral 321
sacred 321
sacrifice 321
sacrilege 321, 483
sacr(o)− 321
sacrum 321

sad 327
saddle 469
safe 338
safety 338
saffron 838
safranine(s) (safranin(s)) 838
sagacious 328
sagacity 328
sage[1] 338
sage[2] 598
saginate 113
sagittal 113
Sagittarius 113
sagittate 113
saint 321
sake 328
sal 193
salad 193

salamander 821
salami 193
salary 193
salicin 830
salicylate 830
salicylic acid 830
salient 606
saline 193, 372
salinity 193
saliva 890
salivary 890
salivate 890
sallow 830, 890
sally 606
salmon 607
Salmonella enteritidis 929
Salmonella typhi 929
salon 169

scapular 266

scar 691

scarce 495

scarification 440

scarify 440

scarlatina 113

scarlet 113

scatacratia 162, 891

scat(o)- (skat(o)-) 891

scatol (skatole) 891

scatology 891

scatter 435

scavenger 455

scenario 114

scene 114

scenery 114

scenic 114

scent 607

scepter (sceptre) 774

sceptic (skeptic) 600

sceptical (skeptical) 600

scepticism (skepticism) 600

schedule 437

schema 124

schematic 124

scheme 124

scherzo 179

-schisis 437

schism 437

schist(o)- 437

Schistosoma 437

schiz(o)- 437

schizogony 523

schizont 437, 632, 759

schizophrenia 437, 718

schizophrenic 437, 718

schizosaccharomyces 138

Schizosaccharomyces pombe 936

schizozoite (merozoite) 463, 571

scholar 123

scholastic 123

school[1] 123

school[2] 545

sciatic 174

sciatica 174

science 436

scientific 436

Scientology 436

sci-fi 436

scilicet (scil., sc.) 435, 462

scinti- 113

scintigram 113, 767

scintilla 113

scintillation 113

scintiscan 113

sciology 435

scirrhous 735

scissile 436

scission 436

scissor 494

sciurus 114

Sciurus 876

sclera 177

scleral 177

scleredema (scleroedema) 177

sclerema 177

scler(o)- 177

scleroderma 177

scleroedema (scleredema) 177

sclerose 177

sclerosed 177

sclerosis 177

-sclerosis 177

sclerotherapy 692

sclerotic 177

sclerotome 171

sclerous 177

scolex 229

scoliosis 229

scoliotic 229

scoop 266

scope[1] 600

scope[2] 600

-scopic 600

-scopy 600

scorbutic 437

scorch 306

score 437

scoria 891

scorpion 824

scot(o)- 707

scotochromogen 707

scotoma 707

scotomatous 707

scotophilia 707, 777

scotophobia 707, 729

scotopia 143, 707

scotopsin 144, 707

scour 102

scourge 102

scout 236

scrabble 437

scrap 437

scrape 437

screak 818

scream 818

screech 818

screen 437

screw 438, 812

scribe 439

scrimmage (scrummage) 437

script 439

scriptorium 439

scripture 439

scrobiculate 438

scrobiculus

scrofula 438, 813

scroll 438

scrotal 438

scrotum 438

scrub 437

scrum 437

scrummage (scrimmage) 437

scruple 440

scrupulous 440

scrutinize 439

scrutiny 439

sculpt 545

sculptor 545

sculpture 545

scum 862

scurf 437

scurvy 437

scutate 437

scuttle 437

scutum 436

scythe 435

se- (sed-) 285, 794

seal 622

seam 553

sear (sere) 317

search 306

season 906

seasonal 906

seat 469

seaweed 915

sebaceous 885

seborrheic 157, 885

seborrhoea (seborrhea) 157, 885

sebum 885

secant 434

secede 496

secession 496

seclude 499

seclusion 499

seclusive 499

second[1] 621

second[2] 621

secondary 621

secret 498, 794

secreta 498

secretagogue 489

secretary 498

secrete 498

secretin 498

secretion 498

secretory 498

sect 621

sectarian 621

sectile 434

section 434

sectional 434

sectionalism 434

sector 434

sectorial 434

secular 375

secund 621

secundigravida 324

secure 103

securi— 435

securiform 435

security 103

sedate 469

sedation 470

sedative 469

sedentary 468

sediment 468

sedimentation 468

sedition 635, 794

seduce 508

seduction 508

seductive 508

seed 907

seek 328

seem 382

seemingly 382

seep 885

segment 435

segmental 435

segmentate 435

segmentation 435

segregate 653

segregation 653

seism 774

seismic (seismal) 774

seismograph (seismometer) 774

seize 328

seizure 328

select 484, 794

selectin 483

selection 484

selective 484

Selene 697

selenium (Se) 697

selenography 697

self 285

sell 650

sella 468

sellar 468

sella turcica 468

semanteme 715

semantic 715

semantics 715

semaphore 715

semasiology 715

sematic 715

semblance 382

semeiology (semiology) 715

semen 906

semester 388, 630

semestral 388, 630

semi— 331, 793

semiannual 129

semicircle 305

semicircular 306

semicolon 230

semilunar 201

semimembranosus (muscle) 362

semimembranous 362

seminal 906

seminar 906

seminary 906

seminiferous 638, 906

semiology (semeiology) 715

semiotic 715

semipermeability 424

semipermeable 424

semitendinosus (muscle) 476

semitendinous 476

semivowel 199

sempiternal 245

senate 244

send 608

senescence 244

senescent 244

senile 244, 358

senility 244

senior 244, 358

sensation 607

sensational 607

sense 607

sensibility 607

sensible 607

sensitive 607

sensitivity 607

sensitize 607

sensor 607

sensorial 279, 607

sensorium 279, 607

sensory 279, 607

sensual 607

sensualism 607

sensuality 607

sensu lato 607

sensuous 607

sensu stricto 607

sentence 607

sentential 607

sententious 607

sentient 607

sentiment 607

sentimental 607

sentinel 607

sentry 607

sepal 779

separable 427

separate 427, 794

separation 427

skeptic (sceptic) 600

skeptical (sceptical) 600

skepticism (scepticism) 600

ski 435

skiascope 114

skid 435

skill 545

skim 862

skimmer 862

skin 435, 862

skirmish 437

skirt 437

skoal 545

skull 545

sky 862

slack 655

slander 546

Slav 146

slave 146

slavery 146

sled 339

sledge 339

sleek 339

sleep 655

sleeve 656

sleigh 339

slick 339

slide 339

slight 339

slime 339

slimy 339

sling 330

slink 330

slip 339

slippage 339

slipper 339

slippery 339

sloe 354

slogan 603

slop 656

sloppy 656

sloven 656

slovenly 656

smallpox 100

smart 627

smear 884

smegma 108

smegmatic 108

smelt 335

smilax 697

smile 310

smilodon 697

smirk 310

smite 108

smith 697

smithery 697

smithy 697

smuggle 137

snail 820

snake 820

snap 158

snare 697

snarl 158

snatch 158

sneak 820

sneer 158, 219

sneeze 219

sniff 158

sniffle 158

snip 158

snivel 158

snore 219

snorkel 158

snort 219

snout 158

snub 158

snuff 158

snuffle 158

soak 553

soap 885

soar 203

sober 307

sobriety 307

soccer 623

sociable 622

social 622

societal 622

society 622

socio— 622

socioeconomic 622

socket 812

Socrates 162, 186

sodium 842

Sodom 169

sodomy 169

soil^1 470

soil^2 812

soiree 315

sojourn 264

sol^1 193

sol^2 (solution) 547

Sol 193

solace 613

solanine 193

solar 193

solarium 193

solder 338

soldier 337

sole^1 169

sole^2 285

solemn 338

solemnity 338

solen 798

solenoid 798

soleus (muscle) 138, 169

solicit 338, 456

solicitous 456

solicitude 456

solid 337

solidarity 338

solidify 337

solidity 338

soliloquy 618

solipsism 290

solitary 285

solitude 285

solo 285

solstice 193, 443

solubility 547

solubilize 547

soluble 547

solute 547

solution (sol^2) 547

solvable 547

solve 547

solvent 547

soma 185, 859

somasthenia 124

somatic 185

somatization 185

somat(o)— 185

somatomedin(s) 185

somatopleure 313

somatostatin 185

somatotopic 155
somatotrope 343
somatotropic 343
somatotropin 185, 343
sombre (somber) 272
some 382
−some[1] 185
−some[2] 382
somersault 606, 673
somite 185
somnambulism 146, 408
somniferous 146, 638
somniloquism (somniloquy) 146
somnolence 146
somnolent 146, 377
Somnus 146
−somy 185
son 812
sonant 146
sonar 146
sonata 146
sone 146
sonic 146
sonicate 146
sonnet 146
sonorant 146
sonority 146
sonorous 146
soot 469
sooth 632
soothe 632
soothsayer 632
Sophia 126
sophism 126
sophist 126
sophisticate 126
Sophocles 769
sophomore 126
soporific 146
soporous 146
soprano 673
sorbefacient 589
sorbic acid 831
sorbitol 831
sorcerer 547
sordid 370
sore 894
sori 185

sororal 195
sorority 195
sorry 894
sort 547
sorter 547
sorus 185
soteriology 185
souffle 418
sough 722
sound 146
soup 553
source 543
south 193
southern 193
souvenir 609
sovereign 672
sovereignty 672
soviet 785
sow[1] 812
sow[2] 907
space 204
spacious 204
spade[1] 901
spade[2] 901
spadix 533
Spain 808
spam 877
Spam[®] 877
span 533
Spaniard 808
Spanish 808
spar 147
spare 204
spareribs 147, 859
sparganosis 798
sparganum 798
sparge 548
sparse 548
spasm 158, 533
spasmodic 533
spasmolytic 533
spastic 533
spasticity 533
spathe 901
spatial 204
spatula 901
spawn 576
spay 901

spear 147
spearmint 147, 834
special 598
specialist 598
speciality (specialty) 598
specialize 598
speciation 598
species (sp.) 598
specific 592, 598
specification 592, 598
specificity 592, 598
specify 592, 598
specimen 598
specious 598
specs 592, 598
spectacle 599
spectacular 599
spectate 599
spectator 599
spectatoritis 599
spectral 599
spectre (specter) 599
spectrin 599
spectrometer 599
spectrophotometer 599
spectroscope 599
spectrum 599
specular 598
speculate 598
speculation 598
speculative 598
speculum 598
speed 204
spend 533
sperm 907
spermatic 907
spermatid 907
spermatocyte 907
spermatogenesis 907
spermatogonium 523, 907, 908
spermatozoon (zoosperm) 571, 907
spermiation 907
spermicide 907
spermi(o)− 907
spermiogenesis 907
spew 170
sphenic 901
sphen(o)− 901

sterile 326

sterility 326

sterilize 326

stern[1] 183

stern[2] 445

sternal 552

stern(o)− 552

sternoclavicular 552

sternocleidomastoid 500, 552, 873

sternum 552

steroid(s) 183, 481

−sterol 183

sterol(s) 183

−sterone 183

stethoscope 721

stew 132

steward 617

sthenia 125

stibium (Sb) 843

stick 549

stiff 651

stigma 549

stigmasterol 112, 549

stigmatic 549

stigmatism 549

stilbene 774

stilbestrol (diethylstilbestrol) 774

stile 707

stiletto 549

still 136

stilt 136

stimulant 549

stimulate 549

stimulation 549

stimulator 549

stimulatory 549

stimulus 549

sting 549

stipe 651

stipel 651

stipend 532

stipes 651

stipple 651

stipulate[1] 651

stipulate[2] 651

stipule 651

stir 116

stirrup 707

stitch 549

stoa 447

stochastic 549

stock 561

stockade 549

Stoic 447

stoicheiometry (stoichiometry) 707

stoke 561

stoker 561

stolid 136

stoma 870

stomach 870

stomachache 894

stomachal 870

stomachic 870

stomachical 870

stomat(o)− 870

−stomia (−stomy) 870

stomodeum 708

−stomy 870

stone 886

stool 445, 891

stoop 561

stop 775

storage 445

store 445

storiform 103, 115

stork 183

storm 116

story 482

stout 136

stove 132

stow 445

strabismus 775

straight 183

strain[1] 550

strain[2] 551

strait 550

strange 669

stranger 669

strangle 697

strangulate 697

strangulation 697

stratagem 490, 553

strategic 490, 553

strategy 490, 553

stratify 552

stratocracy 552

stratosphere 551

stratum 551

stratum basale (stratum germinativum) 552

stratum corneum 552

stratum granulosum 552

stratum lucidum 552

stratum spinosum 552

stratus 552

straw 551

strawberry 551

stray 315

streak 550

stream 157

street 551

strength 698

strenuous 183

strepitus 549

streptococcal 774

streptococcus 774

Streptococcus pneumoniae 181

Streptococcus pyogenes 330

Streptococcus viridans 352

streptomyces 138

streptomycin 138

stress 550

stretch 183

strew 551

stria 550, 796

striae distensae 550

striae gravidarum 324

−strial 376

striate 551

striatum 551

strict 550

stricture 550

strident 550

stridor 550

strigil 550

strike 550

string 698

stringency 550

stringent 550

striola 551

stroboscope 775

stroke 550

stroma 553

stromal 553

syndrome 765, 784
syndromic 765
syne 315
synecdoche 458
synechia 124
synergy 175
synesthesia (synaesthesia) 602
synesthetic 602
syngeneic 523
synod 709
synonym 210
synopsis 144
synoptic 144
synostosis 235
synovia 115

synovial 115
syntactic 252
syntagma 252
syntax 252
synteny 478
synthase 253
synthesis 253
synthesize 253
synthetase 253
synthetic (synthetical) 253
syntripsis 556
synuclein 492
syphilid 240
syphilis 240
syphilitic 240

Syringa 798
syringe 798
syring(o)− 798
syringobulbia 151, 798
syringomyelia 798, 884
syrinx 798
syrup (sirup) 146
syrupy 146
systaltic 136
system 447
systematic 447
systemic 447
systole 136
systolic 136, 784
syzygy 526, 784

T

tabernacle 802
tabes 241
tabes dorsalis 241
tabetic 241
tablature 147
table 147
tablet 147
tabloid 147
tabular 147
tabulate 147
tachistoscope 742
tachometer 742
tachy− 742
tachycardia 233, 742
tachycardiac 233
tachyon 742
tachypnoea (tachypnea) 219, 742
tachyzoite 571
tacit 471
taciturn 471
tack 875
tact 554
tactic 252
tactics 252
tactile 554
tactoid 252, 481
tactual 554
tactus 554
taenia (tenia) 478, 856, 899

taenia coli 856
Taenia saginata 856
Taenia solium 856
taeniola 478
tag 875
tail 875
tailor 115
taint 276
talar 147
talcosis 170
talcum (talc) 170
talent 449
talin 147
talion 449
talipes 147, 188
talisman 502
tally 115
talon 147
talus 147
tame 648
tamoxifen 248
tamper 216
tampon 701
tamponade 701
tan 652
tandem 733
tangent 553
tangential 554
tangible 554

tannin(s) (tannic acid(s)) 652
tansy 896
tantalize 707
tantalum (Ta) 707
Tantalus 707
tantamount 223, 733
tanycyte 478
tap 701
taper 374
tapestry 216
tapetum 216
taphonomy 707
tar 334
tarantella 824
tarantism 824
tarantula 824
tardigrade 625
tardive 340
tardy 340
tardyon 340
targe 782
target 782
tarsal 116
tarsus 116
tart 864
tartar 175
tartaric acid 175
tartrate 175
task 554

tastant 554

taste 554

taurine 447, 810

taurocholic acid 350, 447, 810

Taurus 447, 810

taut 508

taut(o)− 732

tautology 733

tautomer 732

tautomerism 732

tavern 802

tawny 652

tax 554

taxa 251

taxation 554

taxi 554

taxidermy 251

taxis 251

Taxol® (paclitaxel) 711

taxon 251

taxonomy 142, 251

tea 831

teach 506

team 508

teapoy 190, 386

tear[1] 106

tear[2] 864

technetium (Tc) 559

technic 559

technical 559

technique 559

technocracy 559

technocrat 559

technology 559

tectonic 558

tectonism 558

tectorial 555

tectum 554

tedious 472

tedium 472

teem 508

−teen 389

teetotal 331

tegmen 555

tegmentum 555

tegular 555

tegument 555

teich(o)− 800

teichoic acid 800

telamon 449

telangiectasis (telangiectasia) 477

telangiectatic 477

telegram 787

telekinesis 457, 787

telencephalon 878

teleology 502

teleost 235, 501

telepathy 720, 787

telephone (phone) 613, 787

telescope 787

television 787

telic 501

tellurian 147

telluric 147

tellurium (Te) 147

telocentric 173

telogen 522

telomere 463, 501

telophase 247, 501

telpher (telfer) 642

telson 502

temerarious 115

temerity 115

temper 216

tempera 216

temperament 216

temperance 216

temperate 216

temperature 216

tempest 216

Templar 170

template 216

temple[1] 170

temple[2] 216

temple[3] 216

tempo 216

temporal[1] 216

temporal[2] 216

temporary 216

temptation 474

ten 389

tenable 472

tenacious 472

tenacity 472

tenaculum 472

tenant 472

tend[1] 473

tend[2] 474

tendency 473

tender 474

tenderness 474

tendinocyte 475

tendinous 476

tendon 475

tendril 474

−tene 478, 856, 899

tenebrous 115

tenement 472

tenesmus 475

tenet 472

tenia (taenia) 478, 856, 899

tennis 472

tenontoplasty (tenoplasty) 475

tenor 472

tenorrhaphy 475, 569

tenotomy 475

tense[1] 216

tense[2] 473

tensile 473

tension 473

tensive 473

tensor 473

tent 473

tentacle 474

tentative 474

tenth 389

tentorial 279, 473

tentorium 279, 473

tentorium cerebelli 473

tenuity 473

tenuous 348, 473

tenure 472

tepid 370

−ter 726

tera− 715

terabyte 715

terat(o)− 715

teratogen 715

teratology 715

teratoma 715

teratomatous 715

terbium (Tb) 844

terebinth 831

terebinthine 831

title 147
titrate 147
titration 147
titre (titer) 147
tittle 147
titubate 448
titular 147
—tmesis 171
to 668
toast 116
tocology 708
tocolysis 708
tocopherol 641, 708
toe 506, 877
toga 555, 804
togavirus 555, 804
toil 562
toilet 558
toiletry 558
token 506
tolerable 449
tolerance 449
tolerant 448
tolerate 448
toll 449
toluene 845
tomb 185
—tome 171
tomentose (tomentous) 185
tomentum 185
tomography 171, 766
—tomy 171
tone 476
toner 476
tongue 871
—tonic 476
tonic 476
tonicity 476
tonofibril 476
tonofilament 476
tonsil 274
tonsillar 274
tonsorial 170
tonsure 170
tonus 476
too 668
tooth 223
toothache 894

tophaceous 148
tophus 147
topiary 155
topic 155
topical 155
topography 155, 766
topoisomer 155, 738
topology 155
toponym 155, 210
—tor 726
torch 478
toreador 447, 810
torero 447, 810
torment 478
tornado 449
torpedo 183
torpid 183
torpidity 183
torpor 183
torque 478
torrent 116
torrid 116
torsion 478
torticollis 478, 501, 872
tortoise 707
tortuosity 478
tortuous 478
torture 478
torulopsis 478
torulus 478
torus 478
total 331
totalism 331
totalitarian 331
totality 331
totipotent 634
tour 557
tournament 557
tourniquet 557
tow 508
toward 567
tower 240
town 192
toxaemia (toxemia) 711
toxi— (tox(o)—) 711
toxic 711
—toxic 711
toxicant 711

toxication 711
toxicity 711
—toxicity 711
toxic(o)— 711
toxicology 711
toxicosis 711
—toxicosis 711
toxin 711
tox(o)— (toxi—) 711
Toxocara 261, 711
Toxocara canis 939
Toxocara cati 939
toxoid 481, 711
toxophily 711
Toxoplasma 711
Toxoplasma gondii 937
tra— (tetr(a)—) 387
trabecula 802
trabecula carnea 373
trabecular 802
trabeculate 802
trabeculation 802
trace 559
traceable 559
tracer 559
trachea 744
tracheal 744
trachel(o)— 872
trachoma 731, 744
tract 559
tractable 559
traction 559
tractor 559
trade 765
tradition 416, 660
traditor 416
traffic 660
tragacanth 341, 557, 911
tragedy 557, 762, 813
tragic 557, 813
tragus 557, 813
trail 559
trailer 559
train 559
trait 559
traitor 416
traject 596
trajectory 596

trammel 108

tramontane 224

tramp 765

trample 765

trance 637

tranquil 196

tranquillity (tranquility) 196

tranquillize (tranquilize) 196

trans 660

trans- (tran-, tra-) 660

transact 488

transaction 488

transcend 546

transcendent 546

transcendentalism 546

transcribe 440, 660

transcript 440

transcriptase 440

transcription 440

transduce 508

transducer 508

transducin 508

transduction 508

transect 434

transection 434, 591

transfer 640, 660

transference 640

transferrin 841

transfiguration 513

transfigure 513

transfix 512

transform 104

transformant 104

transformation 104

transfuse 517

transfusion 517

transgenic 522

transgress 625

transhumance 178

transient 637

transilluminate 201

transit 637

transition 637

transitional 637

transitive 637

translate 640, 660

translation 640

transliterate 107

translocate 135

translocation 135

translucent 201, 656

translunar 660

transmigrate 424

transmissible 529

transmission 529

transmit 529

transmitter 529

transmural 800

transmute 423

transonic 146

transparency 466

transparent 466

transpicuous 600

transpiration 441

transpire 441

transplant 313

transplantation 313

transport 431

transportation 431

transposable 539

transpose 539

transposition 539

transposon 539

transsexual 435

transsexualism 435

transudate 448

transudation 448

transude 448

transverse 567, 660

transversion 567

transvestism 240

trap^1 765

trap^2 765

trapeze 189

trapezium 189

trapezius (muscle) 189

trapezoid 189

trauma 557

traumatic 557

traumatize 557

traumatology 557

travail 577

travel 577

traverse 567, 660

tray 334

treacherous 557

treachery 557

treacle 307

tread 765

treadle 765

treadmill 765

treason 416

treasure 155

treasury 155

treat 559

treatise 559

treatment 559

treaty 559

tree 334, 909

trefoil 384, 912

trellis 117

trematode 481, 557

tremble 277

tremendous 277

tremor 277

tremulate 277

tremulous 277

trench 661

trenchant 661

trend 864

trepan 556

trepanation 556

trephination 384

trephine 384, 512

trepid 277

trepidation 277

treponema 141, 344

treponemal 141, 344

Treponema pallidum 344

tress 866

tri- 384, 386, 386

triacontanol 389

triad 386, 752

triangle 128

triangular 128

triathlon 699

tribal 385

tribalism 385

tribe 385

triboelectricity 556

tribrach 347

tribulation 555

tribune 385

tributary 385

U

ultimatum 290
ultra 290
ultra– 290, 661
ultradian 264
ultrafiltrate 290, 531
ultrasonic 146, 290
ultrasonography 146
ultrasound 146
ultrastructure 551
ultraviolet (UV) 353
ululate 450
–ulum (–ula) 279
Ulysses 692
–um 749
umbellate 272
umbellifer 272
umbelliferous 272
umbilical 148
umbilicate 148
umbilicus 148
umbo 148
umbra 272
umbrella 272
umlaut 769, 793
umpire 228
un–[1] 659
un–[2] 675, 792
unable 452
unabridged 346
unalienable (inalienable) 290
unanimity 420
unanimous 420
unarmed 226
unary 381
unbalanced 383
unbar 418
uncanny 584
uncial 381
unciform 128
uncinate 128
uncivil 237
uncivilize 237
uncle 129
unconditional 505
unconjugated 525
unconscionable 436
unconscious 436
uncouple 492

uncoupler 492
uncouth 584
uncover 606
unction 887
unctuous 887
uncus 128
undelete 339
under 662
under– 662
underlie 135
underscore 437
understand 445
undesired 215
undifferentiated 639
undue 453
undulant 117
undulate 117
unequal 301
unequivocal 200
uneventful 608
unfathomable 576
unfertilized 326, 638
ungual 240
unguent 887
unguis 240
ungulate 240
uni– 381
unicameral 804
unicellular 97
unicorn 260
unicornuate 260
unidirectional 542
unifocal 804
uniform 103
unilateral 309
unilocular 135
unintentional 475
union 381
unipolar 501
unique 381
unisexual 435
unison 147
unit 381
unitarian 381
unitary 381
unite 381
unity 381
univalent 582

univariate 316
universal 565
universe 565
university 565
unjust 212
unleash 655
unleavened 325
unmyelinated 140, 884
unnamed 210
unnatural 521
unpaired 229
unsatisfied 327
unsaturated 327
unsolicited 456
unstable 442
until 659
unusual 623
unwholesome 857
unwieldy 583
up 673
up– 673
Upanishad 470, 674
upbraid 828
update 415
upgrade 624
upheave 588
upper 673
uppercase 586, 900
upright 543
uproar 781
urachal 124
urachus 124
uracil (U) 118
uraemia (uremia) 119
uranium (U) 706
urate 118
urban 229
urbanity 229
urchin 460
–ure 276
urea 118
ureaplasma 849
uremia (uraemia) 119
uremic 119
ureotelic 501
ureter 118
ureteric (ureteral) 118
urethra 118

urethral 118
urge 479
−urge 174
urgency 479
urgent 479
−urgy 174
−uria 118
uric 118
−uric 118
uric acid 118
uricotelic 501
uridine (U) 118
urinal 118
urinalysis 118, 247
urinary 118
urinate 118
urination 118
urine 118
uriniferous 118, 638
urn 119
urobilinogen 890
urology 118

ur(o)−¹ 118
ur(o)−² 876
uronic acid 118
uroporphyrin 112
urothelial 301
urothelium 301
Ursa Major 816
Ursa Minor 816
ursine 816
ursodeoxycholic acid 350, 816
urticaria 563
urticarial 563
us 284
usage 623
use 623
useful 623
useless 623
usher 869
usquebaugh (whisky, whiskey) 118
ustulation 563
usual 623
usurp 545, 623

usurpation 545
usury 623
ut dictum 675
utensil 623
uterine 148
uterus 148, 881
utilitarian 623
utility 623
utilize 623
utmost 747
Utopia 156, 245
utopian 156
utricle 118, 847
utricular 118, 847
utter 747
uvea 914
uveal 914
uvula 914
uvular 914
uxorial 195
uxoricide 195, 495
uxorious 195

V

vacancy 450
vacant 450
vacation 450
vaccinate 810
vaccination 810
vaccine 810
vaccinia 810
vacciniform 810
vaccinium 833
vacillate 316
vacuity 450
vacuolar 450
vacuolate 450
vacuole 450
vacuolization 450
vacuous 450
vacuum 450
vagabond 315, 371
vagal 315
vagarious 315
vagary 315
vagina 874

vaginal 874
vaginismus 875
vag(o)− 315
vagrant 572
vague 315
vagus 315
vail 573
vain 450
Vaisya 120
vale 573
valediction 504
valence (valency) 583
valeric acid 836
valet 673
valetudinarian 582
valgus 316, 573
Valhalla 215
valiant 582
valid 582
validate 583
validity 583
valine (Val, V) 836

Valkyrie 215
vallecula 573
valley 573
vallum 800
valor (valour) 582
valproic acid 836
valuable 582
value 582
valueless 582
valve 573, 803
valvula 573
valvular 573, 803
vamp 187
vanadium (V) 374
vane 271
vanguard 659
vanilla 875
vanillic acid 875
vanillin 875
vanillylmandelic acid (vanilmandelic
   acid) (VMA) 826, 875
vanish 450

verruca plana 316
verruca vulgaris 316
verruciform 103, 316
verrucose (verrucous) 316
verrucosity 316
versatile 566
versatility 566
verse 565
versicolored (versicolor) 372
version 565
versus (vs., v.) 565
vertebra 565, 859
vertebral 565
vertebrate 565
vertex 565
vertical 565
verticil 565
verticillate 565
vertiginous 282
vertigo 282, 565
verumontanum 224
very 317
vesica 148, 847
vesical 148, 847
vesicant 148, 847
vesicate 148, 847
vesication 148, 847
vesicle 148, 847
vesic(o)- 148, 847
vesicular 148, 847
vesiculate 148, 847
vespa 119
vesper 851
vespertine 851
vespiary 119
vessel 882
vest 240
Vesta 119
vestibular 803
vestibulocochlear 803, 826
vestibulum (vestibule) 803
vestige 844
vestigial 844
vetch 199
veteran 330, 811
veterinarian 330, 811
veterinary 330, 811
veto 450

vex 564
vexation 564
vexillum 171
via 564
viability 570
viable 570
viaduct 564
vial (phiale) 697
viaticum 564
vibrant 450
vibrate 450
vibration 450
vibratory 450
vibrio 450
vibrissae 450
vicar 199
vicarious 199
vice[1] 172
vice[2] (vise) 205
vice- 199
viceroy 193, 542
vice versa 199
vicinage 120
vicinal 120
vicinity 120
vicious 172
vicissitude 199
victim 119
victor 569
victory 569
victual 570
vide infra 479
videlicet (viz.) 462, 479
video 479
vide supra 479
vie[1] 197
vie[2] 570
view 479
vigil 649
vigilant 649
vigor (vigour) 649
vigorous 649
vile 172
vilify 172
vilipend 172, 533
villa 119
village 120
villain 119

villose (villous) 865
villus 865
vim 197
vimentin 205
vinblastine 206
vincible 569
vincristine 206
vinculin 205
vinculum 205
vindicate 505
vindicative 505
vindictive 505
vine 172
vinegar 172, 322, 340
vintage 172, 509
vinyl 172
viola 353
violable 197
violaceous 353
violate 197
violence 197
violent 197
violet 353
viper 427, 569
vir 197
viral 848
virescent 352
virgate 352
virgin 352
virginal 352
Virginia 352
virgule 352
viricide (virucide) 848
viridescent 352
viridity 352
virile 197, 376
virilism 197
virility 197
virilize 197
virion 848
viroid 481, 848
virology 848
virtual 197
virtue 197
virtuosity 197
virtuoso 197
virtuous 197
virucide (viricide) 848

W

정상우

전남대학교(의과대학) 및 대학원(의학과) 졸업, 의학박사
병리과전문의, 진단검사의학과전문의
한국방송통신대학교(영어영문학과) 및 대학원(실용영어학과) 졸업, 문학석사

전남대학교 의과대학 교수 (역임)
대한병리학회 회장 (역임)

「진염색질-이염색질 경계면에서의 mRNA 합성: 경계면 이론의 제안」
「An image analytical study of chromatin pattern in cervical
intraepithelial neoplasia of the uterus」 등

최찬

전남대학교(의과대학)와 전북대학교 대학원(의학과) 졸업, 의학박사
병리과전문의

전남대학교 의과대학 교수 (현)
대한병리학회 회장 (역임)

「Loss of heterozygosity at chromosome segments 8p22 and 8p11.2-21.1
in transitional-cell carcinoma of the urinary bladder」
「Recurrent KRAS mutations identified in papillary renal neoplasm with
reverse polarity - a comparative study with papillary renal cell
carcinoma」 등

이재혁

전남대학교(의과대학) 및 대학원(의학과) 졸업, 의학박사
병리과전문의

전남대학교 의과대학 교수 (현)
전남대학교 의과대학 학장 (역임)
대한병리학회 부회장 (현)

「TACC3 promotes gastric carcinogenesis by promoting epithelial-
mesenchymal transition through the ERK/Atk/cyclin D1 signaling
pathway」
「Proteogenomic characterization of human early-onset gastric cancer」 등